PEDIATRIC ALLERGY

Principles and Practice

DONALD Y.M. LEUNG, MD, PhD
Head, Pediatric Allergy
National Jewish Medical and Research Center
Professor of Pediatrics
University of Colorado Health Sciences Center
Denver, Colorado

HUGH A. SAMPSON, MD
Professor of Pediatrics and Immunobiology
Chief, Pediatric Allergy and Immunology
Director, General Clinical Research Center
Mount Sinai School of Medicine/New York University
Department of Pediatrics
New York, New York

RAIF S. GEHA, MD
Prince Turki bin Abdul Aziz Professor of Pediatrics
Harvard Medical School
Chief, Division of Immunology
Children's Hospital, Boston
Boston, Massachusetts

STANLEY J. SZEFLER, MD
Helen Wohlberg and Herman Lambert Chair in Pharmacokinetics
Head, Pediatric Clinical Pharmacology
National Jewish Medical and Research Center
Professor of Pediatrics and Pharmacology
University of Colorado Health Sciences Center
Denver, Colorado

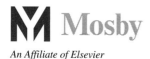

An Affiliate of Elsevier

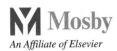

An Affiliate of Elsevier

11830 Westline Industrial Drive
St. Louis, Missouri 63146

Library of Congress Cataloging-in-Publication Data

Pediatric allergy: principles and practice / [edited by] Donald Y.M. Leung . . . [et al.].
    p. ; cm.
  Includes bibliographical references and index.
  ISBN 0-323-01802-5 (alk. paper)
    1. Allergy in children.   2. Immunologic diseases in children.   I. Leung, Donald Y. M.,
1949-
  [DNLM: 1. Immunologic Diseases—physiopathology—Child. 2.
Immunity—physiology—Child. 3. Immunologic Diseases—epidemiology—Child. 4.
Immunologic Diseases—therapy—Child. WD 300 P37125 2003]
  RJ386 .P435 2003
  618.92'97—dc21
                                                                    2002035296

Acquisitions Editor: Cathy Carroll
Developmental Editor: Marla Sussman
Publishing Services Manager: Patricia Tannian
Senior Project Manager: Suzanne C. Fannin

Printed in the United States of America

Last digit is the print number: 9 8 7 6 5 4 3

MARK J. ABZUG, MD
Professor, Pediatric Infectious Diseases, Department of Pediatrics, University of Colorado School of Medicine, Professor of Pediatrics, Department of Pediatric Infectious Disease, The Children's Hospital, Denver, Colorado
Sinusitis

LEONARD B. BACHARIER, MD
Assistant Professor, Department of Pediatrics, Divison of Allergy and Pulmonary Medicine, Washington University School of Medicine, Attending Physician in Allergy and Pulmonary Medicine, Department of Pediatrics, Division of Allergy and Pulmonary Medicine, St. Louis Children's Hospital, St. Louis, Missouri
Infections and Asthma; Asthma in Older Children

MARK BALLOW, MD
Professor, Department of Pediatrics, Director, Allergy/Clinical Immunology Fellowship Training Program, Department of Pediatrics, SUNY Buffalo School of Medicine and Biomedical Sciences, Chief, Division of Allergy/Clinical Immunology and Pediatric Rheumatology, Department of Pediatrics, Children's Hospital of Buffalo, Medical Director of Clinical Laboratories, Department of Pathology, Children's Hospital of Buffalo, Kaleida Health Systems, Buffalo, New York
Intravenous Immune Serum Globulin Therapy

DONALD H. BEEZHOLD, PhD
Senior Scientist, Director, Laboratory of Immunobiology, Guthrie Research Institute, Sayre, Pennsylvania
Latex Allergy

VINCENT S. BELTRANI, MD
Associate Clinical Professor, Department of Dermatology, College of Physicians and Surgeons, Columbia University, New York, New York, Visiting Professor, Department of Medicine, Division of Allergy & Rheumatology, University of Medicine & Dentistry of New Jersey, Newark, New Jersey, Attending Physician, Vassar Brothers Hospital, St. Francis Hospital, Poughkeepsie, New York
Contact Dermatitis

BRUCE G. BENDER, PhD
Professor, Department of Psychiatry, University of Colorado School of Medicine, Head, Pediatric Behavioral Health, Department of Pediatrics, National Jewish Medical and Research Center, Denver, Colorado
Promoting Adherence and Effective Self-Management in Patients with Asthma

STEPHEN D. BETSCHEL, MD
Fellow, Department of Allergy and Clinical Immunology, University of Toronto, Toronto, Ontario, Canada
Latex Allergy

LEONARD BIELORY, MD
Professor, Department of Medicine, Pediatrics, and Ophthalmology, Director, Asthma & Allergy Research Center, Director, Co-Director, Immuno-Ophthalmology Service, Division of Allergy, Immunology, and Rheumatology, Department of Medicine, University of Medicine and Dentistry—New Jersey, Newark, New Jersey
Allergic and Immunologic Eye Disease

S. ALLAN BOCK, MD
Clinical Professor, Department of Pediatrics, University of Colorado Health Sciences Center, Staff Physician, Department of Pediatrics, National Jewish Medical and Research Center, Denver, Colorado
Evaluation of Food Allergy

MARK BOGUNIEWICZ, MD
Professor, Department of Pediatrics, University of Colorado School of Medicine, Division of Pediatric Allergy/Immunology, National Jewish Medical and Research Center, Denver, Colorado
Contact Dermatitis

CATHERINE M. BOLLARD, MBChB, FRACP, RCPA
Assistant Professor, Center for Cell and Gene Therapy, Baylor College of Medicine, Assistant Professor, Texas Children's Cancer Center—Bone Marrow Transplantation, Texas Children's Hospital, Houston, Texas
Gene Therapy and Allergy

FRANCISCO A. BONILLA, MD, PhD
Assistant in Medicine, Department of Medicine/Immunology, Children's Hospital, Assistant Professor of Pediatrics, Department of Pediatrics, Harvard Medical School, Boston, Massachusetts
Antibody Deficiency

DONNA L. BRATTON, MD
Associate Professor, Department of Pediatrics, University of Colorado Health Sciences Center, Associate Staff Physician, Department of Pediatrics, Division of Allergy/Immunology, National Jewish Medical and Research Center, Denver, Colorado
Refractory Childhood Asthma: New Insight into the Pathogenesis, Diagnosis, and Management

MALCOLM K. BRENNER, MB, PhD, FRCP, FRCPath
Director, Center for Cell and Gene Therapy, Baylor College of Medicine, Houston, Texas
Gene Therapy and Allergy

REBECCA H. BUCKLEY, MD
J. Buren Sidbury Professor of Pediatrics and Professor of Immunology, Departments of Pediatrics and Immunology, Chief, Division of Pediatric Allergy and Immunology, Department of Pediatrics, Duke University Medical Center, Durham, North Carolina
Bone Marrow Transplantation

WESLEY BURKS, MD
Professor of Pediatrics, Head, Division of Pediatric Allergy and Immunology, Department of Pediatrics, University of Arkansas for Medical Sciences, Professor, Department of Pediatrics, Arkansas Children's Hospital, Little Rock, Arkansas
Atopic Dermatitis and Food Hypersensitivity

JULIE A. CAKEBREAD, BSc
Doctoral Student, Human Genetics and Infection, Inflammation and Repair Divisions, University of Southampton, Southampton General Hospital, Southampton, Hampshire, United Kingdom
The Genetics of Allergic Disease and Asthma

KENNY H. CHAN, MD
Professor, Department of Otolaryngology, University of Colorado Health Sciences Center, Chief, Department of Pediatric Otolaryngology, The Children's Hospital, Denver, Colorado
Sinusitis

MARTIN D. CHAPMAN, BSc, PhD
Adjunct Professor of Medicine, Asthma and Allergic Diseases Center, University of Virginia Health Sciences Center, President, INDOOR Biotechnologies, Inc., Charlottesville, Virginia
Indoor Allergens

LORAN T. CLEMENT, MD
Professor, Division of Allergy and Immunology, Department of Pediatrics, Los Angeles County and University of Southern California Medical Center, Keck School of Medicine at the University of Southern California, Los Angeles, California
Inner City Asthma

RONINA A. COVAR, MD
Assistant Professor, Department of Pediatrics, University of Colorado Health Sciences Center, Staff Physician, Department of Pediatrics, National Jewish Medical and Research Center, Denver, Colorado
Special Considerations for Infants and Young Children

THOMAS L. CREER, PhD
Professor Emeritus, Department of Psychology, Ohio University, Athens, Ohio
Promoting Adherence and Effective Self-Management in Patients with Asthma

ROSEMARIE H. DeKRUYFF, PhD
Professor, Department of Pediatrics, Division of Immunology and Allergy, Stanford University, Stanford, California
Immunology of the Asthmatic Response

PEYTON A. EGGLESTON, MD
Professor, Department of Pediatrics, Johns Hopkins University, Johns Hopkins Hospital, Baltimore, Maryland
Immunotherapy for Allergic Disease

SAMER FAKHRI, MD
Department of Otolaryngology, Head and Neck Surgery, McGill University Health Center, Jewish General Hospital—Sir Mortimer B. Davis, Fellow, Department of Pathology, Division of Allergy and Immunology, Meakins-Christie Laboratories, Montreal, Quebec, Canada
Sinusitis

HAROLD J. FARBER, MD
Pediatric Pulmonologist, Department of Pediatrics, Kaiser Permanente Medical Center, Vallejo, California, Adjunct Assistant Clinical Investigator, Division of Research, Kaiser Permanente, Oakland, California, Adjunct Assistant Clinical Professor, Touro University College of Osteopathic Medicine, Vallejo, California
Asthma Education Programs for Children

PHILIP FIREMAN, MD
Professor of Pediatrics and Medicine, Departments of Pediatrics and Medicine, University of Pittsburgh School of Medicine, Allergist and Immunologist, Department of Allergy and Immunology, University of Pittsburgh Medical College and Children's Hospital of Pittsburgh, Pittsburgh, Pennsylvania
Otitis Media

THOMAS A. FLEISHER, MD
Chief, Department of Laboratory Medicine, Warren G. Magnuson Clinical Center, National Institutes of Health, Bethesda, Maryland
Autoimmune Lymphoproliferative Syndrome

NOAH J. FRIEDMAN, MD
Staff Allergist, Kaiser Permanente Medical Center, Assistant Clinical Professor of Pediatrics, University of California, San Diego, San Diego, California
Prevention and Natural History of Food Allergy

RAIF S. GEHA, MD
Prince Turki bin Abdul Aziz Professor of Pediatrics, Harvard Medical School, Chief, Division of Immunology, Children's Hospital, Boston, Boston, Massachusetts
Regulation and Biology of Immunoglobulin E

ERWIN W. GELFAND, MD
Professor of Pediatrics and Immunology, University of Colorado Health Sciences Center, Chairman, Department of Pediatrics, National Jewish Medical and Research Center, Professor of Pediatrics, The Children's Hospital, Denver, Colorado
Approach to the Child with Recurrent Infections

DEBORAH A. GENTILE, MD
Assistant Professor of Pediatrics, Department of Pediatrics, University of Pittsburgh School of Medicine, Assistant Professor of Pediatrics, Department of Pediatrics, Children's Hospital of Pittsburgh, Pittsburgh, Pennsylvania
Allergic Rhinitis

JAMES E. GERN, MD
Associate Professor, Department of Pediatrics, University of Wisconsin, Assistant Director for Pediatrics, General Clinical Research Center, University of Wisconsin, Madison, Wisconsin
Infections and Asthma

ALAN M. GERWIRTZ, MD
Doris Duke Distinguished Clinical Professor, Leader-Stem Cell Biology & Therapeutics Program, University of Pennsylvania Cancer Center, Department of Hematology/Oncology, University of Pennsylvania, University of Pennsylvania Hospital, Philadelphia, Pennsylvania
Stem Cell Therapeutics: An Overview

THERESA W. GUILBERT, MD
Assistant Professor of Pediatrics, Pediatric Pulmonary Division, Arizona Respiratory Center, University of Arizona, Tucson, Arizona
Functional Assessment of Asthma

SUSANNE HALKEN, MD
Associate Professor, University of Southern Denmark, Consultant in Pediatrics, Department of Pediatrics, Sønderborg Hospital, Denmark
Approach to Feeding Problems in the Infant and Young Child

QUTAYBA A. HAMID, MD, PhD
James McGill Professor of Medicine and Pathology, Meakins-Christie Laboratories, McGill University, Montreal, Quebec, Canada
Sinusitis

ROBERT G. HAMILTON, PhD, D ABMLI
Professor of Medicine and Pathology, Department of Medicine, Director, Johns Hopkins Dermatology Allergy & Clinical Immunology Reference Laboratory, Johns Hopkins University School of Medicine, Baltimore, Maryland
Laboratory (*In Vitro*) Analyses

IMELDA CELINE HANSON, MD
Professor of Pediatrics, Department of Pediatrics, Baylor College of Medicine, Houston, Texas, Bureau Chief, Bureau of HIV/STD Prevention, Texas Department of Health, Austin, Texas
Immunizations

STEPHEN T. HOLGATE, BSc, MD, DSc, FRCP, FRCPath, FIBiol, FMedSci
Professor, Respiratory Cell and Molecular Biology, Infection, Inflammation and Repair Divisions, University of Southampton School of Medicine, Southampton General Hospital, Southampton, Hampshire, United Kingdom
The Genetics of Allergic Disease and Asthma

STEVEN M. HOLLAND, MD
Head, Immunopathogenesis Unit, Laboratory of Host Defenses, National Institute of Allergy and Infectious Diseases, National Institutes of Health, Bethesda, Maryland
White Blood Cell Defects

J. ROGER HOLLISTER, MD
Professor, Department of Pediatrics, University of Colorado Health Sciences Center, Chief, Division of Rheumatology, The Children's Hospital, Denver, Colorado
Rheumatic Diseases of Childhood: Therapeutic Principles

JOHN W. HOLLOWAY, PhD
Senior Research Fellow, Human Genetics and Infection, Inflammation and Repair Divisions, University of Southampton, Southampton General Hospital, Southampton, Hampshire, United Kingdom
The Genetics of Allergic Disease and Asthma

PATRICK G. HOLT, DSc, FRCPath, FAA
Adjunct Professor, Centre for Child Health Research, The University of Western Australia, Head, Division of Cell Biology, Telethon Institute for Child Health Research, West Perth, Australia
The Developing Immune System and Allergy

ARNE HØST, MD, DMSc
Associate Professor, University of Southern Denmark, Head, Department of Pediatrics, Odense University Hospital, Denmark
Approach to Feeding Problems in the Infant and Young Child

JOHN M. JAMES, MD
Chair, Continuing Medical Education Committee, Department of Pediatrics, Poudre Valley Hospital, Clinician, Colorado Allergy and Asthma Centers, P.C., Fort Collins, Colorado
Food Allergy, Respiratory Disease, and Anaphylaxis

CRAIG A. JONES, MD
Assistant Professor of Clinical Pediatrics, Department of Pediatrics, Keck School of Medicine at the University of Southern California, Director, Division of Allergy and Clinical Immunology, Department of Pediatrics, Los Angeles County and University of Southern California Medical Center, Los Angeles, California
Inner City Asthma

JAMES F. JONES, MD
Professor, Department of Pediatrics, University of Colorado School of Medicine, National Jewish Medical and Reseach Center, The Children's Hospital, Denver, Colorado
Epstein-Barr Virus Infections

STACIE M. JONES, MD
Associate Professor, Department of Pediatrics, University of Arkansas for Medical Sciences, Arkansas Children's Hospital, Little Rock, Arkansas
Atopic Dermatitis and Food Hypersensitivity

GWENDOLYN S. KERBY, MD
Assistant Professor, Department of Pediatrics, Section of Pediatric Pulmonary Medicine, University of Colorado School of Medicine, The Children's Hospital, Denver, Colorado
Functional Assessment of Asthma

GARY L. LARSEN, MD
Professor and Head, Section of Pediatric Pulmonary Medicine, Department of Pediatrics, University of Colorado School of Medicine, Senior Faculty Member and Head, Division of Pediatric Pulmonary Medicine, Department of Pediatrics, National Jewish Medical and Research Center, Professor and Head, Department of Respiratory Medicine, The Children's Hospital, Denver, Colorado
Functional Assessment of Asthma

HOWARD M. LEDERMAN, MD, PhD
Professor of Pediatrics and Medicine, Johns Hopkins University School of Medicine, Director, Immunodeficiency Clinic, Director, Pediatric Immunology Laboratory, Division of Pediatric Allergy and Immunology, Johns Hopkins Hospital, Baltimore, Maryland
Approach to the Child with Recurrent Infections

ROBERT F. LEMANSKE, JR., MD
Professor of Pediatrics and Medicine, Department of Pediatrics and Internal Medicine, University of Wisconsin Medical School, Head, Division of Pediatric Allergy, Immunology, and Rheumatology, University of Wisconsin Hospital and Clinics, Madison, Wisconsin
Infections and Asthma

DONALD Y.M. LEUNG, MD, PhD
Head, Pediatric Allergy, National Jewish Medical and Research Center, Professor of Pediatrics, University of Colorado Health Sciences Center, Denver, Colorado
Atopic Dermatitis

CHRIS A. LIACOURAS, MD
Associate Professor of Pediatrics, Director of Gastrointestinal Endoscopy, Medical Director, Clinical Trials Office, Division of Gastroenterology and Nutrition, The Children's Hospital of Philadelphia, Philadelphia, Pennsylvania
Eosinophilic Esophagitis, Gastroenteritis, and Proctocolitis

ANDREW H. LIU, MD
Associate Professor and Fellowship Program Director, Division of Pediatric Allergy & Immunology, Department of Pediatrics, National Jewish Medical and Research Center, University of Colorado Health Sciences Center, Denver, Colorado
Natural History of Allergic Diseases and Asthma; Sinusitis

CLAUDIA MACAUBAS, PhD
Research Associate, Department of Pediatrics, Stanford University, Stanford, California
Immunology of the Asthmatic Response

JONATHAN E. MARKOWITZ, MD
Assistant Professor, Department of Pediatrics, University of Pennsylvania School of Medicine, Director, Inpatient Gastroenterology, Division of Gastroenterology and Nutrition, The Children's Hospital of Philadelphia, Philadelphia, Pennsylvania
Eosinophilic Esophagitis, Gastroenteritis, and Proctocolitis

FERNANDO D. MARTINEZ, MD
Director, Arizona Respiratory Center, University of Arizona, Swift-McNear Professor of Pediatrics, Arizona Health Sciences Center, Tucson, Arizona
Natural History of Allergic Diseases and Asthma

ELIZABETH C. MATSUI, MD
Fellow, Department of Pediatrics, Division of Allergy and Immunology, Johns Hopkins University, Johns Hopkins Hospital, Baltimore, Maryland
Immunotherapy for Allergic Disease

LLOYD D. MAYER, MD
Professor and Chairman, Immunobiology Center, Dorothy and David Merksamer Professor of Medicine, Chief, Division of Clinical Immunology, Department of Immunobiology, Mount Sinai Medical Center, New York, New York
Mucosal Immunity: An Overview

LOUIS M. MENDELSON, MD
Clinical Professor of Pediatrics, University of Connecticut Health Center, Farmington, Connecticut, Allergist, Connecticut Asthma and Allergy Center, LLC, West Hartford, Connecticut
Drug Allergy

HENRY MILGROM, MD
Professor, Department of Pediatrics, National Jewish Medical and Research Center, Professor, Department of Clinical Science, University of Colorado Health Sciences Center, Denver, Colorado
Chronic Cough

SHIDEH MOFIDI, MS, RD, CSP
Pediatric Dietitian/Instructor, Jaffe Food Allergy Institute, Department of Pediatric Allergy & Immunology, Nutrition Research Manager, General Clinical Research Center, Mount Sinai School of Medicine, New York, New York
Management of Food Allergy

WAYNE J. MORGAN, MD, CM
Professor of Pediatrics and Physiology and Associate Head, Department of Pediatrics, Associate Director for Pediatrics, Arizona Respiratory Center, University of Arizona, Tucson, Arizona
Functional Assessment of Asthma

EDINA H. MOYLETT, MD
Assistant Professor, Department of Pediatrics, Baylor College of Medicine, Assistant Professor, Section of Allergy and Immunology, Texas Children's Hospital, Houston, Texas
Immunizations

HAROLD S. NELSON, MD
Professor of Medicine, University of Colorado Health Sciences Center, Professor of Medicine, National Jewish Medical and Research Center, Denver, Colorado
In Vivo Testing for Immunoglobulin E–Mediated Sensitivity

LUIGI D. NOTORANGELO, MD
Professor of Pediatrics, Head, Department of Pediatrics and Institute of Molecular Medicine "Angelo Nociveli," University of Brescia, Depatment of Pediatrics, Spedali Civilli, Brescia, Italy
T Cell Immunodeficiencies

HANS C. OETTGEN, MD, PhD
Assistant Professor of Pediatrics, Harvard Medical School, Clinical Director, Division of Immunology, Children's Hospital, Boston, Massachussets
Regulation and Biology of Immunoglobulin E

MARY E. PAUL, MD
Assistant Professor of Pediatrics, Department of Pediatric Allergy and Immunology, Baylor College of Medicine, Texas Children's Hospital, Houston, Texas
Pediatric Human Immunodeficiency Virus Infection

ROBERT E. REISMAN, MD
Clinical Professor, Department of Medicine and Pediatrics, State University of New York at Buffalo School of Medicine, Attending Physician, Department of Medicine, Buffalo General Hospital, Attending Allergist, Department of Pediatrics, Buffalo Children's Hospital, Buffalo Medical Group, Buffalo, New York
Insect Sting Anaphylaxis

SERGIO D. ROSENZWEIG, MD
Research Fellow, Laboratory of Host Defenses, National Institute of Allergy and Infectious Diseases, National Institutes of Health, Bethesda, Maryland, Medico Asistente, Servicio de Inmunologia, Hospital Nacional de Pediatria "Juan P. Garrahan," Buenos Aires, Argentina
White Blood Cell Defects

MARC E. ROTHENBERG, MD, PhD
Professor and Endowed Chair, Department of Pediatrics, University of Cincinnati College of Medicine, Director, Division of Allergy and Immunology, Cincinnati Children's Hospital Medical Center, Cincinnati, Ohio
Inflammatory Effector Cells/Cell Migration

JULIE ROWE, PhD
Division of Cell Biology, Telethon Institute for Child Health Research, West Perth, Australia
The Developing Immune System and Allergy

HUGH A. SAMPSON, MD
Professor of Pediatrics and Immunobiology, Chief, Pediatric Allergy and Immunology, Director, General Clinical Research Center, Mount Sinai School of Medicine/New York University, Department of Pediatrics, New York, New York
Evaluation of Food Allergy; Management of Food Allergy

GAIL G. SHAPIRO, MD, FAAP, FAAAAI
Clinical Professor, Department of Pediatrics, University of Washington School of Medicine, Co-Head, Division of Allergy, Attending Physician, Children's Hospital and Regional Medical Center, Partner/Director, Northwest Asthma and Allergy Center and ASTHMA, Inc., Seattle, Washington
Allergic Rhinitis

WILLIAM T. SHEARER, MD, PhD
Professor of Pediatrics and Section Head, Department of Pediatrics— Allergy/Immunology, Baylor College of Medicine, Chief of Service, Department of Allergy and Immunology, Texas Children's Hospital, Houston, Texas
Pediatric Human Immunodeficiency Virus Infection

SCOTT H. SICHERER, MD
Assistant Professor, Department of Pediatrics, Division of Allergy and Immunology, Jaffe Food Allergy Institute, Mount Sinai School of Medicine, New York, New York
Enterocolitis, Proctocolitis, and Enteropathies

DAVID P. SKONER, MD
Associate Professor of Pediatrics and Otolaryngology, Department of Allergy, Immunology, and Infectious Diseases, Children's Hospital of Pittsburgh, Pittsburgh, Pennsylvania
Allergic Rhinitis

ROLAND SOLENSKY, MD
Division of Allergy/Immunology, The Corvallis Clinic, Corvallis, Oregon
Drug Allergy

JOSEPH D. SPAHN, MD
Staff Physician, Department of Pediatrics, National Jewish Medical and Research Center, Associate Professor of Pediatrics, University of Colorado Health Sciences Center, Denver, Colorado
Special Considerations for Infants and Young Children; Refractory Childhood Asthma: New Insight into the Pathogenesis, Diagnosis, and Management

MARISHA A. STANISLAUS, PhD
Division of Hematology/Oncology, University of Pennsylvania School of Medicine, Philadelphia, Pennsylvania, GlaxoSmithKline-Oncology, Collegeville, Pennsylvania
Stem Cell Therapeutics: An Overview

DAVID A. STEMPEL, MD
Clinical Associate Professor of Pediatrics, University of Washington School of Medicine, Children's Hospital and Medical Center, Seattle, Washington
Asthma and the Athlete

ROBERT C. STRUNK, MD
Donald Strominger Professor of Pediatrics, Department of Pediatrics, Washington University School of Medicine, Member, Division of Allergy and Pulmonary Medicine, Department of Pediatrics, St. Louis Children's Hospital, St. Louis, Missouri
Asthma in Older Children

KATHLEEN E. SULLIVAN, MD, PhD
Associate Professor, Department of Pediatrics, University of Pennsylvania School of Medicine, Associate Physician, Department of Immunology, Children's Hospital of Philadelphia, Philadelphia, Pennsylvania
Complement Deficiencies

ROBERT P. SUNDEL, MD
Assistant Professor of Pediatrics, Harvard Medical School, Director of Rheumatology, Department of Rheumatology, Children's Hospital, Boston, Massachussets
Autoimmune Diseases

GORDON L. SUSSMAN, MD, FRCP(C)
Associate Professor, Department of Medicine, Division of Allergy and Immunology, University of Toronto, Staff Physician, Department of Allergy and Immunology, St. Michael's Hospital, Staff Physician, Department of Internal Medicine, Mount Sinai and The Toronto Hospital, Toronto, Ontario, Canada
Latex Allergy

STANLEY J. SZEFLER, MD
Helen Wohlberg and Herman Lambert Chair in Pharmacokinetics, Head, Pediatric Clinical Pharmacology, National Jewish Medical and Research Center, Professor of Pediatrics and Pharmacology, University of Colorado Health Sciences Center, Denver, Colorado
Special Considerations for Infants and Young Children; New Directions in Asthma Management

LYNN M. TAUSSIG, MD
President and Chief Executive Officer, National Jewish Medical and Research Center, Professor of Pediatrics, Department of Pediatrics, University of Colorado Health Sciences Center, Denver, Colorado
Natural History of Allergic Diseases and Asthma

STUART E. TURVEY, MB, BS, D Phil
Clinical Fellow in Pediatrics, Harvard Medical School, Physician, Division of Immunology, Children's Hospital, Boston, Massachussets
Autoimmune Diseases

DALE T. UMETSU, MD, PhD
Professor of Pediatrics, Department of Pediatrics, Division of Immunology and Allergy, Stanford University, Director, Center for Asthma and Allergy Diseases, Lucile Packard Children's Hospital, Stanford, California
Immunology of the Asthmatic Response

ERIKA VON MUTIUS, MD, MSc
Head of the Asthma and Allergy Department, Munich University Children's Hospital, Munich, Germany
Epidemiology of Allergic Diseases

RUDOLPH S. WAGNER, MD
Clinical Associate Professor, Departments of Ophthalmology and Pediatrics, Director of Pediatric Ophthalmology, University of Medicine and Dentistry—New Jersey Medical School, Newark, New Jersey
Allergic and Immunologic Eye Disease

JOHN O. WARNER, MD, FRCP, FRCPCH, FAAAAI
Professor, University Child Health, Allergy & Inflammation Sciences, University of Southampton, Honorary Consultant Paediatrician, Department of Child Health, Southampton University Hospitals NHS Trust, Southampton General Hospital, Southampton, Hampshire, United Kingdom
Guidelines for Treatment of Asthma

SANDRA R. WILSON, PhD
Senior Staff Scientist and Chair, Department of Health Services Research, Palo Alto Medical Foundation Research Institute, Palo Alto, California, Clinical Professor, Departments of Medicine and of Health Research and Policy, Stanford University School of Medicine, Stanford, California
Asthma Education Programs for Children

TODD M. WILSON, DO
Resident, Internal Medicine Department, University of Medicine and Dentistry—New Jersey Medical School, Newark, New Jersey
Allergic and Immunologic Eye Disease

JERRY A. WINKELSTEIN, MD
Professor of Pediatrics, Medicine, and Pathology, Department of Pediatrics, Johns Hopkins University School of Medicine, Johns Hopkins Hospital, Baltimore, Maryland
Complement Deficiencies

ROBERT A. WOOD, MD
Associate Professor of Pediatrics, Department of Pediatrics, Johns Hopkins University School of Medicine, Johns Hopkins Hospital, Baltimore, Maryland
Environmental Control

MICHAEL C. YOUNG, MD
Assistant Clinical Professor, Department of Pediatrics, Harvard Medical School, Assistant in Medicine, Department of Allergy & Immunology, Children's Hospital, Boston, Massachusetts
General Treatment of Anaphylaxis

JOHN W. YUNGINGER, MD
Emeritus Professor of Pediatrics, Mayo Medical School, Rochester, Minnesota
Outdoor Allergens

ROBERT S. ZEIGER, MD, PhD
Clinical Professor, Department of Pediatrics, University of California San Diego, La Jolla, California, Senior Research Investigator, Department of Research and Evaluation, Southern California Permanente Medical Group, Pasadena, California, Director of Allergy Research, Department of Allergy, Kaiser Permanente, San Diego, California
Prevention and Natural History of Food Allergy

BRUCE L. ZURAW, MD
Associate Professor, Molecular & Experimental Medicine, The Scripps Research Institute, Member, Division of Allergy, Asthma, and Immunology, Scripps Clinic/Green Hospital, La Jolla, California
Urticaria and Angioedema

Pediatric allergy-immunology, long the stepchild of academic pediatric subspecialties, has finally come of age, as readers of this new text will appreciate. The editors, Drs. Leung, Sampson, Geha, and Szefler, leading experts in their own area of specific interest, have recruited a formidable group of authors, each of whom can write with authority on their assigned topic. Our specialty has come a long way since Dr. Jerome Glaser, a leading pediatric allergist of his day, published an article entitled *The Menace of Immunology in the Practice of Allergy* in Review of Allergy 1967;21:1120-1131. Dr. Glaser lamented that, during his practice lifetime, immunology had made no significant contribution to the field of clinical allergy. He apparently did not appreciate the fact that pediatricians were there during the earliest days of immunology as a new discipline. Clemens von Pirquet and Bela Schick, both pediatricians, published a classic monograph on serum sickness in 1906, and von Pirquet actually coined the term allergy. In 1908 von Pirquet became the first chairman of the Department of Pediatrics at Johns Hopkins University School of Medicine and Bela Schick became Chairman of the Department of Pediatrics at Mount Sinai Hospital in New York. Oscar Schloss, who served as Chairman of Pediatrics at both Cornell University and Harvard University, was the first to carefully investigate adverse reactions (poisoning) to foods. He also established the feasibility of using scratch skin tests for the diagnosis of hypersensitivity.

Beginning in the 1920s and for two decades, Drs. Bret Ratner and Harry Donnally conducted some fundamental studies on allergic disease in early infancy. Ratner (while in full-time clinical practice), using a guinea pig model, showed that the fetus could be sensitized *in utero* (whether this occurs in humans is still debated). Donnally showed that infants could be sensitized by egg white protein in breast milk.

Pediatric immunology had its roots at the Children's Hospital in Boston. There, in the 1950s, Dr. Charles A. Janeway, who was Physician in Chief and had learned protein electrophoresis from Tiselius and Waldenstrom in Sweden, started a Protein Clinic that followed children with primary immunodeficiency and autoimmune diseases.

The fact that the great majority of authors of this text are pediatricians speaks to the fact that we have a new generation of academicians on the pediatric faculties of leading medical schools. The timing of this new development is very appropriate because epidemiologic data show that the prevalence of asthma in the United States increased from 16.8 million persons in 1980 to 17.3 million persons in 1999, of which 5 million were children. Of these, 1.3 million (26%) were under 5 years of age. In addition, there are 1.9 million Emergency Room visits, 500,000 hospitalizations, 5400 deaths, and 14.5 billion dollars spent in direct costs. Asthma is the leading cause of school absenteeism, with 14 million school absence days—a 50% increase from 1980 to 1996. When one adds the prevalence data for allergic rhinitis and atopic dermatitis, both of which are being diagnosed with increasing frequency, the numbers of children and adults with atopic disorders are truly impressive.

The current generation of pediatric allergy clinical scientists, exemplified by Drs. Leung, Sampson, Geha, and Szefler, has, by their basic science and clinical research, elevated our specialty to a place of substantial respect. It is appropriate to acknowledge that the idea for this text originated with Dr. Leung in Denver where, beginning in 1966 with the discovery of IgE, so much of what we know of the immunology and therapeutics of asthma and allergies was elucidated.

ELLIOT F. ELLIS, MD, FAAAI
EMERITUS PROFESSOR OF PEDIATRICS
STATE UNIVERSITY OF NEW YORK AT BUFFALO

These are exciting times for physicians who treat children and investigators interested in mechanisms underlying diseases in the area of pediatric allergy and clinical immunology. There has been a well-documented rise in prevalence of this group of diseases during the past three decades. Protection against microbial infection and treatment of hypersensitivity reactions to environmental triggers have become primary goals for the practicing pediatrician. As a result, investigators at academic centers and in the pharmaceutical industry have partnered to understand mechanisms underlying these diseases and have developed evidence- and mechanism-based approaches for management and treatment of these illnesses. The need to document and summarize this recent remarkable increase in information justifies this new textbook in the field of pediatric allergy and clinical immunology for practicing physicians and investigators interested in this area.

It is often said, "Children are not simply small adults." In no other subspecialty is this more true than in pediatric allergy and immunology, where the immune system and allergic responses are developing in different host organs. This offers special opportunities for prevention and intervention, which cannot be carried out once disease processes have been established in the older child and adult. Indeed, many diseases that pediatricians see in clinical practice are complex diseases thought to result from a multigene predisposition in combination with exposure to an unknown environmental agent. However, the age at which the host is exposed to a particular environmental agent and the resultant immune response are increasingly being recognized as important factors. Furthermore, determining the appropriate time for intervention will be important in defining a window of opportunity to induce disease remission. For example, endotoxin is a known trigger of established asthma in adults but the "hygiene hypothesis" in children suggests that early exposure to endotoxin prior to the onset of allergies may actually prevent allergic responses and thus account for the low prevalence of allergic disease in children living on farms.

Pediatric Allergy: Principles and Practice is aimed at updating the reader on the pathophysiology of allergic responses and the atopic triad (asthma, allergic rhinitis, and atopic dermatitis), the mechanisms underlying specific allergic and immunologic diseases, and their socioeconomic impact and new treatment approaches that take advantage of emerging concepts of the pathobiology of these diseases. An outstanding group of authors who are acknowledged leaders in their fields has been assembled because of their personal knowledge, expertise, and involvement with their subject matter in children. Every effort has been made to achieve prompt publication of this book, thus ensuring that the content of each chapter is "state of the art."

Section A presents general concepts critical to an understanding of the impact and causes of allergic diseases. These include reviews of the epidemiology and natural history of allergic disease, genetics of allergic disease and asthma, biology of inflammatory-effector cells, regulation of IgE synthesis, and the developing immune system and allergy. Section B reviews an approach to the child with recurrent infection and specific immunodeficiency and autoimmune diseases that pediatricians frequently encounter. Section C updates the reader on a number of important and emerging immune-directed therapies including immunoglobulin therapy, bone marrow transplantation, immunizations, gene therapy, and stem cell therapy. Section D examines the diagnosis and treatment of allergic disease. The remainder of the book is devoted to the management and treatment of asthma and a number of specific allergic diseases such as upper airway disease, food allergy, allergic skin and eye diseases, drug allergy, latex allergy, insect hypersensitivity, and anaphylaxis. In each chapter, the disease is discussed in the context of its differential diagnoses, key concepts, evaluations, environmental triggers, and concepts of emerging and established treatments.

We would like to thank each of the contributors for their time and invaluable expertise, which were vital to the success of this book. The editors are also grateful to Dr. Scott Sicherer for his help in developing the food allergy appendix and to Drs. Francisco Bonilla and Bryce Binstadt for their help on the clinical immunology appendix. We are also indebted to Marla Sussman (Developmental Editor), Cathy Carroll (Acquisitions Editor), and Suzanne Fannin (Senior Project Manager), who have played a major role in editing and organizing this textbook, as well as the production staff at Elsevier Science for their help in the preparation of this book.

DONALD Y.M. LEUNG, MD, PHD
HUGH A. SAMPSON, MD
RAIF S. GEHA, MD
STANLEY J. SZEFLER, MD

CONTENTS

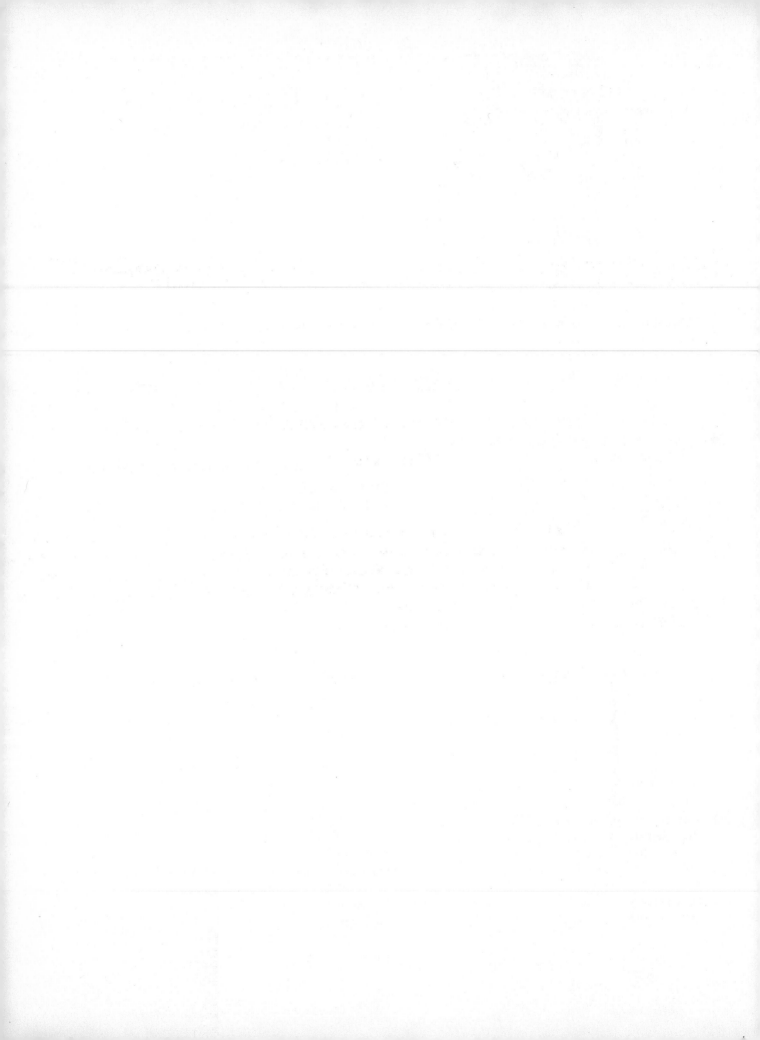

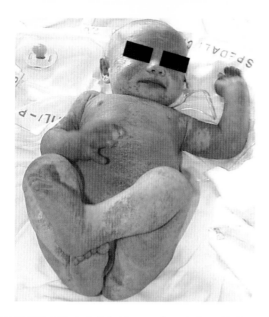

COLOR PLATE 1 Typical clinical features in an infant with Omenn's syndrome. Note generalized erythrodermia with scaly skin, alopecia, and oedema.

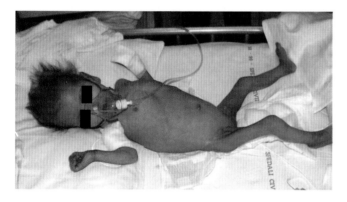

COLOR PLATE 2 Typical appearance of an infant with severe combined immunodeficiency (SCID) [syndrome]. Note severe growth failure and respiratory distress.

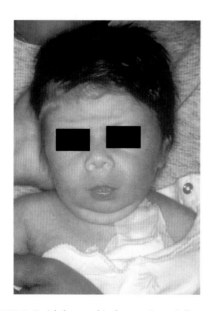

COLOR PLATE 3 Facial dysmorphic features in an infant with DiGeorge syndrome. Note hypertelorism, enlarged nasal root, anteroverted nostrils, low-set ears, and micrognathia.

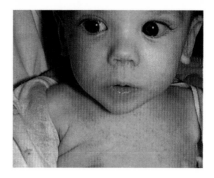

COLOR PLATE 4 Child with Wiskott-Aldrich syndrome. The skin eruptions on the trunk and face are eczematoid and pruritic, but not always similar to atopic dermatitis in flexural distribution. Many of these patients have thrombocytopenia, which results in petechiae of varying distribution and intensity. (From Fireman P, Slavin RG: *Atlas of allergies,* ed 2, London, 1996, Mosby-Wolfe.)

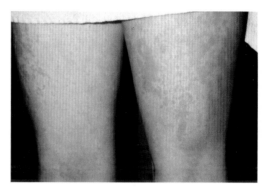

COLOR PLATE 5 Skin eruption in systemic juvenile rheumatoid arthritis.

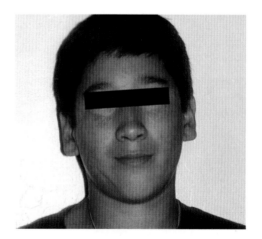

COLOR PLATE 6 Rash in systemic lupus erythematosus.

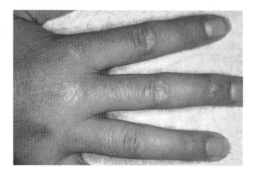

COLOR PLATE 7 Rash in juvenile dermatomyositis.

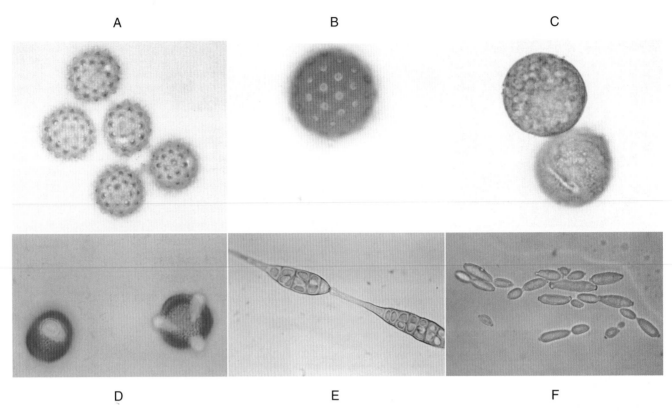

A   B   C

D   E   F

COLOR PLATE 8 Selected examples of common pollen grains and fungal spores (Calberla stain). **A,** Giant ragweed (*Ambrosia trifida*). **B,** Lamb's quarters (*Chenopodium album*). **C,** Sheep sorrel (*Rumex acetosella*). **D,** Common sagebrush (*Artemisia tridentata*). **E,** Alternaria. **F,** *Cladosporium.*

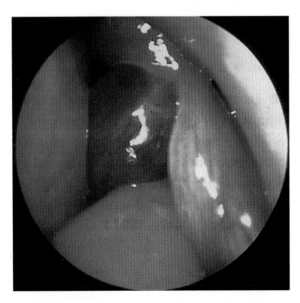

COLOR PLATE 9 Appearance of nasal polyps on rhinoscopy. (Courtesy of Dr. Sylvan Stool, Department of Otolaryngology, Children's Hospital, Denver, Colo.)

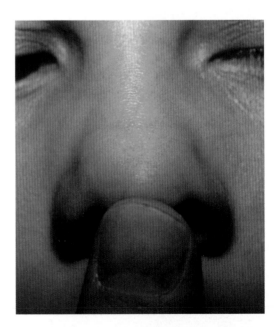

COLOR PLATE 10 The chronic rubbing upward of the nose often results in a nasal crease in patients with allergic rhinitis. (From Fireman P, Slavin R, eds: *Atlas of allergies,* ed 2, London, 1996, Mosby-Wolfe.)

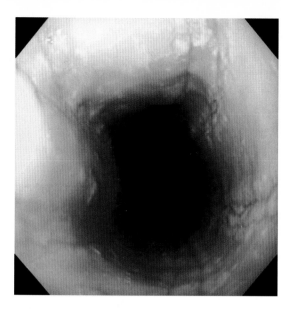

COLOR PLATE 11 Endoscopic photograph of the mid esophagus in a 12-year-old patient with eosinophilic esophagitis. Linear furrows and circumferential rings in the mucosa are prominent.

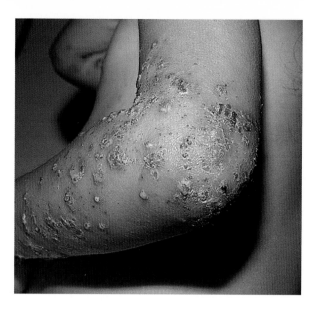

COLOR PLATE 14 Patient with atopic dermatitis who is secondarily infected with *Staphylococcus aureus*. Note multiple pustules and areas of crusting. (From Weston WL, Morelli JG, Lane A, eds: *Color textbook of pediatric dermatology*, ed 3, St Louis, 2002, Mosby.)

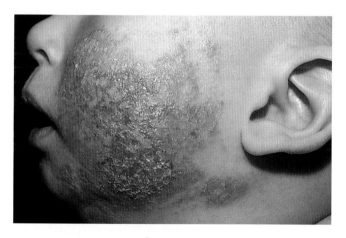

COLOR PLATE 12 Infant with acute atopic dermatitis. Note the oozing and crusting skin lesions. (From Weston WL, Morelli JG, Lane A, eds: *Color textbook of pediatric dermatology*, ed 3, St Louis, 2002, Mosby.)

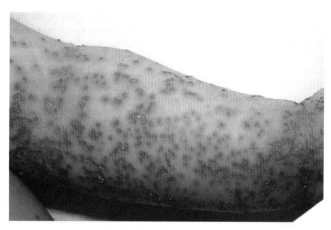

COLOR PLATE 15 Eczema herpeticum, the primary skin manifestation of herpes simplex in atopic dermatitis. (From Fireman P, Slavin R, eds: *Atlas of allergies*, ed 2, London, 1996, Mosby-Wolfe.)

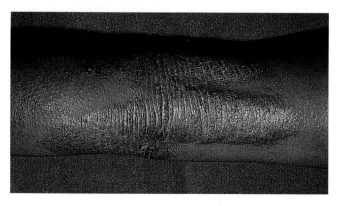

COLOR PLATE 13 Adolescent with lichenification of the popliteal fossa from chronic atopic dermatitis. (From Weston WL, Morelli JG, Lane A, eds: *Color textbook of pediatric dermatology*, ed 3, St Louis, 2002, Mosby.)

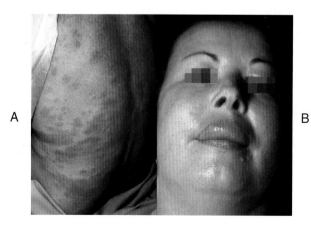

COLOR PLATE 16 Typical examples of swelling. **A,** Diffuse urticaria with areas of confluence. **B,** Angioedema of the upper lip and left eye.

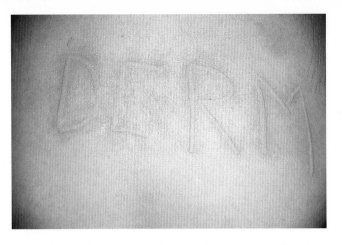

COLOR PLATE 17 Dermatographism. (From Weston WL, Morelli JG, Lane A, eds: *Color textbook of pediatric dermatology,* ed 3, St Louis, 2002, Mosby.)

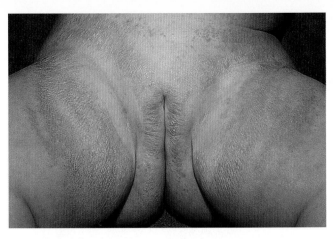

COLOR PLATE 20 Irritant diaper dermatitis. (From Weston WL, Morelli JG, Lane A, eds: *Color textbook of pediatric dermatology,* ed 3, St Louis, 2002, Mosby.)

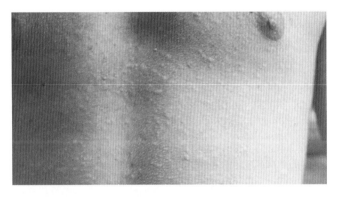

COLOR PLATE 18 Cholinergic urticaria. (From Fireman P, Slavin R, eds: *Atlas of allergies,* ed 2, London, 1996, Mosby-Wolfe.)

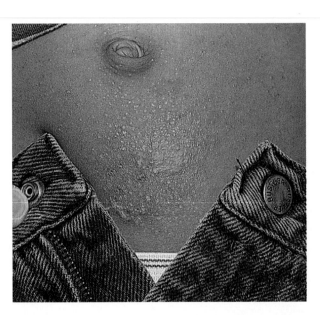

COLOR PLATE 21 Allergic contact dermatitis in a young child to nickel. (From Weston WL, Morelli JG, Lane A, eds: *Color textbook of pediatric dermatology,* ed 3, St Louis, 2002, Mosby.)

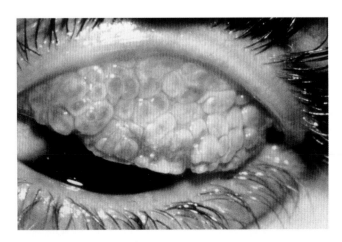

COLOR PLATE 19 Conjunctival hyperemia with papillary hypertrophy (cobblestoning) on an everted palpebral conjunctiva of the upper eyelid in a patient with vernal conjunctivitis.

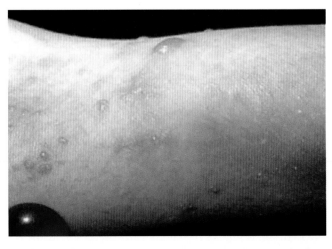

COLOR PLATE 22 Poison ivy dermatitis with characteristic linear vesicles.

CHAPTER 1

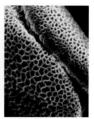

Epidemiology of Allergic Diseases

ERIKA VON MUTIUS

A large proportion of the population in affluent countries reports allergic reactions to a wide range of environmental stimuli. Many of the so-called allergic reactions are nonspecific, barely understood adverse effects of ingestion, inhalation, or other contact to environmental factors and should not be confused with atopic illnesses, which are characterized by the presence of IgE antibodies in affected subjects. Traditionally, asthma, allergic rhinitis, and hay fever, as well as atopic dermatitis, have been categorized as atopic diseases. However, the relation between clinical manifestations of these diseases and the production of IgE antibodies has not been fully clarified. Although in many patients with symptoms sufficiently severe to seek medical advice in tertiary referral centers high levels of total and specific IgE antibodies are found, many individuals in the general population do not show any signs of illness despite elevated IgE levels. Not surprisingly, risk factors and determinants of atopy, defined as the presence of IgE antibodies, differ from those associated with asthma, atopic dermatitis, and hay fever. Moreover, in some individuals various atopic illnesses can be coexpressed, whereas in other subjects only one manifestation of an atopic illness is present. The prevalence of these four atopic entities therefore only partially overlaps in the general population (Figure 1-1).

Asthma had been described in ancient times among Egyptian pharaohs, but hay fever, an easy-to-recognize clinical syndrome, was virtually unknown in Europe and North America until the late nineteenth century, when it was regarded as a rare disease entity. At that time the main causes of infant and adult morbidity were infectious diseases such as tuberculosis, smallpox, dysentery, pneumonia, typhoid fever, and diphtheria.[1] Eighty percent or more of children died from these diseases before reaching adulthood. In these days epidemiological studies were mostly concerned with the observation of the spread of infectious diseases among populations. Since the beginning of the twentieth century improvements in housing conditions, sanitation, water supply, nutrition and medical treatment have drastically reduced infectious diseases as major causes of death in developed countries such as the United States, and increased the average life expectancy from about 50 years in 1900 to nearly 74 years in 1984.[1] This change has been paralleled by the emergence of chronic illnesses such as cancer and heart disease, which are now the main causes of death in developed nations. In addition, many chronic disorders such as autoimmune illnesses and the various manifestations of atopic diseases have emerged.

Asthma, atopic dermatitis, and hay fever are likely to be determined by multiple factors as many other chronic disorders, some of which constitute host characteristics such as gender, race, and genetic predisposition and some of which consist of extrinsic, environmental influences. These influences are likely to interact on many different levels. In addition, environmental exposures may affect susceptible individuals only during certain time windows in which particular organ systems are vulnerable to extrinsic influences, and these windows of opportunity are likely to differ between types of atopic conditions. Therefore the timing of the exposure may be the third important dimension determining the potential of a risk factor to affect the onset, progression, or remission of an allergic disorder. Both the search for genes and for environmental determinants will rely on increasing knowledge about the mutual co-factors, taking into account the timing of exposure.

PREVALENCE OF CHILDHOOD ASTHMA AND ALLERGIES

Asthma is a complex syndrome rather than a single disease entity. Different phenotypes with varying prognoses and determinants have been described, particularly during childhood years,[2] and are discussed in detail in the next chapter. For example, transient early wheezing is characterized by the occurrence of wheezing in infants up to the age of 2 to 3 years, which disappears thereafter. The main predictor of these wheezing illnesses is premorbid reduced lung function before the manifestation of any wheeze.[3,4] These decrements in

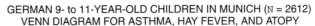

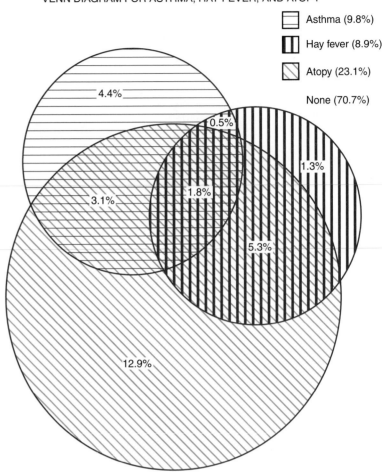

GERMAN 9- to 11-YEAR-OLD CHILDREN IN MUNICH (N = 2612)
VENN DIAGRAM FOR ASTHMA, HAY FEVER, AND ATOPY

Asthma (9.8%)

Hay fever (8.9%)

Atopy (23.1%)

None (70.7%)

4.4%

0.5%

1.3%

3.1%

1.8%

5.3%

12.9%

Percentages calculated for all non-missing cases (N = 1729)

FIGURE 1-1 The prevalence of asthma, hay fever, and atopic sensitization only partially overlaps on a population level. Description of findings from the International Study of Asthma and Allergies in Childhood Phase II study in Munich of German children aged 9 to 11 years. The Writing Committee of the ISAAC Steering Committee consists of Beasley R, Keil U, von Mutius E, and Pearce N. (From The International Study of Asthma and Allergies in Childhood [ISAAC]: *Lancet* 351:1225, 1998.)

pulmonary function are in part determined by passive smoke exposure in utero[5] and result in symptoms of airway obstruction when infants get infected with respiratory viruses. Atopy and a family history of asthma and atopy do not influence the incidence of this wheezing phenotype.

In contrast, wheeze among school-aged children is most often associated with atopic sensitization, bronchial hyperreactivity (BHR), and a familial predisposition for asthma.[2] Furthermore, the severity of symptoms and the degree of atopic sensitization and airway responsiveness determine the prognosis of this wheezing phenotype.[6] Finally, it seems likely that among preschool-aged children, a third wheezing phenotype exists that is mostly triggered by viral infections.[7] These children have a better prognosis than do atopic wheezers and often lose their symptoms around school age.

Most epidemiologic studies have used cross-sectional designs and thereby do not allow disentanglement of the different wheezing phenotypes. Only prospective studies following infants from birth up to school age and adolescence will identify different wheezing phenotypes and enable the differential analysis of risk factors and determinants for certain wheezing

phenotypes. These limitations must be borne in mind when discussing and interpreting findings from cross-sectional surveys. The relative proportion of different wheezing phenotypes is likely to vary among age groups, and therefore the strength of association between different risk factors and wheeze is also likely to vary across age groups.

Similarly, limitations apply with respect to the epidemiology of atopic dermatitis.[8] The definition of atopic eczema varies from study to study, and validations of questionnaire-based estimates have been few. Skin examinations by trained field workers that can add an objective parameter to questionnaire-based data do reflect a point prevalence of skin symptoms at the time of examination and therefore can corroborate estimates of lifetime prevalence only in limited ways, such as assessments by questions inquiring about whether a physician ever made a diagnosis of eczema. In all cross-sectional surveys, identified risk factors relate to the prevalence of the condition, that is, the incidence and persistence of the disease. It is therefore often difficult to disentangle aggravating from causal factors in such studies. There are very few prospective surveys that aim to identify environmental exposures before the onset of clinical manifestations of atopic dermatitis.

Western versus Developing Countries

In general, reported rates of asthma, hay fever, and atopic dermatitis are higher in affluent Western countries than in developing countries. The worldwide prevalence of allergic diseases was assessed in the 1990s by the large-scale International Study of Asthma and Allergies in Childhood (ISAAC).[9] A total of 463,801 children in 155 collaborating centers in 56 countries were studied. Children self-reported, through one-page questionnaires, symptoms of these three atopic disorders. Between twentyfold and sixtyfold differences were found among centers in the prevalence of symptoms of asthma, allergic rhinoconjunctivitis, and atopic eczema. The highest 12-month prevalence of asthma symptoms was reported from centers in the United Kingdom, Australia, New Zealand, and the Republic of Ireland (Figure 1-2). These were followed by most centers in North, Central, and South America. The lowest prevalence was reported by centers in several Eastern European countries, Indonesia, Greece, China, Taiwan, Uzbekistan, India, and Ethiopia. In general, centers with low asthma rates also showed low levels of other atopic diseases. However, countries with the highest prevalence of allergic rhinitis and atopic eczema were not identical to those with the highest asthma rates.

The European Community Respiratory Health Survey (ECRHS) studied young adults aged 20 to 44 years.[10] A highly standardized and comprehensive study instrument including questionnaires, lung function, and allergy testing was used by 35 to 48 centers in 22 countries predominantly in Western Europe but also included centers in Australia, New Zealand, and the United States of America. The ECRHS has shown large geographic differences in the prevalence of respiratory symptoms, asthma, BHR, and atopic sensitization with high prevalence in English-speaking countries and low prevalence rates in the Mediterranean region and Eastern Europe.[11] The geographic pattern emerging from questionnaire findings was consistent with the distribution of atopy and BHR, supporting the conclusion that the geographic variation in asthma is true and not attributable to methodologic factors such as the questionnaire phrasing, the skin testing technique, or the type of assay for the measurement of specific IgE.

Moreover, a strong correlation was found between the findings from children as assessed in the ISAAC Study and the

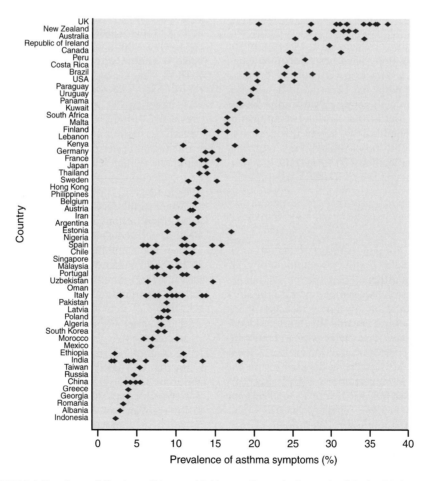

FIGURE 1-2 Prevalence of allergic conditions worldwide according to the International Study of Asthma and Allergies in Childhood Phase I study. (From The International Study of Asthma and Allergies in Childhood [ISAAC]: *Lancet* 351:1225, 1998.)

rates in adults as reported with the ECRHS questionnaire.[12] Sixty-four percent of variation at the country level and 74% of variation at the center level in the prevalence of "wheeze in the last 12 months" in the ECRHS data were explained by the variation rates reported for children in the ISAAC Study. Thus, although there were differences in the absolute prevalences observed in the two surveys, there was good overall agreement, adding support to the validity of both studies.

Within this global perspective some comparisons seem particularly informative. For example, studies of populations with comparable ethnic backgrounds but striking differences in environmental exposures were performed in China among children living in Hong Kong and mainland China, namely Beijing and Urumqi.[13] Beijing children reported significantly more asthma symptoms than did those living in Urumqi, but Hong Kong children had the highest prevalence of asthma and other allergic symptoms. Urumqui, Beijing, and Hong Kong represent communities at increasing stages of affluence and westernization, and the findings from these three cities can be interpreted as a reflection of a worldwide trend for increasing prevalence of asthma and allergies as westernization intensifies.

The prevalence of symptoms, diagnosis, and management of asthma in school-aged children in Australia was compared with that for Nigerian children by using another standardized methodology.[14] Wheeze, asthma, and asthma medication use were less prevalent in Nigeria than in Australia. No significant difference was found in the overall prevalence of atopy between the two countries, although atopy was a strong risk factor for asthma in both countries. Dissociations between the prevalence of asthma and atopy have been documented in other developing countries, such as in Ethiopia.[15,16] In these areas a high prevalence of atopy has been found despite low rates of asthma. Infestation with parasites has been proposed as a potential explanation, but further work must confirm or refute these hypotheses. The findings, however, suggest that "asthma" and "atopy" are only loosely linked phenotypes and that the strength of association between these traits is dependent on the environmental conditions in which the individuals live.

Migration Studies

As proposed earlier, the timing of exposure to certain environments may play a crucial role in the development of allergic diseases, particularly for asthma. Therefore the relation between the prevalence of respiratory symptoms and time since arrival in Australia was studied in immigrant teenagers living in Melbourne. In subjects born outside Australia, residence for 5 to 9 years in Australia was associated with a twofold increase in the odds of self-reported wheeze; after 10 to 14 years, this risk increased threefold. This "time-dose" effect on the prevalence of symptoms in subjects born outside Australia and living in Melbourne was independent of age and country of birth.[17] The findings can be interpreted as suggestive of duration of exposure being the important determinant of incidence of illness. Alternatively, the results indicate that exposure early in life is more important than exposure later in life.

Likewise, in children migrating from the Pacific Islands of Tokelau to New Zealand, a large increase has been documented in the prevalence of atopic eczema compared with that in children of similar ethnic groups in their country of origin.[18] Furthermore, Asian children born in Australia have been reported to be at higher risk of atopic eczema than those who recently immigrated to Australia.[19]

The East-West Gradient Across Europe

A number of reports have demonstrated large differences between east and west European areas in the prevalence of bronchitis, asthma, BHR, hay fever, and atopy in children and adults.[20-25] Studies that investigated infection-associated symptoms such as the frequency of colds,[21] the prevalence of coughing bouts for more than 2 weeks with common cold,[21] or the prevalence of ever having bronchitis[20] found higher prevalences in the Baltic area compared with Sweden or in East Germany compared with West Germany. In contrast, the prevalence of asthma was significantly lower in all study areas in eastern Europe than in western Europe.[20,24] Furthermore, all except one investigator reported significantly lower prevalences of hay fever, nasal allergies, and atopy as measured by skin prick tests or specific serum IgE antibodies to environmental allergens among children and adults living in eastern European areas compared with subjects living in western European areas.[21-25]

Differences in the observed prevalence rates of physician-diagnosed asthma and bronchitis between western and eastern Europe may reflect previous and ongoing differences in diagnostic labeling. However, when considering the relations among atopic sensitization, BHR, and respiratory illnesses in the German studies,[20] wheezing illnesses other than those labeled as asthma were more strongly associated with atopy and BHR in West Germany than in East Germany. Furthermore, the prevalence of bronchitis associated with atopy and BHR was higher in the western part of the country. Finally, the prevalence of BHR was significantly higher in western than in eastern Germany among both children and adults. Cough and bronchitis in Eastern Europe are likely to be at least in part attributable to high levels of exposure to ambient air pollution or to infectious stimuli encountered in the day care centers early in life.

Data from the East European ISAAC studies have corroborated these notions and expanded findings to areas such as Georgia and Uzbekistan.[26] Among the older age group of 13- to 14-year-old children, the prevalence of wheezing was 11.2% to 19.7% in Finland and Sweden; 7.6% to 8.5% in Estonia, Latvia, and Poland; and 2.6% to 5.9% in Albania, Romania, Russia, Georgia, and Uzbekistan (except Samarkand). The prevalence of itchy eyes and flexural dermatitis varied in a similar manner among the three regions.

In contrast to hay fever, atopy, asthma, and BHR, the prevalence of atopic dermatitis is likely to be higher in East Germany than in West Germany. In the studies of preschool-aged children[25] in which children also underwent skin examination by dermatologists, the prevalence of atopic eczema was 17.5% in the east German area and 5.7% to 15.3% in the west German regions. Furthermore, Schäfer et al[25] recently reported that the excess of atopic eczema in East Germany is likely to be related to an intrinsic, nonatopic phenotype of the disease. Although half of the West German children with atopic eczema were sensitized according to skin prick test results, only one third of the East German children had positive skin prick test reactions.

Differences Between Rural and Urban Populations

Studies of children living in urban and rural areas of Africa documented that asthma and BHR were almost nonexistent in some rural areas in the late 1980s and early 1990s.[27] In turn, among the more affluent urban populations of South Africa and Zimbabwe, BHR reached a prevalence of 3.2% and 5.9%, respectively. Similar results were reported from other African regions. However, during the past decade, airway responsiveness seems to have increased in rural Africa.[27] In Saudi Arabia, similar urban-rural differences were reported[28]; a significantly lower prevalence of allergic symptoms was found among rural compared with urban children.

In western European countries, urban-rural differences seem to be less pronounced. In a large British study, only marginal differences were observed in the prevalence of childhood asthma between rural and urban areas.[29] In contrast, data from Sweden indicated a higher prevalence of atopic sensitization to aeroallergens among children from urban centers compared with those living in rural areas.[21] Recent findings from Austria,[30] Finland,[31] Canada,[32] southern Germany,[33] and Switzerland[34] suggested that the lower prevalence of atopic diseases in rural populations may in part be attributable to the presence of protective factors in a farm environment rather than to the absence of urban risk factors. Interestingly, the prevalence of atopic dermatitis did not differ between farm and nonfarm children.

Growing up on a farm confers significant protection against the development of asthma, hay fever, and atopy.[30-32,34] Several investigators observed that the "farming effect" was attributable to frequent contact with livestock and the consumption of nonpasteurized cow's milk. A dose-response relation between exposure to farm animals and the prevalence of atopic disease was reported in one of these studies.[33] The effects were most pronounced when exposure to stables and nonpasteurized milk occurred in the first year of life[35]; the prevalence of asthma was reduced to 1.4% if infants were exposed to stables and farm milk in the first year of life compared with 11.8% in the nonexposed group.[35] This supports the importance of timing with respect to the impact of environmental exposures on the subsequent development of disease; exposures to stables and nonpasteurized milk after the first year of life did not significantly influence the development of asthma, hay fever, and atopy.[35]

Inner-City Areas of the United States

In contrast to the protective factors encountered in pediatric farming populations of rural areas, living conditions of inner-city areas in the United States are associated with a markedly increased risk of asthma.[36] Several potential risk factors are being investigated, such as race and poverty, adherence to asthma treatment,[37] and factors related to the disproportionate exposures associated with socioeconomic disadvantage such as indoor and outdoor exposure to pollution and cockroach infestation.[38] At least early in life, cockroach exposure has been associated with the development of sensitization to cockroach allergen[39] and wheeze[40] in infants living in inner-city areas of the United States. Problems related to inner-city asthma are discussed in more detail in Chapter 37.

TIME TRENDS IN THE PREVALENCE OF ALLERGIC DISEASES

Numerous studies have investigated the trends in the occurrence of allergic disorders.[41] Data collected during the past 40 years in industrialized countries indicate a significant increase in the prevalence of asthma, hay fever, and atopic dermatitis. All of the investigators used identical questionnaires in similar population samples at different times. Therefore these studies are reliable indicators of changes in prevalence over time. Most studies lack objective measurements such as BHR and atopic sensitization. However, the consistent and strong increase in the prevalence of allergic conditions indicates that a true increase in the prevalence has occurred. A well-documented study from Australia that used airway histamine challenges, skin prick tests, and questionnaires supports this notion by showing a doubling of the prevalence of current wheeze and BHR between 1982 and 1992.[42]

Despite the use of different methods and definitions of asthma, most studies from industrialized countries suggest an overall increase in the prevalence of asthma and wheezing between 1960 and 1990. Most studies have been performed among children, and little is known about time trends among adults. Twenty-year trends of the prevalence of treated asthma among pediatric and adult members of a large U.S. health maintenance organization were recently reported.[43] During the period of 1967 through 1987, the treated prevalence of asthma increased significantly in all age-sex categories except males aged 65 and older. In the United States, the greatest increase was detected among children and young adults living in inner cities.[44] Likewise, the prevalence of asthma increased in children and adults from 1981 through 1990 in Saskatchewan, Canada.[45]

Recent studies suggest that in some areas this trend continues unabated. Kuehni et al[46] reported from the United Kingdom that among preschool children, the prevalence of all types of wheezing increased from 1990 through 1998. In contrast, studies for Italy showed that among school-aged children surveyed in 1974, 1992, and 1998, the prevalence of asthma increased significantly during the period of 1974 to 1992, whereas it remained stable during the past 4 years.[47] Further observations are needed to document population morbidity over the years to come.

ENVIRONMENTAL RISK FACTORS FOR ALLERGIC DISEASES

Air Pollution

The weight of evidence argues against a causal relationship between air pollution levels and the initiation of asthma and allergic diseases. The geographic variation in the prevalence of asthma in children does not coincide with variations in air pollution levels. The increase in the prevalence of asthma and allergies seen during the past decades was paralleled by a decrease in emissions of sulfur dioxide and particles from coal combustions and an increase in emissions from motor vehicle traffic. The results from epidemiologic surveys do not, however, support a causal link between exposure to these traffic-related pollutants and the incidence of asthma and allergic illnesses. Because most studies so far have used cross-sectional designs with all of the limitations discussed, there is a need for prospective studies that on a personal level, such as using geographic information systems, link pollution data to the incidence of various wheezing phenotypes.

In panel and time-series studies, air pollutants such as fine particles and ozone reduce lung function among children already affected by asthma and increase symptoms and medication use. Likewise, emergency department visits, general practitioner visits, and hospital admissions for asthma and wheeze are positively associated with ambient air pollution levels. Thus there is ample evidence to suggest that increasing pollutant concentrations and exposure to traffic emissions can trigger and exacerbate preexisting disease, even when taking pollen and mould counts as well as influenza epidemics into account.

Besides pollution, environmental factors such as domestic water supply may be relevant for the inception of atopic dermatitis. An ecologic study of the relation between domestic water hardness and the prevalence of atopic eczema among British school-aged children was performed.[48] Geographic information systems were used to link the geographic distribution of eczema in the study area to four categories of domestic water-hardness data. Among the primary-school children aged 4 to 16 years, a significant relation was found between the prevalence of atopic eczema and water hardness both before and after adjustment for potential confounding factors. The 1-year period prevalence was 17.3% in the highest water-hardness category and 12.0% in the lowest category (adjusted odds ratio, 1.54; 95% confidence interval, 1.19 to 1.99). The effect on recent eczema symptoms was stronger than on lifetime prevalence, which may indicate that water hardness acts more on existing dermatitis by exacerbating the disorder or prolonging its duration than as a cause of new cases.

Environmental Tobacco Smoke

The effects of exposure to environmental tobacco smoke (ETS) on children have been extensively studied, and numerous surveys have consistently reported an association between ETS exposure and respiratory diseases. Strong evidence exists that passive smoking increases the risk of lower respiratory tract illnesses such as bronchitis, wheezy bronchitis, and pneumonia in infants and young children. Maternal smoking during pregnancy and early childhood has been shown to be strongly associated with impaired lung growth and diminished lung function,[3,5,49] which, in turn, may predispose infants to develop transient early wheezing. In children with asthma, parental smoking increases symptoms and the frequency of asthma attacks. A series of epidemiologic studies has also been performed to determine the effect of ETS exposure on the inception, prevalence, and severity of asthma. In most cross-sectional and longitudinal studies, ETS exposure appears to be an important risk factor for the development of childhood asthma. Conversely, no unequivocal association was seen among ETS exposure, atopic sensitization, and atopic dermatitis.

Nutrition

The rise in childhood asthma prevalence during the past 30 years in developed countries has coincided with an increase in affluence in these countries. Increasing affluence is marked by

a substantial change in dietary habits, and therefore the hypothesis was proposed that these changes may contribute to the observed increase in asthma prevalence. However, no consistent findings have emerged from recent surveys that investigated the role of salt and magnesium intake as well as the consumption of saturated and unsaturated fatty acids, antioxidants, and vitamins. Based on the current knowledge, limited evidence exists that a diet low in sodium and rich in fish and vitamin C has a positive effect on the course of asthma symptoms. However, intervention studies are needed to test the hypothesis that nutrition may be involved in the development of childhood asthma and allergies.

Allergen Exposure

There is some evidence to suggest that the level of allergen exposure is a risk factor for the development of atopic sensitization in children.[50,51] In the German Multicentre Atopy Study, a large birth cohort following newborn children up to the age of 7 years, house dust mite and cat allergen concentrations in domestic carpet dust were strongly related to the development of atopic sensitization toward that specific allergen in the first 3 years of life and up to the age of 7 years.[50] A clear dose-response relation was found as well as a strong effect modification by the familial background.

Whether environmental allergen exposure affects the incidence of asthma in ways similar to the development of atopic sensitization is doubtful. If the level of exposure to house dust mites early in life was indeed crucial for the expression of asthma, children brought up in a mite-free environment at high altitude should have a significantly lower prevalence of asthma and wheeze than children from humid, mite-infested areas. The results of two studies performed in the Alps and in New Mexico failed, however, to document such spatial variation.[52,53] Furthermore, in desert areas such as Tucson, Arizona, and inland Australia, where house dust mites are rarely detected, the prevalence of asthma is rather high.[54,55] Furthermore, a recent report from the German Multicentre Study clearly pointed out that although allergen levels were a strong predictor of sensitization toward that specific allergen, the incidence of asthma up to the age of 7 years was not.[56] Thus in contrast to the immunologic processes involved with the production of specific IgE antibodies, the mechanisms inducing an asthmatic condition might not be susceptible to changes in allergen exposure levels.

Family Size

Strachan[57] first reported that sibship size is inversely related to the prevalence of childhood atopic diseases. This observation has since been confirmed by numerous studies showing that atopy, hay fever, and atopic eczema were inversely related to increasing numbers of siblings.[58-60] In contrast, the relation between family size and childhood asthma and BHR is less clear.[61]

Several hypotheses have been proposed in an effort to explain this consistent, strong inverse association. Having more (older) siblings increases the exposure to infections passed on among children. Therefore having (older) siblings may contribute to a higher infectious burden, thereby directing the development of the immune system in a nonatopic direction. However, it is also conceivable that multiple pregnancies alter the immune status of the mother in a way that protects a child from the development of atopic illnesses.

Infections and Hygiene

Viral infections of both the upper and the lower respiratory tract are very common during infancy and early childhood. Nevertheless, most children do not experience any aftermath relating to those infections, including infections with respiratory syncytial virus (RSV).[62] This, therefore, suggests that there is at least one host factor that determines the development of bronchiolitis and recurrent wheeze after RSV infection.

Several investigators have followed children with proved RSV bronchiolitis for several years. Most clinical studies[62-64] reported reductions in lung function and increased prevalence of BHR in cases compared with controls. A recent report from a population-based birth cohort study in Tucson, Arizona, showed that RSV lower respiratory tract illnesses were indeed associated with a diminishing risk of recurrent wheezing over the school years starting with a fourfold increased risk at age 6 years that then reduced to no risk at age 13.[65] The occurrence of RSV lower respiratory tract illnesses was unrelated to the development of atopic sensitization. These findings suggest that an underlying predisposition to wheeze may be unmasked by RSV infections early in life, which is, however, unrelated to the development of atopic asthma.

An inverse relation between asthma and the overall burden of respiratory infections may exist. Evidence for this assumption is derived from a number of sources. First, it had been observed that in developing countries such as in Papua, New Guinea, and the Fiji Islands, as well as in eastern European countries, asthma is inversely related to the overall burden of respiratory infections. The results of other studies substantiate the potential protective effect of infections on the development of asthma and allergies in later childhood. A recent report from southern Italy showed that military recruits who were seropositive for hepatitis A, *Toxoplasma gondii*, or *Helicobacter pylori* had a significantly lower prevalence of atopic sensitization to common aeroallergens, allergic rhinitis, and allergic asthma compared with their peers who did not have antibodies.[66] A dose-response relation was observed: the more orofecal infections that these recruits had, the lower was the prevalence of allergic diseases. Two large studies investigating children in day care early in life have shown that children who are in day care during the first 6 to 12 months of life were at a significantly reduced risk of wheezing, hay fever, and atopic sensitization at school age and adolescence.[67,68]

A potential protective effect of parasitic infections, such as in areas of the developing world, has not yet been explored sufficiently. Microbial stimulation, from both normal commensals and pathogens through the gut, may be another route of exposure that may have altered the normal intestinal colonization pattern in infancy. In this way, the induction and maintenance of oral tolerance of innocuous antigens, such as food proteins and inhaled allergens, may be substantially hampered.[69,70] These hypotheses, although intriguing, have to date not been supported by epidemiologic evidence because significant methodologic difficulties arise when attempting to measure the microbial pattern of the intestinal flora.

Exposure to microbes does, however, occur not only through invasive infection of human tissues. Viable germs and nonviable parts of microbial organisms are ubiquitous in nature and can be found in varying concentrations in daily indoor and outdoor environments. These microbial products are recognized by the innate immune system as strong danger signals even in the absence of overt infection and induce a potent inflammatory response. Therefore environmental exposure to microbial products may play a crucial role in the maturation of a child's immune response, enabling tolerance of other components of its natural environment such as pollen and animal dander.

Findings from a longitudinal survey of infants in Denver, Colorado, support this notion, showing that infants exposed to high concentrations of endotoxin in dust collected from their homes were less likely to develop IgE antibodies to local allergens and have stronger cytokine responses of the Th-1 type by peripheral blood mononuclear cells.[71] Furthermore, exposure to microbial products is likely to explain the protective effects associated with growing up on a farm, in that characteristics of a farming lifestyle, namely exposure to stables and nonpasteurized cow's milk early in life, were found to result in very low prevalence of atopic and nonatopic asthma, hay fever, and IgE-mediated sensitization. Furthermore, indoor levels of endotoxin, a cell wall component of gram-negative bacteria, were found to be higher in dust samples from mattresses and living room floors of farm children, supporting the notion that exposure to microbial products is higher among farm children compared with rural controls.[72] In these subjects, endotoxin exposure was strongly inversely related to the prevalence of atopic asthma and allergies.[73] Interestingly, the effect of endotoxin exposure was independent of and in addition to the strong protection conferred by early farming exposures.

The findings therefore support the notion that endotoxin may not be the only microbial product associated with the lower prevalence of asthma and allergies in subjects living on animal farms. Individuals who are more heavily exposed to endotoxin are likely to be co-exposed to other pathogen-associated molecular patterns, which may also influence the development of immune responses.[74] Recent work suggests that different pathogen-associated molecular patterns, such as lipoproteins, lipopeptides, lipoarabinomannan, lipotechoic acid, and glucans, act as ligands for pattern recognition receptors that are present on the surface of innate immunity cells.

CONCLUSIONS

Large variations have been reported in the prevalence of childhood and adult asthma and allergies (Box 1-1). In affluent countries, prevalences are generally higher than those in poorer countries. Lower levels are seen especially in some rural areas in Africa, Saudi Arabia, and China and among farmers' children in Europe. Overall an increasing trend is reported in the prevalence of asthma, hay fever, and atopic dermatitis in recent decades. Numerous environmental factors have been scrutinized, but no conclusive explanation for the rising trends has been found. Future challenges are to tackle the complex interplay between environmental factors and genetic determinants. The search for genes and for environmental determinants will rely on an increasing knowledge about the mutual co-factors eventually contributing to a better understanding and, it is hoped, to better prevention strategies for asthma and allergies.

BOX 1-1	KEY CONCEPTS *Variation in the Prevalence of Asthma and Allergy*

- Large geographic variations in the prevalence of allergic diseases exist worldwide among children and adults.
- Lower prevalences have been reported from some developing countries, eastern European areas, and rural areas in Africa, China, and Saudi Arabia.
- The prevalence of asthma and allergies has increased during the past decades. It remains to be seen whether this trend is ongoing. Some studies from Europe suggest that a plateau has been reached.
- Allergic diseases are multifactorial illnesses determined by a complex interplay between genetic and environmental factors.

REFERENCES

1. Hennekens C, Buring J: *Epidemiology in medicine*, Boston, 1987, Little, Brown.
2. Martinez F, Wright A, Taussig L, et al: Asthma and wheezing in the first six years of life, *N Engl J Med* 332:133, 1995.
3. Martinez F, Morgan W, Wright A, et al: Diminished lung function as a predisposing factor for wheezing respiratory illness in infants, *N Engl J Med* 319:1112, 1988.
4. Dezateux C, Stocks J, Dundas I, et al: Impaired airway function and wheezing in infancy: the influence of maternal smoking and a genetic predisposition to asthma, *Am J Respir Crit Care Med* 159:403, 1999.
5. Hanrahan J, Tager I, Segal M, et al: The effect of maternal smoking during pregnancy on early infant lung function, *Am Rev Respir Dis* 145:1129, 1992.
6. von Mutius E: Paediatric origins of adult lung disease, *Thorax* 56:153, 2001.
7. Stein R, Holberg C, Morgan W, et al: Peak flow variability, methacholine responsiveness and atopy as markers for detecting different wheezing phenotypes in childhood, *Thorax* 52:946, 1997.
8. von Mutius E: Risk factors for atopic dermatitis. In Bieber T, Leung S, editors: *Atopic dermatitis*, New York/Basel, 2002, Marcel Dekker.
9. Isaacc SC: Worldwide variations in the prevalence of asthma symptoms: the International Study of Asthma and Allergies in Childhood (ISAAC), *Eur Respir J* 12:315, 1998.
10. Burney P, Luczynska C, Chinn S, et al: The European Community Respiratory Health Survey, *Eur Respir J* 7:954, 1994.
11. Janson C, Anto J, Burney P, et al: The European Community Respiratory Health Survey: what are the main results so far? *Eur Respir J* 18:598, 2001.
12. Pearce N, Sunyer J, Cheng S, et al: Comparison of asthma prevalence in the ISAAC and the ECRHS, *Eur Respir J* 16:420, 2000.
13. Zhao T, Wang A, Chen Y, et al: Prevalence of childhood asthma, allergic rhinitis and eczema in Urumqi and Beijing, *J Paediatr Child Health* 36:128, 2000.
14. Faniran A, Peat J, Woolcock A: Prevalence of atopy, asthma symptoms and diagnosis, and the management of asthma: comparison of an affluent and a non-affluent country, *Thorax* 54:606, 1999.
15. Scrivener S, Yemaneberhan H, Zebenigus M, et al: Independent effects of intestinal parasite infection and domestic allergen exposure on risk of wheeze in Ethiopia: a nested case-control study, *Lancet* 358:1493, 2001.
16. Pearce N, Pekkanen J, Beasley R: How much asthma is really attributable to atopy? *Thorax* 54:268, 1999.
17. Powell C, Nolan T, Carlin J, et al: Respiratory symptoms and duration of residence in immigrant teenagers living in Melbourne, Australia, *Arch Dis Child* 81:159, 1999.
18. Waite D, Eyles E, Tonkin S, et al: Asthma prevalence in Tokelauan children in two environments, *Clin Allergy* 10:71, 1980.
19. Leung R: Asthma, allergy and atopy in South-East Asian immigrants in Australia, *Austral N Z J Med* 24:255, 1994.
20. von Mutius E, Martinez FD, Fritzsch C, et al: Prevalence of asthma and atopy in two areas of West and East Germany, *Am J Respir Crit Care Med* 149:358, 1994.
21. Braback L, Breborowicz A, Dreborg S, et al: Atopic sensitization and respiratory symptoms among Polish and Swedish school children, *Clin Exp Allergy* 24:826, 1994.
22. Braback L, Breborowicz A, Julge K, et al: Risk factors for respiratory symptoms and atopic sensitisation in the Baltic area, *Arch Dis Child* 72:487, 1995.
23. Nicolai T, Bellach B, von Mutius E, et al: Increased prevalence of sensitisation against aeroallergens in adults in West- compared to East-Germany, *Clin Exp Allergy* 27:886, 1997.
24. Nowak D, Heinrich J, Jorres R, et al: Prevalence of respiratory symptoms, bronchial hyperresponsiveness and atopy among adults: West and East Germany, *Eur Respir J* 9:2541, 1996.
25. Schäfer T, Vieluf D, Behrendt H, et al: Atopic eczema and other manifestations of atopy: results of a study in East and West Germany, *Allergy* 51:532, 1996.
26. Björksten B, Dumitrascu D, Foucard T, et al: Prevalence of childhood asthma, rhinitis and eczema in Scandinavia and Eastern Europe, *Eur Respir J* 12:432, 1998.
27. Weinberg E: Urbanization and childhood asthma: an African perspective, *J Allergy Clin Immunol* 105:224, 2000.
28. Hijazi N, Abalkhail B, Seaton A: Asthma and respiratory symptoms in urban and rural Saudi Arabia, *Eur Respir J* 12:41, 1998.
29. Strachan DP, Anderson HR, Limb ES, et al: A national survey of asthma prevalence, severity, and treatment in Great Britain, *Arch Dis Child* 70:174, 1994.
30. Riedler J, Eder W, Oberfeld G, et al: Austrian children living on a farm have less hay fever, asthma and allergic sensitization, *Clin Exp Allergy* 30:194, 2000.
31. Kilpelainen M, Terho E, Helenius H, et al: Farm environment in childhood prevents the development of allergies, *Clin Exp Allergy* 30:201, 2000.
32. Ernst P, Cormier Y: Relative scarcity of asthma and atopy among adolescents raised on a farm, *Am J Respir Crit Care Med* 161:1563, 2000.
33. von Ehrenstein O, von Mutius E, Illi S, et al: Reduced risk of hay fever and asthma among children of farmers, *Clin Exp Allergy* 30:187, 2000.
34. Braun-Fahrländer C, Gassner M, Grize L, et al: Prevalence of hay fever and allergic sensitization in farmer's children and their peers living in the same rural community. SCARPOL team. Swiss Study on Childhood Allergy and Respiratory Symptoms with Respect to Air Pollution, *Clin Exp Allergy* 29:28, 1999.
35. Riedler J, Eder W, Schreuer M, et al, and the ALEX Study Team: Early life exposure to farming provides protection against the development of asthma and allergy, *Lancet* 358:1129, 2001.
36. Webber M, Carpiniello K, Oruwariye T, et al: Prevalence of asthma and asthma-like symptoms in inner-city elementary schoolchildren, *Pediatr Pulmonol* 34:105, 2002.
37. Bauman L, Wright E, Leickly F, et al: Relationship of adherence to pediatric asthma morbidity among inner-city children, *Pediatrics* 110:1, 2002.
38. Rauh V, Chew G, Garfinkel R: Deteriorated housing contributes to high cockroach allergen levels in inner-city households, *Environ Health Perspect* 110:323, 2002.
39. Alp H, Yu B, Grant E, et al: Cockroach allergy appears early in life in inner-city children with recurrent wheezing, *Ann Allergy Asthma Immunol* 86:51, 2001.
40. Litonjua A, Carey V, Burge H, et al: Exposure to cockroach allergen in the home is associated with incident doctor-diagnosed asthma and recurrent wheezing, *J Allergy Clin Immunol* 107:41, 2001.
41. von Mutius E: Environmental factors and rising time trends in prevalence and severity. In Holgate S, Boushey H, Fabbri L, editors: *Difficult asthma*, London, 1999, Martin Dunitz.
42. Peat JK, van den Berg RH, Green WF, et al: Changing prevalence of asthma in Australian children, *Br Med J* 308:1591, 1994.
43. Vollmer W, Osborne M, Buist A: 20-Year trends in the prevalence of asthma and chronic airflow obstruction in an HMO, *Am J Respir Crit Care Med* 157:1079, 1998.
44. Eggleston P, Buckley T, Breysse P, et al: The environment and asthma in U.S. inner cities, *Environ Health Perspect* 107:439, 1999.
45. Senthilselvan A: Prevalence of physician-diagnosed asthma in Saskatchewan, 1981 to 1990, *Chest* 114:388, 1998.
46. Kuehni C, Davis A, Brooke A, et al: Are all wheezing disorders in very young (preschool) children increasing in prevalence? *Lancet* 357:1821, 2001.
47. Ronchetti R, Villa M, Barreto M, et al: Is the increase in childhood asthma coming to an end? Findings from three surveys of schoolchildren in Rome, Italy, *Eur Respir J* 17:881, 2001.

48. McNally N, Williams H, Phillips D, et al: Atopic eczema and domestic water hardness, *Lancet* 352:527-531, 1998.

49. Tager IB, Hanrahan JP, Tosteson TD, et al: Lung function, pre- and postnatal smoke exposure, and wheezing in the first year of life, *Am Rev Respir Dis* 147:811-817, 1993.

50. Lau S, Falkenhorst A, Weber I, et al: High mite-allergen exposure increases the risk of sensitization in atopic children and young adults, *J Allergy Clin Immunol* 84:718-725, 1989.

51. Kuehr J, Frischer T, Meinert R, et al: Mite allergen exposure is a risk for the incidence of specific sensitization, *J Allergy Clin Immunol* 94:44-52, 1994.

52. Charpin D, Birnbaum J, Haddi E, et al: Altitude and allergy to house-dust mites: a paradigm of the influence of environmental exposure on allergic sensitization, *Am Rev Respir Dis* 143:983-986, 1991.

53. Sporik R, Ingram JM, Price W, et al: Association of asthma with serum IgE and skin test reactivity to allergens among children living at high altitude: tickling the dragon's breath, *Am J Respir Crit Care Med* 151: 1388-1392, 1995.

54. Halonen M, Stern DA, Wright AL, et al: Alternaria as a major allergen for asthma in children raised in a desert environment, *Am J Respir Crit Care Med* 155:1356-1361, 1997.

55. Peat JK, Woolcock AJ: Sensitivity to common allergens: relation to respiratory symptoms and bronchial hyper-responsiveness in children from three different climatic areas of Australia, *Clin Exp Allergy* 21:573-581, 1991.

56. Lau S, Illi S, Sommerfeld C, et al: Early exposure to house dust mite and cat allergens and the development of childhood asthma, *Lancet* 356: 1392-1397, 2000.

57. Strachan D: Hay fever, hygiene, and household size, *Br Med J* 299: 1259-1260, 1989.

58. Strachan DP, Taylor EM, Carpenter RG: Family structure, neonatal infection, and hay fever in adolescence, *Arch Dis Child* 74:422-426, 1996.

59. Jarvis D, Chinn S, Luczynska C, et al: The association of family size with atopy and atopic disease, *Clin Exp Allergy* 27:240-245, 1997.

60. von Mutius E, Martinez FD, Fritzsch C, et al: Skin test reactivity and number of siblings [see comments], *Br Med J* 308:692-695, 1994.

61. von Mutius E: The environmental predictors of allergic disease, *J Allergy Clin Immunol* 105:9-19, 1994.

62. Long C, McBride J, Hall C: Sequelae of respiratory syncytial virus infections: a role for intervention studies, *Am J Respir Crit Care Med* 151: 1678-1680, 1995.

63. Sims DG, Downham MA, Gardner PS, et al: Study of 8-year-old children with a history of respiratory syncytial virus bronchiolitis in infancy, *Br Med J* 1:11-14, 1978.

64. Pullan CR, Hey EN: Wheezing, asthma, and pulmonary dysfunction 10 years after infection with respiratory syncytial virus in infancy, *Br Med J Clin Res Ed* 284:1665-1669, 1982.

65. Stein R, Sherrill D, Morgan W, et al: Respiratory syncytial virus in early life and risk of wheeze and allergy by age 13 years, *Lancet* 354:541-545, 1999.

66. Matricardi PM, Rosmini F, Riondino S, et al: Exposure to foodborne and orofecal microbes versus airborne viruses in relation to atopy and allergic asthma: epidemiological study, *Br Med J* 320:412-417, 2000.

67. Ball T, Castro-Rodriguez J, Griffith K, et al: Siblings, day-care attendance, and the risk of asthma and wheezing during childhood, *N Engl J Med* 343:538-543, 2000.

68. Krämer U, Heinrich J, Wjst M, et al: Age of entry to day nursery and allergy in later childhood, *Lancet* 352:450-454, 1998.

69. Wold A: The hygiene hypothesis revised: is the rising frequency of allergy due to changes in the intestinal flora? *Allergy* 53:20-25, 1998.

70. Holt P: Mucosal immunity in relation to the development of oral tolerance/sensitization, *Allergy* 53:16-19, 1998.

71. Gereda J, Leung D, Thatayatikom A, et al: Relation between house-dust endotoxin exposure, type 1 T-cell development, and allergen sensitisation in infants at high risk of asthma, *Lancet* 355:1680-1683, 2000.

72. von Mutius E, Braun-Fahrländer C, Schierl R, et al: Exposure to endotoxin or other bacterial components might protect against the development of atopy, *Clin Exp Allergy* 30:1230-1234, 2000.

73. Braun-Fahrländer C, Riedler J, Herz U, et al: Environmental exposure to endotoxin, atopy and asthma in school-aged children, *N Engl J Med* 347:869-877, 2002.

74. Lauener R, Birchler T, Adamski J, et al: Expression of CD14 and Toll-like receptor 2 differs between farmer's and non-farmer's children, *Lancet* 360:465-466, 2002.

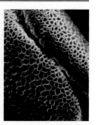

Natural History of Allergic Diseases and Asthma

ANDREW H. LIU ■ FERNANDO D. MARTINEZ ■ LYNN M. TAUSSIG

Natural history studies of allergic diseases are fundamental to our understanding of disease prognosis—for predicting disease onset, progression, and remittance. Such studies reveal a developmental "allergic march" in childhood, from the early onset of atopic dermatitis and food allergies in infancy, to asthma, allergic rhinitis, and inhalant allergen sensitization in later childhood. Allergy and asthma of earlier onset and greater severity are generally associated with disease persistence. By adulthood, remission in allergic rhinitis and asthma are rare. Therefore allergy and asthma commonly develop during the early childhood years, the period of greatest immune maturation and lung growth. This highlights the importance of growth and development in a conceptual framework for allergy and asthma pathogenesis.

This chapter reviews the allergic march of childhood and its different clinical manifestations: food allergies, atopic dermatitis, inhalant allergies, allergic rhinitis, and asthma. Asthma, the best studied of these conditions, is reviewed in depth. The natural history of anaphylaxis, an allergic condition not currently implicated in the allergic march, is also covered. Interventions that reduce the prevalence of allergy and asthma are reviewed toward the end of the chapter. The findings and conclusions presented in this chapter are largely based on long-term prospective (i.e., "natural history") studies. A complementary review of the epidemiology of allergic diseases in childhood can be found in Chapter 1.

It is important to acknowledge current investigational deficits in our understanding of natural history. So far, childhood natural history studies have largely investigated modern metropolitan cohorts and may, therefore, be relevant only for people living in modernized locales. Epidemiologic findings that (1) allergic rhinitis, asthma, and aeroallergen sensitization are less common in children raised in rural areas of developing countries and in farming communities and (2) increased asthma severity occurs in asthmatic children of low-income families in U.S. inner-city communities suggest that the natural history of allergic diseases and asthma is strongly influenced by environment, lifestyle, and disease management factors.

ALLERGIC MARCH OF CHILDHOOD

Natural history studies with the following design features provide a firm epidemiologic foundation for risk factor assessments and etiologic hypotheses: (1) long-term cohort studies of a prospective design minimize biases resulting from poor parental recall; (2) multiple evaluations over time provide important checkpoints during the dynamic period of childhood growth and development; and (3) the inclusion of objective disease measurements strengthens these studies by validating subjective disease assessments (i.e., questionnaire data).

Three prospective, longitudinal, birth cohort studies exemplify optimized natural history studies and are rich resources for our current understanding of the development and outcome of allergy and asthma in childhood: (1) the Tucson Children's Respiratory Study (CRS) in Tucson, Arizona (begun in 1980); (2) a Kaiser-based study in San Diego, California (begun in 1981); and the German Multicentre Allergy Study (MAS) in Germany (begun in 1990). The major findings of these studies have been consistent and reveal a common pattern of allergy and asthma development that begins in infancy.

1. The highest incidence of atopic dermatitis and food allergies is in the first 2 years of life (Figures 2-1, *A*, and 2-2). It is generally believed that infants rarely manifest allergic symptoms in the first month of life. By 3 months of age, however, atopic dermatitis, food allergies, and wheezing problems are common.
2. This is paralleled by a high prevalence of food allergen sensitization in the first 2 years of life (see Figure 2-1, *B*).[1] Early food allergen sensitization is an important risk factor for food allergies, atopic dermatitis, and asthma.
3. Allergic airways diseases generally begin slightly later in childhood (see Figures 2-1, *A*, and 2-2). Most persistent asthma begins before 12 years of age.[2] Childhood asthma often initially manifests with a lower respiratory tract infection or an episode of bronchiolitis in the first few years of life.
4. Allergic rhinitis commonly begins in childhood, although there is also good evidence that allergic rhinitis often develops in early adulthood.[3,4]
5. The development of allergic rhinitis and persistent asthma is paralleled by a rise in inhalant allergen sensitization (see Figure 2-1, *B*). Perennial inhalant allergen sensitization (i.e., cat dander, dust mites) emerges between 2 to 5 years of age, and seasonal inhalant allergen sensitization becomes apparent slightly later in life (ages 3 to 5 years).

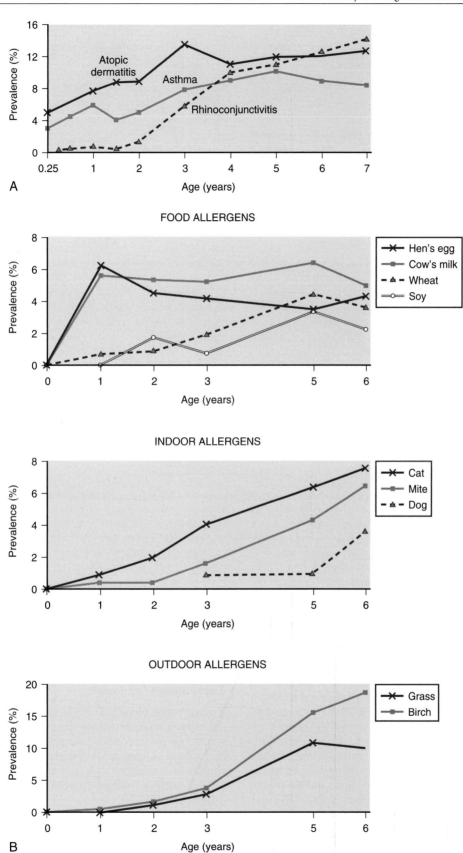

FIGURE 2-1 Allergic march of early childhood. Prevalence of allergic diseases, asthma, and allergen sensitization in a large birth cohort study (Multicentre Allergy Study; Germany). **A,** Period prevalence of atopic dermatitis, asthma, and allergic rhinoconjunctivitis at different ages. **B,** Point prevalence of sensitization to common food allergens, indoor allergens, and outdoor allergens. Based on serum allergen-specific IgE (cutoff level 0.7 kU/L). (**A** From Wahn U: *Allergy* 55:591-599, 2000; **B** From Kulig M, Bergmann R, Klettke U, et al: *J Allergy Clin Immunol* 103:1173-1179, 1999.)

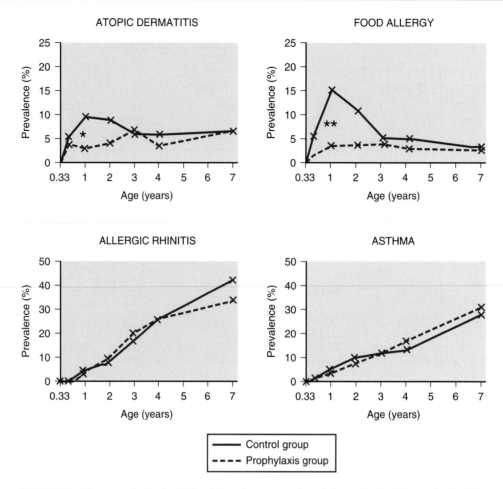

FIGURE 2-2 Allergic march of early childhood. Period prevalence of atopic dermatitis, food allergy, allergic rhinitis, and asthma from birth to 7 years in prophylactic-treated (allergenic food avoidance) and untreated (control) groups (Kaiser Permanente; San Diego). $*P \leq 0.05$; $**P < 0.01$. (Data from Zeiger RS, Heller S: *J Allergy Clin Immunol* 95:1179-1190, 1995; Zeiger RS, Heller S, Mellon MH, et al: *J Allergy Clin Immunol* 84:72-89, 1989.)

EARLY IMMUNE DEVELOPMENT UNDERLYING ALLERGIES

A paradigm of immune development underlies allergy development and progression in early childhood and is the subject of Chapter 6. Briefly, the immune system of the fetus is maintained in a tolerogenic state, preventing adverse immune responses and rejection between the mother and fetus. Placental interleukin-10 (IL-10) suppresses the production of immune-potentiating interferon gamma (IFN-γ) by fetal immune cells. IFN-γ also downregulates the production of pro-allergic cytokines, such as IL-4 and IL-13. The reciprocal relationship between these cytokines and the immune cells that produce them defines "T-helper 2" (Th2), pro-allergic immune responses (i.e., IL-4, IL-13), and anti-allergic, counter-regulatory, "T-helper 1" (Th1) immune development (i.e., IFN-γ). Thus the conditions that favor immune tolerance *in utero* may also foster allergic immune responses. Current studies suggest that newborn immune responses to ubiquitous ingested and inhaled proteins are Th2-biased.[5] Postnatally, repeated encounters with these common allergenic proteins lead to the development of mature immune responses to them. The underlying immune characteristics of allergic diseases—allergen-specific memory Th2 cells and IgE—can be viewed as

aberrant manifestations of immune maturation that can develop during these early years.

Longitudinal prospective studies in young children have provided evidence for this pro-allergic immune developmental process.

Total Serum IgE Levels

At birth, cord blood IgE levels are almost undetectable, but these levels increase during the first 6 years of life. Elevated serum IgE levels in infancy have been associated with persistent asthma in later childhood.[6] High serum IgE levels in later childhood (i.e., after 11 years of age) have also been well correlated with bronchial hyperresponsiveness (BHR) and asthma.[7,8]

Allergen-Specific IgE

In two birth cohort (up to 5 years old) studies of IgG and IgE antibody development to common food and inhalant allergens, IgG antibodies to milk and egg proteins were detectable in nearly all subjects in the first 12 months of life, implying that the infant immune system sees and responds to commonly ingested proteins.[9,10] In comparison, food allergen-specific IgE (especially to egg) was measurable in approximately 30% of subjects at 1 year of age. Low-level IgE responses to food allergens in infancy were common and transient, and sometimes occurred before introduction of the foods into the diet. In children who developed clinical allergic conditions, higher levels and persistence of food allergen-specific IgE were typical.

Of seasonal inhalant allergens, ragweed and grass allergen-specific IgGs were detectable in approximately 25% of subjects at 3 to 6 months of age, and steadily increased to 40% to 50% by 5 years of age.[9,10] In comparison, allergen-specific IgE was detected in < 5% of subjects from 3 to 12 months of age, and increased in prevalence to approximately 20% by 5 years of age. Therefore allergen-specific IgE production emerges in the preschool years and persists in those who develop clinical allergies.

Allergen-Specific Th2 Lymphocytes

The development of allergen-specific antibody production is indicative of allergen-specific T lymphocytes that are guiding the development and differentiation of B lymphocytes to produce IgE through secreted Th2-type cytokines (i.e., IL-4, IL-13) and cell surface molecular interactions (i.e., CD40/CD40 ligand). T cell–derived IL-4, IL-5, and GM-CSF also support eosinophil and mast cell development and differentiation in allergic inflammation. A current paradigm for allergic disease asserts that pro-allergic Th2 cells are (1) differentiated to produce cytokines that direct allergic responses and inflammation and (2) opposed by Th1 cells that produce counter-regulatory cytokines (e.g., IFN-γ) that inhibit Th2 differentiation. As an example of this Th2/Th1 paradigm, peripheral blood mononuclear cells from infants who ultimately manifest allergic disease at 2 years of age produce more pro-allergic Th2 cytokines (i.e., IL-4) to allergen-specific stimulation *in vitro*.[11] In comparison, infants who continue to be non-allergic (i.e., no allergic disease and/or no allergen sensitization in later childhood) produce more counter-regulatory IFN-γ to nonspecific[6,12] and allergen-specific[11] stimuli.

Infants with diminished Th1 responses may be more susceptible to developing asthma for additional reasons. Bronchiolitic infants who continued to have persistent wheezing and airflow obstruction also produce less IFN-γ.[13] This suggests that infants who produce less IFN-γ to ubiquitous allergens and to airway viral infections are susceptible to chronic allergic diseases and asthma because (1) they are less able to impede the development of allergen-specific T cells and IgE and (2) they are more likely to manifest persistent airways abnormalities following respiratory viral infections.

CHILDHOOD ASTHMA

The natural history of childhood asthma has been thoroughly investigated. Approximately 80% of asthmatic patients report disease onset before 6 years of age.[14] However, of all young children who experience recurrent wheezing, only a minority will go on to have persistent asthma in later life. The most common form of recurrent wheezing in preschool children occurs primarily with viral infections (Box 2-1). These "transient wheezers" or "wheezy bronchitics" are not at an increased risk of having asthma in later life. Transient wheezing

| BOX 2-1 | **KEY CONCEPTS** |
| *Childhood Wheezing and Asthma Groups* |

- Transient early wheezing or wheezy bronchitis: most common in infancy and preschool years
- Persistent allergy-associated asthma: most common in school-age children, adults, and elderly
- Nonallergic wheezing: associated with bronchial hyper-responsiveness at birth; continues into childhood
- Asthma associated with obesity, female gender, and early-onset puberty: emerges between 6 and 11 years of age
- Asthma mediated by occupational-type exposures: a probable type of childhood asthma in children living in particular locales, although not yet demonstrated
- Triad asthma: asthma associated with chronic sinusitis, nasal polyposis, and/or hypersensitivity to nonsteroidal antiinflammatory medications (e.g., aspirin, ibuprofen); rarely begins in childhood.

is associated with airways viral infections, smaller airways and lung size, male gender, low birth weight, and prenatal environmental tobacco smoke (ETS) exposure.

Persistent asthma commonly begins and coexists with the large population of transient wheezers (see Box 2-1). Persistent asthma is strongly associated with allergy, which is evident in the early childhood years as clinical conditions (i.e., atopic dermatitis, allergic rhinitis, food allergies) or by testing for allergen sensitization to inhalant and food allergens (e.g., IgE, allergy skin testing). Severity of childhood asthma, determined clinically or by lung function impairment, also predicts asthma persistence into adulthood.

EARLY CHILDHOOD: TRANSIENT VS. PERSISTENT ASTHMA

To study the natural history of asthma, the Tucson CRS began in 1980 and continues today. The remarkable contribution of this extensive longitudinal study to the understanding of the natural course of asthma attests to the commitment of the investigators and subjects in this study. In the first 6 years of life, 49% of their birth cohort reported symptoms of wheezing.[15] These early-childhood wheezers were further subdivided into (1) "transient early wheezers," with wheezing only < 3 years; (2) "persistent wheezers," with manifestations both < 3 years and between 3 and 6 years; and (3) "late-onset wheezers," with manifestations only between 3 and 6 years. Transient wheezers comprised the largest proportion of the group at 20%. Persistent wheezers and late-onset wheezers made up slightly smaller proportions, 14% and 15%, respectively. Of these three groups, persistent wheezers had the greatest likelihood of persistent asthma in later childhood (i.e., over age 11 years) (F.D. Martinez, personal communication) (Figure 2-3). Late-onset wheezers also had an increased likelihood of persistent childhood asthma. In contrast, the likelihood of persistent asthma in the transient wheezer group was not different from non-wheezers.

Lung function in the Tucson CRS was measured in the first year of life (before the occurrence of lower respiratory tract infections) and at 6 years of age. Interestingly, transient wheezers had the lowest airflow measures in infancy, suggesting that they had the narrowest airways and/or the smallest lungs at birth.[15] Their reduced lung function improved significantly by 6 years of age. In comparison, persistent wheezers demonstrated normal lung function in the first few months of

life but a significant decline in airflow measures by 6 years of age. Therefore alterations in lung function were consistent with clinical disease manifestations in the first 6 years of life.

Some children with BHR from birth are also more likely to have asthma in later childhood. Investigators of a birth cohort in Perth, Australia, found that BHR at 1 month of age was associated with lower lung function (i.e., FEV1 and FVC) and a higher likelihood of asthma at 6 years of age.[16] Interestingly, congenital BHR was not associated with total serum IgE, eosinophilia, allergen sensitization, or BHR at 6 years of age and was independent of gender, family history of asthma, and maternal smoking. Congenital BHR alone can be a risk factor for asthma in some children and is consistent with children in the Tucson CRS who manifest a distinct "nonallergic wheezing" phenotype: (1) excessive variability in daily peak flows at 11 years of age; (2) no BHR at 11 years; (3) wheezing to 6 years but not at 11 years; and (4) not associated with IgE or allergen sensitization (see Figure 2-3).[17]

ASTHMA FROM CHILDHOOD TO ADULTHOOD

A cohort of asthmatic 7-year-old children living in Melbourne, Australia, was restudied for persistence and severity of asthma at 10, 14, 21, 28, and 35 years of age. At 35 years of age, 70% of the asthmatics and 90% of the severe asthmatics continued to have asthma symptoms; 75% of the severe asthmatics reported frequent or persistent asthma.[18] In comparison, 24% of "wheezy bronchitics" (i.e., wheezing only with colds at 7 years of age) reported frequent or persistent asthma. These observations—that many asthmatic children experience disease remission or improvement in early adulthood but that

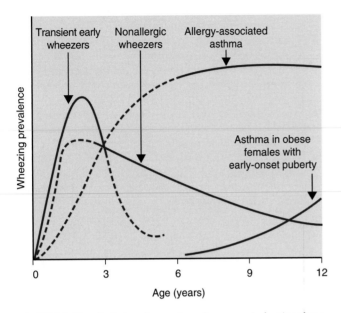

FIGURE 2-3 Hypothetical yearly prevalence for recurrent wheezing phenotypes in childhood (Tucson Children's Respiratory Study, Tucson, Arizona). This classification does not imply that the groups are exclusive. Dashed lines suggest that wheezing can be represented by different curve shapes resulting from many different factors, including overlap of groups. (Modified from Stein RT, Holberg CJ, Morgan WJ, et al: *Thorax* 52:946-952, 1997.)

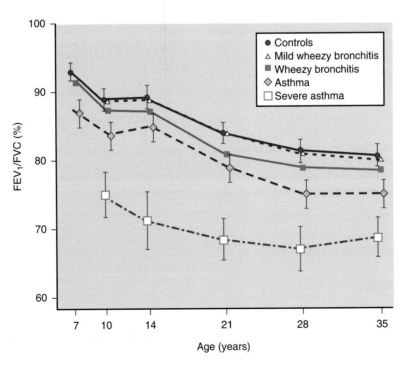

FIGURE 2-4 Natural history of lung function from childhood to adulthood (Melbourne Longitudinal Study of Asthma, Melbourne, Australia). Subjects were classified according to their diagnosis at time of enrollment: nowheezing control; mild wheezy bronchitis; wheezy bronchitis; asthma; and severe asthma. Lung function is represented as FEV1 corrected for lung volume (FEV1/FVC ratio). Mean values and standard error bars are shown. (From Oswald H, Phelan PD, Lanigan A, et al: *Pediatr Pulmonol* 23:14-20, 1997.)

severe asthma persists with age—are remarkably similar to those of several other natural history studies of childhood asthma into adulthood (e.g., in Aberdeen, Scotland[19]; Tasmania, Australia[20]; and a national British study[21]).

Objective measures of lung function both validate and bring further insights to these natural history studies. Spirometric measures of lung function of the Melbourne study children initially revealed that asthmatics (especially severe asthmatics) had lung function impairment, whereas wheezy bronchitics (i.e., "transient" wheezers) had lung function that was not different from that of nonasthmatics. Over the ensuing years these differences in lung function impairment between groups persisted in parallel, without a greater rate of decline in lung function in any group (Figure 2-4).[22] In the Aberdeen study, greater lung function impairment in asthmatics versus those with wheezy bronchitis or controls was complemented by a greater proportion of asthmatic subjects with BHR than the wheezy bronchitis or control groups.[19] These findings support the importance of the early childhood years in asthma development; the establishment of chronic disease and lung function impairment in school-age children appears to predict persistent asthma well into adulthood.

RISK FACTORS FOR PERSISTENT ASTHMA

Natural history studies of asthma have identified biologic, genetic, and environmental risk factors for persistent asthma (Box 2-2). From the Tucson CRS, a statistical optimization of the major risk factors for persistent asthma was recently published.[23] In 2- to 3-year-old children with recurrent wheezing in the past year, risk factor assessment provided 97% specificity and 77% positive predictive value for persistent asthma in later childhood[23] (Figure 2-5).

Allergy

Essentially all of the current natural history studies have found that allergic disease and evidence of pro-allergic immune development are significant risk factors for persistent asthma. In the Tucson CRS, early atopic dermatitis, allergic rhinitis, elevated serum IgE levels in the first year of life, and peripheral blood eosinophilia were all significant risk factors for persistent asthma.[15,23] In the Berlin MAS study, additional risk factors for asthma and BHR at age 7 years included persistent sensitization to foods (i.e., hen's egg, cow's milk, wheat and/or soy) and perennial inhalant allergens (i.e., dust mite, cat dander), especially in early life.[24,25] In the Kaiser San Diego study, milk or peanut allergen sensitization was a risk factor for asthma.[26] Natural history studies of asthma that have extended into adulthood continue to find allergy to be a risk factor for persistent asthma.[18,20,21] Since the eight-center

Childhood Asthma Management Program (CAMP) study of 1041 asthmatic children ages 5 to 12 years found that 88% were sensitized to at least one inhalant allergen at study enrollment, allergy-associated asthma appears to be the most common form of asthma in elementary school-age children in the United States.[27] Furthermore, in the International Study of Asthma and Allergies in Childhood (ISAAC), strong correlations between high asthma prevalence and both high allergic rhinoconjunctivitis and high atopic dermatitis prevalence in different sites throughout the world suggest that allergy-associated asthma is also the most common form of childhood asthma worldwide.[28]

Gender

Male gender is a risk factor for both transient wheezing and persistent asthma in childhood.[15,26] This is generally believed to be caused by the smaller airways of young boys when compared with girls.[29,30] Later in childhood, BHR and inhalant allergen sensitization are more prevalent in boys than in girls.[31,32] For asthma persistence from childhood to adulthood, female gender is a risk factor for greater asthma severity[20] and BHR.[19] These observations are consistent with the higher

---

BOX 2-2	**KEY CONCEPTS**
	Risk Factors for Persistent Asthma

Allergy
Atopic dermatitis
Allergic rhinitis
Elevated total serum IgE levels (first year of life)
Peripheral blood eosinophilia > 4% (2 to 3 years of age)
Food and inhalant allergen sensitization

Gender
Males
■ Transient wheezing
■ Persistent allergy-associated asthma
Females
■ Asthma associated with obesity and early-onset puberty
■ "Triad" asthma (adulthood)

Parental Asthma

Lower Respiratory Tract Infections
Respiratory syncytial virus, parainfluenza
Severe bronchiolitis (i.e., requiring hospitalization)
Pneumonia

Environmental Tobacco Smoke Exposure: (Including Prenatal)

Major criteria	Minor criteria
Parent asthma	Allergic rhinitis
Eczema	Wheezing apart from colds
	Eosinophils > 4%

FIGURE 2-5 Predictive Index for children (Tucson Children's Respiratory Study, Tucson, Arizona). Through a statistically optimized model for 2- to 3-year-old children with frequent wheezing in the past year, one major criterion or two minor criteria provided 77% positive predictive value and 97% specificity for asthma in later childhood (i.e., at 6, 8, 11, and/or 13 years of age). (From Castro-Rodriguez JA, Holberg CJ, Wright AL, et al: *Am J Respir Crit Care Med* 162:1403-1406, 2000.)

prevalence of asthma in males in childhood and in females in adulthood.[14]

Parental History of Asthma

Infants whose parents report a history of childhood asthma have lower lung functions and are more likely to wheeze in early life,[33,34] in later childhood,[15,26] and in adulthood.[20] However, in a two-generation, longitudinal study in Aberdeen, Scotland, the children of well-characterized subjects without atopy or asthma were found to have a surprisingly high prevalence of allergen sensitization (56%) and wheezing (33%).[35] Similarly, in the MAS study, the majority of children with atopic dermatitis and/or asthma in early childhood were born to nonallergic parents.[36] For example, of the study's asthmatic children at 5 years of age, 57% were born to parents without an atopic history. Therefore allergen sensitization and asthma seem to be occurring at high rates, even in persons considered to be at low genetic risk for allergy and asthma.

Lower Respiratory Tract Infections

Certain respiratory viruses have been associated with persistent wheezing problems in children. It is not known if persistent airways abnormalities are primarily the result of virus-induced damage, vulnerable individuals revealing their airway susceptibility to virus-induced airflow obstruction, or airways injury with aberrant repair. In long-term studies, infants hospitalized with respiratory syncytial virus (RSV) bronchiolitis (most occurred by 4 months of age) were significantly more likely to have recurrent wheezing episodes up to 3 years of age.[37] In the Tucson CRS birth cohort, lower respiratory tract infections (LRTIs; manifest as wheezing, deep or wet chest cough, hoarseness, stridor, shortness of breath) were cultured for common pathogens in the first 3 years of life.[38] Ninety-one percent of LRTIs were cultured: 44% were RSV-positive, 14% were parainfluenza-positive, 14% were culture-positive for other respiratory pathogens, and 27% were culture-negative. Followed prospectively, infants with RSV LRTI were more likely to have wheezing symptoms at 6 years of age but not at later ages (i.e., 11 and 13 years old). None of the other LRTI groups were different from non-LRTI children in their prevalence of asthma symptoms at these follow-up time. There were also no differences in prevalence of allergen sensitization or lung function among the RSV group, other LRTI groups, and the non-LRTI group at later times. However, young children who had radiographic evidence of pneumonia or croup symptoms accompanying wheezing were more likely to have persistent asthma symptoms and lung function impairment at 6 and 11 years of age.[39,40] This supports the premise that individuals with lower airway vulnerability to common respiratory virus pathogens are at risk for persistent airways disease.

Environmental Tobacco Smoke Exposure

ETS exposure is a risk factor for wheezing problems at all ages. Prenatal ETS exposure is associated, in a dose-dependent manner, with wheezing manifestations and decreased lung function in infancy and early childhood.[41-43] Postnatal ETS exposure is associated with a greater likelihood of wheezing in infancy,[34] transient wheezing, and persistent asthma in child-

hood.[15] Cigarette smoking has also been strongly associated with persistent asthma and asthma relapses in adulthood.[21]

ETS exposure is also associated with food allergen sensitization,[44] allergic rhinitis, hospitalization for LRTIs, BHR, and elevated serum IgE levels.[45,46] In a 7-year prospective study, ETS exposure was associated with greater inhalant allergen sensitization and reduced lung function.[26]

ASTHMA- AND ALLERGY-PROTECTIVE INFLUENCES

Some lifestyle differences may impart asthma- and/or allergy-protective effects. Natural history studies have started to contribute some epidemiologic evidence in support of these hypotheses.

Breast-Feeding

Numerous studies have investigated the potential of early breast-feeding as a protective influence against the development of allergy and asthma. Meta-analyses of prospective studies of exclusive breast-feeding for 4 or more months from birth have been associated with less atopic dermatitis (AD) and asthma (summary odds ratios of 0.68 and 0.70, respectively).[47,48] In the Tucson CRS, breast-feeding generally reduced the risk of recurrent wheezing up to 2 years of age (odds ratio 0.45); however, in a subgroup of atopic children who were exclusively breast-fed for 4 months by asthmatic mothers, the risk of persistent asthma between 6 and 13 years of age was increased (odds ratio 8.7).[49] This surprising finding was corroborated by findings that infants breast-fed by mothers with lower IgE levels also had lower IgE levels at later ages (i.e., 6 and 11 years) than infants who were not breast-fed, whereas infants breast-fed by mothers with higher IgE levels also had higher IgE levels.[50] Although a potential mechanism for this transmission of increased IgE levels is unclear, the benefit of breast-feeding for allergy and asthma prevention may be confounded for the atopic asthmatic mother: protection in the early years but increased likelihood of asthma in later childhood. However, when considered with many other health and developmental attributes of breast-feeding, prolonged breast-feeding should still be recommended.

Microbial Exposures

Numerous epidemiologic studies have found that a variety of microbial exposures are associated with a lower likelihood of allergen sensitization, allergic disease, and asthma. This has led to a "hygiene" hypothesis, which proposes that the reduction of microbial exposures in childhood in modernized countries has led to the rise in allergy and asthma.[51] This hypothesis is actually based on immune development. Common microbial exposures—viral and bacterial infections and exposure to certain microbial components such as bacterial endotoxin and DNA—are potent inducers of Th1-type immune development and immune memory. Theoretically, microbial exposures in early life, by promoting Th1-type immune memory, might prevent the development of allergen sensitization and strengthen the immune response to respiratory viral infections.

To address this hypothesis, natural history studies have begun to explore the relationships between certain microbial/

microbial component exposures and the development of allergies and asthma. Mostly, such studies have reported on the relationship between viruses that can afflict the lower respiratory tract (e.g., RSV and parainfluenza virus) and a predisposition for persistent wheezing problems (see previous section on Risk Factors for Persistent Asthma). More recently, natural history studies have reported the following observations:

1. In the Tucson CRS, children raised in larger families or in day care from an early age (i.e., < 6 months old) were less likely to have asthma symptoms in later childhood.[52] Children placed in day care in the first 2 years of life experience more infections, generally common colds.

2. In the German MAS, more runny nose colds in the first 3 years of life were associated with a lower likelihood of allergen sensitization, asthma, and BHR at 7 years of age.[53] A dose-dependent effect was observed, such that children who experienced at least 8 colds by age 3 years had an adjusted odds ratio of 0.16 for asthma at age 7 years.

3. In infants with a history of recurrent wheezing, greater exposure levels of naturally occurring bacterial endotoxin were associated with a lack of early allergen sensitization, and correlated with increased proportions of Th1-type lymphocytes.[54] Therefore natural endotoxin exposure may promote early Th1-type immune development, thereby preventing the development of allergen sensitization, allergic airways conditions, and asthma.

4. In a different German birth cohort study, Lifestyle-Related Factors on the Immune System and the Development of Allergies (LISA), early childhood endotoxin exposure was associated with a lower likelihood of atopic dermatitis in the first 6 months of life.[55] Greater endotoxin exposure in the first year of life, however, was reported, in this and another birth cohort study, to be associated with more wheezing in the first year of life.[55,56] Whether endotoxin exposure will be associated with a lower likelihood of allergen sensitization and persistent asthma in later childhood has yet to be determined.

5. In two birth cohort studies of infants followed through the first year of life, allergic infants (i.e., those with allergic disease or allergen sensitization) had less gastrointestinal tract colonization with enterococci and bifidobacteria and more colonization with *Clostridia* and *Staphylococcus aureus*.[57,58] Such alterations in the gut flora of infants from dietary differences (i.e., breast versus formula feeding, semi-sterile food, antibiotic use) may have an allergy-protective effect on the developing immune system.

Pet Ownership

In the Tucson CRS, dog ownership in childhood has been associated with a lower likelihood of asthma.[59] This finding is consistent with other recent epidemiologic studies that have associated pet ownership in childhood with a lower likelihood of allergy and asthma.[60-63] Similarly, in farming and rural locales, a lower likelihood of allergy and asthma has been associated with animal contact or the keeping of domestic animals in the home.[64] Although the mechanism(s) for this potential protective influence are unclear, one possibility is that greater bacterial endotoxin exposure occurs with animal contact and/or animal/pet-keeping in the home. Recent studies have reported that indoor pets are a major factor associated with higher indoor endotoxin levels in metropolitan homes.[64]

OTHER TYPES OF CHILDHOOD ASTHMA

Although males are more likely to experience childhood asthma, the incidence of new-onset cases of asthma becomes more common in females in early adolescence. One contributor to this gender shift in asthma onset was recently described in the Tucson CRS. Female children who became overweight between 6 and 11 years of age (defined as body mass index ≥ 85th percentile) were more likely to develop new-onset asthma between 11 and 13 years of age (see Figure 2-3).[65] This effect was strongest in females with early-onset puberty (i.e., before age 11 years) and was not observed in males.

Asthma mediated by occupational-type exposures is often not considered in children, and yet some children are raised in settings where occupational-type exposures can mediate asthma in adults (e.g., children raised on farms or with farm animals in the home). Children with hypersensitivity and exposure to other common airways irritants or air pollutants such as ETS, endotoxin, ozone, sulphur dioxide, or cold air may also contribute to the pool of non-atopic children with persistent asthma.

"Triad" asthma, characteristically associated with hyperplastic sinusitis/nasal polyposis and/or hypersensitivity to nonsteroidal antiinflammatory medications (e.g., aspirin, ibuprofen), rarely occurs in childhood.

ATOPIC DERMATITIS

AD usually begins during the preschool years and persists throughout childhood. Two prospective birth cohort studies have found the peak incidence of AD to be in the first 2 years of life (see Figures 2-1, *A*, and 2-2).[26,66] Although 66% to 90% of patients with AD have clinical manifestations before 7 years of age,[67,68] eczematous lesions in the first 2 months of life are rare. Natural history studies of AD have reported a wide variation (35% to 82%) in disease persistence throughout childhood.[68,69] The greatest remission in AD seems to occur between 8 and 11 years of age and, to a lesser extent, between 12 and 16 years.[68] Natural history studies of AD may have underestimated the persistent nature of the disease for reasons that include (1) AD definition—some studies have included other forms of dermatitis that have a better prognosis over time (i.e., seborrheic dermatitis),[70] (2) AD recurrence—a recent 23-year birth cohort study found that many patients who went into disease remission in childhood had an AD recurrence in early adulthood,[68] and (3) AD manifestation—it is generally believed that patients with childhood AD will often evolve to manifest hand and/or foot dermatitis as adults. Although adults with AD commonly have hand/foot dermatitis, the relationship between childhood AD and adult hand/foot dermatitis has not yet been demonstrated in natural history studies.

Parental history of AD is an important risk factor for childhood AD.[71,72] This apparent heritability complements studies revealing a high concordance rate of AD among monozygotic versus dizygotic twins (0.72 vs. 0.23, respectively).[73] In a risk

FIGURE 2-6 Atopic dermatitis *(AD)* in young children (2 months to 3 years of age) and allergen sensitization (to food and inhalant allergens), asthma, and allergic rhinoconjunctivitis *(AR)* 4 years later. At enrollment, AD severity was determined, and no subjects had AR or asthma. Four years later, 88% of subjects had a marked improvement or complete resolution of AD. However, all children with severe AD at enrollment were sensitized to inhalant allergens, and 75% had asthma and/or AR. (From Patrizi A, Guerrini V, Ricci G, et al: *Pediatr Dermatol* 17:261-265, 2000.)

	Initial examination		4 years later		
AD severity	Inhalant ± food	Food only	Inhalant ± food	Food only	Asthma and/or AR
Mild	15%	20%	31%	6%	15%
Moderate	18%	26%	52%	6%	32%
Severe	20%	45%	100%	0%	75%

factor assessment for AD in the first 2 years of life, higher levels of maternal education and living in less crowded homes were risk factors for early-onset AD.[74] The environmental/lifestyle risk factors reported for allergic rhinitis and asthma are similar. A meta-analysis of prospective breast-feeding studies concluded that exclusive breast-feeding of infants with a family history of atopy for at least the first 3 months of life is associated with a lower likelihood of childhood AD (odds ratio 0.58). This protective effect was not observed, however, in children without a family history of atopy.[47]

Initial AD disease severity seems predictive of later disease severity and persistence. Of adolescents with moderate to severe AD, 77% to 91% continued to have persistent disease in adulthood.[75] In comparison, of adolescents with mild AD, 50% had AD in adulthood. Food allergen sensitization and exposure in early childhood also contribute to AD development and disease severity. Food allergen sensitization is associated with greater AD severity.[26,76] Furthermore, elimination of common allergenic foods in infancy (i.e., soy, milk, egg, peanuts) is associated with a lower prevalence of allergic skin conditions up to age 2 years (see Figure 2-2).[26]

Natural history studies have found early childhood AD to be a major risk factor for food allergen sensitization in infancy,[77] inhalant allergen sensitization,[77,78] and persistent asthma in later childhood.[15,23] In particular, severe AD in early childhood is associated with a high prevalence of allergen sensitization and airways allergic disease in later childhood (i.e., 4 years later; Figure 2-6). Indeed, in young patients with severe AD, 100% developed inhalant allergen sensitization and 75% developed an allergic respiratory disease (mostly asthma) over 4 years. In contrast to severe AD, patients with mild to moderate AD were not as likely to develop allergen sensitization (36%) or an allergic respiratory disease (26%).

ALLERGIC RHINITIS

Many people develop allergic rhinitis (AR) during childhood. Two prospective birth cohort studies reported a steady rise in total (i.e., seasonal and perennial) AR prevalence, reaching 35% to 40% by age 7 years.[26,79] Seasonal AR emerged after 2 years of age and increased steadily to 15% by age 7 years.[79]

AR also commonly begins in early adulthood. In a 23-year cohort study of Brown University students beginning in their freshman year, perennial AR developed in 4.8% at 7 years and 14% at 23 years of follow-up.[3,4] The incidence increase for seasonal AR was substantially greater: 13% at 7 years and 41% at 23 years of follow-up.[3,4] Allergen skin test sensitization and asthma were prognostic risk factors for the development of AR.

AR persistence has been evaluated in adult patients. Three follow-up studies of adult AR patients have found a disease remission rate of 5% to 10% by 4 years[80] and 23% by 23 years.[3] In the 23-year follow-up study, 55% of the follow-up subjects reported improvement in rhinitis. Onset of disease in early childhood was associated with greater improvement.[3]

FOOD ALLERGY

Food-adverse reactions in childhood include food hypersensitivity that is IgE-mediated and manifests as classic allergic symptoms of immediate onset. Other food-allergic reactions, such as eosinophilic gastroenteropathy and delayed-onset reactions, have variable associations with foods and lack natural history studies.

Natural history studies reveal that the prevalence of food hypersensitivity is greatest in the first few years of life, affecting 5% to 15% of children in their first year of life.[81,82] Most children become tolerant of or seem to "outgrow" their food allergies to milk, soy, and egg within a few years. In a prospective study of young children with milk allergy, most became nonallergic within a few years: 50% by 1 year of age, 70% by 2 years, and 85% by 3 years.[83] Older children and adults with food allergies are less likely to become tolerant (26% to 33%).[84,85] Two recent long-term follow-up studies of peanut-allergic children found that loss of clinical hypersensitivity was uncommon, especially in children with anaphylactic symptoms in addition to urticaria and/or atopic dermatitis.[86,87] Allergies to other nuts, fish, and shellfish are also believed to be more persistent. It is purported that allergen avoidance diets in food-allergic children increase their likelihood of losing clinical hypersensitivity, but this has not been well-studied.[85]

Hypersensitivity to milk at 1 year of age was a risk factor for additional food allergies in later childhood.[88,89] Furthermore, food hypersensitivity in early life (i.e., to milk, egg, peanut) was found to be a risk factor for atopic dermatitis[90,91] and, later, asthma.[24,26] More information on the natural history of food allergy can be found in Chapter 45.

ANAPHYLAXIS

It is generally believed that children are less likely than adults to have anaphylactic reactions. Anaphylaxis in children can result from numerous possible exposures (e.g., foods, antibiotics, insulin, insect venoms, latex) and is sometimes anaphylactoid (clinically similar but non–IgE-mediated reaction, such as occurs with radio-contrast media and aspirin/

nonsteroidal antiinflammatory drugs) or idiopathic. A history of allergic rhinitis or asthma is a risk factor for anaphylaxis to foods and latex.[92] A history of asthma, pollenosis, or food and/or drug allergy is a surprising risk factor for anaphylactoid reactions to radio-contrast media, with a higher prevalence of adverse reactions to ionic versus non-ionic contrast media observed.[93] In contrast, atopy is not a risk factor for anaphylaxis to insulin,[94] penicillin,[95] or insect stings.[96] The natural history of anaphylactic reactions in children has been studied prospectively only for food-induced anaphylaxis (described previously) and bee sting anaphylaxis.

In a Johns Hopkins study examining the natural history of bee venom allergy in children, venom-allergic children with a history of mild generalized reactions were randomly assigned to venom immunotherapy or no treatment and then subjected to a repeat sting in a medical setting 4 years later.[97] Systemic allergic reactions occurred in 1.2% of the treated group and 9.2% of the untreated group. Moreover, no systemic reactions that occurred were more severe than the original incidents. In a smaller study of children and adults with venom hypersensitivity, repeat sting challenges, at least 5 years after the original incidents, induced no systemic reactions in those who originally presented with only urticaria/angioedema but did induce systemic reactions in 21% of those who originally had respiratory and/or cardiovascular complications.[98]

These studies suggest that insect sting anaphylaxis is often self-limited in children, with spontaneous remission usually occurring within 4 years. Those at greatest risk of persistent hypersensitivity include those with previous severe anaphylactic episodes. Conversely, those children with mild systemic reactions to bee stings are less likely to have an allergic reaction on re-sting, and any future anaphylactic episodes from bee stings are not likely to be severe. Finally, in a re-challenge study of subjects with no clinical response to a first sting challenge, 21% experienced anaphylaxis to the second challenge, and, of those, one half developed symptomatic hypotension requiring epinephrine.[99] Therefore even the well-performed studies described previously should be interpreted with caution.

PREVENTION STUDIES

Early-intervention studies to prevent the development of allergic disease and asthma have had limited success so far. Nevertheless, because of their prospective design, such studies can add valuable insights to the natural history of allergic diseases. Although it is difficult to modify some of the risk factors in young children, investigators have attempted to do so.

Avoidance of Allergenic Foods

Perhaps the best-studied intervention so far has been a 7-year follow-up of a randomized, controlled intervention study performed at Kaiser Permanente in San Diego, California, in which the common allergenic foods (cow's milk, peanut, egg, fish) were eliminated from the diets of at-risk infants (i.e., with one parent with an atopic disorder and allergen sensitization) from the third trimester of pregnancy to 24 months of life[82] (see Figure 2-2). Although this intervention significantly

reduced the prevalence of food allergen sensitization, atopic dermatitis, and urticarial rash in the first year of life,[82] a lower prevalence of allergic disease did not persist at either age 4 or 7 years[26] (see Figure 2-2). Furthermore, no effect was observed on inhalant allergen sensitization or allergic airways conditions.

Inhalant Allergen Elimination/Reduction

Addition of thorough dust mite reduction measures to food allergen avoidance for 1 year reduced the likelihood of atopic dermatitis from 1 to 4 years of age and reduced the incidence of allergen sensitization at age 4 years.[100-102] Decreased asthma was observed in the first year of life but not at age 2 or 4 years. Randomized, controlled studies of the influence of indoor allergen reduction alone on the development of allergies and asthma have generally not shown any benefit. One challenge of such studies has been the difficulty of substantially lowering perennial allergen exposure through home mitigation, although recent improvements in this area (i.e., dehumidification) make such studies feasible.[103]

Natural history birth cohort studies, however, suggest that, although lower household mite and cat allergen exposure reduces the likelihood of specific allergen sensitization, it is not associated with less asthma.[25] In homes with lower mite allergen levels in house-dust samples, mite allergen sensitization is less common.[104,105] On the other hand, high levels of household cat allergen exposure has been associated with less cat allergen sensitization.[104] Similarly, in the Tucson CRS, dog ownership in childhood was associated with a lower risk of developing asthma.[59] In contrast, in allergen-sensitized children, chronic allergen exposure (especially to perennial allergens) is associated with greater asthma severity. In a study of cat-sensitive asthmatic children without cats at home, greater cat allergen exposure in public schools (as a result of more cat-owning classmates) was associated with asthma worsening after the start of school.[106] Further strengthening the value of allergen reduction/elimination in allergen-sensitized asthmatic children are studies of mite-sensitive asthmatic children who have been moved to high-altitude locales without dust mite allergen[107,108] or whose bedrooms have undergone extensive mite reduction measures,[47,48,109] resulting in significant improvement.

Breast-Feeding

This has been best addressed in prospective, controlled studies and is discussed earlier in this chapter.

Environmental Tobacco Smoke Elimination/Reduction

The acquisition of definitive proof of the preventive value of reducing or eliminating ETS exposure in infancy and childhood has been hindered by the difficulties in achieving long-term smoking cessation in randomized, controlled studies. ETS exposure at all ages, from prenatal exposure of mothers to smoking in asthmatic adults, is associated with more wheezing problems and more severe disease and is discussed earlier in this chapter. When considered with other health benefits of ETS exposure avoidance, this is strongly recommended.

Pharmacologic Intervention

Several studies represent first attempts to determine if conventional therapy for allergy and asthma may be able to alter the natural course of the allergic march or to prevent persistent allergic disease and chronic asthma.

Antihistamines

In the Early Treatment of the Atopic Child (ETAC) study, the antihistamine cetirizine was administered for 18 months to young children at high risk for asthma because of a history of atopic dermatitis and/or a family history of asthma. Of subjects receiving cetirizine, only young children with early allergen sensitization to mites or grass pollen were less likely to develop asthma symptoms during the treatment period.[110] Eighteen months after cetirizine discontinuation, a slightly lower incidence of asthma symptoms continued for the cetirizine-treated, grass-allergic subjects only.[111]

Conventional "Controller" Pharmacotherapy for Asthma

In the CAMP study, 5- to 12-year-old children were treated with either daily inhaled corticosteroid (budesonide), daily inhaled nonsteroidal antiinflammatory medication (nedocromil), or placebo for more than 4 years.[27] Study medication was then discontinued. The budesonide-treated subjects demonstrated significant improvement in most of the clinical outcomes and lung function measures of asthma, including BHR to methacholine. After discontinuation of budesonide, however, the mean BHR of the budesonide-treated group regressed to that of the placebo group. Nedocromil-treated subjects did not improve BHR when compared with placebo. This suggests that, although long-term administration of inhaled corticosteroids in school-age asthmatic children significantly improves asthma severity, it might not increase the likelihood of asthma remission in later childhood or adulthood. However, the outcome of asthma remission was not the intent of the CAMP study, and, therefore, forthcoming studies designed to determine the influence of asthma pharmacotherapy on asthma persistence or remittance in childhood will be valuable.

Allergen-Specific Immunotherapy

Allergen-specific immunotherapy (AIT) has been studied to determine if it can reduce the likelihood of asthma development in children with AR. A recently published randomized, controlled study found that a 3-year AIT course administered to children with birch and/or grass pollen AR reduced the likelihood of asthma symptom development, and was associated with less BHR to methacholine.[112] Moreover, the clinical benefit and immune-modifying effects of AIT can persist for years after its administration. For example, completion of a 3-year AIT course can induce sustained clinical improvement in AR and asthma for at least 3 additional years.[113] AIT has also been associated with a lack of progression of inhalant allergen sensitization in asthmatic children. This prevention of new sensitization to inhalant allergens has persisted for several years after AIT discontinuation.[114,115] These studies suggest that AIT may alter the allergic march of inhalant allergen sensitization and asthma, but the difficulties and risks of conventional AIT in children warrant careful consideration.

Lactobacillus

Oral lactobacillus has been used to treat diarrheal illnesses in children (e.g., infectious, antibiotic-associated). Some studies suggest that lactobacillus supplementation may also prevent allergies and asthma by promoting Th1-type and/or regulatory T lymphocyte (i.e., antiinflammatory) immune development.[116] A randomized, controlled trial of daily lactobacillus given to at-risk infants (i.e., those of mothers with at least one first-degree relative or partner with AD, allergic rhinitis, or asthma) for the first 6 months of life was recently reported.[116] At age 2 years, a lower AD incidence was observed in the treated group. This observation did not extend, however, to other allergic conditions or measures of allergen sensitization. Other early-intervention studies with oral lactobacillus supplementation are ongoing.

To summarize, allergic diseases and asthma commonly develop in the early childhood years. Current paradigms of immune development and lung growth shape the understanding of disease pathogenesis. The systemic nature of these conditions is such that manifestations of one allergic condition are often risk factors for others (e.g., AD and allergen sensitization are risk factors for persistent asthma). Although many allergy and asthma sufferers improve and can even become disease-free as adults, those with severe disease and some particular conditions (e.g., peanut allergy) are likely to have lifelong disease.

ACKNOWLEDGMENTS

Dr. Liu's work was supported by NIH #K23-HL-04272 and the American Academy of Allergy, Asthma & Immunology (Education & Research Trust).

REFERENCES

1. Kulig M, Bergmann R, Klettke U, et al: Natural course of sensitization to food and inhalant allergens during the first 6 years of life, *J Allergy Clin Immunol* 103:1173-1179, 1999.
2. Rhodes HL, Thomas P, Sporik R, et al: A birth cohort study of subjects at risk of atopy, *Am J Respir Crit Care Med* 165:176-180, 2002.
3. Greisner WA, Settipane RJ, Settipane GA: Co-existence of asthma and allergic rhinitis: a 23-year follow-up study of college students, *Allergy Asthma Proc* 19:185-188, 1998.
4. Hagy GW, Settipane GA: Risk factors for developing asthma and allergic rhinitis: a 7-year follow-up study of college students, *J Allergy Clin Immunol* 58:330-336, 1976.
5. Prescott SL, Macaubas C, Holt BJ, et al: Transplacental priming of the human immune system to environmental allergens: universal skewing of initial T cell responses toward the Th2 cytokine profile, *J Immunol* 160:4730-4737, 1998.
6. Martinez FD, Stern DA, Wright AL, et al: Association of interleukin-2 and interferon-g production by blood mononuclear cells in infancy with parental allergy skin tests and with subsequent development of atopy, *J Allergy Clin Immunol* 96:652-660, 1995.
7. Burrows B, Sears MR, Flannery EM, et al: Relation of the course of bronchial responsiveness from age 9 to age 15 to allergy, *Am J Respir Crit Care Med* 152:1302-1308, 1995.
8. Sears MR, Burrows B, Flannery EM, et al: Relation between airway responsiveness and serum IgE in children with asthma and in apparently normal children, *N Engl J Med* 325:1067-1071, 1991.
9. Hattevig G, Kjellman B, Johansson SG, et al: Clinical symptoms and IgE responses to common food proteins in atopic and healthy children, *Clin Allergy* 14:551-559, 1984.
10. Rowntree S, Cogswell JJ, Platts-Mills TAE, et al: Development of IgE and IgG antibodies to food and inhalant allergens in children at risk of allergic disease, *Arch Dis Child* 60:727-735, 1985.

11. Prescott SL, Macaubas C, Smallacombe TB, et al: Development of allergen-specific T-cell memory in atopic and normal children, *Lancet* 353:196-200, 1999.

12. Tang ML, Kemp AS, Thorburn J, et al: Reduced interferon-gamma secretion in neonates and subsequent atopy, *Lancet* 344:983-985, 1994.

13. Renzi PM, Turgeon JP, Marcotte JE, et al: Reduced interferon-g production in infants with bronchiolitis and asthma, *Am J Resp Crit Care Med* 159:1417-1422, 1999.

14. Yunginger JW, Reed CE, O'Connell, et al: A community-based study of the epidemiology of asthma: incidence rates, 1964-1983, *Am Rev Respir Dis* 146:888-894, 1992.

15. Martinez FD, Wright AL, Taussig LM, et al: Asthma and wheezing in the first six years of life, *N Engl J Med* 332:133-138, 1995.

16. Palmer LJ, Rye PJ, Gibson NA, et al: Airway responsiveness in early infancy predicts asthma, lung function, and respiratory symptoms by school age, *Am J Respir Crit Care Med* 163:37-42, 2001.

17. Stein RT, Holberg CJ, Morgan WJ, et al: Peak flow variability, methacholine responsiveness and atopy as markers for detecting different wheezing phenotypes in childhood, *Thorax* 52:946-952, 1997.

18. Oswald H, Phelan PD, Lanigan A, et al: Outcome of childhood asthma in mid-adult life, *Br Med J* 309:95-96, 1994.

19. Godden DJ, Ross S, Abdalla M, et al: Outcome of wheeze in childhood, *Am J Respir Crit Care Med* 149:106-112, 1994.

20. Jenkins MA, Hopper JL, Bowes G, et al: Factors in childhood as predictors of asthma in adult life, *Br Med J* 309:90-93, 1994.

21. Strachan DP, Butland BK, Anderson HR: Incidence and prognosis of asthma and wheezing illness from early childhood to age 33 in a national British cohort, *Br Med J* 312:1195-1199, 1996.

22. Oswald H, Phelan PD, Lanigan A, et al: Childhood asthma and lung function in mid-adult life, *Pediatr Pulmonol* 23:14-20, 1997.

23. Castro-Rodriguez JA, Holberg CJ, Wright AL, et al: A clinical index to define risk of asthma in young children with recurrent wheezing, *Am J Respir Crit Care Med* 162:1403-1406, 2000.

24. Kulig M, Bergmann R, Tacke U, et al: Long-lasting sensitization to food during the first two years precedes allergic airway disease: the MAS Study Group, Germany, *Pediatr Allergy Immunol* 9:61-67, 1998.

25. Lau S, Illi S, Sommerfeld C, et al: Early exposure to house-dust mite and cat allergens and development of childhood asthma: a cohort study—Multicentre Allergy Study Group, *Lancet* 356:1392-1397, 2000.

26. Zeiger RS, Heller S: The development and prediction of atopy in high-risk children: follow-up at age seven years in a prospective randomized study of combined maternal and infant food allergen avoidance, *J Allergy Clin Immunol* 95:1179-1190, 1995.

27. The Childhood Asthma Management Program Research Group: Long-term effects of budesonide or nedocromil in children with asthma, *N Engl J Med* 343:1054-1063, 2000.

28. ISAAC Steering Committee: Worldwide variation in prevalence of symptoms of asthma, allergic rhinoconjunctivitis, and atopic eczema: ISAAC, *Lancet* 351:1225-1232, 1998.

29. Taussig LM: Maximal expiratory flows at functional residual capacity: a test of lung function for young children, *Am Rev Respir Dis* 116:1031-1037, 1977.

30. Tepper RS, Morgan WJ, Cota K, et al: Physiologic growth and development of the lung during the first year of life, *Am Rev Respir Dis* 134:513-519, 1986.

31. Peat JK, Salome CM, Xuan W: On adjusting measurements of airway responsiveness for lung size and airway caliber, *Am J Respir Crit Care Med* 154:870-875, 1996.

32. Sears MR, Burrows B, Flannery EM, et al: Atopy in childhood. I. Gender and allergen-related risks for development of hay fever and asthma, *Clin Exp Allergy* 23:941-948, 1993.

33. Camilli AE, Holberg CJ, Wright AL, et al: Parental childhood respiratory illness and respiratory illness in their infants: Group Health Medical Associates, *Pediatr Pulmonol* 16:275-280, 1993.

34. Dezateux C, Stocks J, Dundas I, et al: Impaired airway function and wheezing in infancy, *Am J Respir Crit Care Med* 159:403-410, 1999.

35. Christie GL, Helms PJ, Godden DJ, et al: Asthma, wheezy bronchitis, and atopy across two generations, *Am J Respir Crit Care Med* 159:125-129, 1999.

36. Wahn U: Review Series VI: The immunology of fetuses and infants. What drives the allergic march? *Allergy* 55:591-599, 2000.

37. Sigurs N, Bjarnason R, Sigurbergsson F, et al: Asthma and immunoglobulin E antibodies after respiratory syncytial virus bronchiolitis: a prospective cohort study with matched controls, *Pediatrics* 95:500-505, 1995.

38. Stein RT, Sherrill D, Morgan WJ, et al: Respiratory syncytial virus in early life and risk of wheeze and allergy by age 13 years, *Lancet* 354:541-545, 1999.

39. Castro-Rodriguez JA, Holberg CJ, Wright AL, et al: Association of radiologically ascertained pneumonia before age 3 yr with asthma-like symptoms and pulmonary function during childhood: a prospective study, *Am J Respir Crit Care Med* 159:1891-1897, 1999.

40. Castro-Rodriguez JA, Holberg CJ, Morgan WJ, et al: Relation of two different subtypes of croup before age three to wheezing atopy, and pulmonary function during childhood: a prospective study, *Pediatrics* 107:512-518, 2001.

41. Stein RT, Holberg CJ, Sherrill D, et al: Influence of parental smoking on respiratory symptoms during the first decade of life: the Tucson Children's Respiratory Study, *Am J Epidemiol* 149:1030-1037, 1999.

42. Hanrahan JP, Tager IB, Segal MR, et al: The effect of maternal smoking during pregnancy on early infant lung function, *Am Rev Respir Dis* 145:1129-1135, 1992.

43. Young S, Sherrill DL, Arnott J, et al: Parental factors affecting respiration function during the first year of life, *Pediatr Pulmonol* 29:331-340, 2000.

44. Kulig M, Luck W, Lau S, et al: Effect of pre- and postnatal tobacco smoke exposure on specific sensitization to food and inhalant allergens during the first 3 years of life. Multicenter Allergy Study Group, Germany, *Allergy* 54:220-228, 1999.

45. Barbee RA, Halonen M, Kaltenborn W, et al: A longitudinal study of serum IgE in a community cohort: correlations with age, sex, smoking, and atopic status, *J Allergy Clin Immunol* 79:919-927, 1987.

46. Sherrill DL, Halonen M, Burrows B: Relationships between total serum IgE, atopy, and smoking: a twenty-year follow-up analysis, *J Allergy Clin Immunol* 94:954-962, 1994.

47. Gdalevich M, Mimouni D, David M, et al: Breast-feeding and the onset of atopic dermatitis in childhood: a systematic review and meta-analysis of prospective studies, *J Am Acad Dermatol* 45:520-527, 2001.

48. Gdalevich M, Mimouni D, Mimouni M: Breast-feeding and the risk of bronchial asthma in childhood: a systematic review with meta-analysis of prospective studies, *J Pediatr* 139:261-266, 2001.

49. Wright AL, Holberg CJ, Taussig LM, et al: Factors influencing the relation of infant feeding to asthma and recurrent wheeze in childhood, *Thorax* 56:192-197, 2001.

50. Wright AL, Sherrill D, Holberg CJ, et al: Breast-feeding, maternal IgE, and total serum IgE in childhood, *J Allergy Clin Immunol* 104:589-594, 1999.

51. Liu AH: The hygiene hypothesis of allergy and asthma: from barn to bench to bedside, *Ann Allergy,* In press.

52. Ball TM, Castro-Rodriguez JA, Griffith KA, et al: Siblings, day-care attendance, and the risk of asthma and wheezing during childhood, *N Engl J Med* 343:538-543, 2000.

53. Illi S, von Mutius E, Lau S, et al: Early childhood infectious diseases and the development of asthma up to school age: a birth cohort study, *Br Med J* 322:390-395, 2001.

54. Gereda JE, Leung DYM, Thatayatikom A, et al: Relation between house-dust endotoxin exposure, type 1 T-cell development, and allergen sensitization in infants at high risk of asthma, *Lancet* 355:1680-1683, 2000.

55. Gehring U, Bolte G, Borte M, et al: Exposure to endotoxin decreases the risk of atopic eczema in infancy: a cohort study, *J Allergy Clin Immunol* 108:847-854, 2001.

56. Park JH, Gold DR, Spiegelman DL, et al: House dust endotoxin and wheeze in the first year of life, *Am J Respir Crit Care Med* 163:322-328, 2001.

57. Bjorksten B, Sepp E, Julge K, et al: Allergy development and the intestinal microflora during the first year of life, *J Allergy Clin Immunol* 108:516-520, 2001.

58. Kalliomaki M, Kirjavainen P, Eerola E, et al: Distinct patterns of neonatal gut microflora in infants in whom atopy was and was not developing, *J Allergy Clin Immunol* 107:129-134, 2001.

59. Remes ST, Castro-Rodriguez JA, Holberg CJ, et al: Dog exposure in infancy decreases the subsequent risk of frequent wheeze but not of atopy, *J Allergy Clin Immunol* 108:509-515, 2001.

60. Hesselmar B, Aberg N, Aberg B, et al: Does early exposure to cat or dog protect against later allergy development? *Clin Exp Allergy* 29:611-617, 1999.

61. Nafstad P, Magnus P, Gaarder PI, et al: Exposure to pets and atopy-related diseases in the first 4 years of life, *Allergy* 56:307-312, 2001.

62. Reijonen TM, Kotaniemi-Syrjanen A, Korhonen K, et al: Predictors of asthma three years after hospital admission for wheezing in infancy, *Pediatrics* 106:1406-1412, 2000.

63. Svanes C, Jarvis D, Chinn S, et al: Childhood environment and adult atopy: results from the European Community Respiratory Health Survey, *J Allergy Clin Immunol* 103:415-420, 1999.

64. Liu AH: Endotoxin exposure in allergy and asthma: reconciling a paradox, *J Allergy Clin Immunol* 109:379-392, 2002.

65. Castro-Rodriguez JA, Holberg CJ, Morgan WJ, et al: Increased incidence of asthma-like symptoms in girls who become overweight or obese during the school years, *Am J Respir Crit Care Med* 163:1344-1349, 2001.

66. Bergmann RL, Bergmann KE, Lau-Schadensdorf S, et al: Atopic diseases in infancy. The German multicenter atopy study (MAS-90), *Pediatr Allergy Immunol* 5:19-25, 1994.

67. Hanifin JM, Rajka G: Diagnostic features of atopic dermatitis, *Acta Dermatol Venereol (suppl)* 92:44-47, 1980.

68. Williams HC, Strachan DP: The natural history of childhood eczema: observations from the British 1958 cohort study, *Br J Dermatol* 139:834-839, 1998.

69. Linna O: Ten-year prognosis for generalized infantile eczema, *Acta Pediatr* 81:1013, 1992.

70. Vickers CFH: The natural history of atopic eczema, *Acta Dermatol Venereal* 92:113-115, 1980.

71. Berth-Jones J, George S, Graham-Brown RA: Predictors of atopic dermatitis in Leicester children, *Br J Dermatol* 136:498-501, 1997.

72. Dold S, Wjst M, von Mutius E, et al: Genetic risk for asthma, allergic rhinitis, and atopic dermatitis, *Arch Dis Child* 67:1018-1022, 1992.

73. Schultz Larsen F: Atopic dermatitis: a genetic-epidemiologic study in a population-based twin sample, *J Am Acad Dermatol* 28:719-723, 1993.

74. Harris JM, Cullinan P, Williams HC, et al: Environmental associations with eczema in early life, *Br J Dermatol* 144:795-802, 2001.

75. Lammintausta K: Prognosis of atopic dermatitis: a prospective study in early adulthood, *Int J Dermatol* 30:563-568, 1991.

76. Guillet G, Guillet MH: Natural history of sensitizations in atopic dermatitis, *Arch Dermatol* 128:187-192, 1992.

77. Patrizi A, Guerrini V, Ricci G, et al: The natural history of sensitizations to food and aeroallergens in atopic dermatitis: a 4-year follow-up, *Pediatr Dermatol* 17:261-265, 2000.

78. Bergmann RL, Edenharter G, Bergmann KE, et al: Atopic dermatitis in early infancy predicts allergic airway disease at 5 years, *Clin Exp Allergy* 28:965-970, 1998.

79. Kulig M, Klettke U, Wahn V, et al: Development of seasonal allergic rhinitis during the first 7 years of life, *J Allergy Clin Immunol* 106:832-839, 2000.

80. Broder I: Epidemiology of asthma and allergic rhinitis in a total community, Tecumseh, Michigan. IV. Natural history, *J Allergy Clin Immunol* 54:100, 1974.

81. Bock SA: Prospective appraisal of complaints of adverse reactions to foods in children during the first 3 years of life, *Pediatrics* 79:683-688, 1987.

82. Zeiger RS, Heller S, Mellon MH, et al: Effect of combined maternal and infant food-allergen avoidance on development of atopy in early infancy: a randomized study, *J Allergy Clin Immunol* 84:72-89, 1989.

83. Host A: Cow's milk protein allergy and intolerance in infancy: some clinical, epidemiological and immunological aspects, *Pediatr Allergy Immunol* 5:1-36, 1994.

84. Bock SA: The natural history of food sensitivity, *J Allergy Clin Immunol* 69:173-177, 1982.

85. Sampson HA, Scanlon SM: Natural history of food hypersensitivity in children with atopic dermatitis, *J Pediatr* 115:23-27, 1989.

86. Spergel JM, Beausoleil JL, Pawlowski NA: Resolution of childhood peanut allergy, *Ann Allergy Asthma Immunol* 85:435-437, 2000.

87. Vander Leek TK, Liu AH, Stefanski K, et al: The natural history of peanut allergy in young children and its association with serum peanut-specific IgE, *J Pediatr* 137:749-755, 2000.

88. Hill DJ, Bannister DG, Hosking CS, et al: Cow milk allergy within the spectrum of atopic disorders, *Clin Exp Allergy* 24:1137-1143, 1994.

89. Host A, Halken S: A prospective study of cow milk allergy in Danish infants during the first 3 years of life: clinical course in relation to clinical and immunological type of hypersensitivity reaction, *Allergy* 45:587-596, 1990.

90. Cogswell JJ, Halliday DF, Alexander JR: Respiratory infections in the first year of life in children at risk of developing atopy, *Br Med J* 284:1011-1013, 1982.

91. Van Asperen PP, Kemp AS, Mellis CM: Skin test reactivity and clinical allergen sensitivity in infancy, *J Allergy Clin Immunol* 73:381-386, 1984.

92. Fernandez de Corres L, Moneo I, Munoz D, et al: Sensitization from chestnuts and bananas in patients with urticaria and anaphylaxis from contact with latex, *Ann Allergy* 70:35-39, 1993.

93. Katayama H, Yamaguchi K, Kozuka T, et al: Adverse reactions to ionic and nonionic contrast media. A report from the Japanese Committee on the Safety of Contrast Media, *Radiology* 175:621-628, 1990.

94. Lieberman P, Patterson R, Metz R, et al: Allergic reactions to insulin, *JAMA* 215:1106-1112, 1971.

95. Green GR, Rosenblum A: Report of the Penicillin Study Group—American Academy of Allergy, *J Allergy Clin Immunol* 48:331-343, 1971.

96. Settipane GA, Klein DE, Boyd GK: Relationship of atopy and anaphylactic sensitization: a bee sting allergy model, *Clin Allergy* 8:259-265, 1978.

97. Valentine MD, Schuberth KC, Kagey-Sobotka A, et al: The value of immunotherapy with venom in children with allergy to insect stings, *N Engl J Med* 323:1601-1603, 1990.

98. Savliwala MN, Reisman RE: Studies of the natural history of stinging-insect allergy: long-term follow-up of patients without immunotherapy, *J Allergy Clin Immunol* 80:741-745, 1987.

99. Franken HH, Dubois AE, Minkema HJ, et al: Lack of reproducibility of a single negative sting challenge response in the assessment of anaphylactic risk in patients with suspected yellow jacket hypersensitivity, *J Allergy Clin Immunol* 93:431-436, 1994.

100. Arshad SH, Matthews S, Gant C, et al: Effect of allergen avoidance on development of allergic disorders in infancy, *Lancet* 339:1493-1497, 1992.

101. Hide DW, Matthews S, Matthews L, et al: Effect of allergen avoidance in infancy on allergic manifestations at age two years, *J Allergy Clin Immunol* 93:842-846, 1994.

102. Hide DW, Matthews S, Tariq S, et al: Allergen avoidance in infancy and allergy at 4 years of age, *Allergy* 51:89-93, 1996.

103. Arlian LG, Neal JS, Morgan MS, et al.: Reducing relative humidity is a practical way to control dust mites and their allergens in homes in temperate climates, *J Allergy Clin Immunol* 107:99-104, 2001.

104. Platts-Mills T, Vaughan J, Squillace S, et al: Sensitization, asthma, and a modified Th2 response in children exposed to cat allergen: a population-based cross-sectional study, *Lancet* 357:752-756, 2001.

105. Sporik R, Holgate ST, Platts-Mills TAE, et al: Exposure to house-dust mite allergen (*Der p* I) and the development of asthma in childhood, *N Engl J Med* 323:502-507, 1990.

106. Almqvist C, Wickman M, Perfetti L, et al: Worsening of asthma in children allergic to cats, after indirect exposure to cat at school, *Am J Respir Crit Care Med* 163:694-698, 2001.

107. Boner AL, Niero E, Antolini I, et al: Pulmonary function and bronchial hyperreactivity in asthmatic children with house dust mite allergy during prolonged stay in the Italian Alps (Misurina, 1756 m), *Ann Allergy* 54:42-45, 1985.

108. Grootendorst DC, Dahlen SE, Van Den Bos JW, et al: Benefits of high-altitude allergen avoidance in atopic adolescents with moderate to severe asthma, over and above treatment with high-dose inhaled steroids, *Clin Exp Allergy* 31:400-408, 2001.

109. Murray AB, Ferguson AC: Dust-free bedrooms in the treatment of asthmatic children with house dust or house dust mite allergy: a controlled trial, *Pediatrics* 71:418-422, 1983.

110. ETAC Study Group: Allergic factors associated with the development of asthma and the influence of cetirizine in a double-blind, randomized, placebo-controlled trial: first results of ETAC. Early treatment of the atopic child, *Pediatr Allergy Immunol* 9:116-124, 1998.

111. Warner JO: A double-blinded, randomized, placebo-controlled trial of cetirizine in preventing the onset of asthma in children with atopic dermatitis: 18 months' treatment and 18 months' posttreatment follow-up, *J Allergy Clin Immunol* 108:929-937, 2001.

112. Moller C, Dreborg S, Ferdousi HA, et al: Pollen immunotherapy reduces the development of asthma in children with seasonal rhinoconjunctivitis (the PAT-study), *J Allergy Clin Immunol* 109:251-256, 2002.

113. Durham SR, Walker SM, Varga EM, et al: Long-term clinical efficacy of grass-pollen immunotherapy, *N Engl J Med* 341:468-475, 1999.

114. Purello-D'Ambrosio F, Gangemi S, Merendino RA, et al: Prevention of new sensitizations in monosensitized subjects submitted to specific immunotherapy or not: a retrospective study, *Clin Exp Allergy* 31:1295-1302, 2001.

115. Des Roches A, Paradis L, Menardo JL, et al: Immunotherapy with a standardized *Dermatophagoides pteronyssinus* extract. VI. Specific immunotherapy prevents the onset of new sensitizations in children, *J Allergy Clin Immunol* 99:450-453, 1997.

116. Kalliomaki M, Salminen S, Arvilommi H, et al: Probiotics in primary prevention of atopic disease: a randomized placebo-controlled trial, *Lancet* 357:1076-1079, 2001.

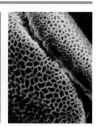

CHAPTER **3**

The Genetics of Allergic Disease and Asthma

JOHN W. HOLLOWAY ■ JULIE A. CAKEBREAD ■ STEPHEN T. HOLGATE

Considerable effort has been made since the first report of linkage of a region of the human genome with allergic disease[1] to identify the genetic factors that modify susceptibility to allergic disease, the severity of disease in affected individuals, and response to treatment. Since the report of linkage between chromosome 11q13 and atopy in 1989, there have been hundreds of published studies of the genetics of asthma and other allergic diseases. Our knowledge of how genetics contributes to the pathophysiology of these complex disorders has expanded considerably, yet the field of genetic analysis of allergic disease still remains on the cusp of success with few genes underlying susceptibility identified with any certainty. In this chapter we outline the approaches used to undertake genetic studies and the complexities of genetic analysis of complex disease and provide examples of how these approaches are beginning to reveal new insights into the pathophysiology of allergic disease.

WHY UNDERTAKE GENETIC STUDIES OF ALLERGIC DISEASE?

The ongoing research into genetic factors behind the development and pathogenesis of atopy and allergic disease will in due course provide a greater understanding of the fundamental mechanisms of these disorders. The study of these genetic factors in large longitudinal cohorts with extensive environmental information will allow the identification of both the environmental factors that in susceptible individuals trigger allergic disease and the periods of life in which this occurs, potentially leading to the prevention of disease through environmental modification. Identification of genetic variants that predispose to allergic disease will result in several outcomes. First, the greater understanding of the susceptibility factors for the disease will allow the development of specific new drugs to both relieve and prevent symptoms. In addition, different genetic variants may also influence the response to therapy, and the identification of individuals with altered response to current drug therapies will allow optimization of current therapeutic measures. Second, the identification of susceptibility factors for allergic disease will allow early identification of susceptible children, allowing them to be targeted at an early age for both preventative therapy and environmental intervention such as avoidance of allergen exposure. Genetic screening in early life may thus become a practical and cost-effective option in preventing allergic disease.

APPROACHES TO GENETIC STUDIES OF COMPLEX GENETIC DISEASES

What Is a Complex Genetic Disease?

The use of genetic analysis to identify genes responsible for simple mendelian traits such as cystic fibrosis[2] and Huntington's disease[3] has become almost routine in the 20 years since it was recognized that genetic inheritance can be traced with naturally occurring DNA sequence variation.[4] Since then over 500 such genes have been mapped to specific chromosomal locations and more than 100 have been positionally cloned. However, many of the most common medical conditions known to have a genetic component to their etiology, including diabetes, hypertension, heart disease, schizophrenia, and asthma, have much more complex inheritance patterns.

Complex disorders show a clear hereditary pattern, but the mode of inheritance does not follow any simple mendelian pattern such as autosomal dominant, recessive, or sex linked. Also, unlike single-gene disorders, they tend to have an extremely high prevalence. Asthma occurs in at least 10% of children in the United Kingdom, and atopy is as high as 40% in some population groups.[5] This compares with a frequency of one of the most common mendelian disorders, cystic fibrosis, of 1:2000 live white births. There are a number of different factors that influence whether a disorder is inherited in a mendelian fashion. There may be a number of different genes that predispose individuals to the disease, either more than one gene in an individual (polygenic inheritance) or different genes in different individuals (genetic heterogeneity). There may also be a number of environmental factors necessary for the expression of the disease phenotype.

How to Identify Genes Underlying Complex Disease

There are a number of different factors that need to be considered before any genetic study of a complex disease can be initiated. These include assessing the heritability of a disease of interest to establish whether there is indeed a genetic component to the disease in question; defining the phenotype of physical characteristics to be measured in a population and comparing it with the genetic data, size, and nature of the population to be studied; and determining which genetic markers are going to be typed in the DNA samples obtained from the population, how the relationships between the genetic data and the phenotypes measure in individuals are to be analyzed, and how this data can be used to identify the genes underlying the disease.

One of the most important considerations in genetic studies of complex disease susceptibility is the choice of the methods of genetic analysis to be used. This choice will reflect and be reflected in the design of the study; that is, will it be a population study or a family-based study? What numbers of subjects will be needed? Susceptibility to asthma is likely to result from the inheritance of one or more mutant genes. Unfortunately, in asthma, as in many other disorders, the specific biochemical defect that causes the disease is unknown. Consequently, these mutant genes and their abnormal gene products can be recognized solely by the anomalous phenotypes they produce. Identifying the chromosomal location of, and subsequently the genes themselves that produce these disease phenotypes, will allow a better understanding of the pathogenic mechanisms of the disease process.

Inheritance

The first step in any genetic analysis of a complex disease is to determine whether genetics contribute at all to an individual's susceptibility to disease. The fact that a disease has been observed to "run in families" is insufficient evidence to begin molecular genetic studies because this can occur for a number of reasons, including common environmental exposure and biased ascertainment, as well as a true genetic disposition. There are a number of approaches that can be taken to determine if genetics contributes to a disease or disease phenotype of interest including family studies, segregation analysis, twin and adoption studies, heritability studies, and population-based relative risk to relatives of probands.

There are three main steps involved in the identification of genetic mechanisms for a disease.[6,7]

1. Determine whether there is familial aggregation of the disease—does the disease occur more frequently in relatives of cases than of controls?
2. If there is evidence for familial aggregation, is this because of genetic effects or other factors such as environmental or cultural effects?
3. If there are genetic factors, which specific genetic mechanisms are operating?

The exact methods used in this process will vary depending on a number of disease-specific factors. For example, is the disease of early or late onset, and is the phenotype in question discrete or continuous (e.g., blood pressure or insulin resistance)?

Family studies involve the estimation of the frequency of the disease in relatives of affected compared with unaffected individuals. The strength of the genetic effect can be measured as λ_R, where λ_R is the ratio of risk to relatives of type R (e.g., sibs, parents, offspring, etc.) compared with the population risk ($\lambda_R = \kappa_R/\kappa$, where κ_R is the risk to relatives of type R and κ is the population risk). The stronger the genetic effect, the higher the value of λ. For example, for a single gene recessive mendelian disorder such as cystic fibrosis, the λ_S is about 500; for a dominant one such as Huntington's disease, it is about 5000. For complex disorders the values of λ are much lower, such as 20 to 30 for multiple sclerosis, 15 for insulin-dependent diabetes mellitus (IDDM), and 4 to 5 for Alzheimer's disease. It is important to note though that λ is a function of both the strength of the genetic effect and the frequency of the disease in the population. Therefore a disease with a λ of 3 to 4 does not mean that genes are less important in that trait than in a trait with a λ of 30 to 40. A strong effect in a very common disease will have a smaller λ than the same strength of effect in a rare disease.

Determining the relative contribution of common genes versus common environment to clustering of disease within families can be undertaken using twin studies where the concordance of a trait in monozygotic and dizygotic twins is assessed. Monozygotic twins have identical genotypes, whereas dizygotic twins share on average only one half of their genes. Therefore a disease that has a genetic component is expected to show a higher rate of concordance in monozygotic than in dizygotic twins. Another approach to disentangling the effects of nature versus nurture in a disease is in adoption studies, where, if the disease has a genetic basis, the frequency of the disease should be higher in biologic relatives of probands than in their adopted family.

Once familial aggregation with a probable genetic etiology for a disease has been established, the mode of inheritance can be determined by observing the pattern of inheritance of a disease or trait by observing how it is distributed within families. For example, is there evidence of a single major gene, and is it dominantly or recessively inherited? Segregation analysis is the most established method for this purpose. The observed frequency of a trait in offspring and siblings is compared with the distribution expected with various modes of inheritance. If the distribution is significantly different than predicted, that model is rejected. The model that cannot be rejected is therefore considered the most likely. However, for complex disease, it is often difficult to undertake segregation analysis because of the multiple genetic and environmental effects making any one model hard to determine. This has implication for the methods of analysis of genetic data in studies because some method, such as the parametric lod score approach, require a model to be defined to obtain estimates of parameters such as gene frequency and penetrance (see later).

Phenotype

Studies of a genetic disorder require that a phenotype be defined, to which genetic data are compared. Phenotypes can be classified in two ways. They may be complex, such as asthma or atopy, and are likely to involve the interaction of a number of genes. Alternatively, intermediate phenotypes may be used, such as bronchial hyperresponsiveness (BHR) for asthma and serum IgE levels and specific IgE responsiveness to particular allergens for atopy. These phenotypes contribute to an individual's expression of the overall complex disease phenotype but are likely to involve the interaction of fewer genetic influences, thus increasing the chances of identifying specific genetic factors predisposing toward the disease. Phenotypes may also be discrete or qualitative, such as the presence or absence of wheeze, atopy, or asthma, or quantitative. Quantitative phenotypes, such as blood pressure (mm Hg) and serum IgE levels, are phenotypes that can be measured as a continuous variable. With quantitative traits, no arbitrary cut off point has to be assigned (making quantitative trait analysis important) because clinical criteria used to define an affected or an unaffected phenotype may not reflect whether an individual is a gene carrier or not. In addition, the use of quantitative phenotypes allows the use of alternative methods of genetic analysis that, in some situations, can be more powerful.

Population

Having established that the disease or phenotype of interest does have a genetic component to its etiology, the next step is to recruit a study population in which to undertake molecular genetic analyses to identify the gene(s) responsible. The type and size of study population recruited depend heavily on a number of interrelated factors, including the epidemiology of the disease, the method of genetic epidemiologic analysis being used, and the class of genetic markers typed. For example, the recruitment of families is necessary to undertake linkage analysis, whereas association studies are better suited to either a randomly selected or case-control cohort. In family-based linkage studies, the age of onset of a disease will determine whether it is practical to collect multigenerational families or affected sib-pairs for analysis. Equally, if a disease is rare, then actively recruiting cases and matched controls will be a more practical approach than recruiting a random population that would need to be very large to have sufficient power.

Genetic Markers

Genetic markers used can be any identifiable site within the genome (locus) where the DNA sequence is variable (polymorphic). The most common genetic markers used for linkage analysis are microsatellite markers. These comprise short lengths of DNA consisting of repeats of a specific sequence (e.g., CA_n). The number of repeats varies between individuals, thus providing polymorphic markers that can be used in genetic analysis to follow the transmission of a chromosomal region from one generation to the next. The locations of well over 5000 microsatellite markers in the human genome have been identified, spanning the whole genome at an average of 2 cM.[8]

Single-nucleotide polymorphisms (SNPs) are the simplest class of polymorphism in the genome resulting from a single base mutation that substitutes one nucleotide for another: cytosine substituted for thymidine. As a result there are only two possible "classes" or alleles at a given SNP. This makes SNPs less useful as markers for linkage because they are less informative than microsatellite markers, where there can be many alleles (e.g., 10 copies of a repeat, 12 copies, 16 copies, etc.). However, SNPs are much more frequent in the human genome, occurring in introns, exons, promoters, and intergenic regions, with several hundred thousand SNPs now having been identified and mapped. SNPs are more suited to mapping by association and linkage disequilibrium than microsatellites.[9]

Analysis

The method chosen to analyze the molecular genetic data obtained by the typing of genetic markers within a study cohort, like the cohort recruited and the selection of genetic markers, is interdependent on the other parameters of the study. There are two main approaches. Linkage analysis involves proposing a model to explain the inheritance pattern of phenotypes and genotypes observed in a pedigree. Linkage is evident when a gene that produces a phenotypic trait (and its surrounding markers) are inherited together. In contrast, those markers not associated with the anomalous phenotype of interest will be randomly distributed among affected family members as a re-

sult of the independent assortment of chromosomes and crossing over during meiosis.

Parametric lod score analyses for testing linkage between phenotypes and polymorphic DNA markers involve assuming a model of inheritance and comparing the probability that the observed family data would arise under one hypothesis, such as linkage between a disease causing gene and the marker, to an alternative hypothesis—no linkage. The evidence for one hypothesis over the other is measured by the ratio of their odds, the likelihood ratio (LR), or more equivalently by the lod score, $Z = \log10(LR)$.[10] Generally, linkage is confirmed when the odds ratio drops to 1000:1 in favor of linkage ($Z = 3.0$) and rejected when the odds ratio drops to 100:1 in favor of no linkage ($Z = -2.0$),[11] giving a false-positive rate of 5%. However, this does not always hold true in the analysis of more complex traits, and it has been suggested that a higher lod score ($Z = 3.3$) should be taken as evidence of linkage.[12] However, an estimation of all the relevant parameters is difficult, and this has made assigning a standard level of significance difficult; interpretation of lod scores for complex disease remains controversial.[11,13] Parametric linkage analysis is the method of choice for simple mendelian traits because the allowable models are few and easily tested. However, it is more difficult to apply to complex traits, because it may be hard to find a precise model that adequately explains the inheritance pattern, although models have been developed to account for genetic heterogeneity.[14]

An alternative approach involves allele-sharing methods that test whether the inheritance pattern of a particular chromosomal region is not consistent with random mendelian segregation by showing that pairs of affected relatives inherit identical copies of the region more often than would be expected by chance. Because allele-sharing methods are nonparametric, it is not necessary to define a model for the inheritance of the trait, making allele-sharing methods more robust than linkage analysis: affected relatives should show excess sharing even in the presence of incomplete penetrance, phenocopy, genetic heterogeneity, and high-frequency disease alleles. However, allele-sharing methods are often less powerful and, therefore, require more subjects than correctly specified linkage models.[15] Affected sib-pair analysis is the simplest form of allele-sharing analysis. Because both siblings are affected, the disease genes are assumed to have acted and therefore nonpenetrant individuals are excluded from the analysis. Two sibs can show identical-by-descent (IBD) sharing for no, one, or two copies of any locus (with a 1:2:1 distribution expected under random segregation). Excess allele sharing can be measured with a simple χ^2 test. Allele sharing can also be applied to quantitative traits. One method for doing this involves performing regression analysis of the squared difference in a trait between two relatives and the number of alleles shared IBD at a locus.[16]

Association studies do not examine inheritance patterns of alleles; rather, they are case-control studies based on a comparison of allele frequencies between groups of affected and unaffected individuals from a population. A particular allele is said to be associated with the trait if it occurs at a significantly higher frequency among affected individuals as compared with those in the control group. The relative risk of the trait in individuals is then assessed as the ratio of the frequency of the allele in the affected population compared with the unaffected population. The greatest problem in association studies is the selection of a suitable control group to compare with the affected population group. Although association studies can be performed with any random DNA polymorphism, they have the most significance when applied to polymorphisms that have functional consequences in genes relevant to the trait (candidate genes).

It is important to remember with association studies that there are a number of reasons leading to an association between a phenotype and a particular allele.

- A positive association between the phenotype and the allele will occur if the allele is the cause of, or contributes to, the phenotype. This association would be expected to be replicated in other populations with the same phenotype, unless there are several different alleles at the same locus contributing to the same phenotype, in which case association would be difficult to detect, or if the trait was predominantly the result of different genes in the other population (genetic heterogeneity).

- Positive associations may also occur between an allele and a phenotype if the particular allele is in linkage disequilibrium with the phenotype-causing allele. That is, the allele tends to occur on the same parental chromosome that also carries the trait-causing mutation more often than would be expected under mendelian segregation. Linkage disequilibrium will occur when most causes of the trait are the result of relatively few ancestral mutations at a trait-causing locus and the allele is present on one of those ancestral chromosomes and lies close enough to the trait-causing locus that the association between them has not been eroded away through recombination between chromosomes during meiosis.

- Positive association between and an allele and a trait can also be artefactual as a result of recent population admixture. In a mixed population, any trait present in a higher frequency in a subgroup of the population (e.g., an ethnic group) will show positive association with an allele that also happens to be more common in that population subgroup. Thus to avoid spurious association arising through admixture, studies should be performed in large, relatively homogeneous populations. An alternative method to test for association in the presence of linkage is the "transmission test for linkage disequilibrium" (transmission/disequilibrium test [TDT]).[17,18] The TDT uses families with at least one affected child, and the transmission of the associated marker allele from a heterozygous parent to an affected offspring is evaluated. If a parent is heterozygous for an associated allele *A1* and a nonassociated allele *A2*, then *A1* should be passed on to the affected child more often than *A2*. When a disease is found to be associated with such a marker, the TDT may detect linkage even when haplotype-sharing tests do not.

Currently, association studies are not well suited to whole genome searches in large mixed populations. Because linkage disequilibrium extends over very short genetic distances in an old population, many more markers would need to be typed to "cover" the whole genome. Therefore genomic searches for association might be more favorable in young, genetically isolated populations because linkage disequilibrium extends over greater distances and the number of disease-causing alleles is likely to be fewer.

Identify Gene

If, as in most complex disorders, the exact biochemical or physiologic basis of the disease is unknown, there are two main approaches to finding the disease gene(s). One method is to test markers randomly spaced throughout the entire genome for linkage with the disease phenotype. If linkage is found between a particular marker and the phenotype, then further typing of genetic markers including SNPs and association analysis will enable the critical region to be further narrowed; the genes positioned in this region can be examined for possible involvement in the disease process and the presence of disease-causing mutations in affected individuals. This approach is often termed *positional cloning*, or *genome scanning* if the whole genome is examined in this manner. Although this approach requires no assumptions to be made as to the particular gene involved in genetic susceptibility to the disease in question, it does require considerable molecular genetic analysis to be undertaken, involving considerable time and expense. Alternatively, in the candidate gene approach individual genes can be directly tested for their involvement in the disease process. Genes are selected for this approach because of the function of the gene product being involved in the disease process. The gene is then screened for polymorphism, which is tested for association with the disease or phenotype in question. A hybrid of the two approaches is the selection of candidate genes based not only on their function but also on their position within a genetic region previously linked to the disease (positional candidate), which may help to reduce the considerable work required to narrow a large genetic region of several megabases of DNA identified through linkage containing tens to hundreds of genes to one single gene associated with the disease.

A means for identifying genes for complex diseases, both the association and the affected sib-pair approaches have limitations. Population association between a disease and a genetic marker can arise as an artefact of population structure, even in the absence of linkage, and linkage studies with modest numbers of affected sib-pairs may fail to detect linkage, especially if there is genetic heterogeneity. Linkage analysis has been used successfully to identify genes underlying single-gene disorders, but in complex diseases it is very difficult to sufficiently narrow a region of linkage to just a single gene. Association and linkage equilibrium analyses using SNPs are more useful in this final stage of gene identification.[9] This approach was successful in the identification of two genes underlying the complex genetic diseases of Crohn's disease and the *NOD2* gene[19] and non-IDDM (NIDDM) and the calpain 10 (*CAPN10*) gene.[20]

Once a gene has been identified, it is really only the beginning of the work required to understand its role in the disease pathogenesis. Further molecular genetic studies may help to identify the precise genetic polymorphism that is having functional consequences for the gene's expression or function as opposed to those that are merely in linkage disequilibrium with the causal SNP. Often the gene identified may be completely novel and cell and molecular biology studies will be needed to understand the gene product's role in the disease and to define genotype/phenotype correlations. By using cohorts with information available on environmental exposures, it may be possible to define how the gene product may interact with the environment to cause disease. Ultimately, knowledge of the gene's role in disease pathogenesis may lead to the development of novel therapeutics.

Asthma and Allergy as Complex Genetic Diseases

From studies of the epidemiology and heritability of allergic diseases, it is clear that they are complex diseases in which the interaction between genetic and environmental factors plays a fundamental role in the development of IgE-mediated sensitivity and the subsequent development of clinical symptoms. The development of IgE responses by an individual, and therefore allergies, is the function of several genetic factors. These include the regulation of basal serum immunoglobulin production, the regulation of the switching of Ig-producing B cells to IgE, and the control of the specificity of responses to antigens. Furthermore, the genetic influences on allergic diseases such as asthma are more complex than those on atopy alone, involving not only genes controlling the induction and level of an IgE-mediated response to allergen but also "lung"- or "asthma"-specific genetic factors that result in the development of asthma. This also applies equally to other clinical manifestations of atopy such as rhinitis and atopic dermatitis.

PHENOTYPES FOR ALLERGY AND ALLERGIC DISEASE: WHAT SHOULD WE MEASURE?

The term *atopy* (from the Greek word for "strangeness") was originally used by Coca and Cooke[21] in 1923 to describe a particular predisposition to develop hypersensitivity to common allergens associated with an increase of circulating reaginic antibody, now defined as IgE, and with clinical manifestations such as whealing-type reactions, asthma, and hay fever. Today, even if the definition of *atopy* is not yet precise, the term is commonly used to define a disorder that involves IgE antibody responses to ubiquitous allergens that is associated with a number of clinical disorders such as asthma, allergic dermatitis, allergic conjunctivitis, and allergic rhinitis.

In industrialized countries atopy is usually correlated with an increased total serum IgE level, which is considered the most reliable index of atopy. However, because not all atopic subjects have an increased total serum IgE level, atopy can also be measured by the presence of antigen-specific IgE antibodies and/or a positive skin test to common allergens. Furthermore, because of their complex clinical phenotype, atopic diseases can be studied using intermediate or surrogate disease-specific measurements, such as BHR for asthma. Phenotypes can be defined in several ways, ranging from subjective measures (e.g., symptoms), objective measures (e.g., BHR or serum IgE level), or both. In addition, some studies have used quantitative scores that are derived from both physical measures such as serum IgE and BHR and questionnaire data.[22,23] The use of scores as phenotypes enables the quantitative evaluation of complex traits such as asthma affection, allowing the use of potentially more powerful methods that rely on the use of a quantitative rather than dichotomous trait for genetic analysis. It is a lack of a clear definition of atopic phenotypes that presents the greatest problem when reviewing studies of the genetic basis of atopy, with multiple definitions of the same intermediate phenotype often being used in different studies.

THE HERITABILITY OF ATOPIC DISEASE: ARE ATOPY AND ATOPIC DISEASE HERITABLE CONDITIONS?

In 1916 the first comprehensive study of the heritability of atopy was undertaken by Robert Cooke and Albert Vander Veer[24] at the Department of Medicine of the Postgraduate Hospital and Medical School of New York. Although the atopic conditions they included, as well as those excluded (e.g., eczema), may be open for debate today, the conclusions nonetheless remain the same. There is a high heritable component to the development of atopy and atopic disease and, as is more clearly understood biologically now, this is an inheritance of a tendency to generate specific IgE responses to common proteins.

Subsequent to the work of Cooke and Vander Veer, the results of many studies have established that atopy and atopic disease such as asthma, rhinitis, and eczema have strong genetic components. Family studies have shown an increased prevalence of atopy, and phenotypes associated with atopy, among the relatives of atopic compared with nonatopic subjects.[25-27] In a study of 176 normal families, Gerrard et al[28] found a striking association between asthma in the parent and asthma in the child, between hay fever in the parent and hay fever in the child, and between eczema in the parent and eczema in the child. These studies suggest that "end-organ sensitivity" or which allergic disease an allergic individual will develop is controlled by specific genetic factors, differing from those that determine susceptibility to atopy per se. This hypothesis is borne out by a questionnaire study involving 6665 families in southern Bavaria. Children with atopic diseases had a positive family history in 55% of cases compared with 35% in children without atopic disease ($P < 0.001$).[29] Subsequent researchers used the same population to investigate familial influences unique to the expression of asthma and found that the prevalence of asthma alone (i.e., without hay fever or eczema) increased significantly if the nearest of kin had asthma alone (4.7% vs. 11.7%, $P < 0.0001$). A family history of eczema or hay fever (without asthma) was unrelated to asthma in the offspring.[30]

Numerous twin studies[31-37] have shown a significant increase in concordance among monozygotic twins compared with dizygotic twins, providing evidence for a genetic component to atopy. Atopic asthma has also been widely studied, and both twin and family studies have shown a strong heritable component to this phenotype.[31,35,36,38-40] In a recent study using a twin-family model, Laitinen et al[41] reported that in families with asthma in successive generations, genetic factors alone accounted for as much as 87% of the development of asthma in offspring, and the incidence of the disease in twins with affected parents is fourfold compared with the incidence in twins without affected parents. This indicates that asthma is recurring in families as a result of shared genes rather than shared environmental risk factors. This has been further substantiated in a recent study of 11,688 Danish twin pairs. Using additive genetic and nonshared environmental modeling, it was suggested that 73% of susceptibility to asthma was the result of the genetic component. However, a substantial part of the variation liability of asthma was the result of environmental factors; there also was no evidence for genetic dominance or shared environmental effects.[42]

Segregation analysis has been applied to IgE and BHR as phenotypes as well as to disease phenotypes such as asthma and eczema. Several different modes of inheritance of high IgE levels have been suggested, including autosomal recessive, autosomal dominant, and polygenic inheritance.[43-49] A study by Lawrence et al[22] looked at eight traits—log IgE, BHR, skin prick test, eczema, hay fever, wheeze, asthma, and atopy—on a cohort of 131 families recruited at random from the population of Wessex. Complex segregation analysis showed it to be unlikely that any major genes are involved in the production of any of these traits, with the data favoring a two-locus model.

MOLECULAR REGULATION OF ATOPY AND ATOPIC DISEASE, I: SUSCEPTIBILITY GENES

Positional Cloning by Genome-wide Screens

Many genome-wide screens for atopy and atopic disorder susceptibility genes have been completed (Table 3-1). The first genome scan to be completed was a study of Australian and U.K. populations by Daniels et al.[50] This study identified six regions of potential linkage on chromosomes 4, 6, 7, 11, 13, and 16 with atopy and BHR. Recently, the same group has shown positive linkage of serum IgA levels to a marker on chromosome 13 previously linked to atopy.[51] The Collaborative Study on Genetics of Asthma (CSGA) is a large, multicenter, ongoing study in the United States. In its first report, describing the analysis of 237 affected sib-pairs, the linkage between asthma and six novel regions in three racial groups was described: 5p15 and 17p11.1-11.2 in blacks, 11p15 and 19q13 in whites, and 2q13 and 21q12 in Hispanics. They also detected linkage in five regions previously reported to be linked to asthma phenotype: 5q, 6p, 12q, 13q, and 14q in whites and 12q in Hispanics.[52] An additional report from the CSGA study[53] using 199 single pedigrees and 67 extended pedigrees with ethnicity-specific analyses, which allowed for different frequencies of asthma-susceptibility genes in each ethnic population, provided the strongest evidence for linkage at 6p21 in the white population, at 11q21 in the black population, and at 1p32 in the Hispanic population. Conditional analysis and affected sib-pair two-locus analysis provided further evidence for linkage at 5q31, 8p23, 12q22, and 15q13.[53] Genome scans have also been completed in a sample of German and Swedish families, French families,[54] Dutch families,[55] a large cohort of 533 families from China,[56] and a Japanese cohort.[57]

Three genome scans for asthma have been undertaken in genetically isolated populations. The advantage of genetically isolated populations is that being relatively homogeneous, the molecular mechanisms underlying a complex disease such as asthma might also have reduced heterogeneity and therefore be easier to dissect than in mixed populations. In the Hutterites, a genetically isolated population of European ancestry, an initial sample of 361 individuals and a replication sample of 292 individuals were evaluated for asthma phenotypes, and 12 markers in 10 regions were identified that showed possible linkage to asthma or an associated phenotype. Linkage was found in both the initial and replication samples in four regions (5q23-31, 12q15-24.1, 19q13, and 21q21) that have also shown linkage to asthma phenotypes in other samples. In addition, one novel region linked to asthma phenotypes, 3p24.2-22, was also identified.[58] A study of a population from eastern central Finland (Kainuu province) found strong evidence for linkage in a 20-cM region of chromosome 7p14-p15 for three phenotypes: asthma, a high level of total serum IgE (>100 kU/L), and the combination of the two phenotypes (i.e., asthma and high serum IgE levels). The strongest linkage was seen for high serum IgE (nonparametric linkage = score 3.9, $P = 0.0001$).[59]

Three genome scans have also been completed for childhood atopic dermatitis and allergic rhinitis, resulting in the identification of four candidate loci: 3q21,[60] 1q21, 17q25,[61] and 4q24-27.[62] These loci overlap closely with loci previously identified as susceptibility loci for psoriasis.[61] This suggests that atopic dermatitis may be influenced by genes with general effects on dermal inflammation and immunity.

The results of the genome-wide screens for allergy and allergic disease susceptibility genes reflect the genetic and environmental heterogeneity seen in allergic disorders. Multiple regions of the genome have been observed to be linked to varying phenotypes with differences between cohorts recruited from both similar and different populations. This illustrates the difficulty of identifying susceptibility genes for complex genetic diseases. Different genetic loci will show linkage in populations of different ethnicities and different environmental exposures. Identification of the gene(s) underlying the linkage observed is therefore a major challenge. As discussed earlier, in studies of complex disease, the real challenge has not been identification of regions of linkage but rather identification of the precise gene and genetic variant underlying the observed linkage. To date, *ADAM33* is the only gene to be identified as the result of positional cloning using a genome-wide scan for allergic disease phenotypes.[63]

ADAM33 and Asthma

The A Disintegrin And Metalloprotease 33 *(ADAM33)* gene is a member of a subgroup of the zinc-dependent metalloprotease family. ADAM family members are involved in a wide range of biologic processes, including the shedding of cell-surface proteins such as cytokines and cytokine receptors. In a genome-wide scan of 460 white families for physician-diagnosed asthma, suggestive evidence for linkage (likelihood ratio, 2.24) was found on chromosome 20 at 9.99 cM. The addition of 13 more markers at 1 to 2 cM increased the likelihood ratio to 2.94 at D20S482 (12.1 cM), which further increased to 3.93 when BHR was included in the definition of asthma, thereby exceeding the threshold for genome-wide significance.[11] In contrast, when asthma was conditioned for serum total IgE and allergen-specific IgE, the maximum lod score fell to 2.3 at 11.6 cM and 1.87 at 12.1 cM, respectively, indicating the presence of genes more closely linked to altered airway function than to allergic inflammation per se.

Physical mapping and direct cDNA selection identified 40 genes in the region under the peak of linkage at 20p13.[63] Single-stranded conformational polymorphism analysis and direct sequencing were used to identify SNPs in the region, and 135 polymorphisms in 23 genes that lay in the 2.5-Mb 90% confidence interval around the peak of linkage were typed. Twenty-five SNPs were localized to a cluster of five genes showing significant association with both asthma and BHR. Fourteen of these lay within a single gene identified as

TABLE 3-1 Summary of Genome Scans for Atopy and Allergic Disease Phenotypes

Chromosome	Position	Phenotype	Population	Author, Year
1	1p21-1p22	Asthma (strict/loose) and atopy[a]	U.S. Hutterites	Ober et al, 1998[58]
	1p31	Asthma[b]	France	Dizier et al, 2000[54]
	1p32	Asthma[c]	U.S. Hispanics	Xu et al, 2001[53]
	1q21	Atopic dermatitis	United Kingdom	Cookson et al, 2001[61]
	1q25	Atopy and asthma[d]	China	Xu et al, 2001[56]
2	2pter	Asthma, BHR, IgE, and RAST	Germany	Wjst et al, 1999[87]
	2p25	Atopy and asthma[d]	China	Xu et al, 2001[56]
	2q21-q23	Der p−specific IgE	U.S. whites	CSGA, 1998[140]
	2q33	Asthma	U.S. Hispanics	CSGA, 1997[52]
	2q	Atopy and IgE	Holland	Koppelman et al, 2002[55]
3	3p24.2-22	Asthma symptoms	U.S. Hutterites	Ober et al, 1998[58]
	3q21	Atopic dermatitis	Europe	Lee et al, 2000[60]
4	4p15.3	Atopy and asthma[d]	China	Xu et al, 2001[56]
	4q24-27	Allergic rhinitis	Denmark	Haagerup et al, 2001[62]
	4q35	Asthma[e]	Australia	Daniels et al, 1996[50]
	4q35	Mite-sensitive atopic asthma[f]	Japan	Yokouchi et al, 2000[57]
5	5p15	Asthma	U.S. blacks	CSGA, 1997[52]
	5q23-31	Asthma	U.S. whites	CSGA, 1997[52]
	5q31-33	Asthma, BHR, and symptoms	U.S. Hutterites	Ober et al, 1998[58]
	5q31[g]	Asthma[c]	U.S. total	Xu et al, 2001[53]
	5q31	IgE	Holland	Xu et al, 2000[86]
	5q31-33	Mite-sensitive atopic asthma[f]	Japan	Yokouchi et al, 2000[57]
6	6p21	Asthma[c]	U.S. whites	CSGA, 1997[52] and Xu et al, 2001[53]
	6p21	Atopy[a]	U.S. Hutterites	Ober et al, 2000[141]
	6p21.3	Asthma, IgE, RAST, and eosinophils	Germany	Wjst et al, 1999[87]
	6p22-p21.3	Mite-sensitive atopic asthma	Japan	Yokouchi et al, 2000[57]
	6p	Atopy and IgE	Holland	Koppelman et al, 2002[55]
	6q16.3-6q25.2	Asthma[e]	Australia	Daniels et al, 1996[50]
7	7p21-7p15	Asthma[e]	Australia	Daniels et al, 1996[50]
	7p14-15	Asthma, IgE	Finland	Laitinen, 2001[59]
	7q	Total and specific IgE	Holland	Xu et al, 2000[86]
	7q	Atopy and IgE	Holland	Koppelman et al, 2002[55]
8p	8p23[g]	Asthma	U.S. total	Xu et al, 2001[53]
	8p23-21	Der p−specific IgE	U.S. blacks	CSGA, 1998[140]
9	9p	Asthma, IgE, and RAST	Germany	Wjst et al, 1999[87]
10	10p25	Atopy and asthma[d]	China	Xu et al, 2001[56]
11	11p13	Asthma[b]	France	Dizier et al, 2000[54]
	11p15	Asthma	U.S. whites	CSGA, 1997[52]
	11q13	Asthma[e]	United Kingdom and Australia	Daniels et al, 1996[50]
	11q13	Asthma[b]	France	Dizier et al, 2000[54]
	11q21	Asthma[c]	U.S. blacks	CSGA, 2001[52]
	11q	Atopy	Holland	Koppelman et al, 2002[55]
12	12q	Total IgE	Holland	Xu et al, 2000[86]
	12q13	Asthma	Germany	Wjst et al, 1999[87]
	12q 15-24.1	Asthma, BHR, and symptoms	U.S. Hutterites	Ober et al, 1998[58]
	12q14-24.2	Asthma, BHR, and IgE	U.S. whites and Hispanics	Xu et al, 2001[53]
	12q21-q23	Mite-sensitive atopic asthma, BHR	Japan	Yokouchi et al, 2000[57]
	12q24	Asthma[b]	France	Dizier et al, 2000[54]

BHR, Bronchial hyperresponsiveness; *CSGA,* Collaborative Study on the Genetics of Asthma; *RAST,* radioallergosorbent test.
The results of the genome-wide screens for susceptibility genes reflect the genetic and environmental heterogeneity seen in allergic disorders. Multiple regions of the genome have been linked to varying phenotypes with differences between cohorts recruited from different populations; this illustrates the difficulty of identifying susceptibility genes for complex genetic diseases.
[a]Five intermediate phenotypes associated with atopy.
[b]Asthma and four intermediate phenotypes.
[c]Asthma intermediate phenotypes.
[d]Intermediate phenotypes (quantitative trait loci) include BHR, forced expiratory volume in 1 second, forced vital capacity, total IgE, eosinophils, skin-prick test wheal size, and specific IgE.
[e]Four intermediate phenotypes associated with asthma.
Ober, 1998: "loose asthma" phenotype = BHR and/or asthma symptoms; "strict asthma" = asthma.
Ober, 2000: cough, wheeze, sob (2/3), and BHR = strict asthma; either symptoms or BHR = loose asthma.

Continued

TABLE 3-1 Summary of Genome Scans for Atopy and Allergic Disease Phenotypes—cont'd

Chromosome	Position	Phenotype	Population	Author, Year
13	13q11	Mite-sensitive atopic asthma[f]	Japan	Yokouchi et al, 2000[57]
	13q12-13	IgE	Holland	Koppelman et al, 2002[55]
	13q14.1-13q14.3	Asthma[e]	Australia and United Kingdom	Daniels et al, 1996[50]
	13q14.1-q14.3	Mite-sensitive atopic asthma, BHR	Japan	Yokouchi et al, 2000[57]
	13q21.3	Asthma	Whites	CSGA, 1997[52]
	13q31	Asthma[b]	France	Dizier et al, 2000[50]
14	14q11-13	Asthma	U.S. whites	CSGA, 1997[52]
	14q32	IgE and BHR	U.S. total	CSGA, 1997[52]; 2001[53]
15	15q13[g]	Asthma[c]	United States	Xu et al, 2001[53]
16	16p12	Atopy[a]	U.S. Hutterites	Ober et al, 1998[62]
	16p12	Atopy and asthma[d]	China	Xu et al, 2001[56]
	16q24.1	Asthma[e]	Australia and United Kingdom	Daniels et al, 1996[50]
17	17p11.1-q11.2	Asthma	U.S. blacks	CSGA, 1997[52]
	17q12-21	Asthma[b]	France	Dizier et al, 2000[54]
	17q25	Atopic dermatitis	United Kingdom	Cookson et al, 2001[61]
	17q25	Eosinophils	Holland	Koppelman et al, 2002[55]
19	19q13	Asthma	U.S. Hutterites	Ober et al, 1998[58]
	19q13	Asthma[b]	France	Dizier et al, 2000[54]
	19q13	Asthma	Whites	CSGA, 1997[52]
	19q13.1	Atopy and asthma[d]	China	Xu et al, 2001[56]
20	20p12	Atopic dermatitis and asthma	United Kingdom	Cookson et al, 2001[61]
21	21q21	Asthma	U.S. Hutterites	Ober et al, 1998[58]
	21q21	Asthma	U.S. Hispanics	CSGA, 1997[52]
22	22q11.2	Atopy and asthma[d]	China	Xu et al, 2001[56]
	22q	Atopy	Holland	Koppelman et al, 2002[55]

[f]House dust mite–sensitive asthma.
[g]Significant only after conditioning for another locus (see Xu et al, 2001).[53]

ADAM33, a novel member of the ADAM family,[63] achieving significance of $P = 0.005$ to 0.05. Both in the combined populations and in the U.K. and U.S. samples analyzed separately, additional SNP typing strengthened the location of the signal to ADAM33, and this was further confirmed by both haplotype analysis (5 to 7 SNP combinations at $P = 0.000001$ to 0.005) and TDT testing (10 SNP combinations at $P < 0.005$).

ADAM33 is the most recently reported member of the ADAM gene family of zinc-dependent matrix metalloproteases.[64] ADAM genes have a complex organization that involves eight domains, with the first six encoding signal sequence and pro-, catalytic, disintegrin, cysteine-rich, and EGF domains,[65] which are anchored at the cell surface or Golgi apparatus by a transmembrane domain followed by a cytoplasmic domain with signaling-specific sequences. ADAM33 belongs to the ADAM 12, 15, 19, and 28 subfamily, all of which possess proteolytic activity.[65,66] ADAM33 is expressed in a number of lung cell types, including bronchial smooth muscle, myofibroblasts, and fibroblasts, but not in bronchial epithelial cells, T cells, or inflammatory leukocytes. The significance of ADAM33 for asthma is strengthened by the existence of a syntenic region on mouse chromosome 2 at 74 cM that has been linked to BHR[67] overlying an orthologue of ADAM33 that exhibits approximately 70% homology with its human counterpart.

Asthma is a chronic disorder in which T cell–mediated inflammation causes thickening of airway walls, smooth muscle contraction, and narrowing of the airways. Epithelial damage, smooth muscle hyperplasia, and increased matrix deposition are important characteristics of asthmatic airways that are thought to contribute to airway responsiveness.[68] This remodeling process has been linked to activation of the epithelial-mesenchymal trophic unit, leading to the proliferation of biosynthetically active fibroblasts, myofibroblasts, and smooth muscle, a feature of BHR.[69] A role for ADAM33 in airway remodeling and BHR is supported by its expression in human lung fibroblasts and bronchial smooth muscle. The pattern of expression of ADAM33 suggests that alterations in the activity or expression levels of ADAM33 may underlie abnormalities in airway function rather than the immunologic components of asthma. In addition, the known functions of ADAM family members in promoting myogenic fusion[70] and the release of proliferative growth factors[66] further support a role for ADAM33 in airway remodeling. The identification of ADAM33 as a susceptibility gene for asthma and BHR illustrates that the positional cloning approach for complex disease can be successful, leading to the identification of novel genes and pathways involved in disease pathogenesis.

Candidate Gene/Gene Region Studies

A large number of candidate regions have been studied for both linkage to and association with a range of atopy-related phenotypes. In addition, SNPs in the promoter and coding regions of a wide range of candidate genes have been examined. These genes have been chosen because of both their chromosomal location and their products' known function in allergic disease processes. There are now more than 200 studies that have examined polymorphism in more than 100 genes for association with asthma and allergy phenotypes. A more comprehensive summary of all studies of the genetic basis of allergy and asthma can be found on the Asthma Gene Database website (http://cooke.gsf.de/asthmagen/main.cfm).[71] When assessing the significance of association studies, it is important to consider several things. For example, was the size of the study adequately powered if negative results are reported? Were the cases and controls appropriately matched? Could population stratification account for the associations observed? In the definitions of the phenotypes, which phenotypes have been measured (and which have not)? How were they measured? Regarding correction for multiple testing, have the authors taken multiple testing into account when assessing the significance of association? Recent publications by Weiss,[72] Hall,[73] and Tabor et al[74] review these issues in depth. Many candidate gene regions and genes have been examined in detail since the first report of linkage between a chromosomal region and atopy in 1989 (chromosome 11q13[1]). To illustrate the difficulties in identification of causal SNPs underlying positive linkage of a candidate region, the example of the Th2 cytokine cluster on chromosome 5q31 is used later.

Chromosome 5q31-35

The first reported linkage of atopy with chromosome 5 was made by Marsh et al.[75] In this study of 11 large Amish pedigrees, selected on the basis of serum IgE antibodies to common allergens in at least one child, there was linkage between five markers located on chromosome 5q31 and total serum IgE, with the linkage being centered around the interleukin (IL)-4 locus. No linkage was seen between allergen-specific IgE and the same markers. There are a number of genes on chromosome 5q that may be important in the development or progression of inflammation associated with atopy and atopic disease, including the cytokines IL-3, IL-4, IL-5, IL-9, IL-12 (β-chain), IL-13, and granulocyte-macrophage colony-stimulating factor. Further evidence for the role of this Th2 cytokine cluster was provided by Meyers et al.[49] Using a similar phenotype, linkage was reported between several markers on 5q31-33 and total IgE in 92 Dutch families. Further segregation analysis of these families provided evidence for a second major locus regulating serum IgE levels[76] unlinked to that on 5q31-33. In addition, a positive linkage between several markers on 5q and BHR[77] was seen in this population, with the strongest linkage evidence for both phenotypes being centered around the β$_2$-adrenergic receptor.

Many other studies have also confirmed linkage between 5q markers and a wide variety of allergic phenotypes, including IgE in a random U.K. population,[78] atopy in Japanese families,[79] total serum IgE and allergen-specific IgE antibody levels but not BHR in Australian families,[80] and asthma in U.K. families.[81] Equally, many studies have reported negative linkage with this genetic region.[82-85]

In the genome-wide scans that have been undertaken, several have identified linkage between 5q13-33 and a number of phenotypes, including asthma,[52,53] asthma and BHR,[58] IgE,[86] and mite-sensitive atopic asthma.[57] Equally, several scans have provided no evidence of 5q31-33 being linked to allergic disease phenotypes.[50,59,87]

The inconsistency of the results of linkage studies on 5q13-33 may be attributable to differences in populations, such as ethnicity and ascertainment of the families studied, and/or to differences in the definition of phenotype. In addition, many of the published studies may have had insufficient power to detect genes of small effect. However, the linkage between 5q31 and atopy and asthma phenotypes is one of the most reproduced of all the linkages reported. Based on this evidence, studies have begun to identify polymorphisms in candidate genes at this locus and to examine possible associations of these polymorphisms with disease traits.

Interleukin-4

IL-4 plays an essential role in the IgE-mediated immune response; it induces IgE synthesis in B cells and differentiation to the Th2 phenotype in T cells. This makes the *IL4* gene itself, or factors that regulate its expression, a strong candidate gene for atopy and asthma. A polymorphism in the promoter of *IL4*, a C-to-T substitution at −589 bp from the open reading frame, in 20 asthmatic and 5 control families has been identified. This polymorphism has been shown to be associated with high serum IgE levels and to increase the transcriptional levels of the *IL4* gene in a chloramphenicol acetyltransferase assay.[88] However, the role of this polymorphism is still controversial. Two large populations, consisting of 230 nuclear families from Australia and 124 unrelated atopic asthmatic patients and 59 unrelated nonatopic, nonasthmatic control subjects from the United Kingdom, have been studied. Only a weak association of this polymorphism with IgE antibody specific to house dust mite and to wheeze was found in the first population, whereas no association with any measure of asthma or atopy was found in the U.K. population.[89] A study of two populations, one of families ascertained through an asthmatic child and one a randomly ascertained population as a control, found no significant difference in the prevalence of the polymorphism between the two groups. No difference was observed in total IgE or IgE antibody levels, whether the individual was homozygous for the C allele or heterozygous or homozygous for the T allele. However, using the TDT, a significant association between the T allele and asthma was found in the family sample.[90] Finally, a recent study has shown an association between C589T polymorphism and the severity of asthma measured by FEV$_1$.[91] The *IL4* C589T polymorphism has also been studied in patients with atopic dermatitis. The T allele has been found to be transmitted preferentially to the affected offspring, and the number of T allele homozygotes was significantly increased in the patients with atopic dermatitis compared with controls.[92]

Interleukin-13

The cytokine IL-13 is closely related to IL-4, which is also produced by Th2 cells. IL-13 along with IL-4 can switch B cells to produce IgE; however, unlike IL-4, IL-13 cannot induce Th2 cell differentiation. In adults, only 50% of asthma is associated with atopy, yet all forms of the disease are characterized by enhanced T cell secretion of Th2 cytokines in the airways. In addition, severe chronic asthma is characterized by the deposition of interstitial collagens in the lamina reticularis beneath the epithelial basement membrane associated with an increased number of myofibroblasts, epithelial damage, and increased mucus production and airway remodeling. Of importance in asthma, IL-4 and IL-13 are also key regulators of this response, with wide-ranging effects on epithelial cells, fibroblasts, and smooth muscle. Evidence suggesting a critical role for IL-13 in asthma comes from well-characterized experimental models of allergic asthma. Sensitization and subsequent challenge of mice with allergen result in airway hyperresponsiveness, an increase in specific IgE, mucus secretion, and airway eosinophilia. Daily administration of IL-13 to the airways of mice has been shown to induce airway hyperresponsiveness, increased total IgE, mucus secretion, goblet cell metaplasia, and airway eosinophilia.[93,94] Similarly, transgenic expression of IL-13 in the lungs of mice has been shown to cause similar phenotypes.[95]

IL-13, like IL-4, is encoded in the Th2 cytokine gene cluster on chromosome 5q31 (Figure 3-1). It is located within 12 kb of IL-4,[96] with which it shares 40% homology. A number of polymorphisms have now been identified in the *IL13* gene. Van der Pouw-Kraan et al[97] identified a single–base pair substitution in the promoter of IL-13 adjacent to a consensus nuclear factor of activated T cell binding sites. Using a sample of 101 asthmatics and 107 controls, they observed an increased frequency of homozygotes in the asthmatic group (13 of 107 vs. 2 of 107, $P = 0.002$, odds ratio = 8.3). Additional in vitro experiments demonstrated that the polymorphism was associated with reduced inhibition of IL-13 production by cyclosporin and increased binding of nuclear factor of activated T cells. In addition to promoter polymorphisms of IL-13, an amino acid polymorphism of IL-13 has been identified: R110Q.[98-100] Protein modeling suggests that this polymorphism may influence binding of IL-13 to its receptor. The

work of Graves et al[98] and, more recently, the publication of Liu et al[101] show strong associations between this IL-13 polymorphism and atopy in children. However, neither study examined associations with asthma. In contrast, the study of Heinzmann et al[99] shows that in adults, polymorphisms in IL-13 are associated with asthma and not with atopy. Howard et al[102] also recently showed that the −1112 C/T variant of IL-13 contributes significantly to BHR susceptibility ($P = 0.003$) but not to total serum IgE levels. Thus it is possible that polymorphisms in IL-13 may confer susceptibility to airway remodeling in persistent asthma, as well as to allergic inflammation in early life.

The conflicting reports of positive and negative associations between polymorphisms in the *IL4* and *IL13* genes highlight a number of issues that need to be addressed when interpreting the results of association studies. Polymorphisms that are physically close to one another in the genome are often in association with each other (linkage disequilibrium) and therefore are not inherited independently. Consequently, association seen between polymorphism A and a disease phenotype may not indicate that polymorphism A is affecting gene function but rather that it is merely in linkage disequilibrium with polymorphism B that is exerting an effect on gene function or expression. Given that both IL-13 and IL-4 are good functional candidates for atopy and asthma, polymorphism in either or both of them may be affecting disease

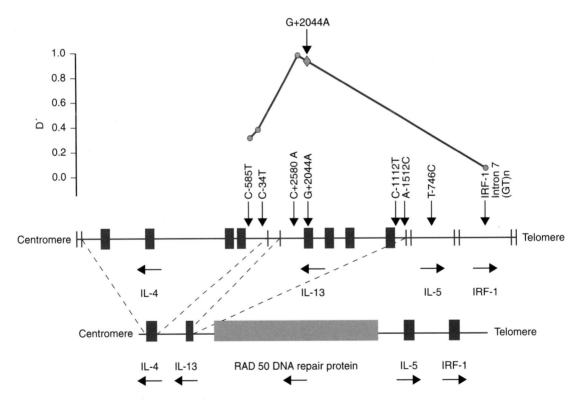

FIGURE 3-1 Diagram of the *IL4/IL13* gene region on chromosome 5q31 showing the location of a number of polymorphisms that have been associated with atopy and asthma phenotypes. The physical proximity of the candidate genes means that a positive association observed between a single polymorphism and a phenotype may result from linkage disequilibrium between that polymorphism and another nearby causal polymorphism. The graph shows the degree of linkage disequilibrium (measured as D′, relative to the G2044A arginine-to-glutamine polymorphism of IL-13) between candidate polymorphisms in a white U.K. cohort. The lack of linkage disequilibrium between the *IL4* and *IL13* polymorphisms and between the *IRF1* and *IL13* polymorphisms suggests that the previously observed association of each of these genes may reflect independent causal single-nucleotide polymorphisms, each affecting the disease.

susceptibility. Therefore to gain a true understanding of the roles of individual polymorphisms, it will be necessary to type polymorphism across the two genes in a single population and to assess the significance of association for the different haplotypes (combinations of polymorphisms).

Furthermore, Noguchi et al[103] demonstrated in a Japanese population that haplotypes consisting of IL-4 promoter polymorphisms and polymorphism lying in the intergenic region between the *IL4* and *IL13* genes show significant association with asthma.

β_2-Adrenergic Receptor

The β_2-adrenergic receptor is a transmembrane protein that, after agonist binding, activates G protein−mediated signal transduction, leading to airway smooth muscle relaxation and protection of the airways from bronchoconstriction. It has long been hypothesized that a defective β_2-adrenergic receptor may be a pathogenic factor in asthma, and a linkage between IgE and BHR and markers on chromosome 5q around the β_2-adrenergic receptor has been shown.[77] The two most common polymorphisms[104] are at amino acid 16 (R16G) and at amino acid 27 (Q27E). Studies in vitro have shown that the Gly16 increases down-regulation of the β_2-adrenergic receptor after exposure to a β_2-agonist. In contrast, the Glu27 polymorphism appears to protect against agonist-induced down-regulation and desensitization of the β_2-adrenergic receptor.[105,106] Although a number of studies have indicated that β_2-adrenergic receptor polymorphism may have disease-modifying effects in asthmatic patients, the contribution to the heritable component of atopy or asthma susceptibility is still not clear. The Glu27 polymorphism has been associated with elevated IgE levels in asthmatic families,[107] and the haplotype Gly16-Gln27 has been associated with BHR.[108] However, an association between either the Gly16 or Glu27 β_2-adrenergic receptor polymorphism and an increased risk of asthma or atopy per se is not clear.[109-112] A recent study by Wang et al[113] suggests, however, that there is a gene environment interaction between cigarette smoking and β_2-adrenergic receptor genotype in determining susceptibility to asthma.

CD14

Atopy is the result of interaction between genetic and environmental factors. Recent studies have suggested that bacterial infections in infancy may protect against the development of allergy, possibly by promoting Th1 immune responses and thereby suppressing the Th2 responses, which regulate IgE production. CD14 is a multifunctional receptor with specificity for lipopolysaccharides and other bacterial wall−derived components, and its engagement is associated with an increased production of IL-12 and thus a Th1 differentiation of T cells. Recently, Jones, et al[114] showed that reduced soluble CD14 levels in amniotic fluid and breast milk are associated with the subsequent development of atopy, eczema, or both.

The *CD14* gene is located on chromosome 5q31.1. A C-to-T substitution in the promoter region at position −159 from the transcription has been identified and associated with a higher level of soluble CD14 and a lower level of IgE but not atopy per se in school-aged children from the United States.[115] Subsequent studies in an adult Dutch population have shown that although sCD14 C-149T is not associated with allergy per se, it is associated with the number of positive skin tests and total serum IgE levels in skin test−positive individuals.[116] This suggests that sCD14 is not a susceptibility gene for atopy but may predispose to a more severe atopic phenotype. Equally, polymorphisms of other genes whose products play an important role in neonatal immune responses to bacteria may also play a role in determining atopy severity and susceptibility.

The 5q13-33 region provides an excellent example of the difficulties of the candidate gene−gene region approach to identify the causal polymorphism(s) underlying a region of linkage. With several good functional candidates and many reports of association of SNPs in these candidates with disease phenotypes, it is unclear to what extent each of the different genes contributes to the genetic susceptibility to allergy and asthma. It will be necessary for more comprehensive studies of this region to untangle the respective contributions of each gene. These studies have begun to be undertaken by several investigators[59,117]; recently one of these studies of linkage and association with multiple makers concluded that there may be as many as three asthma/"atopy" loci in the 5q13-33 region, each with a relatively small effect.[117]

Analysis of Clinically Defined Subgroups

One approach to genetic analysis of complex disease that has proved successful in other complex genetic disorders such as type 2 diabetes is to identify genes in rare, severely affected subgroups of patients in whom disease appears to follow a pattern of inheritance that indicates the effect of a single major gene. The assumption is that mutations (polymorphisms) of milder functional effect in the same gene in the general population may play a role in susceptibility to the complex genetic disorder. For example, researchers investigating the genetic basis of NIDDM have used families with maturity-onset diabetes of the young (MODY) to identify genes that may play a role in NIDDM.

Although it appears that most of the genes involved in MODY play a very limited role in "normal" type 2 diabetes with the exception of the gene encoding the transcription factor PDX1, they have been shown to result in MODY when there is a single copy of a severe mutation with other mutations in the *PDX1* gene with milder effects on gene function predisposing to type 2 diabetes.[118,119] Nonetheless, genetic analysis of MODY has provided a number of insights into the molecular mechanisms underlying glucose regulation and as such has helped in understanding the pathogenesis of diabetes.

SPINK5/LEKTI

The only example of this approach in studies of atopic disease has been the identification of the gene *SPINK5* encoding the serine proteinase inhibitor LEKT1 on chromosome 5q32 as the cause of Netherton's syndrome. Netherton's syndrome is a severe autosomal recessive disorder characterized by congenital ichthyosis with defective cornification, a specific hair shaft defect, and severe atopic manifestations including atopic dermatitis, hay fever, high total serum IgE, and hypereosinophilia. The Netherton gene was localized to 5q32 through a combination of linkage analysis and homozygosity mapping,[120] in a region where the serine protease inhibitor LEKT1 had previously been mapped. *LEKT1* was considered a good candidate gene for Netherton syndrome as a result of its proteolytic activity because proteolysis has been shown to be important in cell activation and communication and serine protease inhibitors have previously been shown to down-regulate the proinflammatory nuclear factor kappa (NF-κB) pathway. In addition, steady state mRNA levels encoding *LEKT1* were shown to be lower in cultured keratinocytes from patients,[121] suggesting nonsense-mediated decay of mutated transcripts, as is often seen in recessive diseases.[122]

The previously observed linkage of atopy to 5q31-33 (see section on "Chromosome 5q31-35") and severe atopic manifestations, including atopic dermatitis being a component of the Netherton phenotype, led Walley et al[123] to screen the *SPINK5* gene for common polymorphism and to test association of identified polymorphism with atopic dermatitis. Six coding polymorphisms were identified in *SPINK5*, and one, E420K, was shown to be significantly associated with atopy and atopic dermatitis in two independent family cohorts.

The role of *SPINK5* in rare and common skin disease demonstrates the value of studying rare but less genetically complex diseases to gain insight into the mechanisms underlying the more common complex traits. From the identification of the genes involved in monogenic disorders and the cellular pathways involved in their clinical manifestation, parallels can be drawn to similar but more prevalent complex genetic diseases.

MOLECULAR REGULATION OF ATOPY AND ATOPIC DISEASE, II: DISEASE-MODIFYING GENES

The concept of genes interacting to alter the effects of mutations in susceptibility genes is not unknown. A number of genetic disorders caused by mutations in single genes are known to exhibit interfamilial and intrafamilial variability.[124] A proportion of interfamilial variability can be explained by differences in environmental factors and differences in the effect of different mutations in the same gene. Intrafamilial variability, especially in siblings, cannot be so readily accredited to these types of mechanisms. There is increasing evidence that many genetic disorders are influenced by "modifier" genes that are distinct from the disease susceptibility locus. For example, not all individuals with IDDM develop diabetic nephropathy, but the relative risk of this complication is increased twofold in relatives of IDDM patients with nephropathy.[125]

Genetic Influences on Disease Severity

Very few studies of the heritability of IgE-mediated disease have examined phenotypes relating to severity. Sarafino and Goldfedder[126] studied 39 monozygotic twin pairs and 55 same-sex dizygotic twin pairs for the heritability of asthma and asthma severity. Asthma severity (as measured by frequency and intensity of asthmatic episodes) was examined in twin pairs concordant for asthma. Severity was significantly correlated for monozygotic pairs but not for dizygotic pairs. In contrast, a more recent study[127] examined the family prevalence of "atopy" and IgE-mediated diseases, including asthma. Although the prevalence of asthma in children of parents with asthma was significantly increased compared with children whose parents did not have asthma (55% vs. 29% for the eldest child), when the severity of a child's asthma was compared with that of the parents, there was no correlation between the severity of the child's asthma and either the severity of the parents' asthma or the number of parents with asthma.

A number of studies have examined associations between asthma severity and polymorphisms in candidate genes; these have included the genes encoding tumor necrosis factor α,[128] IL-4,[91,129] and IL-4Rα,[129] but the conclusive identification of genetic factors contributing to asthma severity has been hampered by the lack of clear, easily applied, accurate phenotype definitions for asthma severity that distinguish between underlying severity and level of therapeutic control. For example, it has been shown that β₂-adrenergic receptor polymorphisms could influence asthma severity, because Gly16 polymorphism is overexpressed in patients with nocturnal asthma[130] and in steroid-dependent asthmatics.[104] It is not clear whether this reflects β₂-adrenergic receptor polymorphism affecting patients' responses to β₂-agonists and hence leading to poor therapeutic control or whether, regardless of their effects on treatment, polymorphism of the β₂-adrenergic receptor leads to more severe chronic asthma. The development of such phenotypes in conjunction with more extensive studies of the genetics of asthma severity may allow identification of at-risk individuals and targeting of prophylactic therapy.

Genetic Regulation of Response to Therapy: Pharmacogenomics

Genetic variability may not only play a role in influencing susceptibility to atopy but may also modify its severity or influence the effectiveness of therapy.[131] Clinical studies have shown that β₂-adrenergic receptor polymorphisms influence the response to bronchodilator treatment. Asthmatic patients carrying Gly16 have been shown to be more prone to develop a bronchodilator desensitization,[132] whereas children who are homozygous or heterozygous for Arg16 are more likely to show positive responses to bronchodilators.[133] However, some studies have shown that response to bronchodilator treatment is genotype independent.[134,135]

A study of 190 asthmatics examined whether β₂-adrenergic receptor genotype affects the response to regular versus as-needed albuterol use.[136] During a 16-week treatment period, there was a small but significant decline in morning peak flow in patients homozygous for the Arg16 polymorphism who used albuterol regularly. The effect was magnified during the 4-week run-out period when all patients returned to albuterol as needed, with Arg16 homozygotes on regular albuterol having a morning peak flow 30.5 ± 12.1 L/min lower than that of the Arg16 homozygotes, who took albuterol only as needed ($P = 0.012$). These findings are difficult to explain in the light of the studies discussed linking the Gly16 allele with BHR, β₂-agonist effectiveness, and asthma severity.

Genetic polymorphism may also play a role in regulating responses to the class of antiasthma drug known as the antileukotrienes. A repeat length polymorphism in the promoter of the 5-lipoxygenase (*ALOX5*) gene has been reported to modify transcription factor binding and reporter gene expression.[137] This polymorphism also seems to be associated with a reduced response to 5-LO inhibitor therapy.[138]

CONCLUSIONS

The varying and sometimes conflicting results of studies to identify allergic disease susceptibility genes reflect the genetic and environmental heterogeneity seen in allergic disorders and illustrate the difficulty of identifying susceptibility genes for complex genetic diseases. This is the result of a number of factors, including difficulties in defining phenotypes and population heterogeneity with different genetic loci showing linkage in populations of differing ethnicity and differing environmental exposure. Identifying the gene or genes underlying the linkage observed is therefore a major challenge.

It is clear from genetic studies that the propensity to develop atopy is influenced by factors different than those that influence disease. However, these disease factors require interaction with atopy (or something else) to trigger disease. For example, in asthma, bronchoconstriction is triggered mostly by an allergic response to inhaled allergen accompanied by an eosinophilic inflammation in the lungs, but in some people who may have "asthma susceptibility genes" but not the atopy, asthma is triggered by other factors, such as toluene diisocyanate, for example (Box 3-1).

In the past 10 years, there have been many linkage and association studies examining genetic susceptibility to atopy and allergic disease. Further research is needed to confirm previous studies. Larger family-based cohorts and the pooling of data across studies, as well as more specific markers for IgE-mediated allergy, should help in the enormous task of identifying the gene or genes that underlie regions of linkage. Large population samples including longitudinal cohorts will prove essential in determining not only the contribution of identified polymorphisms to susceptibility but also how these polymorphisms interact with the environment to initiate allergic disease.

In reality we know little more in genetic terms that we did in 1916—namely, that atopy and atopic disease are heritable disorders, that there are separate genetic influences determining susceptibility to atopy and development of specific atopic disease, and that interaction with environmental exposures is important. Despite intensive effort and the advances of molecular biology over recent years, few genes involved in the pathogenesis of atopy and asthma have been clearly identified with any certainty. The major difficulties in genetic studies of atopy and other IgE-mediated disorders have included phenotype definition and sample ascertainment. Examples such as the association studies of the IL-13 R110Q polymorphism also illustrate that the same polymorphisms may be associated with different phenotypes at different stages of life (atopy in childhood and asthma in adulthood). Thus studies of the same polymorphism or genetic region that use different methods of subject ascertainment (atopy vs. asthma or atopic dermatitis, adult vs. child probands, atopy defined as high total IgE or based only on case history, etc.) and different measures of the same phenotype are unlikely to replicate one another.

These issues are now being addressed seriously, and much effort is being directed at consensus between groups and cooperation in research efforts. An attempt to address some of these issues has been undertaken in the form of COAG.[139] Another such project can be found in the asthma gene database[71] (http://cooke.gsf.de/), which is a database of studies (both published and unpublished) relating to asthma genetics.

Despite all of these difficulties and complexities in identification of genes, the prospects for the future are bright. The discovery of genes such as *ADAM33* and *SPINK5* that appear to be involved in the pathogenesis of BHR and atopic dermatitis, respectively, show that genetic approaches can lead to identification of new biologic pathways involved in the pathogenesis of allergic disease, the development of new therapeutic approaches, and the identification of at-risk individuals (Box 3-2).

BOX 3-2   KEY CONCEPTS

Genetic Effects on Allergy and Allergic Disease

Determine Susceptibility Atopy
- "Th2" or "IgE switch" genes
  Determine specific target-organ disease in atopic individuals
- Asthma susceptibility genes
  "Lung-specific factors" that regulate susceptibility of lung epithelium/fibroblasts to remodeling in response to allergic inflammation, such as *ADAM33*
- Atopic dermatitis susceptibility genes
  Genes that regulate dermal inflammation and immunity, such as *SPINK5*

Influence the Interaction of Environmental Factors with Atopy and Allergic Disease
- Regulation of specific IgE responses (which allergen will you respond to?), such as MHC class II alleles, TCR V gene use
- Determining immune responses to factors that drive Th1/Th2 skewing of the immune response, such as CD14 polymorphism and early childhood infection
- Altering interaction between environmental factors and established disease, such as genetic polymorphism regulating responses to respiratory syncytial virus infection and asthma symptoms

Modify Severity of Disease
Examples are tumor necrosis factor α polymorphisms and asthma severity

Regulate Response to Therapy
- Pharmacogenetics
- Examples are β_2-adrenergic receptor polymorphism and response to β_2-agonists

---

BOX 3-1   KEY CONCEPTS

What Can Genetics Studies of Allergic Disease Tell Us?

Greater Understanding of Disease Pathogenesis
- Identification of novel genes and pathways leading to new pharmacologic targets for developing therapeutics

Identification of Environmental Factors that Interact with an Individual's Genetic Make-up to Initiate Disease
- Prevention of disease by environmental modification

Identification of Susceptible Individuals
- Early-in-life screening and targeting of preventative therapies to at-risk individuals to prevent disease

Targeting of Therapies
- Subclassification of disease on the basis of genetics and targeting of specific therapies based on this classification
- Determination of the likelihood of an individual responding to a particular therapy (pharmacogenetics) and individualized treatment plans

REFERENCES

1. Cookson WO, Sharp PA, Faux JA, et al: Linkage between immunoglobulin E responses underlying asthma and rhinitis and chromosome 11q, *Lancet* 1:1292, 1989.
2. Kerem B, Rommens JM, Buchanan JA, et al: Identification of the cystic fibrosis gene: genetic analysis, *Science* 245:1073, 1989.
3. The Huntington's Disease Collaborative Research Group. A novel gene containing a trinucleotide repeat that is expanded and unstable on Huntington's disease chromosomes. The Huntington's Disease Collaborative Research Group, *Cell* 72:971, 1993.
4. Botstein D, White RL, Skolnick M, et al: Construction of a genetic linkage map in man using restriction fragment length polymorphisms, *Am J Hum Genet* 32:314, 1980.
5. Pearce N, Weiland S, Keil U, et al: Self-reported prevalence of asthma symptoms in children in Australia, England, Germany and New Zealand: an international comparison using the ISAAC protocol, *Eur Respir J* 6:1455, 1993.
6. King MC, Lee GM, Spinner NB, et al: Genetic epidemiology, *Annu Rev Public Health* 5:1, 1984.
7. Farrer LA, Cupples LA: Determining the genetic component of a disease. In Haines JL, Pericak-Vance MA, editors: *Approaches to gene mapping in complex human diseases*, New York, 1998, Wiley-Liss.
8. Dib C, Faure S, Fizames C, et al: A comprehensive genetic map of the human genome based on 5,264 microsatellites, *Nature* 380:152, 1996.
9. Palmer LJ, Cookson WO: Using single nucleotide polymorphisms as a means to understanding the pathophysiology of asthma, *Respir Res* 2:102, 2001.
10. Morton N: Major loci for atopy? *Clin Exp Allergy* 22:1041, 1992.
11. Lander E, Kruglyak L: Genetic dissection of complex traits: guidelines for interpreting and reporting linkage results, *Nat Genet* 11:241, 1995.
12. Risch N: Genetic linkage: interpreting lod scores, *Science* 255:803, 1992.
13. Risch N, Merikangas K: The future of genetic studies of complex human diseases, *Science* 273:1516, 1996.
14. Schork NJ, Boehnke M, Terwilliger JD, et al: Two-trait-locus linkage analysis: a powerful strategy for mapping complex genetic traits, *Am J Hum Genet* 53:1127, 1993.
15. Lander ES, Schork NJ: Genetic dissection of complex traits [published erratum appears in *Science* 266:353, 1994], *Science* 265:2037, 1994.
16. Haseman JK, Elston RC: The investigation of linkage between a quantitative trait and a marker locus, *Behav Genet* 2:3, 1972.
17. Spielman RS, McGinnis RE, Ewens WJ: Transmission test for linkage disequilibrium: the insulin gene region and insulin-dependent diabetes mellitus (IDDM), *Am J Hum Genet* 52:506, 1993.
18. Spielman RS, Ewens WJ: The TDT and other family-based tests for linkage disequilibrium and association, *Am J Hum Genet* 59:983, 1996.
19. Hugot JP, Chamaillard M, Zouali H, et al: Association of NOD2 leucine-rich repeat variants with susceptibility to Crohn's disease, *Nature* 411:599, 2001.
20. Horikawa Y, Oda N, Cox NJ, et al: Genetic variation in the gene encoding calpain-10 is associated with type 2 diabetes mellitus, *Nat Genet* 26:163, 2000.
21. Coca A, Cooke R: On the classification of the phenomena of hypersensitiveness, *J Immunol* 8:163, 1923.
22. Lawrence S, Beasley R, Doull I, et al: Genetic analysis of atopy and asthma as quantitative traits and ordered polychotomies, *Ann Hum Genet* 58:359, 1994.
23. Wilkinson J, Grimley S, Collins A, et al: Linkage of asthma to markers on chromosome 12 in a sample of 240 families using quantitative phenotype scores, *Genomics* 53:251, 1998.
24. Cooke RA, Vander Veer A: Human sensitisation, *J Immunol* 16:201, 1916.
25. Hayashi T, Kawakami N, Kondo N, et al: Prevalence of and risk factors for allergic diseases: comparison of two cities in Japan, *Ann Allergy Asthma Immunol* 75:525-529, 1995.
26. Jenkins MA, Hopper JL, Giles GG: Regressive logistic modeling of familial aggregation for asthma in 7,394 population-based nuclear families, *Genet Epidemiol* 14:317, 1997.
27. Bazaral M, Orgel HA, Hamburger RN: IgE levels in normal infants and mothers and an inheritance hypothesis, *J Immunol* 107:794, 1971.
28. Gerrard JW, Vickers P, Gerrard CD: The familial incidence of allergic disease, *Ann Allergy* 36:10, 1976.
29. Dold S, Wjst M, von Mutius E, et al: Genetic risk for asthma, allergic rhinitis, and atopic dermatitis, *Arch Dis Child* 67:1018, 1992.
30. von Mutius E, Nicolai T: Familial aggregation of asthma in a South Bavarian population, *Am J Respir Crit Care Med* 153:1266, 1996.
31. Duffy DL, Martin NG, Battistutta D, et al: Genetics of asthma and hay fever in Australian twins, *Am Rev Respir Dis* 142:1351, 1990.
32. Wuthrich B, Baumann E, Fries RA, et al: Total and specific IgE (RAST) in atopic twins, *Clin Allergy* 11:147, 1981.
33. Sarafino EP, Goldfedder J: Genetic factors in the presence, severity, and triggers of asthma, *Arch Dis Child* 73:112, 1995.
34. Husby S, Holm NV, Christensen K, et al: Cord blood immunoglobulin E in like-sexed monozygotic and dizygotic twins, *Clin Genet* 50:332, 1996.
35. Hopp RJ, Bewtra AK, Watt GD, et al: Genetic analysis of allergic disease in twins, *J Allergy Clin Immunol* 73:265, 1984.
36. Harris JR, Magnus P, Samuelsen SO, et al: No evidence for effects of family environment on asthma: a retrospective study of Norwegian twins, *Am J Respir Crit Care Med* 156:43, 1997.
37. Hanson B, McGue M, Roitman-Johnson B, et al: Atopic disease and immunoglobulin E in twins reared apart and together, *Am J Hum Genet* 48:873, 1991.
38. Sibbald B, Horn ME, Gregg I: A family study of the genetic basis of asthma and wheezy bronchitis, *Arch Dis Child* 55:354, 1980.
39. Sibbald B, Turner-Warwick M: Factors influencing the prevalence of asthma among first degree relatives of extrinsic and intrinsic asthmatics, *Thorax* 34:332, 1979.
40. Longo G, Strinati R, Poli F, et al: Genetic factors in nonspecific bronchial hyperreactivity: an epidemiologic study, *Am J Dis Child* 141:331, 1987.
41. Laitinen T, Rasanen M, Kaprio J, et al: Importance of genetic factors in adolescent asthma: a population-based twin-family study, *Am J Respir Crit Care Med* 157:1073, 1998.
42. Skadhauge LR, Christensen K, Kyvik KO, et al: Genetic and environmental influence on asthma: a population-based study of 11,688 Danish twin pairs, *Eur Respir J* 13:8, 1999.
43. Blumenthal MN, Namboodiri K, Mendell N, et al: Genetic transmission of serum IgE levels, *Am J Med Genet* 10:219, 1981.
44. Dizier MH, Hill M, James A, et al: Detection of a recessive major gene for high IgE levels acting independently of specific response to allergens, *Genet Epidemiol* 12:93, 1995.
45. Gerrard JW, Rao DC, Morton NE: A genetic study of immunoglobulin E, *Am J Hum Genet* 30:46, 1978.
46. Hasstedt SJ, Meyers DA, Marsh DG: Inheritance of immunoglobulin E: genetic model fitting, *Am J Med Genet* 14:61, 1983.
47. Meyers DA, Beaty TH, Freidhoff LR, et al: Inheritance of total serum IgE (basal levels) in man, *Am J Hum Genet* 41:51, 1987.
48. Meyers DA, Beaty TH, Colyer CR, et al: Genetics of total serum IgE levels: a regressive model approach to segregation analysis, *Genet Epidemiol* 8:351, 1991.
49. Meyers DA, Postma DS, Panhuysen C, et al: Evidence for a locus regulating total serum IgE levels mapping to chromosome 5, *Genomics* 23:464, 1994.
50. Daniels SE, Bhattacharyya S, James A, et al: A genome-wide search for quantitative trait loci underlying asthma, *Nature* 383:247, 1996.
51. Wiltshire S, Bhattacharyya S, Faux JA, et al: A genome scan for loci influencing total serum immunoglobulin levels: possible linkage of IgA to the chromosome 13 atopy locus, *Hum Mol Genet* 7:27, 1998.
52. Collaborative Study on the Genetics of Asthma: A genome-wide search for asthma susceptibility loci in ethnically diverse populations, *Nat Genet* 15:389, 1997.
53. Xu J, Meyers DA, Ober C, et al: Genomewide screen and identification of gene-gene interactions for asthma-susceptibility loci in three U.S. populations: collaborative study on the genetics of asthma, *Am J Hum Genet* 68:1437, 2001.
54. Dizier MH, Besse-Schmittler C, Guilloud-Bataille M, et al: Genome screen for asthma and related phenotypes in the French EGEA study, *Am J Respir Crit Care Med* 162:1812, 2000.
55. Koppelman GH, Stine OC, Xu J, et al: Genome-wide search for atopy susceptibility genes in Dutch families with asthma, *J Allergy Clin Immunol* 109:498, 2002.
56. Xu X, Fang Z, Wang B, et al: A genomewide search for quantitative-trait loci underlying asthma, *Am J Hum Genet* 69:1271, 2001.
57. Yokouchi Y, Nukaga Y, Shibasaki M, et al: Significant evidence for linkage of mite-sensitive childhood asthma to chromosome 5q31-q33 near the interleukin 12 B locus by a genome-wide search in Japanese families, *Genomics* 66:152, 2000.
58. Ober C, Cox NJ, Abney M, et al: Genome-wide search for asthma susceptibility loci in a founder population, *Hum Mol Genet* 7:1393, 1998.
59. Laitinen T, Daly MJ, Rioux JD, et al: A susceptibility locus for asthma-related traits on chromosome 7 revealed by genome-wide scan in a founder population, *Nat Genet* 28:87, 2001.

60. Lee YA, Wahn U, Kehrt R, et al: A major susceptibility locus for atopic dermatitis maps to chromosome 3q21, *Nat Genet* 26:470, 2000.

61. Cookson WOCM, Ubhi B, Lawrence R, et al: Genetic linkage of childhood atopic dermatitis to psoriasis susceptibility loci, *Nat Genet* 27:372, 2001.

62. Haagerup A, Bjerke T, Schoitz PO, et al: Allergic rhinitis: a total genome-scan for susceptibility genes suggests a locus on chromosome 4q24-q27, *Eur J Hum Genet* 9:945, 2001.

63. Van Eerdewegh P, Little RD, Dupuis J, et al: Association of the ADAM33 gene with asthma and bronchial hyperresponsiveness, *Nature* 418: 426-430, 2002; DOI:10.1038/NATURE 00878, Nature AOP, published online July 10, 2002.

64. Yoshinaka T, Nishii K, Yamada K, et al: Identification and characterization of novel mouse and human ADAM33s with potential metalloprotease activity, *Gene* 282:227, 2002.

65. Primakoff P, Myles DG: The ADAM gene family: surface proteins with adhesion and protease activity, *Trends Genet* 16:83, 2000.

66. Black RA, White JM: ADAMs: focus on the protease domain, *Curr Opin Cell Biol* 10:654, 1998.

67. De Sanctis GT, Merchant M, Beier DR, et al: Quantitative locus analysis of airway hyperresponsiveness in A/J and C57BL/6J mice, *Nat Genet* 11:150, 1995.

68. Holgate ST, Lackie PM, Howarth PH, et al: Activation of the epithelial mesenchymal trophic unit in the pathogenesis of asthma, *Int Arch Allergy Immunol* 124:253, 2001.

69. Richter A, Puddicombe SM, Lordan JL, et al: The contribution of interleukin (IL)-4 and IL-13 to the epithelial-mesenchymal trophic unit in asthma, *Am J Respir Cell Mol Biol* 25:385, 2001.

70. Yagami-Hiromasa T, Sato T, Kurisaki T, et al: A metalloprotease-disintegrin participating in myoblast fusion, *Nature* 377:652, 1995.

71. Wjst M, Immervoll T: An Internet linkage and mutation database for the complex phenotype asthma, *Bioinformatics* 14:827, 1998.

72. Weiss ST: Association studies in asthma genetics, *Am J Respir Crit Care Med* 164:2014, 2001.

73. Hall I: Candidate gene studies in respiratory disease: avoiding the pitfalls, *Thorax* 57:377, 2002.

74. Tabor HK, Risch NJ, Myers RM: Candidate gene approaches for studying complex genetic traits: practical considerations, *Nat Rev Genet* 3:391, 2002.

75. Marsh DG, Neely JD, Breazeale DR, et al: Linkage analysis of IL-4 and other chromosome 5q31.1 total serum immunoglobulin E concentrations, *Science* 264:1152, 1994.

76. Xu J, Levitt RC, Panhuysen C, et al: Evidence for two unlinked loci regulating total serum IgE levels, *Am J Hum Genet* 57:425, 1995.

77. Postma DS, Bleecker ER, Amelung PJ, et al: Genetic susceptibility to asthma: bronchial hyperresponsiveness coinherited with a major gene for atopy, *N Engl J Med* 333:894, 1995.

78. Doull IJM, Lawrence S, Watson M, et al: Allelic association of gene markers on chromosomes 5q and 11q with atopy and bronchial hyperresponsiveness, *Am J Respir Crit Care Med* 153:1280, 1996.

79. Noguchi E, Shibasaki M, Arinami T, et al: Evidence for linkage between asthma/atopy in childhood and chromosome 5q31-q33 in a Japanese population, *Am J Respir Crit Care Med* 156:1390, 1997.

80. Palmer LJ, Daniels SE, Rye PJ, et al: Linkage of chromosome 5q and 11q gene markers to asthma-associated quantitative traits in Australian children, *Am J Respir Crit Care Med* 158:1825, 1998.

81. Holloway J, Lonjou C, Beghé B, et al: Suggestion for linkage between markers on chromosome 5q31-33 and asthma in 240 UK families, *Genes Immun* 2:20-24, 2001.

82. Blumenthal MN, Wang Z, Weber JL, et al: Absence of linkage between 5q markers and serum IgE levels in four large atopic families, *Clin Exp Allergy* 26:892, 1996.

83. Kamitani A, Wong ZYH, Dickson P, et al: Absence of genetic linkage of chromosome 5q31 with asthma and atopy in the general population, *Thorax* 52:816, 1997.

84. Laitinen T, Kauppi P, Ignatius J, et al: Genetic control of serum IgE levels and asthma: linkage and linkage disequilibrium studies in an isolated population, *Hum Mol Genet* 6:2069, 1997.

85. Mansur AH, Bishop DT, Markham AF, et al: Association study of asthma and atopy traits and chromosome 5q cytokine cluster markers, *Clin Exp Allergy* 28:141, 1998.

86. Xu J, Postma DS, Howard TD, et al: Major genes regulating total serum immunoglobulin E levels in families with asthma, *Am J Hum Genet* 67:1163, 2000.

87. Wjst M, Fischer G, Immervoll T, et al: A genome-wide search for linkage to asthma. German Asthma Genetics Group, *Genomics* 58:1, 1999.

88. Rosenwasser LJ, Klemm DJ, Dresback JK, et al: Promoter polymorphisms in the chromosome 5 gene cluster in asthma and atopy, *Clin Exp Allergy* 25:74, 1995.

89. Walley AJ, Cookson WOCM: Investigation of an interleukin-4 promoter polymorphism for associations with asthma and atopy, *J Med Genet* 33:689, 1996.

90. Noguchi E, Shibasaki M, Arinami T, et al: Association of asthma and the interleukin-4 promoter gene in Japanese, *Clin Exp Allergy* 28:449, 1998.

91. Burchard EG, Silverman EK, Rosenwasser LJ, et al: Association between a sequence variant in the IL-4 gene promoter and FEV in asthma, *Am J Respir Crit Care Med* 160:919, 1999.

92. Kawashima T, Noguchi E, Arinami T, et al: Linkage and association of an interleukin 4 gene polymorphism with atopic dermatitis in Japanese families, *J Med Genet* 35:502, 1998.

93. Grunig G, Warnock M, Wakil AE, et al: Requirement for IL-13 independently of IL-4 in experimental asthma, *Science* 282:2261, 1998.

94. Wills-Karp M, Luyimbazi J, Xu X, et al: Interleukin-13: central mediator of allergic asthma, *Science* 282:2258, 1998.

95. Zhu C, Homer RJ, Wang Z, et al: Pulmonary expression of interleukin-13 causes inflammation, mucus hypersecretion, subepithelial fibrosis, physiologic abnormalities, and eotaxin production, *J Clin Invest* 103:779, 1999.

96. Frazer KA, Ueda Y, Zhu Y, et al: Computational and biological analysis of 680 kb of DNA sequence from the human 5q31 cytokine gene cluster region, *Genome Res* 7:495, 1997.

97. van der Pouw Kraan T, van Veen A, Boeije L, et al: An IL-13 promoter polymorphism associated with increased risk of allergic asthma, *Genes Immun* 1:61, 1999.

98. Graves PE, Kabesch M, Halonen M, et al: A cluster of seven tightly linked polymorphisms in the IL-13 gene is associated with total serum IgE levels in three populations of white children, *J Allergy Clin Immunol* 105:506, 2000.

99. Heinzmann A, Mao XQ, Akaiwa M, et al: Genetic variants of IL-13 signalling and human asthma and atopy, *Hum Mol Genet* 9:549, 2000.

100. Pantelidis P, Jones MG, Welsh KI, et al: Identification of four novel interleukin-13 gene polymorphisms, *Genes Immun* 1:341, 2000.

101. Liu X, Nickel R, Beyer K, et al: An IL-13 coding region variant is associated with a high total serum IgE level and atopic dermatitis in the German Multicenter Atopy Study (MAS-90), *J Allergy Clin Immunol* 106:167, 2000.

102. Howard TD, Whittaker PA, Zaiman AL, et al: Identification and association of polymorphisms in the interleukin-13 gene with asthma and atopy in a Dutch population, *Am J Respir Cell Mol Biol* 25:377, 2001.

103. Noguchi E, Nukaga-Nishio Y, Jian Z, et al: Haplotypes of the 5' region of the IL-4 gene and SNPs in the intergene sequence between the IL-4 and IL-13 genes are associated with atopic asthma, *Hum Immunol* 62:1251, 2001.

104. Reihsaus E, Innis M, MacIntyre N, et al: Mutations in the gene encoding for the β₂-adrenergic receptor in normal and asthmatic subjects, *Am J Respir Cell Mol Biol* 8:334, 1993.

105. Green SA, Turki J, Innis M, et al: Amino-terminal polymorphisms of the human β₂-adrenergic receptor impart distinct agonist-promoted regulatory properties, *Biochemistry* 33:9414, 1994.

106. Green SA, Turki J, Bejarano P, et al: Influence of β₂-adrenergic receptor genotypes on signal transduction in human airway smooth muscle cells, *Am J Respir Cell Mol Biol* 13:25, 1995.

107. Dewar JC, Wilkinson J, Wheatley A, et al: The glutamine 27 β₂-adrenoceptor polymorphism is associated with elevated IgE levels in asthmatic families, *J Allergy Clin Immunol* 100:261, 1997.

108. D'Amato M, Vitiani LR, Petrelli G, et al: Association of persistent bronchial hyperresponsiveness with beta2-adrenoceptor (ADRB2) haplotypes: a population study, *Am J Respir Crit Care Med* 158:1968, 1998.

109. Dewar JC, Wheatley AP, Venn A, et al: β₂-Adrenoceptor polymorphisms are in linkage disequilibrium, but are not associated with asthma in an adult population, *Clin Exp Allergy* 28:442, 1998.

110. Hopes E, McDougall C, Christie G, et al: Association of glutamine 27 polymorphism of β₂-adrenoceptor with reported childhood asthma: population based study, *Br Med J* 316:664, 1998.

111. Ramsay CE, Hayden CM, Tiller KJ, et al: Polymorphisms in the beta2-adrenoreceptor gene are associated with decreased airway responsiveness, *Clin Exp Allergy* 29:1195, 1999.

112. Deichmann KA, Schmidt A, Heinzmann A, et al: Association studies on β2-adrenoceptor polymorphisms and enhanced IgE responsiveness in an atopic population, *Clin Exp Allergy* 29:794, 1999.

113. Wang Z, Chen C, Niu T, et al: Association of asthma with beta-adrenergic receptor gene polymorphism and cigarette smoking, *Am J Respir Crit Care Med* 163:1404, 2001.

114. Jones CA, Holloway JA, Popplewell EJ, et al: Reduced soluble CD14 levels in amniotic fluid and breast milk are associated with the subsequent development of atopy, eczema, or both, *J Allergy Clin Immunol* 109:858, 2002.

115. Baldini M, Lohman IC, Halonen M, et al: A polymorphism in the 5′ flanking region of the CD14 gene is associated with circulating soluble CD14 levels and with total serum immunoglobulin E, *Am J Respir Cell Mol Biol* 20:976, 1999.

116. Koppelman GH, Reijmerink NE, Colin Stine O, et al: Association of a promoter polymorphism of the CD14 gene and atopy, *Am J Respir Crit Care Med* 163:965, 2001.

117. Walley AJ, Wiltshire S, Ellis CM, et al: Linkage and allelic association of chromosome 5 cytokine cluster genetic markers with atopy and asthma associated traits, *Genomics* 72:15, 2001.

118. Macfarlane WM, Frayling TM, Ellard S, et al: Missense mutations in the insulin promoter factor-1 gene predispose to type 2 diabetes, *J Clin Invest* 104:R33, 1999.

119. Hani EH, Stoffers DA, Chevre JC, et al: Defective mutations in the insulin promoter factor-1 (IPF-1) gene in late-onset type 2 diabetes mellitus, *J Clin Invest* 104:R41, 1999.

120. Chavanas S, Garner C, Bodemer C, et al: Localization of the Netherton syndrome gene to chromosome 5q32, by linkage analysis and homozygosity mapping, *Am J Hum Genet* 66:914, 2000.

121. Chavanas S, Bodemer C, Rochat A, et al: Mutations in SPINK5, encoding a serine protease inhibitor, cause Netherton syndrome, *Nat Genet* 25:141, 2000.

122. Culbertson MR: RNA surveillance: unforeseen consequences for gene expression, inherited genetic disorders and cancer, *Trends Genet* 15:74, 1999.

123. Walley AJ, Chavanas S, Moffatt MF, et al: Gene polymorphism in Netherton and common atopic disease, *Nat Genet* 29:175, 2001.

124. Houlston RS, Tomlinson IP: Modifier genes in humans: strategies for identification, *Eur J Hum Genet* 6:80, 1998.

125. Quinn M, Angelico MC, Warram JH, et al: Familial factors determine the development of diabetic nephropathy in patients with IDDM, *Diabetologia* 39:940, 1996.

126. Sarafino EP, Goldfedder J: Genetic factors in the presence, severity, and triggers of asthma, *Arch Dis Child* 73:112, 1995.

127. Sarafino EP: Connections among parent and child atopic illnesses, *Pediatr Allergy Immunol* 11:80, 2000.

128. Chagani T, Paré P, Wier T, et al: TNFα and IL-4 promoter polymorphisms and asthma, *Am J Respir Crit Care Med* 157:A875, 1998.

129. Sandford AJ, Chagani T, Zhu S, et al: Polymorphisms in the IL-4, IL-4RA, and FCERIB genes and asthma severity, *J Allergy Clin Immunol* 106:135, 2000.

130. Turki J, Pak J, Green SA, et al: Genetic polymorphisms of the beta 2-adrenergic receptor in nocturnal and nonnocturnal asthma: evidence that Gly16 correlates with the nocturnal phenotype, *J Clin Invest* 95:1635, 1995.

131. Palmer LJ, Silverman ES, Weiss ST, et al: Pharmacogenetics of asthma, *Am J Respir Crit Care Med* 165:861, 2002.

132. Tan S, Hall IP, Dewar J, et al: Association between β_2-adrenoceptor polymorphism and susceptibility to bronchodilator desensitisation in moderately severe stable asthmatics, *Lancet* 350:995, 1997.

133. Martinez FD, Graves PE, Baldini M, et al: Association between genetic polymorphisms of the β_2-adrenoceptor and response to albuterol in children with and without a history of wheezing, *J Clin Invest* 100:3184, 1997.

134. Lipworth BJ, Hall IP, Tan S, et al: Effects of genetic polymorphism on ex vivo and in vivo function of beta2-adrenoceptors in asthmatic patients, *Chest* 115:324, 1999.

135. Hancox RJ, Sears MR, Taylor DR: Polymorphism of the β_2-adrenoceptor and the response to long-term β_2-agonist therapy in asthma, *Eur Respir J* 11:589, 1998.

136. Israel E, Drazen JM, Liggett SB, et al: The effect of polymorphisms of the β_2-adrenergic receptor on the response to regular use of albuterol in asthma, *Am J Respir Crit Care Med* 162:75, 2000.

137. In KH, Asano K, Beier D, et al: Naturally occurring mutations in the human 5-lipoxygenase gene promoter that modify transcription factor binding and reporter gene transcription, *J Clin Invest* 99:1130, 1997.

138. Drazen JM, Yandava CN, Dube L, et al: Pharmacogenetic association between ALOX5 promoter genotype and the response to anti-asthma treatment, *Nat Genet* 22:168, 1999.

139. Palmer LJ, Lonjou C, Barnes K, et al: Special report: a retrospective collaboration on chromosome 5 by the International Consortium on Asthma Genetics (COAG), *Clin Exp Allergy* 31:152-154, 2001.

140. Hizawa N, Freidhoff LR, Chiu YF, et al: A genome-wide screening for genes influencing Dermatophagoides pteronyssinus (Der p)-specific IgE responsiveness, *J Allergy Clin Immunol* 101:772, 1998.

141. Ober C, Tsalenko A, Parry R, et al: A second-generation genomewide screen for asthma-susceptibility alleles in a founder population, *Am J Hum Genet* 67:1154, 2000.

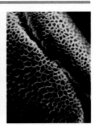

CHAPTER **4**

Regulation and Biology of Immunoglobulin E

HANS C. OETTGEN ■ RAIF S. GEHA

Normally present at very low levels in plasma, antibodies of the immunoglobulin E (IgE) isotype were first discovered in 1967, decades after the description of IgG, IgA, and IgM. IgE antibodies are produced primarily by plasma cells in mucosal-associated lymphoid tissue and their levels are uniformly elevated in patients suffering from atopic conditions like asthma, allergic rhinitis, and atopic dermatitis. Production of allergen-specific IgE in atopic individuals is driven both by a genetic predisposition to the synthesis of this isotype as well as by environmental factors, including chronic allergen exposure. The lineage commitment by B cells to produce IgE involves irreversible genetic changes at the immunoglobulin heavy chain gene locus and is very tightly regulated. It requires both cytokine signals (interleukin [IL]-4 and IL-13) and interaction of B cell CD40 with its ligand on activated T cells.

IgE antibodies exert their biologic functions via the high-affinity IgE receptor, FcεRI, and the low-affinity receptor, CD23. In the classic "immediate hypersensitivity" reaction, the interaction of polyvalent allergens with IgE bound to mast cells via FcεRI triggers receptor aggregation, which initiates a series of signals that result in the release of vasoactive and chemotactic mediators of acute tissue inflammation. Clinical manifestations of IgE-induced immediate hypersensitivity include systemic anaphylaxis (triggered by foods, drugs, and insect stings), acute airflow obstruction in asthmatic patients (following allergen inhalation), and cutaneous wheal and flare responses in allergen skin testing.

Although best known for their critical function in mediating antigen-specific immediate hypersensitivity reactions, IgE antibodies have several antigen-independent effects on IgE receptor expression and cellular function. IgE antibodies directly up-regulate the surface expression of their receptors FcεRI and CD23 on mast cells and B cells, respectively, in a positive feedback loop that may augment ongoing allergic responses. Antigen-independent monomeric IgE signaling via FcεRI provides a survival signal for mast cells. CD23-bound IgE facilitates allergen uptake by B cells that can present captured antigen to specific T cells resulting in augmented secondary immune responses. Occupancy of CD23 by its ligand also inhibits proteolytic shedding of sCD23, a soluble fragment with immunomodulatory properties. This chapter will describe in detail the regulation of IgE synthesis and provide an overview of the biologic actions of IgE antibodies and their role in allergic pathogenesis.

COMPONENTS OF THE IMMUNE RESPONSE

Immunoglobulin E Protein Structure and Gene Organization

Immunoglobulin E (IgE) antibodies are tetramers consisting of two light chains (κ or λ) and two ε-heavy chains (Figure 4-1 and Box 4-1). The heavy chains each contain a variable (V_H) region and four constant region domains. The V_H domain, together with the V-regions of the light chains (V_L), confers antibody specificity and the $C_ε$ domains confer isotype-specific functions, including interaction with FcεRI and CD23. IgE antibodies are relatively heavily glycosylated and contain numerous intrachain and interchain disulfide bonds. The exons encoding the ε-heavy chain domains are located near the 3′ end of the immunoglobulin heavy chain locus (IgH) (Figure 4-2).[1] Additional exons, M1 and M2, encode hydrophobic sequences present in the ε-heavy chain mRNA splice isoform encoding transmembrane IgE in IgE⁺ B cells. In contrast to IgG antibodies, which have a half-life of about three weeks, IgE antibodies have a very short life in plasma ($T_{1/2}$ less than 1 day) and they can remain fixed to mast cells in tissues for weeks or months.

The assembly of a functional IgE gene requires two sequential processes of DNA excision and ligation.[2-4] In the first, which occurs in pre-B cells, individual V_H, D, and J_H exons randomly combine, using very precise joins, to generate a V_HDJ_H cassette encoding an antigen-specific V_H domain. In B cells that have undergone "productive" V_HDJ_H rearrangements (e.g., no stop codons have been introduced during assembly), this V_HDJ_H cassette is situated just upstream of the $C_μ$ exons so that functional μ-heavy chain protein transcripts can be produced. A second DNA excision and ligation process, called *class switch recombination* (CSR), must occur before B cells can produce antibodies of other isotypes, including IgE. These antibodies retain the original V_HDJ_H cassette and antigenic specificity but exchange C_H cassettes of various isotypes to construct different heavy chains and effect distinct biologic functions. In this tightly regulated and irreversible process sometimes referred to as *deletional switch recombination*, a long stretch of genomic DNA spanning from the Sμ region between V_HDJ_H and $C_μ$ to Sε upstream of the $C_ε$ locus is excised (see Figure 4-2). The DNA products of this reaction include an extrachromosomal circle of intervening DNA and

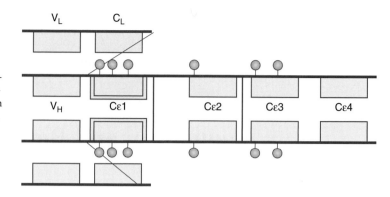

FIGURE 4-1 IgE antibody structure. IgE antibodies are tetramers containing two immunoglobulin light chains and two immunoglobulin ε-heavy chains connected by interchain disulfide bonds as indicated. Each light chain contains one V_L and one C_L immunoglobulin domain and each ε-heavy chain contains an N-terminal V_H domain and four Cε domains. Intrachain disulfide bonds are contained within each of these immunoglobulin domains. The Cε domains contain IgE isotype-specific sequences important for interactions with IgE receptors FcεRI and CD23. IgE antibodies are relatively heavily glycosylated; glycosylation sites are indicated with circles.

BOX 4-1

KEY CONCEPTS

Components of the Immune Response

IgE Antibodies, Genes, and Receptors
- **IgE structure** — IgE protein
  — IgE gene arrangement
- **IgE class switch recombination** — Germline transcription
  — Structure of the Iε promoter
  — Cytokine regulation of germline transcription
  — CD40/CD154 signaling
  — Activation-induced cytidine deaminase
  — DNA double strand breaks and repair
- **IgE receptors** — FcεRI
  — CD23

the contiguous $V_H DJ_H$ and Cε sequences, joined by Sμ-Sε ligation (which is imprecise and heterogeneous), to generate a functional IgE gene. A complex series of cytokine signals and cell surface interactions collaborate to trigger deletional switch recombination in B cells destined for IgE production.

Regulation of IgE Isotype Switching

ε-Germline Transcription Precedes Isotype Switch Recombination

Before the initiation of deletional isotype switch recombination, RNA transcription is activated in B cells at the unrearranged or "germline" ε-heavy chain locus driven from a promoter 5′ of the Iε exon, located just upstream of the Sε switch recombination region and the four Cε exons (Figure 4-3). This is referred to as *ε-germline RNA* and the transcripts include a 140-bp Iε exon as well as exons Cε1-Cε4.[5,6] As Iε contains several stop codons, germline transcripts do not encode functional proteins and have been referred to as "sterile."[7] B cells in which the I exon or its promoter have been mutated are unable to undergo isotype switching, indicating that germline transcription is a prerequisite of deletional switch recombination.[8-10] Conversely, introduction of an active promoter upstream of the I exon not only promotes germline transcription but also promotes isotype switching.[11]

Regulation of Germline Transcription, the Iε Promoter

Initiation of germline transcription is regulated by the Iε promoter that contains binding sites for several known transcription factors including STAT-6, NFκB, BSAP (Pax5), C/EBP, and PU.1 (see Figure 4-3). Translocation of activated STAT-6 to the nucleus is triggered by IL-4 and IL-13 signaling. STAT-6 activation appears to be the key regulator of ε-germline transcription. Although neither BSAP nor NFκB nuclear-binding activities have been shown to be altered by cytokine signaling, these promoter elements must be present for normal Iε promoter function.[12,13] The requirement for NFκB may be related to a physical interaction and resultant synergism in promoter activation between NFκB and STAT-6.[14] CD40 signaling also stimulates NFκB activation and may enhance cytokine-driven germline transcription by activating the NFκB promoter elements. Isotype switching is impaired in NFκB p50[-/-] mice[15] and enhanced in mice lacking the NFκB inhibitor IkB-α.[16] BSAP overexpression can drive Iε transcription and promote IgE isotype switching.[17] PU.1, like NFκB, may synergize with STAT-6 in activating the promoter.[18]

BCL-6, a POZ/zinc-finger transcription factor expressed in B cells, is an important *negative* regulator of the Iε promoter. BCL-6 binds to STAT-6 sites and can repress the induction of ε-germline transcripts by IL-4.[19] Consistent with this model, BCL-6[-/-] mice have enhanced IgE isotype switching, whereas BCL-6[-/-] STAT-6[-/-] animals do not produce IgE. As IL-4– and IL-13–induced STAT-6 activation supports not only IgE germline transcription but also Th2 differentiation, expression of CD23, and up-regulation of VCAM, alterations in the regulation or function of BCL-6 are likely to have a great impact on allergy pathogenesis.

Cytokines IL-4 and IL-13 Activate STAT-6

The cytokines IL-4 and IL-13 are potent inducers of ε-germline transcription in B cells.[5,20,21] The multimeric receptors for these two cytokines share the IL-4R-α chain. The IL-4 receptor is composed of the ligand-binding IL-4Rα and the signal-transducing common cytokine receptor γ-chain γc. The IL-13 receptor contains the IL-4R-α chain along with an IL-13 binding chain (IL-13Rα1 or IL-13Rα2). IL-4 receptor signaling triggers the activation of Janus family tyrosine kinases Jak-1 (via IL-4Rα) and Jak-3 (via γc).[22,23] IL-13Rα associates with Jak-2 and TYK2.[24,25] These activated Jaks then phosphorylate tyrosine residues in the intracellular domains of the receptor chain. These phosphotyrosines serve as binding sites for STAT-6, which is in turn phosphorylated and then dimerizes and translocates to the nucleus.[26,27]

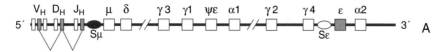

VDJ RECOMBINATION

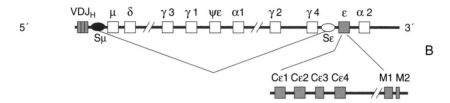

DELETIONAL ISOTYPE SWITCH

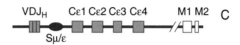

ε-HEAVY CHAIN GENE

FIGURE 4-2 The human immunoglobulin heavy chain gene locus; deletional class switch recombination. **A,** The human immunoglobulin heavy chain locus contains clusters of V_H, D_H, and J_H cassettes that are stochastically rearranged during B cell ontogeny. This process, which involves DNA excision and repair, results in the assembly of a complete VDJ exon encoding an antigen-binding V_H domain. Pre-B cells that have completed this rearrangement are capable of producing intact μ-heavy chains and, following an analogous process of light chain rearrangements, can produce intact IgM antibodies. **B,** Production of other antibody isotypes, bearing the original antigenic specificity, requires an additional excision and repair process, deletional "class switch recombination" (CSR). For IgE isotype switching, this process involves the excision of a large piece of genomic DNA spanning from Sμ switch sequences just upstream of the μ-heavy chain exons to the Sε sequence 5′ of the Cε exons. **C,** Ligation of the VDJ sequences to the Cε locus then gives rise to an intact ε-heavy chain gene containing a V_H-encoding VDJ exon and exons Cε1-4 encoding the constant region domains of ε-heavy chain. The M1 and M2 exons encode transmembrane sequences that are present in RNA splice isoforms encoding the membrane IgE of IgE+ B cells.

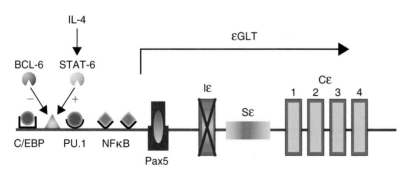

FIGURE 4-3 ε-Germline transcription (εGLT). Class switch recombination is invariably preceded by a process of RNA transcription at the C_H locus being targeted by specific cytokine signals. ε-Germline transcripts originate at a promoter upstream of the Iε exon. This promoter contains binding sites for transcription factors C/EBP, PU.1, STAT-6, NFκB (2 sites), and Pax5. STAT-6 activation is triggered by IL-4 and IL-13 receptor signaling and is the critical regulatory factor in ε-germline transcription. BCL-6 is a transcriptional repressor that binds to the STAT-6 target site and inhibits εGLT. Germline transcripts contain Iε and Cε1-4 exons but, because the Iε exon contains stop codons ("X"), these RNAs do not encode a functional protein.

CD40/CD154 Provides Second Signal for Isotype Switch Recombination

The cytokines IL-4 and IL-13 are very efficient inducers of ε-germline transcription, and this transcription is an absolute prerequisite for isotype switching. However, cytokine-induced germline transcription alone is not sufficient to drive B cells to complete the genomic deletional switch recombination reaction that gives rise to a functional IgE gene. A second signal, provided by the interaction of CD40 on B cells with its ligand, CD154, on activated T cells, is required to bring the process to completion.

CD154 is transiently expressed on antigen/MCH-stimulated T cells.[28] T cell CD154 induces CD40 aggregation on B cells, triggering signal transduction via four intracellular proteins belonging to the TRAF family of TNF-receptor associated factors.[29,30] TRAF-2, -5, and -6 promote the dissociation of NFκB from its inhibitor, IκB, allowing NFκB to translocate to the nucleus and synergize with STAT-6 to activate the Iε promoter as described above.[31,32] In addition to inducing TRAF association and signaling, aggregation of CD40 activates protein tyrosine kinases (PTKs) including Jak-3, which play an important role in immunoglobulin class switching.[33,34] CD154 is encoded on the X chromosome. Boys with X-linked immunodeficiency with hyper-IgM (XHIM) are deficient in CD154. Consequently, their B cells are unable to produce IgG, IgA, or IgE.[35-39] Mice with a targeted disruption of the CD154 or CD40 genes have the same defect in antibody production.[40-42]

Cytokine-Stimulated Germline Transcripts and CD40-Induced AID Collaborate to Execute Switch Recombination

It has been known for some time that deletional class switch recombination stimulated by cytokines and CD40/CD154 requires the synthesis of new proteins and it has been inferred that these proteins might constitute the enzymatic apparatus required for the excision of intervening genomic DNA and ligation of V_HDJ_H cassette to the $C\epsilon$ locus in CSR. In 1999 a subtractive approach was used to identify one of these proteins as activation-induced cytidine deaminase (AID), which is expressed in activated splenic B cells and in the germinal centers of lymph nodes.[43,44] AID-deficient mice have elevated IgM levels and a major defect in isotype switching with absent IgG, IgE, and IgA. A rare autosomal form of hyper-IgM syndrome (HIGM2), which is associated with striking lymphoid hypertrophy, has now been attributed to mutations in the AID gene.[45] An unanticipated phenotype of both mice and humans with AID mutations is a decrease in somatic V region hypermutation during active antibody responses.

The mechanisms whereby AID participates in switch recombination are the subject of speculation at present. AID has homology to APOBEC, an RNA editing enzyme, which modifies specific sites in ApoB precursor RNA to give rise to a transcript encoding the functional apoB48 protein. AID might execute a similar RNA-editing function in B cells, processing pre-RNA(s) encoding proteins such as nucleases or ligases involved in deletional class switch recombination or hypermutation. Alternatively, AID might mediate the construction of ribozymes, complex RNA structures with their own nuclease activity, or it could act directly on DNA substrates in the heavy chain locus. Transfection of AID into fibroblasts is adequate to confer switch recombination in an artificial switch construct.[46] B cells from AID-deficient mice exhibit diminished recruitment of Nbs1 and γ-H2AX, enzymes associated with DNA damage, to the IgH locus following stimulation for isotype switching, consistent with a role for AID in focal assembly at the IgH locus of a complex of proteins responsible for generating DNA breaks.[47]

ϵ-Germline Transcripts Hybridize with S-region DNA and Target Nucleases to IgE Locus in Switch Recombination

As "sterile" ϵ-germline transcripts do not encode functional protein, their mechanistic role in isotype switching has, until recently, been mysterious. Structural analyses of their association with template DNA suggest that they mediate the assembly of DNA/RNA hybrid structures, called *R-loops,* which serve as substrates for nucleases in the initial DNA cleavage in the "cut-and-paste" reaction of deletional switch recombination (Figure 4-4). In deletional class switch recombination at the ϵ-locus, the initial DNA cleavage occurs within the $S\epsilon$ region located between the $I\epsilon$ and $C\epsilon$ exons. ϵ-Germline transcripts, originating just upstream of $I\epsilon$, pass through the $S\epsilon$ region and continue into the $C\epsilon$ exons. In *in vitro* transcription experiments the S region–containing RNA does not separate from its genomic template but rather remains associated to form a DNA-RNA hybrid.[48-50] These hybrids generate R-loops, in which the S transcript hybridizes to the template DNA, leaving the opposite strand as single-stranded DNA.[51]

Endogenous excision repair nucleases have been shown to be capable of cleaving these R-loops. These observations have led to speculation that R-loops formed by the association of $S\epsilon$ RNA with its $S\epsilon$ genomic template serve as substrates for nucleases that generate double-strand the DNA breaks in the first step of deletional switching. In subsequent steps of the process, these breaks would be annealed by the DNA end joining analogous breaks, located at $S\mu$ between V_HDJ_H and the $C\mu$ exons. The resultant juxtaposition of the V_HDJ_H and $C\epsilon$ sequences would generate a functional IgE gene. Just as the mechanisms for introduction of DNA double-strand breaks at $S\mu$ and $S\epsilon$ are speculative at this point, the enzymatic reactions leading to the ligation of the resultant breaks are also uncertain.[52] The heterogeneous nature of the $S\mu$-$S\epsilon$ junctions suggests a nonhomologous end-joining mechanism. Consistent with this possibility, B cells lacking Ku70, Ku80, and DNA-PKcs, all of which are involved in nonhomologous end joining, cannot execute isotype switching normally.[53-55]

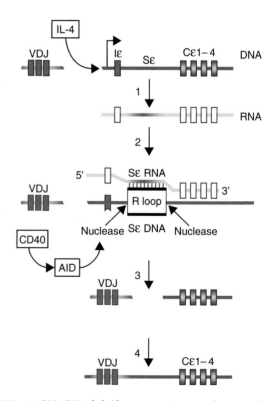

FIGURE 4-4 DNA/RNA hybrid structures target nucleases to cleave sequences. ϵ-Germline transcription (ϵGLT) RNA is a transcribed response to IL-4 or IL-13 at the germline ϵ-heavy chain locus originating at the $I\epsilon$ promoter. $S\epsilon$ RNA hybridizes to one of the strands of $S\epsilon$ DNA, creating an "R-loop" structure, a substrate for endogenous nucleases that introduce double-stranded DNA breaks. Joining can then occur between $S\epsilon$ and $S\mu$ breaks upstream of the $C\epsilon$ cluster of exons and downstream of the VDJ exons, giving rise to an intact IgE heavy chain gene.

Regulation of Allergen-Specific T Cell Responses

The execution of IgE isotype switch recombination in B cells, as detailed previously, requires that cytokine (IL-4 and IL-13) signals and the CD40 ligand, CD154, be delivered in a coordinated fashion. Both these stimuli are provided by Th2-type allergen-specific T-helper cells. Thus, the mechanisms that regulate expansion and survival of Th2 cells are crucial in regulating IgE responses.

Th2 Helper T Cell Development

CD4+ T cells can be segregated based on their constellation of cytokine secretion into Th1 (which makes interferon [IFN]-γ and IL-2) and Th2 (which produces IL-4, IL-5, IL-6, IL-9, IL-10, IL-13, and GM-CSF).[56] Th2 cells express cell surface receptors, which target their trafficking to allergic sites and trigger activation in settings of allergic inflammation, including the chemokine receptors CCR3 (eotaxin/CCL11 receptor), CCR4 (a receptor for TARC/CCL17 and MDC/CCL22), CRTh2, and CCR8 (I309/CCL1 receptor) and an orphan receptor of the IL-1 receptor family, T1/ST2.[57-60]

Following the initial antigen encounter, naive T cells produce abundant quantities of IL-2 but relatively insignificant amounts of the Th1- and Th2-specific cytokines, IFN-γ and IL-4. This initial antigenic contact also triggers a differentiating phase in which cytokine genes (both Th1 and Th2) become accessible for transcription.[61] This is followed by three stages of cytokine expression that eventually drive Th cells to definitive commitment to either Th1 or Th2 phenotypes (Figure 4-5). In the case of Th2 development, the first phase, which is that of *initiation,* is highly dependent on antigen and IL-4 signaling via STAT-6. Initiation is associated with changes in chromatin structure induced by a selective pattern of histone acetylation.[62-64] In the *commitment* phase that follows, accessibility for transcription of the Th2 constellation of cytokines is fixed by the action of Th2-specific transcription factors, including GATA-3 and c-Maf. Th1 cells express T-bet. These factors may bind to regulatory sequences, recruit chromatin remodeling enzymes, and lead to stably inherited changes.[65] Subsequent activation of the committed Th2 cells by antigen triggers acute gene transcription driven by the transcription factor NFAT1, which now has restricted access to the precommitted cytokine promoters relevant to the lineage.

Genetic Influences on Th2 Development

Both host and environmental factors promote the Th2 shift observed in allergic individuals. Some inbred mouse strains have a propensity for Th2-dominated responses to particular antigens, whereas others are characterized by Th1-dominant responses indicating a significant genetic contribution to T-helper cell differentiation. It is possible that specific evolutionary pressures exerted by particular pathogen exposures might account for this; mice with a dominant Th1 response mount effective attacks against intracellular pathogens such as *Leishmania.*[66,67] In contrast, those with enhanced Th2 responsiveness may be at an advantage in the elimination of parasites.[68] In humans it is clear that the tendency to develop allergic responses to antigens also varies greatly among individuals raised within nearly identical environments and that this allergic tendency is familial.

Genetic predispositions toward Th1 or Th2 are partly accounted for by T cell autonomous tendencies to transcribe

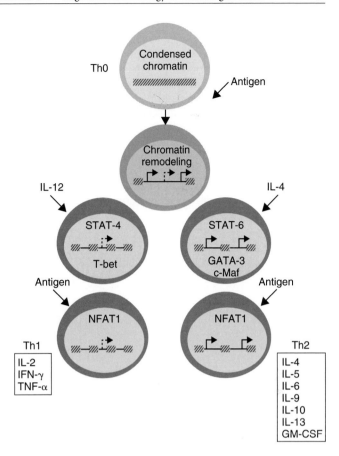

FIGURE 4-5 CD4+ T-helper cell differentiation into Th1 and Th2 lineages. *CD4+ T-helper cells undergo a process of differentiation to Th1 (producing IL-2, IFN-γ, and TNF-α) or Th2 (producing IL-4, IL-5, IL-6, IL-9, IL-10, IL-13, and GM-CSF) phenotypes. Following initial antigen encounter, uncommitted Th0 cells produce relatively small amounts of cytokines. Persistent activation and cell division, however, drive chromatin remodeling that is permissive for transcription of a range of cytokines. Differentiation into preferential expression of Th1 versus Th2 cytokines occurs under the influence of IL-4 (Th2) and IL-12 (Th1). Exposure to these cytokines is accompanied by expression of Th1- (T-bet) and Th2- (GATA-3, c-Maf) specific transcription and stable chromatin changes that favor transcriptional access for the Th1 and Th2 cytokines, respectively. Fully differentiated Th1 or Th2 cells activated by antigen are thus committed to NFAT-driven transcription of specific cytokines.*

Th1 versus Th2 cytokines, but are also the result of a wide range of influences external to T cells.[69] Perhaps the most potent Th1/Th2-polarizing effect is exerted by the cytokine milieu, particularly tissue levels of IL-4, IL-12, and IFN-γ. IL-4 promotes Th2 responses and suppresses Th1 development. IL-12 drives Th1 differentiation (an effect that is greatly potentiated by the presence of IFN-γ) and can inhibit and even reverse Th2 development. In ongoing immune responses these cytokines can be provided by existing T cells already committed to a particular Th phenotype. In *de novo* allergen encounters cytokines produced by cells of the "innate" immune response may tip the balance.

Antigen-Presenting Cell Function in Th Differentiation

Naive T cells initially encounter antigens as MHC-bound processed peptides on the surface of antigen-presenting cells (APCs). The most potent APCs are dendritic cells (DCs), which reside in tissues as immature sentinels and sample antigens in their milieu. Upon activation, these cells acquire mature APC function and migrate to regional lymphoid tissues where they efficiently activate antigen-specific T helper cells via MHC-peptide complexes. Dendritic cells obtained from various lymphoid tissues *in vivo* or cultured *ex vivo* under a range of conditions all express MHC II and, following activation, express costimulatory molecules, including CD80/86. However, there is some functional heterogeneity among DC, especially with respect to the ability to induce Th1 versus Th2 T helper responses.[70] "DC1" cells favor the induction of Th1 responses, whereas "DC2" cells preferentially stimulate Th2 responses. The critical distinguishing feature of DC1s is their capacity to produce relatively large amounts of IL-12, a critical Th1-inducing cytokine.

Microbial Products and Dendritic Cell Phenotype

The recent understanding that Th polarity may be determined by DC polarity obviously begs the following question: what determines DC polarity? IFN-γ favors DC1 development, whereas histamine and PGE$_2$ promote the development of DC2.[71-73] Recent data suggest that conserved microbial structures, which signal via the Toll-like receptor (TLR) family of receptors, can shift DC polarity. These receptors, which bind microbial lipid and polysaccharide structures, are conserved from *Drosophila* to humans and are critical in the early "innate" response to pathogens. Dendritic cells express a range of TLR family receptors and the specific effects of ligand binding by each of these receptors on DC phenotype remain to be fully elucidated. It has recently been demonstrated that DCs from

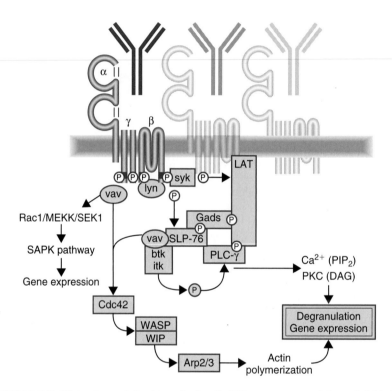

FIGURE 4-6 FcεRI structure and signal transduction. FcεRI is a tetramer containing an IgE-binding α-chain (with two extracellular immunoglobulin-type domains), a disulfide-linked, signal-transducing dimer of γ-chains, each of which contains an intracellular immunoreceptor tyrosine-based activation motif (ITAM *[black squares]*) and a tetramembrane spanner β-chain that also contains a cytosolic ITAM and serves to augment FcεRI surface expression and signal transduction intensity. Trimeric forms of the receptor, lacking the β-chain, can be expressed on some cell types.

Aggregation of the receptor by the interaction of its ligand, IgE, with polymeric antigens induces signal transduction. The β-chain—associated protein tyrosine kinase, lyn, in aggregated receptor complexes phosphorylates *(P)* the β- and γ-chain ITAMs, generating docking sites for the SH2-domain containing kinase, syk. Activated syk phosphorylates the membrane-associated scaffolding protein LAT as well as the adapter, SLP-76 (which is also bound to LAT via the Grb-2 homolog, Gads). These proteins have no inherent enzymatic activity but serve to assemble a membrane-associated supramolecular complex of proteins that brings together a number of signaling molecules. LAT and SLP-76 both recruit PLC-γ, whose activity is enhanced by the SLP-76–associated kinases btk and itk. PLC-γ activation results in the production of phosphatidyl inositol bisphosphate *(PIP$_2$)* and diacyl glycerol *(DAG)* with resultant increases in intracellular Ca^{2+} and activation of protein kinase C *(PKC)*.

Alongside this protein tyrosine kinase pathway, FcεRI aggregation triggers a vav/cytoskeletal signaling cascade. The guanine nucleotide exchange factor, vav, which is directly associated with FcεRI-γ as well as with SLP-76, activates the GTPase Cdc42 which, in turn, induces a conformational change in a complex of proteins, WASP and WIP, associated with the cytoskeleton. This exposes binding sites for Arp2/3, a complex of proteins that mediates actin polymerization. Vav activation also drives the stress-activated protein kinase *(SAPK)* pathway. The combined effects of elevated Ca^{2+}, PKC activation, actin polymerization, and SAPK activation drive mast cell degranulation and induction of gene expression.

mice deficient in TLR-4 are defective in inducing Th2 responses.[74]

Non-T Cell Sources of IL-4: Mast Cells, NK1.1 T Cells, and NK Cells

Although allergen-specific T-helper cells committed to the Th2 lineage are a major source of IL-4 in allergic tissues, several other cell types can provide IL-4 and IL-13. Mast cells, which are abundant in the respiratory and gastrointestinal mucosa, are excellent producers of both IL-4 and IL-13 following activation via IgE/FcεRI.[75,76] NK1.1+ CD4+ T cells are another source of IL-4. These cells express a very restricted repertoire of αβ T cell receptors and interact with the nonclassical MHC class I molecule, CD1.[77] The intravenous injection of anti-CD3 in mice induces large amounts of IL-4, derived primarily from these NK1.1+ T cells. Mice with abundant NK1.1 cells have enhanced IL-4 production and IgE synthesis, whereas those depleted of the same population show suppressed Th2 responses.[78] NK cells may also provide IL-4 early in immune responses to allergens. Both cultured and freshly isolated human NK cells have been shown to be differentiated to produce either IL-10 and IFN-γ (NK1) or IL-5 and IL-13 (NK2), a polarity analogous to that observed in Th1 versus Th2 T-helper cells.[79-81] In light of the strong association between asthma flares and viral respiratory infections, particularly in the first 2 to 3 years of life, the NK contribution to tissue cytokine levels may be important.

IgE Receptors

FcεRI Structure

The high-affinity IgE receptor FcεRI is a multimeric complex expressed in two isoforms, a tetrameric αβγ$_2$ receptor present on mast cells and basophils and a trimeric αγ$_2$ receptor expressed, albeit at levels tenfold to one hundredfold lower, by several cell lineages including eosinophils, platelets, monocytes, dendritic cells, and cutaneous Langerhans cells[82] (Figure 4-6). The α chain contains two extracellular immunoglobulin-related domains and is responsible for binding IgE. The β-subunit of the receptor contains four transmembrane-spanning domains with both N- and C-terminal ends on the cytosolic side of the plasma membrane. FcεRI-β appears to have two functions that result in enhanced receptor activity. β-chain expression both enhances cell surface density of FcεRI and amplifies the signal transduced following activation of the receptor by IgE aggregation.[83-85] The γ-chains (which have homology to the ζ and η chains important in T cell receptor signaling) exist as disulfide-linked dimers with transmembrane domains and cytoplasmic tails. The β and γ chains perform critical signal transduction functions and their intracellular domains contain immunoreceptor tyrosine-based activation motifs (ITAMs), 18 amino acid long tyrosine-containing sequences that constitute docking sites for SH2 domain-containing signaling proteins.

CD23 Expression and Structure

Although its common designation as the "low-affinity" IgE receptor implies differently, CD23 actually has a fairly high affinity for IgE with a K_A of about 10^8.[86,87] A wide variety of cell types express CD23 in humans, including B cells, Langerhans cells, follicular dendritic cells, T cells, and eosinophils.[88] It is a type II transmembrane protein with a C-type lectin domain,

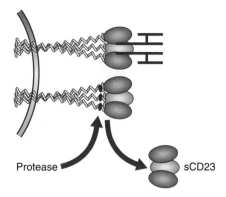

FIGURE 4-7 CD23 structure. CD23 is a type II transmembrane protein (with intracellular N-terminus) that contains α-helical coiled stalks and oligomerizes at the cell surface. Occupancy of the receptor by IgE stabilizes the receptor. In the absence of the IgE ligand, protease-sensitive sites appear *(ovals)* and endogenous proteases as well as proteases present in allergens such as *Der p 1* cleave CD23, shedding soluble sCD23 into the milieu.

making it the only immunoglobulin receptor that is not in the Ig superfamily.[89,90] Adjacent to its lectin domain, CD23 has sequences that are predicted to give rise to α-helical coiled-coil stalks (Figure 4-7). As a result, CD23 is known to have a tendency to multimerize and only oligomeric CD23 will bind IgE.[91] CD23 has homology to the asialo glycoprotein receptor, suggesting a role for CD23 in endocytosis.

PRINCIPLES OF DISEASE MECHANISM

Once produced, allergen-specific IgE antibodies engage their receptors and trigger a wide variety of tissue-specific responses. The cellular and molecular mechanisms of pathogenesis giving rise to specific allergic disorders are presented in great detail later in this textbook. This section will provide a general overview of the consequences of IgE interaction with its receptors, including immediate hypersensitivity, late-phase reactions, regulation of IgE receptor expression, and immune modulation (Box 4-2).

BOX 4-2	KEY CONCEPTS
	Principles of Disease Mechanism

Effector Functions of IgE

■ **Mast cell activation/FcεRI**	FcεRI signaling—antigen dependent
	Immediate hypersensitivity reactions
	Late-phase reactions
	FcεRI signaling—antigen independent
■ **IgE regulation of IgE receptors**	FcεRI
	CD23
■ **CD23 functions**	IgE antigen capture
	Regulation of IgE synthesis by CD23 and by CD23

Mast Cell Activation and Homeostasis

FcεRI Signaling

FcεRI has high affinity for IgE (Kd 10^{-8} M) and under physiologic conditions mast cell and basophil FcεRI is fully occupied by IgE antibodies. Aggregation of this receptor-bound IgE by an encounter with polyvalent allergen triggers a cascade of signaling events[92] (see Figure 4-6). Receptor aggregation induces transphosphorylation of intracellular ITAMs on FcεRI-β and FcεRI-γ by receptor-associated lyn tyrosine kinase, providing docking sites for the SH2-containing syk protein tyrosine kinase. Lyn phosphorylation of these ITAMs is also favored by recruitment of aggregated FcεRI into lipid rafts, domains of the plasma membrane that are relatively rich in lyn. Receptor-associated syk phosphorylates a series of scaffolding and adapter molecules leading to the assembly of a supramolecular plasma membrane-localized signaling complex, focused around the scaffolding molecules LAT and SLP-76, which recruits and activates PLCγ with resultant changes in cytosolic calcium, degranulation, and activation of gene transcription. Mast cells from animals with mutations in several key components of this signaling complex, including LAT and SLP-76, have markedly inhibited FcεRI-mediated mast cell activation following receptor cross-linking.[93,94] Cytoskeletal reorganization provides a critical parallel signaling pathway driven by FcεRI aggregation in mast cells and basophils. This cytoskeletal signaling is driven by the guanine nucleoside exchange factor vav.[95] Vav associates both with the SLP-76/LAT complex and directly with FcεRI-γ.[96] Vav activates Cdc42, a GTPase, which binds to Wiskott-Aldrich syndrome protein (WASP) and induces a conformational change in the cytoskeletal WASP/WASP-interacting protein (WIP) protein complex, allowing interaction with the actin-polymerizing Arp2/3 complex. Vav, via a series of intermediates, also leads to the activation of the stress-activated protein kinase (SAPK) pathway.

In the classic immediate hypersensitivity reaction, cross-linking of IgE induces the complex signaling cascade just described, resulting in the release of preformed mediators including histamine, proteoglycans, and proteases; transcription of cytokines (IL-4, TNF, IL-6); and de novo synthesis of prostaglandins (PGD_2) and leukotrienes (LTD_4). In the airways of asthmatic patients, these mediators rapidly elicit bronchial mucosal edema, mucus production, and smooth muscle constriction and, eventually, recruit an inflammatory infiltrate. In asthmatic patients subjected to allergen inhalation, these cellular and molecular events result in an acute obstruction of airflow with a drop in FEV_1.[97]

In many subjects exposed to allergens by inhalation, ingestion, cutaneous exposure, or injection, immediate responses are followed 8 to 24 hours later by a second, delayed-phase reaction, designated the *late-phase response (LPR)*. LPR can manifest as delayed or repeated onset of airflow obstruction, gastrointestinal symptoms, skin inflammation, or anaphylaxis hours after initial allergen exposure and after the acute response has completely subsided. In animal models IgE antibodies can transfer both acute and LPR sensitivity to allergen challenge.[98] Interference with mast cell activation or inhibition of the mast cell mediators blocks the onset of both acute-phase and late-phase responses.[99] It has been proposed that chronic obstructive symptoms in asthma patients subjected to recurrent environmental allergen exposure result from persistent late-phase responses.[100,101]

Monomeric IgE Signaling via FcεRI

Although IgE-mediated signaling via FcεRI has long been believed to be dependent on antigen-mediated receptor aggregation, some recent evidence suggests that the binding of IgE *per se*, in the absence of antigen, provides a signal to mast cells and basophils. Experiments using cultured bone marrow mast cells have revealed that monomeric IgE has a survival-enhancing effect, protecting these cells from apoptosis following the withdrawal of growth factor.[102,103] This effect is mediated via FcεRI; no antiapoptotic effect is observed in FcεRI-deficient mast cells exposed to IgE. One group has reported that this antigen-independent pathway activates intracellular signaling molecules and cytokine production. Phosphorylation of members of the MAPK and SAPK pathways is induced by monomeric IgE via an FcεRI/lipid raft-dependent pathway, and the transcription of several mast cell cytokines, including TNF and IL-6 (also IL-4 and IL-13), is enhanced.

IgE Regulation of Receptors

The expression of both FcεRI and CD23 is positively regulated by their mutual ligand, IgE. FcεRI expression is markedly diminished on peritoneal mast cells from IgE-deficient mice and this defect can be reversed *in vivo* by injection of IgE antibodies.[104-106] Low FcεRI expression in IgE$^{-/-}$ mice is associated with diminished mast cell activation following IgE sensitization and allergen exposure. Treatment with anti-IgE has been shown to induce a decrease in IgE receptor expression.[107]

CD23 expression on cultured B cells is enhanced in the presence of IgE, which, by occupancy of its receptor, prevents proteolytic degradation of CD23 and shedding into the medium.[87,108] This regulatory interaction between IgE and CD23 is operative *in vivo* as well; B cells from IgE$^{-/-}$ animals have markedly diminished CD23 levels and intravenous injection of IgE induces normal CD23 expression.[109] Restoration of CD23 expression can be induced using monomeric IgE and is antigen independent. Exposure to IgE does not alter transcription of mRNA encoding CD23 or the FcεRI subunits but rather modulates receptor turnover and proteolytic shedding.[110] The positive feedback interaction between IgE and its receptors may have implications in terms of augmenting allergic responses in atopic individuals with high IgE levels.

CD23 Function: Antigen Capture

Several investigators have now shown that the binding of allergen by specific IgE facilitates allergen uptake by CD23-bearing cells for processing and presentation to T cells.[111-113] Mice immunized intravenously with antigen produce stronger IgG responses when antigen-specific IgE is provided at the time of immunization.[114,115] As expected, CD23$^{-/-}$ mice cannot display augmentation of immune responses by IgE but acquire responsiveness to IgE following reconstitution with cells from CD23$^+$ donors.[116,117] These findings suggest a scenario in which preformed allergen-specific IgE present in the bronchial and gut mucosa of patients with recurrent allergen exposure would enhance immune responses upon repeated allergen inhalation or ingestion.

CD23 Function: IgE Regulation

In addition to its role in allergen uptake, CD23 appears to have regulatory influences on IgE synthesis and allergic inflammation. Although the data in this area have seemed to be conflicting at times, the emerging consensus from human and animal studies is that ligation of membrane-bound CD23 on B cells suppresses IgE production. Ligation of CD23 on human B cells by activating antibodies inhibits IgE synthesis[118] and transgenic mice overexpressing CD23 have suppressed IgE responses.[119,120] Conversely, mice rendered CD23-deficient by targeted gene disruption have increased and sustained specific IgE titers following immunization, also consistent with a suppressive effect of membrane-bound CD23.[121] This enhanced tendency toward IgE synthesis in CD23-/- mice is also observed following allergen inhalation and is accompanied by increased eosinophilic inflammation of the airways.[122-125]

In contrast, there have been reports that soluble CD23 (sCD23) fragments, which are generated by proteolytic cleavage, may enhance IgE production, either by direct interaction with B cells (via CD21) or by binding to IgE, thereby blocking its interaction with membrane-bound CD23.[126] The IgE-enhancing effects of crude sCD23 have not yet been reproduced with recombinant sCD23[127] and it is unclear whether this discrepancy arises from IgE-inducing activity attributable to other components of sCD23-containing culture supernatants or whether the lack of activity of recombinant sCD23 is the consequence of a nonphysiologic structure. Recent data implicate a role for allergens, some of which are proteases, as

effectors of CD23 cleavage and for IgE itself as a stabilizer of membrane CD23 and inhibitor of proteolytic shedding.[128] Two possible consequences of such allergen-mediated cleavage would be decreased suppressive signaling to the B cell via CD23, along with increased production of activating sCD23 fragments, both promoting IgE production. Inhibition of proteolytic activity of *Der p 1* blocks its ability to induce IgE responses *in vivo* both in normal and humanized scid mice.[129,130] Similar effects are observed in culture systems. Metalloproteinase inhibitors block sCD23 shedding in cultures of tonsillar B cells or peripheral blood mononuclear cells and this is accompanied by decreased IgE production following stimulation with IL-4.[131]

To summarize, IgE antibodies are invariably elevated in individuals affected by the atopic conditions of asthma, allergic rhinitis, and atopic dermatitis. The production of IgE follows a series of complex genomic rearrangements in B cells, called *deletional class switch recombination,* a process that is tightly regulated by the cytokines IL-4 and IL-13 along with T-B cell interaction and CD40/CD154 signaling. IgE antibodies exert their biologic effects via receptors FcεRI and CD23. It is now clear that, in addition to mediating the classic immediate hypersensitivity reactions by inducing acute mediator release by mast cells, IgE antibodies have a number of immunomodulatory functions (Figure 4-8). These include up-regulation of IgE receptors, enhancement of allergen uptake by B cells for antigen presentation, and induction of Th2 cytokine expression by mast cells and may all collaborate to amplify and perpetuate allergic responses in susceptible individuals. Thus blockade of IgE effects, using novel anti-IgE therapies, may ultimately prove to have a broad benefit.

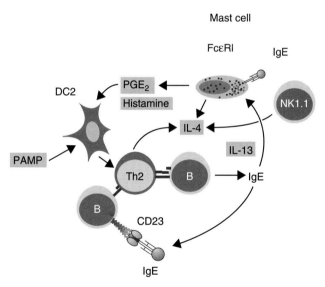

FIGURE 4-8 The IgE network: cellular and cytokine control of IgE production in allergic tissues and amplification of allergic responses by preformed IgE. A confluence of cellular and molecular stimuli supports IgE synthesis in the tissues of asthmatic patients. Tissue DCs are driven toward a Th2-promoting DC2 phenotype by a variety of environmental influences, including exposure to microbial "pathogen-associated molecular patterns" *(PAMPs)* and histamine and PGE2 (both of which can be provided by mast cells). Activated DC2s translocate to mucosal- or skin-associated lymphoid tissues where they attain competence as antigen-presenting cells (APCs) and drive the generation of Th2 expansion. B cells also serve as APCs, a function that is augmented when preformed IgE (generated during previous allergen encounter) is present and can facilitate B cell antigen uptake via CD23.

IL-4 and IL-13 are derived from numerous cellular sources. In the setting of recurrent allergen challenge, pre-existing, allergen-specific Th2 T cells are likely to provide a major source of IL-4. Additional producers of IL-4 include NK1.1 cells (both NK1.1 T cells and "NK2" NK cells) and mast cells. Mast cell IL-4 synthesis can be triggered via FcεRI in the presence of preformed IgE. IL-4 and IL-13 along with cognate T-B interactions involving antigen presentation and CD40 signaling then support IgE isotype switching in B cells.

REFERENCES

1. Liu FT: Gene expression and structure of immunoglobulin epsilon chains, *Crit Rev Immunol* 6:47, 1986.
2. Bacharier LB, Jabara H, Geha RS: Molecular mechanisms of immunoglobulin E regulation, *Int Arch Allergy Immunol* 115:257, 1998.
3. Oettgen HC: Regulation of the IgE isotype switch: new insights on cytokine signals and the functions of epsilon germline transcripts, *Curr Opin Immunol* 12:618, 2000.
4. Oettgen HC, Geha RS: IgE regulation and roles in asthma pathogenesis, *J Allergy Clin Immunol* 107:429, 2001.
5. Vercelli D, Jabara H, Arai K-I, et al: Induction of human IgE synthesis requires interleukin 4 and T/B interactions involving the T cell receptor/CD3 complex and MHC class II antigens, *J Exp Med* 169:1295, 1989.
6. Del Prete G, Maggi E, Parronchi P, et al: IL-4 is an essential factor for the IgE synthesis induced in vitro by human T cell clones and their supernatants, *J Immunol* 140:4193, 1988.
7. Gauchat J-F, Lebman D, Coffman R, et al: Structure and expression of germline transcripts in human B cells induced by interleukin 4 to switch to IgE production, *J Exp Med* 172:463, 1990.
8. Jung S, Rajewsky K, Radbruch A: Shutdown of class switch recombination by deletion of a switch region control element, *Science* 259:984, 1993.
9. Zhang J, Bottaro A, Li S, et al: A selective defect in IgG2b switching as a result of targeted mutation of the I gamma 2b promoter and exon, *EMBO J* 12:3529, 1993.
10. Lorenz M, Jung S, Radbruch A: Switch transcripts in immunoglobulin class switching, *Science* 267:1825, 1995.
11. Bottaro A, Lansford R, Xu L, et al: S region transcription per se promotes basal IgE class switch recombination but additional factors regulate the efficiency of the process, *EMBO J* 13:665, 1994.
12. Thienes CP, de Monte L, Monticelli S, et al: The transcription factor B cell-specific activator protein (BSAP) enhances both IL-4- and CD40-mediated activation of the human epsilon germline promoter, *J Immunol* 158:5874, 1997.

13. Monticelli S, De Monte L, Vercelli D: Molecular regulation of IgE switching: let's walk hand in hand, *Allergy* 53:6, 1998.

14. Shen CH, Stavnezer J: Interaction of stat6 and NF-kappaB: direct association and synergistic activation of interleukin-4-induced transcription, *Mol Cell Biol* 18:3395, 1998.

15. Sha WC, Liou HC, Tuomanen EI, et al: Targeted disruption of the p50 subunit of NF-kappa B leads to multifocal defects in immune responses, *Cell* 80:321, 1995.

16. Chen CL, Singh N, Yull FE, et al: Lymphocytes lacking kappaB-alpha develop normally, but have selective defects in proliferation and function, *J Immunol* 165:5418, 2000.

17. Qiu G, Stavnezer J: Overexpression of BSAP/Pax-5 inhibits switching to IgA and enhances switching to IgE in the 1.29 mu B cell line, *J Immunol* 161:2906, 1998.

18. Stutz AM, Woisetschlager M: Functional synergism of STAT6 with either NF-kappa B or PU.1 to mediate IL-4-induced activation of IgE germline gene transcription, *J Immunol* 163:4383, 1999.

19. Harris MB, Chang CC, Berton MT, et al: Transcriptional repression of Stat6-dependent interleukin-4-induced genes by BCL-6: specific regulation of epsilon transcription and immunoglobulin E switching, *Mol Cell Biol* 19:7264, 1999.

20. Punnonen J, Aversa G, Cocks B, et al: Interleukin 13 induces interleukin 4-independent IgG4 and IgE synthesis and CD23 expression by human B cells, *Proc Natl Acad Sci U S A* 90:3730, 1993.

21. Defrance T, Carayon P, Billian G, et al: Interleukin 13 is a B cell stimulating factor, *J Exp Med* 179:135, 1994.

22. Witthuhn B, Silvennoinen O, Miura O, et al: Involvement of the Jak-3 Janus kinase in signalling by interleukins 2 and 4 in lymphoid and myeloid cells, *Nature* 370:153, 1994.

23. Rolling C, Treton D, Beckmann P, et al: JAK3 associates with the human interleukin 4 receptor and is tyrosine phosphorylated following receptor triggering, *Oncogene* 10:1757, 1995.

24. Palmer-Crocker P, Hughes C, Pober J: IL-4 and IL-13 activate the JAK2 tyrosine kinase and STAT6 in cultured human vascular endothelial cells through a common pathway that does not involve the gc chain, *J Clin Invest* 98:604, 1996.

25. Welham M, Learmonth L, Bone H, et al: Interleukin-13 signal transduction in lymphohemopoietic cells, *J Biol Chem* 270:12286, 1995.

26. Schindler C, Kashleva H, Pernis A, et al: STF-IL-4: a novel IL-4-induced signal transducing factor, *EMBO J* 13:1350, 1994.

27. Ivashkiv L: Cytokines and STATs: how can signals achieve specificity? *Immunity* 3:1, 1995.

28. Grewal I, Flavell R: A central role of CD40 ligand in the regulation of CD4+ T-cell responses, *Immunol Today* 17:410, 1996.

29. Cheng G, Cleary AM, Ye Z, et al: Involvement of CRAF1, a relative of TRAF, in CD40 signaling, *Science* 267:494, 1995.

30. Ishida T, Mizushima S, Azuma S, et al: Identification of TRAF6, a novel tumor necrosis factor receptor-associated protein that mediates signaling from an amino-terminal domain of the CD40 cytoplasmic region, *J Biol Chem* 271:28745, 1996.

31. Messner B, Stutz A, Albrecht B, et al: Cooperation of binding sites for STAT6 and NFkB/rel in the IL-4-induced up-regulation of the human IgE germline promoter, *J Immunol* 159:3330, 1997.

32. Iciek LA, Delphin SA, Stavnezer J: CD40 cross-linking induces Ig epsilon germline transcripts in B cells via activation of NF-kappaB: synergy with IL-4 induction, *J Immunol* 158:4769, 1997.

33. Ren C, Morio T, Fu S, et al: Signal transduction via CD40 involves activation of lyn kinase and phosphatidylinositol-3-kinase, and phosphorylation of phospholipase C gamma 2, *J Exp Med* 179:673, 1994.

34. Faris M, Gaskin F, Geha R, et al: Tyrosine phosphorylation defines a unique transduction pathway in human B cells mediated via CD40, *Trans Assoc Am Phys* 106:187, 1993.

35. Allen RC, Armitage RJ, Conley ME, et al: CD40 ligand gene defects responsible for X-linked hyper-IgM syndrome [see comments], *Science* 259:990, 1993.

36. Aruffo A, Farrington M, Hollenbaugh D, et al: The CD40 ligand, gp39, is defective in activated T cells from patients with X-linked hyper-IgM syndrome, *Cell* 72:291, 1993.

37. Fuleihan R, Ramesh N, Loh R, et al: Defective expression of the CD40 ligand in X chromosome-linked immunoglobulin deficiency with normal or elevated IgM, *Proc Natl Acad Sci U S A* 90:2170, 1993.

38. DiSanto JP, Bonnefoy JY, Gauchat JF, et al: CD40 ligand mutations in x-linked immunodeficiency with hyper-IgM [see comments], *Nature* 361:541, 1993.

39. Korthauer U, Graf D, Mages HW, et al: Defective expression of T-cell CD40 ligand causes X-linked immunodeficiency with hyper-IgM [see comments], *Nature* 361:539, 1993.

40. Xu J, Foy T, Laman J, et al: Mice deficient for CD40 ligand, *Immunity* 1:423, 1994.

41. Castigli E, Alt FW, Davidson L, et al: CD40-deficient mice generated by recombination-activating gene-2-deficient blastocyst complementation, *Proc Natl Acad Sci U S A* 91:12135, 1994.

42. Kawabe T, Naka T, Yoshida K, et al: The immune responses in CD40-deficient mice: impaired immunoglobulin class switching and germinal center formation, *Immunity* 1:167, 1994.

43. Muramatsu M, Sankaranand VS, Anant S, et al: Specific expression of activation-induced cytidine deaminase (AID), a novel member of the RNA-editing deaminase family in germinal center B cells, *J Biol Chem* 274:18470, 1999.

44. Muramatsu M, Kinoshita K, Fagarasan S, et al: Class switch recombination and hypermutation require activation-induced cytidine deaminase (AID), a potential RNA editing enzyme [see comments], *Cell* 102:553, 2000.

45. Revy P, Muto T, Levy Y, et al: Activation-induced cytidine deaminase (AID) deficiency causes the autosomal recessive form of the Hyper-IgM syndrome (HIGM2) [see comments], *Cell* 102:565, 2000.

46. Okazaki IM, Kinoshita K, Muramatsu M, et al: The AID enzyme induces class switch recombination in fibroblasts, *Nature* 416:340, 2002.

47. Petersen S, Casellas R, Reina-San-Martin B, et al: AID is required to initiate Nbs1/gamma-H2AX focus formation and mutations at sites of class switching, *Nature* 414:660, 2001.

48. Reaban ME, Griffin JA: Induction of RNA-stabilized DNA conformers by transcription of an immunoglobulin switch region [see comments], *Nature* 348:342, 1990.

49. Stavnezer J: Triple helix stabilization? [letter; comment], *Nature* 351:447, 1991.

50. Daniels GA, Lieber MR: RNA:DNA complex formation upon transcription of immunoglobulin switch regions: implications for the mechanism and regulation of class switch recombination, *Nucleic Acids Res* 23:5006, 1995.

51. Tian M, Alt FW: Transcription-induced cleavage of immunoglobulin switch regions by nucleotide excision repair nucleases in vitro, *J Biol Chem* 275:24163, 2000.

52. Manis JP, Tian M, Alt FW: Mechanism and control of class-switch recombination, *Trends Immunol* 23:31, 2002.

53. Rolink A, Melchers F, Andersson J: The SCID but not the RAG-2 gene product is required for S mu-S epsilon heavy chain class switching, *Immunity* 5:319, 1996.

54. Manis JP, Gu Y, Lansford R, et al: Ku70 is required for late B cell development and immunoglobulin heavy chain class switching, *J Exp Med* 187:2081, 1998.

55. Manis JP, Dudley D, Kaylor L, et al: IgH class switch recombination to IgG1 in DNA-PKcs-deficient B cells, *Immunity* 16:607, 2002.

56. Mossman TR, Cherwinski H, Bond MW, et al: Two types of murine helper T cell clone: definition according to profiles of lymphokine activities and secreted proteins, *J Immunol* 136:2348, 1986.

57. Sallusto F, Mackay CR, Lanzavecchia A: Selective expression of the eotaxin receptor CCR3 by human T helper 2 cells, *Science* 277:2005, 1997.

58. Annunziato F, Galli G, Cosmi L, et al: Molecules associated with human Th1 or Th2 cells, *Eur Cytokine Netw* 9:12, 1998.

59. Coyle AJ, Lloyd C, Tian J, et al: Crucial role of the interleukin 1 receptor family member T1/ST2 in T helper cell type 2-mediated lung mucosal immune responses, *J Exp Med* 190:895, 1999.

60. Sallusto F, Mackay CR, Lanzavecchia A: The role of chemokine receptors in primary, effector, and memory immune responses, *Annu Rev Immunol* 18:593, 2000.

61. Avni O, Rao A: T cell differentiation: a mechanistic view, *Curr Opin Immunol* 12:654, 2000.

62. Young HA, Ghosh P, Ye J, et al: Differentiation of the T helper phenotypes by analysis of the methylation state of the IFN-gamma gene, *J Immunol* 153:3603, 1994.

63. Melvin AJ, McGurn ME, Bort SJ, et al: Hypomethylation of the interferon-gamma gene correlates with its expression by primary T-lineage cells, *Eur J Immunol* 25:426, 1995.

64. Fitzpatrick DR, Shirley KM, McDonald LE, et al: Distinct methylation of the interferon gamma (IFN-gamma) and interleukin 3 (IL-3) genes in newly activated primary CD8+ T lymphocytes: regional IFN-gamma promoter demethylation and mRNA expression are heritable in CD44(high)CD8+ T cells, *J Exp Med* 188:103, 1998.

65. Viola JP, Rao A: Molecular regulation of cytokine gene expression during the immune response, *J Clin Immunol* 19:98, 1999.

66. Sadick MD, Locksley RM, Tubbs C, et al: Murine cutaneous leishmaniasis: resistance correlates with the capacity to generate interferon-gamma in response to *Leishmania* antigens in vitro, *J Immunol* 136:655, 1986.

67. Sadick MD, Heinzel FP, Shigekane VM, et al: Cellular and humoral immunity to Leishmania major in genetically susceptible mice after in vivo depletion of L3T4+ T cells, *J Immunol* 139:1303, 1987.

68. Pritchard DI, Hewitt C, Moqbel R: The relationship between immunological responsiveness controlled by T-helper 2 lymphocytes and infections with parasitic helminths, *Parasitology* 115:S33, 1997.

69. Murphy KM, Ouyang W, Szabo SJ, et al: T helper differentiation proceeds through Stat1-dependent, Stat4-dependent and Stat4-independent phases, *Curr Top Microbiol Immunol* 238:13, 1999.

70. Kalinski P, Hilkens CM, Wierenga EA, et al: T-cell priming by type-1 and type-2 polarized dendritic cells: the concept of a third signal, *Immunol Today* 20:561, 1999.

71. Kalinski P, Schuitemaker JH, Hilkens CM, et al: Prostaglandin E2 induces the final maturation of IL-12-deficient CD1a+ CD83+ dendritic cells: the levels of IL-12 are determined during the final dendritic cell maturation and are resistant to further modulation, *J Immunol* 161:2804, 1998.

72. Vieira PL, de Jong EC, Wierenga EA, et al: Development of Th1-inducing capacity in myeloid dendritic cells requires environmental instruction, *J Immunol* 164:4507, 2000.

73. Mazzoni A, Young HA, Spitzer JH, et al: Histamine regulates cytokine production in maturing dendritic cells, resulting in altered T cell polarization, *J Clin Invest* 108:1865, 2001.

74. Dabbagh K, Dahl ME, Stepick-Biek P, et al: Toll-like receptor 4 is required for optimal development of Th2 immune responses: role of dendritic cells, *J Immunol* 168:4524, 2002.

75. Galli SJ: Complexity and redundancy in the pathogenesis of asthma: reassessing the roles of mast cells and T cells, *J Exp Med* 186:343, 1997.

76. Toru H, Pawankar R, Ra C, et al: Human mast cells produce IL-13 by high-affinity IgE receptor cross-linking: enhanced IL-13 production by IL-4-primed human mast cells, *J Allergy Clin Immunol* 102:491, 1998.

77. Yoshimoto T, Bendelac A, Hu-Li J, et al: Defective IgE production by SJL mice is linked to the absence of CD4+, NK1.1+ T cells that promptly produce interleukin 4, *Proc Natl Acad Sci U S A* 92:11931, 1995.

78. Bendelac A, Hunziker RD, Lantz O: Increased interleukin 4 and immunoglobulin E production in transgenic mice overexpressing NK1 T cells, *J Exp Med* 184:1285, 1996.

79. Peritt D, Robertson S, Gri G, et al: Differentiation of human NK cells into NK1 and NK2 subsets, *J Immunol* 161:5821, 1998.

80. Hoshino T, Winkler-Pickett RT, Mason AT, et al: IL-13 production by NK cells: IL-13-producing NK and T cells are present in vivo in the absence of IFN-gamma, *J Immunol* 162:51, 1999.

81. Deniz G, Akdis M, Aktas E, et al: Human NK1 and NK2 subsets determined by purification of IFN-gamma-secreting and IFN-gamma-nonsecreting NK cells, *Eur J Immunol* 32:879, 2002.

82. Kinet JP: The high-affinity IgE receptor (Fc epsilon RI): from physiology to pathology, *Annu Rev Immunol* 17:931, 1999.

83. Lin S, Cicala C, Scharenberg AM, et al: The Fc (epsilon) RI beta subunit functions as an amplifier of Fc (epsilon) RI gamma-mediated cell activation signals, *Cell* 85:985, 1996.

84. Dombrowicz D, Lin S, Flamand V, et al: Allergy-associated FcRbeta is a molecular amplifier of IgE- and IgG-mediated in vivo responses, *Immunity* 8:517, 1998.

85. Donnadieu E, Jouvin MH, Kinet JP: A second amplifier function for the allergy-associated Fc (epsilon) RI-beta subunit, *Immunity* 12:515, 2000.

86. Vander-Mallie R, Ishizaka T, Ishizaka K: Lymphocyte bearing Fc receptors for IgE. VIII: affinity of mouse IgE for FceR on mouse B lymphocytes, *J Immunol* 128:2306, 1982.

87. Lee WT, Conrad DH: Murine B cell hybridomas bearing ligand-inducible Fc receptors for IgE, *J Immunol* 136:4573, 1986.

88. Delespesse G, Sarfati M, Hofstetter H, et al: Structure, function and clinical relevance of the low-affinity receptor for IgE, *Immunol Invest* 17:363, 1988.

89. Kikutani H, Inui S, Sato R, et al: Molecular structure of human lymphocyte receptor for immunoglobulin E, *Cell* 47:657, 1986.

90. Bettler B, Hofstetter H, Rao M, et al: Molecular structure and expression of the murine lymphocyte low-affinity receptor for IgE (Fc epsilon RII), *Proc Natl Acad Sci U S A* 86:7566, 1989.

91. Dierks SE, Bartlett WC, Edmeades RL, et al: The oligomeric nature of the murine Fc epsilon RII/CD23: implications for function, *J Immunol* 150:2372, 1993.

92. Rivera J, Gonzalez-Espinosa C, Kovarova M, et al: The architecture of IgE-dependent mast cell signalling, *ACI International* 14:25, 2002.

93. Pivniouk VI, Martin TR, Lu-Kuo JM, et al: SLP-76 deficiency impairs signaling via the high-affinity IgE receptor in mast cells, *J Clin Invest* 103:1737, 1999.

94. Saitoh S, Arudchandran R, Manetz TS, et al: LAT is essential for Fc(epsilon)RI-mediated mast cell activation, *Immunity* 12:525, 2000.

95. Manetz TS, Gonzalez-Espinosa C, Arudchandran R, et al: Vav1 regulates phospholipase cgamma activation and calcium responses in mast cells, *Mol Cell Biol* 21:3763, 2001.

96. Song JS, Gomez J, Stancato LF, et al: Association of a p95 Vav-containing signaling complex with the Fc epsilonRI gamma chain in the RBL-2H3 mast cell line: evidence for a constitutive in vivo association of Vav with Grb2, Raf-1, and ERK2 in an active complex, *J Biol Chem* 271:26962, 1996.

97. Howarth PH, Durham SR, Kay AB, et al: The relationship between mast cell-mediator release and bronchial reactivity in allergic asthma, *J Allergy Clin Immunol* 80:703, 1987.

98. Shampain MP, Behrens BL, Larsen GL, et al: An animal model of late pulmonary responses to Alternaria challenge, *Am Rev Respir Dis* 126:493, 1982.

99. Cockcroft DW, Murdock KY: Comparative effects of inhaled salbutamol, sodium cromoglycate and beclomethasone dipropionate on allergen-induced early asthmatic responses, late asthmatic responses and increased bronchial responsiveness to histamine, *J Allergy Clin Immunol* 79:734, 1987.

100. Cartier A, Thomson NC, Frith PA, et al: Allergen-induced increase in bronchial responsiveness to histamine: relationship to the late asthmatic response and change in airway caliber, *J Allergy Clin Immunol* 70:170, 1982.

101. McFadden ER, Gilbert IA: Asthma, *N Engl J Med* 327:1928, 1992.

102. Asai K, Kitaura J, Kawakami Y, et al: Regulation of mast cell survival by IgE, *Immunity* 14:791, 2001.

103. Kalesnikoff J, Huber M, Lam V, et al: Monomeric IgE stimulates signaling pathways in mast cells that lead to cytokine production and cell survival, *Immunity* 14:801, 2001.

104. Yamaguchi M, Lantz CS, Oettgen HC, et al: IgE enhances mouse mast cell FceRI expression in vitro and in vivo: evidence for a novel amplification mechanism for IgE-dependent reactions, *J Exp Med* 185:663, 1997.

105. Lantz CS, Yamaguchi M, Oettgen HC, et al: IgE regulates mouse basophil Fc epsilon RI expression in vivo, *J Immunol* 158:2517, 1997.

106. Yamaguchi M, Sayama K, Yano K, et al: IgE enhances Fc epsilon receptor I expression and IgE-dependent release of histamine and lipid mediators from human umbilical cord blood-derived mast cells: synergistic effect of IL-4 and IgE on human mast cell Fc epsilon receptor I expression and mediator release, *J Immunol* 162:5455, 1999.

107. Saini SS, MacGlashan DW Jr, Sterbinsky SA, et al: Down-regulation of human basophil IgE and FC epsilon RI alpha surface densities and mediator release by anti-IgE-infusions is reversible in vitro and in vivo, *J Immunol* 162:5624, 1999.

108. Lee WT, Rao M, Conrad DH: The murine lymphocyte receptor for IgE. IV. The mechanism of ligand-specific receptor upregulation on B cells, *J Immunol* 139:1191, 1987.

109. Kisselgof AB, Oettgen HC: The expression of murine B cell CD23, in vivo, is regulated by its ligand, IgE, *Int Immunol* 10:1377, 1998.

110. Borkowski TA, Jouvin MH, Lin SY, et al: Minimal requirements for IgE-mediated regulation of surface Fc epsilon RI, *J Immunol* 167:1290, 2001.

111. Kehry MR, Yamashita LC: Low-affinity IgE receptor (CD23) function on mouse B cells: role in IgE-dependent antigen focusing, *Proc Natl Acad Sci U S A* 86:7556, 1989.

112. Pirron U, Schlunck T, Prinz JC, et al: IgE-dependent antigen focusing by human B lymphocytes is mediated by the low-affinity receptor for IgE, *Eur J Immunol* 20:1547, 1990.

113. van der Heijden FL, Joost van Neerven RJ, van Katwijk M, et al: Serum-IgE-facilitated allergen presentation in atopic disease, *J Immunol* 150:643, 1993.

114. Heyman B, Liu T, Gustavsson S: In vivo enhancement of the specific antibody response via the low-affinity receptor for IgE, *Eur J Immunol* 23:1739, 1993.

115. Gustavsson S, Hjulstrom S, Liu T, et al: CD23/IgE-mediated regulation of the specific antibody response in vivo, *J Immunol* 152:4793, 1994.

116. Fujiwara H, Kikutani H, Suematsu S, et al: The absence of IgE antibody-mediated augmentation of immune responses in CD23-deficient mice, *Proc Natl Acad Sci U S A* 91:6835, 1994.

117. Gustavsson S, Wernersson S, Heyman B: Restoration of the antibody response to IgE/antigen complexes in CD23-deficient mice by CD23+ spleen or bone marrow cells, *J Immunol* 164:3990, 2000.

118. Sherr E, Macy E, Kimata H, et al: Binding the low-affinity Fc epsilon R on B cells suppresses ongoing human IgE synthesis, *J Immunol* 142:481, 1989.

119. Payet ME, Woodward EC, Conrad DH: Humoral response suppression observed with CD23 transgenics, *J Immunol* 163:217, 1999.
120. Payet-Jamroz M, Helm SL, Wu J, et al: Suppression of IgE responses in CD23-transgenic animals is due to expression of CD23 on nonlymphoid cells, *J Immunol* 166:4863, 2001.
121. Yu P, Kosco-Vilbois M, Richards M, et al: Negative feedback regulation of IgE synthesis by murine CD23, *Nature* 369:753, 1994.
122. Haczku A, Takeda K, Hamelmann E, et al: CD23 deficient mice develop allergic airway hyperresponsiveness following sensitization with ovalbumin, *Am J Respir Crit Care Med* 156:1945, 1997.
123. Cernadas M, De Sanctis GT, Krinzman SJ, et al: CD23 and allergic pulmonary inflammation: potential role as an inhibitor, *Am J Respir Cell Mol Biol* 20:1, 1999.
124. Haczku A, Takeda K, Hamelmann E, et al: CD23 exhibits negative regulatory effects on allergic sensitization and airway hyperresponsiveness, *Am J Respir Crit Care Med* 161:952, 2000.
125. Riffo-Vasquez Y, Spina D, Thomas M, et al: The role of CD23 on allergen-induced IgE levels, pulmonary eosinophilia and bronchial hyperresponsiveness in mice, *Clin Exp Allergy* 30:728, 2000.
126. Saxon A, Ke Z, Bahati L, et al: Soluble CD23 containing B cell supernatants induce IgE from peripheral blood B-lymphocytes and costimulate with interleukin-4 in induction of IgE, *J Allergy Clin Immunol* 86:333, 1990.
127. Uchibayashi N, Kikutani H, Barsumian EL, et al: Recombinant soluble Fc epsilon receptor II (Fc epsilon RII/CD23) has IgE binding activity but no B cell growth promoting activity, *J Immunol* 142:3901, 1989.
128. Schulz O, Sutton BJ, Beavil RL, et al: Cleavage of the low-affinity receptor for human IgE (CD23) by a mite cysteine protease: nature of the cleaved fragment in relation to the structure and function of CD23, *Eur J Immunol* 27:584, 1997.
129. Gough L, Schulz O, Sewell HF, et al: The cysteine protease activity of the major dust mite allergen Der p 1 selectively enhances the immunoglobulin E antibody response, *J Exp Med* 190:1897, 1999.
130. Mayer RJ, Bolognese BJ, Al-Mahdi N, et al: Inhibition of CD23 processing correlates with inhibition of IL-4-stimulated IgE production in human PBL and hu-PBL-reconstituted SCID mice, *Clin Exp Allergy* 30:719, 2000.
131. Christie G, Barton A, Bolognese B, et al: IgE secretion is attenuated by an inhibitor of proteolytic processing of CD23 (Fc epsilonRII), *Eur J Immunol* 27:3228, 1997.

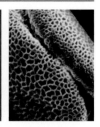

CHAPTER 5

Inflammatory Effector Cells/Cell Migration

MARC E. ROTHENBERG

One of the hallmarks of allergic disorders is the accumulation of an abnormally large number of leukocytes, including eosinophils, neutrophils, lymphocytes, basophils, and macrophages, in the inflammatory tissue. There is substantial evidence that inflammatory cells are major effector cells in the pathogenesis of allergic disorders. Therefore understanding the mechanisms by which leukocytes accumulate and are activated in tissues is very relevant to allergic diseases. During the past decade, substantial progress has been made in understanding the specific molecules involved in leukocyte migration and the specific mechanisms by which effector cells participate in disease pathogenesis. In particular, cellular adhesion proteins, integrins, and chemoattractant cytokines (chemokines) have emerged as critical molecules in these processes. Chemokines are potent leukocyte chemoattractants, cellular activating factors, and histamine-releasing factors, making them attractive new therapeutic targets for the treatment of allergic disease. This chapter focuses on recently emerging data on the mechanisms by which specific leukocyte subsets are recruited into allergic tissues and the mechanisms by which they participate in disease pathogenesis.

ALLERGIC INFLAMMATION

Experimentation in the allergy field has largely focused on analysis of the cellular and molecular events induced by allergen exposure in sensitized animals (primarily mice) and humans.[1-3] In patient studies, naturally sensitized individuals are challenged by exposure to allergen (e.g., segmental antigen challenge for analysis of asthmatic responses).[4] In the animal models, mice are typically subjected to sensitization with antigen (e.g., ovalbumin [OVA]) in the presence of adjuvant (e.g., alum) via intraperitoneal injection.[5] Subsequently, mice are challenged by exposure to mucosal allergen (via intratracheal, intranasal, nebulized, or cutaneous routes) and pathologic responses are monitored. In other animal models, nonsensitized mice are repeatedly exposed to mucosal allergens (e.g., extracts of *Aspergillus fumigatus*) and the development of experimental allergy is monitored.[6] Although no animal model adequately mimics human disease, experimentation in animals has provided a framework to dissect key cells and molecules involved in the pathogenesis of allergic responses.

The animal and human experimental systems have demonstrated that allergic inflammatory responses are often biphasic. For example, asthma is characterized by a biphasic bronchospasm response, consisting of an early-phase asthmatic response (EAR) and a late-phase asthmatic response (LAR)[7] (Figure 5-1). The EAR phase is characterized by immediate bronchoconstriction in the absence of pronounced airway inflammation or morphologic changes in the airway tissue.[7,8] The EAR phase has been shown to directly involve IgE mast cell–mediated release of spasmogens (histamine, prostaglandin D_2, and cysteinyl-peptide leukotrienes [LTC_4, LTD_4, LTE_4]), which are potent mediators of bronchoconstriction. After the immediate response, individuals with asthma often experience an LAR, which is characterized by more persistent bronchoconstriction associated with extensive airway inflammation and morphologic changes to the airways.[7,9-11] Clinical investigations have demonstrated that the LAR is associated with increased levels of inflammatory cells, in particular activated T-lymphocytes and eosinophils (see Figure 5-1). The elevated levels of T-lymphocytes and eosinophils correlate with increased levels of eosinophilic constituents in the bronchoalveolar lavage fluid (BALF), the degree of airway epithelial cell damage, enhanced bronchial responsiveness to inhaled spasmogens, and disease severity.[7,10-17] Analysis of tissue biopsy samples from patients with allergic disorders has revealed that chronic inflammation is associated with a variety of processes, including tissue remodeling. For example, asthmatic tissue is characterized by the accumulation of a large number of inflammatory cells (e.g., eosinophils, neutrophils, basophils, mast cells), increased mucus production, epithelial shedding and hypertrophy, mucus and smooth muscle cell hyperplasia/metaplasia, hyperplasia and metaplasia of submucosal mucus glands, and fibrosis (with deposition of collagen types I, III, and V).[2,18-23]

In summary, allergic responses involve a complex interplay of diverse cells including infiltrating leukocytes (under the regulation of chemokines) and residential cells including endothelial, epithelial, and smooth muscle cells.[2,18,21] This interface results in elevated production of IgE, mucus, eosinophils, complement proteins, and enhanced tissue reactivity to stimulants (e.g., hyperresponsiveness to spasmogens in the case of asthma).[22,23]

Effector Cells

T cells

T cells are specialized leukocytes distinguished by their expression of antigen-specific receptors that arise from somatic gene rearrangement. Two major subpopulations were originally

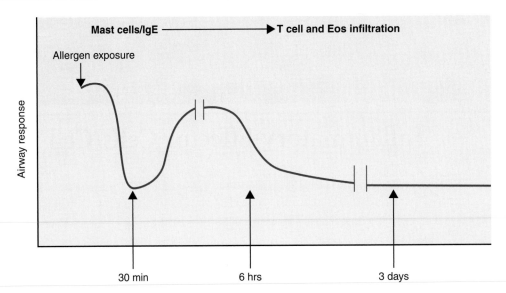

FIGURE 5-1 Early- and late-phase allergic responses. Animal and human experimental systems have demonstrated that allergic inflammatory responses are often biphasic. The airway response (e.g., forced expiratory volume in the first second [FEV$_1$]) is illustrated when an allergen-sensitized individual is experimentally exposed to an allergen; a biphasic bronchospasm response, consisting of an early-phase asthmatic response (EAR) and a late-phase asthmatic response (LAR), is shown. The EAR phase is characterized by immediate bronchoconstriction in the absence of pronounced airway inflammation or morphologic changes in the airways tissue. The EAR phase has been shown to directly involve IgE mast cell–mediated release of spasmogens (histamine, prostaglandin D$_2$, and cysteinyl-peptide leukotrienes [LTC$_4$, LTD$_4$, LTE$_4$]), which are potent mediators of bronchoconstriction. After the immediate response, the airway recovers but later undergoes marked decline in function, which is characterized by more persistent bronchoconstriction associated with extensive airway inflammation (involving T cells and eosinophils).

defined based on the expression of the CD4 and CD8 antigens and their associated function. CD4+ T cells recognize antigen in association with MHC class II molecules and are primarily involved in orchestrating immune responses (e.g., B cell antibody secretion), whereas CD8+ cells recognize antigen in association with MHC class I molecules and are primarily involved in cytotoxicity. More recently, populations of regulatory T cells have been characterized. Regulatory T cells include a subpopulation of natural killer (NK) T cells (generally CD1a+), as well as CD4+ CD25+ T cells; both populations appear to be chief sources of regulatory cytokines, including interleukin (IL)-4 and IL-10.[24]

Extensive characterization of the immunopathogenesis of allergic disorders and studies in animal models of allergic airway inflammation suggest that CD4+ T-lymphocytes have central roles in allergic responses by regulating the production of IgE and the effector function of mast cells and eosinophils.[25] CD4+ T-lymphocytes can be divided into two distinct subsets, which are primarily based on their restricted cytokine profiles and different immune functions (Figure 5-2). CD4+ Th1-type T-lymphocytes produce IL-2, tumor necrosis factor (TNF)-β (lymphotoxin), and interferon (IFN)-γ and are involved in delayed-type hypersensitivity responses. Th2-lymphocytes (Th2 cells) secrete IL-4, IL-5, IL-9, IL-10, and IL-13 and promote antibody responses and allergic inflammation (see Figure 5-2).

Both subsets produce IL-3 and granulocyte-macrophage colony-stimulating factor (GM-CSF). Clinical investigations indicate that CD4+ T-lymphocytes are activated and are predominantly of the Th2-type subclass in allergic disorders. Notably, there is a strong correlation between the presence of

CD4+ Th2 lymphocytes and disease severity, suggesting an integral role for these cells in the pathophysiology of allergic diseases.[26,27] Th2 cells are thought to induce asthma through the secretion of an array of cytokines that activate inflammatory and residential effector pathways both directly and indirectly.[28] In particular, IL-4 and IL-13 are produced at elevated levels in the allergic tissue and are thought to be central regulators of many of the hallmark features of the disease.[29] However, in addition to Th2 cells, inflammatory cells (e.g., eosinophils, basophils, and mast cells) within the allergic tissue also produce IL-4, IL-13, and a variety of other cytokines.[30,31] IL-4 promotes Th2 cell differentiation, IgE production, tissue eosinophilia, and, in the case of asthma, morphologic changes to the respiratory epithelium and airway hyperreactivity.[32,33] IL-13 induces IgE production, mucus hypersecretion, eosinophil recruitment and survival, airway hyperreactivity, the expression of CD23, adhesion systems, and chemokines (e.g., eotaxin-1).[29,34,35] IL-4 and IL-13 share similar signaling requirements such as utilization of the IL-4 receptor (R) α chain and the induction of Janus kinase 1 and signal transducer and activator of transcription (STAT)-6.[36-38] A critical role for IL-13 in orchestration of experimental asthma has been suggested by the finding that a soluble IL-13 receptor homologue blocks many of the essential features of experimental asthma.[39,40] Furthermore, mice deficient in the IL-4Rα chain have impaired development of certain features of asthma (e.g., eosinophil recruitment and mucus production) but still develop airway hyperreactivity.[41] Mice with the targeted deletion of STAT-6 have impaired development of asthma including inflammatory cell infiltrates, IL-13 production, and airway hyperreactivity.[42-45] Collectively, these studies

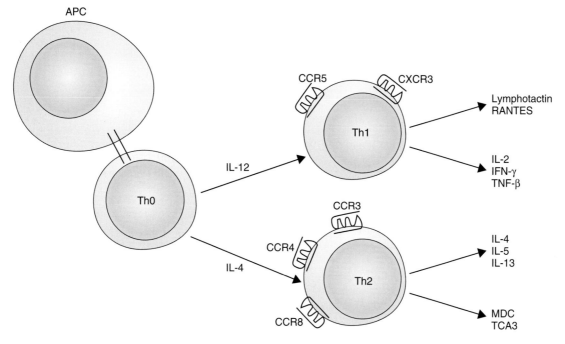

FIGURE 5-2 Chemokine and chemokine receptor expression by Th1 and Th2 cells. Th0 cells differentiate into Th1 or Th2 cells following their activation by antigen-presenting cells *(APCs)*. IL-12 promotes the development of Th1 cells that preferentially express CCR5 and CXCR3. IL-4 promotes the development of Th2 cells that preferentially express CCR3, CCR4, and CCR8. In addition to expressing distinct cytokines (IL-2, IL-4, IL-5, IL-13, and IFN-γ), murine T cells have recently been shown to express a unique panel of chemokines, as indicated.

have provided the rationale for the development of multiple therapeutic agents that interfere with specific inflammatory pathways.[46,47] We are in the early stages of clinical trials with therapeutic agents that block effector phases of allergic responses such as anti-IgE, anti-IL-4, and anti-IL-5[21] (Box 5-1).

Eosinophils
Eosinophils are multifunctional proinflammatory leukocytes implicated in the pathogenesis of numerous inflammatory processes, especially allergic disorders.[48,49] In addition, it was recently recognized that eosinophils may have a physiologic role in organ morphogenesis (e.g., postgestational mammary gland development).[50] Eosinophils selectively express the receptor for IL-5, a cytokine that regulates eosinophil expansion (during allergic states) and eosinophil survival (by inhibition of eosinophil apoptosis) and primes eosinophils to respond to appropriate activating signals. Mice deficient in IL-5 have markedly reduced allergen-induced bone marrow and blood eosinophilia and eosinophil recruitment to the lung. In addition, IL-5−deficient mice have impaired development of airway hyperreactivity in certain strains of mice. Eosinophils also express numerous receptors (for chemokines [e.g., eotaxin, an eosinophil-selective chemoattractant], immunoglobulin, and complement proteins) that when engaged lead to eosinophil activation, resulting in several processes, including the release of toxic secondary granule proteins[31] (Figure 5-3). The secondary granule contains a crystalloid core composed of major basic protein (MBP) and a granule matrix that is mainly composed of eosinophil cationic protein (ECP), eosinophil neurotoxin (EDN), and eosinophil peroxidase (EPO). These proteins elicit potent cytotoxic effects on a variety of host tissues

BOX 5-1	**KEY CONCEPTS**
	T Cells

- Mature T cells are primarily divided into CD4+ and CD8+ cells.
- T cells express antigen-specific T cell receptors (TCR) that recognize antigen in the context of major histocompatibility molecules (MHC).
- CD4+ T cells are engaged by antigen in the context of class II molecules.
- CD4+ T cells are divided into Th1 and Th2 cells.
- Th1 cells are major producers of Th1 cytokines (e.g., interferon-gamma) and Th2 cells are major producers of Th2 cytokines (e.g., IL-4, IL-5, IL-13).

at concentrations similar to those found in biologic fluid from patients with eosinophilia. The cytotoxic effects of eosinophils may be elicited through multiple mechanisms including degrading cellular ribonucleic acid because ECP and EDN have substantial functional and structural homology to a large family of ribonuclease genes.[51,52] Notably, ECP and EDN are the most divergent family of coding sequences in the human genome (compared with other species), even though their homologues have conserved RNase activity. The strong positive evolutionary pressure to modulate this family of proteins suggests a critical role for these enzymes and eosinophils in host survival, perhaps related to the antiviral activity of these molecules. ECP also inserts ion-nonselective pores into the mem-

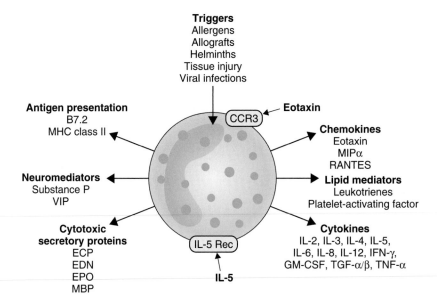

Triggers
Allergens
Allografts
Helminths
Tissue injury
Viral infections

Antigen presentation
B7.2
MHC class II

Eotaxin

CCR3

Chemokines
Eotaxin
MIPα
RANTES

Neuromediators
Substance P
VIP

Lipid mediators
Leukotrienes
Platelet-activating factor

Cytotoxic secretory proteins
ECP
EDN
EPO
MBP

IL-5 Rec

IL-5

Cytokines
IL-2, IL-3, IL-4, IL-5,
IL-6, IL-8, IL-12, IFN-γ,
GM-CSF, TGF-α/β, TNF-α

FIGURE 5-3 Schematic diagram of an eosinophil and its diverse properties. Eosinophils are bilobed granulocytes that respond to diverse stimuli including allergens, helminths, viral infections, allografts, and nonspecific tissue injury. Eosinophils express the receptor for IL-5, a critical eosinophil growth, differentiation, activating, and survival factor, as well as the receptor for eotaxin and related chemokines (CCR3). The secondary granules contain four primary cationic proteins designated eosinophil peroxidase *(EPO)*, major basic protein *(MBP)*, eosinophil cationic protein *(ECP)*, and eosinophil derived neurotoxin *(EDN)*. All four proteins are cytotoxic molecules; in addition, ECP and EDN are ribonucleases. In addition to releasing their preformed cationic proteins, eosinophils can release a variety of cytokines (e.g., IL-2, IL-3, IL-4, IL-5, IL-6, IL-8, IL-12, IFN-γ, GM-CSF, TGF-α/β, and TNF-α), chemokines (e.g., eotaxin, RANTES, and MIP-1α), and neuromediators (substance P and vasoactive intestinal peptide *[VIP]*) and generate large amounts of LTC₄. Last, eosinophils can be induced to express MHC class II and costimulatory (e.g., B7.2) molecules and may be involved in propagating immune responses by presenting antigen to T cells.

branes of target cells, which may allow the entry of the cytotoxic proteins.[53] Further proinflammatory damage is caused by the generation of unstable oxygen radicals formed by the respiratory burst oxidase apparatus and EPO. Furthermore, direct degranulation of mast cells and basophils is triggered by MBP. In addition to being cytotoxic, MBP directly increases smooth muscle reactivity by causing dysfunction of vagal muscarinic M2 receptors.[54] By acting as a competitive inhibitor of M2 receptors, MBP increases acetylcholine release that is likely to be at least one mechanism for induction of airway hyperresponsiveness.[55] Vagal dysfunction induced by eosinophil MBP may be an important pathway involved in asthma where eosinophils frequently cluster around airway nerves, and the release of MBP is seen in fatal asthma.[55] Activation of eosinophils also leads to the generation of large amounts of LTC₄, which induces increased vascular permeability, mucous secretion, and smooth muscle constriction.[56] Also, activated eosinophils generate a wide range of cytokines including IL-1, -3, -4, -5, and -13; GM-CSF; transforming growth factor (TGF)-α/β; TNF-α; RANTES (regulated on activation, normal T cells expressed and secreted); macrophage inflammatory protein (MIP)-1α; and eotaxin, indicating that they have the potential to sustain or augment multiple aspects of the immune response, inflammatory reaction, and tissue repair process.[30] Eosinophils also produce neuroactive mediators (e.g., substance P and vasoactive intestinal peptide [VIP]).[57] Interestingly, specimens from pa-

tients with eosinophilic disorders often display eosinophils undergoing marked degranulation near nerves, suggesting that they may indeed be involved in promoting inflammatory changes to neurons.[58,59] The gastric dysmotility during experimental oral antigen–induced gastrointestinal inflammation is associated with eosinophils in the proximity of damaged nerves, suggesting a causal role for eosinophils in nerve dysfunction.[60] Also, experimental eosinophil accumulation in the gastrointestinal tract is associated with the development of weight loss, which is attenuated in eotaxin-deficient mice that have a deficiency in gastrointestinal eosinophils.[61] Finally, eosinophils have the capacity to initiate antigen-specific immune responses by acting as antigen-presenting cells. Consistent with this, eosinophils express relevant co-stimulatory molecules (CD40, CD28, CD86, B7),[62,63] secrete cytokines capable of inducing T cell proliferation and maturation (IL-2, IL-4, IL-6, IL-10, IL-12),[30,64,65] and can be induced to express MHC class II molecules.[64] Interestingly, experimental adoptive transfer of antigen-pulsed eosinophils induces antigen-specific T cell responses *in vivo*[66] (Box 5-2).

Mast Cells
Mast cells are major effector cells involved in allergic responses; in addition, they are important cytokine-producing cells that are involved in nonallergic processes such as the innate immune responses (Figure 5-4). In contrast to other hematopoietic cells that complete their differentiation in the

bone marrow, mast cell progenitors leave the bone marrow and complete their differentiation in tissues (e.g., skin, gastrointestinal tract, respiratory mucosa, and conjunctiva). Elegant studies in mice have demonstrated that mast cell development from bone marrow cells is dependent on IL-3, and their tissue differentiation is primarily dependent on stem cell factor (SCF). These studies have been primarily conducted in two mast cell–deficient strains of mice: one strain has a homozygous deficiency in the white spotting locus (*W*), whereas the other strain has deficiencies at the steel locus (*Sl*).[67] Mice deficient in the *W* locus can be cured by adoptive transfer of normal bone marrow because they are deficient in the SCF receptor (*c-kit*), whereas mice deficient in the *Sl* locus cannot be cured with adaptive transfer of bone marrow because they are deficient in SCF itself.[68,69] Mast cell–deficient mice have been instrumental in defining the critical role of mast cells in experimental anaphylaxis and bacterial peritonitis.[70-72] In addition, mast cells have been shown to contribute to the chronic inflammation associated with the LAR in experimental asthma.[72] In contrast to the mast cell culture conditions in the murine system (which depend on IL-3), mature human mast cells are obtained by culturing progenitor cells (e.g., cord blood mononuclear cells) with SCF, IL-6, and IL-10. Furthermore, treatment of mature human mast cells with IL-4 induces further maturation, including enhancing their capacity for IgE-dependent activation and their enzymatic machinery for synthesizing PGD_2 and cysteinyl leukotrienes.[73]

Mast cells exist as heterogeneous populations depending on the tissue microenvironment in which they reside and on the immunologic status of the individual. In work with rodents, the terms *mucosal mast cell* (MMC) and *connective tissue mast cell* (CTMC) have emerged, but designating these two populations of mast cells by tissue location alone is an oversimplification. In general, MMCs express less sulfated proteoglycans (chondroitin sulfate) in their granules than CTMCs (heparin proteoglycans) and hence have different staining characteristics with metachromatic stains. In addition, mast cell populations express distinct granule proteases; in humans, the mast cell nomenclature is based on neutral protease expression. Human cells that express only tryptase (MC_T) are distinguished from mast cells that express tryptase, chymase, carboxypeptidase, and cathepsin G (MC_{TC}). In normal tissues, MC_T cells are the predominant cells in the lung and small intestine mucosa, whereas MC_{TC} cells are the predominant types found in the skin and gastrointestinal submucosa.

Mast cell activation occurs through several pathways; classically, a multivalent allergen cross-links IgE molecules bound to the high-affinity IgE receptor (FcεRI), exclusively expressed by mast cells and basophils. In addition, mast cells directly respond to a variety of other agents including calcium ionophore A23187, basic polypeptides (polylysine, polyarginine), eosinophil granule proteins (e.g., MBP), morphine sulfate, chemokines, formyl-methionyl-leucyl-phenylalanine (fMLP) peptides, complement degradation products (e.g., C5a), and substance P. After engagement of receptors with their ligands, mast cells undergo regulated exocytosis of their granules resulting in the release of preformed mediators; in addition, activated mast cells undergo *de novo* synthesis and release of a variety of potent mediators (such as prostaglandin D_2 and LTC_4). Preformed mediators in mast cells include biogenic amines such as histamine (a vasodilator), various neutral proteases, a variety of cytokines, acid hydrolases (e.g., β-hexosaminidase), and proteoglycans. Notably, nearly 20% of the protein of human mast cells is composed of tryptase, a proinflammatory protease with a wide range of activities (e.g., cleavage of complement proteins).[74] Mast cells store a variety of cytokines in their granules (e.g., TNF-α, IL-1, IL-4, IL-5, and IL-6 and chemokines including IL-8) and, after activation with allergens or cytokines, mast cells can increase their synthesis and secretion of these cytokines. It is well established that mast cell products (e.g., histamine) contribute to the

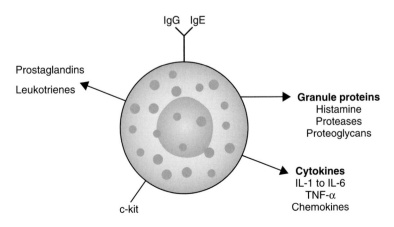

FIGURE 5-4 Schematic diagram of a mast cell and its products. Mast cells are mononuclear cells that express high-affinity IgE receptors (as well as IgG receptors) and contain a large number of metachromatic granules. Mast cells express c-*kit*, the receptor for stem cell factor (SCF), a critical mast cell growth and differentiation factor. The secondary granule of a mast cell also contains abundant levels of proteases, proteoglycans, and histamine. In addition to releasing their preformed proteins, mast cells can also release a variety of cytokines (e.g., IL-1 to IL-6, TNF-α, and chemokines) and generate large amounts of prostaglandins (PGD_2) and leukotrienes (LTC_4).

early phase of allergic responses, but the contribution of mast cell products such as cytokines has been less clear. Although the exact contribution of mast cell–derived cytokines compared with lymphocyte-derived cytokines has been debated, mast cells appear to be a chief source of TNF-α in asthmatic lung and in experimental bacterial peritonitis[75] (Box 5-3).

Basophils

Basophils are hematopoietic cells that arise from a lineage shared with eosinophils; in fact, there is evidence for a common eosinophil/basophil precursor cell.[76] Basophils complete their development in the bone marrow and circulate as mature cells, representing less than 2% of blood leukocytes. Similar to mast cells, basophils express substantial levels of FcεRI and store histamine in their granules. They are distinguished from mast cells by their segmented nuclei, ultrastructural features, growth factor requirements, granule constituents, and surface marker expression (c-$kit-$, FcεRI$^+$).[77] In the human system, they develop largely in response to IL-3 (not SCF) in a process augmented by TFG-β. Mature basophils maintain expression of the IL-3 receptor, and IL-3 is a potent basophil priming and activating cytokine.[78]

Several processes activate basophils; notably, on crosslinking of their surface-bound IgE, basophils release preformed mediators including histamine and proteases and synthesize LTC$_4$. Basophils do not express mast cell proteases, except for trace amounts of tryptase, which is generally not detectable by immunochemical means. In addition, they secrete cytokines such as IL-4 and IL-13; notably, the amount of IL-4 secreted by basophils appears to be substantial compared with Th2 cells.[79] Similar to eosinophils, basophils are also activated by IgA (by expressing FcαR) and by CCR3 ligands. Basophils also express several other chemokine receptors, including CCR2, whose ligands are potent histamine-releasing factors (e.g., macrophage chemoattractant protein [MCP]-1). Recently, two monoclonal antibodies that specifically recognize basophils (the respective antigens recognized are 2D7 and basogranin)[80,81] have been developed, and they have permitted detection and analysis of basophils in allergic tissue. Using these reagents, basophils have been demonstrated to be recruited in allergen-induced, late-phase skin reactions and to

be associated with induction of the chemokines RANTES and MCP-3[82,83] (Box 5-4).

Macrophages

Macrophages are tissue-dwelling cells that originate from hematopoietic stem cells in the bone marrow and are subsequently derived from circulating blood monocytes.[84,85] Under healthy conditions, bone marrow colony-forming cells rapidly progress through monoblast and promonocyte stages to monocytes, which subsequently enter the bloodstream for about 3 days, where they account for about 5% of circulating leukocytes in most species. On entering various tissues, monocytes terminally differentiate into morphologically, histochemically, and functionally distinct tissue macrophage populations that have the capacity to survive for several months.[86] Tissue-specific populations of macrophages include dendritic cells (skin, gut), Kupfer cells (liver), and alveolar macrophages (lung). Under healthy conditions, macrophages have an important role in end-organ function. For example, they are required for eye and breast gland development,[50,87] and in the lung, they are required for normal lung surfactant metabolism by contributing to the catabolism of both surfactant lipids and surfactant proteins.[88]

Macrophage colony-stimulating factor (M-CSF) 1 promotes monocyte differentiation into macrophages, and mice with a genetic mutation in CSF1 (op/op mice) have a deficiency of tissue macrophages.[89] In addition, GM-CSF promotes the survival, differentiation, proliferation, and function of myeloid progenitors as well as the proliferation and function of macrophages.[90] An unexpected but critical role for GM-CSF in lung homeostasis was revealed by ablation of murine loci for GM-CSF (GM$^{-/-}$ mice)[91] or its receptor (GM Rc$^{-/-}$ mice),[90] both of which result in pulmonary alveolar proteinosis (PAP) and abnormalities of alveolar macrophage function. Interestingly, the ability of GM-CSF to regulate macrophage differentiation is dependent on PU.1, an ETS-family transcription factor that also regulates myeloid and B cell lineage development.[92]

Tissue macrophages contribute to innate immunity by virtue of their ability to migrate, phagocytose, and kill microorganisms and to recruit and activate other inflammatory cells. By expressing Toll-like receptor-mediated pathogen recognition molecules that induce the release of cytokines capable of programming adaptive immune responses (e.g., IL-12 and IL-18 production), macrophages provide important links between innate and adaptive immunity.[93] Macrophages

---

BOX 5-3	**KEY CONCEPTS**
	Mast Cells

- Mast cells are bone marrow–derived, tissue-dwelling cells.
- Mast cells do not normally exist in the circulation.
- Mast cell development is critically dependent on the cytokine stem cell factor and its receptor c-kit.
- Mast cells express a high-affinity IgE receptor (FcεR) that is normally occupied with IgE.
- Mast cell activation results in the release of preformed mediators (e.g., histamine and proteases) and newly synthesized mediators such as prostaglandins and leukotrienes.
- Mast cells also produce cytokines such as tumor necrosis factor-α and have an important role in innate immune responses (e.g., by attracting neutrophils).

BOX 5-4	**KEY CONCEPTS**
	Basophils

- Basophils are bone marrow leukocytes that normally account for less than 2% of circulating leukocytes.
- Basophils express the high-affinity IgE receptor FcεR.
- Basophils and eosinophils share a common lineage during their development.
- Basophils are distinguished from mast cells by their separate lineage, bilobed nuclei, and distinct granule proteins.
- Basophils accumulate in tissues during late-phase responses.

also express high- and low-affinity receptors for IgG (FcγRI/II) and complement receptors (CR1) that promote their activation. Activated macrophages produce a variety of pleiotropic proinflammatory cytokines such as IL-1, TNF-α, and IL-8, as well as lipid mediators (e.g., leukotrienes and prostaglandins). Notably, macrophages express costimulatory molecules (e.g., CD86) and are potent antigen-presenting cells capable of efficiently activating antigen-specific T cells. In addition, macrophages actively metabolize arginine via two competing pathways, depending on their cytokine polarization.[94] For example, IFN-γ and lipopolysaccharide (LPS) augment the expression of inducible nitric oxide synthase (iNOS), which results in the production of NO, a potent smooth muscle and endothelial cell regulator (e.g., bronchodilator in the lung). Alternatively, the treatment of macrophages with IL-4 or IL-13 induces the expression of arginase, which preferentially shunts arginine away from NOS (thus promoting bronchoconstriction). Arginase metabolizes arginine into ornithine, a precursor for polyamines and proline, critical regulators of cell growth and collagen deposition, respectively.

A substantial body of evidence has revealed that macrophages are critical effector cells in allergic responses. For example, peripheral blood monocytes from asthmatic individuals secrete elevated levels of superoxide anion and GM-CSF.[95] In addition, the lung tissue and BALF from asthmatic individuals have elevated levels of macrophages compared with healthy control individuals.[96] Consistent with this, the asthmatic lung has overexpression of macrophage-active chemokines (e.g., MCP-1).[97]

Dendritic Cells

Dendritic cells are unique antigen-presenting cells that have a pivotal role in innate and acquired immune responses. These cells originate in the bone marrow and subsequently migrate into the circulation before they assume tissue locations as immature dendritic cells, incidentally at locations where maximum allergen encounter occurs (e.g., skin, gastrointestinal tract, and airways). Immature dendritic cells are potent in antigen uptake, efficient in capturing pathogens, and producers of potent cytokines (e.g., IFN-α and IL-12). By expressing pattern recognition receptors (e.g., Toll-like receptors), dendritic cells directly recognize a variety of pathogens. Immature dendritic cells express the CC chemokine receptor (CCR) 6 that binds to MIP-3α and β-defensin, which are produced locally in tissues such as those in the lung.[98] After antigen uptake, dendritic cells rapidly cross into the lymphatic vessels and migrate into draining secondary lymphoid tissue. During this migration, the dendritic cells undergo maturation, which in turn is characterized by down-regulation in their capacity to capture antigen, up-regulation of antigen processing and presentation capabilities (including expression of co-stimulatory molecules [e.g., CD80 and CD86]), and up-regulation of CCR7, which likely promotes dendritic cell recruitment to secondary lymphoid organs (which express CCR7 ligands).[99] After presentation of antigen to antigen-specific T cells in the T cell–rich areas of secondary lymphoid organs, dendritic cells mainly undergo apoptosis.

Dendritic cells are composed of heterogeneous populations based on ultrastructural features, surface molecule expression, and function. In human blood, dendritic cells are divided into three types including two myeloid-derived subpopulations and another lymphoid-derived population (plasmacytoid dendritic cells).[100] The myeloid populations are divided into CD1+ and CD1−. CD1 is a molecule involved in the presentation of glycolipids to T cells. CD1c+ myeloid dendritic cells also express high levels of CD11c (complement receptor-4 [iC3b receptor]), whereas the CD1c− population expresses lower levels of CD11c. The plasmacytoid dendritic cell population is CD1c−, CD11c−, but is distinguished by its high levels of CD123 (the IL-3 receptor) expression. This population of dendritic cells (mainly studied in mice) appears to be a primary source of IFN-α. Dendritic cells can be cultured from freshly isolated human cord or peripheral blood; myeloid dendritic cells are primarily derived in response to stimulation with GM-CSF, TNF-α, and IL-4, whereas plasmacytoid dendritic cells develop in culture with IL-3.

Dendritic cells have a potent ability to prime naïve CD4+ T cells and naïve CD8+ T cells. Dendritic cells can differentially influence Th cell differentiation preferentially by induction of Th1 or Th2 cell responses (see Figure 5-2). There is evidence that the same population of dendritic cells can influence Th1 and Th2 differentiation depending on several factors. For example, the ratio between dendritic cells and T cells has profound effects on influencing Th1 and Th2 differentiation.[101] In addition, Th1 polarized effector dendritic cells (matured with IFN-γ) induce Th1 responses, whereas Th2 polarized dendritic cells (matured in the presence of prostaglandin E₂) induce Th2 responses.[100] Also, plasmacytoid dendritic cells stimulated first with the IL-3 and then with CD40 ligand (before adding naive T cells) induce strong Th1 responses but no Th2 cytokine production. Finally, dendritic cells that express specific co-stimulatory molecules may promote distinct Th differentiation; for example, expression of B7-related protein (ICOS ligand) promotes Th2 development.[102] As such, dendritic cells are likely to have critical roles in the development of allergic responses. Recent studies indicate that dendritic cells are required for the development of eosinophilic airway inflammation in response to inhaled antigen.[103] Importantly, adoptive transfer of antigen-pulsed dendritic cells has been shown to be sufficient for the induction of Th2 responses and eosinophilic airway inflammation to inhaled antigen.[99,104] There also is experimental evidence that injection of allergenic peptides into the skin of strongly allergic asthmatics can induce specific late-phase reactions in the lung apparently mediated by migrating skin dendritic cells.[105] Finally, elevated levels of CD1a+, MHC class II+ dendritic cells, are found in the lung of atopic asthmatics compared with nonasthmatics[99] (Box 5-5).

BOX 5-5 | **KEY CONCEPTS**
Dendritic Cells

- Dendritic cells normally exist as tissue surveillance cells.
- On contact with antigen (e.g., invading pathogen), dendritic cells migrate via lymphatics to secondary lymphoid organs.
- Immature dendritic cells are chief sources of innate cytokines (e.g., interferon-α).
- Mature dendritic cells are potent antigen-presenting cells.
- Dendritic cells can preferentially activate Th1 or Th2 responses.

Neutrophils

Neutrophils are bone marrow−derived granulocytes that account for the largest proportion of cells in most inflammatory sites. Neutrophils develop in the bone marrow by the sequential differentiation of progenitor cells into myeloblasts, promyelocytes, and then myelocytes, an ordered process regulated by growth factors such as GM-CSF. Granulocyte-CSF promotes the terminal differentiation of neutrophils, which normally reside in the bloodstream for only 6 to 8 hours. A significant pool of marginated neutrophils exists in select tissues (e.g., there are 280×10^8 neutrophils in the lungs versus 5×10^6 in the blood),[106] allowing rapid mobilization of neutrophils in response to a variety of triggers (e.g., chemoattractant signals, including the chemokine IL-8 and the lipid mediators LTB_4 and platelet-activating factor [PAF]).

Activated neutrophils have the capacity to release a variety of products at inflammatory sites, which may induce tissue damage. These products include those of primary (azurophilic), secondary (or specific), and tertiary granules, including proteolytic enzymes, oxygen radicals, and lipid mediators (LTB_4, PAF, and thromboxane A2). Neutrophil granules contain more than 20 enzymes; of these, elastase, collagenase, and gelatinase have the greatest potential for inducing tissue damage. Neutrophil-derived defensins, lysozyme, and cathepsin G have well-defined roles in antibacterial defense. In fact, recent studies have suggested that the major function of superoxide release into the phagocytic vesicle is not its direct bactericidal activity; rather, superoxide raises the concentrations of intravesicle H^+ and K^+, permitting conditions for optimal protease-mediated bacterial killing.[107]

Although neutrophils are not the predominant cell type associated with allergic disorders, there are several studies that have demonstrated a correlation and possible for role for neutrophils in the pathogenesis of allergic disease.[108] There also is evidence that individuals who die within 1 hour of the onset of an acute asthma attack have neutrophil-dominant airway inflammation,[109] suggesting that neutrophils may have a pathogenic role in some clinical situations. Finally, neutrophil-depletion experiments (with the use of cytotoxic drugs in animals) have suggested an effector role for neutrophils in asthma, although these depletion strategies are not necessarily cell specific.[110]

LEUKOCYTE RECRUITMENT

The trafficking of leukocytes into various tissues is regulated by a complex network of signaling events between leukocytes in the circulation and endothelial cells lining blood vessels. These interactions involve a multistep process including (1) leukocyte rolling (mediated by endothelial selectin and specific leukocyte ligands), (2) rapid activation of leukocyte integrins, (3) firm adhesion between endothelial molecules and counterligands on leukocytes, and (4) transmigration of leukocytes through the endothelial layer (Figure 5-5). Chemokines are thought to have a central role in modulating this multistep process by (1) activating both the leukocytes and the endothelium and (2) increasing leukocyte integrin and adhesion molecule interaction affinity. The multistep signaling cascade must occur rapidly (seconds to minutes) to allow for the leukocytes to reduce rolling velocity, mediate ad-

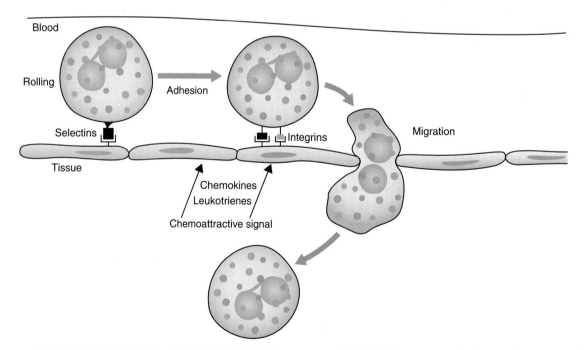

FIGURE 5-5 Overview of leukocyte migration. The trafficking of leukocytes into various tissues is regulated by a complex network of signaling events between leukocytes in the circulation and endothelial cells lining blood vessels. These interactions involve a multistep process including (1) leukocyte rolling (mediated by endothelial selectin and specific leukocyte ligands), (2) rapid activation of leukocyte integrins, (3) firm adhesion between endothelial molecules and counterligands on leukocytes, and (4) transmigration of leukocytes through the endothelial layer. Chemoattractive mediators (e.g., chemokines and leukotrienes) are thought to have a central role in modulating this multistep process by activating both the leukocyte and the endothelium and by increasing leukocyte integrin and adhesion molecule interaction affinity.

herence, and extravasate into tissues in response to a chemokine gradient (see Figure 5-5). In addition to mediating leukocyte movement from the bloodstream into tissues, chemokines use similar steps to mediate leukocyte-directed motion across other tissue barriers such as respiratory epithelium. The ultimate distribution of leukocytes in particular tissue locations represents a balance between cell recruitment and cell death, the latter occurring via necrosis or regulated apoptosis (Box 5-6).

Leukocyte Chemoattraction

Chemokine and chemokine receptor families

Chemokines represent a large family of chemotactic cytokines that have been divided into four groups, designated CXC, CC, C, and CX3C, depending on the spacing of conserved cysteines (Figure 5-6). These four families of chemokines are grouped into distinct chromosomal loci (see Figure 5-6). The CXC and CC groups, in contrast to the C and CX3C chemokines, contain many members and have been studied in greatest detail. The CXC chemokines mainly target neutrophils, whereas the CC chemokines target a variety of cell types including macrophages, eosinophils, and basophils. Due to the complexity of the system, a new nomenclature was recently proposed,[111] which is based on the current chemokine receptor nomenclature that uses CC, CXC, XC, or CX3C (to designate chemokine group) followed by R (for receptor) and then a number. The new chemokine nomenclature substitutes the R for L (for ligand) and the number is derived from the one already assigned to the gene encoding the chemokine from the SCY (small secreted cytokine) nomenclature. Thus a given gene has the same number as its protein ligand (e.g., the gene encoding eotaxin-1 is *SCYA11*, and the chemokine is referred to as CCL11). Table 5-1 summarizes the chemokine family using this nomenclature.

Chemokines induce leukocyte migration and activation by binding to specific G protein–coupled, seven-transmembrane–spanning cell surface receptors (GPCRs).[112] Although chemokine receptors are similar to many GPCRs, they have unique structural motifs such as the amino acid sequence DRYLAIV in the second intracellular domain.[112,113] There have been five CXCR receptors identified, which are referred to as CXCR1 through CXCR5, and 10 human CC chemokine receptor genes cloned, which are known as CCR1 through CCR10 (Figure 5-7). The chemokine and leukocyte selectivities of chemokine receptors overlap extensively; a given leukocyte often expresses multiple chemokine receptors, and more than one chemokine typically binds to the same receptor (see Figure 5-7). For example, monocytes express the CC chemokine receptors CCR1, CCR2, CCR4, and CCR5; eosinophils express CCR1 and CCR3; and basophils express CCR1, CCR2, and CCR3. All of the MCP proteins characterized to date are ligands for CCR2. In addition, MCP-2, -3, and -4 are also ligands for CCR3. In contrast, the eotaxin chemokines signal only through CCR3.

Chemokine Receptor Signal Transduction

Chemokine receptors are, for the most part, inhibited by pertussis toxin, indicating that they are primarily coupled to G proteins.[112] Receptor activation leads to a cascade of intracellular signaling events that in turn lead to activation of phos-

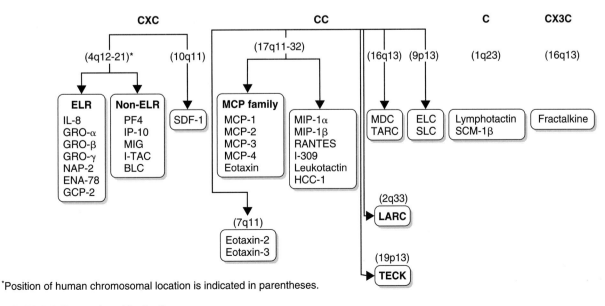

*Position of human chromosomal location is indicated in parentheses.

FIGURE 5-6 Human chemokine family.

TABLE 5-1 Systematic Names for Human and Mouse Ligands

Systematic Name	Human Ligand	Mouse Ligand
CXC family		
CXCL1	GRO-α/MGSA-α	GRO/KC?*
CXCL2	GRO-β/MGSA-β	GRO/KC?
CXCL3	GRO-γ/MGSA-γ	GRO/KC?
CXCL4	PF4	PF4
CXCL5	ENA-78	LIX?
CXCL6	GCP-2	Ckα-3
CXCL7	NAP-2	?
CXCL8	IL-8	?
CXCL9	Mig	Mig
CXCL10	IP-10	IP-10
CXCL11	I-TAC	?
CXCL12	SDF-1α/β	SDF-1
CXCL13	BLC/BCA-1	BLC/BCA-1
CXCL14	BRAK/bolekine	BRAK
CXCL15	?	Lungkine
CC family		
CCL1	I-309	TCA-3, P500
CCL2	MCP-1/MCAF	JE ?
CCL3	MIP-1α/LD78α	MIP-1α
CCL4	MIP-1β	MIP-1β
CCL5	RANTES	RANTES
CCL6	?	C10, MRP-1
CCL7	MCP-3	MARC?
CCL8	MCP-2	MCP-2?
CCL9/10	?	MRP-2, CCF18, MIP-1γ
CCL11	Eotaxin	Eotaxin
CCL12	?	MCP-5
CCL13	MCP-4	?
CCL14	HCC-1	?
CCL15	HCC-2/Lkn-1/MIP-1δ	?
CCL16	HCC-4/LEC	LCC-1
CCL17	TARC	TARC
CCL18	DC-CK1/PARC/AMAC-1	?
CCL19	MIP-3β/ELC/exodus-3	MIP-3β/ELC/exodus-3
CCL20	MIP-3α/LARC/exodus-1	MIP-3α/LARC/exodus-1
CCL21	6Ckine/SLC/exodus-2	6Ckine/SLC/exodus-2/TCA-4
CCL22	MDC/STCP-1	ABCD-1
CCL23	MPIF-1	?
CCL24	MPIF-2/Eotaxin-2	Eotaxin-2
CCL25	TECK	TECK
CCL26	Eotaxin-3	?
CCL27	CTACK/ILC	ALP/CTACK/ILC/ESkine
CCL28	MEC	MEC
C family		
XCL1	Lymphotactin/SCM-1α/ATAC	Lymphotactin
XCL2	SCM-1β	?
CX3C family		
CX3CL1	Fractalkine	Neurotactin

*A question mark indicates that the mouse and human homologues are ambiguous.

phatidylinositol-specific phospholipase C, protein kinase C, small GTP-ases, Src-related tyrosine kinases, phophatidylinositol-3-OH kinases, and protein kinase B. Phospholipase C delivers two secondary messengers, inositol-1,4,5 triphosphate, which releases intracellular calcium, and diacylglycerol, which activates protein kinase C. Multiple phosphorylation events are triggered by chemokines. Phosphatidylinositol-3-OH kinase can be activated by the βγ subunit of G proteins, small GTP-ases or Src-related tyrosine kinases. Phosphorylation of the tyrosine kinase, RAFTK, a member of the focal adhesion kinase family, has been shown to be induced by signaling through CCR5.[114] Recently, mitogen-activated protein kinases have also been shown to be phosphorylated and activated within 1 minute after exposure of leukocytes to chemokines.[115] In addition to triggering intracellular events, engagement with ligand induces rapid chemokine receptor internalization. For example, in human eosinophils, after only 15 minutes of exposure to eotaxin or RANTES, CCR3 expression is reduced to only 20% to 40% of the original level. Internalized CCR3 enters an early endosome compartment shared with the transferrin receptor and is subsequently recycled or targeted to the lysozyme for protein degradation. Ligand-induced internalization of most chemokine receptors occurs independent of calcium transients, G protein coupling, and protein kinase C, indicating a mechanism different from that with the induction of chemotaxis. Thus chemokine receptor internalization may provide a mechanism for chemokines to also halt leukocyte trafficking *in vivo*.

Regulation of Chemokine and Chemokine Receptor Expression

The main stimuli for the secretion of chemokines are the early proinflammatory cytokines, such as IL-1 and TNF-α, bacterial products such as LPS, and viral infection[116-118] (Figure 5-8). Thus chemokine induction is associated with initial innate immune response. In addition, products of the adaptive arm of the immune system, including both Th1 and Th2 cells, IFN-γ and IL-4, respectively, also induce the production of chemokines independently and in synergy with IL-1 and TNF-α. Although there are many similarities in the regulation of chemokines, important differences that may have implications for asthma are beginning to be appreciated. For example, in the healthy lung, epithelial cells are the primary source of chemokines; however, in the inflamed lung, infiltrating cells (especially macrophages) within the submucosa are a major cellular source of chemokines.[119] Furthermore, the induced expression of chemokines by TNF-α or IL-1 treatment of epithelial cells is suppressed by the steroid dexamethasone.[120] This may be relevant to the clinical effectiveness of inhaled glucocorticoids at decreasing the eosinophil-rich inflammatory exudate characteristically seen in the respiratory tract of individuals with asthma.

Analysis of the 5′ flanking regions of most chemokines reveals several conserved regulatory elements that may explain the observed regulation of the chemokine genes by cytokines and glucocorticoids[121,122] (see Figure 5-8). Of note, nuclear factor kappa B (NFκB), glucocorticoid response element (GRE), gamma interferon response element (γIRE), Sp1, and E2A binding site motifs are well conserved in both human and mouse chemokine promoters. For example, the eotaxin promoter in mice and humans has NFκB and STAT-6 sequences;

A

CCR1	CCR2	CCR3	CCR4	CCR5	CCR6	CCR7	CCR8	CCR9	CCR10
		CCL5							
		CCL7							
		CCL8							
CCL3		CCL11							
CCL5		CCL13							
CCL7	CCL2	CCL15							
CCL14	CCL7	CCL24		CCL3					CCL27
CCL15	CCL8	CCL26	CCL17	CCL4		CCL19			
CCL23	CCL13	CCL28	CCL22	CCL5	CCL20	CCL21	CCL1	CCL25	CCL28

B

CXCR1	CXCR2	CXCR3	CXCR4	CXCR5
	CXCL1			
	CXCL2			
	CXCL3			
	CXCL5			
	CXCL6	CXCL9		
CXCL6	CXCL7	CXCL10		
CXCL8	CXCL8	CXCL11	CXCL12	CXCL13

FIGURE 5-7 Ligands for CC (**A**) and CXC (**B**) receptor families.

mutation of the NFκB and STAT-6 sites impairs eotaxin promoter activity in response to TNF-α and IL-4, respectively.[123] NFκB is a nuclear factor that is activated after the stimulation of cells with various immunologic agents, such as LPS, IL-1, and TNF-α. NFκB has been shown to be important for the transcriptional activation of selected chemokines. For example, a single NFκB binding site is essential for TNF-α– and IL-1–induced expression of the MCP-1[124] and growth-regulated oncogene-α (GRO-α)[125] genes and LPS-induced expression of the *MIP-2* gene.[126] GRE mediates glucocorticoid regulation of transcription.[127] Interestingly, IL-5, an eosinophil-specific growth and differentiation factor, and the chemokine IL-8 also contain a GRE sequence in their promoters. Furthermore, deletion analysis of the GRE from the IL-8 promoter revealed that this element participated in dexamethasone suppression of IL-8 expression.[128] *In vitro*, the glucocorticoid budesonide inhibits eotaxin promoter-driven reporter gene activity and accelerates the decay of eotaxin mRNA.[129] These studies indicate that glucocorticoids inhibit chemokine expression through multiple mechanisms of action.

Chemokine receptors are constitutively expressed on some cells, whereas they are inducible on others. For example, CCR1 and CCR2 are constitutively expressed on monocytes but are expressed on lymphocytes only after IL-2 stimulation.[130,131] Activated lymphocytes are then responsive to multiple CC chemokines that use these receptors, including the MCPs. In addition, some constitutive receptors can be down-modulated by biologic response modifiers. For example, IL-10 was shown to modify the activity of CCR1, CCR2, and CCR5 on dendritic cells and monocytes.[132] Normally, dendritic cells mature in response to inflammatory stimuli, and shift from expressing CCR1, CCR2, CCR5, and CCR6 to CCR7 expression. However, IL-10 blocks the chemokine receptor switch. Importantly, although CCR1, CCR2, and CCR5 remain detectable on the cell surface and bind appropriate ligands, they do not signal in calcium mobilization and chemotaxis assays. Thus IL-10 converts chemokine receptors to functional decoy receptors, thereby serving a down-regulatory function (Box 5-7).

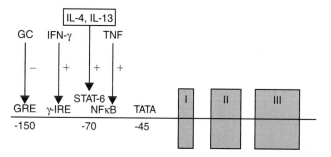

FIGURE 5-8 Regulatory elements in chemokine promoter. Depicted are the positions of the transcription factor motifs and the regulatory cytokines of the eotaxin-1 promoter. The three exons of the gene are depicted with rectangles. Positive signals are indicated with (+), whereas inhibitory signals are indicated with (−). Notably, IL-4/IL-13 via STAT-6 induces transcription; IFN-γ induces transcription through an IFN response element (γ-IRE), *and TNF-α induces transcription through NFκB. Glucocorticoids (GC) inhibit transcription via the glucocorticoid response element (GRE).*

BOX 5-7

KEY CONCEPTS
Chemokines

- Chemokines are chemoattractive cytokines.
- Chemokines are functionally divided into molecules that are constitutively expressed and those that are inducible.
- Chemokines are divided into several families depending on the spacing of the first two cysteines (e.g., CC and CXC families).
- Chemokines bind to seven-transmembrane–spanning, G protein–linked receptors.
- Chemokine receptors are genetically polymorphic.
- Chemokine receptors often bind to more than one chemokine ligand (e.g., they are promiscuous).

Chemokine Regulation of Leukocyte Effector Function

Chemoattraction

Structural motifs in the primary amino acid sequence of chemokines have an important impact on their chemoattractive ability. For example, CXC chemokines are mainly chemoattractants for neutrophils and lymphocytes. Furthermore, ELR (Glu-Leu-Arg)-containing CXC chemokines (e.g., IL-8) are mainly chemoattractive on neutrophils, whereas non-ELR CXC chemokines (e.g., IP-10) chemoattract selected populations of lymphocytes. In contrast to cellular specificity of CXC chemokines, CC chemokines are active on a variety of leukocytes, including dendritic cells, monocytes, basophils, lymphocytes, and eosinophils. For example, as their names imply, all MCPs have strong chemoattractive activity for monocytes. However, they display partially overlapping chemoattractant activity on basophils and eosinophils. In particular, MCP-2, MCP-3, and MCP-4 have basophil and eosinophil chemoattractive activity, but MCP-1 is only active on basophils. In distinction to the MCPs, the eotaxin subfamily of chemokines (e.g., eotaxin-1, -2, and -3) has limited activity on macrophages but are potent eosinophil and basophil chemoattractants.[133,134] For example, the administration of eotaxin intranasally or subcutaneously induces a rapid selective tissue accumulation of eosinophils in the murine lung or skin. Chemokines also work in concert with other cytokines to promote leukocyte trafficking. For example, the activity of eotaxin is greatly enhanced when it is codelivered with IL-5.[135-137] IL-5 collaborates with eotaxin in promoting tissue eosinophilia by (1) increasing the pool of circulating eosinophils (by stimulating eosinophilopoiesis and bone marrow release) and (2) priming eosinophils to have enhanced responsiveness to eotaxin. The ability of two cytokines (IL-5 and eotaxin) that are relatively eosinophil selective to cooperate in promoting tissue eosinophilia offers a molecular explanation for the occurrence of selective tissue eosinophilia in human allergic diseases.

Cellular Activation

In addition to promoting leukocyte accumulation, chemokines are potent cell activators. After binding to the appropriate G protein−linked, seven-transmembrane−spanning receptor, chemokines elicit transient intracellular calcium flux, actin polymerization, oxidative burst with release of superoxide free radicals, the exocytosis of secondary granule constituents, and increased avidity of integrins for their adhesion molecules.[138-140] For example, in basophils, chemokine-induced cellular activation results in degranulation with the release of histamine and the *de novo* generation of LTC₄.[117,141,142] Notably, basophil activation by chemokines requires cellular priming with IL-3, IL-5, or GM-CSF for the maximal effect of each chemokine, highlighting the cooperativity between cytokines and chemokines.

Hematopoiesis

In addition to being involved in leukocyte accumulation during inflammatory reactions, chemokines also have a role in regulating hematopoiesis. These functions include (1) chemotaxis of hematopoietic progenitor cells (HPC), (2) suppression and enhancement activity on HPC proliferation and differentiation, and (3) mobilization of HPCs to the peripheral blood (reviewed in Kim and Broxmeyer[143]). For example, stromal cell−derived factor (SDF)-1, a CXC chemokine, is critical for B cell lymphopoiesis and bone marrow myelopoiesis as demonstrated by gene targeting.[144] Furthermore, eotaxin has been shown to directly stimulate the release of eosinophilic progenitor cells and mature eosinophils from the bone marrow.[145] Eotaxin synergizes with stem cell factor in stimulating yolk sac development into mast cells *in vitro*[146] and has been shown to function as a GM-CSF after allergic challenge in the lungs.[147] In contrast, MIP-1α appears to be an inhibitor of hematopoiesis.[148]

Regulation of Dendritic Cells

A central question in allergy research is to understand the mechanism for initial allergen recognition in mucosal surfaces. Tissue resident dendritic cells are believed to have a fundamental role in this process because they are able to efficiently take up, process, and deliver antigens to lymphoid tissues. The migration pattern of dendritic cells is complex and is thought to involve a coordinated chemokine-signaling network. Dendritic cell progenitors from the bone marrow migrate into nonlymphoid tissues where they develop into immature dendritic cells that have an active role in antigen uptake and processing. Antigen stimulation and the production of inflammatory cytokines promote the differentiation of immature dendritic cells into mature presenting dendritic cells (as discussed earlier in this chapter). This promotes dendritic cell trafficking from the periphery to regional lymph nodes via afferent lymphatics. On reaching the lymph nodes, dendritic cells home in on T cell−rich regions where they present the processed antigen to naive T cells and generate an antigen-specific primary T cell response. As part of the maturation program, immature dendritic cells up-regulate the expression of CCR7 and become responsive to ELC and SLC, chemokines responsible for their trafficking to lymph nodes. At the same time, they decrease the expression of CCR1, CCR2, and CCR5, the receptors for inflammatory chemokines.[149-151]

Modulation of T Cell Immune Responses

Recently there was rapid progress in understanding the effects of chemokines on T-lymphocyte biology.[152] T-lymphocytes have been shown to express a majority of chemokine receptors, thus making them potentially responsive to a large number of different chemokines. Characterization of chemokine receptor expression has shown that T-lymphocytes display a dynamic expression pattern of chemokine receptors, and it is the differential expression of receptors during T-lymphocyte maturation and differentiation that is thought to allow for individual chemokine-specific functionality on T-lymphocytes.[152] As mentioned previously, CCR7 plays an important role in trafficking of naive T cells into lymph nodes.[153] On activation, T cells may express an array of chemokine receptors, including CCR1, CCR2, CCR5, CXCR1, and CXCR4. They thus become sensitive to inflammatory chemokines, including MIP-1α, MIP-1β, MCP-3, and RANTES, which are thought to mediate T cell trafficking to sites of inflammation.[154] Also, specific subsets of memory T cells can be distinguished based on their expression of CCR7 and the propensity to migrate into lymph nodes.[155] Chemokines have an important role in the induction of inflammatory responses and are central in selecting the type of immune response (Th1 vs. Th2). During bacterial or viral infections IP-10, Mig, IL-8, and I-TAC production correlates with the presence of CD4+ Th1-type T cells. In contrast, during allergic inflammatory responses, eotaxin, RANTES, MCP-2, MCP-3, and MCP-4 are induced, and the majority of the CD4+ T-lymphocytes are of the Th2-type phenotype. The characterization of chemokine receptor expression on T-lymphocytes suggests that this may be explained by the expression of CXCR3 and CCR5 predominantly on Th1-type T cells, whereas CCR3, CCR4, and CCR8 have been associated with Th2-type T cells (see Figure 5-2). In addition, Th1 and Th2 cells secrete distinct chemokines[156] (see Figure 5-2). In mice, Th1 cells preferentially secrete RANTES and lymphotactin, whereas Th2 cells secrete MDC and TCA3. Interestingly, supernatants from Th2 cells preferentially attract Th2 cells. These data suggest that the presence of specific patterns of chemokine receptors on T cell subsets predicts which subset will be preferentially accumulated at sites of inflammation. Alternatively, chemokines may directly influence the differentiation of naïve T cells to the Th1 or Th2 phenotype. MIP-1α and MCP-1 have been described as capable of inducing the differentiation of Th1 and Th2 cells,[157] and MCP-1–deficient mice have defective Th2 responses.[158] Consistent with this, Bcl-6–deficient animals express high levels of chemokines, including MCP-1, and have systemic Th2-type inflammation.[159]

Chemokines and Chemokine Receptors Strongly Implicated in Allergic Disorders

Eotaxin/CCR3

Because eosinophilia is a hallmark feature of allergic inflammation, a large body of research has focused on the analysis of chemokine receptors and signaling pathways on eosinophils. Eosinophils from most healthy donors express CCR3 at the highest level[134,160,161] and have significantly lower levels of CCR1. Consistent with the expression of CCR1 and CCR3, eosinophils respond to MIP-1α, RANTES, MCP-2, MCP-3, MCP-4, eotaxin-1, eotaxin-2, and eotaxin-3. CCR3 appears to function as the predominant eosinophil chemokine receptor because CCR3 ligands are generally more potent eosinophil chemoattractants. Furthermore, an inhibitory monoclonal antibody specific for CCR3 blocks the activity of RANTES, a chemokine that could signal through CCR1 or CCR3 in eosinophils.[162] Also, cytokine-primed human eosinophils respond to IL-8,[163] and eosinophils have the capacity to express CXCR2, the low-affinity IL-8 receptor, when they are cultured in IL-5.[162] IL-5 also primes eosinophils to respond to CCR3 ligands.[164] The importance of eotaxin and CCR3 in orchestrating eosinophil recruitment into allergic tissue is highlighted from results with eotaxin- and CCR3-deficient mice. Eotaxin-deficient mice have a major impairment in the baseline level of tissue eosinophils and a reduction in early eosinophil recruitment into the asthmatic lung.[165] In addition, CCR3-deficient mice have impaired eosinophil recruitment into the skin and lung in a model of allergy induced via cutaneous allergen sensitization.[166] Interestingly, in this latter model, CCR3-deficient mice are resistant to the induction of airway hyperreactivity, implicating CCR3 as an important therapeutic target. The eotaxin/CCR3 pathway is not the only signaling system important for eosinophil tissue recruitment; eosinophils have recently been shown to express or respond to ligands of CCR6, CXCR3, and CXCR4.[167-169] For instance, eosinophils isolated from allergic donors responded to MIP-

- Chemokines regulate leukocyte recruitment.
- Chemokines are potent cellular activating factors.
- Chemokines are potent histamine-releasing factors.
- Th2 cytokines (e.g., IL-4 and IL-13) are potent inducers of allergy-associated chemokines (e.g., eotaxin).
- In allergic tissue, chemokines are frequently produced by epithelial cells.

3α in chemotaxis and calcium mobilization assays; FACS analysis revealed that about 20% of eosinophils express low levels of CCR6. Importantly, eosinophils isolated from nonallergic donors failed to respond to MIP-3α.[167] In contrast, in this study, 50% of eosinophils from nonallergic donors express CXCR3 by FACS analysis and these cells respond in functional assays. The significance of these chemokine receptors in eosinophil accumulation in healthy and diseased states remains to be elucidated (Box 5-8).

Genetic Polymorphisms Affecting Cellular Migration in Allergic Responses

Polymorphisms in individual chemokines and chemokine receptor genes are likely to influence the course of allergic disorders. For example, CCR5Δ32 is a 32-bp deletion in the *CCR5* gene that is associated with protection against HIV strains that are tropic for this receptor. Notably, this genetic polymorphism also appears to protect against asthma.[170] Also, a polymorphism in the RANTES promoter (G→A at position bp401) appears to have an effect on atopic dermatitis.[171] The polymorphism confers higher transcriptional activity and a new GATA transcription binding site. Also, it is associated with increased susceptibility to atopic dermatitis because the proportion of individuals carrying the mutant allele is higher in children with atopic dermatitis. Furthermore, the polymorphism has a higher frequency in individuals of African descent than in white subjects. A similar mutation (G→A at position bp403 of the RANTES promoter) is associated with increased susceptibility to both asthma and atopy because the proportion of individuals carrying the mutant allele is higher in atopic and nonatopic asthma patients.[172] In addition, the polymorphism is associated with increased aeroallergen skin test positivity, and homozygosity is associated with increased risk of airway obstruction.

THERAPEUTIC APPROACH TO INTERFERING WITH CHEMOKINES

One of the actions of glucocorticoids is to inhibit the transcription and/or stability of chemokine mRNA (see Figure 5-8). However, the ideal pharmaceutical agent would interfere with the selective function of critical chemokines and/or their receptors in the pathophysiology of disease but not in protective immune responses. CCR3 represents such a potential target because preliminary studies indicate that it is likely to be critically involved in allergic inflammation and antagonizing CCR3 would selectively target eosinophils, basophils, and Th2 cells. Also, CCR4 and CCR8 may be potential targets because both are reported to be Th2 specific and involved in recruitment of Th2 cells in allergic inflammation.[173,174] CCR8 represents a potentially attractive target; recent studies with CCR8-deficient mice have shown impaired antigen-driven Th2 responses and pulmonary eosinophilia.[174]

Chemokine and/or chemokine receptor inhibition has thus been an active area of research. Studies have also been fueled by the finding that natural chemokine receptor mutations block the HIV co-receptor function of selected chemokine receptors (e.g., CCR2 and CCR5), suggesting that pharmaceutical targeting of chemokine receptors is a promising strategy for treatment of HIV infection.[175,176] There are several potential approaches for blockade of chemokines and their receptors. One approach is to develop humanized monoclonal antibodies against chemokines and/or their receptors, an approach already validated in animal models.[177] Specifically, an antibody directed against a chemokine receptor (e.g., CCR3) would offer an advantage over antibodies against chemokines because actions of multiple chemokines through a single receptor would be affected. Another approach involves developing receptor antagonists based on chemokine protein modifications. One such agent has been derived by the addition of a single methionine to the amino terminus of RANTES (designated Met-RANTES).[178,179] This agent acts as a strong competitive inhibitor of CCR1, CCR3, and CCR5. In vivo studies have demonstrated significant reduction in eosinophil numbers after Met-RANTES administration in a murine model of allergic airway inflammation.[180] The success of protein antagonists has already been recognized by viruses, some of which have developed their own chemokine antagonists. For example, the human herpes simplex virus-8 genome encodes for two chemokine-related proteins, and one of these, vMIP-II, is a potent broad-spectrum antagonist against both CXC and CC chemokine receptors.[181,182] Another example is a potent CCR8 antagonist encoded by the poxvirus molluscum contagiosum, termed MC148.[183] Also, small molecule inhibitors of chemokine receptors have recently been described and display potent inhibition at nanomolar concentrations in vitro.[184,185] Three companies have reported the development of small-molecule CCR3 antagonists[186,187]; these compounds share the presence of a hydrophobic group some distance from a basic nitrogen group. It has been postulated that the basic nitrogen group interacts with a key anionic residue in or near the seven-transmembrane region of the receptor, as found with antagonists of the monoamine receptors, which

are seven-transmembrane—spanning receptors. However, no in vivo data are yet available (Box 5-9).

An additional approach to inhibiting chemokines can be induction of prolonged desensitization to chemokine stimulation.[188] It may be possible to induce cellular desensitization by promoting chemokine receptor internalization.[189] Alternatively, the transcription or translation of specific chemokines or chemokine receptors could be blocked. For example, antisense oligonucleotides and transcription factor inhibitors specifically designed to interact with regulatory regions in chemokine receptors may have clinical use. A more detailed understanding of the regulation of chemokine and chemokine receptor genes is necessary for the development of these approaches.

CONCLUSIONS

Allergic disorders involve the complex interplay of a large number of leukocytes (especially mast cells, eosinophils, neutrophils, lymphocytes, basophils, and dendritic cells) and structural tissue cells (especially epithelial and smooth muscle cells). A combination of mouse and human studies has been used to define the specific mechanisms involved in leukocyte activation, migration, and effector function. Although the exact contribution of each cell type has not been fully elucidated, there is now substantial evidence that each of these cells (to various degrees) has a contributory role in disease pathogenesis. In particular, cellular adhesion proteins, integrins, and chemokines have emerged as critical molecules involved in leukocyte accumulation and activation. Also, a combination of innate activation pathways (involving mast cells, dendritic cells, and eosinophils) that induce proinflammatory pathways and adaptive immune pathways (involving antigen-specific Th2 cells) have been elucidated. Although we are in the early phases of analysis of disease pathogenesis, we have already identified critical pathways that are currently being therapeutically targeted (e.g., anticytokine therapeutics) in patients. It is the author's hope that this chapter has provided the appropriate framework for the reader to understand (and contribute to) the next generation of clinical intervention strategies for the treatment of allergic disorders.

Acknowledgments

The editorial assistance of Andrea Lippelman is appreciated. This work was supported in part by National Institutes of Health grants R01-AI42242 and R01-AI45898, a grant from the Human Frontiers Science Program, and the Translational Research Grant from the Burroughs Wellcome Fund.

BOX 5-9 · KEY CONCEPTS
Chemokine Blockade

- Experimental models (e.g., knockouts and neutralizing antibodies) have demonstrated an essential role for chemokines in allergic responses.
- Chemokine receptors can be blocked with small-molecule inhibitors (e.g., receptor antagonists).
- Chemokine inhibition can be accomplished with humanized neutralizing antibodies.
- The treatment of allergic diseases with chemokine inhibitors is not likely to be accomplished unless several receptors and/or ligand groups are simultaneously blocked.

REFERENCES

1. Leong KP, Huston DP: Understanding the pathogenesis of allergic asthma using mouse models, *Ann Allergy Asthma Immunol* 87:96-109, 2001.
2. Wills-Karp M: Immunologic basis of antigen-induced airway hyperresponsiveness, *Annu Rev Immunol* 17:255-281, 1999.
3. O'Byrne PM, Inman MD, Parameswaran K: The trials and tribulations of IL-5, eosinophils, and allergic asthma, *J Allergy Clin Immunol* 108:503-508, 2001.
4. Makker HK, Montefort S, Holgate S: Investigative use of fibreoptic bronchoscopy for local airway challenge in asthma, *Eur Respir J* 6:1402-1408, 1993.
5. Lloyd CM, Gonzalo JA, Coyle AJ, et al: Mouse models of allergic airway disease, *Adv Immunol* 77:263-295, 2001.

6. Kurup VP, Mauze S, Choi H, et al: A murine model of allergic bronchopulmonary aspergillosis with elevated eosinophils and IgE, *J Immunol* 148:3783-3788, 1992.

7. Wardlaw AJ, Dunnette S, Gleich GJ, et al: Eosinophils and mast cells in bronchoalveolar lavage in subjects with mild asthma. Relationship to bronchial hyperreactivity, *Am Rev Respir Dis* 137:62-69, 1988.

8. Broide DH, Firestein GS: Endobronchial allergen challenge in asthma, *J Clin Invest* 88:1048-1053, 1991.

9. Lam S, LeRiche J, Phillips D, et al: Cellular and protein changes in bronchial lavage fluid after late asthmatic reaction in patients with red cedar asthma, *J Allergy Clin Immunol* 80:44-50, 1987.

10. Beasley R, Roche WR, Roberts JA, et al: Cellular events in the bronchi in mild asthma and after bronchial provocation, *Am Rev Respir Dis* 139: 806-817, 1989.

11. De Monchy JG, Kauffman HF, Venge P, et al: Bronchoalveolar eosinophilia during allergen-induced late asthmatic reactions, *Am Rev Respir Dis* 131:373-376, 1985.

12. Fukuda T, Dunnette SL, Reed CE, et al: Increased numbers of hypodense eosinophils in the blood of patients with bronchial asthma, *Am Rev Respir Dis* 132:981-985, 1985.

13. Frick WE, Sedgwick JB, Busse WW: The appearance of hypodense eosinophils in antigen-dependent late phase asthma, *Am Rev Respir Dis* 139:1401-1408, 1989.

14. Gleich GJ, Flavahan NA, Fujisawa T, et al: The eosinophil as a mediator of damage to respiratory epithelium: a model for bronchial hyperreactivity, *J Allergy Clin Immunol* 81:637-648, 1988.

15. Walker C, Kaegi MK, Braun P, et al: Activated T cells and eosinophilia in bronchoalveolar lavages from subjects with asthma correlated with disease severity, *J Allergy Clin Immunol* 88:935-942, 1991.

16. Bousquett J, Chanes P, Lacoste JY, et al: Eosinophilic inflammation in asthma, *N Engl J Med* 323:1033-1039, 1990.

17. Broide DH, Gleich GJ, Cuomo AJ, et al: Evidence of ongoing mast cell and eosinophil degranulation in symptomatic asthma airway, *J Allergy Clin Immunol* 88:637-648, 1991.

18. Bochner BS, Undem BJ, Lichtenstein LM: Immunological aspects of allergic asthma, *Annu Rev Immunol* 12:295-335, 1994.

19. Wilson JW, Li X: The measurement of reticular basement membrane and submucosal collagen in the asthmatic airway, *Clin Exp Allergy* 27:363-371, 1997.

20. Muro S, Minshall EM, Hamid QA: The pathology of chronic asthma, *Clin Chest Med* 21:225-244, 2000.

21. Barnes PJ: New directions in allergic diseases: mechanism-based anti-inflammatory therapies, *J Allergy Clin Immunol* 106:5-16, 2000.

22. Broide DH: Molecular and cellular mechanisms of allergic disease, *J Allergy Clin Immunol* 108:S65-S71, 2001.

23. Humbles AA, Lu B, Nilsson CA, et al: A role for the C3a anaphylatoxin receptor in the effector phase of asthma, *Nature* 406:998-1001, 2000.

24. Annacker O, Pimenta-Araujo R, Burlen-Defranoux O, et al: On the ontogeny and physiology of regulatory T cells, *Immunol Rev* 182:5-17, 2001.

25. Hogan SP, Foster PS: Cytokines as targets for the inhibition of eosinophilic inflammation, *Pharmacol Ther* 74:259-283, 1997.

26. Robinson DS, Hamid Q, Ying S, et al: Predominant TH2-like bronchoalveolar T-lymphocyte population in atopic asthma, *N Engl J Med* 326:298-304, 1992.

27. Hogan SP, Koskinen A, Mattaei KI, et al: Interleukin-5-producing CD4+ T cells play a pivotal role in aeroallergen-induced eosinophilia, bronchial hyperreactivity, and lung damage in mice, *Am J Respir Crit Care Med* 157:210-218, 1998.

28. Ray A, Cohn L: Th2 cells and GATA-3 in asthma: new insights into the regulation of airway inflammation, *J Clin Invest* 104:985-993, 1999.

29. Wills-Karp M: IL-12/IL-13 axis in allergic asthma, *J Allergy Clin Immunol* 107:9-18, 2001.

30. Kita H: The eosinophil: a cytokine-producing cell? *J Allergy Clin Immunol* 97:889-892, 1996.

31. Rothenberg ME: Eosinophilia, *N Engl J Med* 338:1592-1600, 1998.

32. Brusselle GG, Kips JC, Tavernier JH, et al: Attenuation of allergic airway inflammation in IL-4 deficient mice, *Clin Exp Allergy* 24:73-80, 1994.

33. Rankin JA, Picarella DE, Geba GP, et al: Phenotypic and physiologic characterization of transgenic mice expressing interleukin 4 in the lung: lymphocytic and eosinophilic inflammation without airway hyperreactivity, *Proc Natl Acad Sci U S A* 93:7821-7825, 1996.

34. Bochner BS, Klunk DA, Sterbinsky SA, et al: IL-13 selectively induces vascular cell adhesion molecule-1 expression in human endothelial cells, *J Immunol* 154:799-803, 1995.

35. Zhu Z, Homer RJ, Wang Z, et al: Pulmonary expression of interleukin-13 causes inflammation, mucus hypersecretion, subepithelial fibrosis, physiologic abnormalities, and eotaxin production, *J Clin Invest* 103:779-788, 1999.

36. Murata T, Noguchi PD, Puri RK: IL-13 induces phosphorylation and activation of JAK2 Janus kinase in human colon carcinoma cell lines: similarities between IL-4 and IL-13 signaling, *J Immunol* 156:2972-2978, 1996.

37. Takeda K, Tanaka T, Shi W, et al: Essential role of Stat6 in IL-4 signalling, *Nature* 380:627-630, 1996.

38. Takeda K, Kamanaka M, Tanaka T, et al: Impaired IL-13-mediated functions of macrophages in STAT6-deficient mice, *J Immunol* 157: 3220-3222, 1996.

39. Grunig G, Warnock M, Wakil AE, et al: Requirement for IL-13 independently of IL-4 in experimental asthma, *Science* 282:2261-2263, 1998.

40. Wills-Karp M, Luyimbazi J, Xu X, et al: Interleukin-13: central mediator of allergic asthma, *Science* 282:2258-2261, 1998.

41. Mattes J, Yang M, Siqueira A, et al: IL-13 induces airways hyperreactivity independently of the IL-4R alpha chain in the allergic lung, *J Immunol* 167:1683-1692, 2001.

42. Mathew A, MacLean JA, DeHaan E, et al: Signal transducer and activator of transcription 6 controls chemokine production and T helper cell type 2 cell trafficking in allergic pulmonary inflammation, *J Exp Med* 193:1087-1096, 2001.

43. Akimoto T, Numata F, Tamura M, et al: Abrogation of bronchial eosinophilic inflammation and airway hyperreactivity in signal transducers and activators of transcription (STAT)6-deficient mice, *J Exp Med* 187:1537-1542, 1998.

44. Kuperman D, Schofield B, Wills-Karp M, et al: Signal transducer and activator of transcription factor 6 (Stat6)-deficient mice are protected from antigen-induced airway hyperresponsiveness and mucus production, *J Exp Med* 187:939-948, 1998.

45. Yang M, Hogan SP, Henry PJ, et al: Interleukin-13 mediates airways hyperreactivity through the IL-4 receptor-alpha chain and STAT-6 independently of IL-5 and eotaxin, *Am J Respir Cell Mol Biol* 25:522-530, 2001.

46. Barnes PJ: Therapeutic strategies for allergic diseases, *Nature* 402:B31-B38, 1999.

47. Standiford TJ: Anti-inflammatory cytokines and cytokine antagonists, *Curr Pharm Res* 6:633-649, 2000.

48. Gleich GJ, Adolphson CR: The eosinophilic leukocyte: structure and function, *Adv Immunol* 39:177-253, 1986.

49. Weller PF: The immunobiology of eosinophils, *N Engl J Med* 324: 1110-1118, 1991.

50. Gouon-Evans V, Rothenberg ME, Pollard JW: Postnatal mammary gland development requires macrophages and eosinophils, *Development* 127:2269-2282, 2000.

51. Slifman NR, Loegering DA, McKean DJ, et al: Ribonuclease activity associated with human eosinophil-derived neurotoxin and eosinophil cationic protein, *J Immunol* 137:2913-2917, 1986.

52. Rosenberg HF, Dyer KD, Tiffany HL, et al: Rapid evolution of a unique family of primate ribonuclease genes, *Nat Genet* 10:219-223, 1995.

53. Young JD, Peterson CG, Venge P, et al: Mechanism of membrane damage mediated by human eosinophil cationic protein, *Nature* 321:613-616, 1986.

54. Jacoby DB, Gleich GJ, Fryer AD: Human eosinophil major basic protein is an endogenous allosteric antagonist at the inhibitory muscarinic M2 receptor, *J Clin Invest* 91:1314-1318, 1993.

55. Jacoby DB, Costello RM, Fryer AD: Eosinophil recruitment to the airway nerves, *J Allergy Clin Immunol* 107:211-218, 2001.

56. Lewis RA, Austen KF, Soberman RJ: Leukotrienes and other products of the 5-lipoxygenase pathway. Biochemistry and relation to pathobiology in human diseases, *N Engl J Med* 323:645-655, 1990.

57. Metwali A, Blum AM, Ferraris L, et al: Eosinophils within the healthy or inflamed human intestine produce substance P and vasoactive intestinal peptide, *J Neuroimmunol* 52:69-78, 1994.

58. Stead RH: Innervation of mucosal immune cells in the gastrointestinal tract, *Reg Immunol* 4:91-99, 1992.

59. Dvorak AM, Onderdonk AB, McLeod RS, et al: Ultrastructural identification of exocytosis of granules from human gut eosinophils in vivo, *Int Arch Allergy Immunol* 102:33-45, 1993.

60. Hogan SP, Mishra A, Brandt EB, et al: A pathological function for eotaxin and eosinophils in eosinophilic gastrointestinal inflammation, *Nat Immunol* 2:353-360, 2001.

61. Hogan SP, Mishra A, Brandt EB, et al: The chemokine eotaxin is a central mediator of experimental eosinophilic gastrointestinal allergy, *J Allergy Clin Immunol* 105:S379, 1999.

62. Ohkawara Y, Lim KG, Xing Z, et al: CD40 expression by human peripheral blood eosinophils, *J Clin Invest* 97:1761-1766, 1996.

63. Woerly G, Roger N, Loiseau S, et al: Expression of CD28 and CD86 by human eosinophils and role in the secretion of type 1 cytokines (interleukin 2 and interferon gamma). Inhibition by immunoglobulin a complexes, *J Exp Med* 190:487-496, 1999.

64. Lucey DR, Nicholson WA, Weller PF: Mature human eosinophils have the capacity to express HLA-DR, *Proc Natl Acad Sci U S A* 86:1348-1351, 1989.

65. Lacy P, Levi-Schaffer F, Mahmudi Azer S, et al: Intracellular localization of interleukin-6 in eosinophils from atopic asthmatics and effects of interferon gamma, *Blood* 91:2508-2516, 1998.

66. Shi HZ, Humbles A, Gerard C, et al: Lymph node trafficking and antigen presentation by endobronchial eosinophils, *J Clin Invest* 105:945-953, 2000.

67. Kitamura Y, Go S, Hatanaka K: Decrease of mast cells in W/Wv mice and their increase by bone marrow transplantation, *Blood* 52:447-452, 1978.

68. Geissler EN, Ryan MA, Housman DE: The dominant-white spotting (W) locus of the mouse encodes the c-kit proto-oncogene, *Cell* 55:185-192, 1988.

69. Flanagan JG, Leder P: The kit ligand: a cell surface molecule altered in steel mutant fibroblasts, *Cell* 63:185-194, 1990.

70. Echtenacher B, Mannel DN, Hultner L: Critical protective role of mast cells in a model of acute septic peritonitis, *Nature* 381:75-77, 1996.

71. Malaviya R, Ikeda T, Ross E, et al: Mast cell modulation of neutrophil influx and bacterial clearance at sites of infection through TNF-alpha, *Nature* 381:77-80, 1996.

72. Williams CM, Galli SJ: The diverse potential effector and immunoregulatory roles of mast cells in allergic disease, *J Allergy Clin Immunol* 105: 847-859, 2000.

73. Hsieh FH, Lam BK, Penrose JF, et al: T helper cell type 2 cytokines coordinately regulate immunoglobulin E-dependent cysteinyl leukotriene production by human cord blood-derived mast cells: profound induction of leukotriene C(4) synthase expression by interleukin 4, *J Exp Med* 193:123-133, 2001.

74. Oh SW, Pae CI, Lee DK, et al: Tryptase inhibition blocks airway inflammation in a mouse asthma model, *J Immunol* 168:1992-2000, 2002.

75. Bradding P, Roberts JA, Britten KM, et al: Interleukin-4, -5, and -6 and tumor necrosis factor-alpha in normal and asthmatic airways: evidence for the human mast cell as a source of these cytokines, *Am J Respir Cell Mol Biol* 10:471-480, 1994.

76. Boyce JA, Friend D, Matsumoto R, et al: Differentiation in vitro of hybrid eosinophil/basophil granulocytes: autocrine function of an eosinophil developmental intermediate, *J Exp Med* 182:49-57, 1995.

77. Schwartz LB: Mast cells and basophils, *Clin Allergy Immunol* 16:3-42, 2002.

78. Miura K, Saini SS, Gauvreau G, et al: Differences in functional consequences and signal transduction induced by IL-3, IL-5, and nerve growth factor in human basophils, *J Immunol* 167:2282-2291, 2001.

79. Devouassoux G, Foster B, Scott LM, et al: Frequency and characterization of antigen-specific IL-4- and IL-13-producing basophils and T cells in peripheral blood of healthy and asthmatic subjects, *J Allergy Clin Immunol* 104:811-819, 1999.

80. Kepley CL, Craig SS, Schwartz LB: Identification and partial characterization of a unique marker for human basophils, *J Immunol* 154:6548-6555, 1995.

81. McEuen AR, Buckley MG, Compton SJ, et al: Development and characterization of a monoclonal antibody specific for human basophils and the identification of a unique secretory product of basophil activation, *Lab Invest* 79:27-38, 1999.

82. Irani AM, Huang C, Xia HZ, et al: Immunohistochemical detection of human basophils in late-phase skin reactions, *J Allergy Clin Immunol* 101:354-362, 1998.

83. Ying S, Robinson DS, Meng Q, et al: C-C chemokines in allergen-induced late-phase cutaneous responses in atopic subjects: association of eotaxin with early 6-hour eosinophils, and of eotaxin-2 and monocyte chemoattractant protein-4 with the later 24-hour tissue eosinophilia, and relationship to basophils and other C-C chemokines (monocyte chemoattractant protein-3 and RANTES), *J Immunol* 163:3976-3984, 1999.

84. Thomas ED, Ramberg RE, Sale GE, et al: Direct evidence for a bone marrow origin of the alveolar macrophage in man, *Science* 192:1016-1018, 1976.

85. Kennedy DW, Abkowitz JL: Mature monocytic cells enter tissues and engraft, *Proc Natl Acad Sci U S A* 95:14944-14949, 1998.

86. Hume DA, Robinson AP, MacPherson GG, et al: The mononuclear phagocyte system of the mouse defined by immunohistochemical localization of antigen F4/80. Relationship between macrophages, Langerhans cells, reticular cells, and dendritic cells in lymphoid and hematopoietic organs, *J Exp Med* 158:1522-1536, 1983.

87. Lang RA, Bishop JM: Macrophages are required for cell death and tissue remodeling in the developing mouse eye, *Cell* 74:453-462, 1993.

88. Yoshida M, Ikegami M, Reed JA, et al: GM-CSF regulates protein and lipid catabolism by alveolar macrophages, *Am J Physiol Lung Cell Mol Physiol* 280:L379-L386, 2001.

89. Begg SK, Radley JM, Pollard JW, et al: Delayed hematopoietic development in osteopetrotic (op/op) mice, *J Exp Med* 177:237-242, 1993.

90. Trapnell BC, Whitsett JA: GM-CSF regulates pulmonary surfactant homeostasis and alveolar macrophage-mediated innate host defense, *Annu Rev Physiol* 64:775-802, 2002.

91. Dranoff G, Crawford AD, Sadelain M, et al: Involvement of granulocyte-macrophage colony-stimulating factor in pulmonary homeostasis, *Science* 264:713-716, 1994.

92. Shibata Y, Berclas PY, Chroneos ZC, et al: GM-CSF regulates alveolar macrophage differentiation and innate immunity in the lung through PU.1, *Immunity* 15:557-567, 2001.

93. Aderem A, Ulevitch RJ: Toll-like receptors in the induction of the innate immune response, *Nature* 406:782-787, 2000.

94. Mills CD: Macrophage arginine metabolism to ornithine/urea or nitric oxide/citrulline: a life or death issue, *Crit Rev Immunol* 21:399-425, 2001.

95. Rivier A, Pene J, Rabesandratana H, et al: Blood monocytes of untreated asthmatics exhibit some features of tissue macrophages, *Clin Exp Immunol* 100:314-318, 1995.

96. Poston RN, Chanez P, Lacoste JY, et al: Immunohistochemical characterization of the cellular infiltration in asthmatic bronchi, *Am Rev Respir Dis* 145:918-921, 1992.

97. Sousa AR, Lane SJ, Nakhosteen JA, et al: Increased expression of the monocyte chemoattractant protein-1 in bronchial tissue from asthmatic subjects, *Am J Respir Cell Mol Biol* 10:142-147, 1994.

98. Randolph GJ: Dendritic cell migration to lymph nodes: cytokines, chemokines, and lipid mediators, *Semin Immunol* 13:267-274, 2001.

99. Lambrecht BN: The dendritic cell in allergic airway diseases: a new player to the game, *Clin Exp Allergy* 31:206-218, 2001.

100. Keller R: Dendritic cells: their significance in health and disease, *Immunol Lett* 78:113-122, 2001.

101. Tanaka H, Demeure CE, Rubio M, et al: Human monocyte-derived dendritic cells induce naive T cell differentiation into T helper cell type 2 (Th2) or Th1/Th2 effectors. Role of stimulator/responder ratio, *J Exp Med* 192:405-412, 2000.

102. Hutloff A, Dittrich AM, Beier KC, et al: ICOS is an inducible T-cell costimulator structurally and functionally related to CD28, *Nature* 397:263-266, 1999.

103. Lambrecht BN, Salomon B, Klatzmann D, et al: Dendritic cells are required for the development of chronic eosinophilic airway inflammation in response to inhaled antigen in sensitized mice, *J Immunol* 160:4090-4097, 1998.

104. Lambrecht BN, De Veerman M, Coyle AJ, et al: Myeloid dendritic cells induce Th2 responses to inhaled antigen, leading to eosinophilic airway inflammation, *J Clin Invest* 106:551-559, 2000.

105. Haselden BM, Barry Kay A, Larche M: Immunoglobulin E-independent major histocompatibility complex-restricted T cell peptide epitope-induced late asthmatic reactions, *J Exp Med* 189:1885-1894, 1999.

106. Cartwright GE, Athens JW, Winthrobe MM: The kinetics of granulopoiesis in normal man, *Blood* 24:780-803, 1964.

107. Reeves EP, Lu H, Jacobs HL, et al: Killing activity of neutrophils is mediated through activation of proteases by K+ flux, *Nature* 416:291-297, 2002.

108. Kelly C, Ward C, Stenton CS, et al: Number and activity of inflammatory cells in bronchoalveolar lavage fluid in asthma and their relation to airway responsiveness, *Thorax* 43:684-692, 1988.

109. Sur S, Crotty TB, Kephart GM, et al: Sudden-onset fatal asthma. A distinct entity with few eosinophils and relatively more neutrophils in the airway submucosa? *Am Rev Respir Dis* 148:713-719, 1993.

110. O'Byrne PM, Walters EH, Gold BD, et al: Neutrophil depletion inhibits airway hyperresponsiveness induced by ozone exposure, *Am Rev Respir Dis* 130:214-219, 1984.

111. Zlotnik A, Yoshie O: Chemokines: a new classification system and their role in immunity, *Immunity* 12:121-127, 2000.

112. Murphy PM: The molecular biology of leukocyte chemoattractant receptors, *Annu Rev Immunol* 12:593-633, 1994.

113. Gerard C, Gerard NP: The pro-inflammatory seven-transmembrane segment receptors of the leukocyte, *Curr Opin Immunol* 6:140-145, 1994.

114. Ganju RK, Dutt P, Wu L, et al: Beta-chemokine receptor CCR5 signals via the novel tyrosine kinase RAFTK, *Blood* 91:791-797, 1998.

115. Boehme SA, Sullivan SK, Crowe PD, et al: Activation of mitogen-activated protein kinase regulates eotaxin-induced eosinophil migration, *J Immunol* 163:1611-1618, 1999.

116. Proost P, Wuyts A, Van Damme J: Human monocyte chemotactic proteins-2 and -3: structural and functional comparison with MCP-1, *J Leukoc Biol* 59:67-74, 1996.

117. Garcia-Zepeda EA, Rothenberg ME, Ownbey RT, et al: Human eotaxin is a specific chemoattractant for eosinophil cells and provides a new mechanism to explain tissue eosinophilia, *Nat Med* 2:449-456, 1996.

118. Stellato C, Collins P, Ponath PD, et al: Production of the novel C-C chemokine MCP-4 by airway cells and comparison of its biological activity to other C-C chemokines, *J Clin Invest* 99:926-936, 1997.

119. Minshall EM, Cameron L, Lavigne F, et al: Eotaxin mRNA and protein expression in chronic sinusitis and allergen-induced nasal responses in seasonal allergic rhinitis, *Am J Respir Cell Mol Biol* 17:683-690, 1997.

120. Lilly CM, Nakamura H, Kesselman H, et al: Expression of eotaxin by human lung epithelial cells: induction by cytokines and inhibition by glucocorticoids, *J Clin Invest* 99:1767-1773, 1997.

121. Nelson PJ, Kim HT, Manning WC, et al: Genomic organization and transcriptional regulation of the RANTES chemokine gene, *J Immunol* 151:2601-2612, 1993.

122. Garcia-Zepeda EA, Rothenberg ME, Weremowicz S, et al: Genomic organization, complete sequence, and chromosomal location of the gene for human eotaxin (SCYA11), an eosinophil-specific CC chemokine, *Genomics* 41:471-476, 1997.

123. Matsukura S, Stellato C, Plitt JR, et al: Activation of eotaxin gene transcription by NF-kappaB and STAT6 in human airway epithelial cells, *J Immunol* 163:6876-6883, 1999.

124. Ueda A, Okuda K, Ohno S, et al: NF-kappa B and Sp1 regulate transcription of the human monocyte chemoattractant protein-1 gene, *J Immunol* 153:2052-2063, 1994.

125. Anisowicz A, Messineo M, Lee SW, et al: An NF-kappa B-like transcription factor mediates IL-1/TNF-alpha induction of gro in human fibroblasts, *J Immunol* 147:520-527, 1991.

126. Widmer U, Manogue KR, Cerami A, et al: Genomic cloning and promoter analysis of macrophage inflammatory protein (MIP)-2, MIP-1 alpha, and MIP-1 beta, members of the chemokine superfamily of proinflammatory cytokines, *J Immunol* 150:4996-5012, 1993.

127. Beato M: Gene regulation by steroid hormones, *Cell* 56:335-344, 1989.

128. Mukaida N, Gussella GL, Kasahara T, et al: Molecular analysis of the inhibition of interleukin-8 production by dexamethasone in a human fibrosarcoma cell line, *Immunology* 75:674-679, 1992.

129. Stellato C, Matsukura S, Fal A, et al: Differential regulation of epithelial-derived C-C chemokine expression by IL-4 and the glucocorticoid budesonide, *J Immunol* 163:5624-5632, 1999.

130. Loetscher P, Seitz M, Baggiolini M, et al: Interleukin-2 regulates CC chemokine receptor expression and chemotactic responsiveness in T lymphocytes, *J Exp Med* 184:569-577, 1996.

131. Loetscher M, Gerber B, Loetscher P, et al: Chemokine receptor specific for IP10 and mig: structure, function, and expression in activated T-lymphocytes, *J Exp Med* 184:963-969, 1996.

132. D'Amico G, Frascaroli G, Bianchi G, et al: Uncoupling of inflammatory chemokine receptors by IL-10: generation of functional decoys, *Nat Immunol* 1:387-391, 2000.

133. Yamada H, Hirai K, Miyamasu M, et al: Eotaxin is a potent chemotaxin for human basophils, *Biochem Biophys Res Commun* 231:365-368, 1997.

134. Luster AD, Rothenberg ME: Role of monocyte chemoattractant protein and eotaxin subfamily of chemokines in allergic inflammation, *J Leukoc Biol* 62:620-633, 1997.

135. Rothenberg ME, Ownbey R, Mehlhop PD, et al: Eotaxin triggers eosinophil-selective chemotaxis and calcium flux via a distinct receptor and induces pulmonary eosinophilia in the presence of interleukin 5 in mice, *Mol Med* 2:334-348, 1996.

136. Collins PD, Marleau S, Griffiths-Johnson DA, et al: Cooperation between interleukin-5 and the chemokine eotaxin to induce eosinophil accumulation in vivo, *J Exp Med* 182:1169-1174, 1995.

137. Mould AW, Matthaei KI, Young IG, et al: Relationship between interleukin-5 and eotaxin in regulating blood and tissue eosinophilia in mice, *J Clin Invest* 99:1064-1071, 1997.

138. Bischoff SC, Krieger M, Brunner T, et al: Monocyte chemotactic protein 1 is a potent activator of human basophils, *J Exp Med* 175:1271-1275, 1992.

139. Dahinden CA, Geiser T, Brunner T, et al: Monocyte chemotactic protein 3 is a most effective basophil- and eosinophil-activating chemokine, *J Exp Med* 179:751-756, 1994.

140. Elsner J, Hochstetter R, Kimmig D, et al: Human eotaxin represents a potent activator of the respiratory burst of human eosinophils, *Eur J Immunol* 26:1919-1925, 1996.

141. Alam R, Lett-Brown MA, Forsythe PA, et al: Monocyte chemotactic and activating factor is a potent histamine-releasing factor for basophils, *J Clin Invest* 89:723-728, 1992.

142. Alam R, Forsythe P, Stafford S, et al: Monocyte chemotactic protein-2, monocyte chemotactic protein-3, and fibroblast-induced cytokine. Three new chemokines induce chemotaxis and activation of basophils, *J Immunol* 153:3155-3159, 1994.

143. Kim CH, Broxmeyer HE: Chemokines for immature blood cells: effects on migration, proliferation, and differentiation. In Rothenberg ME, ed: *Chemokines in allergic disease*, New York, 2000, Marcel Dekker.

144. Nagasawa T, Hirota S, Tachibana K, et al: Defects of B-cell lymphopoiesis and bone-marrow myelopoiesis in mice lacking the CXC chemokine PBSF/SDF-1, *Nature* 382:635-638, 1996.

145. Palframan RT, Collins PD, Williams TJ, et al: Eotaxin induces a rapid release of eosinophils and their progenitors from the bone marrow, *Blood* 91:2240-2248, 1998.

146. Quackenbush EJ, Aguirre V, Wershil BK, et al: Eotaxin influences the development of embryonic hematopoietic progenitors in the mouse, *J Leukoc Biol* 62:661-666, 1997.

147. Peled A, Gonzalo JA, Lloyd C, et al: The chemotactic cytokine eotaxin acts as a granulocyte-macrophage colony-stimulating factor during lung inflammation, *Blood* 91:1909-1916, 1998.

148. Graham GJ, Wright EG, Hewick R, et al: Identification and characterization of an inhibitor of haemopoietic stem cell proliferation, *Nature* 344:442-444, 1990.

149. Sallusto F, Schaerli P, Loetscher P, et al: Rapid and coordinated switch in chemokine receptor expression during dendritic cell maturation, *Eur J Immunol* 28:2760-2769, 1998.

150. Sozzani S, Luini W, Borsatti A, et al: Receptor expression and responsiveness of human dendritic cells to a defined set of CC and CXC chemokines, *J Immunol* 159:1993-2000, 1997.

151. Dieu-Nosjean MC, Vicari A, Lebecque S, et al: Regulation of dendritic cell trafficking: a process that involves the participation of selective chemokines, *J Leukoc Biol* 66:252-262, 1999.

152. Rollins BJ: Chemokines, *Blood* 90:909-928, 1997.

153. Gunn MD, Tangemann K, Tam C, et al: A chemokine expressed in lymphoid high endothelial venules promotes the adhesion and chemotaxis of naive T lymphocytes, *Proc Natl Acad Sci U S A* 95:258-263, 1998.

154. Ward SG, Bacon K, Westwick J: Chemokines and T lymphocytes: more than an attraction, *Immunity* 9:1-11, 1998.

155. Sallusto F, Lenig D, Forster R, et al: Two subsets of memory T lymphocytes with distinct homing potentials and effector functions, *Nature* 401:708-712, 1999.

156. Zhang S, Lukacs NW, Lawless VA, et al: Cutting edge: differential expression of chemokines in Th1 and Th2 cells is dependent on Stat6 but not Stat4, *J Immunol* 165:10-14, 2000.

157. Karpus WJ, Kennedy KJ: MIP-1alpha and MCP-1 differentially regulate acute and relapsing autoimmune encephalomyelitis as well as Th1/Th2 lymphocyte differentiation, *J Leukoc Biol* 62:681-687, 1997.

158. Gu L, Tseng S, Horner RM, et al: Control of TH2 polarization by the chemokine monocyte chemoattractant protein-1, *Nature* 404:407-411, 2000.

159. Toney LM, Cattoretti G, Graf JA, et al: BCL-6 regulates chemokine gene transcription in macrophages, *Nat Immunol* 1:214-220, 2000.

160. Ponath PD, Qin S, Post TW, et al: Molecular cloning and characterization of a human eotaxin receptor expressed selectively on eosinophils, *J Exp Med* 183:2437-2448, 1996.

161. Daugherty BL, Siciliano SJ, DeMartino JA, et al: Cloning, expression, and characterization of the human eosinophil eotaxin receptor, *J Exp Med* 183:2349-2354, 1996.

162. Heath H, Qin SX, Rao P, et al: Chemokine receptor usage by human eosinophils—the importance of CCR3 demonstrated using an antagonistic monoclonal antibody, *J Clin Invest* 99:178-184, 1997.

163. Warringa RAJ, Koenderman L, Kok PTM, et al: Modulation and induction of eosinophil chemotaxis by granulocyte-macrophage colony-stimulating factor and interleukin-3, *Blood* 77:2694-2700, 1991.

164. Lamkhioued B, Renzi PM, Abi-Younes S, et al: Increased expression of eotaxin in bronchoalveolar lavage and airways of asthmatics contributes to the chemotaxis of eosinophils to the site of inflammation, *J Immunol* 159:4593-4601, 1997.

165. Rothenberg ME: Eotaxin. An essential mediator of eosinophil trafficking into mucosal tissues, *Am J Respir Cell Mol Biol* 21:291-295, 1999.

166. Ma W, Bryce PJ, Humbles AA, et al: CCR3 is essential for skin eosinophilia and airway hyperresponsiveness in a murine model of allergic skin inflammation, *J Clin Invest* 109:621-628, 2002.

167. Sullivan SK, McGrath DA, Liao F, et al: MIP-3alpha induces human eosinophil migration and activation of the mitogen-activated protein kinases (p42/p44 MAPK), *J Leukoc Biol* 66:674-682, 1999.

168. Nagase H, Miyamasu M, Yamaguchi M, et al: Expression of CXCR4 in eosinophils: functional analyses and cytokine-mediated regulation, *J Immunol* 164:5935-5943, 2000.

169. Jinquan T, Jing C, Jacobi HH, et al: CXCR3 expression and activation of eosinophils: role of IFN-gamma-inducible protein-10 and monokine induced by IFN-gamma, *J Immunol* 165:1548-1556, 2000.

170. Gerard C, Rollins BJ: Chemokines and disease, *Nat Immunol* 2:108-115, 2001.

171. Nickel RG, Casolaro V, Wahn U, et al: Atopic dermatitis is associated with a functional mutation in the promoter of the C-C chemokine RANTES, *J Immunol* 164:1612-1616, 2000.

172. Fryer AA, Spiteri MA, Bianco A, et al: The −403 G→A promoter polymorphism in the RANTES gene is associated with atopy and asthma, *Genes Immunol* 1:509-514, 2000.

173. Lloyd CM, Delaney T, Nguyen T, et al: CC chemokine receptor (CCR)3/eotaxin is followed by CCR4/monocyte-derived chemokine in mediating pulmonary T helper lymphocyte type 2 recruitment after serial antigen challenge in vivo, *J Exp Med* 191:265-274, 2000.

174. Chensue SW, Lukacs NW, Yang TY, et al: Aberrant in vivo T helper type 2 cell response and impaired eosinophil recruitment in CC chemokine receptor 8 knockout mice, *J Exp Med* 193:573-584, 2001.

175. Dean M, Carrington M, Winkler C, et al: Genetic restriction of HIV-1 infection and progression to AIDS by a deletion allele of the CKR5 structural gene. Hemophilia Growth and Development Study, Multicenter AIDS Cohort Study, Multicenter Hemophilia Cohort Study, San Francisco City Cohort, ALIVE Study, *Science* 273:1856-1862, 1996.

176. Smith MW, Dean M, Carrington M, et al: Contrasting genetic influence of CCR2 and CCR5 variants on HIV-1 infection and disease progression. Hemophilia Growth and Development Study (HGDS), Multicenter AIDS Cohort Study (MACS), Multicenter Hemophilia Cohort Study (MHCS), San Francisco City Cohort (SFCC), ALIVE Study, *Science* 277:959-965, 1997.

177. Sabroe I, Conroy DM, Gerard NP, et al: Cloning and characterization of the guinea pig eosinophil eotaxin receptor, C-C chemokine receptor-3: blockade using a monoclonal antibody in vivo, *J Immunol* 161:6139-6147, 1998.

178. Proudfoot AE, Power CA, Hoogewerf AJ, et al: Extension of recombinant human RANTES by the retention of the initiating methionine produces a potent antagonist, *J Biol Chem* 271:2599-2603, 1996.

179. Elsner J, Petering H, Hochstetter R, et al: The CC chemokine antagonist Met-RANTES inhibits eosinophil effector functions through the chemokine receptors CCR1 and CCR3, *Eur J Immunol* 27:2892-2898, 1997.

180. Gangur V, Oppenheim JJ: Are chemokines essential or secondary participants in allergic responses? *Ann Allergy Asthma Immunol* 84:569-579, 2000.

181. Moore PS, Boshoff C, Weiss RA, et al: Molecular mimicry of human cytokine and cytokine response pathway genes by KSHV, *Science* 274:1739-1744, 1996.

182. Kledal TN, Rosenkilde MM, Coulin F, et al: A broad-spectrum chemokine antagonist encoded by Kaposi's sarcoma-associated herpesvirus, *Science* 277:1656-1659, 1997.

183. Luttichau HR, Stine J, Boesen TP, et al: A highly selective CC chemokine receptor (CCR)8 antagonist encoded by the poxvirus molluscum contagiosum, *J Exp Med* 191:171-180, 2000.

184. White JR, Lee JM, Young PR, et al: Identification of a potent, selective non-peptide CXCR2 antagonist that inhibits interleukin-8-induced neutrophil migration, *J Biol Chem* 273:10095-10098, 1998.

185. Hesselgesser J, Ng HP, Liang M, et al: Identification and characterization of small molecule functional antagonists of the CCR1 chemokine receptor, *J Biol Chem* 273:15687-15692, 1998.

186. Bertrand CP, Ponath PD: CCR3 blockade as a new therapy for asthma, *Expert Opin Invest Drugs* 9:43-52, 2000.

187. Sabroe I, Peck MJ, Van Keulen BJ, et al: A small molecule antagonist of chemokine receptors CCR1 and CCR3. Potent inhibition of eosinophil function and CCR3-mediated HIV-1 entry, *J Biol Chem* 275:25985-25992, 2000.

188. Rutledge BJ, Rayburn H, Rosenberg R, et al: High level monocyte chemoattractant protein-1 expression in transgenic mice increases their susceptibility to intracellular pathogens, *J Immunol* 155:4838-4843, 1995.

189. Zimmermann N, Conkright JJ, Rothenberg ME: CC chemokine receptor-3 undergoes prolonged ligand-induced internalization, *J Biol Chem* 274:12611-12618, 1999.

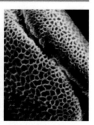

CHAPTER 6

The Developing Immune System and Allergy

PATRICK G. HOLT ■ JULIE ROWE

The prevalence of allergic diseases has risen markedly since the 1960s, particularly in the developed countries of the western world. The diseases manifest initially during childhood, and are apparently becoming more persistent in successive birth cohorts. The importance of genetic susceptibility in the disease process is widely recognized, and it is further recognized that the ultimate expression of the disease is the result of complex interactions between genetic and environmental factors, neither of which have yet been comprehensively characterized. There is increasing evidence that the level of complexity inherent in the pathogenesis of allergic diseases may be even greater than is currently contemplated, as an additional set of crucial factors appear to be involved. Notably, it appears likely that the ultimate effect(s) of these "gene x environment" interactions within individuals may also be related to the developmental status of the relevant target tissues at the time the interactions occur. Examples of the latter, discussed below, are elements of innate and adaptive immune function and aspects of airways function relevant to atopic asthma.

The following discussion is presented in two major subsections. First, our current understanding of the maturation of the immune system is broadly summarized. Second, recent findings relating to the etiology of allergic disease in general (and atopic asthma in particular) are presented, with a particular focus upon the role of immune developmental factors during infancy and early childhood.

IMMUNE FUNCTION DURING FETAL LIFE

The initial stage of hematopoiesis in the human fetus occurs in extraembryonic mesenchymal tissue and in the mesoderm of the yolk sac, and pluripotent erythroid and granulomacrophage progenitors are detectable in the latter at around the fourth week of gestation (Box 6-1). These cells appear subsequently in the fetal circulation and by weeks 5 to 6 in the liver, which at that stage of development is the major site of hematopoiesis. The spleen and thymus are seeded from the liver, and by the eighth week of development CD7+ precursor cells are found in the thymus[1-3]; stem cells do not appear in bone marrow until around the twelfth week of gestation.[4] T cells recognizable by expression of characteristic TcR/CD3 are found in peripheral lymphoid organs from weeks 13 to 15 of gestation onwards,[5-7] despite the lack of well-defined thymic cortical and medullary regions and mature epithelial components.[1] These early T cells also express CD2 and CD5.[3] The maturation of nonlymphoid components within peripheral lymphoid tissues progresses even more slowly and takes up to 20 weeks.[7-10]

It is feasible that the fetal gastrointestinal tract may be an additional site for extrathymic T cell differentiation in the human fetus, as has been reported in the mouse.[11] T cells are detectable in the intestinal mucosa by 12 weeks of gestation,[12] and many of these express the CD8αα phenotype, in particular within Peyer's patches.[13] In the mouse, CD8αα cells appear to be thymus independent and are believed to develop in the gut. Although there is no direct evidence for this in humans, it is noteworthy initially that fetal gut lamina propria lymphocytes are an actively proliferating population as indicated by constitutive expression of Ki67, and there is little or no overlap between gut-derived and blood-derived TcRβ transcripts.[14]

The gut mucosa may also be a major site for differentiation of TcRγ/δ cells during fetal life. Rearranged TcRδ genes are first detectable in the gut at 6 to 9 weeks of gestation,[15] which is earlier than is observed in the thymus. The liver is another significant extrathymic site for TcRγ/δ differentiation in humans, including a unique subset expressing CD4.[16]

The capacity to respond to polyclonal stimuli such as phytohemagglutinin (PHA) is first seen at 15 to 16 weeks of gestation.[17] The degree to which the fetal immune system can respond to foreign antigens has not been clearly established. On the one hand, the offspring of mothers infected during pregnancy with a range of pathogens including measles,[18] ascaris,[19] malaria,[20] schistosomes,[21] and helminths[22] display evidence of pathogen-specific T cell reactivity at birth, whereas infection with other organisms such as toxoplasma[23] may induce tolerance. Additionally, vaccination of pregnant women with tetanus toxoid results in the appearance of IgM in the fetal circulation that is indicative of fetal T cell sensitization.[24] Also, there is a variety of evidence based on *in vitro* lymphoproliferation of cord blood mononuclear cells, which suggests that environmental antigens (including dietary and inhalant allergens) to which pregnant women are exposed may in some circumstances prime T cell responses transplacentally.

It is also noteworthy that, despite the lack of significant numbers of CD4+ and CD8+ CD45RO+ T cells in cord blood, fetal spleen and cord blood samples from premature infants contain these cells in relatively high frequency.[25] These "postactivated or memory" T cells were unresponsive to

- Weeks 5-6 of gestation: pluripotent erythroid and granulomacrophage progenitors are detected in the liver
- Week 8 of gestation: CD7+ precursor cells found in the thymus
- Week 12 of gestation: stem cells appear in bone marrow
- Weeks 13-15 of gestation: T cells found in peripheral lymphoid organs
- Weeks 15-16 of gestation: fetal T cells respond to mitogen
- IgM responses develop in fetus following maternal vaccination
- Infant T cells express CD1, PNA, and CD38, indicative of mature thymocytes
- Proportion of CD45RO+ CD4+ T cells increase from <10% at birth to >65% in adulthood, reflecting progressive antigenic exposure
- Adult peripheral blood T cells express CCR-1, -2, -5, and -6 and CXCR-3 and CXCR-4, whereas cord blood expresses only CXCR-4, reflecting decreased capacity to respond to proinflammatory signals at birth
- At infancy, cytotoxic effector functions and capacity to drive B cell immunoglobulin production are attenuated

recombinant IL-2, suggesting they may have been anergized by earlier contact with self- or environmental antigens.[25]

These findings collectively suggest that the fetal immune system develops at least partial functional competence before birth but lack the full capacity to generate sustained immune responses; although IgM responses develop in the fetus following maternal tetanus vaccination, there is no evidence of class-switching in the offspring until they are actively vaccinated.[24] Given the fact that the fetal immune system can generate at least primary immune responses against external stimuli, the question arises as to how immune responses within or in close contact with the fetal compartment are regulated. The necessity for tight control of these responses becomes obvious in light of findings that a variety of T cell cytokines are exquisitely toxic to the placenta.[26] It is also pertinent to question how potential immunostimulatory interactions between cells derived from fetal and maternal bone marrow are regulated at the fetomaternal interface. In particular, it has been clearly demonstrated that fetal cells readily traffic into the maternal circulation,[27-31] potentially sensitizing the maternal immune system against paternal HLA antigens present on the fetal cells. However, it is clear from recent studies[32] that the maternal immune system in the vast majority of circumstances successfully eradicates fetal cells from the peripheral circulation while remaining functionally tolerant of the fetus. This suggests that tolerance of the fetal allograft is a regionally controlled process that is localized to the fetomaternal interface.

The mechanisms that regulate the induction and expression of immune responses in this milieu are complex and multilayered. The first line of defense appears to be a local immunosuppressive "blanket" maintained via the local production within the placenta by trophoblasts and macrophages of metabolites of tryptophan generated via indolamine 2,3-dioxygenase, which are markedly inhibitory against T cell activation and proliferation.[33] Constitutive production of high levels of IL-10 by placental trophoblasts provides a second broad-spectrum immunosuppressive signal to dampen local T cell responses.[34]

A second line of defense operates to protect against T cell activation events that evade suppression via these pathways. One such mechanism involves expression of FasL on cells within the placenta, providing a potential avenue for apoptosis-mediated elimination of locally activated T cells.[35,36] The latter is complemented by a series of mechanisms that operate to selectively dampen production at the fetomaternal interface of Th1 cytokines, in particular, of interferon (IFN)-γ. This cytokine plays an important role in implantation,[37] but if produced in suprathreshold levels at later stages of pregnancy, triggered, for example, by local immune responses against microbial or alloantigens, IFN-γ (and other Th1 cytokines) can potentially cause placental detachment and fetal resorption.[38,39] These Th2-trophic mechanisms involve local production of a range of immunomodulators including IL-10,[34] which programs antigen-presenting cells (APCs) for Th2 switching[40]; progesterone, which directly inhibits IFN-γ gene transcription[41-43]; and PGE2, which promotes Th2 switching via effects upon APCs, dendritic cells in particular.[40]

RESISTANCE TO INFECTION DURING INFANCY

It is well established that infancy represents a period of high susceptibility to infection with a range of pathogens including bacteria and fungi[44] and, in particular, viruses.[45-47] The expression of cell-mediated immunity during active viral infection is attenuated in infants as compared to older age groups,[48-50] and the subsequent generation of virus-specific immunologic memory is also inefficient[51] (see following discussion on vaccine immunity). These findings suggest that a range of developmentally related deficiencies in innate and adaptive immunologic mechanisms are operative in the immediate postnatal period, and the nature and clinical significance of the latter are the subject of increasingly intensive research. Some of the salient findings from this evolving literature are reviewed next.

SURFACE PHENOTYPE OF T CELLS IN EARLY LIFE

Total lymphocyte counts in peripheral blood are higher in infancy than in adulthood,[52] and at birth T cell levels are twice those of adults. Longitudinal studies on individual infants indicate a further, rapid doubling in T cell numbers in the circulation during the first 6 weeks of life, which is maintained throughout infancy.[53] Surface marker expression on infant T cells differs markedly from that observed in adults. The most noteworthy characteristics are frequent expression of CD1[54] and PNA[55] antigens and CD38.[53,56,57] These three antigens are considered to mark mature thymocytes as opposed to circulating "mature" naive T cells.

Recent analyses performed on CD38+ cord blood cells have reinforced this view. In particular, animal model studies on thymic output have led to the development of an accurate technique for phenotypic identification of recent thymic emigrants (RTE), which are newly produced peripheral naive T cells that retain a distinct phenotypic signature of recent thymic maturation that distinguishes them from long-lived naive T cells produced at remote sites. This approach involves the measurement of T cell receptor excision circles (TRECs), which are stable extrachromosomal products generated during the process of variable/diverse/joining (VDJ) TcR gene rearrangement. These excision DNA circles are not replicated during mitosis and as a consequence become diluted with each round of cell division. Employing this procedure, Hassan and Reen[57] have demonstrated that the majority of circulating CD4+ CD45R+ human T cells at birth are RTE as reflected by their high level of expression of TRECs. These researchers also demonstrated that analogous to thymocytes the RTE were highly susceptible to apoptosis,[57] and unlike mature adult-derived CD4+ CD45RA+ naive T cells they were uniquely responsive to common γ-chain cytokines, particularly IL-7.[57,58] Whereas IL-7 promotes their proliferation and survival, IL-7−exposed RTE could not reexpress recombination-activating gene-2 gene expression *in vitro*. These findings suggest that postthymic naive peripheral T cells in early infancy are at a unique stage in ontogeny as RTEs, during which they can undergo homeostatic regulation including survival and antigen-independent expansion while maintaining their preselected TcR repertoire.[57]

The patterns of postnatal change in T cell surface marker expression have been analyzed in several recent studies. Of relevance to the preceding conclusions are observations noting the presence of relatively high numbers of T cells coexpressing both CD4 and CD8 during infancy, which is also a hallmark of immaturity.[53,59,60] In contrast, expression of CD57 on T cells, which marks non–MHC-restricted cytotoxic cells, is infrequent, as are T cells coexpressing IL-2 and HLA-DR, which is indicative of recent activation.[59] The expression of other activation markers such as CD25, CD69, and CD154, is also low.[53]

Of particular interest in relation to the understanding of overall immune competence during postnatal life are changing patterns of surface CD45RA and CD45RO on T cells. T cells exported from the thymus express the CD45RA isoform of the leukocyte common antigen CD45, and after activation switch to CD45RO expression. Most postactivated neonatal CD4+ CD45RO+ T cells are short-lived and die within a matter of days, but a subset of these is believed to be programmed to enter the long-lived recirculating T cell compartment as T memory cells.[61] The proportion of CD45RO+ cells within the CD4+ T cell compartment progressively increases from a baseline of less than 10% at birth up to 65% in adulthood, reflecting age-dependent accumulation of antigenic exposure.[53,59,61-66] The rate of increase within the TcR α/β and TcRγ/δ populations is approximately equivalent and is slightly more rapid for CD4+ T cells relative to CD8+ T cells.[66] The relative proportion of CD45RO+ putative memory T cells attain adult-equivalent levels within the teen years,[59,66] but it is noteworthy that the population spread during the years of childhood is very wide.[66] This suggests substantial heterogeneity within the pediatric population in the efficiency of mechanisms regulating the generation of T helper memory, an issue that is discussed next in more detail.

FUNCTIONAL PHENOTYPE OF T CELLS DURING INFANCY AND EARLY CHILDHOOD

T cell function during infancy exhibits a variety of qualitative and quantitative differences relative to that observed in adults. Of particular note, when employing a limiting dilution analytic system it has been demonstrated that at least 90% of peripheral blood CD4+ T cells from adults can give rise to stable T cell clones, whereas the corresponding (mean) figure for immunocompetent T cell precursors in infants was less than 35%.[67] It was also observed that cloning frequencies within the infant population were bimodally distributed, with a significant subset of ostensibly normal healthy subjects displaying particularly low cloning frequencies of no more than 20%.[67]

In apparent contrast to these findings, the kinetics of initial T cell proliferation induced by polyclonal T cell mitogens such as PHA in short-term cultures is higher at birth than subsequently during infancy and adulthood.[68,69] However, proliferation is not sustained, which may reflect the greater susceptibility of neonatal T cells to apoptosis postactivation[57] and/or decreased production of IL-2.[70,71] In contrast, activation induced by TcR stimulation[72] and cross-linking CD2[70,73] or CD28[74] is reduced.

In addition to these deficiencies, neonatal T cells are hyperresponsive to IL-4[75] and hyporesponsive to IL-12[76] relative to adults, the latter being associated with reduced receptor expression.[77] They also exhibit heightened susceptibility to anergy induction poststimulation with bacterial superantigen, employing protocols that do not tolerise adult T cells.[78,79] The latter has been ascribed to deficient IL-2 production,[78] but may alternatively be related to developmentally related deficiencies in the Ras signaling pathway, which have been associated with secondary unresponsiveness to alloantigen stimulation by T cells from neonates.[80] Additional aberrations in intracellular signaling pathways reported in neonatal T cells include phospholipase C and associated Lck expression,[81] protein kinase C,[82] and CD28, which is associated with dysfunction in FasL-mediated cytotoxicity[83] and reduced NFκB production.[74]

A recent study also reported distinct profiles of chemokine receptor expression and responsiveness in neonatal T cells. In particular, adult peripheral blood T cells expressed CCR-1, -2, -5, -6 and CXCR-3 and CXCR-4, whereas those from cord blood expressed only CXCR-4, reflecting markedly attenuated capacity to respond to signals from inflammatory foci.[84]

Evidence from a range of studies indicates that both cytotoxic effector functions[85,86] and capacity to provide help for B cell immunoglobulin production[85-89] are attenuated during infancy. These functional deficiencies are likely to be the result of a combination of factors that include decreased expression of CD40L,[85,87,88] reduced expression of cytokine receptors,[77,90] and decreased production of a wide range of cytokines following stimulation.[67,71,91-97] The mechanism(s) underlying these reduced cytokine responses are unclear, but factors intrinsic to the T cells themselves,[67,98] as well as those involving accessory cell functions,[98-100] appear to be involved. Issues relating to accessory cells are discussed next. In relation to the T cells, it is pertinent to note a recent report from this laboratory demonstrating hypermethylation at multiple CpG sites in the proximal promoter region of the IFN-γ gene in CD4+ CD45RA+ T cells in cord blood relative to their adult counterparts.[101] Hypermethylation of this nature in gene promoters is associated with reduced capacity for gene expression in several systems; it is additionally noteworthy that similar patterns of hypermethylation were not observed in the IL-4 promoter in neonates, suggesting that this mechanism is not universal.

B CELL FUNCTION IN EARLY LIFE

Certain aspects of B cell function in neonates appear unique in relation to adults. In particular, large numbers of neonatal B cells express CD5,[102,103] together with activation markers such as IL-2R and CD23.[102] It has been postulated that these CD5+ B cells act as a "first line of defense" in primary antibody responses in neonates utilizing a preimmune repertoire, in contrast to CD5− B cells in which response patterns are acquired following antigen contact.[104] Unlike adult B cells, these neonatal B cells proliferate readily in the presence of IL-2 or IL-4 without requirement of further signals.[102,105-107] An additional (albeit less frequent) neonatal B cell subset that expresses IgD, IgM, CD23, and CD11b and is CD5 variable spontaneously secretes IgM antibodies against a range of autoantigens.[102]

Conventional B cell function, that is, antibody production following infection or vaccination, is reduced in infants relative to adults,[51] and some in vitro studies suggest that this may be related to a defect in isotype switching.[108] The relative contributions of the T cell and B cell compartments to this deficiency in immunoglobulin production are widely debated, but the consensus is that both cell types play a role.

As noted previously, T cells in infants do not readily express high levels of CD40L[85-89] unless provided with particularly potent activating stimuli.[109] CD40L represents a critical signal for T helper cell-induced class switching[110] and the generally low expression on neonatal T cells may thus be a limiting factor in the process. Reduced T cell cytokine production[67,71,91-97] may further exacerbate the problem. However, although immunoglobulin production by neonatal B cells is low in the presence of neonatal T helper cells, production levels can be markedly improved if mature T helper cells or adequate soluble signals are provided.[89,105,111] However, the neonatal B cells still fail to reach adult-equivalent levels of production, suggesting that an intrinsic defect also exists.

ANTIGEN-PRESENTING CELL POPULATIONS

The key "professional" antigen-presenting cell (APC) populations in this context are the mononuclear phagocytes (MPCs), dendritic cells (DCs), and B cells. The precise role of each cell type in different types of immune response is not completely clear, although it is evident that DCs represent the most potent APC for priming the naive T cell system against antigens encountered at low concentrations (e.g., virus and environmental allergens).

Ontogenic studies on human MPCs have been essentially limited to blood monocytes. Neonatal populations appear comparable to the adult in number and phagocytic activity[112,113] and display reduced chemotactic responses[114] and reduced capacity for secretion of inflammatory cytokines such

as tumor necrosis factor-α.[115] Their capacity to present alloantigen to T cells is reportedly normal,[116] but they display reduced levels of MHC class II expression.[117] Several studies have implicated poor accessory cell function of infant blood monocytes as cofactors in the reduced IFN-γ responses of infant T cells to polyclonal mitogens such as PHA,[98-100] possibly as a result of diminished elaboration of co-stimulator signals. Macrophage populations at mucosal sites such as the lung and airways have important immunoregulatory roles in adults,[118] but it is not clear whether these mechanisms are operative in early life. One recent murine study from our group indicates lower levels of expression of immunomodulatory molecules including IL-10 and N0 by lung macrophages during the neonatal period.[119]

B cells are also recognized as important APCs, in particular for secondary immune responses.[120,121] In murine systems it has been demonstrated that neonatal B cells function poorly as APCs relative to their adult counterparts and do not reach adult-equivalent levels of activity until after weaning.[112,122] No direct information is available on the APC function of human neonatal B cells.

As noted previously, DCs are the most potent APC population in adult experimental animals for initiation of primary immunity and in this regard have been designated as the "gatekeepers" of the immune response.[123] The distribution and phenotypes of these cells appear comparable in murine and human tissues, and it is accordingly reasonable to speculate that the proposed role of murine DCs as the link between the innate and adaptive arms of the immune system[123-126] is also applicable to man. Importantly, in the context of allergic disease comparative studies on DCs from mucosal sites in humans and experimental animals suggest very similar functional characteristics.[127]

DCs commence seeding into peripheral tissues relatively early in gestation,[128] and at birth recognizable networks of these cells can be detected in a variety of tissues including epidermis,[128-130] intestinal mucosa,[131,132] and the upper and lower respiratory tract.[133,134] The cells within these DC networks in perinatal tissues are typically present at lower densities and express lower levels of surface MHC class II relative to adults,[129,130,134] hinting at developmentally related variations in function phenotype. Recent murine studies have emphasized these differences. Notably, the phenomenon of neonatal tolerance in mice has recently been ascribed to the relative inability of neonatal DCs from central lymphoid organs to present Th1-inducing signals to T cells, leading to the preferential generation of Th2-biased immune responses.[135] Of particular relevance to studies on susceptibility to infectious and allergic diseases in infancy, our group has demonstrated that in the rat, the airway mucosal DC compartment develops postnatally very slowly, and does not obtain adult-equivalent levels of tissue density, MHC class II expression, and capacity to respond to local inflammatory stimuli until after biologic weaning.[134,136]

Direct functional data on mucosal DC populations in humans are lacking, but indirect data based on immunohistochemical studies of autopsy tissues suggest that the kinetics of postnatal maturation of airway DC networks in humans may be comparably slow.[137,138] Recent reports suggest that the numbers of circulating HLA-DR+ DCs are reduced at birth relative to adults[139] and these cells display diminished APC activity.[140] Additionally, analysis of cord blood monocyte-derived DC functions indicates diminished expression of HLA-DR, CD80, and CD40 and attenuated production of IL-12p35 in response to stimuli such as LPS, poly (I:C), and CD40 ligation.[141]

EOSINOPHILS AND MAST CELLS

Eosinophils and mast cells play key roles in the pathogenesis of allergic disease, perform important functions in relation to host resistance to certain pathogens, and are thus of particular relevance to this discussion.

Eosinophilia at 3 months of age has been linked to enhanced risk for later development of atopic disease,[142] but little additional data on disease association are available. Several earlier observations are suggestive of developmentally related problems in eosinophil trafficking in early life. In particular, inflammatory exudates in neonates frequently contain elevated numbers of eosinophils,[143-145] and eosinophilia is common in premature infants.[146,147] The mechanism(s) underlying these developmental variations in eosinophil function are unclear, but some evidence suggests a role for integrin expression including Mac-1[148] and L-selectin.[149]

Adult mucosal tissues contain discrete populations of mucosal mast cells (MMCs) and connective tissue mast cells (CTMCs), respectively, within epithelia and underlying lamina propria. No direct information is available on the ontogeny of these MC, in human tissues, but indirect evidence suggests that they seed into gut tissues during infancy in response to local inflammatory stimulation.[150] Our group has examined the kinetics of postnatal development of MCs in the rat respiratory tract, and has reported that both MMC and CTMC populations develop slowly between birth and weaning.[151] MC-derived proteases appear transiently in serum around the time of weaning in the rat, suggesting that the immature MC populations may be unstable or are undergoing local stimulation at this time,[152] and a similar transient peak of MC-tryptase is observed in human serum during infancy.[153]

Direct functional studies on MCs from immature subjects are lacking. However, a recent report has employed oligonucleotide microarray technology to examine IL-4–induced gene expression in cultured MCs derived from cord blood versus adult peripheral blood, and the results indicate that expression of FcεR1α is tenfold higher in adult-derived MCs.[154] This suggests that during infancy the capacity to express IgE-mediated immunity may be restricted, but confirmation of this possibility must await further detailed studies.

VACCINE IMMUNITY IN EARLY LIFE

Investigations on vaccine immunity during infancy and early childhood are of intrinsic importance in their own right. In addition, they provide a unique experimental window through which to study the postnatal development of human adaptive immune function and are thus of particular relevance to this review; some recent key findings are summarized below.

As discussed previously, significant aspects of immune function are immature at birth, not reaching adult capacity for several years. For example, the *in utero* generation of tetanus-specific IgM following maternal immunization with tetanus toxoid demonstrates the ability of the fetus to generate an active, albeit immature, immune response because no switch from IgM to IgG is evident until later during infancy, following boosting.[155]

After birth, there is a progressive maturation of the capacity to generate adult-like responses, both quantitatively and qualitatively. After measles-mumps-rubella vaccination, the seroconversion rate against measles is age-dependent, with those vaccinated between 9 and 11 months having significantly lower antibody titers than those vaccinated between 15 and 17 months.[156] In another study, Gans and colleagues[157] observed that while antibody responses were lower in infants receiving the measles vaccine at 6 months than those vaccinated at 9 or 12 months, there was no significant difference in *in vitro* antigen-specific IFN-γ or IL-12 production. However, when these responses were compared to those of adults, the infants produced significantly lower levels of IL-12 after *in vitro* stimulation with measles antigen.[157] In mice, significant B and T cell vaccine responses were obtained as early as the first year of life. However, neonatal responses differed qualitatively from those in adults, with neonates having a decreased ratio of IgG2a/IgG1 and higher *in vitro* vaccine-specific IL-5 and decreased IFN-γ.[158]

In a prospective cohort of 132 infants, we have examined the response to the tetanus component of the diphtheria/tetanus/acellular pertussis (DTaP) vaccine and compared these responses to age-related changes in systemic Th1 and Th2 cytokine function. Our results indicate early Th1 and Th2 cytokine responses to the vaccine antigen. Although Th2 vaccine-specific responses persisted throughout the study period, Th1 responses were transient.[159,160] These results are similar to those observed in mice, with balanced Th1/Th2 vaccine responses generated in neonatal animals. However, Th2 secondary responses predominated in mice first vaccinated as neonates, suggesting that Th1 cells may not be well maintained early in life.[161]

Interestingly, in our study, although vaccine-specific IFN-γ production declined after the final priming DTaP dose at 6 months, between 12 and 18 months in the absence of further vaccination there was a marked resurgence in these responses, coinciding with a parallel increase in overall IFN-γ production capacity.[160] Ausiello and colleagues[162] reported a similar finding in relation to increased pertussis-specific IFN-γ responses in the absence of further vaccination, which was attributed to boosting by covert infection with *Bordetella pertussis*. With regard to our findings, we hypothesize that the vaccine-independent upswing of Th1 responses may reflect boosting by environmental antigens that cross-react with tetanus toxoid. However, given the parallel increase in polyclonal IFN-γ–secreting capacity over the same period, a more likely explanation is that changes in accessory cell function permit more efficient *in vitro* expression of IFN-γ memory responses by previously primed tetanus toxoid-specific Th1 cells. In this context, it is pertinent to note that it has been demonstrated that given a mature source of accessory cells, peripheral blood T cell IFN-γ production in response to polyclonal mitogen stimulation can be boosted to approximate those of adults.[98,99] Similarly, vaccination with the use of powerful stimuli such as BCG[63,164] or selective Th1-driving agents such as IL-12,[165] plasmid DNA,[166] and CpG-containing oligonucleotides[167] can all induce adult-like Th1 responses in early life, presumably through activation of accessory cell function.

As discussed in more detail later, slow postnatal maturation of IFN-γ production capacity is linked to genetic risk for atopy. There is some evidence to suggest that delayed Th1 maturation may reduce the capacity of children at high risk of atopy to respond to vaccination efficiently in infancy. In response to BCG vaccination in infancy, for example, failure to develop long-lasting delayed-type hypersensitivity responses to tuberculin was associated with increased risk of atopy at 12 years.[168] In addition, children who develop atopic dermatitis had a reduced ability to respond to pneumococcal vaccination.[169] With regard to the DTP vaccine, we also have observed that infants at high risk of atopy had specific responses to tetanus toxoid that were consistently more Th2 skewed, displaying higher Th2/Th1 ratios.[160] This difference was no longer evident in these subjects at 18 months.[160] Furthermore, in another study we have shown that *in vitro* proliferative responses to tetanus toxoid during infancy were inversely related to the atopic phenotype.[170] It is important to stress that in our experience these differences appear transient, and after the completion of the standard priming/boosting vaccine schedule at age 6 years there was no significant difference in vaccine response when comparing atopic patients to their non-atopic counterparts.[171] However, the possibility remains that transient hyporesponsiveness to vaccines during infancy in subjects genetically at high risk of developing atopy may confer significant risk for infection from the organisms targeted by the vaccines, and further work needs to be done to clarify this issue.

VARIATIONS IN KINETICS OF POSTNATAL MATURATION OF IMMUNE FUNCTIONS

Recent studies from a number of groups have highlighted the importance of the early postnatal period in relation to the development of long-lasting response patterns to environmental allergens. In particular, it is becoming clear that initial priming of the naive immune system typically occurs before weaning and may consolidate into stable immunologic memory before the end of the preschool years. Given that the underlying immunologic processes involve the coordinate operations of the full gamut of innate and adaptive immune mechanisms, issues relating to developmentally determined functional competence during this life phase may be predicted to be of major importance.

In relation to initial priming of the T cell system against allergens, reports from numerous groups indicate the presence of T cells responsive to food and inhalant allergens in cord blood.[172-176] Cloning of these cells and subsequent DNA genotyping indicated fetal as opposed to maternal origin,[177] and the array of cytokines produced *in vitro* in their responses are dominated by Th2 cytokines, although IFN-γ is also observed, suggestive of a Th0-like pattern.[177] The issue of how initial priming of these cells occurs remains to be resolved. It is possible that transplacental transport of allergen, perhaps conjugated with maternal IgG, may be responsible, and some indirect supporting evidence based on *in vitro* perfusion studies has been published recently to support this notion.[178] Alternatively, initial T cell priming may be against cross-reacting antigens as opposed to native allergen, and the uncertain relationship between maternal allergen exposure and newborn T cell reactivity is consistent with this view.[179,180] The mucosal T cell epitope map of the typical cord blood T cell response to ovalbumin (OVA), involving multiple regions of the OVA molecule,[181] suggests major qualitative differences relative to conventional adult T cell responses.

Regardless of how initial T cell responses are primed, it is clear that direct exposure to environmental allergens during infancy drives the early responses down one of two alternate pathways. In the majority of (nonatopic) subjects, the Th2 cytokine component of these early responses progressively diminishes, and by age 5 years *in vitro* T cell responses to allergens comprise a combination of low-level IFN-γ and IL-10 production.[181-183] In contrast, a subset of children develop positive skin prick test (SPT) reactivity to one or more allergens, and *in vitro* stimulation of PBMC with the latter elicits a mixed or Th0-like response pattern comprising IL-4, IL-5, IL-9, IL-10, IL-13, and IFN-γ.[183] This latter pattern closely resembles that seen in the majority of adult atopic patients, and much more commonly develops in atopic family history–positive (AFH[+]) children than in their AFH[-] counterparts.

It is increasingly debated whether it remains useful to describe these differing responses in human atopic and nonatopic patients within the framework of the murine Th1/Th2 paradigm, which was based upon the concept of reciprocal and/or antagonistic patterns of Th-memory expression. In this context, recent studies from our group[184,185] indicate that reciprocal patterns of expression of the transcription factor GATA-3, analogous to those that distinguish Th1 from Th2 polarized cell lines (with regard to down-regulation versus up-regulation, respectively, poststimulation), are reiterated during the allergen-specific recall responses of CD4+ T cells from nonatopic versus atopic subjects. This suggests that the Th1/Th2 model still provides a potentially useful framework for the study of allergic responses, despite the strong likelihood of significant interspecies differences.

The central issue in relation to understanding the initial phase of allergic sensitization in childhood concerns the molecular basis for genetic susceptibility to development of Th2-polarized memory against inhalant allergens, and the key to the resolution of this puzzle may lie in a more comprehensive understanding of the mechanisms that drive postnatal maturation of adaptive immune function. In this regard we have reported earlier that genetic risk for atopy was associated with delayed postnatal maturation of Th-cell function, in particular Th1 function, and that this may increase risk for consolidating Th2-polarized memory against allergens during childhood. The evidence originally presented was based on decreased peripheral blood T cell cloning frequency and diminished IFN-γ production by T cell clones in AFH[+] infants relative to their counterparts,[67] and these findings have been substantiated in several independent laboratories employing bulk culture studies with neonatal PBMC.[186-191] We have proposed that this phenomenon may derive from inappropriate postnatal persistence of one or more of the mechanisms responsible for selective damping of Th1 immunity during fetal life.[192] Alternatively, given that the postnatal maturation of adaptive immunity is essentially driven by microbial signals from the outside environment,[192-194] one or more deficiencies in relevant receptors or downstream signaling pathways may retard this process. The recently described genetic variations in CD14 may be an archetypal example,[195] and similar variants in one or more of the Toll receptor genes constitute additional likely candidates. These possibilities are of particular interest in light of recent reports that environmental exposure to airborne bacterial lipopolysaccharide in childhood may be protective against Th2-mediated sensitization to inhalant allergens.[196,197]

Further research is required to elucidate the complex regulatory mechanisms that govern generation of different patterns of allergen-specific Th memory during childhood. However, it is also becoming clear that an additional, and related, set of complexities needs to be considered. It is now evident that only a subset of atopic patients progress to development of severe persistent allergic diseases, in particular atopic asthma,[198] and it is likely that these subjects suffer additional and/or particularly intense inflammatory insults to target tissues. In this context, epidemiologic evidence suggests that risk for development of persistent asthma is most marked in children who display early allergic sensitization to inhalants[199,200] and who develop severe wheezing and lower respiratory tract infections during infancy.[200-202] This has given rise to the suggestion that susceptibility to development of the airways remodeling characteristic of chronic asthma[203] may in many circumstances be the long-term result of inflammation-induced changes in lung and airway differentiation during critical stages of early growth during childhood. It is additionally noteworthy that resistance to respiratory infections is also mediated by the same Th1 mechanisms just identified as attenuated in children at risk of atopy,[204] suggesting that the same set of genetic mechanisms may be responsible for airways inflammation induced via the viral infection and atopic pathways in children at high risk of asthma (Box 6-2).

An additional variable that merits more detailed research is the role of airway DC populations in this complex equation. In the adult these cells regulate the Th1/Th2 balance in immune responses to airborne antigens[205] and also mediate primary and secondary immunity to viral pathogens.[123] However, airway DC networks develop very slowly postnatally, apparently "driven" by exposure to inhaled airborne irritants,[134] in particular bacterial lipopolysaccharides.[206,207] Hence the rate at which this key cell population gains competence to respond to maturation-inducing stimuli, and then to orchestrate appropriately balanced T cell responses against viral pathogens and allergens, may be a key determinant of overall susceptibility to allergic disease. Variations in the genes that govern the functions of these cells in early life are thus likely to be of major importance in the etiology of a variety of disease processes, in particular atopic asthma and related syndromes.

BOX 6-2

KEY CONCEPTS

Role of Immune Developmental Factors on Allergic Response

- Dendritic cells (DCs) are the most potent antigen-presenting cells for priming naive T cells against antigens encountered at low concentrations.
- Neonatal DCs present weak Th1-inducing signals to T cells, leading to preferential generation of Th2 immune responses.
- Slow postnatal maturation of interferon-gamma production capacity is linked to genetic risk for atopy.
- Postnatal maturation of adaptive immunity is driven by microbial signals.
- A deficiency in microbial receptors (e.g., CD14, Toll receptors) or downstream signaling pathways may prevent the development of polarized Th1 responses.

REFERENCES

1. Haynes BF, Martin ME, Kay HH, et al: Early events in human T cell ontogeny: phenotypic characterization and immunohistologic localization of T cell precursors in early human fetal tissues, *J Exp Med* 168:1061-1080, 1988.
2. Compana D, Janossy G, Coustan-Smith E, et al: The expression of T cell receptor-associated proteins during T cell ontogeny in man, *J Immunol* 142:57-66, 1989.
3. Haynes BF, Singer KH, Dennning SM, et al: Analysis of expression of CD2, CD3, and T cell antigen receptor molecules during early human fetal thymic development, *J Immunol* 141:3776-3784, 1988.
4. Migliaccio G, Migliaccio AR, Petti S, et al: Human embryonic hemopoiesis: kinetics of progenitors and precursors underlying the yolk sac to liver transition, *J Clin Invest* 78:51-60, 1986.
5. Asma GEM, Van Den Bergh RL, Vossen JM: Use of monoclonal antibodies in a study of the development of T lymphocytes in the human fetus, *Clin Exp Immunol* 53:429-436, 1983.
6. Royo C, Touraine J-L, De Bouteiller O: Ontogeny of T lymphocyte differentiation in the human fetus: acquisition of phenotype and functions, *Thymus* 10:57-73, 1987.
7. Timens W, Rozeboom T, Poppema S: Fetal and neonatal development of human spleen: an immunohistological study, *Immunology* 60:603-609, 1987.
8. Markgraf R, von Gaudecker B, Muller-Hermelink H-K: The development of the human lymph node, *Cell Tissue Res* 225:387-413, 1982.
9. Vellguth S, von Gaudecker B, Muller-Hermelink H-K: The development of the human spleen: ultrastructural studies in fetuses from the 14th to 24th week of gestation, *Cell Tissue Res* 242:579-592, 1985.
10. Namikawa R, Mizuno T, Matsuoka H, et al: Ontogenic development of T and B cells and non-lymphoid cells in the white pulp of human spleen, *Immunology* 57:61-69, 1986.
11. Fichtelius KE: The gut epithelium—a first level lymphoid organ? *Exp Cell Res* 49:87-104, 1968.
12. Spencer J, MacDonald TT, Finn T, et al: The development of gut-associated lymphoid tissue in the terminal ileum of fetal human intestine, *Clin Exp Immunol* 64:536-543, 1986.
13. Latthe M, Terry L, MacDonald TT: High frequency of CD8 alpha alpha homodimer-bearing T cells in human fetal intestine, *Eur J Immunol* 24:1703-1705, 1994.
14. Howie D, Spencer J, DeLord D, et al: Extrathymic T cell differentiation in the human intestine early in life, *J Immunol* 161:5862-5872, 1998.
15. McVay LD, Jaswal SS, Kennedy C, et al: The generation of human gamma delta T cell repertoires during fetal development, *J Immunol* 160:5851-5860, 1998.
16. Wucherpfennig KW, Liao YJ, Prendergast M, et al: Human fetal liver gamma/delta T cells predominantly use unusual rearrangements of the T cell receptor delta and gamma loci expressed on both CD4+ CD8- and CD4- CD8- gamma/delta T cells, *J Exp Med* 177:425-432, 1993.
17. Stites DP, Carr MC, Fudenberg HH: Ontogeny of cellular immunity in the human fetus: development of responses to phytohaemagglutinin and to allogeneic cells, *Cell Immunol* 11:257-271, 1974.
18. Aase JM, Noren GR, Reddy DV, et al: Mumps-virus infection in pregnant women and the immunologic response of their offspring, *N Engl J Med* 286:1379-1382, 1972.
19. Sanjeevi CB, Vivekanandan S, Narayanan PR: Fetal response to maternal ascariasis as evidenced by anti-*Ascaris lumbricoides* IgM antibodies in the cord blood, *Acta Pediatr Scand* 80:1134-1138, 1991.
20. Fievet N, Ringwald P, Bickii J: Malaria cellular immune responses in neonates from Cameroon, *Parasite Immunol* 18:483-490, 1996.
21. Novato-Silva E, Gazzinelli G, Colley DG: Immune responses during human schistosomiasis mansoni. XVIII. Immunologic status of pregnant women and their neonates, *Scand J Immunol* 35:429-437, 1992.
22. King CL, Malhotra I, Mungai P, et al: B cell sensitization to helminthic infection develops in utero in humans, *J Immunol* 160:3578-3584, 1998.

23. McLeod R, Mack DG, Boyer K, et al: Phenotypes and functions of lymphocytes in congenital toxoplasmosis, *J Lab Clin Med* 116:623-635, 1990.

24. Gill TJ, Repetti CF, Metlay LA: Transplacental immunisation of the human fetus to tetanus by immunisation of the mother, *J Clin Invest* 72:987-996, 1983.

25. Byrne JA, Stankovic AK, Cooper MD: A novel subpopulation of primed T cells in the human fetus, *J Immunol* 152:3098-3106, 1994.

26. Wegmann TG, Lin H, Guilbert L, et al: Bidirectional cytokine interactions in the maternal-fetal relationship: is successful pregnancy a Th2 phenomenon? *Immunol Today* 14:353-356, 1993.

27. Herzenberg LA, Bianchi DW, Schroder J, et al: Fetal cells in the blood of pregnant women: detection and enrichment by fluorescence-activated cell sorting, *Proc Natl Acad Sci U S A* 76:1453-1455, 1979.

28. Lo Y-MD, Wainscoat JS, Gillmer MDG, et al: Prenatal sex determination by DNA amplification from maternal peripheral blood, *Lancet* 9:1363-1365, 1989.

29. Bianchi DW, Zickwolf GK, Yih MC, et al: Erythroid-specific antibodies enhance detection of fetal nucleated erythrocytes in maternal blood, *Prenat Diagn* 13:293-300, 1993.

30. Wachtel S, Elias S, Price J, et al: Fetal cells in the maternal circulation: isolation by multiparameter flow cytometry and confirmation by polymerase chain reaction, *Hum Reprod* 6:1466-1469, 1991.

31. Price JO, Elias S, Wachtel SS, et al: Prenatal diagnosis with fetal cells isolated from maternal blood by multiparameter flow cytometry, *Am J Obstet Gynecol* 165:1731-1737, 1994.

32. Bonney EA, Matzinger P: The maternal immune system's interaction with circulating fetal cells, *J Immunol* 158:40-47, 1997.

33. Munn DH, Zhou M, Attwood JT, et al: Prevention of allogeneic fetal rejection by tryptophan catabolism, *Science* 281:1191-1193, 1998.

34. Roth I, Corry DB, Locksley RM, et al: Human placental cytotrophoblasts produce the immunosuppressive cytokine interleukin 10, *J Exp Med* 184:539-548, 1996.

35. Guller S, LaChapelle L: The role of placental Fas ligand in maintaining immune privilege at maternal-fetal interface, *Semin Reprod Endocrinol* 17:39-44, 1999.

36. Hammer A, Blaschitz A, Daxbock C, et al: Gas and Fas-ligand are expressed in the uteroplacental unit of first-trimester pregnancy, *Am J Reprod Immunol* 41:41-51, 1999.

37. Ashkar AA, Di Santo JP, Croy BA: Interferon gamma contributes to initiation of uterine vascular modification, decidual integrity, and uterine natural killer cell maturation during normal murine pregnancy, *J Exp Med* 192:259-269, 2000.

38. Krishnan L, Guilbert LJ, Wegmann TG, et al: T helper 1 response against *Leishmania major* in pregnant C57BL/6 mice increases implantation failure and fetal resorptions, *J Immunol* 156:653-662, 1996.

39. Krishnan L, Guilbert LJ, Russell AS, et al: Pregnancy impairs resistance of C57BL/6 mice to *Leishmania major* infection and causes decreased antigen-specific IFN-g responses and increased production of T helper 2 cytokines, *J Immunol* 156:644-652, 1996.

40. Hilkens CM, Vermeulen H, Joost van Neerven RJ, et al: Differential modulation of T helper type 1 (Th1) and T helper type 2 (Th2) cytokine secretion by prostaglandin E_2 critically depends on interleukin-2, *Eur J Immunol* 25:59-63, 1995.

41. Piccinni M-P, Giudizi M-G, Biagiotti R, et al: Progesterone favours the development of human T helper cells producing Th2-type cytokines and promotes both IL-4 production and membrane CD30 expression in established Th1 cell clones, *J Immunol* 155:128-133, 1995.

42. Szekeres-Bartho J, Faust Z, Varga P, et al: The immunological pregnancy-protective effect of progesterone is manifested via controlling cytokine production, *Am J Reprod Immunol* 35:348-351, 1996.

43. Szekeres-Bartho J, Wegmann TG: A progesterone-dependent immunomodulatory protein alters the Th1/Th2 balance, *J Reprod Immunol* 31:81-95, 1996.

44. Miller ME: Phagocyte function in the neonate: selected aspects, *Pediatrics* 64:709-712, 1979.

45. Wilson CB: Immunologic basis for increased susceptibility of the neonate to infection, *J Pediatr* 108:1-12, 1986.

46. Burchett SK, Corey L, Mohan KM, et al: Diminished interferon-g and lymphocyte proliferation in neonatal and postpartum primary herpes simplex virus infection, *J Infect Dis* 165:813-818, 1992.

47. Siegrist CA: Vaccination in the neonatal period and early infancy, *Int Rev Immunol* 19:195-219, 2000.

48. Friedmann PS: Cell-mediated immunological reactivity in neonates and infants with congenital syphilis, *Clin Exp Immunol* 30:271-276, 1977.

49. Starr SE, Tolpin MD, Friedman HM, et al: Impaired cellular immunity to cytomegalovirus in congenitally infected children and their mothers, *J Infect Dis* 140:500-505, 1979.

50. Hayward AR, Herberger M, Saunders D: Herpes simplex virus-stimulated gamma-interferon production by newborn mononuclear cells, *Pediatr Res* 20:398-400, 1986.

51. Hayward AR, Groothuis J: Development of T cells with memory phenotype in infancy, *Adv Exp Med Biol* 310:71-76, 1991.

52. Comans-Bitter WM, de Groot R, van den Beemd R, et al: Immunophenotyping of blood lymphocytes in childhood: reference values for lymphocyte subpopulations, *J Pediatr* 130:388-393, 1997.

53. de Vries E, de Bruin-Versteeg S, Comans-Bitter WM, et al: Longitudinal survey of lymphocyte subpopulations in the first year of life, *Pediatr Res* 47:528-537, 2000.

54. Griffiths-Chu S, Patterson JAK, Berger CL, et al: Characterization of immature T cell subpopulations in neonatal blood, *Blood* 64:296-300, 1984.

55. Maccario R, Nespoli L, Mingrat G, et al: Lymphocyte subpopulations in the neonate: identification of an immature subset of OKT8-positive, OKT3-negative cells, *J Immunol* 130:1129-1131, 1983.

56. Clement LT, Vink PE, Bradley GE: Novel immunoregulatory functions of phenotypically distinct subpopulations of CD4+ cells in the human neonate, *J Immunol* 145:102-108, 1990.

57. Hassan J, Reen DJ: Human recent thymic emigrants—identification, expansion and survival characteristics, *J Immunol* 167:1970-1976, 2001.

58. Hassan J, Reen DJ: IL-7 promotes the survival and maturation but not differentiation of human post-thymic CD4[+] T-cells, *Eur J Immunol* 28:3057-3065, 1998.

59. Hannet I, Erkeller-Yuksel F, Lydyard P, et al: Developmental and maturational changes in human blood lymphocyte subpopulations, *Immunol Today* 13:215-218, 1992.

60. Calado RT, Garcia AB, Falcao RP: Age-related changes of immunophenotypically immature lymphocytes in normal human peripheral blood, *Cytometry* 38:133-137, 1999.

61. Hassan J, Reen DJ: Neonatal CD4+ CD45RA+ T cells: precursors of adult CD4+ CD45RA+ T cells? *Res Immunol* 144:87-92, 1993.

62. Sanders ME, Makgoba MW, Shaw S: Human naive and memory T cells: reinterpretation of helper-inducer and suppressor-inducer subsets, *Immunol Today* 9:195-199, 1988.

63. Gerli R, Bertotto A, Spinozzi F, et al: Phenotypic dissection of cord blood immunoregulatory T-cell subsets by using a two-color immunofluorescence study, *Clin Immunol Immunopathol* 40:429-435, 1986.

64. Kingsley G, Pitzalis C, Waugh A, et al: Correlation of immunoregulatory function with cell phenotype in cord blood lymphocytes, *Clin Exp Immunol* 73:40-45, 1988.

65. Bradley L, Bradley J, Ching D, et al: Predominance of T cells that express CD4[+] in the CD4[+] helper/inducer lymphocyte subset of neonates, *Clin Immunol Immunopathol* 51:426-435, 1989.

66. Hayward A, Lee J, Beverley PCL: Ontogeny of expression of UCHL1 antigen on TcR-1[+] (CD4/8) and TcR delta[+] T cells, *Euro J Immunol* 19:771-773, 1989.

67. Holt PG, Clough JB, Holt BJ, et al: Genetic 'risk' for atopy is associated with delayed postnatal maturation of T-cell competence, *Clin Exp Allergy* 22:1093-1099, 1992.

68. Pirenne H, Aujard Y, Eljaafari A, et al: Comparison of T cell functional changes during childhood with the ontogeny of CDw29 and CD45RA expression on CD4+ T cells, *Pediatr Res* 32:81-86, 1992.

69. Stern DA, Hicks MJ, Martinez FD, et al: Lymphocyte subpopulation number and function in infancy, *Dev Immunol* 2:175-179, 1992.

70. Hassan J, Reen DJ: Cord blood CD4[+] CD45RA[+] T cells achieve a lower magnitude of activation when compared with their adult counterparts, *Immunology* 90:397-401, 1997.

71. Hassan J, Reen DJ: Reduced primary antigen-specific T-cell precursor frequencies in neonates is associated with deficient interleukin-2 production, *Immunology* 87:604-608, 1996.

72. Bertotto A, Gerli R, Lanfrancone L, et al: Activation of cord T lymphocytes. II. Cellular and molecular analysis of the defective response induced by anti-CD3 monoclonal antibody, *Cell Immunol* 127:247-259, 1990.

73. Gerli R, Agea E, Muscat C, et al: Activation of cord T lymphocytes. III. Role of LFA-1/ICAM-1 and CD2/LFA-3 adhesion molecules in CD3-induced proliferative response, *Cell Immunol* 148:32-47, 1993.

74. Hassan J, O'Neill S, O'Neill LAJ, et al: Signaling via DC28 of human naive neonatal T lymphocytes, *Clin Exp Immunol* 102:192-198, 1995.

75. Early EM, Reen DJ: Antigen-independent responsiveness to interleukin-4 demonstrates differential regulation of newborn human T cells, *Eur J Immunol* 26:2885-2889, 1996.

76. Shu U, Demeure CE, Byun D-G, et al: Interleukin 12 exerts a differential effect on the maturation of neonatal and adult human CD45RO− CD4 T cells, *J Clin Invest* 94:1352-1358, 1994.

77. Zola H, Fusco M, Weedon H, et al: Reduced expression of the inter-leukin-2-receptor g chain on cord blood lymphocytes: relationship to functional immaturity of the neonatal immune response, *Immunology* 87:86-91, 1996.

78. Takahashi N, Imanishi K, Nishida H, et al: Evidence for immunologic immaturity of cord blood T cells, *J Immunol* 155:5213-5219, 1995.

79. Macardle PJ, Wheatland L, Zola H: Analysis of the cord blood T lym-phocyte response to superantigen, *Hum Immunol* 60:127-139, 1999.

80. Porcu P, Gaddy J, Broxmeyer HE: Alloantigen-induced unresponsiveness in cord blood T lymphocytes is associated with defective activation of Ras, *Proc Natl Acad Sci U S A* 95:4538-4543, 1998.

81. Miscia S, Du Baldassarre A, Sabatino G, et al: Inefficient phospholipase C activation and reduced Lck expression characterize the signaling de-fect of umbilical cord T lymphocytes, *J Immunol* 163:2416-2424, 1999.

82. Whisler RL, Newhouse YG, Grants IS, et al: Differential expression of the a- and b-isoforms of protein kinase C in peripheral blood T and B cells from young and elderly adults, *Mech Ageing Dev* 77:197-211, 1995.

83. Sato K, Nagayama H, Takahasji TA: Aberrant CD3- and CD28-mediated signaling events in cord blood T cells are associated with dysfunctional regulation of Fas ligand-mediated cytotoxicity, *J Immunol* 162:4464-4471, 1999.

84. Sato K, Kawasaki H, Nagayama H, et al: Chemokine receptor expressions and responsiveness of cord blood T cells, *J Immunol* 166:1659-1666, 2001.

85. Andersson U, Bird AG, Britten S, et al: Human and cellular immunity in humans studied at the cellular level from birth to two years, *Immunol Rev* 57:5-19, 1981.

86. Hayward AR: Development of lymphocyte responses in humans, the fetus and newborn, *Immunol Rev* 57:43-61, 1981.

87. Durandy A, De Saint Basile G, Lisowska-Grospierre B, et al: Unde-tectable CD40 ligand expression on T cells and low B cell responses to CD40 binding antagonists in human newborns, *J Immunol* 154:1560-1568, 1995.

88. Fuleihan R, Ahern D, Geha RS: Decreased expression of the ligand for CD40 in newborn lymphocytes, *Eur J Immunol* 24:1925-1928, 1994.

89. Splawski JB, Lipsky PE: Cytokine regulation of immunoglobulin secre-tion by neonatal lymphocytes, *J Clin Invest* 88:967-977, 1991.

90. Zola H, Fusco M, MacArdle PJ, et al: Expression of cytokine receptors by human cord blood lymphocytes: comparison with adult blood lympho-cytes, *Pediatr Res* 38:397-403, 1995.

91. Lee SM, Suen Y, Chang L, et al: Decreased interleukin-12 (IL-12) from activated cord versus adult peripheral blood mononuclear cells and up-regulation of interferon-g, natural killer, and lymphokine-activated killer activity by IL-12 in cord blood mononuclear cells, *Blood* 88:945-954, 1996.

92. Chheda S, Palkowetz KH, Garofalo R, et al: Decreased interleukin-10 production by neonatal monocytes and T cells: relationship to decreased production and expression of tumor necrosis factor-a and its receptors, *Pediatr Res* 40:475-483, 1996.

93. Qian JX, Lee SM, Suen Y, et al: Decreased interleukin-15 from activated cord versus adult peripheral blood mononuclear cells and the effect of interleukin-15 in upregulating antitumor immune activity and cytokine production in cord blood, *Blood* 90:3106-3117, 1997.

94. Scott ME, Kubin M, Kohl S: High level interleukin-12 production, but diminished interferon-g production, by cord blood mononuclear cells, *Pediatr Res* 41:547-553, 1997.

95. Kotiranta-Ainamo A, Rautonen J, Rautonen N: Interleukin-10 produc-tion by cord blood mononuclear cells, *Pediatr Res* 41:110-113, 1997.

96. Chalmers IMH, Janossy G, Contreras M, et al: Intracellular cytokine profile of cord and adult blood lymphocytes, *Blood* 92:11-18, 1998.

97. Adkins B: T-cell function in newborn mice and humans, *Immunol Today* 20:330-335, 1999.

98. Wilson CB, Westall J, Johnston L, et al: Decreased production of inter-feron gamma by human neonatal cells: intrinsic and regulatory defi-ciencies, *J Clin Invest* 77:860-867, 1986.

99. Taylor S, Bryson YJ: Impaired production of gamma-interferon by new-born cells *in vitro* is due to a functionally immature macrophage, *J Immunol* 134:1493-1498, 1985.

100. Lewis DB, Yu CC, Meyer J, et al: Cellular and molecular mechanisms for reduced interleukin 4 and interferon-gamma production by neonatal T cells, *J Clin Invest* 87:194-202, 1991.

101. White GP, Watt PM, Holt BJ, et al: Differential patterns of methylation of the IFNγ promoter at CpG and non-CpG sites underlie differences in IFNγ gene expression between human neonatal and adult CD45RO− T-cells, *J Immunol* 168:2820-2827, 2002.

102. Barbouche R, Forveille M, Fischer A, et al: Spontaneous IgM autoanti-body production in vitro by B lymphocytes of normal human neonates, *Scand J Immunol* 35:659-667, 1992.

103. Durandy A, Thuillier L, Forveille M, et al: Phenotypic and functional characteristics of human newborns' B lymphocytes, *J Immunol* 144:60-65, 1990.

104. Casali P, Notkins AL: CD5+ B lymphocytes polyreactive antibodies and the human B-cell repertoire, *Immunol Today* 10:364-367, 1989.

105. Watson W, Oen K, Ramdahin R, et al: Immunoglobulin and cytokine production by neonatal lymphocytes, *Clin Exp Immunol* 83:169-174, 1991.

106. Caligaris-Cappio F, Riva M, Tesio L, et al: Human normal CD5+ B lym-phocytes can be induced to differentiate to CD5− B lymphocytes with germinal center cell features, *Blood* 73:1259-1264, 1989.

107. Punnonen J: The role of interleukin-2 in the regulation of proliferation and IgM synthesis of human newborn mononuclear cells, *Clin Exp Im-munol* 75:421-425, 1989.

108. Lewis DB, Wilson CB: Developmental immunology and role of host de-fenses in fetal and neonatal susceptibility to infection. In Remington JS, Klein JO, eds: *Infectious diseases of the fetus and newborn infant*, Philadelphia, 2001, WB Saunders.

109. Splawski JB, Nishioka J, Nishioka Y, et al: CD40 ligand is expressed and functional on activated T cells, *J Immunol* 156:119-127, 1996.

110. Stavnezer J: Antibody class switching, *Adv Immunol* 61:79-146, 1996.

111. Gauchat J-F, Gauchat D, De Weck AL, et al: Cytokine mRNA levels in antigen-stimulated peripheral blood mononuclear cells, *Eur J Immunol* 7:804-810, 1989.

112. Morris JF, Hoyer JT, Pierce SK: Antigen presentation for T cell inter-leukin-2 secretion is a late acquisition of neonatal B cells, *Eur J Immunol* 22:2923-2928, 1992.

113. Van Tol MJD, Ziljstra J, Thomas CMG, et al: Distinct role of neonatal and adult monocytes in the regulation of the *in vitro* antigen-induced plaque-forming cell response in man, *J Immunol* 134:1902-1908, 1984.

114. Serushago B, Issekutz AC, Lee SH, et al: Deficient tumour necrosis fac-tor secretion by cord blood mononuclear cells upon in vitro stimulation with *Listeria monocytogenes*, *J Interferon Cytokine Res* 16:381-387, 1996.

115. Weston WL, Carson BS, Barkin RM, et al: Monocyte-macrophage func-tion in the newborn, *Am J Dis Child* 131:1241-1242, 1977.

116. Clerici M, DePalma L, Roilides E, et al: Analysis of T helper and antigen-presenting cell functions in cord blood and peripheral blood leukocytes from healthy children of different ages, *J Clin Invest* 91:2829-2836, 1993.

117. Stiehm ER, Sztein MB, Oppenheim JJ: Deficient DR antigen expression on human cord blood monocytes: reversal with lymphokines, *Clin Immunol Immunopathol* 30:430-436, 1984.

118. Holt PG: Regulation of antigen-presenting cell function(s) in lung and airway tissues, *Eur Respir J* 6:120-129, 1993.

119. Lee PT, Holt PG, McWilliam AS: Ontogeny of rat pulmonary alveolar function: evidence for a selective deficiency in IL-10 and nitric oxide production by newborn alveolar macrophages, *Cytokine* 15:53-57, 2001.

120. Chesnut RW, Grey HM: Antigen presentation by B cells and its signifi-cance in T-B interactions, *Adv Immunol* 39:51-82, 1986.

121. Pierce SK, Morris JF, Grusby MJ, et al: Antigen-presenting function of B lymphocytes, *Immunol Rev* 106:149-156, 1988.

122. Muthukkumar S, Goldstein J, Stein KE: The ability of B cells and den-dritic cells to present antigen increases ontogeny, *J Immunol* 165:4803-4813, 2000.

123. Steinman RM: The dendritic cell system and its role in immunogenicity, *Annu Rev Immunol* 9:271-296, 1991.

124. Janeway CA: The immune response evolved to discriminate infectious nonself from noninfectious self, *Immunol Today* 13:11-16, 1992.

125. McWilliam AS, Napoli S, Marsh AM, et al: Dendritic cells are recruited into the airway epithelium during the inflammatory response to a broad spectrum of stimuli, *J Exp Med* 184:2429-2432, 1996.

126. Matzinger P: Tolerance, danger, and the extended family, *Annu Rev Immunol* 12:991-1045, 1994.

127. Holt PG, Stumbles PA: Regulation of immunologic homeostasis in pe-ripheral tissues by dendritic cells: the respiratory tract as a paradigm, *J Allergy Clin Immunol* 105:421-429, 2000.

128. Foster CA, Holbrook KA: Ontogeny of Langerhans cells in human em-bryonic and fetal skin: cell densities and phenotypic expression relative to epidermal growth, *Am J Anat* 184:157-164, 1989.

129. Mizoguchi S, Takahashi K, Takeya M, et al: Development, differentiation and proliferation of epidermal Langerhans cells in rat ontogeny studied by a novel monoclonal antibody against epidermal Langerhans cells, RED-1, *J Leukoc Biol* 52:52-61, 1992.

130. Romani N, Schuler G, Fritsch P: Ontogeny of Ia-positive and Thy-1-positive leukocytes of murine epidermis, *J Invest Dermatol* 86:129-133, 1986.

131. Mayrhofer G, Pugh CW, Barclay AN: The distribution, ontogeny and origin in the rat of Ia-positive cells with dendritic morphology and of Ia antigen in epithelia, with special reference to the intestine, *Eur J Immunol* 13:112-122, 1983.

132. Brandtzaeg P, Halstensen TS, Huitfeldt HS, et al: Epithelial expression of HLA, secretory component (poly-Ig receptor), and adhesion molecules in the human alimentary tract, *Ann N Y Acad Sci* 664:157-179, 1992.

133. McCarthy KM, Gong JL, Telford JR, et al: Ontogeny of Ia+ accessory cells in fetal and newborn rat lung, *Am J Respir Cell Mol Biol* 6:349-356, 1992.

134. Nelson DJ, McMenamin C, McWilliam AS, et al: Development of the airway intraepithelial dendritic cell network in the rat from class II MHC (Ia) negative precursors: differential regulation of Ia expression at different levels of the respiratory tract, *J Exp Med* 179:203-212, 1994.

135. Ridge JP, Fuchs EJ, Matzinger P: Neonatal tolerance revisited: turning on newborn T cells with dendritic cells, *Science* 271:1723-1726, 1996.

136. Nelson DJ, Holt PG: Defective regional immunity in the respiratory tract of neonates is attributable to hyporesponsiveness of local dendritic cells to activation signals, *J Immunol* 155:3517-3524, 1995.

137. Stoltenberg L, Thrane PS, Rognum TO: Development of immune response markers in the trachea in the fetal period and the first year of life, *Pediatr Allergy Immunol* 4:13-19, 1993.

138. Holt PG: Dendritic cell ontogeny as an aetiological factor in respiratory tract diseases in early life, *Thorax* 56:419-420, 2001.

139. Sorg RV, Kogler G, Wernet P: Identification of cord blood dendritic cells as an immature CD11c- population, *Blood* 93:2302-2307, 1999.

140. Hunt DW, Huppertz HI, Jiang HJ, et al: Studies of human cord blood dendritic cells: evidence for functional immaturity, *Blood* 84:4333-4343, 1994.

141. Goriely S, Vincart B, Stordeur P, et al: Deficient IL-12(p35) gene expression by dendritic cells derived from neonatal monocytes, *J Immunol* 166:2141-2146, 2001.

142. Borrese MP, Odelram H, Irander K, et al: Peripheral blood eosinophilia in infants at three months of age is associated with subsequent development of atopic disease in early childhood, *J Allergy Clin Immunol* 95:694-698, 1995.

143. Bullock JD, Robertson AF, Bodenbender JG, et al: Inflammatory response in the neonate re-examined, *Pediatrics* 44:58-61, 1969.

144. Eitzman DV, Smith RT: The nonspecific inflammatory cycle in the neonatal infant, *Am J Dis Child* 97:326-334, 1959.

145. Roberts RL, Ank BJ, Salusky IB, et al: Purification and properties of peritoneal eosinophils from pediatric dialysis patients, *J Immunol Methods* 126:205-211, 1990.

146. Bhat AM, Scanlon JW: The pattern of eosinophilia in premature infants, *J Pediatr* 98:612-616, 1981.

147. Gibson EL, Vaucher Y, Corrigan JJ: Eosinophilia in premature infants: relationship to weight gain, *J Pediatr* 95:99-101, 1979.

148. Smith JB, Kunjummen RD, Raghavender BH: Eosinophils and neutrophils of human neonates have similar impairments of quantitative up-regulation of Mac-1 (CD11b/CD18) expression *in vitro*, *Pediatr Res* 30:355-361, 1991.

149. Smith JB, Kunjummen RD, Kishimoto TK, et al: Expression and regulation of L-selectin on eosinophils from human adults and neonates, *Pediatr Res* 32:465-471, 1992.

150. Spencer J, Isaacson PG, Walker-Smith JA, et al: Heterogeneity in intraepithelial lymphocyte subpopulations in fetal and postnatal human small intestine, *J Pediatr Gastroenterol Nutr* 9:173-177, 1989.

151. Wilkes LK, McMenamin C, Holt PG: Postnatal maturation of mast cell subpopulations in the rat respiratory tract, *Immunology* 75:535-541, 1992.

152. Cummins AG, Munro GH, Miller HRP, et al: Association of maturation of the small intestine at weaning with mucosal mast cell activation in the rat, *J Cell Biol* 66:417-423, 1988.

153. Cummins AG, Eglinton BA, Gonzalez A, et al: Immune activation during infancy in healthy humans, *J Clin Immunol* 14:107-115, 1994.

154. Iida M, Matsumoto K, Tomita H, et al: Selective down-regulation of high-affinity IgE receptor (FcεRI) α-chain messenger RNA among transcriptome in cord blood-derived versus adult peripheral blood-derived cultured human mast cells, *Blood* 97:1016-1022, 2001.

155. Dastur FD, Shastry P, Iyer E, et al: The foetal immune response to maternal tetanus toxoid immunization, *J Assoc Physicians India* 41:94-96, 1993.

156. Klinge J, Lugauer S, Korn K, et al: Comparison of immunogenicity and reactogenicity of a measles, mumps and rubella (MMR) vaccine in German children vaccinated at 9-11, 12-14 or 15-17 months of age, *Vaccine* 18:3134-3140, 2000.

157. Gans HA, Maldonado Y, Yasukawa LL, et al: IL-12, IFN-g, and T cell proliferation to measles in immunized infants, *J Immunol* 162:5569-5575, 1999.

158. Barrios C, Brawand P, Berney M, et al: Neonatal and early life immune responses to various forms of vaccine antigens qualitatively differ from adult responses: predominance of a Th2-biased pattern which persists after adult boosting, *Eur J Immunol* 26:1489-1496, 1996.

159. Rowe J, Macaubas C, Monger T, et al: Antigen-specific responses to diphtheria-tetanus-acellular pertussis vaccine in human infants are initially Th2 polarized, *Infect Immun* 68:3873-3877, 2000.

160. Rowe J, Macaubas C, Monger T, et al: Heterogeneity in diphtheria-tetanus-acellular pertussis vaccine-specific cellular immunity during infancy: relationship to variations in the kinetics of postnatal maturation of systemic Th1 function, *J Infect Dis* 184:80-88, 2001.

161. Adkins B, Du R-Q: Newborn mice develop balanced Th1/Th2 primary effector responses *in vivo* but are biased to Th2 secondary responses, *J Immunol* 160:4217-4224, 1998.

162. Ausiello CM, Lande R, Urbani F, et al: Cell-mediated immune responses in four-year-old children after primary immunization with acellular pertussis vaccines, *Infect Immol* 67:4064-4071, 1999.

163. Marchant A, Goetghebuer T, Ota M, et al: Newborns develop a Th1-type immune response to *Mycobacterium bovis* bacillus Calmette-Guérin vaccination, *J Immunol* 163:2249-2255, 1999.

164. Vekemans J, Amedei A, Ota MO, et al: Neonatal bacillus Calmette-Guérin vaccination induced adult-like IFN-γ production by CD4+ T lymphocytes, *Eur J Immunol* 31:1531-1535, 2001.

165. Arulanandam BP, Van Cleave VH, Metzger DW: IL-12 is a potent neonatal vaccine adjuvant, *Eur J Immunol* 29:256-264, 1999.

166. Martinez X, Brandt C, Saddallah F, et al: DNA immunization circumvents deficient induction of T helper type 1 and cytotoxic T lymphocyte responses in neonates and during early life, *Proc Natl Acad Sci U S A* 94:8726-8731, 1997.

167. Kovarik J, Bozzotti P, Love-Homan L, et al: CpG oligodeoxynucleotides can circumvent the Th2 polarization of neonatal responses to vaccines but may fail to fully direct Th2 responses established by neonatal priming, *J Immunol* 162:1611-1617, 1999.

168. Shirakawa T, Enomoto T, Shimazu S, et al: Inverse association between tuberculin responses and atopic disorder, *Science* 275:77-79, 1997.

169. Arkwright PD, Patel L, Moran A, et al: Atopic eczema is associated with delayed maturation of the antibody response to pneumococcal vaccine, *Clin Exp Immunol* 122:16-19, 2000.

170. Prescott SL, Sly PD, Holt PG: Raised serum IgE associated with reduced responsiveness to DPT vaccination during infancy, *Lancet* 351:1489, 1998.

171. Holt PG, Rudin A, Macaubas C, et al: Development of immunologic memory against tetanus toxoid and pertactin antigens from the diphtheria-tetanus-pertussis vaccine in atopic versus nonatopic children, *J Allergy Clin Immunol* 105:1117-1122, 2000.

172. Kondo N, Kobayashi Y, Shinoda S, et al: Cord blood lymphocyte responses to food antigens for the prediction of allergic disorders, *Arch Dis Child* 67:1003-1007, 1992.

173. Piccinni M-P, Mecacci F, Sampognaro S, et al: Aeroallergen sensitization can occur during fetal life, *Int Arch Allergy Immunol* 102:301-303, 1993.

174. Piastra M, Stabile A, Fioravanti G, et al: Cord blood mononuclear cell responsiveness to beta-lactoglobulin: T-cell activity in "atopy-prone" and "non-atopy-prone" newborns, *Int Arch Allergy Immunol* 104:358-365, 1994.

175. Miles EA, Warner JA, Jones AC, et al: Peripheral blood mononuclear cell proliferative responses in the first year of life in babies born to allergic parents, *Clin Exp Allergy* 26:780-788, 1996.

176. Holt PG, O'Keeffe PO, Holt BJ, et al: T-cell "priming" against environmental allergens in human neonates: sequential deletion of food antigen specificities during infancy with concomitant expansion of responses to ubiquitous inhalant allergens, *Ped Allergy Immunol* 6:85-90, 1995.

177. Prescott SL, Macaubas C, Holt BJ, et al: Transplacental priming of the human immune system to environmental allergens: universal skewing of initial T-cell responses towards the Th-2 cytokine profile, *J Immunol* 160:4730-4737, 1998.

178. Szépfalusi Z, Loibichler C, Pichler J, et al: Direct evidence for transplacental allergen transfer, *Pediatr Res* 48:404-407, 2000.
179. Björkstén B, Holt BJ, Baron-Hay MJ, et al: Low-level exposure to house dust mites stimulates T-cell responses during early childhood independent of atopy, *Clin Exp Allergy* 26:775-779, 1996.
180. Smillie FI, Elderfield AJ, Patel F, et al: Lymphoproliferative responses in cord blood and at one year: no evidence for the effect of *in utero* exposure to dust mite allergens, *Clin Exp Allergy* 31:1194-1204, 2001.
181. Yabuhara A, Macaubas C, Prescott SL, et al: Th-2-polarised immunological memory to inhalant allergens in atopics is established during infancy and early childhood, *Clin Exp Allergy* 27:1261-1269, 1997.
182. Prescott SL, Macaubas C, Smallacombe T, et al: Development of allergen-specific T-cell memory in atopic and normal children, *Lancet* 353:196-200, 1999.
183. Macaubas C, Sly PD, Burton P, et al: Regulation of Th-cell responses to inhalant allergen during early childhood, *Clin Exp Allergy* 29:1223-1231, 1999.
184. Macaubas C, Holt PG: Regulation of cytokine production in T-cell responses to inhalant allergen: GATA-3 expression distinguishes between Th1- and Th2-polarized immunity, *Int Arch Allergy Immunol* 124:176-179, 2001.
185. Macaubas C, Lee PT, Smallacombe TB, et al: Reciprocal patterns of allergen-induced GATA-3 expression in peripheral blood mononuclear cells from atopics vs. non-atopics, *Clin Exp Allergy* 32:97-106, 2002.
186. Rinas U, Horneff G, Wahn V: Interferon-gamma production by cord-blood mononuclear cells is reduced in newborns with a family history of atopic disease and is independent from cord blood IgE-levels, *Pediatr Allergy Immunol* 4:60-64, 1993.
187. Tang MLK, Kemp AS, Thorburn J, et al: Reduced interferon-g secretion in neonates and subsequent atopy, *Lancet* 344:983-986, 1994.
188. Liao SY, Liao TN, Chiang BL, et al: Decreased production of IFNg and increased production of IL-6 by cord blood mononuclear cells of newborns with a high risk of allergy, *Clin Exp Allergy* 26:397-405, 1996.
189. Martinez FD, Stern DA, Wright AL, et al: Association of interleukin-2 and interferon-g production by blood mononuclear cells in infancy with parental allergy skin tests and with subsequent development of atopy, *J Allergy Clin Immunol* 96:652-660, 1995.
190. Warner JA, Miles EA, Jones AC, et al: Is deficiency of interferon gamma production by allergen-triggered cord blood cells a predictor of atopic eczema? *Clin Exp Allergy* 24:423-430, 1994.
191. Williams TJ, Jones CA, Miles EA, et al: Fetal and neonatal IL-13 production during pregnancy and at birth and subsequent development of atopic symptoms, *J Allergy Clin Immunol* 105:951-959, 2000.
192. Holt PG, Macaubas C: Development of long-term tolerance versus sensitisation to environmental allergens during the perinatal period, *Curr Opin Immunol* 9:782-787, 1997.
193. Holt PG: Environmental factors and primary T-cell sensitisation to inhalant allergens in infancy: reappraisal of the role of infections and air pollution, *Pediatr Allergy Immunol* 6:1-10, 1995.
194. Martinez FD, Holt PG: The role of microbial burden in the aetiology of allergy and asthma, *Lancet* 354:12-15, 1999.
195. Baldini M, Lohman IC, Halonen M, et al: A polymorphism in the 5′ flanking region of the CD14 gene is associated with circulating soluble CD14 levels with total serum IgE, *Am J Resp Cell Mol Biol* 20:976-983, 1999.
196. Von Ehrenstein OS, Von Mutius E, Illi S, et al: Reduced risk of hay fever and asthma amongst children of farmers, *Clin Exp Allergy* 30:187-193, 2000.
197. Gereda JE, Leung DYM, Thatayatikom A, et al: Relation between house-dust endotoxin exposure, type 1 T-cell development, and allergen sensitisation in infants at high risk of asthma, *Lancet* 355:1680-1683, 2000.
198. Woolcock AJ, Peat JK, Trevillion LM: Is the increase in asthma prevalence linked to increase in allergen load? *Allergy* 50:935-940, 1995.
199. Peat JK, Salome CM, Woolcock AJ: Longitudinal changes in atopy during a 4-year period: relation to bronchial hyperresponsiveness and respiratory symptoms in a population sample of Australian schoolchildren, *J Allergy Clin Immunol* 85:65-74, 1990.
200. Martinez FD, Wright AL, Taussig LM, et al: Asthma and wheezing in the first six years of life, *N Engl J Med* 332:133-138, 1995.
201. Welliver RC, Duffy L: The relationship of RSV-specific immunoglobulin E antibody responses in infancy, recurrent wheezing, and pulmonary function at age 7-8 years, *Pediatr Pulmonol* 15:19-27, 1993.
202. Oddy WH, de Klerk N, Sly PD, et al: Antecedents of childhood asthma: respiratory infections, atopy and breast-feeding have independent and multiplicative effects, *Eur Respir J.* In press.
203. Holgate ST: The inflammation-repair cycle in asthma: the pivotal role of the airway epithelium, *Clin Exp Allergy* 28 (suppl 5):97-103, 1998.
204. Holt PG, Sly PD: Interactions between respiratory tract infections and atopy in aetiology of asthma, *Eur Respir J* 19:1-8, 2002.
205. Stumbles PA, Thomas JA, Pimm CL, et al: Resting respiratory tract dendritic cells preferentially stimulate Th2 responses and require obligatory cytokine signals for induction of Th1 immunity, *J Exp Med* 188:2019-2031, 1998.
206. Schon-Hegrad MA, Oliver J, McMenamin PG, et al: Studies on the density, distribution, and surface phenotype of intraepithelial class II major histocompatibility complex antigen (Ia)-bearing dendritic cells (DC) in the conducting airways, *J Exp Med* 173:1345-1356, 1991.
207. McWilliam AS, Nelson D, Thomas JA, et al: Rapid dendritic cell recruitment is a hallmark of the acute inflammatory response at mucosal surfaces, *J Exp Med* 179:1331-1336, 1994.

IMMUNOLOGIC DISEASES

RAIF S. GEHA

CHAPTER **7**

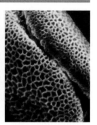

Approach to the Child with Recurrent Infections

HOWARD M. LEDERMAN ■ ERWIN W. GELFAND

Many children who present for allergy evaluation have chronic/recurrent infections of the upper and lower respiratory tracts. Allergy may predispose the patient to such symptoms because swelling of the nasal mucosa causes obstruction of the sinus ostia and the eustachian tubes. However, one must be alert to the possibility of other underlying problems, including primary immunodeficiency diseases, secondary immunodeficiency caused by human immunodeficiency virus (HIV) or Epstein-Barr virus (EBV) infection, cystic fibrosis, disorders of ciliary structure and function, swallowing dysfunction and pulmonary aspiration caused by anatomic or physiologic abnormalities, and aspirated foreign body. Environmental factors such as exposure to cigarette smoke, day care, and the number of household members must also be considered. This chapter provides an approach to evaluating children for these disorders.

DEFINITION OF RECURRENT INFECTIONS

It is difficult to assign a precise frequency of infections that defines increased susceptibility to infection (Table 7-1). For example, chronic/recurrent otitis media is very common in the first 2 years of life but thereafter decreases in frequency. Rather than defining an arbitrary number of ear infections that is too many, the nature and pattern of those infections provide a more reliable guide to identify the child who deserves further evaluation.[1] Ear infections that increase in frequency after the age of 2 years, ear infections associated with mastoiditis, ear infections associated with infections at other sites, and ear infections occurring in the context of failure to thrive should raise the suspicion of an underlying disorder. Similarly, it is unusual for a child to have more than one

episode of pneumonia per decade of life, chronic sinusitis, or chronic bronchitis.

Other clues to an abnormal susceptibility to infection include a history of infections at multiple anatomic locations or relatively unusual infections such as sepsis, mastoiditis, septic arthritis, osteomyelitis, and meningitis. In some instances, patients may present with one or more infections that are unusually severe, lead to an unexpected complication (e.g., empyema or fistula formation), or are caused by an organism of relatively low virulence (e.g., *Aspergillus* or *Pneumocystis carinii*).

Sometimes, the most challenging aspect of evaluating the past medical history is assessing the reliability of the data. It may be difficult to distinguish pneumonia from atelectasis with fever in children with reactive airway disease. Sinusitis is easily mistaken for purulent rhinitis, unless a computed tomography scan documents sinus involvement. Diarrhea may be the result of infection or an adverse effect of antibiotic therapy.

It is also important to account for environmental exposure. There may be an obvious explanation for frequent infections in an infant attending a large day care center during the winter months, whereas the same number of infections might raise concern if an only child were cared for in his or her home. Similarly, exposure to cigarette smoke and drinking from a bottle in a supine position are known risk factors for respiratory tract symptoms.

Early diagnosis of an underlying disorder is critical because it may lead to more effective approaches to therapy and appropriate anticipatory guidance. Furthermore, because some underlying disorders are inherited in mendelian fashion, early diagnosis is essential for making genetic information available to the families of affected individuals.

TABLE 7-1 Guidelines for Identifying Children with Increased Susceptibility to Infections

Frequency
More than one episode of pneumonia per decade of life
Increasing frequency of otitis media in children older than 2 years
Persistent otitis media and drainage despite patent tympanostomy tubes
Persistent sinusitis despite medical and, when appropriate, surgical treatment

Severity
Pneumonia with empyema
Bacterial meningitis, arthritis, or osteomyelitis
Sepsis
Mastoiditis

Infection with opportunistic pathogens
Pneumocystis carinii pneumonia
Mucocutaneous candidiasis
Invasive fungal infection
Vaccine-acquired poliomyelitis
Bacille Calmette-Guérin infection after vaccination

Infections at multiple anatomic locations

Lack of other epidemiologic explanations (e.g., day care center, exposure to cigarette smoke, environmental allergies)

Anatomic or physiologic features suggestive of a syndrome complex

Failure to thrive

THE CLINICAL PRESENTATION OF UNDERLYING DISORDERS

Allergy

Patients with allergic disease, rhinitis, and/or asthma often have symptoms of both acute and chronic sinusitis.[2] There is little to distinguish the symptoms or mucopurulent discharge in patients with immunodeficiency compared with those with allergic disease. Similarly, radiographic studies do not discriminate between the two. Often, allergic patients with sinusitis have negative cultures. History is important because flare-ups of sinusitis often accompany exacerbations of the underlying allergic symptoms. Patients may report more symptomatic improvement when treated with corticosteroids than when treated with antibiotics. In general, a history of atopy makes a diagnosis of antibody deficiency less likely because the ability to produce specific IgE antibodies usually indicates normal B and T cell function.

Recurrent sinopulmonary infection is the most frequent illness associated with selective IgA deficiency. IgA deficiency and allergy may also be associated. Even in blood bank donors in whom IgA deficiency was accidentally discovered, allergy may be twice as common as in healthy donors.[3] The most common allergic disorders in IgA-deficient individuals are rhino/sinusitis, eczema, conjunctivitis, and asthma.[4]

Because of this association between allergy and sinusitis, a careful history may often be sufficient, obviating the need for extensive testing for immunodeficiency. Screening for IgA deficiency may be of some help in understanding the association between the two in IgA-deficient individuals. Management of sinusitis should be medical with avoidance of surgery, unless all else fails. Improvement in asthma symptoms after sinus surgery is questionable and only transient at best.

Immunodeficiency

The primary immunodeficiency diseases were originally viewed as rare disorders, characterized by severe clinical expression early in life. However, it has become clear that these diseases are not as uncommon as originally suspected, that their clinical expression can sometimes be relatively mild, and that they are seen nearly as often in adolescents and adults as they are in infants and children.[5-7] In fact, the presentation of immunodeficiency may be so subtle that the diagnosis will be made only if the physician is alert to that possibility.

Patients with primary immunodeficiency diseases most often are recognized because of their increased susceptibility to infection, but these patients may also present with a variety of other clinical manifestations (Table 7-2). In fact, noninfectious manifestations, such as autoimmune disease, may be the first or the predominant clinical symptom of the underlying immunodeficiency. Other immunodeficiency diseases may be diagnosed because of their known association with syndrome complexes.

Infection

An increased susceptibility to infection is the hallmark of the primary immunodeficiency diseases. In most patients, the striking clinical feature is the chronic or recurring nature of the infections rather than the fact that individual infections are unusually severe.[1] However, not all immunodeficient patients are diagnosed after recurrent infections. In some, the first infection may be sufficiently unusual to raise the question of immunodeficiency. For example, a patient who presents with infection caused by *P. carinii* or another opportunistic pathogen is likely to be immunodeficient even if it is his or her first recognized infection.

Autoimmune/Chronic Inflammatory Disease

Immunodeficient patients can present with autoimmune or chronic inflammatory diseases. It is thought that the basic abnormality leading to immunodeficiency may also lead to faulty discrimination between self and nonself and thus to autoimmune disease. The manifestations of these disorders may be limited to a single target cell or organ (e.g., autoimmune

TABLE 7-2 Clinical Features of Immunodeficiency

Increased susceptibility to infection
Chronic/recurrent infections without other explanations
Infection with organism of low virulence
Infection of unusual severity

Autoimmune or inflammatory disease
Target cells (e.g., hemolytic anemia, immune thrombocytopenia, thyroiditis)
Target tissues (e.g., rheumatoid arthritis, vasculitis, systemic lupus erythematosus)

Syndrome complexes

hemolytic anemia or thrombocytopenia, autoimmune thyroiditis) or may involve a number of different target organs (e.g., vasculitis, systemic lupus erythematosus, or rheumatoid arthritis). The autoimmune and inflammatory diseases are more commonly seen in particular primary immunodeficiency diseases, most notably common variable immunodeficiency,[8] selective IgA deficiency, chronic mucocutaneous candidiasis,[9] and deficiencies of early components (C1 through C4) of the classic complement pathway.[10]

Occasionally a disorder that appears to be autoimmune in nature may in fact be due to an infectious agent. For example, the dermatomyositis that is sometimes seen in patients with X-linked agammaglobulinemia is actually a manifestation of chronic enterovirus infection and not autoimmune disease.

Syndrome Complexes

Immunodeficiency can also be seen as one part of a constellation of signs and symptoms in a syndrome complex.[11] In fact, the recognition that a patient has a syndrome in which immunodeficiency occurs may allow a diagnosis of immunodeficiency to be made before there are any clinical manifestations of that deficiency (Table 7-3). For example, children with the DiGeorge syndrome are usually identified initially because of the neonatal presentation of congenital heart disease, hypocalcemic tetany, or both. This should lead to T-lymphocyte evaluation before the onset of opportunistic infections. Similarly, a diagnosis of Wiskott-Aldrich syndrome can often be made in young boys with eczema and thrombocytopenia even before the onset of infections.

Cystic Fibrosis

Cystic fibrosis (CF) is one of the most common autosomal recessive disorders among white populations, occurring with an incidence of almost 1:3000 live newborns.[12] The classic presentation of CF with chronic/recurrent sinopulmonary infections caused by *Pseudomonas* and *Staphylococcus,* diarrhea with malabsorption, and failure to thrive is easy to recognize. New methods for diagnosis have led to the recognition of a broader clinical phenotype, including patients whose first or only manifestation is chronic/recurrent sinusitis.[13,14] The diagnosis of CF should be considered in any patient with chronic/recurrent sinopulmonary infections, especially if *Pseudomonas, Staphylococcus,* nontypable *Haemophilus influenzae,* or *Burkholderia cepacia* are identified as pathogens.

Abnormalities of Airway Anatomy and Physiology

A variety of anatomic abnormalities may increase a child's susceptibility to upper and lower respiratory tract infections. Some anatomic abnormalities, such as craniofacial anomalies involving the palate and the nose, may be readily apparent on physical examination. Others, such as bronchogenic cysts and extralobar pulmonary sequestrations, may be suspected when recurrent infections occur at a single anatomic site.[15] Unilateral otitis media and sinusitis in a young child should prompt an investigation for a nasal foreign body.

Abnormalities of airway muscle function may cause similar symptoms. Swallowing dysfunction with aspiration may be obvious in a child with cerebral palsy who coughs and gags when eating. More subtle clues are a history of drooling or the presence of dysarthria.

Disorders of Ciliary Structure and Function

Primary ciliary dyskinesia (PCD) is a rare problem, estimated to occur with an incidence of less than 1:10,000 in the general population.[16] In most cases, it is inherited as an autosomal recessive trait, but PCD is genetically and clinically heterogeneous. Affected individuals have chronic/recurrent rhinitis, otitis media, sinusitis, pneumonia, and bronchiectasis that begins at an early age. In approximately half of the cases, there are accompanying abnormalities of laterality such as situs inversus or heterotaxy, and complex congenital heart disease has been reported in approximately 10% of individuals with PCD. The presence of abnormal ciliary function of spermatozoa can cause infertility in males, and abnormal ciliary function in the fallopian tubes can result in ectopic pregnancy.

Cilia are complex structures formed from a set of nine peripheral microtubular doublets surrounding two single central microtubules. PCD can be caused by abnormalities of any of the structural proteins: inner or outer dynein arms, radial spokes, or microtubules. PCD can also be caused by disordered orientation of cilia on mucosal surfaces, preventing them from beating in a synchronized wave that clears mucus from the airways.[17]

TABLE 7-3 Examples of Immunodeficiency Syndromes that May Increase Susceptibility to Sinopulmonary Infections

Syndrome	Clinical Presentation	Immunologic Abnormality	Other Contributing Factors
Ataxia telangiectasia	Ataxia, telangiectasia	Variable B- and T-lymphocyte dysfunction	Dysfunctional swallow with pulmonary aspiration
DiGeorge syndrome	Congenital heart disease, hypoparathyroidism, abnormal facies	Thymic hypoplasia or aplasia	Craniofacial anomalies including cleft palate; physiologic abnormalities including dysfunction of soft palate
Dysmotile cilia syndromes	Situs inversus, male infertility, ectopic pregnancy, upper and lower respiratory tract infections	Immotile cilia	
Hyper-IgE syndrome	Coarse facies, eczematoid rash, retained primary teeth, bone fractures, pneumonia	Elevated serum IgE, eosinophilia	
Wiskott-Aldrich syndrome	Thrombocytopenia, eczema	Variable B- and T-lymphocyte dysfunction	

Secondary Immunodeficiency

Immunodeficiency may occur secondary to other illnesses or medications.[18] A variety of infections, particularly viruses, may cause either temporary or long-lived abnormalities of humoral and/or cell-mediated immunity. Such viruses include HIV, measles, and EBV, among others. Malnutrition or malabsorption can cause hypogammaglobulinemia and impaired cell-mediated immunity. A number of medications, most notably corticosteroids and chemotherapeutic agents, are immunosuppressive; phenytoin therapy has been associated with secondary IgA deficiency. Posttraumatic splenectomy, or the "autosplenectomy" that occurs at an early age in sickle cell anemia, leads to an increased risk of sepsis. Susceptibility to infection is dependent on the secondary immunodeficiency that is caused by these or other agents; that is, patients with acquired deficiency of humoral immunity are at highest risk for infections with encapsulated bacteria and enteroviruses, whereas patients with acquired deficiency of cell-mediated immunity are at risk for infection by a wide variety of bacterial, fungal, and viral pathogens.

LABORATORY TESTS FOR UNDERLYING DISORDERS

Immunodeficiency

Although the clinician can suspect immune system dysfunction after a careful review of the history and physical examination, specific diagnoses are rarely evident without use of the laboratory. However, the types of infections and other symptoms should help to focus the laboratory work-up on specific parts of the immune system (Table 7-4). For example, patients with antibody deficiency typically have sinopulmonary infections as a prominent presenting feature.[19] Deficiency of cell-mediated immunity predisposes individuals to develop infections caused by *P. carinii*, other fungi, and a variety of viruses.[20] Abnormalities of phagocytic function should be suspected when patients have recurrent skin infections or visceral abscesses,[21] whereas patients with complement deficiency most often present with bacterial sepsis or immune complex–mediated diseases.[22]

Screening tests that should be performed in almost all patients include a complete blood count with differential and quantitative measurement of serum immunoglobulins. Other tests should be guided by the clinical features of the patient

(Table 7-5). Finally, whenever primary immunodeficiency is suspected, consideration must also be given to secondary causes of immunodeficiency, including HIV infection, therapy with antiinflammatory medications (e.g., corticosteroids), and other underlying illnesses (e.g., lymphoreticular neoplasms and viral infections such as infectious mononucleosis).

Examination of the Peripheral Blood Smear

The complete blood count with examination of the blood smear is an inexpensive and readily available test that provides important diagnostic information relating to a number of immunodeficiency diseases. Neutropenia most often occurs secondary to immunosuppressive drugs, infection, malnutrition, or autoimmunity but may be a primary problem (congenital or cyclic neutropenia). In contrast, persistent neutrophilia is characteristic of leukocyte adhesion molecule deficiency,[23] and abnormal cytoplasmic granules may be seen in the peripheral blood smear of patients with Chediak-Higashi syndrome.[24]

The blood is predominantly a "T cell organ;" that is, the majority (50% to 70%) of peripheral blood lymphocytes are T cells, whereas only 5% to 15% are B cells. Therefore lymphopenia is sometimes a presenting feature of T cell or combined immunodeficiency disorders such as severe combined immunodeficiency disease or DiGeorge syndrome.

Thrombocytopenia may occur as a secondary manifestation of immunodeficiency but is often a presenting manifestation of the Wiskott-Aldrich syndrome. A unique finding in the latter group of patients is an abnormally small platelet (and lymphocyte) volume,[25] a measurement that is easily made with automated blood counters.

Examination of red blood cell morphology can yield clues about splenic function. Howell-Jolly bodies may be visible in peripheral blood in cases of splenic dysfunction or asplenia.[26] However, the converse is not always true, and the absence of Howell-Jolly bodies does not ensure that splenic function is normal.

Evaluation of Humoral Immunity

Measurement of serum immunoglobulin levels is an important screening test to detect immunodeficiency for three reasons: (1) more than 80% of patients with primary disorders

---

TABLE 7-4 Patterns of Illness Associated with Primary Immunodeficiency

	Illnesses	
Disorder	*Infection*	*Other*
Antibody	Sinopulmonary (pyogenic, encapsulated bacteria) Gastrointestinal (enteroviruses, *Giardia lamblia*)	Autoimmune disease (autoantibodies, inflammatory bowel disease)
Cell-mediated immunity	Pneumonia (pyogenic bacteria, *Pneumocystis carinii*, viruses) Gastrointestinal (viruses) Skin, mucous membranes (fungi)	
Complement	Sepsis and other blood-borne encapsulated bacteria (*Streptococcus, Pneumococcus, Neisseria*)	Autoimmune disease (systemic lupus erythematosus, glomerulonephritis)
Phagocytosis	Skin, reticuloendothelial system, abscesses (*Staphylococcus,* enteric bacteria, fungi, mycobacteria)	

TABLE 7-5 Screening Tests for Underlying Disorders

Suspected Abnormality	Diagnostic Tests
Antibody	Quantitative immunoglobulins (IgG, IgA, IgM)
	Antibody response to immunization
Cell-mediated immunity	Lymphocyte count
	T-lymphocyte enumeration (CD3, CD4, CD8)
	Human immunodeficiency virus serology
	Delayed-type hypersensitivity tests
Complement	Total hemolytic complement (CH_{50})
Phagocytosis	Neutrophil count
	Nitroblue tetrazolium dye test

of immunity will have abnormalities of serum immunoglobulins; (2) immunoglobulin measurements yield indirect information about several disparate aspects of the immune system because immunoglobulin synthesis requires the coordinated function of B-lymphocytes, T-lymphocytes, and monocytes; and (3) the measurement of serum immunoglobulin levels is readily available, highly reliable, and relatively inexpensive. The initial screening test for humoral immune function is the quantitative measurement of serum immunoglobulins. Neither serum protein electrophoresis nor immunoelectrophoresis is sufficiently sensitive or quantitative to be useful for this purpose. Quantitative measurements of serum IgG, IgA, and IgM will identify patients with panhypogammaglobulinemia as well as those with deficiencies of an individual class of immunoglobulins, such as selective IgA deficiency. Interpretation of results must be made in view of the marked variations in normal immunoglobulin levels with age[27]; therefore age-related normal values must always be used for comparison.

A clue to immunodeficiency may be a low-normal IgG level in an individual with recurrent infections. In such cases, it is critical to assess antibody function in addition to immunoglobulin level. Antibody levels generated in response to childhood immunization with tetanus toxoid or the *H. influenzae* protein conjugate vaccines are usually the most convenient to measure. In children over the age of 18 to 24 months, it is also important to assess antibody responses to polysaccharide antigens because these responses may be deficient in some patients who can respond normally to protein antigens.[28] Antibody can be measured in response to immunization with pneumococcal capsular polysaccharide vaccine. (The pneumococcal polysaccharide/protein conjugate vaccines can be used but may not be a direct reflection of pure polysaccharide responsiveness.) Alternatively, because the ABO blood group antigens are polysaccharides, quantifying isoagglutinin titers (usually of the IgM class) can assess antipolysaccharide antibody. However, the value of this test in the young child is limited because many normal children do not have significant isoagglutinin titers.[29] Live viral (e.g., oral polio, measles, mumps, rubella, varicella) and bacterial (e.g., bacille Calmette-Guérin) vaccines should never be used for the evaluation of suspected immunodeficiency because they

may cause disseminated infection in an immunocompromised host.

The role for IgG subclass measurements is controversial.[30] There are four subclasses of IgG, and selective deficiencies of each of these have been described. However, the significance of an IgG subclass deficiency in the presence of normal antibody responses to protein and polysaccharide antigens is not known. Many physicians therefore rely on antibody measurements and find that information about IgG subclass levels adds to the expense but not to the diagnosis.

Evaluation of Cell-Mediated Immunity

Testing for defects of cell-mediated immunity is relatively difficult because of the lack of good screening tests. Lymphopenia is suggestive of T-lymphocyte deficiency because T lymphocytes constitute the majority (50% to 70%) of peripheral blood mononuclear cells. However, lymphopenia is not always present in patients with T-lymphocyte functional defects. Similarly, the lack of a thymus silhouette on chest radiography is rarely helpful in the evaluation of T lymphocyte disorders because the thymus of normal children may involute after stress and provide the appearance of thymic hypoplasia.

Indirect information about T cell function may be obtained by enumerating peripheral blood T lymphocytes with appropriate monoclonal antibodies (anti-CD2 or CD3 for total T cells, anti-CD4 for T helper cells, and anti-CD8 for T-cytotoxic cells).[31] Patients with severe combined immunodeficiency and DiGeorge syndrome generally have decreased numbers of CD3+, CD4+, and CD8+ T lymphocytes. In contrast, patients infected with HIV have decreased T-lymphocyte levels because there are decreased numbers of CD4+ lymphocytes.

Delayed-type hypersensitivity (DTH) skin testing with a panel of antigens is an excellent screening method for older children and adults. A standardized panel of antigens prepared for DTH testing should be used.[32,33] The presence of one or more positive delayed-type skin tests is generally indicative of intact cell-mediated immunity. However, there are significant limitations to this testing[34]: (1) prior exposure to antigen is a prerequisite, (2) normal patients may have transient depression of DTH with acute viral infections such as infectious mononucleosis, (3) a positive skin test to some antigens does not ensure that the patient has normal cell-mediated immunity to all antigens (e.g., patients with chronic mucocutaneous candidiasis have a limited defect in which cell-mediated immunity is generally intact except for their response to *Candida*), and (4) normal children under the age of 12 months frequently are unresponsive to all of the antigens in the panel.[35,36] When negative, DTH skin tests are therefore generally not helpful for the evaluation of suspected T-lymphocyte abnormalities that present early in life (e.g., severe combined immunodeficiency or DiGeorge syndrome).

Evaluation of the Complement System

Most of the genetically determined deficiencies of complement can be detected with the total serum hemolytic complement (CH_{50}) assay.[37] Because this assay depends on the functional integrity of the classic complement pathway (C1 through C9), a severe deficiency of any of these components leads to a marked reduction or absence of total hemolytic complement activity. Alternative pathway deficiencies (e.g., factor H, factor I, and properdin) are extremely rare; they may be suspected if the CH_{50} is in the low range of normal and the serum C3 level is low. The final identification of the specific complement component that is deficient usually rests on both functional and immunochemical tests, and highly specific assays have been developed for each of the individual components.

Evaluation of Phagocytic Cells

Evaluation of phagocytic cells usually entails assessment of both their number and function. Disorders such as congenital agranulocytosis or cyclic neutropenia that are characterized by a deficiency in phagocytic cell number can be easily detected by using a white blood cell count and differential. Beyond that, assessment of phagocytic cell function is relatively specialized because it depends on a variety of *in vitro* assays, including measurement of directed cell motility (chemotaxis), ingestion (phagocytosis), and intracellular killing (bactericidal activity). The most common of the phagocyte function disorders, chronic granulomatous disease, can be identified by the nitroblue tetrazolium (NBT) dye test, which measures the oxidative metabolic response of neutrophils and monocytes.[38]

Evaluation of Cilia

For suspected ciliary dyskinesia, ciliary structure and function must be assessed. Structure is assessed by electron microscopy of tissue obtained from the nasal mucosa, tonsils, adenoids, or bronchial mucosa. Because tobacco smoke, other pollutants, and infection may cause secondary abnormalities of cilia, it is sometimes difficult to find an appropriate tissue to sample. The microscopic examination should look for the presence of an anatomic defect that is consistent from cilia to cilia, such as the absence of dynein arms, and assess the orientation of cilia on the epithelium. With secondary causes, the structural abnormalities vary from cilia to cilia.[39] At the same time that tissue is obtained for electron microscopy, epithelial cell brushings from the nasal turbinates or bronchi can be examined for ciliary waveform and beat frequency. Assessments of mucociliary clearance are usually made by placing a small particle of saccharin on the anterior portion of the middle turbinate and then measuring the time until the patient tastes the saccharin.[40] For this test, the subject must sit quietly without sniffing or sneezing, and it is therefore difficult to perform in young children. A sweet taste should be evident within 1 hour in normal subjects, but this test has a very high rate of false-positive results.

Cystic Fibrosis

In most cases, the diagnosis of CF can be made by measuring the chloride concentration in sweat after iontophoresis of pilocarpine.[41] A minimum acceptable volume or weight of sweat must be collected to ensure an average sweat rate of greater than 1 g/m²/min, and the diagnosis can be made with certainty if the sweat chloride concentration is greater than 60 mmol/L. However, this test may be falsely negative, especially among those patients who have an atypical clinical presentation. If the clinical suspicion of CF is high, other useful diagnostic tests include mutation analysis of the CF trans-

membrane conductance regulator (CFTR) gene and/or measurement of potential difference across the nasal epithelium (nasal PD). The genetic testing is commercially available; the measurement of nasal PD is not widely available and should still be considered a research tool.

Evaluation for Human Immunodeficiency Virus and Other Immunosuppressive Virus Infections

Many techniques for the diagnosis of viral infection focus on the serologic detection of antibodies to viral proteins. There are, however, several problems with sole reliance on antibody detection techniques. First, antibody tests will not detect infection in patients during the "window period" between the time of infection and seroconversion. For HIV infections, 95% of infected individuals will seroconvert within 6 months of infection, although "window periods" of as long as 35 months have been reported.[42,43] Second, if the virus induces immunodeficiency, it may inhibit the production of antiviral antibodies.[44] Thus in a patient with known or suspected immunodeficiency, viral cultures as well as tests to detect viral antigens and nucleic acids should be performed in addition to serologic tests.[45]

CONCLUSIONS

The majority of children with recurrent respiratory tract infections will have environmental risk factors such as exposure to day care or cigarette smoke or an associated problem with allergies. It is the task of the allergist to identify the individuals who are most likely to have an underlying deficiency of host defense and to perform appropriate screening tests for such disorders. Early identification is critical for optimal clinical management and genetic counseling (Box 7-1).

HELPFUL WEBSITE

Immune Deficiency Foundation website (www.primaryimmune.org)

BOX 7-1

KEY CONCEPTS

Identification of Underlying Disorders in Children with Recurrent Infections

Children with chronic/recurrent infections may have one of the following underlying defects
- Allergy
- Immunodeficiency (primary or secondary)
- Cystic fibrosis
- Ciliary dysmotility
- Localized abnormalities of anatomy or physiology

Immunodeficient patients present with a variety of symptoms
- Increased susceptibility to infection
- Autoimmune or inflammatory disorders
- Syndrome complexes

Recurrent infections at a single anatomic site should prompt investigation of the anatomy and physiology of that site

REFERENCES

1. Johnston RB Jr: Recurrent bacterial infections in children, *N Engl J Med* 310:1237-1243, 1989.
2. Rachelefsky GS, Katz RM, Siegel SC: Chronic sinus disease with associated reactive airway disease in children, *Pediatrics* 73:526-529, 1984.
3. Kaufman HS, Hobbs JR: Immunologic deficiencies in an atopic population, *Lancet* 2:1061-1063, 1970.
4. Cunningham-Rundles C: Disorders of the IgA system. In Stiehm ER, ed: *Immunologic disorders in infants and children,* ed 4, Philadelphia, 1996, WB Saunders.
5. International Union of Immunological Societies: Primary immunodeficiency diseases: report of an IUIS scientific committee, *Clin Exp Immunol* 118(suppl 1):1-28, 1999.
6. Puck JM: Primary immunodeficiency diseases, *JAMA* 278:1835-1840, 1997.
7. Sicherer SH, Winkelstein JA: Primary immunodeficiency diseases in adults, *JAMA* 279:5861, 1998.
8. Cunningham-Rundles C, Bodian C: Common variable immunodeficiency: clinical and immunologic features of 248 patients, *Clin Immunol* 92:34-48, 1999.
9. Herrod HG: Chronic mucocutaneous candidiasis and complications of non-*Candida* infection: a report of the Pediatric Immunodeficiency Collaborative Study Group, *J Pediatr* 116:377-382, 1990.
10. Sullivan KE: Complement deficiency and autoimmunity, *Curr Opin Pediatr* 10:600-606, 1998.
11. Ming JE, Stiehm ER, Graham JM Jr: Syndromes associated with immunodeficiency, *Adv Pediatr* 46:271-351, 1999.
12. Mickle JE, Cutting GR: Genotype-phenotype relationships in cystic fibrosis, *Med Clin North Am* 84:597-607, 2000.
13. Wiatrak BJ, Meyer CM III, Cottin RT: Cystic fibrosis presenting with sinus disease in children, *Am J Dis Child* 147:258-260, 1993.
14. Wang X-J, Maylan B, Leopold DA, et al: Mutation in the gene responsible for cystic fibrosis and predisposition to chronic rhinosinusitis in the general population, *JAMA* 284:1814-1819, 2000.
15. Winters WD, Effmann EL: Congenital masses of the lung: prenatal and postnatal imaging evaluation, *J Thorac Imaging* 16:196-206, 2001.
16. Meeks M, Buch A: Primary ciliary dyskinesia (PCD), *Pediatr Pulmonol* 29:307-316, 2000.
17. Rutland J, de Iongh RU: Random ciliary orientation: a cause of respiratory tract disease, *N Engl J Med* 323:1681-1684, 1990.
18. Sandberg ET, Kline MW, Shearer WT: The secondary immunodeficiencies. In Stiehm ER, ed: *Immunologic disorders in infants and children,* ed 4, Philadelphia, 1996, WB Saunders.
19. Lederman HM, Winkelstein JA: X-linked agammaglobulinemia: an analysis of 96 patients, *Medicine* 64:145-156, 1985.
20. Buckley RH: Primary cellular immunodeficiencies, *J Allergy Clin Immunol* 109:747-757, 2002.
21. Holland SM, Gallin JI: Evaluation of the patient with recurrent bacterial infections, *Annu Rev Med* 49:185-199, 1998.
22. Walport MJ. Complement, *N Engl J Med* 344:1058-1066, 1140-1144, 2001.
23. Anderson DC, Springer TA: Leukocyte adhesion deficiency: an inherited defect in the Mac-1, LFA-1, and p150,95 glycoproteins, *Annu Rev Med* 38:175-194, 1987.
24. Introne W, Boissy RE, Gahl WA: Clinical, molecular, and cell biological aspects of Chediak-Higashi syndrome, *Mol Genet Metab* 68:283-303, 1999.
25. Corash L, Shafer B, Blaese RM. Platelet-associated immunoglobulin, platelet size, and the effect of splenectomy in the Wiskott-Aldrich syndrome, *Blood* 65:1439-1443, 1985.
26. Pearson HA, Gallagher D, Chilcote R, et al: Developmental pattern of splenic dysfunction in sickle cell disorders, *Pediatrics* 76:392-397, 1985.
27. Jolliff CR, Cost KM, Stivrins PC, et al: Reference intervals for serum IgG, IgA, IgM, C3 and C4 as determined by rate nephelometry, *Clin Chem* 28:126-128, 1982.
28. Ambrosino DM, Siber GR, Chilmonczyk BA, et al: An immunodeficiency characterized by impaired antibody responses to polysaccharides, *N Engl J Med* 316:790-793, 1987.
29. Auf de Maur C, Hodel M, Nydegger UE, et al: Age dependency of ABO histo-blood group antibodies: reexamination of an old transfusion dogma, *Transfusion* 33:915-918, 1993.
30. Herrod HG: Clinical significance of IgG subclasses, *Curr Opin Pediatr* 5:696-699, 1993.
31. Comans-Bitter WM, de Groot R, van den Beemd R, et al: Immunophenotyping of blood lymphocytes in childhood, *J Pediatr* 130:388-393, 1997.
32. Gordon EH, Krouse HA, Kinney JL, et al: Delayed cutaneous hypersensitivity in normals: choice of antigens and comparison to in vitro assays of cell-mediated immunity, *J Allergy Clin Immunol* 72:487-494, 1983.
33. Palmer DL, Reed WP: Delayed hypersensitivity skin testing. II. Clinical correlates and anergy, *J Infect Dis* 130:138-143, 1974.
34. Centers for Disease Control and Prevention: Anergy skin testing and preventive therapy for HIV-infected persons: revised recommendations, *MMWR Morb Mortal Wkly Rep* 46(RR-15):1-19, 1997.
35. Kniker WT, Anderson CT, McBryde JL, et al: Multitest CMI for standardized measurement of delayed cutaneous hypersensitivity and cell-mediated immunity: normal values and proposed scoring system for healthy adults in the USA, *Ann Allergy* 52:75-82, 1984.
36. Kniker WT, Lesourd BM, McBryde JL, et al: Cell-mediated immunity assessed by multitest CMI skin testing in infants and preschool children, *Am J Dis Child* 139:840-845, 1985.
37. Sullivan KE, Winkelstein JA: Genetically determined deficiencies of the complement system, *Pediatr Allergy Immunol* 3:97-109, 1992.
38. Baehner RL, Nathan DG: Quantitative nitroblue tetrazolium test in chronic granulomatous disease, *N Engl J Med* 278:971-976, 1968.
39. Carson JL, Collier AM, Hu S-CS: Acquired ciliary defects in nasal epithelium of children with acute viral upper respiratory infections, *N Engl J Med* 312:463-468, 1985.
40. Stanley P, MacWilliam L, Greenstone M, et al: Efficacy of a saccharin test for screening to detect abnormal mucociliary clearance, *Br J Dis Chest* 78:62-65, 1984.
41. Rosenstein BJ, Cutting GR, for the Cystic Fibrosis Foundation Consensus Panel: The diagnosis of cystic fibrosis: a consensus statement, *J Pediatr* 132:589-595, 1998.
42. Horsburgh CH Jr, Jason J, Longini IM Jr, et al: Duration of human immunodeficiency virus infection before detection of antibody, *Lancet* 2:637-640, 1989.
43. Imagawa DT, Lee MH, Wolinsky SM, et al: Human immunodeficiency virus type 1 infection in homosexual men who remain seronegative for prolonged periods, *N Engl J Med* 320:1458-1462, 1989.
44. Saulsbury FT, Wykoff RF, Boyle RJ: Transfusion-acquired human immunodeficiency virus infection in twelve neonates: epidemiologic, clinical and immunologic features, *Pediatr Infect Dis J* 6:544-549, 1987.
45. Centers for Disease Control and Prevention: Revised guidelines for HIV counseling, testing, and referral and revised recommendations for HIV screening of pregnant women, *MMWR Morb Mortal Wkly Rep* 50(RR-19):1-110, 2001.

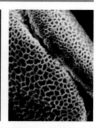

CHAPTER 8

Antibody Deficiency

FRANCISCO A. BONILLA

Primary immunodeficiency diseases are those disorders resulting from inherited or spontaneous genetic lesions that affect immune system function. These are frequently subdivided into the humoral, cellular, and combined immunodeficiencies as a result of lymphocyte dysfunction and disorders that result from defects of phagocytes or the complement system.[1] Humoral immunodeficiencies, which are also called antibody deficiencies, are characterized by low serum levels of one or more immunoglobulin classes and/or relative impairment of antibody responses to various forms of antigen challenge. This may arise as the result of a defect intrinsic to the antibody-producing cells (B cells) or of a failure of communication between T cells and B cells (T cell help for antibody production). Cell-mediated immunity is intact.

The most common complications of humoral immunodeficiency are recurrent bacterial infections of the upper and lower respiratory tract. Pyogenic skin infections, meningitis, osteomyelitis, and sepsis are also seen with increasing frequency in these disorders. These infections are generally caused by the same organisms virulent in immunocompetent hosts, predominantly encapsulated bacteria such as *Streptococcus pneumoniae, Haemophilus influenzae, Staphylococcus aureus,* and *Neisseria meningitidis.* Viral infections are usually cleared normally by these patients, although they will have a higher frequency of recurrence with the same agent, since they often do not produce neutralizing antibodies or B cell memory. Additional infectious diseases may be associated with particular syndromes.

The most severely affected patients will have treatment-resistant recurrent otitis media, sinusitis, and pneumonia in rapid succession. Those with less severe disease fall into a gray area with respect to the severity and frequency of infections. Unfortunately, there are no clinically based criteria that have been well validated for predicting which children with recurrent otitis media or sinusitis or one or two episodes of pneumonia will have an identifiable immunologic defect. A high index of suspicion for antibody deficiency should be maintained in cases of recurrent, refractory, or severe infections. Retrospective studies of patients with refractory sinusitis have revealed immunoglobulin abnormalities in up to 20%.[2] Up to 67% of a small group of patients older than 1 year who presented with overwhelming sepsis had low serum IgG levels.[3]

Table 8-1 contains a classification of humoral immunodeficiencies according to known gene defects, as well as clinically defined entities.

EPIDEMIOLOGY AND ETIOLOGY

Estimates of the incidence of immunodeficiency overall range from about 1:10,000 to 1:2000 (see, for example, Stray-Pedersen et al[4] and Zelazko et al[5] and references therein). These studies are based on survey or registry data. The estimated prevalence of immunodeficiency overall is about 8 to 9:100,000. Because antibody deficiencies account for roughly half of all immune defects, the incidence should be about 1:20,000 to 1:4000. The prevalence should be about 4 to 5:100,000 overall, although it may be higher in the pediatric population because perhaps more than half of diagnoses are transient antibody deficiencies that will resolve during mid to late childhood.[6]

X-Linked Agammaglobulinemia

Ogden Bruton[7] published what is considered the classic description of this disorder in 1952; therefore this condition is often called "Bruton's agammaglobulinemia." It is caused by a defect in a signal transducing protein known as Bruton's tyrosine kinase (Btk).[8,9] Btk is expressed in B cells at all stages of development, as well as in monocytes, macrophages, mast cells, erythroid cells, and platelets; it transduces signals from the B cell immunoglobulin receptor.[10] In its absence, B cell development is impeded at an early stage (the pro-B cell–pre-B cell transition).[11]

Only males are affected, and they are often asymptomatic during infancy. During this period, they are protected by maternal antibodies acquired through placental transfer during gestation. Maternal IgG gradually disappears, and infectious complications usually begin by the age of 9 to 18 months. The absence of visible tonsils or palpable lymph nodes is notable on examination. Laboratory investigation reveals absent or very low serum levels of immunoglobulins and B cells. Neutropenia is not uncommon and may occur in up to 25% of patients.[12]

Despite normal cellular immunity, patients with X-linked agammaglobulinemia (XLA) are prone to certain viral infections, including chronic enteroviral meningoencephalitis and vaccine-associated paralytic poliomyelitis. Chronic nonprogressive myelitis caused by coxsackievirus has also been reported.[13] This susceptibility suggests the importance of specific antibody for control of these infections. Additional infections described in these patients include mycoplasma or ureaplasma arthritis.[14] Opportunistic infections such as

Classification of Humoral Immunodeficiencies

Disease	Gene
Known genetic basis	
X-linked (Bruton's) agammaglobulinemia (XLA) due to mutation of Bruton's tyrosine kinase	*BTK*
Autosomal recessive agammaglobulinemia (AR AGAM) due to:	
Mutation of IgM constant region (C_μ)	*IGHM*
Mutation of signal transducing molecule Ig-α	*CD79A*
Mutation of surrogate light chain	*CD179B*
Mutation of B cell linker protein	*BLNK*
Hyper-IgM syndrome (HIM)	
X-linked (XHIM, HIM1) due to mutation of tumor necrosis factor superfamily member 5 (CD154, CD40 ligand)	*TNFSF5*
Autosomal recessive (HIM2) due to mutation of activation-induced cytidine deaminase	*AICDA*
Unknown genetic basis	
Common variable immunodeficiency	
IgA deficiency	
IgG subclass deficiency	
Specific antibody deficiency with normal immunoglobulins	
Transient hypogammaglobulinemia of infancy	
Hypogammaglobulinemia, unspecified	

Pneumocystis carinii pneumonia are seen only very rarely.[15] Autoimmune manifestations are not characteristic of XLA. However, a patient with XLA was recently reported to have developed insulin-dependent diabetes mellitus, presumably because of cell-mediated autoimmune destruction of pancreatic β cells.[16]

XLA may not be diagnosed definitively by the clinical and laboratory criteria described earlier. About half of patients will have a family history of affected male relatives on the maternal side.[8] The remainder will not, and autosomal recessive forms of agammaglobulinemia with a virtually identical phenotype (see later) must be distinguished. It is desirable to confirm the diagnosis at the molecular level in all cases. Btk is expressed in platelets and may be detected by flow cytometry.[17] Some have suggested that this is a convenient screening test. It is also useful for detecting carrier females, who have random X-chromosome inactivation in megakaryocytes and two platelet populations: Btk+ and Btk−. Identical methods may be used to assess Btk expression in monocytes with essentially indistinguishable results.[18]

Some patients with Btk mutations have an "atypical" phenotype with low numbers of B cells and low-level antibody production.[9] Some have even recovered from wild-type poliovirus infection.[19] Some of these atypical XLA cases were misdiagnosed as having common variable immunodeficiency (see later) before the recognition of the Btk kinase defect.[20] There is no consistent genotype-phenotype correlation in XLA.[21] Even siblings with identical mutations may show divergent clinical features.[22] Female carriers of XLA show nonrandom X chromosome inactivation in their B cells, and this can be used for carrier detection.[8]

A few patients have agammaglobulinemia with autosomal recessive inheritance. Mutations of the immunoglobulin (Ig)-μ heavy-chain locus *(IGHM)* prevent formation of Ig receptors on pre-B cells and mature B cells.[23] Defects of the λ5 (surrogate light chain) gene similarly prevent formation of the pre-B cell Ig receptor.[24] Igα (CD79a) is a signal transducer for Ig receptors; absence of this protein prevents Ig receptor signaling.[25] Finally, mutations in the gene encoding the signal transduction adapter protein BLNK (B cell linker protein) have been described.[26] This molecule is also required for normal Ig receptor signaling in B cells. All of these mutations arrest B cell development at an early stage.

The diagnosis of common variable immunodeficiency (CVID) encompasses an unknown number of potentially genetically and etiologically distinct conditions having in common a (relatively) late-onset humoral immunodeficiency, most often in the first or third decade of life.[27,28] Hypogammaglobulinemia and impaired specific antibody production are universal by definition. IgA deficiency is also common in CVID. These patients have the recurrent sinopulmonary bacterial infections characteristic of antibody deficiency. One detailed study of lung involvement in 19 patients showed bronchiectasis in 11, which was multilobar in 8.[29] About half had airway obstruction, and 11 had reduced carbon monoxide diffusion capacity.

Additional manifestations of CVID include asthma, chronic rhinitis, chronic giardiasis, and recurrent or chronic arthropathy.[27] Chronic enteroviral infections, including meningoencephalitis, may also be seen in CVID. The apparent "atopic" symptoms found in about 10% of patients occur in the absence of allergen-specific IgE. Malabsorption, inflammatory bowel disease, and autoimmune syndromes such as pernicious anemia and autoimmune cytopenias (thrombocytopenia, anemia, and neutropenia) also occur with increased frequency. Other autoimmune diseases such as autoimmune polyglandular syndrome type 2 have also been described in association with CVID.[30] In addition, noncaseating granulomatous disease resembling sarcoidosis may be encountered in the skin or viscera, even in children.[27] It often responds well to immunosuppressive therapy such as steroids or cyclosporine A.

Widespread lymphoproliferation may cause splenomegaly, adenopathy, and intestinal lymphonodular hyperplasia, and patients with CVID also have a higher incidence of gastrointestinal and lymphoid malignancy. The relative risk of lymphoma has been estimated to be as much as 30- to 400-fold greater than that for the general population.[31] Stated another way, between 1.4% and 7% of patients with CVID develop lymphoma. Most of these are B cell non-Hodgkin's lymphomas, and some may arise in lymphocytes in mucosa-associated lymphoid tissue (MALT).[32,33]

The levels of particular Ig isotypes in a given patient with CVID are often static over time, but fluctuations may occur. B cells appear to be normal in most patients and produce antibody on stimulation *in vitro*.[34] Some patients have low numbers of poorly functional B cells.[35] Reduction in the ratio of CD4+ to CD8+ T cells is common in CVID.

No well-defined molecular defects have been identified in any significant proportion of patients with a diagnosis of CVID. Most cases of CVID appear to be sporadic. A few cases have been noted to occur after solid organ transplantation.[36]

X-linked lymphoproliferative disease (XLP) results from mutations in the SH2D1A signal transducing molecule.[37] Some of these patients have dysgammaglobulinemias of various types, and a few had been classified as having CVID before the discovery of the genetic basis of XLP.[38] It is important to rule out XLP in males with a CVID phenotype because prognosis and therapy are distinct for these disorders. Very few male patients with Btk mutations may also have been misdiagnosed as having CVID.[39]

The occurrence of thymoma in the context of a clinical and immunologic picture very similar to CVID with low B cell numbers has been designated Good's syndrome.[40] It is not clear whether these patients exhibit as yet undiscovered specific genetic or immunologic abnormalities that distinguish them from the larger group of patients with CVID. It appears that disseminated and opportunistic infections (such as *P. carinii* pneumonia) occur more frequently in Good's syndrome and that the prognosis may be worse than that for the typical CVID patient.

IgA Deficiency

Human IgA is divided into two subclasses: IgA1 and IgA2. These are encoded by separate genes on the heavy-chain C region locus on chromosome 14. IgA1 constitutes 80% to 90% of serum IgA; both contribute equally to secretory IgA. Both subclasses are affected in IgA deficiency (IGAD). Low levels of IgA are found in about 1:700 whites.[41] Most individuals with low serum levels of IgA are asymptomatic. Some have clinical manifestations similar to those of patients with CVID or IgG subclass deficiency[42] (see later). In a population of patients with chronic bacterial sinusitis, IGAD is more prevalent than in healthy individuals.[43] Furthermore, 20 years of prospective follow-up of IgA-deficient blood donors showed an increased incidence of respiratory infections and autoimmune disease.[44]

Atopic disease is found frequently among IgA-deficient patients.[42] In addition, autoimmune syndromes such as rheumatoid arthritis, systemic lupus erythematosus, Sjögren's syndrome, insulin-dependent diabetes mellitus and other endocrinopathies, pernicious anemia, hemolytic anemia, and autoimmune hepatitis are not uncommon. Other inflammatory disorders, such as Crohn's disease, have also been noted in patients with low serum IgA.[45] Finally, the forms of malignancy associated with CVID also occur with greater frequency in IGAD. Rare cases of IGAD may evolve into CVID or improve over time.[46] About one third of IGAD patients have a concomitant IgG subclass deficiency (see later). This association is more frequently accompanied by deficits in specific antibody production and significant infectious complications.[47]

In vitro studies suggest some heterogeneity in the immunologic defects underlying IgA deficiency.[48] Four principal forms have been noted: (1) an intrinsic B cell defect, (2) an IgA suppressor T cell effect, (3) a combination of forms 1 and 2, and (4) a selective lack of T cell help in IgA production. No genetic defects underlying IGAD have been defined. In whites,

IGAD and CVID are associated with the HLA haplotype A1,B8,DR3.[49] An "IGAD susceptibility" locus (*IGAD1*) has been mapped to the boundary region between HLA class II and class III. One case of phenytoin-induced IGAD has been reported[50]; the serum IgA levels rose after the drug was discontinued.

IgG Subclass Deficiency

Human IgG is divided into four subclasses designated IgG1, 2, 3, and 4, each encoded by different Ig constant region genes. Each represents approximately 67%, 23%, 7%, and 3% of the total, respectively. IgG subclasses are produced in different relative amounts depending on the antigenic stimulus.[51] For example, IgG1 predominates in responses to soluble protein antigens, and responses to pneumococcal capsular polysaccharides consist almost entirely of the IgG2 subclass.

A disproportionately low level of one or more IgG subclasses with a normal total serum IgG constitutes an IgG subclass deficiency (IGGSD). Individuals with IGGSD may present with recurrent sinopulmonary infections of varying severity caused by common respiratory bacterial pathogens.[52] Frequent viral infections and recurrent diarrhea (infectious or allergic in nature) may also be seen. Additional clinical manifestations often include atopic diseases such as asthma and allergic rhinitis. Also, rheumatologic disorders such as vasculitis or other autoimmune diseases may be seen, as is the case in IGAD and CVID. IGGSD has been reported in patients with HIV infection/AIDS,[53] combined immunodeficiencies such as Wiskott-Aldrich syndrome and ataxia-telangiectasia,[54,55] and after bone marrow transplantation.[56] As is true of IGAD, IGGSD is not commonly the result of genetic lesions in the human Ig heavy-chain locus. Mutations preventing expression of cell surface IgG2 have been found in a few reported cases of IgG2 deficiency.[57]

Considerable diagnostic controversy arises due to variations in immunoglobulin subclass determinations depending on laboratory methods, as well as significant differences in normal ranges depending on age and ethnicity. Furthermore, most individuals with isolated low IgG subclass levels are asymptomatic, rendering its significance questionable in patients with recurrent infections. However, several studies show a higher prevalence of subclass deficiency in groups of patients with chronic or recurrent sinopulmonary bacterial infections.[58-60] Not all of these patients have demonstrably impaired specific antibody responses to vaccines or infectious challenge. Thus the connection between IgG subclass deficiency and susceptibility to infection or other disease may be difficult to appreciate.

IgG subclass deficiencies occur in various patterns. A low level of IgG2 is most common in children, where it is found most often in males. It may occur in isolation but is also frequently associated with IgG4 and/or IgA deficiency.[47] Selective deficiency of IgG3 is found more commonly in women and may be associated with low levels of IgG1.[61] Recurrent infections may also occur in some patients with only a deficiency of IgG4.[62] Patients with IGGSDs in childhood often improve with time, although the IgG subclass abnormality may never normalize completely. When IGGSD is diagnosed in adulthood, resolution is much less likely.

Specific Antibody Deficiency with Normal Immunoglobulins

There exists a population of patients with recurrent infections and poor antibody responses (mainly to polysaccharide antigens) who have normal levels of antibody classes and subclasses. This has been called "specific antibody deficiency with normal immunoglobulins" (SADNI), or "functional antibody deficiency."[63] In a retrospective study of 90 patients evaluated for immunodeficiency in one tertiary care center, SADNI was the most frequent diagnosis (23% of patients).[64] The relationship of SADNI to other humoral immunodeficiencies is unclear, although these patients are clinically very similar to those with IGGSD and recurrent infections.

Transient Hypogammaglobulinemia of Infancy

In humans, IgG is actively transported from the maternal to the fetal circulation during gestation, mainly during the third trimester. Maternal antibody has a half-life in the infant's circulation between 20 and 30 days. A physiologic nadir of serum IgG occurs at 3 to 9 months of age as maternal Ig is cleared and newborn IgG production gradually begins. Transient hypogammaglobulinemia of infancy (THI) is an IgG deficiency that begins in infancy and resolves spontaneously by 36 to 48 months of age.[65] Thus, the diagnosis can be confirmed only after IgG levels normalize. By definition, the serum IgG is lower than is normal for age (approximately 3 g/L in the first year of life). As is the case in IGAD and IGGSD, many of these children are asymptomatic. Beginning at about 6 months of age, some of these IgG-deficient children manifest the types of recurrent infections associated with hypogammaglobulinemia. Some cases may also be associated with food allergy. Severe infections are not often seen, but vaccine strain polio meningoencephalitis has been reported in one case of THI.[66]

The reasons for delayed rise in serum IgG in THI are not known. The numbers of B and T cells are normal, as are various measures of lymphocyte function *in vitro*. Some studies suggest there may be a delay in the development of highly efficient T cell help for antibody production.[67] However, most children with THI have normal antibody responses to immunization and other antigen challenges well before their serum antibody levels enter the normal range.[68] Inadequate antibody responses do not exclude the diagnosis of THI but should prompt further investigation for other forms of immunodeficiency.

Hyper-IgM Syndrome

The eponym "hyper-IgM syndrome" has been applied to a pattern of immunodeficiency with a prominent defect in Ig class switching. In normal primary antibody responses, IgM is produced initially, with IgG and other isotypes being produced later. This is called *class switching* and requires genetic rearrangement at the immunoglobulin locus to bring the variable region gene into juxtaposition with a new heavy-chain gene. If this process is impaired, IgM production predominates in antibody responses with very few, if any, other isotypes being produced (hence the term *hyper-IgM syndrome*). The X-linked hyper-IgM syndrome (sometimes abbreviated XHIM or HIM1) is a combined immunodeficiency resulting from mutation of the *TNFSF5,* or *tumor necrosis factor super-family member 5 gene.*[69] This molecule is also called CD154 or CD40 ligand. Many would consider this to be truly a combined immunodeficiency because the interactions of T cells with antigen-presenting cells and effector mononuclear cells are significantly impaired. However, HIM1 is often classified with antibody deficiencies because hypogammaglobulinemia is such a prominent feature.

Usually within the first 2 years of life, patients with HIM1 develop the types of recurrent bacterial infections generally seen in hypogammaglobulinemia.[69] They are also prone to opportunistic infections from protozoan or fungal pathogens such as *Pneumocystis* or *Histoplasma*. Additional infections noted most frequently include anemia due to parvovirus and sclerosing cholangitis due to *Cryptosporidium*. Noninfectious complications include neutropenia and liver and certain hematologic malignancies.

Laboratory evaluation shows a normal number of B cells in the circulation. IgG is usually low and IgM high; more than half of patients lack IgA. Specific antibody formation is often impaired. Patients make IgM antibody in response to immunization or infection but little, if any, IgG is produced. Antibody levels wane rapidly, and there are no memory responses. Secondary lymphoid tissues are poorly developed and do not contain germinal centers. The diagnosis may be established by demonstrating a failure of T cells to express CD154 on mitogenic stimulation. The diagnosis should be confirmed with molecular genetic study.

An autosomal recessive form of hyper-IgM syndrome (sometimes abbreviated HIM2) results from mutations of the gene encoding activation-induced cytidine deaminase.[70] Bacterial sinopulmonary infections occur in the majority of patients. Less frequent complications include diarrhea with failure to thrive and massive lymphadenopathy.

Another autosomal recessive form of hyper-IgM syndrome has been described in one male and two female patients having a clinical presentation identical to that of the X-linked form. These individuals were found to carry mutations in the gene encoding TNFRSF5, also known as CD40.[71] Because this is the ligand for TNFSF5, the molecule affected in HIM1, all of the same cellular interactions are affected, and the pathophysiology is identical.

DIFFERENTIAL DIAGNOSIS

Clinical entities that may mimic (or even coexist with) antibody deficiency are listed in Table 8-2. The most frequent presentation of antibody deficiency includes recurrent, frequent, and severe upper and lower respiratory tract infections with encapsulated bacteria. As described earlier, additional bacterial infections may occur in other sites, as well as frequent viral infections, and a variety of noninfectious complications. Of course, antibody deficiency may accompany cellular immunodeficiency (i.e., combined immunodeficiency). If the cellular immune defect is not profound, the manifestations related to the antibody deficiency component may predominate in the clinical presentation. Normal cellular immune function should be confirmed in all cases of significant abnormalities of humoral immunity (see next section and Figure 8-1).

Complement deficiency may present with the infectious complications characteristic of antibody deficiency. Patients with phagocyte defects frequently present with distinct infec-

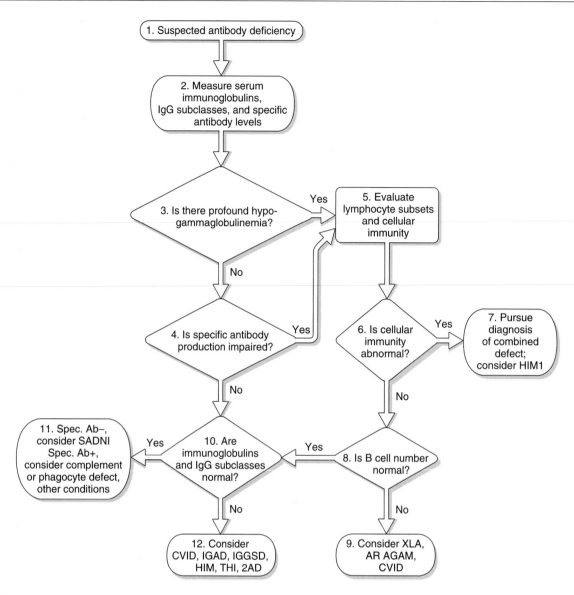

FIGURE 8-1 Algorithm for evaluation of the patient with suspected antibody deficiency (see text for annotations and abbreviations).

tious complications, such as deep-seated abscesses or cellulitis, which are not as often seen in antibody deficiencies although they do occur occasionally.

Some "nonimmune" disorders of host defense may mimic antibody deficiencies, such as CF. Similarly, ciliary dysmotility syndromes may have a presentation identical to that of antibody deficiency. Nasopharyngeal anatomic defects or hyperplasia of lymphoid tissue may lead to Eustachian tube or ostiomeatal obstruction and lead to recurrent or chronic otitis media and/or sinusitis. Allergic rhinosinusitis may also lead to sinus and nasopharyngeal mucosal inflammation, promoting mucous stasis and infection. As mentioned, atopic disease (or clinically similar pathology) may accompany antibody deficiencies such as CVID, IGAD, and IGGSD. Based on other clinical features of the case in question, some or all of these disorders should be investigated in patients with normal humoral immunity in the setting of infections characteristic of antibody deficiency.

EVALUATION

Figure 8-1 shows an algorithm that may be applied to patients suspected of having humoral immunodeficiency. Some combined immunodeficiencies have characteristic clinical features that should prompt investigation of cellular immune function, even if the history of infections at the time of evaluation is more suggestive of antibody deficiency. Examples include the eczema and thrombocytopenia of Wiskott-Aldrich syndrome, ataxic gait in ataxia-telangiectasia, etc. This algorithm assumes that there are no such features because evaluation of cellular immunity would be undertaken immediately in such cases. The following annotations correspond to the numbered elements in Figure 8-1.

1. The descriptions of the various diseases mentioned point out the characteristic elements of a medical history that should arouse suspicion of impaired anti-

TABLE 8-2 Differential Diagnosis of Antibody Deficiency

Primary humoral immunodeficiency
Secondary or acquired humoral immunodeficiency (immunosuppression, cancer)
Primary combined immunodeficiency
    Severe combined immunodeficiency
    Wiskott-Aldrich syndrome
    DiGeorge syndrome
    Ataxia-telangiectasia
    Other
Secondary or acquired combined immunodeficiency (HIV/AIDS)
Complement deficiency
Phagocytic cell defect
    Chronic granulomatous disease
    Leukocyte adhesion defect
    Chédiak-Higashi syndrome
    Neutropenia
Allergic rhinosinusitis
Anatomic obstruction of Eustachian tube or sinus ostia (tumor, foreign body, lymphoid hyperplasia)
Cystic fibrosis
Ciliary dysfunction

body production, with the main element being recurrent upper and lower respiratory tract bacterial infections. Physical examination is generally not specific, often showing only the presence or sequelae of microbial infections. Visible or palpable lymphoid tissue may be scarce or absent in some cases, especially in areas rich in B cells (e.g., tonsils). This is most often the case in the agammaglobulinemias. Specific diagnosis rests entirely on the laboratory evaluation.

2. The initial laboratory examination of humoral immunity consists of measuring the levels of various Ig isotypes (IgG, IgA, IgM, and IgG subclasses) in serum, as well as a measure of function or specific antibody production (Table 8-3). Specific antibody titers both to protein and polysaccharide antigens should be measured. These substances differ in how they stimulate antibody production, and clinically significant disease may result from a selective inability to respond to polysaccharide antigens (see earlier). Antibody levels for protein vaccine antigens such as tetanus and diphtheria are often determined. Antibodies against the capsular polysaccharide (polyribose phosphate [PRP]) of *H. influenzae* type B (HIB) may also be measured. It is important to note that current HIB vaccines couple the PRP to a protein carrier, and PRP titers in immunized children, although specific for a polysaccharide, are indicative of immune response to a protein. Similar considerations apply to measurement of antibodies against pneumococcal capsular polysaccharides. Antibody levels measured after natural exposure or immunization with unconjugated pneumococcal vaccines are indicative of polysaccharide responses. Newer pneumococcal vaccines also couple the polysaccharide to a protein carrier, and responses to these vaccines are

indicative of protein antigen response. If initial measurements of specific antibodies are low, response to booster immunization should be assessed. Postvaccination levels may be determined after 4 to 6 weeks. One must bear in mind that polysaccharide antibody responses are not reliable in normal children under the age of 2 years, and negative responses to these antigens in these patients should be interpreted with caution.[72] Serum isohemagglutinins are naturally occurring antibodies against ABO blood group antigens. They are produced in response to polysaccharide antigens of gut flora, and measurement is a useful indicator of polysaccharide immunity.[73]

3. Profound hypogammaglobulinemia with serum IgG of less than 100 mg/dl in an infant or less than 200 to 300 mg/dl in an older child or adult should prompt additional evaluation of lymphocyte populations and cellular immune function to investigate combined immunodeficiency and B cell number.

4. Specific antibody responses may be impaired as a result of the failure of T cell help for antibody production, even if serum Ig levels are normal or near normal. This situation should also prompt an evaluation of cellular immunity.

5. Cellular immunity is evaluated because of either severe hypogammaglobulinemia or impaired specific antibody production.

6. and 7. If cellular immunity is abnormal, then the eventual diagnosis will be a form of combined immunodeficiency. Recall that some classify HIM1 as a combined immunodeficiency.

8. Cellular immunity is normal; it is important to determine whether there appears to be a significant impairment of B cell development.

9. B cells are usually absent or severely reduced in X-linked or autosomal recessive agammaglobulinemia (XLA or AR AGAM). A positive family history of affected male relatives on the mother's side establishes the diagnosis of XLA.[8] Demonstration of maternal carrier status (nonrandom inactivation of X chromosomes in maternal B cells) is presumptive evidence; the diagnosis should be confirmed by molecular analysis. B cells may also be low in some cases of CVID.

10. At this point, either there is no severe hypogammaglobulinemia and specific antibody formation is not significantly impaired or specific antibody is reduced, a cellular immunologic evaluation is normal, and the B cell number is normal. Most of the remaining diagnoses are clinically defined, in part by the serum Ig profile.

11. If specific antibody formation is impaired (Spec. Ab−) and serum immunoglobulins are normal, then the diagnosis is SADNI. Otherwise, all measurements are normal (Spec. Ab+), and alternative explanations for recurrent infections should be sought. See the discussion on differential diagnosis.

12. There is an immunoglobulin abnormality, with or without demonstrable impairment of specific antibody production. Possible diagnoses include CVID and either form of HIM, IGAD, IGGSD, THI, and possibly secondary antibody deficiency.

TABLE 8-3 Reference Ranges for Serum Immunoglobulins and Specific Antibody Levels*

Age	IgG (mg/dl)	IgA (mg/dl)	IgM (mg/dl)	
0-1 mo	700-1300	0-11	5-30	
1-4 mo	280-750	6-50	15-70	
4-7 mo	200-1200	8-90	10-90	
7-13 mo	300-1500	16-100	25-115	
13 mo-3 yr	400-1300	20-230	30-120	
3-6 yr	600-1500	50-150	22-100	
6 yr-adult	639-1344	70-312	56-352	

Age	IgG1 (mg/dl)	IgG2 (mg/dl)	IgG3 (g/dl)	IgG4 (mg/dl)
Cord	435-1084	143-453	27-146	1-47
0-3 mo	218-496	40-167	4-23	1-120
3-6 mo	143-394	23-147	4-100	1-120
6-9 mo	190-388	37-60	12-62	1-120
9 mo-2 yr	286-680	30-327	13-82	1-120
2-4 yr	381-884	70-443	17-90	1-120
4-6 yr	292-816	83-513	8-111	2-112
6-8 yr	422-802	113-480	15-133	1-138
8-10 yr	456-938	163-513	26-113	1-95
10-12 yr	456-952	147-493	12-179	1-153
12-14 yr	347-993	140-440	23-117	1-143
Adult	422-1292	117-747	41-129	10-67

	Tetanus toxoid (IU/ml)	PRP (HIB) (ng/ml)	Pneumococcus
Protective level	0.15	1000	1000
Adequate response	Fourfold rise	Fourfold rise	Fourfold rise

	Isohemagglutinin Titer	
Age	Anti-A	Anti-B
0-6 mo	Unpredictable	Unpredictable
6 mo-2 yr	≥1:4-8	≥1:4-8
2-10 yr	1:4-256	1:16-256
10 yr-adult	≥1:4-8	≥1:4-8

*These are normal ranges from the laboratories of Children's Hospital, Boston, Mass. (except isohemagglutinins, see Fong SW, Qaqundah BY, Taylor WF: *Transfusion* 14:551, 1974.) Normal ranges are method-dependent and should be validated for each laboratory. These reference ranges are intended for educational purposes only.

TREATMENT

There are two principal modalities used to treat patients with antibody deficiencies: antimicrobial therapy (and prophylaxis) and intravenous immunoglobulin (IVIG) (Box 8-1). Agammaglobulinemia, CVID, and HIM are clear indications for immediate replacement therapy with IVIG.[8,27,69] Antibiotics are used as necessary to treat infectious complications before or during IVIG replacement. The choice of antibiotic depends on the site of infection, severity, past history of infections and antibiotic use, and microbiologic data, where available. Doses do not need to be adjusted for immunodeficiency; however, resolution may be slower in comparison with immunocompetent patients, and treatment may need to be prolonged.

The role of IVIG in the therapy of IGAD, IGGSD, and specific antibody deficiency is not as clear. These patients are probably best managed initially with therapeutic and prophylactic antibiotics and thorough evaluation to rule out other potential predisposing factors (e.g., anatomic defects, environmental allergies). If standard preventive regimens[74] are not effective, prophylaxis may be attempted by using half of the therapeutic daily dose of the antibiotic of choice. If infections continue to occur with unacceptable frequency or severity, and especially if antibody responses to immunization are poor, gamma globulin replacement is indicated.

Human immunoglobulin was first administered in the 1950s as an intramuscular injection for patients with XLA.[7] These treatments quickly and dramatically reduced the frequency and severity of infections. Modern IVIG preparations may provide some of these patients with an almost normal lifestyle. Studies in patients with agammaglobulinemia (serum IgG of less than 100 mg/ml) have clearly shown that relatively high-dose regimens of monthly IVIG (600 mg/kg) versus low-dose (200 mg/kg) replacement are superior, as determined by subjective criteria such as chest radiographs, pulmonary function, and rates of major or minor infections.[75] Maintaining a trough serum IgG level of greater than 500 to 600 mg/dl is beneficial. Most patients do well with about 300 to 500 mg/kg, usually at 2- to 4-week intervals. Adjustment of both the dose and the infusion interval is empirical. A retrospective study of bacterial infections in XLA patients showed

THERAPEUTIC PRINCIPLES
Care of Patients with Antibody Deficiency

THERAPY FOR EXISTING INFECTIONS

Antimicrobial chemotherapy, standard-dose regimens are appropriate

Intravenous immunoglobulin, doses range from 300-800 mg/kg q2-4wks (see text)

PREVENTION OF FURTHER INFECTIONS

Intravenous immunoglobulin

Antimicrobial chemoprophylaxis	CHILDREN	ADULTS
Amoxicillin	20 mg/kg qd or ÷ bid	500 mg qd/bid
Trimethoprim (TMP)/ sulfamethoxazole (dosing for TMP)	5 mg/kg qd	160 mg qd
Azithromycin	10 mg/kg qwk	500 mg qwk

SUPPORTIVE CARE

Fluid and nutritional support, enteral, parenteral

Cardiopulmonary support

a reduction in incidence from 0.4 to 0.06 episode per patient per year with IVIG therapy.[76] Some viral infections, including enteroviral meningoencephalitis, may occur in patients even while receiving IVIG.

The great majority of patients with CVID should be treated with IVIG infusions.[27] In one recent study, IVIG therapy (see later) was associated with a 43% reduction in lower respiratory tract infection (from 0.28 to 0.16 episode per patient per year).[29] Another randomized crossover study in 41 hypogammaglobulinemic patients compared low-dose (300 mg/kg in adults, 400 mg/kg in children) with high-dose (double the low dose) monthly IVIG therapy.[77] High-dose therapy was associated with significant reduction in both number (3.5 versus 2.5 per patient over 9 months) and duration (median, 33 days versus 21 days) of infections.

Most patients with CVID do well with IVIG replacement therapy (see later). Occasionally, antibiotic prophylaxis is also required. Additional therapies have also been studied in CVID. One report compared 15 CVID patients treated for 18 months with polyethylene glycol–conjugated interleukin-2 with 39 untreated CVID controls.[78] After 12 months, treated patients had significant increases in T cell responses to mitogens and antigens *in vitro*, as well as enhanced antibody responses to a bacteriophage neoantigen. Treated patients also recorded reduced occurrence of bronchitis, diarrhea, and joint pain in comparison with controls, but differences were not statistically significant.

Autoimmune cytopenias in CVID have been treated with steroids, IVIG, and anti-D (rho) antibodies.[79] One adult male patient with arthritis and scarring alopecia with granulomatous scalp inflammation was successfully treated with a human IgG–tumor necrosis factor receptor fusion protein.[80]

Some have reported anaphylactoid reactions to IgA-containing blood products (including IVIG) in IgA-deficient CVID patients with circulating anti-IgA antibodies.[81] However, other reports suggest that anti-IgA antibodies may not be pathogenic in a significant proportion of patients,[82] and IVIG containing IgA may be administered safely at least to some patients with CVID having circulating anti-IgA antibodies.[83,84]

There are no randomized trials of IVIG therapy in IGAD, IGGSD, specific antibody deficiency, or THI. One open trial of IVIG in 12 patients with IgG3 subclass deficiency for whom antibiotic prophylaxis failed found significant reductions in the frequency of acute sinusitis and otitis media.[61] Patients with IGGSD and SADNI have also been included in some clinical trials of IVIG products. One such study compared IVIG with equivalent cumulative monthly doses administered by subcutaneous infusion on a weekly basis.[85] There were no differences in efficacy or rate of adverse events. Symptomatic IGGSD or THI should be managed initially with antibiotic prophylaxis. Failure of preventive antibiotic treatment may justify a period of gamma globulin replacement. After 6 to 12 months, infusions should be stopped and antibody production reevaluated. Children with recurrent infections, regardless of immunoglobulin class or subclass levels, and normal responses to immunization may be difficult to manage. The benefit of gamma globulin replacement is less predictable, although an attempt is probably warranted in patients with significant infectious complications in the absence of other predisposing factors for whom antibiotic prophylaxis fails.

HIM1 is usually treated with IVIG and trimethoprim/sulfamethoxazole prophylaxis of *P. carinii* pneumonia.[69] Neutropenia in this disorder sometimes responds to granulocyte colony-stimulating factor (G-CSF, or filgrastim). HIM1 is curable with bone marrow transplantation. Successful sequential liver and bone marrow transplantation has also been reported. IVIG therapy alone with or without the use of antibiotic prophylaxis is generally adequate therapy for otherwise uncomplicated HIM2.

CONCLUSIONS

There are no prospective studies that define the "true" incidence of clinically significant antibody deficiency. Some diagnostic controversy still exists with respect to what constitutes "clinically significant" rates or severity of infection, and there are no criteria regarding such histories that have proven sensitivity or specificity leading toward diagnosis of antibody deficiency. Thus it is important to maintain an index of suspicion in cases where an infectious predisposition appears to exist (see Box 8-2).

One prospective analysis of patients presenting with hypogammaglobulinemia under the age of 4 years showed three distinct patterns over time.[6] In group 1, composed of 29 patients (83%), IgG and its subclass levels and antibody responses all became normal and infections ceased; in group 2 (3 patients, or 9%) IgG levels remained low, and antibody production was poor; and in the remaining 3 patients (group 3), IgG levels became normal, but antibody production remained poor. Group 1 would be classified as THI and group 3 as SADNI. Group 2 consists of uncharacterized, persistent hypogammaglobulinemia. This could include atypical XLA, CVID, HIM1 or HIM2, or undefined conditions. Invasive infections and low tetanus antibody level at presentation were

KEY CONCEPTS
Antibody Deficiencies

■ A clinician must maintain an index of suspicion for immunodeficiency when confronted with patients with infections considered unusual with respect to organism, frequency, severity, or response to treatment.

■ The possibility of antibody deficiency in particular should be considered when the history includes pyogenic upper and lower respiratory tract infections.

■ Early diagnosis is critical for reducing morbidity and mortality rates for immunodeficiency diseases.

■ To provide the most efficient and complete approach to diagnosis and management, referral to a clinical immunology specialist is indicated where there is clear evidence for, or suspicion of, antibody or other immunodeficiency syndrome.

■ Intravenous immunoglobulin (IVIG) replacement therapy and antibiotic prophylaxis are the main modalities for management of antibody deficiency disorders.

■ With IVIG and antibiotics, many patients with agammaglobulinemia/hypogammaglobulinemia may lead normal or near-normal lives.

the most significant predictors of persistent hypogammaglobulinemia.

Although it may be reassuring that a large proportion of these patients appear to improve with time, this will certainly not be the case for all. Even for patients who are destined to recover completely, early diagnosis is critical for preventing significant morbidity and mortality (Box 8-2).

HELPFUL WEBSITES

The American Academy of Allergy, Asthma and Immunology website (www.aaaai.org/)

The Clinical Immunology Society website (www.clinimmsoc. org/)

The Immune Deficiency Foundation website (www. primaryimmune.org/)

The Immunodeficiency Resource website (www.uta.fi/imt/bioinfo/idr/)

The Immunology Link website (www.immunologylink. com/)

REFERENCES

1. Rosen FS, Wedgwood RJP, Eibl M, et al: Primary immunodeficiency diseases: report of a WHO scientific group, *Clin Exp Immunol* 109(suppl 1):1, 1997.

2. Chee L, Graham SM, Carothers DG, et al: Immune dysfunction in refractory sinusitis in a tertiary care setting, *Laryngoscope* 111:233, 2001.

3. Lantz A, Armstrong J, Truemper E, et al: Immunoglobulin deficiency in children with a sudden overwhelming infection, *Ann Allergy Asthma Immunol* 86:55, 2001.

4. Stray-Pedersen A, Abrahamsen TG, Froland SS: Primary immunodeficiency diseases in Norway, *J Clin Immunol* 20:477, 2000.

5. Zelazko M, Carneiro-Sampaio M, Cornejo de Luigi M, et al: Primary immunodeficiency diseases in Latin America: first report from eight countries participating in the LAGID. Latin American Group for Primary Immunodeficiency Diseases, *J Clin Immunol* 18:161, 1998.

6. Dalal I, Reid B, Nisbet-Brown E, et al: The outcome of patients with hypogammaglobulinemia in infancy and early childhood, *J Pediatr* 133:144, 1998.

7. Bruton OC: Agammaglobulinemia, *Pediatrics* 9:722, 1952.

8. Conley ME, Rohrer J, Minegishi Y: X-linked agammaglobulinemia, *Clin Rev Allergy Immunol* 19:183, 2000.

9. Stewart DM, Lian L, Nelson DL: The clinical spectrum of Bruton's agammaglobulinemia, *Curr Allergy Asthma Rep* 1:558, 2001.

10. Petro JB, Rahman SM, Ballard DW, et al: Bruton's tyrosine kinase is required for activation of IkappaB kinase and nuclear factor kappaB in response to B cell receptor engagement, *J Exp Med* 191:1745, 2000.

11. Noordzij JG, de Bruin-Versteeg S, Comans-Bitter WM, et al: Composition of precursor B-cell compartment in bone marrow from patients with X-linked agammaglobulinemia compared with healthy children, *Pediatr Res* 51:159, 2002.

12. Cham B, Bonilla MA, Winkelstein J: Neutropenia associated with primary immunodeficiency syndromes, *Semin Hematol* 39:107, 2002.

13. Katamura K, Hattori H, Kunishima T, et al: Non-progressive viral myelitis in X-linked agammaglobulinemia, *Brain Dev* 24:109, 2002.

14. Furr PM, Taylor-Robinson D, Webster AD: Mycoplasmas and ureaplasmas in patients with hypogammaglobulinaemia and their role in arthritis: microbiological observations over twenty years, *Ann Rheum Dis* 53:183, 1994.

15. Alibrahim A, Lepore M, Lierl M, et al: Pneumocystis carinii pneumonia in an infant with X-linked agammaglobulinemia, *J Allergy Clin Immunol* 101:552, 1998.

16. Martin S, Wolf-Eichbaum D, Duinkerken G, et al: Development of type 1 diabetes despite severe hereditary B-lymphocyte deficiency, *N Engl J Med* 345:1036, 2001.

17. Futatani T, Watanabe C, Baba Y, et al: Bruton's tyrosine kinase is present in normal platelets and its absence identifies patients with X-linked agammaglobulinaemia and carrier females, *Br J Haematol* 114:141, 2001.

18. Kanegane H, Futatani T, Wang Y, et al: Clinical and mutational characteristics of X-linked agammaglobulinemia and its carrier identified by flow cytometric assessment combined with genetic analysis, *J Allergy Clin Immunol* 108:1012, 2001.

19. Sarpong S, Skolnick HS, Ochs HD, et al: Survival of wild polio by a patient with XLA, *Ann Allergy Asthma Immunol* 88:59, 2002.

20. Stewart DM, Tian L, Nelson DL: A case of x-linked agammaglobulinemia diagnosed in adulthood, *Clin Immunol* 99:94, 2001.

21. Tao L, Boyd M, Gonye G, et al: Btk mutations in patients with X-linked agammaglobulinemia: lack of correlation between presence of peripheral B lymphocytes and specific mutations, *Hum Mutat* 16:528, 2000.

22. Bykowsky MJ, Haire RN, Ohta Y, et al: Discordant phenotype in siblings with X-linked agammaglobulinemia, *Am J Hum Genet* 58:477, 1996.

23. Yel L, Minegishi Y, Coustan-Smith E, et al: Mutations in the mu heavy-chain gene in patients with agammaglobulinemia, *N Engl J Med* 335:1486, 1996.

24. Minegishi Y, Coustan-Smith E, Wang YH, et al: Mutations in the human lambda5/14.1 gene result in B cell deficiency and agammaglobulinemia, *J Exp Med* 187:71, 1998.

25. Minegishi Y, Coustan-Smith E, Rapalus L, et al: Mutations in Igalpha (CD79a) result in a complete block in B-cell development, *J Clin Invest* 104:1115, 1999.

26. Minegishi Y, Rohrer J, Coustan-Smith E, et al: An essential role for BLNK in human B cell development, *Science* 286:1954, 1999.

27. Cunningham-Rundles C: Common variable immunodeficiency, *Curr Allergy Asthma Rep* 1:421, 2001.

28. Cunningham-Rundles C, Bodian C: Common variable immunodeficiency: clinical and immunological features of 248 patients, *Clin Immunol* 92:34, 1999.

29. Martinez Garcia MA, de Rojas MD, Nauffal Manzur MD, et al: Respiratory disorders in common variable immunodeficiency, *Respir Med* 95:191, 2001.

30. Topaloglu AK, Yuksel B, Yilmaz M, et al: Coexistence of common variable immunodeficiency and autoimmune polyglandular syndrome type 2, *J Pediatr Endocrinol Metab* 14:565, 2001.

31. Cunningham-Rundles C, Lieberman P, Hellman G, et al: Non-Hodgkin lymphoma in common variable immunodeficiency, *Am J Hematol* 37:69, 1991.

32. Cunningham-Rundles C, Cooper DL, Duffy TP, et al: Lymphomas of mucosal-associated lymphoid tissue in common variable immunodeficiency, *Am J Hematol* 69:171, 2002.

33. Reichenberger F, Wyser C, Gonon M, et al: Pulmonary mucosa-associated lymphoid tissue lymphoma in a patient with common variable immunodeficiency syndrome, *Respiration* 68:109, 2001.

34. Nonoyama S, Farrington M, Ishida H, et al: Activated B cells from patients with common variable immunodeficiency proliferate and synthesize immunoglobulin, *J Clin Invest* 92:1282, 1993.

35. Denz A, Eibel H, Illges H, et al: Impaired up-regulation of CD86 in B cells of "type A" common variable immunodeficiency patients, *Eur J Immunol* 30:1069, 2000.

36. Miller BW, Brennan DC, Korenblat PE, et al: Common variable immunodeficiency in a renal transplant patient with severe recurrent bacterial infection: a case report and review of the literature, *Am J Kidney Dis* 25:947, 1995.

37. Sayos J, Wu C, Morra M, et al: The X-linked lymphoproliferative-disease gene product SAP regulates signals induced through the co-receptor SLAM, *Nature* 395:462, 1998.

38. Morra M, Silander O, Calpe S, et al: Alterations of the X-linked lymphoproliferative disease gene SH2D1A in common variable immunodeficiency syndrome, *Blood* 98:1321, 2001.

39. Weston SA, Prasad ML, Mulligan CG, et al: Assessment of male CVID patients for mutations in the Btk gene: how many have been misdiagnosed? *Clin Exp Immunol* 124:465, 2001.

40. Tarr PE, Sneller MC, Mechanic LJ, et al: Infections in patients with immunodeficiency with thymoma (Good syndrome): report of 5 cases and review of the literature, *Medicine (Baltimore)* 80:123, 2001.

41. Ropars C, Muller A, Paint N, et al: Large scale detection of IgA deficient blood donors, *J Immunol Methods* 54:183, 1982.

42. Cunningham-Rundles C: Physiology of IgA and IgA deficiency, *J Clin Immunol* 21:303, 2001.

43. Tahkokallio O, Seppala IJ, Sarvas H, et al: Concentrations of serum immunoglobulins and antibodies to pneumococcal capsular polysaccharides in patients with recurrent or chronic sinusitis, *Ann Otol Rhinol Laryngol* 110:675, 2001.

44. Koskinen S, Tolo H, Hirvonen M, et al: Long-term follow-up of anti-IgA antibodies in healthy IgA-deficient adults, *J Clin Immunol* 15:194, 1995.

45. Iizuka M, Itou H, Sato M, et al: Crohn's disease associated with selective immunoglobulin a deficiency, *J Gastroenterol Hepatol* 16:951, 2001.

46. Johnson ML, Keeton LG, Zhu ZB, et al: Age-related changes in serum immunoglobulins in patients with familial IgA deficiency and common variable immunodeficiency (CVID), *Clin Exp Immunol* 108:477-483, 1997.

47. French MA, Denis KA, Dawkins R, et al: Severity of infections in IgA deficiency: correlation with decreased serum antibodies to pneumococcal polysaccharides and decreased serum IgG2 and/or IgG4, *Clin Exp Immunol* 100:47, 1995.

48. Inoue T, Okubo H, Kudo J, et al: Selective IgA deficiency: analysis of Ig production in vitro, *J Clin Immunol* 4:235, 1984.

49. Schroeder HW: Genetics of IgA deficiency and common variable immunodeficiency, *Clin Rev Allergy Immunol* 19:127, 2000.

50. Braconier JH: Reversible total IgA deficiency associated with phenytoin treatment, *Scand J Infect Dis* 31:515, 1999.

51. Ferrante A, Beard LJ, Feldman RG: IgG subclass distribution of antibodies to bacterial and viral antigens, *Pediatr Inf Dis J* 9:S16, 1990.

52. Umetsu DT, Ambrosino DM, Quinti I, et al: Recurrent sinopulmonary infection and impaired antibody response to bacterial capsular polysaccharide antigen in children with selective IgG-subclass deficiency, *N Engl J Med* 313:1247, 1985.

53. Bartmann P, Grosch-Worner I, Wahn V, et al: IgG2 deficiency in children with human immunodeficiency virus infection, *Eur J Pediatr* 150:234, 1991.

54. Aucouturier P, Bremard-Oury C, Griscelli C, et al: Serum IgG subclass deficiency in ataxia telangiectasia, *Clin Exp Immunol* 68:392, 1987.

55. Ochs HD: The Wiskott-Aldrich syndrome, *Clin Rev Allergy Immunol* 20:61, 2001.

56. Kristinsson VH, Kristinsson JR, Jonmundsson GK, et al: Immunoglobulin class and subclass concentrations after treatment of childhood leukemia, *Pediatr Hematol Oncol* 18:167, 2001.

57. Terada T, Kaneko H, Fukao T, et al: Fate of the mutated IgG2 heavy chain: lack of expression of mutated membrane-bound IgG2 on the B cell surface in selective IgG2 deficiency, *Int Immunol* 13:249, 2001.

58. Karaman O, Uguz A, Uzuner N: IgG subclasses in wheezing infants, *Indian J Pediatr* 66:345, 1999.

59. May A, Zielen S, von Ilberg C, et al: Immunoglobulin deficiency and determination of pneumococcal antibody titers in patients with therapy-refractory recurrent rhinosinusitis, *Eur Arch Otorhinolaryngol* 256:445, 1999.

60. Ojuawo A, Milla PJ, Lindley KJ: Serum immunoglobulin and immunoglobulin G subclasses in children with allergic colitis, *West Afr J Med* 17:206, 1998.

61. Barlan IB, Geha RS, Schneider LC: Therapy for patients with recurrent infections and low serum IgG3 levels, *J Allergy Clin Immunol* 92:353, 1993.

62. Schur PH: IgG human subclasses: a review, *Ann Allergy* 58:89, 1987.

63. Antall PM, Meyerson H, Kaplan D, et al: Selective antipolysaccharide antibody deficiency associated with peripheral blood CD5+ B-cell predominance, *J Allergy Clin Immunol* 103:637, 1999.

64. Javier FC, III, Moore CM, Sorensen RU: Distribution of primary immunodeficiency diseases diagnosed in a pediatric tertiary hospital, *Ann Allergy Asthma Immunol* 84:25, 2000.

65. Kilic SS, Tezcan I, Sanal O, et al: Transient hypogammaglobulinemia of infancy: clinical and immunologic features of 40 new cases, *Pediatr Int* 42:647, 2000.

66. Inaba H, Hori H, Ito M, et al: Polio vaccine virus-associated meningoencephalitis in an infant with transient hypogammaglobulinemia, *Scand J Infect Dis* 33:630, 2001.

67. Siegal RL, Issekutz T, Schwaber J, et al: Deficiency of helper T cells in transient hypogammaglobulinemia of infancy, *N Engl J Med* 305:1307, 1981.

68. Dressler F, Peter HH, Muller W, et al: Transient hypogammaglobulinemia of infancy: five new cases, review of the literature and redefinition, *Acta Pediatr Scand* 78:767, 1989.

69. Bonilla FA, Geha RS: CD154 deficiency and related syndromes, *Immunol Allergy Clin North Am* 21:65, 2001.

70. Arakawa H, Hauschild J, Buerstedde JM: Requirement of the activation-induced deaminase (AID) gene for immunoglobulin gene conversion, *Science* 295:1301, 2002.

71. Ferrari S, Giliani S, Insalaco A, et al: Mutations of CD40 gene cause an autosomal recessive form of immunodeficiency with hyper IgM, *Proc Natl Acad Sci U S A* 98:12614, 2001.

72. Leinonen M, Sakkinen A, Kalliokoski R, et al: Antibody response to 14-valent pneumococcal capsular polysaccharide vaccine in pre-school age children, *Pediatr Infect Dis* 5:39, 1986.

73. Carneiro-Sampaio MM, Grumach AS, Manissadjian A: Laboratory screening for the diagnosis of children with primary immunodeficiencies, *J Invest Allergol Clin Immunol* 1:195, 1991.

74. De Diego JI, Prim MP, Alfonso C, et al: Comparison of amoxicillin and azithromycin in the prevention of recurrent acute otitis media, *Int J Pediatr Otorhinolaryngol* 58:47, 2001.

75. Roifman CM, Levison H, Gelfand EW: High-dose versus low-dose intravenous immunoglobulin in hypogammaglobulinaemia and chronic lung disease, *Lancet* 1:1075, 1987.

76. Quartier P, Debre M, De Blic J, et al: Early and prolonged intravenous immunoglobulin replacement therapy in childhood agammaglobulinemia: a retrospective survey of 31 patients, *J Pediatr* 134:589, 1999.

77. Eijkhout HW, van Der Meer JW, Kallenberg CG, et al: The effect of two different dosages of intravenous immunoglobulin on the incidence of recurrent infections in patients with primary hypogammaglobulinemia: a randomized, double-blind, multicenter crossover trial, *Ann Intern Med* 135:165, 2001.

78. Cunningham-Rundles C, Bodian C, Ochs HD, et al: Long-term low-dose IL-2 enhances immune function in common variable immunodeficiency, *Clin Immunol* 100:181, 2001.

79. Longhurst HJ, O'Grady C, Evans G, et al: Anti-D immunoglobulin treatment for thrombocytopenia associated with primary antibody deficiency, *J Clin Pathol* 55:64, 2002.

80. Smith KJ, Skelton H: Common variable immunodeficiency treated with a recombinant human IgG, tumour necrosis factor-alpha receptor fusion protein, *Br J Dermatol* 144:597, 2001.

81. Cunningham-Rundles C, Zhou Z, Mankarious S, et al: Long-term use of IgA-depleted intravenous immunoglobulin in immunodeficient subjects with anti-IgA antibodies, *J Clin Immunol* 13:272, 1993.

82. Sandler SG, Mallory D, Malamut D, et al: IgA anaphylactic transfusion reactions, *Transfus Med Rev* 9:1, 1995.

83. Limaye S, Walls RS, Riminton S: Safe and effective use of chromatographically purified intravenous immunoglobulin despite profound anti-IgA sensitization, *Intern Med J* 31:256, 2001.

84. de Albuquerque Campos R, Sato MN, da Silva Duarte AJ: IgG anti-IgA subclasses in common variable immunodeficiency and association with severe adverse reactions to intravenous immunoglobulin therapy, *J Clin Immunol* 20:77, 2000.

85. Chapel HM, Spickett GP, Ericson D, et al: The comparison of the efficacy and safety of intravenous versus subcutaneous immunoglobulin replacement therapy, *J Clin Immunol* 20:94, 2000.

CHAPTER 9

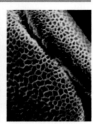

T Cell Immunodeficiencies

LUIGI D. NOTARANGELO

T lymphocytes are an essential component of adaptive immunity. Through cytolytic activity and release of Th1 cytokines (such as interferon [IFN]-γ) they mediate resistance to intracellular pathogens. In addition, interaction of T cells with B lymphocytes and antigen-presenting cells on the one hand, and release of soluble mediators such as interleukin (IL)-4 and IL-10 on the other, is essential in order to mount T-dependent antibody responses to soluble and particulate antigens, thus contributing to defense against extracellular pathogens. Consequently, severe defects in T cell development and/or function result in severe combined immunodeficiency (SCID) [syndrome], a heterogeneous group of disorders characterized by increased susceptibility to severe infections since early in life.[1] The overall frequency of these disorders is estimated to be 1 in 50,000 to 100,000 live births.

In addition, T lymphocytes play a crucial role in maintaining peripheral immune homeostasis. In keeping with this, it has been demonstrated that defects that do not severely compromise T cell development but impair T cell function in the periphery often result in immune dysregulation and autoimmunity. Because of the differences in clinical presentation, this chapter will discuss SCID and other congenital T cell disorders separately. For a more detailed discussion of some topics related to this issue (e.g., bone marrow transplantation, gene therapy) the reader is referred to Chapters 18 and 20, respectively.

SEVERE COMBINED IMMUNODEFICIENCY

Etiology

SCID includes a heterogeneous group of disorders that present with a distinct immunologic phenotype, and are caused by mutations of different genes (Table 9-1). The causes of SCID so far known in humans are discussed below.

X-Linked Severe Combined Immunodeficiency (SCIDX1, γ_c Deficiency)

SCIDX1 is the most common form of SCID in humans, with an estimated incidence of 1:150,000 live births. Inherited as an X-linked trait, in its typical form it is characterized by complete absence of both T and NK lymphocytes, with a preserved development of B lymphocytes (T⁻ B⁺ NK⁻ SCID). The disease is caused by mutations in the gene that encodes for the IL-2 receptor common gamma chain (IL-2Rγ_c, γ_c), located on the X-chromosome at Xq12-13.1.[2] The γ_c-chain is constitutively expressed by T, B, and NK cells, as well as myeloid cells and erythroblasts. γ_c, together with the IL-2R α and β subunits generates the high-affinity receptor for IL-2, which plays a major role in signal transduction through activation of its associated tyrosine kinase Janus kinase 3 (Jak-3).[3] Several studies have shown that γ_c is not only a member of the IL-2 receptor but also of the IL-4, IL-7, IL-9, IL-15, and IL-21 receptors. The SCID-X1 phenotype therefore appears to be the complex association of defects in all of these cytokine receptors' signaling pathways. In particular, lack of circulating T cells in SCIDX1 males is mainly caused by defective signaling through the IL-7R, as shown by targeting of the *IL7* and *IL7R* genes in mice,[4,5] and also by findings in infants with SCID caused by mutation of the IL-7Rα chain.[6] Furthermore, lack of circulating NK cells is likely the result of defective signaling through the IL-15R. Altogether, a variety of genetic defects in the *IL2RG* gene have been identified in SCIDX1.[7] Whereas in most cases defects in the *IL2RG* gene result in T⁻ B⁺ NK⁻ SCID, some mutations may impair, but do not completely abolish, cytokine-mediated signaling, possibly resulting in atypical presentations.

Jak-3 Deficiency

Jak-3 is a cytoplasmic tyrosine kinase that is associated with the γ_c in all of the γ_c-containing cytokine receptors, and mediates signaling through IL-2R, IL-4R, IL-7R, IL-9R, IL-15R, and IL-21R.[8] Jak-3 deficiency was first suspected as a possible cause of SCID after X-linked SCID patients were identified whose mutations of γ_c were demonstrated to result in impaired interaction between γ_c and Jak-3.[9] A series of patients affected with autosomal recessive T⁻ B⁺ SCID and mutations of Jak-3 were subsequently described.[10,11] Because γ_c and Jak-3 are physically and functionally associated, SCID caused by Jak-3 deficiency is clinically and immunologically undistinguishable from SCIDX1; however, it follows an autosomal recessive pattern of inheritance, the *Jak-3* gene being located on chromosome 19.

IL-7Rα Deficiency

IL-7Rα deficiency results in an autosomal recessive form of SCID characterized by selective absence of circulating T lymphocytes, with preserved development of B and NK cells (T⁻ B⁺ NK⁺ SCID).[6,12] IL-7 is produced by stromal cells in bone marrow and in the thymus. The IL-7 receptor consists of two subunits, the γ_c chain shared with the IL-2, -4, -9, -15 and

TABLE 9-1 Genetic and Immunologic Features of Combined Immune Deficiency

Disease	Gene	Inheritance	Circulating Lymphocytes T	B	NK
B⁻ SCID					
Reticular dysgenesis	?	AR	↓↓	↓↓	↓↓
RAG deficiency, T⁻ B⁻ SCID	*RAG1, RAG2*	AR	↓↓	↓↓	N
Omenn syndrome	*RAG1, RAG2*	AR	↓/N	↓↓	N/↑
Radiation-sensitive T⁻ B⁻ SCID	*Artemis*	AR	↓↓	↓↓	N
T⁻ B⁺ SCID					
X-linked SCID	*IL2RG*	XL	↓↓	N/↑	↓↓
Jak-3 deficiency	*Jak-3*	AR	↓↓	N/↑	↓↓
IL-7R deficiency	*IL7RA*	AR	↓↓	N/↑	N
CD45 deficiency	*CD45*	AR	↓↓	↑	↓
Purine metabolism deficiency					
Adenosine deaminase deficiency	*ADA*	AR	↓↓	↓	↓
Nucleoside phosphorylase deficiency	*PNP*	AR	↓↓	↓/N	↓/N
ZAP-70 deficiency	*ZAP70*	AR	↓(↓↓ CD8)	N	N
CD25 deficiency	*IL2RA*	AR	↓	N	N
CD3 deficiency					
CD3γ deficiency	*CD3G*	AR	N (↓ CD3)	N	N
CD3ε deficiency	*CD3E*	AR	N (↓ CD3)	N	N
T cell activation defects	?	AR	N	N	N
Multiple cytokine defects	?	AR (?)	N	N	N
Human nude phenotype	*Whn*	AR	↓↓	N	N
TAP deficiency	*TAP1, TAP2*	AR	↓(↓↓ CD8)	N	N
MHC class II deficiency	*CIITA, RFXANK, RFX5, RFXAP*	AR	↓(↓↓ CD4)	N	N
X-linked hyper-IgM syndrome	*CD40L (TNFS5)*	XL	N	N	N
ID + multiple intestinal atresia	?	AR (?)	↓	↓	N

T, T lymphocytes; *B*, B lymphocytes; *NK*, natural killer lymphocytes; *AR*, autosomal recessive; *XL*, X-linked; *N*, normal.

-21 receptors (see SCID-X1) and the α chain, which is specific for IL-7R. The IL-7 receptor is expressed by lymphoid precursor cells, including a fraction of marrow CD34+ cells. IL-7 provides survival and proliferative signals to IL-7R+ cells. Consequently, mutations that impair expression of IL-7R result in an early block in T cell development. Moreover, signaling through IL-7R is not essential in humans for B cell development, whereas it is essential in mice.[4]

CD45 Deficiency

Two unrelated patients have been reported in whom SCID was caused by the complete absence of the CD45 protein, a phosphatase that modulates signaling through the TCR/CD3 complex.[13,14] The immunologic phenotype is characterized by complete lack of T cells, with normal to increased B cell counts.

T⁻ B⁻ SCID Caused by Defective VDJ Recombination

B and T lymphocytes recognize foreign antigen through specialized receptors: the immunoglobulin (Ig) and the T cell receptor (TCR), respectively. The highly polymorphic antigen-recognition regions of these receptors are composed of variable/diverse/joining (VDJ) gene segments that undergo somatic rearrangement prior to their expression by a mechanism known as VDJ recombination.[15] The process of VDJ recombination is initiated when the lymphoid-specific recombinase activating gene 1 (RAG1) and RAG2 proteins recognize specific recombination signal sequences (RSS) that flank each of the V, D, and J gene elements, and introduce a DNA double-strand break in this region.[16,17] Subsequently, a variety of

ubiquitously expressed proteins (including Ku70, Ku80, DNA-PKcs, XRCC4, DNA ligase IV, and Artemis) involved in recognition and repair of DNA damage mediate the final steps of the VDJ recombination process.

In humans, the second most common phenotype of SCID (after T⁻ B⁺ SCID) is characterized by a complete absence of both T and B lymphocytes in the periphery.[18] A subgroup of these patients have a defect in VDJ recombination. These patients can be further divided into two subgroups according to their cellular response *in vitro* to ionizing radiations. The first group of patients is defective in the early steps of VDJ recombination, and does not exhibit an increased radiosensitivity. These patients carry severe mutations in either the *RAG1* or the *RAG2* genes.[19] In contrast, the second subgroup of patients shows increased cellular radiosensitivity and is mutated in the recently cloned *Artemis* gene, which participates in the later phases of VDJ recombination.[20] This latter form of T⁻ B⁻ SCID is more common among Athabascan-speaking Native Americans, with an estimated incidence of approximately 1 in 2000 live births.

Omenn's Syndrome

Omenn's syndrome (OS) is a SCID that affects infants of both sexes who present with generalized exudative erythroderma, enlarged lymph nodes, hepatosplenomegaly, severe respiratory infections, diarrhea, failure to thrive, hypoproteinemia with edema, and eosinophilia[21] (Figure 9-1). This clinical phenotype may mimic histiocytosis or graft-versus-host disease, and may in fact occasionally be seen in SCID infants with transplacental passage of alloreactive maternal T cells.

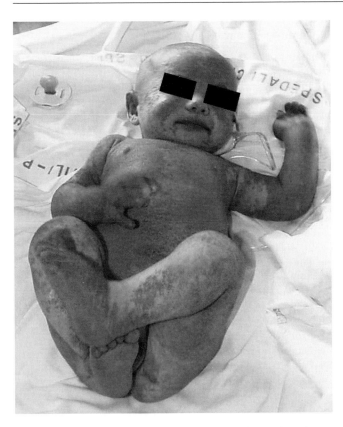

FIGURE 9-1 Typical clinical features in an infant with Omenn's syndrome. Note generalized erythrodermia with scaly skin, alopecia, and oedema.

Although the latter condition is also referred to as *Omenn's-like syndrome,* the term *Omenn's syndrome* is reserved for cases in which presence of alloreactive T cells has been ruled out.

The molecular pathogenesis of OS has long remained obscure. However, the demonstration of oligoclonal, activated T cells in OS infants and the simultaneous occurrence of OS and of T⁻ B⁻ SCID in two siblings[22] suggest that OS may be genetically related to T⁻ B⁻ SCID and may reflect defective T and B lymphocyte differentiation. This hypothesis was proved when mutations in *RAG1* and *RAG2* genes were demonstrated in OS patients.[23] Although the disease follows an autosomal recessive pattern of inheritance, each patient carries at least one mutant allele that allows for partial RAG protein expression and function.[24] This results in a leaky VDJ rearrangement defect and permits some intrathymic T cell differentiation, with generation of oligoclonal T cells that undergo peripheral expansion, possibly in response to autoantigens.

SCID Caused by Adenosine Deaminase Deficiency

Adenosine deaminase (ADA) is a ubiquitously expressed enzyme that mediates conversion of adenosine into inosine, and of deoxyadenosine into deoxyinosine. The *ADA* gene maps to chromosome 20. Deficiency of ADA, inherited as an autosomal recessive trait, results in intracellular accumulation of deoxyadenosine and of its phosphorylated metabolites, among which dATP is particularly toxic to lymphoid precursors.[25] Consequently, patients with complete ADA deficiency are affected by T⁻ B⁻ SCID. Partial defects of the enzyme may result in less severe clinical presentation (delayed or late-onset forms) that may even present in adulthood.[26] *In vitro* expres-

sion studies of the mutant alleles in *Escherichia coli* have enabled the recognition that these different degrees of clinical severity correspond to variability of residual enzymatic activity.[27]

Nucleoside Phosphorylase Deficiency

Purine nucleoside phosphorylase (PNP) is another purine metabolism enzyme that converts guanosine into guanine and deoxyguanosine to deoxyguanine. The *PNP* gene maps to chromosome 20. Deficiency of PNP activity, inherited as an autosomal recessive trait, results in accumulation of phosphorylated deoxyguanosine metabolites (and of dGTP in particular) that inhibit ribonucleotide reductase, whose activity is essential to DNA synthesis. Although PNP is widely expressed, its deficiency is particularly deleterious to lymphoid development, and especially to T cell generation. Consequently, patients with PNP deficiency experience a dramatic and progressive T cell lymphopenia during the first years of life, thus accounting for the SCID phenotype.[28]

SCID Caused by ZAP-70 Deficiency

ZAP-70 is an intracellular tyrosine kinase that is required for T cell activation following engagement of the CD3/T cell receptor (CD3/TCR) complex. Stimulation of T cells through TCR results in activation of the p56lck kinase, which mediates tyrosine phosphorylation of immunoreceptor tyrosine–based activation motifs (ITAMs) in the CD3-γ, -δ, -ε, and -ζ chains. ZAP-70 is then recruited into the CD3/TCR complex through binding of its SH2 domains to phosphorylated ITAM motifs of the ζ chain.[29] ZAP-70 itself then becomes phosphorylated by Src-family protein tyrosine kinases, and this phosphorylation triggers ZAP-70 activation, allowing phosphorylation of downstream signaling molecules such as linker for activation of T cells (LATs) and SLP-76.[30]

Defects in ZAP-70 are inherited as an autosomal recessive trait, and result in impaired T cell development and function.[31-33] In fact, in humans ZAP-70 is required for development of single positive CD8+ T cells in the thymus; moreover, a normal ZAP-70 functional activity is necessary in order for peripheral blood T cells to proliferate normally in response to mitogens and antigens. Consequently, infants with ZAP-70 deficiency present with typical clinical features of SCID and a peculiar immunologic phenotype with virtual absence of CD8+ T cells and nonfunctional CD4+ T lymphocytes.

p56lck Deficiency

p56lck in a src-tyrosine kinase that is critically involved in TCR-mediated signaling, contributing to phosphorylation of the ITAM motifs of the proteins of the CD3/TCR complex. Defective expression of p56lck has been found in a SCID infant, whose immunologic phenotype consisted of panhypogammaglobulinemia, lymphopenia with a reduced proportion of CD4+ T cells, and reduced *in vitro* proliferative responses to CD3 cross-linking.[34]

Reticular Dysgenesis

This rare form of SCID is characterized by a combined defect in lymphoid and myeloid differentiation.[35] Autosomal recessive inheritance is presumed. It is not clear whether some forms of SCID with neutropenia truly represent a unique syndrome or whether, in some cases, the block in hematopoiesis could be secondary to persistent viral infections or to deleterious effects of maternally derived T cells on the bone marrow.

MHC Class II Deficiency

Although this is not strictly a T cell deficiency (the defect lying in the inability of thymic epithelial cells and antigen-presenting cells to express major histocompatibility complex (MHC) class II molecules), it is included in this chapter because it results in profound abnormalities in T cell development and function. In fact, MHC class II molecules are crucial for numerous aspects of immune function, including antibody production, T cell–mediated immunity, induction of tolerance, and inflammatory responses. The primary basis for the immunodeficiency resides in the inability of T cells to recognize antigens in the context of self-MHC class II molecules expressed by antigen-presenting cells.

MHC class II deficiency has an autosomal recessive pattern of inheritance. The disease is not caused by mutations in the genes that encode MHC class II molecules, but rather in transcription factors that control MHC class II gene expression.[36] Genetic heterogeneity within MHC class II deficiency was demonstrated by means of somatic cell fusion studies. Four complementation groups (A, B, C, and D) of patients have been identified. The genes responsible for each of these complementation groups have been recently identified. In particular, mutations of the Class II transactivator (CIITA) account for complementation group A, whereas RFXANK/RFX-B, RFX5, and RFXAP (the three components of the RFX transcription factor) are mutated in complementation groups B, C, and D, respectively.[37-39] At variance with RFX (which is a true DNA-binding multimolecular complex), CIITA does not bind DNA, but rather interacts with other factors on the MHC class II promoter, as well as with the transcriptional machinery, to drive transcription of MHC class II genes. CIITA expression correlates directly with MHC class II expression and is regulated by IFN-γ, a cytokine known to increase expression of MHC class II molecules. Thus, CIITA acts as a molecular switch for MHC class II regulation.

Differential Diagnosis of SCID

All forms of SCID are characterized by typical clinical signs (Box 9-1), consisting of early-onset severe infections (interstitial pneumonia, chronic diarrhea, persistent candidiasis), that lead to growth failure[18,40] (Figure 9-2). Infections are sustained by bacteria, viruses, and fungi. Demonstration that the infection is sustained by an opportunistic pathogen (*Pneumocystis*

BOX 9-1

KEY CONCEPTS

Clinical and Laboratory Elements in the Diagnosis of SCID

Clinical Features
- Positive family history (X-linked, parental consanguinity)
- Presentation early in life (within the first 4-6 months of age)
- Severe respiratory infections (interstitial pneumonia)
- Protracted diarrhea
- Failure to thrive
- Persistent candidiasis (oral thrush)
- Skin rash, erythrodermia

Laboratory Elements
- Lymphopenia (ALC: <2000/μL)
- Reduced number (>1500/μL) of circulating CD3+ T cells
- Very low to undetectable levels of serum immunoglobulins*
- Very low to absent *in vitro* proliferative response to mitogens

---

SCID, Severe combined immunodeficiency [syndrome].
*IgG serum levels may initially be normal because of transplacental passage of maternal IgG.

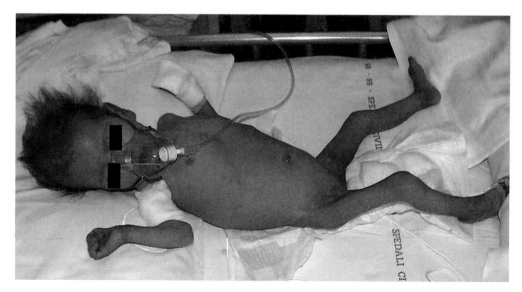

FIGURE 9-2 Typical appearance of an infant with severe combined immunodeficiency (SCID) [syndrome]. Note severe growth failure and respiratory distress.

carinii, cytomegalovirus) should immediately raise the suspicion of SCID. Skin manifestations are also common (rash, generalized erythroderma, alopecia). These may reflect the presence of autoreactive T cell clones (such as in OS), or may represent manifestations of a true graft-versus-host disease (GVHD) caused by transplacental passage of alloreactive maternal T lymphocytes. Maternal T cell engraftment is a common finding in SCID (it involves up to 50% of all cases), but is only observed in those forms of SCID with complete lack of T cell immunity (such as γ_c deficiency, Jak-3 deficiency, RAG, or *Artemis* gene defects).[41] No cases of maternal T cell engraftment have been reported in infants with residual T cell immunity, such as adenosine deaminase deficiency, MHC class II deficiency, or ZAP-70 defect. Most often asymptomatic, transplacental passage of maternal T lymphocytes may occasionally result in clinical signs of GVHD other than skin manifestations alone: an increase of liver enzymes with hepatomegaly, anemia, thrombocytopenia and leukopenia (as the result of bone marrow aggression), and eosinophilia.[41]

Some forms of SCID may present with additional typical clinical and laboratory features. Adenosine deaminase deficiency is often characterized by cupping and flaring of the ribs and by liver dysfunction that in most cases is caused by accumulation of toxic metabolites in the liver, and not by infections.[42] In addition, the clinical onset of PNP deficiency is often marked by autoimmune hemolytic anemia; furthermore, progressive and severe neurodegeneration, with regression of psychomotor skills, is typically observed in this disease.[43]

Because infections mark the clinical onset of SCID, the differential diagnosis should be focused to consider alternative causes of severe infections. Congenital heart disease, pulmonary defects, cystic fibrosis, and secondary immune deficiencies (such as perinatal HIV infection) should be included in the differential diagnosis. However, it is important to remember that SCID is a medical emergency. Because of this, all infants with a possible diagnosis of SCID need to be carefully and rapidly evaluated by means of appropriate laboratory assays (see Box 9-1 and below).

Infants with SCID may also present as "red babies," with generalized erythroderma (caused by transplacental passage of maternal T cells or by OS). The differential diagnosis in this case includes severe allergy, various forms of ichthyosis, IPEX (*immune dysregulation, polyendocrinopathy, enteropathy, X-linked*), a recently identified X-linked disorder with immune dysregulation,[44] and Netherton's syndrome. In the latter, hair shaft anomalies are frequently observed. More than a skin biopsy, demonstration of typical immunologic abnormalities will most often lead to a correct diagnosis of immune deficiency.

Finally, SCID disorders are inherited; therefore, in the general approach to infants with possible SCID it is important to collect adequate information on the family history. The most common form of SCID, SCIDX1, is inherited as an X-linked trait; consequently, it is important to pay attention to other putatively affected males along the maternal side. However, even for SCIDX1 a substantial proportion of cases represent sporadic presentation. All other forms of SCID are autosomal recessive. In these forms, affected infants would belong to the same sibship; furthermore, parental consanguinity is a common finding.

Evaluation and Management

A correct diagnosis of SCID should be established as soon as possible in order to offer an optimal perspective on treatment. The most rapid tool to consolidate the diagnosis of SCID is represented by accurate evaluation of a complete WBC count; lymphopenia is observed in most SCID infants.[45] Importantly, in normal infants the lymphocyte count tends to be high (2000 to 10,000 cells/μL) as compared to later periods in life; thus, values below 2000 lymphocytes/μL have been proposed to identify at birth infants at risk of SCID.[45] In spite of this concept, a proportion of SCID infants are not lymphopenic. This may reflect the presence of a reasonable number of autologous lymphocytes (as observed in OS, MHC class II deficiency, ZAP-70 deficiency) or the transplacental passage of maternal T cells. Consequently, and regardless of the total lymphocyte count, all infants with a putative diagnosis of SCID should be evaluated for the distribution of lymphocyte subsets by flow cytometry (see Box 9-1). This should include characterization and enumeration of total (CD3+) T lymphocytes, CD4+ and CD8+ T cell subsets, B (CD19+) lymphocytes, and NK (CD16+) cells, as well as analysis of MHC class II molecule expression on the surface of B lymphocytes and monocytes. In most cases, such a panel of immunophenotyping will reveal the diagnosis of SCID, and also orient towards specific gene defects. More subtle analysis may then be applied to selected cases. For instance, differential diagnosis between a γ_c or a Jak-3 defect in a male infant with T$^-$ B$^+$ NK$^-$ SCID may often be resolved by analyzing γ_c expression on the surface of lymphocytes by flow cytometry.[46] However, even investigation of lymphocyte subpopulations may not lead to a final diagnosis in selected cases, such as SCID with maternal T cell engraftment or atypical presentations of SCID. In such instances, should the clinical signs strongly suggest a possible diagnosis of SCID, the infant ought to be evaluated by means of functional assays, such as *in vitro* proliferation to mitogens. Low or undetectable levels of IgA and IgG may support the diagnosis of SCID; however, IgG serum levels may initially be normal because of transplacental passage of maternally derived antibodies.

Extreme lymphopenia associated with difficulty in phenotyping the few circulating lymphoid cells is often observed in ADA deficiency. For a final diagnosis of ADA and PNP deficiency, measurement of enzymatic ADA and PNP activity in red cells is required. Determination of plasma levels of toxic phosphorylated metabolites of adenosine (dAXP) may help in the diagnosis. Importantly, whenever ADA or PNP deficiencies are suspected, use of red cell transfusions should be delayed, if possible, until determination of enzymatic activity has been performed.

Ultimately, now that the genes responsible for most forms of SCID have been identified, mutation analysis represents an important diagnostic tool.[47] All infants with a probable diagnosis of SCID should be evaluated for specific gene defects (see Table 9-1), as this may not only allow definitive diagnosis but also provides important information for accurate genetic counseling and possible future prenatal diagnosis in the family. However, it is important to emphasize that the diagnosis of SCID should not be based strictly on demonstration of a specific gene defect, as this would often require too much time. In contrast, careful evaluation of clinical and laboratory (hematology/immunology) data is sufficient to pose a diagnosis of SCID, and so to immediately initiate the procedures for definitive treatment.

The main therapeutic strategies for SCID are illustrated in Box 9-2. Optimal treatment of SCID is based on bone marrow transplantation (BMT). Transplantation from an HLA-identical family donor can cure > 90% of infants with SCID, and excellent results have also been obtained with transplantation from haploidentical family donors or matched unrelated donors.[48,49] Among these options, HLA-haploidentical transplantation is more commonly used, because of the emergency to treat the patients. In this group of infants, factors influencing survival include the presence of lung infection prior to BMT and the immunologic phenotype of SCID (B⁺ SCID being associated with a more favorable outcome than B⁻ SCID).[50]

These data emphasize the need to protect SCID infants from infections, and offer a rationale for the use of BMT in the neonatal period or even prenatally. Indeed, recent data indicate that hematopoietic stem cell transplantation for SCID leads to superior thymic function and improved survival, if performed early after birth.[45] Furthermore, there have been a few reports that *in utero* transplantation of hematopoietic stem cells from a haploidentical parent can cure fetuses in whom the diagnosis of SCID was established prenatally.[51-53]

Importantly, all infants with a tentative diagnosis of SCID need to receive adequate protection against infection, even while the laboratory work-up is in progress. Prophylactic trimethoprim-sulfametoxazole is effective in preventing *P. carinii* pneumonia (PCP); moreover, intravenous immunoglobulin, regardless of serum IgG levels, should be given to SCID infants. While waiting for BMT, isolation of affected infants in a protected environment and supportive treatment with parenteral nutrition and transfusions may also improve the health status of affected children. However, all blood products need to be irradiated because alloreactive T cells contained in the transfusion would invariably cause rapidly fatal GVHD.[18]

Alternative therapeutic approaches are available in selected cases. Patients affected with ADA deficiency may be treated with weekly intramuscular injections of polyethylene glycole-conjugated ADA (PEG-ADA). In most cases, this treatment results in complete immune reconstitution.[54]

Gene therapy has originally been attempted, with limited success, for ADA deficiency.[55-57] In contrast, very promising results have been recently achieved following transduction of CD34+ hematopoietic stem cells from SCIDX1 infants with a retroviral vector containing the γ_c cDNA.[58]

Originally described in 1965, DiGeorge syndrome (DGS) is a developmental anomaly characterized by thymic hypoplasia, hypoparathyroidism with consequent hypocalcemia, congenital heart disease, and facial dysmorphism.[59] These defects may be variably associated within a spectrum of manifestations that is also referred to as *CATCH22* (*C*ardiac defect, *A*bnormal facies, *T*hymic hypoplasia, *C*left palate, *H*ypocalcemia, chromosome *22*). The vast majority (> 90%) of patients have a partial monosomy of chromosome 22 (haploinsufficiency for the 22q11 region). Only a minority of patients exhibit significant immunologic abnormalities, and only a few of them have a severe T cell defect (so-called complete DiGeorge syndrome). Recent data from gene-targeted mice indicate that haploinsufficiency of the *TBX1* gene, which encodes for a transcription factor, accounts for the heart defect, but the pathogenesis of the thymic defect is still unclear.[60]

Typical cases of DGS should be suspected early after birth because of the association of heart defect (especially interrupted aortic arch type B or truncus arteriosus) with hypocalcemic seizures. Micrognathia, hypertelorism, antimongoloid slant of the eyes, and ear malformation are also common (Figure 9-3). Although these patients show increased susceptibility to infections, immune deficiency is rarely a serious problem. However, persistent candidiasis, chronic diarrhea, and PCP are indicators of a severe thymic defect and require prompt investigation of the immune system, with enumeration of lymphocyte subsets and assessment of *in vitro* proliferative response to mitogens. Dysregulation of thymic function may also result in progressive development of autoimmune manifestations. Infants with these features, even if present only in part, need to be investigated for possible monosomy of the 22q11 region by fluorescent *in situ* hybridization (F.I.S.H.).

Always consider an infant with putative SCID as a medical emergency.

Treat any infections promptly and aggressively.

Take into account the high frequency of *Pneumocystis carinii* pneumonia (PCP). Take appropriate measures to evaluate this possibility (chest x-ray, bronchoalveolar lavage). If PCP is suspected or proven, use trimethoprim-sulfamethoxazole (20 mg/kg/d IV).

If growth failure is present, start parenteral nutrition.

Start prophylaxis of PCP with trimethoprim-sulfamethoxazole (5 mg/kg/d).

Start prophylaxis of fungal infections with fluconazole (5 mg/kg/d).

Give intravenous immunoglobulins regularly (400 mg/kg/21 days).

Isolate the infant in a protected environment (laminar-flow unit).

Always irradiate blood products, if transfusions are necessary.

Avoid administration of live-attenuated vaccines.

Immediately plan for a bone marrow transplantation once the diagnosis of SCID has been established.

SCID, Severe combined immunodeficiency [syndrome].

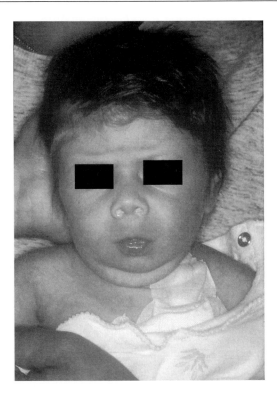

FIGURE 9-3 Facial dysmorphic features in an infant with DiGeorge syndrome. Note hypertelorism, enlarged nasal root, anteroverted nostrils, low-set ears, and micrognathia.

Management and Treatment

Heart defects are the most severe manifestation of the disease, and should be treated aggressively if necessary. Hypocalcemia requires supplementation with calcium and vitamin D; however, in most cases seizures do not recur beyond the neonatal period. If a significant immune defect is present, PCP prophylaxis with trimethoprim-sulfamethoxazole is indicated. Use of live-attenuated vaccines is contraindicated, but intravenous immunoglobulins are often used to prevent infections. Complete DGS may occasionally mimic SCID, with extreme lymphopenia and virtual absence of circulating T cells. These infants may show delayed appearance of T cells that, however, are oligoclonal, activated, and poorly functioning.[61] Thymic transplantation can be corrective in such cases.[62] Alternatively, unmanipulated bone marrow transplantation from HLA-identical donors can be attempted, with the hope that expansion of post-thymic precursors contained in the graft may lead to immune reconstitution.

OTHER T CELL DEFICIENCIES

Immunodeficiency Caused by TAP Deficiency

HLA class I molecules are polymorphic cell surface glycoproteins that play an essential role in presenting antigenic peptides to cytotoxic T lymphocytes, and in modulating the activity of natural killer (NK) cells that bear HLA class I–binding receptors. HLA class I molecules are composed of a polymorphic heavy chain, encoded by HLA-A, -B, and -C genes, associated with β2-microglobulin (β2M). The assembly of HLA class I molecules occurs in the lumen of the endoplasmic reticulum (ER), where they are loaded with peptides derived from the degradation of intracellular organisms. These peptides are transported into the ER via *t*ransporter associated with *a*ntigen *p*resentation (TAP) proteins.[63] TAP consists of two structurally related subunits (TAP1 and TAP2), which interact to form a functional peptide transporter system. Defects in either TAP1 or TAP2 protein result in impaired peptide-HLA class I/β2M complex formation and eventually lead to reduced surface expression of HLA class I molecules.

Overall, nine patients, from seven unrelated families, have been reported with defective HLA class I molecule expression caused by a defect in either TAP1[64,65] or TAP2.[66,67] The clinical phenotype associated with TAP deficiency is far less severe than that observed in MHC class II expression, and mainly consists of recurrent sinopulmonary infections and deep skin ulcers that require treatment with antibiotics and chest physiotherapy.

IL-2Rα (CD25) Deficiency

Deficiency of the α chain of the IL-2 receptor (IL-2Rα, CD25) has been reported in a single patient who presented with early-onset severe and recurrent viral and bacterial infections, oral thrush, and chronic diarrhea. In addition, the child developed signs of lymphoproliferative disease (lymphadenopathy, hepatosplenomegaly), reflecting the role of IL-2–mediated signaling in maintaining peripheral immune homeostasis. Mild lymphopenia, with reduced CD4+ T cell counts, and low *in vitro* proliferative response to mitogens were the main immunologic hallmarks. A thymic biopsy revealed poor cortex/medulla demarcation.[68] The infant was successfully treated with BMT.

CD3 Deficiency

Four patients from three families have been described with immune deficiency related to low expression of the CD3/TCR complex.[69] The clinical manifestations were variable, ranging from complete lack of symptoms to a SCID phenotype (with failure to thrive, pneumonia, chronic diarrhea) to autoimmunity. In all cases, lymphocyte counts were normal, but the density of CD3 molecules at the surface of T cells was reduced (10% to 50% of normal), and *in vitro* proliferative responses to CD3 cross-linking were diminished. Mutations in either the CD3γ- or the CD3ε-encoding genes have been documented.

Human "Nude" Phenotype (*Whn* Defect)

In two siblings a severe T cell immunodeficiency with complete lack of CD8+ T cells was found in association with alopecia.[70] The disease is caused by mutation of the winged-helix-nude *(whn)* gene, whose abnormality accounts for the SCID nude phenotype in mice. *Whn* encodes for a transcription factor that is critical for maturation of the thymic microenvironment. Although thymic transplantation should be the treatment of choice in this disease, HLA-identical bone marrow transplantation in one of the siblings resulted in marked clinical improvement, most likely through maturation and expansion of post-thymic precursors contained in the inoculum.[71]

Combined Immunodeficiency with Multiple Intestinal Atresias

The association of combined immune deficiency with multiple gastrointestinal atresia has been observed in two families.[72,73] The molecular cause of this disease, with a presumed autosomal recessive inheritance, remains unknown.

T Cell Transduction Defects

Some patients have been described, in whom T cells were present in normal numbers, but who were impaired in their proliferative response to CD3 cross-linking or to mitogens. Use of calcium ionophore resulted in normal proliferation, suggesting a proximal defect in TCR-mediated signaling. Most of these patients showed defective antibody responses. In some cases, the signal transduction defect also involved other cell types and was associated with myopathy.[74]

Cytokine Deficiencies

Functional T cell immunodeficiency and hypogammaglobulinemia may also be associated with abnormal cytokine production. In these patients the number and distribution of T cell subsets are normal; however, proliferative response to mitogens is defective, but is normalized following addition of exogenous IL-2. A defect in IL-2 production has been reported.[75] In one case defective production of IL-4, IL-5, and IFN-γ was also present, and was caused by abnormal binding of the NF-AT transcriptional complex to the promoter of cytokine genes.[76]

Cartilage Hair Hypoplasia

Cartilage hair hypoplasia (CHH) is an autosomal recessive disease, in which metaphyseal dysplasia is associated with immune deficiency of variable degree. Short-limbed dwarfism and sparse hair are typical clinical features. The immune deficiency most often involves the T cell compartment; the majority of patients have a limited susceptibility to bacterial and viral infections, but some may present with severe infections and may die early in life. These patients are lymphopenic, and show reduced number and function of T lymphocytes; in such cases, BMT is indicated. The molecular defect has been recently identified in the *RMRP* gene, which encodes for an RNA species with presumed ribozyme activity.[77]

SYNDROMES WITH SIGNIFICANT T CELL DEFICIENCY

Ataxia-Telangiectasia, Nijmegen Breakage Syndromes, and Related Disorders of DNA Repair Etiology

Ataxia-telangiectasia (AT) is an autosomal recessive disorder characterized by telangiectasia, progressive ataxia, recurrent respiratory tract infections, and an increased susceptibility to tumors (leukemia, lymphoma, dysgerminoma, and gonadoblastoma).[78] Cells derived from AT patients show an increased sensitivity to ionizing radiation. The disease is caused by mutations of the *ATM* gene, which maps at 11q22-23. This gene encodes for a large protein that participates in the repair

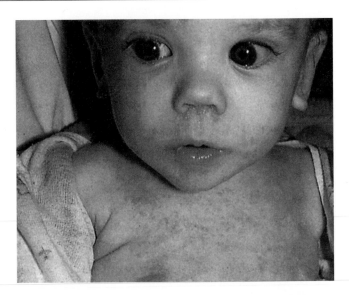

FIGURE 9-4 Child with Wiskott-Aldrich syndrome. The skin eruptions on the trunk and face are eczematoid and pruritic, but not always similar to atopic dermatitis in flexural distribution. Many of these patients have thrombocytopenia, which results in petechiae of varying distribution and intensity. (From Fireman P, Slavin RG: *Atlas of allergies*, ed 2, London, 1996, Mosby-Wolfe.)

of DNA breakage and controls cell cycle and cellular apoptosis.[79]

Nijmegen breakage syndrome (NBS) is characterized by microcephaly, growth retardation, bird-like facies, increased susceptibility to infections, and higher occurrence of tumors. Inherited as an autosomal recessive trait, the disease is caused by mutations of the *NBS1* gene, which encodes for nibrin, another protein involved in DNA repair.[80]

More recently, a subgroup of patients with an AT-like disorder have been identified in whom the defect was in the *hMRE11* gene, which encodes for another component of the DNA repair machinery that associates with nibrin.[81]

Differential Diagnosis

Although these disorders share similar findings (increased susceptibility to infections, higher risk of tumors), they also present typical features that permit differential diagnosis. Ocular telangiectasias and progressive ataxia are early signs of AT, and usually occur within the first few years of life. Confirmation of the diagnosis is provided by the demonstration of increased serum levels of alpha-fetoprotein (AFP) and by the presence of reciprocal chromosomal translocations (mostly involving chromosomes 7 and 14) in lymphocytes. In contrast, patients affected with NBS do not develop telangiectasias or ataxia, and show normal AFP levels; however, they also present chromosomal translocations.[78]

In all these disorders immune deficiency is marked by recurrent sinopulmonary infections that are sustained by bacteria or viruses. However, unlike patients with SCID, patients with AT, AT-like disease, or NBS do not develop opportunistic infections. Laboratory investigations show progressive reduction of the T cell number (particularly the CD4+ subset), with impaired *in vitro* proliferative response to mitogens. IgA deficiency is common and is often associated with low/undetectable IgG2 and IgG4. These defects are more severe in AT than in NBS.[78]

Management and Treatment

At present, there is no definitive cure for these disorders. Use of prophylactic antibiotics, chest physiotherapy, and administration of intravenous immunoglobulins may decrease the risk of infections. Careful monitoring of the clinical conditions may allow early recognition of tumors. However, in spite of these measures, the prognosis remains poor, particularly in AT patients, and infections and tumors are the main causes of death.[78]

WISKOTT-ALDRICH SYNDROME

Etiology

Wiskott-Aldrich syndrome (WAS) is an X-linked disorder characterized by eczema, congenital thrombocytopenia with small-sized platelets, and immune deficiency. The responsible gene, named *WASP*, maps at Xp11.2 and encodes for a protein involved in cytoskeleton reorganization in hematopoietic cells.[82] Most patients with typical WAS have mutations that impair expression and/or function of the WASP protein. However, some missense mutations are associated with a milder phenotype (isolated X-linked thrombocytopenia, XLT) (Figure 9-4).

Differential Diagnosis

The diagnosis of WAS is relatively simple, if all elements of the triad (eczema, thrombocytopenia, and immune deficiency) are present; however, this happens only in one third of the cases. An important and consistent element in the differential diagnosis of WAS/XLT versus other forms of congenital thrombocytopenia simple forms of allergy, or other causes of recurrent infections is represented by the demonstration of reduced mean platelet volume.

The immune deficiency of WAS may manifest as recurrent bacterial and viral infections, autoimmune manifestations, and increased occurrence of tumors (leukemia, lymphoma). Immunologic laboratory abnormalities include progressive decline of T cell numbers and function, reduced serum IgM with increased levels of IgA and IgE, and inability to mount effective antibody responses to T-independent antigens.[82]

Management and Treatment

The only curative approach to WAS is represented by bone marrow transplantation, which gives optimal results only if performed from HLA-identical family donors or early in life from matched unrelated donors.[83,84] Administration of intravenous immunoglobulins, regular antibiotic prophylaxis, topical steroids to control eczema, and use of more vigorous immune suppression for autoimmunity are the hallmarks of conservative treatment. Splenectomy may be indicated in case of severe and refractory thrombocytopenia; however, it carries the risk of overwhelming sepsis.

X-LINKED HYPER-IgM SYNDROME (HIGM1, CD40 LIGAND DEFICIENCY)

Etiology

CD40 ligand (CD40L, CD154) is a cell-surface molecule predominantly expressed by activated CD4+ T lymphocytes. Interaction of CD40L with its counter-receptor CD40 (expressed by B and dendritic cells, macrophages, endothelial cells, and some epithelial cells) is essential for germinal center formation, terminal differential of B lymphocytes, and effective defense against intracellular pathogens. Mutations in the *CD40L (TNFSF5)* gene, mapping at Xq26, result in X-linked hyper-IgM syndrome (HIGM1), characterized by an increased occurrence of bacterial and opportunistic infections, chronic diarrhea (often sustained by *Cryptosporidium*), liver/biliary tract disease, and susceptibility to liver and gut tumors.[85]

Differential Diagnosis

Presentation early in life with opportunistic infections (PCP) requires differential diagnosis with SCID and other forms of severe T cell defects. The typical immunoglobulin profile (undetectable or very low serum IgG and IgA, with normal to increased IgM) may also be observed in common variable immunodeficiency or in autosomal recessive hyper-IgM caused by defects in the *AID* or in the *CD40* genes. Neutropenia is a common finding. The diagnosis of HIGM1 is made based on demonstration of defective expression of CD40L (but not of other activation markers) on the surface of T cells following *in vitro* activation, and is eventually confirmed by mutation analysis.[85]

Management and Treatment

Treatment is based on regular use of intravenous immunoglobulins, prophylactic trimethoprim-sulfamethoxazole, and use of sterile/filtered water to prevent *Cryptosporidium* infection. Monitoring of liver/biliary tract morphology and function by ultrasound scanning, measurement of appropriate laboratory parameters of liver and biliary tract function, and, when indicated, liver biopsy is also advised. Severe neutropenia may be treated with recombinant granulocyte colony-stimulating factor (G-CSF). In spite of these measures, the long-term prognosis is poor because of severe infections and liver disease. For these reasons bone marrow transplantation has been indicated and has proven effective.[86] Use of non-myeloablative regimens may reduce the risk of drug-related toxicity.[87] Combined bone marrow and liver transplantation has been successfully used in patients with terminal liver disease caused by sclerosing cholangitis.[88]

Irrespective of the specific definitive diagnosis, all forms of T cell immunodeficiencies are characterized by significant morbidity and some of them also by high early-onset mortality rates, thus emphasizing the critical role played by T lymphocytes in ensuring effective immune defense mechanisms and in maintaining homeostasis. Consequently, it is a primary physician's responsibility to perform accurate clinical and laboratory evaluation of patients with a putative T cell immunodeficiency. Whereas clinical history and physical examination may disclose the diagnosis in some forms of T cell immunodeficiency (e.g., Wiskott-Aldrich syndrome, ataxia-telangiectasia, cartilage hair hypoplasia), laboratory evaluation is most often required to provide a definitive diagnosis. In spite of the heterogeneity of this group of disorders, simple laboratory assays (total lymphocyte count and subsets distribution, *in vitro* proliferative responses, delayed-type hypersensitivity assays) are usually sufficient to confirm the suspicion. It is noteworthy that some forms of T cell immunodeficiencies (SCID in particular) represent true medical emergencies, and warrant prompt and accurate evaluation, and eventually rapid treatment by hematopoietic stem cell transplantation. Based on recent experience, it is likely that gene therapy may be successfully applied in a broader group of disorders in the near future.

HELPFUL WEBSITES

Online Mendelian Inheritance in Man (OMIM) website (www.ncbi.nlm.nih.gov/omim/)
European Society for Immune Deficiencies (ESID) website (www.esid.org/)
Jeffrey Modell Foundation website (www.jmfworld.com/)

REFERENCES

1. Fischer A: Severe combined immunodeficiencies (SCID), *Clin Exp Immunol* 122:143-149, 2000.
2. Noguchi M, Yi H, Rosenblatt HM, Filipovich AH, et al: Interleukin-2 receptor gamma chain mutation results in X-linked severe combined immunodeficiency in humans, *Cell* 73:147-157, 1993.
3. Leonard WJ, Noguchi M, Russell SM, et al: The molecular basis of X-linked severe combined immunodeficiency: the role of the interleukin-2 receptor gamma chain as a common gamma chain, gamma c, *Immunol Rev* 138:61-86, 1994.
4. Peschon JJ, Morrissey PJ, Grabstein KH, et al: Early lymphocyte expansion is severely impaired in interleukin 7 receptor-deficient mice, *J Exp Med* 180:1955-1960, 1994.
5. von Freeden-Jeffry U, Vieira P, Lucian LA, et al: Lymphopenia in interleukin (IL)-7 gene-deleted mice identifies IL-7 as a nonredundant cytokine, *J Exp Med* 181:1519-1526, 1995.
6. Puel A, Leonard WJ: Mutations in the gene for the IL-7 receptor result in T⁻B⁺NK⁺ severe combined immunodeficiency disease, *Curr Opin Immunol* 12:468-473, 2000.
7. Puck JM: IL2RGbase: a database of γc-chain defects causing human X-SCID, *Immunol Today* 17:507-511, 1996.
8. O'Shea JJ, Notarangelo LD, Johnston JA, et al: Advances in the understanding of cytokine signal transduction: the role of Jaks and STATs in immunoregulation and the pathogenesis of immunodeficiency, *J Clin Immunol* 17:431-447, 1997.
9. Russell SM, Johnston JA, Noguchi M, et al: Interaction of IL-2Rβ and γc chains with Jak1 and Jak3: implications for XSCID and XCID, *Science* 266:1042-1045, 1994.
10. Macchi P, Villa A, Giliani S, et al: Mutations of Jak-3 gene in patients with autosomal severe combined immune deficiency (SCID), *Nature* 377:65-68, 1995.
11. Russell SM, Tayebi N, Nakajima H, et al: Mutation of Jak3 in a patient with SCID: essential role of Jak3 in lymphoid development, *Science* 270:797-800, 1995.
12. Puel A, Ziegler S, Buckley RH, et al: Defective IL7R expression in T⁻B+NK+ severe combined immunodeficiency, *Nat Genet* 20:394-397, 1998.
13. Kung C, Pingel JT, Heikinheimo M, et al: Mutations in the tyrosine phosphatase CD45 gene in a child with severe combined immunodeficiency disease, *Nat Med* 6:343-345, 2000.
14. Tchilian EZ, Wallace DL, Wells RS, et al: A deletion in the gene encoding the CD45 antigen in a patient with SCID, *J Immunol* 166:1308-1313, 2001.
15. Sekiguchi J, Frank K: V(D)J recombination, *Curr Biol* 22:835, 1999.
16. Schatz DG, Oettinger MA, Baltimore D: The V(D)J recombination activating gene, *RAG-1, Cell* 59:1035-1048, 1989.
17. Oettinger MA, Schatz DG, Gorka C, et al: RAG-1 and RAG-2, adjacent genes that synergistically activate V(D)J recombination, *Science* 248:1517-1523, 1990.
18. Stephan JL, Vlekova V, Le Deist F, et al: Severe combined immunodeficiency: a retrospective single-center study of clinical presentation and outcome in 117 patients, *J Pediatr* 123:564-572, 1993.
19. Schwarz K, Gauss GH, Ludwig L, et al: RAG mutations in human B cell-negative SCID, *Science* 274:97-99, 1996.
20. Moshous D, Callebaut I, de Chasseval R, et al: Artemis, a novel DNA double-strand break repair/V(D)J recombination protein, is mutated in human severe combined immune deficiency, *Cell* 105:177-186, 2001.
21. Omenn GS: Familial reticuloendotheliosis with eosinophilia, *N Engl J Med* 273:427-432, 1965.
22. De Saint-Basile G, Le Deist F, de Villartay JP, et al: Restricted heterogeneity of T lymphocytes in combined immunodeficiency with hypereosinophilia (Omenn's syndrome), *J Clin Invest* 87:1352-1359, 1991.
23. Villa A, Santagata S, Bozzi F, et al: Partial V(D)J recombination activity leads to Omenn syndrome, *Cell* 93:885-896, 1998.
24. Villa A, Sobacchi C, Notarangelo LD, et al: V(D)J recombination defects in lymphocytes due to *Rag* mutations: a severe immunodeficiency with a spectrum of clinical presentation, *Blood* 97:81-88, 2001.
25. Apasov SG, Blackburn MR, Kellems RE, et al: Adenosine deaminase deficiency increases thymic apoptosis and causes defective T cell receptor signaling, *J Clin Invest* 108:131-141, 2001.
26. Ozsahin H, Arredondo-Vega FX, Santisteban I, et al: Adenosine deaminase deficiency in adults, *Blood* 89:2849-2855, 1997.
27. Arredondo-Vega FX, Santisteban I, Daniels S, et al: Adenosine deaminase deficiency: genotype-phenotype correlations based on expressed activity of 29 mutant alleles, *Am J Hum Genet* 63:1049-1059, 1998.
28. Markert ML, Finkel BD, McLaughlin TM, et al: Mutations in purine nucleoside phosphorylase deficiency, *Hum Mutat* 9:118-121, 1997.
29. Chan AC, van Oers NSC, Tran A, et al: Differential expression of ZAP-70 and Syk protein tyrosine kinases, and the role of this family of protein tyrosine kinases in TCR signaling, *J Immunol* 152:4758-4764, 1994.
30. van Leeuwen JEM, Samelson LE: T cell antigen-receptor signal transduction, *Curr Opin Immunol* 11:242-248, 1999.
31. Chan AC, Kadlecek TA, Elder ME, et al: ZAP-70 deficiency in an autosomal recessive form of severe combined immunodeficiency, *Science* 264:1599-1601, 1994.
32. Arpaia E, Shahar M, Dadi H, et al: Defective T cell receptor signaling and CD8+ thymic selection in humans lacking Zap-70 kinase, *Cell* 76:947-958, 1994.
33. Elder ME, Lin D, Clever J, et al: Human severe combined immunodeficiency due to a defect in ZAP-70, a T cell tyrosine kinase, *Science* 264:1596-1599, 1994.
34. Goldman FD, Ballas ZK, Schutte BC, et al: Defective expression of p56lck in an infant with severe combined immunodeficiency, *J Clin Invest* 102:421-429, 1998.
35. de Vaal OM, Seynhaeve V: Reticular dysgenesia, *Lancet* ii:1123-1124, 1959.
36. Mach B, Steimle V, Reith W: MHC class II-deficient combined immunodeficiency: a disease of gene regulation, *Immunol Rev* 138:207-221, 1994.
37. Steimle V, Otten LA, Zufferey M, et al: Complementation cloning of an MHC class II transactivator mutated in hereditary MHC class II deficiency (or bare lymphocyte syndrome), *Cell* 75:135-146, 1993.
38. Masternak K, Barras E, Zufferey M, et al: A gene encoding a novel RFX-associated transactivator is mutated in the majority of MHC class II deficiency patients, *Nat Genet* 20:273-277, 1998.
39. Villard J, Lisowska-Gospierre B, van den Elsen P, et al: Mutation of RFXAP, a regulator of MHC class II genes, in primary MHC class II deficiency, *N Engl J Med* 337:748-753, 1997.
40. Buckley RH, Schiff RI, Schiff SE, et al: Human severe combined immunodeficiency: genetic, phenotypic, and functional diversity in one hundred eight infants, *J Pediatr* 130:378-387, 1997.
41. Müller SM, Ege M, Pottharst A, et al: Transplacentally acquired maternal T lymphocytes in severe combined immunodeficiency: a study of 121 patients, *Blood* 98:1847-1851, 2001.
42. Bollinger ME, Arredondo-Vega FX, Santisteban I, et al: Hepatic dysfunction as a complication of adenosine deaminase deficiency, *N Engl J Med* 334:1367-1371, 1996.
43. Carson DA, Carrera CJ: Immunodeficiency secondary to adenosine deaminase deficiency and purine nucleoside phosphorylation deficiency, *Semin Hematol* 27:260-269, 1990.

44. Bennett CL, Ochs HD: IPEX is a unique X-linked syndrome characterized by immune dysfunction, polyendocrinopathy, enteropathy, and a variety of autoimmune phenomena, *Curr Opin Pediatr* 13:533-538, 2001.

45. Myers LA, Patel DD, Puck JM, et al: Hematopoietic stem cell transplantation for severe combined immunodeficiency in the neonatal period leads to superior thymic output and improved survival, *Blood* 99:872-878, 2002.

46. Notarangelo LD, Giliani S, Mazza C, et al: Of genes and phenotypes: the immunological and molecular spectrum of combined immune deficiency. Defects of the γc-JAK3 signaling pathway as a model, *Immunol Rev* 178:39-48, 2000.

47. Fischer A: Primary immunodeficiency diseases: an experimental model for molecular medicine, *Lancet* 357:1863-1869, 2001.

48. Fischer A, Landais P, Friedrich W, et al: European experience of bone-marrow transplantation for severe combined immunodeficiency, *Lancet* 336:850-854, 1990.

49. Buckley RH, Schiff SE, Schiff RI, et al: Hematopoietic stem-cell transplantation for the treatment of severe combined immunodeficiency, *N Engl J Med* 340:508-516, 1999.

50. Bertrand Y, Landais P, Friedrich W, et al: Influence of severe combined immunodeficiency phenotype on the outcome of HLA non-identical, T-cell-depleted bone marrow transplantation: a retrospective European survey from the European group for bone marrow transplantation and the European Society for Immunodeficiency, *J Pediatr* 134:740-748, 1999.

51. Wengler GS, Lanfranchi A, Frusca T, et al: *In utero* transplantation of parental CD34 haematopoietic progenitor cells in a patient with X-linked severe combined immunodeficiency (SCIDXI), *Lancet* 348:1484-1487, 1996.

52. Flake AW, Roncarolo MG, Puck JM, et al: Treatment of X-linked severe combined immunodeficiency by in utero transplantation of paternal bone marrow, *N Engl J Med* 335:1806-1810, 1996.

53. Bartolome J, Porta F, Lanfranchi A, et al: B cell function after haploidentical in utero bone marrow transplantation in a patient with severe combined immunodeficiency, *Bone Marrow Transplant* 29:625-628, 2002.

54. Hershfield MS: Enzyme replacement therapy of adenosine deaminase deficiency with polyethylene glycol-modified adenosine deaminase (PEG-ADA), *Immunodeficiency* 4:93-97, 1993.

55. Blaese RM, Culver KW, Miller AD, et al: T lymphocyte-directed gene therapy for ADA-SCID: initial trial results after 4 years, *Science* 270:475-480, 1995.

56. Bordignon C, Notarangelo LD, Nobili N, et al: Gene therapy in peripheral blood lymphocytes and bone marrow for ADA-immunodeficient patients, *Science* 270:470-475, 1995.

57. Kohn DB, Hershfield MS, Carbonaro D, et al: T lymphocytes with a normal ADA gene accumulate after transplantation of transduced autologous umbilical cord blood CD34+ cells in ADA-deficient SCID neonates, *Nat Med* 4:775-780, 1998.

58. Hacein-Bey S, Le Deist F, Carlier F, et al: Sustained correction of X-linked severe combined immunodeficiency by ex vivo gene therapy, *N Engl J Med* 346:1185-1193, 2002.

59. Greenberg F: DiGeorge syndrome: a historical review of clinical and cytogenetic features, *J Med Genet* 30:803-806, 1993.

60. Lindsay EA, Vitelli F, Su H, et al: Tbx1 haploinsufficiency in the DiGeorge syndrome region causes aortic arch defects in mice, *Nature* 410:97-101, 2001.

61. Markert ML, Hummell DS, Rosenblatt HM, et al: Complete Di George syndrome: persistence of profound immunodeficiency, *J Pediatr* 132:15-21, 1998.

62. Markert ML, Boeck A, Hale LP, et al: Transplantation of thymus tissue in complete DiGeorge syndrome, *N Engl J Med* 341:1180-1189, 1999.

63. Gadola SD, Moins-Teisserenc HT, Trowsdale Jet al: TAP deficiency syndrome, *Clin Exp Immunol* 121:173-178, 2000.

64. Furukawa H, Murata S, Yabe T, et al: Splice acceptor site mutation of the transporter associated with antigen processing-1 gene in human bare lymphocyte syndrome, *J Clin Invest* 103:649-652, 1999.

65. de la Salle H, Zimmer J, Fricker D, et al: HLA class I deficiencies due to mutations in subunit 1 of the peptide transporter TAP1, *J Clin Invest* 103:9-13, 1999.

66. de la Salle H, Hanau D, Fricker D, et al: Homozygous human TAP peptide transporter mutation in HLA class I deficiency, *Science* 265:237-241, 1994.

67. Moins-Teisserenc HT, Gadola SD, Cella M, et al: Association of a syndrome resembling Wegener's granulomatosis with low surface expression of HLA class-I molecules, *Lancet* 354:1598-1603, 1999.

68. Sharfe N, Dadi HK, Shahar M, et al: Human immune disorder arising from mutation of the a chain of the interleukin-2 receptor, *Proc Natl Acad Sci U S A* 94:3168-3171, 1997.

69. Alarcon B, Reguiero JR, Arnaiz-Villena A, et al: Familial defect in the surface expression of the T-cell receptor-CD3 complex, *N Engl J Med* 319:1203-1208, 1988.

70. Frank J, Pignata C, Panteleyev AA, et al: Exposing the human nude phenotype, *Nature* 398:473-474, 1999.

71. Pignata C, Gaetaniello L, Masci AM: Human equivalent of the mouse nude/SCID phenotype: long-term evaluation of immune reconstitution after bone marrow transplantation, *Blood* 97:880-885, 2001.

72. Moreno LA, Gottrand F, Turck D, et al: Severe combined immunodeficiency syndrome associated with autosomal recessive familial multiple gastrointestinal atresias, *Am J Med Genet* 37:143-146, 1990.

73. Walker MW, Lovell MA, Thaddeus EK, et al: Multiple areas of intestinal atresia associated with immunodeficiency and posttransfusion graft-versus-host disease, *J Pediatr* 123:93-95, 1993.

74. Le Deist F, Hivroz C, Partiseti M, et al: A primary T-cell immunodeficiency associated with defective transmembrane calcium influx, *Blood* 85:1053-1062, 1995.

75. Chatila T, Castigli E, Pahwa R, et al: Primary combined immunodeficiency resulting from defective transcription of multiple T-cell lymphokine genes, *Proc Natl Acad Sci U S A* 87:10033-10037, 1990.

76. Castigli E, Pahwa R, Good RA, et al: Molecular basis of a multiple lymphokine deficiency in a patient with severe combined immunodeficiency, *Proc Natl Acad Sci U S A* 90:4728-4731, 1993.

77. Ridanpää M, van Eenennaam H, Pelin K, et al: Mutations in the RNA component of RNase MRP cause a pleiotropic human disease, cartilage-hair hypoplasia, *Cell* 104:195-203, 2001.

78. Gennery AR, Cant AC, Jeggo PA: Immunodeficiency associated with DNA repair defect, *Clin Exp Immunol* 121:1-7, 2000.

79. Savitsky K, Bar-Shira A, Gilad S, et al: A single ataxia-telangiectasia gene with a product similar to PI-3 kinase, *Science* 268:1749-1753, 1995.

80. Varon R, Vissinga C, Platzer M, et al: Nibrin, a novel DNA double-strand break repair protein, is mutated in Nijmegen breakage syndrome, *Cell* 93:467-476, 1998.

81. Stewart GS, Maser RS, Stankovic T, et al: The DNA double-strand break repair gene *hMRE11* is mutated in individuals with an ataxia-telangiectasia-like disorder, *Cell* 99:577-587, 1999.

82. Thrasher AJ, Kinnon C: The Wiskott-Aldrich syndrome, *Clin Exp Immunol* 120:2-9, 2000.

83. Fischer A, Landais P, Friedrich W, et al: Bone marrow transplantation in Europe for primary immunodeficiencies other than severe combined immunodeficiency: a report from the European Group for BMT and the European Group for Immunodeficiency, *Blood* 83:1149-1154, 1994.

84. Filipovich AH, Shapiro RS, Ramsay NKC, et al: Unrelated donor bone marrow transplantation for correction of lethal congenital immunodeficiencies, *Blood* 80:270-276, 1992.

85. Notarangelo LD, Hayward AR. X-linked immunodeficiency with hyper-IgM (X-HIM), *Clin Exp Immunol* 120:349-405, 2000.

86. Thomas C, de Saint-Basile G, Le Deist F, et al: Correction of X-linked hyper-IgM syndrome by allogeneic bone marrow transplantation, *N Engl J Med* 333:426-429, 1995.

87. Amrolia P, Gaspar HB, Hassan A, et al: Nonmyeloablative stem cell transplantation for congenital immunodeficiencies, *Blood* 96:1239-1246, 2000.

88. Hadzic N, Pagliuca A, Rela M, et al: Correction of the hyper-IgM syndrome after liver and bone marrow transplantation, *N Engl J Med* 5:320-324, 2000.

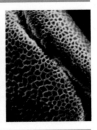

CHAPTER 10

Pediatric Human Immunodeficiency Virus Infection

MARY E. PAUL ■ WILLIAM T. SHEARER

Human immunodeficiency virus (HIV) infection in pediatrics is a chronic infection of infants who are infected for the most part at the time of birth or through breast-feeding or adolescents infected through adult-type high-risk behaviors. Although worldwide mother-to-infant transmission of HIV is a problem of enormous proportions, in the United States transmission from mother to infant is greatly reduced and limited to transmission from mothers who have not received prenatal care, have not followed medical advice, or in whom HIV infection remains undiagnosed. In the past, pediatric HIV infection had been marked by more rapid disease progression than seen in adults. However, with highly active combination antiretroviral therapy (ART), even those with rapid disease progression can be rescued. The key to success with therapy involves meeting the patient's psychosocial needs, providing the understanding and tools necessary for compliance, addressing and correcting formulation and dosing problems when possible, and having the patient or guardian committed to achieving adherence approaching 100% for ART doses.

EPIDEMIOLOGY AND ETIOLOGY

Twenty years after the first clinical evidence of HIV was recognized, HIV infection remains the fourth leading cause of death worldwide. The World Health Organization has estimated that 40 million people around the globe were living with HIV infection at the end of 2001, many of whom were unaware that they were infected.[1] One third of the infected are between the ages of 15 and 24. Of children younger than 15 years of age, 2.7 million children were living with HIV infection at the end of 2001 and 800,000 were newly infected with HIV during the year 2001. In the United States in 2001 the Centers for Disease Control and Prevention reported that there were over 4000 children under the age of 13 years who were living with HIV infection or acquired immunodeficiency syndrome (AIDS).[2] Only a small portion of HIV-infected adolescents have been identified and an even smaller number are receiving care. The number of HIV-positive adolescents required to produce the incident number of AIDS cases in the United States in 13- to 19-year-olds is estimated between 12,000 and 38,000.[3]

Transmission in the pediatric setting is usually secondary to mother-to-infant transmission that can occur during gestation,

at the time of delivery or in the intrapartum period, or postpartum as a result of breast-feeding. In a study conducted in Bangkok, Thailand, *in utero* transmission accounted for approximately 30% of perinatal HIV infection.[4] In the United States, HIV-infected women are counseled to forgo breast-feeding; however, in developing countries, breast-feeding still accounts for a considerable percentage of perinatal infections. However, the majority of perinatal transmission likely occurs close to the time of or during the delivery of the child.[5]

Combination ART is the treatment standard of care for HIV-infected pregnant women for both the prevention of perinatal transmission and for HIV treatment in the mother. In 1994 the Pediatric AIDS Clinical Trials Group (PACTG) 076 protocol showed that a course of zidovudine (ZDV), when given to HIV-infected pregnant women in a regimen that included pregnancy, peripartum, and postpartum dosing in the infant, could reduce transmission of HIV to the infant in a non–breast-feeding population by nearly 70%.[6] Since 1995, universal prenatal HIV testing with consent and counseling has been recommended by the Public Health Service (PHS) for all pregnant women in the United States.[7] Highly active ART including the use of a protease inhibitor (PI) medication has been shown to further reduce transmission with some predictions of transmission rates of less than 2% when used during pregnancy.[8,9] The best-studied combinations and potential toxicities are discussed and updated in the PHS's *Use of Antiretroviral Drugs in Pregnant HIV-1–Infected Women Guidelines* and in *Guidelines for HIV Treatment in Adolescents and Adults*. Table 10-1 lists the medications and the Food and Drug Administration pregnancy category and potential teratogenicity as shown by animal studies.[10,11] The non-nucleoside analogue reverse transcriptase inhibitor (NNRTI), efavirenz, is not used during pregnancy because animal teratology studies have shown possible teratogenic effects with exposure at therapeutic doses in monkeys (see Table 10-1). No epidemiologic studies of congenital anomalies in newborns exposed to efavirenz have been conducted; however, a neural tube defect has been reported in one of three infants of women who conceived during therapy with efavirenz, and myelomeningocele has been separately reported.[12,13]

In the initial reports from the PACTG 076 trial, follow-up of infants was short term and ZDV was well tolerated in

TABLE 10-1 Data Relevant to the Use of Antiretroviral Agents in Pregnancy

Antiretroviral Drug	FDA Pregnancy Category*	Long-Term Animal Carcinogenicity Studies	Animal Teratogen Studies
Nucleoside and nucleotide analogue reverse transcriptase inhibitors			
Zidovudine (Retrovir, AZT, ZDV)	C	Positive (rodent, noninvasive vaginal epithelial tumors)	Positive (rodent; near lethal dose)
Zalcitabine (HIVID, ddC)	C	Positive (rodent, thymic lymphomas)	Positive (rodent; hydrocephalus at high dose)
Didanosine (Videx, ddI)	B	Negative (no tumors, lifetime rodent study)	Negative
Stavudine (Zerit, d4T)	C	Not completed	Negative (but sternal bone calcium decreases in rodents)
Lamivudine (Epivir, 3TC)	C	Negative (no tumors, lifetime rodent study)	Negative
Abacavir (Ziagen, ABC)	C	Not completed	Positive (rodent anasarca and skeletal malformations at 1000 mg/kg (35× human exposure) during organogenesis; not seen in rabbits)
Tenofovir DF (Viread)	B	Not completed	Negative (osteomalacia when given to juvenile animals at high doses)
Non-nucleoside reverse transcriptase inhibitors			
Nevirapine (Viramune)	C	Not completed	Negative
Delavirdine (Rescriptor)	C	Not completed	Positive (rodent; ventricular septal defect)
Efavirenz (Sustiva)	C	Not completed	Positive (cynomologus monkey; anencephaly, anophthalmia, microphthalmia)
Protease inhibitors			
Indinavir (Crixivan)	C	Not completed	Negative (but extra ribs in rodents)
Ritonavir (Norvir)	B	Positive (rodent; liver adenomas and carcinomas in male mice)	Negative (but cryptorchidism in rodents)
Saquinavir (Fortovase)	B	Not completed	Negative
Nelfinavir (Viracept)	B	Not completed	Negative
Amprenavir (Agenerase)	C	Not completed	Negative (but deficient ossification and thymic elongation in rats and rabbits)
Lopinavir/Ritonavir (Kaletra)	C	Not completed	Negative (but delayed skeletal ossification and increase in skeletal variations in rats at maternally toxic doses)

Modified from Centers for Disease Control and Prevention: Public Health Service Task Force recommendation for use of antiretroviral drugs in pregnant women with HIV-1 for maternal health and for reducing HIV-1 transmission in the United States, http://www.hivatis.org, Feb 2002.

*Food and Drug Administration (FDA) pregnancy categories:

A: Adequate and well-controlled studies of pregnant women fail to demonstrate a risk to the fetus during the first trimester of pregnancy (and there is no evidence of risk during later trimesters);

B: Animal reproduction studies fail to demonstrate a risk to the fetus and adequate and well-controlled studies of pregnant women have not been conducted;

C: Safety in human pregnancy has not been determined, animal studies are either positive for fetal risk or have not been conducted, and the drug should not be used unless the potential benefit outweighs the potential risk to the fetus;

D: Positive evidence of human fetal risk based on adverse reaction data from investigational or marketing experiences, but the potential benefits from the use of the drug in pregnant women may be acceptable despite its potential risks;

X: Studies in animals or reports of adverse reactions have indicated that the risk associated with the use of the drug for pregnant women clearly outweighs any possible benefit.

general, with the exception that anemia was a common side effect. However, transplacental carcinogenicity of ZDV in humans is a theoretic concern and noninvasive squamous epithelial vaginal tumors have developed in adult rodents following continuous high-dose ZDV.[14] Also, vaginal epithelial tumors were observed in female offspring of mice who had a lifetime exposure to ZDV.[15] In a study in which ZDV was given to pregnant mice during the last third of the gestation period at a dose equivalent to 25 to 50 times greater than the daily dose given to humans, an increase in tumors of the liver, lung,

and female reproductive organs was observed in the rodent offspring.[16] In a follow-up study of the infants in the PACTG 076 trial, no adverse effects of any kind were observed in HIV-uninfected children with *in utero* or neonatal exposure to ZDV who were followed for as long as 5.6 years.[17,18] In addition, no malignancies have been observed in infants exposed to ZDV in the perinatal period in a large observational study, the Women and Infant Transmission Study.[19] Long-term follow-up of infants exposed to antiretroviral medication *in utero* is recommended by the PHS.

Other concerns regarding the *in utero* exposure to antiretroviral medications include those on the subject of the development of mitochondrial toxicity. Nucleoside analogue reverse transcriptase inhibitor (NRTI) medications have been shown to cause mitochondrial toxicity because of the affinity of these drugs for the mitochondrial gamma DNA polymerase and interference with mitochondrial replication. Clinical disorders linked to mitochondrial toxicity include cardiomyopathy, neuropathy, myopathy, hepatic steatosis, lactic acidosis, and pancreatitis. The concern about mitochondrial toxicity following *in utero* exposure stems from a report from France of eight HIV-uninfected infants, of a cohort of 1754 born to HIV-infected women, who developed indications of mitochondrial dysfunction (two died with severe neurologic disease, three had less severe neurologic symptoms, and three had laboratory abnormalities alone).[20] The two infants who died were exposed to both ZDV and lamivudine (3TC) *in utero*, as were two other infants. The remaining four were exposed to ZDV alone. The association between these findings of possible mitochondrial dysfunction and *in utero* antiretroviral medication exposure has not been clearly established. Other large studies have failed to find similar neurologic events in infants born to HIV-infected women.[18,21]

Although the benefits from the antiretroviral medications in terms of preserving or improving maternal health and preventing transmission of HIV in the infant greatly outweigh the possible risks associated with use of these medications during pregnancy, clearly the infants exposed to these medications should have long-term follow-up and the mothers should be followed by an obstetrician who has experience in treating HIV. Other concerns regarding the use of these medications include issues of mitochondrial toxicity in the mother and conflicting data, some of which suggest an increase in preterm delivery in women receiving combination ART.[22-26]

Most infants infected with HIV acquire the infection around the time of delivery and obstetric factors associated with HIV transmission have been closely examined. Increased transmission risk is associated with more than four hours of ruptured membranes, chorioamnionitis, and maternal bleeding during the pregnancy.[27] Also, mode of delivery influences transmission risk. Scheduled cesarean delivery performed before the onset of labor and rupture of membranes is associated with a reduction in transmission in studies performed before routine viral load monitoring and combination ART were used in pregnant HIV-infected women.[28] However, rates of vertical HIV transmission are similarly low for women who have undetectable viral load late in pregnancy on combination ART and for those who are receiving ZDV alone who undergo scheduled cesarean delivery.[18] The American College of Gynecology recommends scheduled cesarean delivery for women who have viral loads of greater than or equal to 1000 copies per milliliter late in pregnancy as an additional measure to prevent transmission of HIV.[29] Also, HIV-infected women who have viral loads of less than 1000 copies per milliliter may not need ART to preserve their own health. As transmission of HIV to infants has occurred in women with very low viral loads and the protective effect of antiretroviral medication against transmission of HIV in the perinatal setting is not completely caused by the control of viremia, a minimum of ZDV prophylaxis should be given even to mothers who have undetectable viral loads.[30-32] Additionally, shorter

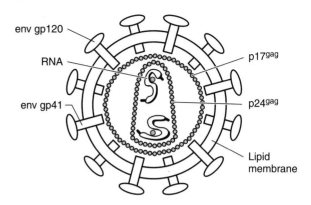

Drawing of human immunodeficiency virus (HIV). HIV is a retrovirus that has an envelope formed of two major viral envelope proteins, gp120 and gp41, and a lipid membrane. Important core proteins are p17^{gag} matrix protein, and p24^{gag} capsid protein. Two nucleocapsid proteins, p6^{gag} and p7^{gag}, are not shown. Within the inner core are two copies of the single-stranded HIV-1 genomic viral RNA that are associated with enzymes including the reverse transcriptase, protease, and integrase enzymes.

courses of ZDV; peripartum nevirapine, an NNRTI medication given to the mother and infant; and the combination of ZDV and lamivudine, a second NRTI medication, have shown efficacy in reducing transmission rates.[33,34] These specific regimens are useful alternatives for transmission reduction in resource-poor countries and for women who are not diagnosed as HIV infected until around the time of delivery.

HIV infection is caused by a retrovirus that has a structure that includes an outer envelope and inner core proteins that surround two copies of single-stranded genomic RNA (Figure 10-1). Within the core is the reverse transcriptase enzyme as well. The HIV surface envelope protein, gp120, allows the virus to attach to the target cell by binding to the target cell surface co-receptors, namely the CD4 molecule and a chemokine receptor, either CCR5 (macrophage tropic virus) or CXCR4 (T cell tropic virus).[35] The viral envelope protein, gp41, then mediates viral envelope fusion with the target cell to gain entry. The core is then injected into the cytoplasm of the target cell where the reverse transcriptase enzyme uses the host cell machinery to make a double-stranded DNA viral copy that is imported into the nucleus and inserted into the host genome by the viral integrase.

HIV infection should be in the differential diagnosis for any infant, child, or adolescent who has recurrent infections including recurrent otitis media or bacterial pneumonia (Box 10-1). Unlike adults, recurrent bacterial infections are considered a sign of disease progression in HIV-infected children. Similar to adults, untreated HIV-infected children not uncommonly have eczematous rashes and wasting or growth failure. Therefore HIV infection should be a diagnosis considered when evaluating failure to thrive. A complete history includes discussion of maternal HIV testing during pregnancy and, for youth, obtaining drug use and sexual histories. Also, opportunistic infection should trigger an evaluation for T cell immunodeficiency, including HIV infection/AIDS.

KEY CONCEPTS
Differential Diagnosis

- Human immunodeficiency virus (HIV) infection should be included in the differential diagnosis of children who have recurrent infection
- Children who have undiagnosed HIV infection can present with recurrent bacterial infection
- Opportunistic infections occur at higher CD4+ T cell counts for children than for adults

EVALUATION AND MANAGEMENT

Testing for HIV infection is routinely done in children who are older than 18 months of age and in youth using the HIV enzyme-linked immunosorbent assay (ELISA), which tests for the presence of specific antibody to HIV. If the ELISA is positive, confirmation of infection is provided most frequently by the HIV Western blot test, which also looks for specific antibody to HIV. As there is a window period between HIV infection and antibody production during which the HIV ELISA may be negative, testing should be repeated until 6 months after the time of suspected exposure or high-risk behavior to confirm infection status.

Infants are diagnosed with HIV by using virologic tests rather than the HIV ELISA because the ELISA may be positive because of antibody obtained through transplacental passage of antibody from the mother (Box 10-2). The HIV DNA polymerase chain reaction (PCR) is most commonly used for diagnosis because its convenience and sensitivity in diagnosis is well known. The sensitivity and specificity of the RNA PCR test for HIV diagnosis has not been as well studied. HIV cultures are more expensive and have a slower turnaround time for results, although cultures are sensitive to diagnosis when specimens are properly handled. The HIV DNA PCR was positive in 38% of 271 HIV-infected infants by age 48 hours in a meta-analysis of published data.[36] Virtually all infected infants can be definitively diagnosed by 6 months of age. Infants should be evaluated with an HIV DNA PCR within the first several days of life and at 1 to 2 and 4 to 6 months of age. If the DNA PCR is negative at two time points, at 2 months of age or older and 4 months of age or older, the infant born to an HIV-infected mother was not infected with HIV.

Monitoring for disease progression and efficacy of ART is performed using CD4+ T cell count and HIV RNA PCR values; these tests are typically followed every 3 to 4 months.

KEY CONCEPTS
Evaluation of the Perinatally HIV-Exposed Infant

- Infants should be evaluated with an HIV DNA PCR within the first several days of life and at 1 to 2 and 4 to 6 months of age. If the DNA PCR is negative at two time points, both at ≥2 months of age and ≥4 months of age, the infant was not infected with HIV perinatally.
- Prophylaxis for PCP is started at 4 to 6 weeks of age and continued until the diagnosis of HIV is excluded. If the infant is HIV infected, PCP prophylaxis is continued until after 1 year of age at which time CD4+ T cell count is used as a guide to determine if prophylaxis should be continue or stopped with monitoring of CD4+ T cell count performed every 3 months.
- HIV ELISA and Western blot testing can be used in diagnosis of HIV infection in infants and children older than 18 months of age, after antibody that was acquired through transplacental passage from the mother has been lost.
- Infants who have been exposed to antiretroviral therapy *in utero* should be followed long term.

HIV, Human immunodeficiency virus; *DNA*, deoxyribonucleic acid; *PCR*, polymerase chain reaction; *PCP*, *Pneumocystis carinii* pneumonia; *ELISA*, enzyme-linked immunosorbent assay.

CD4+ T cell counts are normally higher in infants and children than in adults and these counts decline to adult values by age 6 years. Therefore CD4+ T cell counts indicating immunosuppression and risk for opportunistic infection and malignancy are higher in children than in adults and vary with age (Table 10-2). CD4+ T cell values also vary with intercurrent illness and following immunization; therefore changes should be interpreted with this in mind. Declining CD4+ T cell values may need to be repeated to confirm the change in value before therapy decisions are made.

The amount of HIV RNA in the peripheral blood is an important prognostic indicator and is a sensitive measure of treatment response. Viral burden is typically determined by quantitative HIV RNA PCR measures. HIV-infected infants typically have a rising viral load in the first several months of life that peaks in the first year and slowly declines over the next several years. The viral load peaks are typically very high; the Women and Infants Transmission study reported a mean

TABLE 10-2 1994 Revised HIV Pediatric Classification System: Immune Categories Based on Age-Specific CD4+ T Cell Count and Percentage

Immune Category	<12 Months		1-5 Years		6-12 Years	
	No./mm³	*Percent*	*No./mm³*	*Percent*	*No./mm³*	*Percent*
Category 1: No suppression	≥1500	(≥25)	≥1000	(≥25)	≥500	(≥25)
Category 2: Moderate suppression	750-1499	(15-24)	500-999	(15-24)	200-499	(15-24)
Category 3: Severe suppression	<750	(<15)	<500	(<15)	<200	(<15)

Modified from Centers for Disease Control and Prevention: *MMWR* 43:1-10, 1994.
HIV, Human immunodeficiency virus.

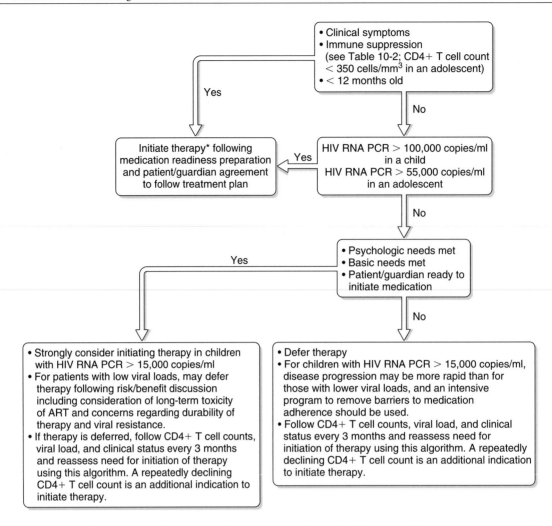

FIGURE 10-2 Algorithm for deciding when to initiate antiretroviral therapy in children and adolescents. Some experts would recommend initiating therapy in most adolescents who have acute primary human immunodeficiency virus *(HIV)* infection because of theoretic advantage of reducing viral set-point, preserving immune function, and reducing the risk for viral transmission. However, the potential risks of initiating therapy for acute HIV infection include indefinite need for therapy, risk for drug resistance if viral replication is not suppressed, early exposure to drugs with potential toxicities, and adverse impact on quality of life resulting from daily medication regimens. *PCR,* Polymerase chain reaction; *ART,* antiretroviral therapy. *The patient is at risk for disease progression. However, short-term deferral of therapy may be necessary to allow for maximizing psychosocial support and medication readiness.

viral load in the first year of life of 185,000 copies per milliliter and most infants had viral loads greater than 100,000 copies per milliliter.[37] Because of the effects of this high viral burden on a developing immune system, infants are usually treated aggressively with combination ART in the first year of life. Adolescents are expected to behave similar to adults following infection; that is, high viral burden is found within the first several months following infection and then, with the establishment of immune responses to HIV, viral burden declines to a lower, stable level within a year after infection. The level of the stable viral burden, or set-point, is a predictor of rapidity of disease progression.[38] Perinatally infected children greater than 3 years of age have chronic HIV infection as well. The viral set-point is a useful value in treatment initiation decisions for older children and adolescents.[10,39] Figure 10-2 demonstrates factors to consider when initiating ART in children and adolescents.

TREATMENT

The approach to treatment of HIV infection in children differs depending upon age and mode of infection. Perinatally infected infants, children, and teens and newly HIV-infected adolescents each have unique issues to consider regarding the decision to begin ART. Perinatally infected infants should begin therapy soon after infection has been identified. This approach is taken to suppress viremia, to allow more normal maturation of immune responses, and to allow for more normal growth and development.

Aging perinatally infected children are more difficult to treat because of their past use of ART. Many of these patients were treated with NRTIs as single- and dual-therapy agents as the medications became available. Therefore, for some, current therapy options are limited. It is difficult to move children who had grown up without available therapy for

HIV infection to a mindset where combination regimens that have side effects are acceptable. Finally, psychosocial issues must be addressed because these issues influence medication adherence. Some of these factors are family disruption resulting from loss of HIV-infected parents and entering into adolescence with a chronic infection, one that can be transmitted to sexual partners and, for the young women, to their infants; patients also may have physical stigmata, such as growth problems, which impact treatment acceptance and adherence.

Newly HIV-infected adolescents are often approached in the same way that HIV-infected adults are approached in that combination ART is offered if acute HIV infection is present. Otherwise, therapy is typically withheld until a threshold HIV RNA level is reached or until the CD4+ T cell count falls to a threshold level, after which disease progression is expected (see Figure 10-2)

Box 10-3 shows the ART combinations that are recommended for the treatment of HIV infection in infants and children by the PHS. These medications differ somewhat from those recommended for HIV-infected adolescents and adults because of the lack of pediatric data for some medications and the formulation difficulties for some medications in infants and children. Efficacy of therapy is monitored by following CD4+ T cell count and viral load.

Both these levels are done at baseline and, after therapy is started, initial monitoring of viral load changes is usually performed at 4 weeks, although some data suggest that 1-week HIV RNA values might be predictive of long-term durability of therapy.[40] Maximum virologic response may not occur until after 8 to 12 weeks of therapy. Virologic indications for change in therapy include less than a $1.0 \log_{10}$ decrease from baseline after 8 to 12 weeks, HIV RNA not suppressed to undetectable levels after 4 to 6 months of therapy, repeated detection of HIV RNA in children who initially had undetectable levels, and an increase in HIV RNA value after an initial response to low levels of detectable HIV RNA. Changes in HIV RNA should be confirmed by repeating the level after at least 1 week and an increase from a low level is indicated by a greater than threefold increase in copy number in children 2 years of age or older or a greater than fivefold increase for children less than 2 years of age. Few data indicate that suppression to undetectable HIV RNA levels is always achievable and an immediate change in therapy may not be warranted if a 1.5 to $2.0 \log_{10}$ decrease in baseline HIV RNA copy number is achieved, especially given the limited number of alternative regimens available for children. Substantial declines in CD4+ T cell counts, changes in immune classification (see Table 10-2), and for children in immune category 3, a decline of five percentiles or more are indications that a change in therapy should be considered. CD4+ T cell count is an independent predictor of disease progression. Clinical changes such as growth failure and neurodevelopmental deterioration are also indications for a consideration of ART change.

When a change in ART is being considered, reasons for therapy failure should be assessed. The goal of therapy is to reduce plasma HIV RNA to less than 50 copies per milliliter to minimize the likelihood that viral resistance to ART will emerge. Measures of viral resistance while the child is still receiving the therapy, that is, before the regimen is discontinued and wild-type virus replaces resistant strains, are likely helpful in directing the choice of new regimens, although data are

---

THERAPEUTIC PRINCIPLES

BOX 10-3

Recommended Antiretroviral Regimens for Initial Therapy for Human Immunodeficiency Virus Infection in Children

STRONGLY RECOMMENDED

One highly active protease inhibitor (nelfinavir or ritonavir) plus two nucleoside analogue reverse transcriptase inhibitors.

Recommended dual nucleoside reverse transcriptase inhibitor (NRTI) combinations: zidovudine (ZDV) and dideoxyinosine (ddI), ZDV and lamivudine (3TC), and stavudine (d4T) and ddI. More limited data are available for the combinations of d4T and 3TC and ZDV and dideoxycitidine (ddC).*

For children who can swallow capsules: the non-nucleoside reverse transcriptase inhibitor (NNRTI) efavirenz† plus two NRTIs or efavirenz plus nelfinavir and one NRTI.

Clinical trial evidence of suppression of HIV replication, but (1) durability may be less in adults and/or children than with strongly recommended regimens or may not yet be defined; or (2) evidence of efficacy may not outweigh potentially adverse consequences (i.e., toxicity, drug interactions, cost, etc); and (3) experience in infants and children is limited.

RECOMMENDED AS AN ALTERNATIVE

Nevirapine (NVP) and two NRTIs.

Abacavir (ABC) in combination with ZDV and 3TC.

Lopinavir/ritonavir with two NRTIs or one NRTI and one NNRTI.‡

Indinavir (IDV) or Saquinavir (SQV) soft gel capsule with two NRTIs for children who can swallow capsules.

Clinical trial evidence of either (1) virologic suppression that is less durable than that for the strongly recommended or alternative regimens; or (2) data are preliminary or inconclusive for use as initial therapy but may be reasonably offered in special circumstances.

OFFERED ONLY IN SPECIAL CIRCUMSTANCES

Two NRTIs.

Amprenavir (APV) in combination with two NRTIs or ABC.

From Centers for Disease Control and Prevention: *MMWR*, 47:1-38, 1998. Taken from http://www.hivatis.org update 12/14/01.
*ddC is not available commercially in a liquid preparation although a liquid formulation is available through a compassionate-use program of the manufacturer (Hoffman-La Roche Inc., http://www.rocheusa.com, Nutley, New Jersey). ZDV and ddC are less preferred choices for use in combination with a protease inhibitor.
†EFV is currently available only in capsule form, although a liquid formulation is available through an expanded-access program of the manufacturer (Bristol-Myers Squibb Company http://www.bms.com). There are currently no data on the appropriate dosage of EFV in children under age 3 years.
‡The data presented to the Food and Drug Administration for review during the drug approval process provided significant data on the pharmacokinetics and safety in children receiving lopinavir/ritonavir (Kaletra) for 24 weeks. The combination of lopinavir/ritonavir with either two NRTIs or one NRTI and one NNRTI may be moved up to the strongly recommended category as experience with this drug is gained by U.S. investigators.

lacking in children to make recommendations regarding the use of resistance testing. The presence of resistance to a drug indicates that the drug is unlikely to suppress viremia. Previous failed regimens may also indicate the presence of strains that are cross-resistant with drugs under consideration for the new regimen. This viral resistance may not be detected on resistance analysis until after the new regimen is started and the resistant viral strains re-emerge; thus history of previous ART is imperative in considering when to change regimens.

Causes of drug failure include noncompliance with the regimen or subtherapeutic drug exposure; each cause should be investigated. Therapeutic drug monitoring through use of measures of plasma drug levels is increasingly becoming a routine part of care, especially when medications with drug-drug interactions caused by common elimination pathways must be used. Resistance is a serious problem given that there is cross-resistance that develops rapidly to the NNRTI medications, and resistance to one of the available PI medications may reduce sensitivity to other PIs. HIV-infected adolescents have many psychosocial barriers to antiretroviral medication adherence that must be addressed before therapy is considered or changed. A therapeutic alliance must be reached between the adolescent and the medical professional that is based on mutual respect and trust. Basic needs including those of shelter, food, clothing, and safety in the environment are minimal criteria for successful therapy. The adolescent or the guardian of the child has to be made aware of the data regarding development of resistance to ART resulting from even small percentages of missed doses of medication so that the reality of the complexity of therapy is clear. Strategies should be discussed to help solve scheduling problems resulting from school, work, socializing, troubleshooting side effects and formulation difficulties, and decreasing missed doses. The patient's transportation needs must also be met. Adolescents who are HIV infected benefit from interaction with HIV-infected peers through support groups or mentorship programs.

Clearly, treatment of HIV infection should be done in consultation with a medical professional who has experience in HIV treatment. Single-drug changes can be made if the change is necessary because of toxicity but not because of therapy failure. Combinations that have similar toxicity profiles should be avoided. Follow-up should include monitoring for toxicity or drug intolerance. Many antiretroviral drugs, especially the PIs, have interactions with other medications that should be avoided. Adverse clinical events associated with combination ART are monitored during therapy and investigations are ongoing regarding the potential long-term effects of these therapies in children. Hyperlactatemia, possibly secondary to the mitochondrial effects of the NRTIs, discussed earlier in this chapter; hyperlipidemia; osteopenia; fat maldistribution; and hyperglycemia or diabetes mellitus, especially associated with PI use, have all been described in children on chronic ART.

The standard of care in treating HIV infection in infants, children, and adolescents includes the use of prophylaxis to prevent opportunistic infection.[41] *Pneumocystis carinii* pneumonia prophylaxis is indicated for HIV-infected or HIV-indeterminate infants aged 1 to 12 months, HIV-infected children aged 1 to 5 years with CD4+ T cell counts less than 500/μl or CD4+ T cell percentage less than 15%, and HIV-infected children and adolescents aged 6 years and above with CD4+ T cell percentage less than 15% (6 to 12 years old) or CD4+ T cell counts less than 200/μl. The first choice of preventive regimens is trimethoprim-sulfamethoxazole (TMP-SMX), with dapsone used as an alternative. TMP-SMX, when used daily, also protects against infection caused by *Toxoplasma gondii*, and prevention is recommended for infants, children, and adolescents who have severe immunosuppression (CD4+ T cell count less than 100/μl for adolescents) and positive IgG antibody to *Toxoplasma*. *Mycobacterium avium* complex (MAC) prophylaxis is indicated as follows: for infants less than 1 year of age, CD4+ T cell count less than 750/μl; for children 1 to 2 years of age, CD4+ T cell count less than 500/μl; for children 2 to 6 years of age, CD4+ T cell count less than 75/μl; and for children at least 6 years of age and adolescents, CD4+ T cell count less than 50/μl. Clarithromycin and azithromycin are the first-choice agents of preventive regimens for MAC and are started following documentation of a negative peripheral blood culture for mycobacterium. The tuberculin skin test (TST) is performed yearly, and antimycobacterial medication is used if the TST reaction is at least 5 mm or in case of contact with any case of active tuberculosis regardless of TST result. *Varicella zoster* immune globulin should be considered for use in infants, children, or adolescents who have significant exposure to varicella or shingles with no prior history of chickenpox or shingles. HIV-infected children should receive routine immunizations with a few exceptions.[41] All inactivated poliovirus vaccine schedules should be used for HIV-infected children and all household contacts. The measles, mumps, and rubella vaccine is not given to severely immunosuppressed (Category 3) children. Vaccination against varicella is indicated only for asymptomatic, nonimmunosuppressed children. HIV-infected children who are eligible to receive the varicella vaccine should receive two doses initially with at least a 3-month interval between doses.

CONCLUSIONS

HIV infection is a worldwide problem with tremendous impact. Although in the United States infection rates in the pediatric setting are markedly reduced by the use of measures to prevent perinatal transmission of HIV, young women, men, and infants continue to become infected with HIV (Box 10-4). Challenges for the future include further management

---

BOX 10-4   **KEY CONCEPTS**
Take-Home Messages

- Human immunodeficiency virus (HIV) infection in the pediatric population occurs through perinatal infection and through new infections in adolescents resulting from sexual or intravenous drug use exposure routes.
- Testing of infants for HIV involves a direct test for virus. After 18 months of age, the tests for HIV antibody, the HIV enzyme-linked immunosorbent assay, and Western blot can be used for diagnosis.
- Management of HIV in children and youth includes consideration of medication formulation, tolerability, and unique adherence issues.

difficulties caused by ART resistance that is a particular concern in the noncompliant patient; in older, treatment-experienced, perinatally infected youth; and in HIV-infected young women who are having repeated pregnancies. Newer approaches to improve compliance and prevention hold promise for the future. Practitioners impact infection risk by providing routine prevention messages to youth in their care and by promoting HIV testing in pregnant youth.

HELPFUL WEBSITES

HIV/AIDS Treatment Information Service website (http://www.hivatis.org)
Centers for Disease Control and Prevention website (http://www.cdc.org)

REFERENCES

1. UNAIDS, WHO: AIDS epidemic update: December 2001. Geneva: Joint United Nations Programme on HIV/AIDS, 2001.
2. Centers for Disease Control and Prevention: HIV/AIDS Surveillance Report 13:1-41, 2001.
3. Rogers AS: Report on NIH-community consultation on including adolescents in HIV prevention vaccine research, 1-12, 2001.
4. Mock PA, Shaffer N, Bhadrakom C, et al: Maternal viral load and timing of mother-to-child HIV transmission, Bangkok, Thailand. Bangkok Collaborative Perinatal HIV Transmission Study Group, AIDS 13:407, 1999.
5. Mofenson LM: Interaction between timing of perinatal human immunodeficiency virus infection and the design of preventive and therapeutic interventions, Acta Paediatr Suppl 421:1-9, 1997.
6. Connor EM, Sperling RS, Gelber R, et al: Reduction of maternal-infant transmission of human immunodeficiency virus type 1 with zidovudine treatment, N Engl J Med 331:1173, 1994.
7. CDC: US Public Health Service recommendations for human immunodeficiency virus counseling and voluntary testing for pregnant women, MMWR 44:1-14, 1995.
8. Cooper ER, Charurat M, Mofenson L, et al: Combination antiretroviral strategies for the treatment of pregnant HIV-1 infected women and prevention of perinatal HIV-1 transmission, J AIDS 29:484-494, 2002.
9. Mandelbrot L, Landreau-Mascaro A, Rekacewicz C, et al: Lamivudine-zidovudine combination for prevention of maternal-infant transmission of HIV-1, JAMA 285:2083-2093, 2001.
10. CDC: Guidelines for the use of antiretroviral agents in HIV-infected adults and adolescents, MMWR 47:39-82, 1998 (and updates most recent 5/18/02 http://www.hivatis.org).
11. CDC: Public health service task force recommendation use of antiretroviral drugs in pregnant women with HIV-1 for maternal health and for reducing HIV-1 transmission in the United States, MMWR 47:1-30, 1998 (and updates http://www.hivatis.org).
12. De Santis M, Carducci B, De Santis L, et al: Periconceptional exposure to efavirenz and neural tube defects, Arch Intern Med 162:355, 2002.
13. Fundaro C, Genovese O, Rendeli C, et al: Myelomeningocele in a child with intrauterine exposure to efavirenz, AIDS 16:299-300, 2002.
14. Ayers KM, Clive D, Tucker WE Jr, et al: Nonclinical toxicology studies with zidovudine: genetic toxicity tests and carcinogenicity bioassays in mice and rats, Fundam Appl Toxicol 32:148, 1996.
15. Ayers KM, Torrey CE, Reynolds DJ: A transplacental carcinogenicity bioassay in CD-1 mice with zidovudine, Fundam Appl Toxicol 38:195, 1997.
16. Olivero OA, Anderson LM, Divan BA, et al: Transplacental effects of 3'-azido-2',3'-dideoxythymidine (AZT): tumorigenicity in mice and genotoxicity in mice and monkeys, J Natl Cancer Inst 89:7, 1997.
17. Culane M, Fowler MG, Lee SS, et al: Lack of long-term effects of in utero exposure to zidovudine among uninfected children born to HIV-infected women, JAMA 281:151-157, 1999.
18. Sperling RS, Shapiro DE, McSherry GD, et al: Safety of the maternal-infant zidovudine regimen utilized in the Pediatric AIDS Clinical Trials Group 076 Study, AIDS 12:1805-1813, 1998.
19. Hanson IC, Antonelli TA, Sperling RS, et al: Lack of tumors in infants with perinatal HIV-1 exposure and fetal/neonatal exposure to zidovudine, J AIDS Hum Retrovirol 20:463-467, 1999.
20. Blanche S, Tardieu M, Rustin P, et al: Persistent mitochondrial dysfunction and perinatal exposure to antiretroviral nucleoside analogues, Lancet 354:1084-1089, 1999.
21. The Perinatal Safety Review Working Group: Nucleoside exposure in the children of HIV-infected women receiving antiretroviral drugs: absence of clear evidence for mitochondrial disease in children who died before 5 years of age in five United States cohorts, J AIDS Hum Retrovirol 25:261-268, 2000.
22. Lorenzi P, Spicher VM, Laubereau B, et al: Antiretroviral therapies in pregnancy: maternal, fetal and neonatal effects. Swiss HIV Cohort Study, the Swiss Collaborative HIV and Pregnancy Study, and the Swiss Neonatal HIV Study, AIDS 12:F241-F247, 1998.
23. The European Collaborative Study and the Swiss Mother + Child HIV Cohort Study: Combination antiretroviral therapy and duration of pregnancy, AIDS 14:2913-2920, 2000.
24. Martin R, Boyer P, Hammill H, et al: Incidence of premature birth and neonatal respiratory disease in infants of HIV-positive mothers: The Pediatric Pulmonary and Cardiovascular Complications of Vertically Transmitted Human Immunodeficiency Virus Infection Study Group, J Pediatr 131:851-856, 1997.
25. Ibdah JA, Bennett MJ, Rinaldo P, et al: A fetal fatty-acid oxidation disorder as a cause of liver disease in pregnant women, N Engl J Med 340:1723-1731, 1999.
26. Sims HF, Brackett JC, Powell CK, et al: The molecular basis of pediatric long-chain 3-hydroxyacyl Co-A dehydrogenase deficiency associated with maternal acute fatty liver of pregnancy, Proc Natl Acad Sci U S A 92:841-845, 1995.
27. Landesman SH, Kalish LA, Burns DN, et al: Obstetrical factors and the transmission of human immunodeficiency virus type 1 from mother to child, N Engl J Med 334:617, 1996.
28. The European Mode of Delivery Collaboration: Elective cesarean-section versus vaginal delivery in prevention of vertical HIV-1 transmission: a randomised clinical trial, Lancet 353:1035-1039, 1999.
29. American College of Obstetricians and Gynecologists Committee Opinion: Scheduled cesarean delivery and the prevention of vertical transmission of HIV infection, 234, May 2000.
30. Garcia PM, Kalish LA, Pitt J, et al: Maternal levels of plasma HIV type 1 RNA and the risk of perinatal transmission, N Engl J Med 341:394-402, 1999.
31. The European Collaborative Study: Maternal viral load and vertical transmission of HIV-1: an important factor but not the only one, AIDS 13:1377-1385, 1999.
32. Ioannidis JPA, Abrams EJ, Ammann A, et al: Perinatal transmission of HIV type 1 by pregnant women with RNA virus loads < 1000 copies/ml, J Infect Dis 183:539-545, 2001.
33. Guay LA, Musoke P, Fleming T, et al: Intrapartum and neonatal single-dose nevirapine compared with zidovudine for prevention of mother-to-child transmission of HIV-1 in Kampala, Uganda: HIVNET 012 randomised trial, Lancet 354:795-802, 1999.
34. Shaffer N, Bulterys M, Simonds RJ: Short courses of zidovudine and perinatal transmission of HIV, N Engl J Med 340:1042-1043, 1999.
35. Kinter A, Arthos J, Cicala C, Fauci AS: Chemokines, cytokines and HIV: a complex network of interactions that influence HIV pathogenesis, Immunol Rev 177:88-98, 2000.
36. Dunn DT, Brandt CD, Kirvine A, et al: The sensitivity of HIV-1 DNA polymerase chain reaction in the neonatal period and the relative contributions of intrauterine and intrapartum transmission, AIDS 9:F7-F11, 1995.
37. Shearer WT, Quinn TC, LaRussa P, et al: Viral load and disease progression in infants infected with human immunodeficiency virus type 1: Women and Infants Transmission Study Group, N Engl J Med 336:1337, 1997.
38. Mellors JW, Kingsley LA, Rinaldo CR, et al: Quantitation of HIV-1 RNA in plasma predicts outcome after seroconversion, Ann Intern Med 122:573-579, 1995.
39. Centers for Disease Control and Prevention: Guidelines for the use of antiretroviral agents in pediatric HIV infection, MMWR 47:1, 1998. Living document on the worldwide web on ATIS website: http://hivatis.org/.
40. Polis MA, Sidorov IA, Yoder C, et al : Correlation between reduction in plasma HIV-1 RNA concentration 1 week after start of antiretroviral treatment and long-term efficacy, Lancet 358:1760-1765, 2001.
41. Centers for Disease Control and Prevention: 1997 USPHS/IDSA guidelines for the prevention of opportunistic infections in persons infected with human immunodeficiency virus, MMWR 46:1, 1997. Living document on the worldwide web on ATIS website: http://hivatis.org/.

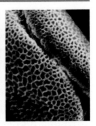

CHAPTER 11

Complement Deficiencies

JERRY A. WINKELSTEIN ■ KATHLEEN E. SULLIVAN

The complement system was first identified at the end of the nineteenth century as a serum activity that "complemented" the action of antibody in the lysis of gram-negative bacteria. During the next 100 years there was a growing appreciation that complement not only played an important role in host defense against infection but also was important in the generation of inflammation, the clearance of immune complexes and apoptotic cells, and the production of a normal humoral immune response.[1]

Deficiencies of the complement system may be genetically determined, secondary to other conditions, or the result of immaturity. In this chapter, we review deficiencies of the complement system in humans with an emphasis on pathophysiology and clinical presentation.

PATHOPHYSIOLOGY AND CLINICAL EXPRESSION

Patients with deficiencies of the complement system may have a variety of clinical presentations, including an increased susceptibility to infection, rheumatic disorders, and angioedema. The pathophysiologic basis for the increased susceptibility to infection and the rheumatic diseases has been elucidated.

Pathophysiologic Basis for an Increased Susceptibility to Infection

An increased susceptibility to infection is a prominent clinical expression of most of the complement deficiency diseases.

The activation of the complement system by microorganisms, through either the classical or alternative pathways, results in the generation of cleavage products and macromolecular complexes that possess opsonic activity (C3b), anaphylatoxic activity (C4a, C3a, and C5a), chemotactic activity (C5a), or bactericidal/bacteriolytic activity (C5b, C6, C7, C8, and C9). All play a role in the host's defense against infection.[1,2] Experiments in complement-deficient experimental animals, whether naturally occurring or genetic "knockouts," have shown that the complement system plays an important role in the host's defense against a wide variety of bacteria, viruses, and fungi. Its protective effects are critical in the generation of the initial inflammatory response to infection, prevention of spread of the infection from the initial site of infection to other areas of the body, and clearance of the microorganism from the bloodstream. Furthermore, it

appears to play its most important role in the early stages of infection, and the generation of opsonic activity is among its most critical functions.

The nature of the infections in complement-deficient individuals generally reflects the specific roles of the deficient component in host defense. For example, C3 is responsible for generating complement-mediated opsonic activity. Thus patients with C3 deficiency are unduly susceptible to infection from encapsulated bacteria (e.g., *Streptococcus pneumoniae*, *Haemophilus influenzae*, and *Streptococcus pyogenes*),[3-5] organisms for which opsonization is a critical host defense mechanism. In contrast, patients with deficiencies of C5, C6, C7, C8, or C9 possess C3 and are not susceptible to these bacteria.[4,5] They are, however, unduly susceptible to neisserial infections because the generation of bactericidal activity, mediated by C5b through C9, is critical to defense against this genus. Interestingly, although a number of gram-negative bacteria are susceptible to the bactericidal activity of complement, the susceptibility of patients with deficiencies of C5 through C9 appears to be limited to *Neisseria* spp.[4,5]

There are some characteristic clinical features of infections in complement-deficient patients. For example, despite the fact that experimental animals with complement deficiencies are susceptible to a variety of different microorganisms, bacterial infections are the most prominent in complement-deficient patients.[4,5] The infections seen in complement-deficient individuals can be localized (e.g., pneumonia or sinusitis), although systemic infections (e.g., bacteremia/sepsis, meningitis, or osteomyelitis) are common and often are recurrent.[4,5]

A number of studies have examined the prevalence of complement deficiencies among patients with characteristic infections. Although complement-deficient patients do not appear to be sufficiently common among patients with single episodes of pneumococcal, streptococcal, or *H. influenzae* sepsis and/or meningitis to justify routine screening of patients with these infections, complement deficiencies are sufficiently common among patients with systemic neisserial infections to make routine screening worthwhile.[6-8] For example, estimates of the prevalence of complement deficiencies among patients with a single episode of meningococcal sepsis have varied from 5% to 15%; the difference probably relates to differences in the populations being studied. Not unexpectedly, the prevalence is as high as 40% if the patient has had recurrent meningococcal sepsis, has an infection with an uncommon serotype, or has a positive family history of meningococcal systemic infections.[9,10]

Pathophysiologic Basis for Rheumatic Disorders

Rheumatic disorders are common in patients with deficiencies of certain specific components, namely C1, C4, C2, and C3.

A variety of pathophysiologic mechanisms exist by which complement deficiencies can lead to the development of rheumatic disorders. The two most attractive relate to the role of the complement system in the processing and clearance of immune complexes and the processing and clearance of apoptotic cells.

The complement system participates significantly in the processing and clearance of immune complexes via a variety of mechanisms. First, immune complexes carrying C3b can be ingested by phagocytic cells. Second, the activation of C3 by immune complexes retards their precipitation, helping to maintain them as soluble complexes, and can solubilize them once they have precipitated.[11] Importantly, there is an excellent correlation between the inability of sera from patients with complement deficiencies to prevent the precipitation of immune complexes and the occurrence of rheumatic diseases in these patients.[12] The sera of patients with deficiencies of C1, C4, C2, and C3 do not prevent precipitation of immune complexes *in vitro*, and rheumatic diseases occur in nearly half of the patients with deficiencies of these components. Conversely, the sera of patients with deficiencies of C5, C6, C7, C8, or C9 do prevent precipitation of immune complexes, and rheumatic diseases are very uncommon in these patients.

Finally, a third mechanism exists in humans and other primates by which immune complexes are cleared and processed. Humans possess receptors (CR1) for cleavage products of C3 on their erythrocytes, and circulating immune complexes containing C3b can reversibly bind to those receptors. As erythrocytes carrying immune complexes pass through the liver, the immune complexes are picked off the surface by Kupffer's cells, ingested, and processed, thus effectively removing them from the circulation and preventing their deposition in other organs such as the kidney.[13]

Recently, another attractive hypothesis to explain the occurrence of rheumatic diseases in patients with deficiencies of early components of the classical pathway was developed. The early components of the classical pathway, especially C1q, participate in the clearance of apoptotic cells.[14,15] As cells undergo apoptosis, intracellular constituents are reorganized and appear on the surface of the cell in blebs. Autoantigens targeted in patients with systemic lupus erythematosus (SLE), such as SSA and/or SSB, are often found on the surface in these blebs, rendering a normally "invisible" antigen "visible." Thus patients deficient in these components may develop rheumatic disorders, especially SLE, because they lack an important mechanism of clearance of apoptotic cells.

The rheumatic diseases seen in complement-deficient patients include SLE, discoid lupus, dermatomyositis, scleroderma, anaphylactoid purpura, vasculitis, and membranoproliferative glomerulonephritis.[4,5] There are some clinical and laboratory features that are characteristic of the rheumatic diseases seen in complement-deficient individuals. For example, the SLE seen in C2-deficient patients is frequently associated with photosensitive dermatitis. It is not uncommon for C2-deficient patients to have low (or absent) titers of antibodies to nuclear antigen and/or native DNA, whereas the prevalence of anti-Ro antibodies in C2-deficient patients with lupus is much greater than in non−C2-deficient patients with lupus.[16,17] Patients deficient in C1 or C4 usually have an early onset of clinical symptoms with prominent cutaneous manifestations.[18,19]

INHERITED COMPLEMENT DEFICIENCIES

Genetically determined deficiencies have been identified for most of the individual components of complement. Most are inherited as autosomal recessive traits, although one is inherited as an X-linked recessive trait (properdin deficiency) and one is inherited as an autosomal dominant trait (C1 esterase deficiency) (Table 11-1).

C1q Deficiency

Molecular Biology and Pathophysiology

C1q is one of the three subcomponents of C1; the other two are C1r and C1s. C1q is composed of six identical subunits, each of which is composed of three different polypeptide chains, C1qA, C1qB, and C1qC, encoded by genes on the long arm of chromosome 1.[20] IgG or IgM, after engaging antigen and forming an immune complex, binds C1q, which then activates C1r, in turn activating C1s. Activated C1s then cleaves

TABLE 11-1 Inherited Complement Deficiency Diseases

Component	Inheritance	Major Clinical Expression
Classical pathway		
C1q	Autosomal recessive	Rheumatic disorders and pyogenic infections
C1r/s	Autosomal recessive	Rheumatic disorders
C4	Autosomal recessive	Rheumatic disorders and pyogenic infections
C2	Autosomal recessive	Rheumatic disorders and pyogenic infections
C3 and terminal components		
C3	Autosomal recessive	Pyogenic infections and rheumatic disorders
C5	Autosomal recessive	Meningococcal sepsis and meningitis
C6	Autosomal recessive	Meningococcal sepsis and meningitis
C7	Autosomal recessive	Meningococcal sepsis and meningitis
C8	Autosomal recessive	Meningococcal sepsis and meningitis
C9	Autosomal recessive	Meningococcal sepsis and meningitis
Control proteins		
C1 inhibitor	Autosomal dominant	Angioedema
Factor I	Autosomal recessive	Pyogenic infections
Properdin	X-linked recessive	Meningococcal sepsis and meningitis

both C4 and C2, creating the bimolecular enzyme C4b,2a, which activates C3 and ultimately the terminal components (C5 through C9) via the classical pathway. Thus C1q plays a critical role in activation of the classical pathway and the generation of the biologic activities of C3 and C5 through C9. In addition, recent studies have shown that C1q recognizes apoptotic cells and targets them for clearance.[14,15]

C1q-deficient individuals have markedly reduced serum total hemolytic activity and C1 functional activity. In most affected individuals, C1q protein level is also markedly reduced, but in some a dysfunctional immunoreactive protein is produced.[21]

Clinical Expression

The most prominent clinical manifestation of C1q deficiency is SLE. Although SLE is also a prominent clinical feature of patients with deficiencies of other components of the classical pathway (e.g., C1r, C1s, C4, and C2) and C3, C1q-deficient patients carry the highest risk (> 90% prevalence).[4,5,21] Deficiencies of all of the early components of the classical pathway, including C1q deficiency, would be expected to have impaired immune complex clearance. However, C1q-deficient patients would also have the additional disadvantage of an impaired ability to clear apoptotic cells. There are some differences between the SLE seen in C1q-deficient patients and that seen in complement-sufficient individuals. For example, the age of onset of the SLE tends to be earlier, usually prepubertal, and the disease tends to be somewhat more severe. In addition, although antinuclear antibodies may be present, they tend to be of low titer, and anti−double-stranded (ds) DNA antibodies are usually negative.

C1q-deficient individuals also have an increased susceptibility to encapsulated bacteria, reflecting their inability to activate the classical pathway and efficiently generate opsonically active C3b. In fact, nearly one third of C1q-deficient patients have significant bacterial infections and 10% have died of infections.[4,5,21]

Molecular Genetics

Multiple mutations have been described in C1q deficiency.[22] The disease is especially prominent in Turkey and is usually the result of a C-to-T transition in exon 2 of C1qA.[23,24] The most common mutations result in a premature stop codon and C1q protein is not detectable.[22-24] Missense mutations may result in the production of a dysfunctional protein that can neither bind to immunoglobulin heavy chains nor activate C1r.[22,25]

C1r/C1s Deficiency

Molecular Biology and Pathophysiology

The C1 complex is composed of six C1q subunits and two subunits each of C1r and C1s. The genes for C1r and C1s are closely linked on chromosome 12 and encode highly homologous serine proteases.[1] As mentioned earlier, C1q, after it binds to an immune complex, activates C1r, which in turn activates C1s. It is C1s that cleaves C4 and C2, resulting in the assembly of the C3 cleaving enzyme C4b,2a.

Patients with C1r/s deficiency have markedly reduced levels of total hemolytic complement activity and C1 functional activity. Typically, C1r levels are reduced to less than 1% of normal values, and C1s levels are between 20% and 50% of

normal values.[21] Interestingly, a few patients have been described in whom C1s levels are markedly reduced, whereas C1r levels are approximately 50% of normal. The observation that deficiency of one component leads to reduced levels of the other suggests that neither is stable in the absence of the other.

Clinical Expression

The most common clinical expression of C1r/s deficiency has been SLE.[4,5,21] Some patients have also presented with glomerulonephritis or bacterial infections.

Molecular Genetic Basis

The mutations responsible for C1s deficiency have been varied. Although the mutations responsible for C1r deficiency have not been identified, 7 of the first 12 patients have been of Puerto Rican descent, suggesting a Founder effect.

C4 Deficiency

Molecular Biology and Pathophysiology

The fourth component of complement (C4) is encoded by two closely linked genes (C4A and C4B) located within the major histocompatibility complex (MHC) on chromosome 6.[1] Although the protein products of the two loci share most of their structure and function, there are four amino acid differences between them that account for differences in their electrophoretic mobility, minor antigenic determinants, functional activity, and molecular weight of the alpha chain. As mentioned, the larger cleavage product of C4, C4b, forms part of the bimolecular enzyme C4b,2a, which is responsible for activation of C3 and C5 through C9 via the classical pathway. It therefore plays an important role in the generation of the biologic activities of C3 and C5 through C9.

Because C4 is encoded by two distinct genes, patients with complete C4 deficiency are homozygous deficient at both loci (C4A*Q0,C4B*Q0/C4A*Q0,C4B*Q0).[19,26] In contrast to the rarity of patients with complete C4 deficiency, individuals who are heterozygous for either C4A or C4B deficiency are relatively common.[19,26] Approximately 13% to 14% of the population is heterozygous for C4A deficiency and 15% to 16% is heterozygous for C4B deficiency, with the corresponding frequencies for homozygous-deficient individuals being 1% and 3%. Individuals who have complete C4 deficiency (i.e., are homozygous deficient for both C4A and C4B) have little, if any, total hemolytic activity in their sera and markedly reduced levels of C4 protein and functional activity. As a result of the absence of C4, these individuals have a markedly decreased ability to generate serum opsonic, chemotactic, and bactericidal activities via activation of the classical pathway.[27,28]

Clinical Expression

Patients with complete C4 deficiency may present with SLE and/or an increased susceptibility to infection.[4,5,19] The onset of SLE is usually early in life and is characterized by prominent cutaneous features such as photosensitive skin rash, vasculitic skin ulcers, and Raynaud's phenomenon. As with other deficiencies of early components of the classical pathway, anti-DNA titers may be absent. Patients with complete C4 deficiency also have an increased susceptibility to bacterial infections; most deaths in C4-deficient patients are the result of infection.

In contrast to the rarity of complete C4 deficiency, individuals who are homozygous deficient at one but not the other locus *(C4A or C4B)* are relatively common in the general population.[19,26] Because of the differences in functional activity between C4A and C4B,[29] individuals who are homozygous deficient in one or the other isotype might be predisposed to certain illnesses. For example, individuals who are homozygous deficient for C4A lack the isotype that is most efficient in interacting with proteins. Therefore they might not be able to process protein-containing immune complexes as well as do individuals who possess C4A and will be at risk for the development of immune complex diseases such as SLE. In fact, the prevalence of homozygous C4A deficiency in patients with SLE is markedly elevated, approaching 10% to 15%, a frequency at least 10 times that in the population at large.[30-32] Interestingly, patients with SLE who have C4A deficiency have some clinical and laboratory features that are different from those of complement-sufficient patients with SLE. They have less neurologic and renal disease but more photosensitivity than other patients with SLE, and they have a lower prevalence of anticardiolipin, anti-Ro, anti-dsDNA, and anti-Sm antibodies.[33,34]

In contrast to individuals with homozygous C4A deficiency, homozygous C4B-deficient individuals lack the C4 isotype that interacts most efficiently with polysaccharides. Therefore they might not be able to activate C3 through the classical pathway and opsonize bacteria possessing a polysaccharide capsule as well as individuals possessing C4B and thereby have an increased risk of infections with encapsulated bacteria. In fact, there is an increased prevalence of homozygous C4B deficiency in children with bacteremia and/or bacterial meningitis.[35,36]

Molecular Genetic Basis

C4A deficiency is often the result of a large gene deletion.[37] In addition, a 2-base pair (bp) insertion in exon 29 is relatively common.[38] Some instances of C4B deficiency are the result of gene deletions.[37] Finally, gene conversions can cause either C4A or C4B deficiency.[39]

C2 Deficiency

Molecular Biology and Pathophysiology

The second component of complement (C2) is encoded by a gene within the MHC on chromosome 6.[1] Like C4, C2 is cleaved by C1s into two fragments, the larger of which (C2a) forms part of the C3-cleaving enzyme of the classical pathway, C4b,2a. Thus C2, like C4, plays a critical role in generating the biologic activities of C3 and the terminal components, C5 through C9.

C2-deficient patients usually have absent total hemolytic activity and less than 1% of the normal levels of C2 protein and function.[40] Those complement-mediated serum activities that can be mediated via activation of the alternative pathway, such as serum opsonic, chemotactic, and bactericidal activities, are usually present but not generated as quickly or to the same degree as those in individuals who possess C2 and have an intact classical pathway.[41-43]

Clinical Expression

Genetically determined C2 deficiency occurs in 1 in 10,000 individuals, making it one of the most common inherited complement deficiencies.[44,45] Its clinical manifestations vary and include a variety of rheumatic disorders and an increased susceptibility to infection.[4,5,44] In addition, there are some C2-deficient individuals who are asymptomatic.[4,5,44]

The most common clinical manifestation of C2 deficiency is lupus, most commonly either SLE or discoid lupus.[4,5,44] Although patients with C2 deficiency manifest many of the typical clinical features of lupus, severe nephritis, cerebritis, and aggressive arthritis are less common, whereas photosensitive cutaneous lesions are more common. They also have a lower prevalence of anti-DNA antibodies than other patients with SLE, but the prevalence of anti-Ro and -La antibodies is higher.[16,17] Other rheumatic diseases have also been described in C2 deficiency and have included glomerulonephritis, inflammatory bowel disease, dermatomyositis, anaphylactoid purpura, and vasculitis.[4,5,44,46-48]

An increased susceptibility to infection is also a prominent clinical presentation of C2 deficiency.[7,8,44] The infections are usually caused by encapsulated pyogenic organisms such as *Pneumococcus, Streptococcus,* and *H. influenzae* and are blood borne, such as sepsis, meningitis, arthritis, and/or osteomyelitis.[4,5,49]

Molecular Genetic Basis

The majority of C2-deficient individuals (> 95%) have the same molecular genetic defect, a 28-bp deletion at the 3′ end of exon 6, which causes premature termination of transcription.[45,50] The deletion is associated with a conserved MHC haplotype consisting of *HLA-B18, C2*Q0, Bf*S, C4A*4, C4B*2,* and *Dr*2.*[45,50,51] As mentioned earlier, C2 deficiency is the most common of the genetically determined complement deficiencies; the gene frequency of this deletion is between 0.05 and 0.007 in individuals of European descent, which translates into a prevalence of homozygotes of approximately 1:10,000.[45,51] Two additional molecular genetic defects have been described in C2 deficiency but neither is nearly as common as the 28-bp deletion.[52,53]

C3 Deficiency

Molecular Biology and Pathophysiology

The third component of complement (C3) is encoded by a gene located on chromosome 19.[1] Like most complement components, the majority of serum C3 is derived from hepatic synthesis, although synthesis by monocytes, fibroblasts, endothelial cells, and epithelial cells may contribute to local tissue content of C3.[54] Whether activated by the classical or alternative pathways, C3 is cleaved into two fragments of unequal sizes. The smaller, C3a, is an anaphylatoxin, whereas the larger, C3b, is an opsonin and also forms part of the classical and alternative pathway enzymes that active C5 and the other terminal components. Thus C3 is not only critical in generating C3-mediated serum opsonizing and anaphylatoxic activities but also in generating the chemotactic and bactericidal activities of C5 through C9.

Patients with the deficiency usually have less than 1% of the normal level of C3 in their sera. Similarly, serum opsonic, chemotactic, and bactericidal activities are also markedly reduced.[3]

Clinical Expression

An increased susceptibility to infection is the most prominent clinical expression of C3 deficiency.[3-5] Patients tend to present with infections in childhood, and recurrent infections are relatively common. Although the most common infections are blood-borne infections caused by pyogenic bacteria such as *Pneumococcus, H. influenzae,* and *Meningococcus,* localized infections such as pneumonia and sinusitis have also been reported.[3-5]

Rheumatic diseases are also relatively common in patients with C3 deficiency.[3-5] Some patients have presented with a syndrome characterized by arthralgias and vasculitic skin rashes, whereas others have developed a clinical picture consistent with SLE. As with patients with deficiencies of other components of complement, they may not have the typical serologic findings of lupus.

Membranoproliferative glomerulonephritis has also been seen in patients with C3 deficiency.[3-5] The lesions are characterized by mesangial cell proliferation, an increase in the mesangial matrix, and electron-dense deposits in both the mesangium and subendothelium of the capillary loops. Immunofluorescent studies have revealed the presence of immunoglobulins in the kidney, and circulating immune complexes may be present in the serum, suggesting that membranoproliferative glomerulonephritis in these patients is the result of immune complex deposition.

Molecular Genetic Basis

The mutations responsible for C3 deficiency in humans have been diverse.[3,55,56] However, there is a relatively common 800-bp deletion found among Afrikaans-speaking South Africans (gene frequency of 0.0057) that has been responsible for C3 deficiency in at least one patient.[55,56]

C5 Deficiency

Molecular Biology and Pathophysiology

The gene encoding the fifth component of complement (C5) is on the short arm of chromosome 9.[1] When C5 is activated by either the classical or alternative pathways, it is cleaved into two fragments of unequal size. The smaller fragment, C5a, is a potent chemotactic fragment, and the larger, C5b, initiates assembly of the membrane attack complex, C5b through C9, and is responsible for bactericidal activity.

Affected individuals have markedly reduced levels of serum total hemolytic activity and C5. As expected, their sera are also unable to generate chemotactic or bactericidal activity.

Clinical Expression

The most common clinical expression of C5 deficiency is an increased susceptibility to systemic neisserial infections.[4,5] In addition, a small number of C5-deficient patients have presented with autoimmune disease.

Molecular Genetic Basis

The mutations causing C5 deficiency are diverse.[57]

C6 Deficiency

Molecular Biology and Pathophysiology

The genes for C6 and C7 are located near each other on the long arm of chromosome 5.[1] C6 participates in the formation of the membrane attack complex and therefore plays a critical role in the generation of bactericidal activity.

The usual form of C6 deficiency is characterized by absent total serum hemolytic activity and very low levels (< 1%) of serum C6. Another form of C6 deficiency, subtotal C6 deficiency (C6SD), is characterized by 1% to 2% of the normal levels of C6 and levels of total hemolytic activity that are reduced but present.[58]

Clinical Expression

C6 deficiency is one of the most common complement deficiencies.[4,5] Among African Americans in the United States, it is reported to be as common as 1:1600 individuals (0.062%).[59] It is thought to be uncommon among individuals of European descent. Like other terminal components, C6 deficiency is associated with systemic neisserial infections such as meningococcal sepsis or meningitis and disseminated gonococcal infections.[4,5]

Molecular Genetic Basis

The most common mutation causing C6 deficiency is a single base-pair deletion at position 879.[59,60] Interestingly, the mutations among African Americans are different from those in the African population.[59,60] C6SD is the result of a loss of the splice donor site of intron 15 and results in a truncated C6 that can support some lytic activity.[58]

C7 Deficiency

Molecular Biology and Pathophysiology

The genes for C6, C7, and C9, all members of the membrane attack complex, are clustered on the short arm of chromosome 5.[1] It participates in the formation of the membrane attack complex and therefore is critical to the generation of serum bactericidal activity.

Patients who are deficient in C7 have markedly reduced serum total hemolytic activity and C7 levels. As expected, their serum bactericidal activity is similarly reduced.

Clinical Expression

Like other patients with deficiencies of the terminal components (C5, C6, C7, C8, and C9), the most prominent clinical manifestation of C7 deficiency is an increased susceptibility to systemic neisserial infections.[4,5] A few patients have presented with SLE, rheumatoid arthritis, pyoderma gangrenosum, and scleroderma, but it is unclear whether these are pathophysiologically related to the C7 deficiency.

Molecular Genetic Basis

A number of different mutations are responsible for C7 deficiency.[61-64]

C8 Deficiency

Molecular Biology and Pathophysiology

Native C8 comprises three different polypeptide chains (α, β, and γ), which are encoded by separate genes (*C8A, C8B,* and *C8G*).[1] The genes *C8A* and *C8B* map to the short arm of chromosome 1, and the gene *C8G* maps to the long arm of chromosome 9.[1] The alpha and gamma chains are covalently linked to form one chain (C8 α,γ), which is joined to the C8 γ chain by noncovalent bonds. C8 is an integral part of the pore-forming membrane attack complex C5b-9 and as such plays a critical role in the generation of complement-mediated bactericidal activity.

There are several forms of C8 deficiency, and each is inherited as an autosomal recessive trait. In one form, patients lack the C8 β subunit, whereas in the other form the α,γ subunit is deficient.[65] In either form, total hemolytic activity is absent from the serum, as is functional C8 activity. However, some C8 antigen can usually be detected in C8 β deficiency because patients possess the C8 α,γ subunit. In contrast, patients with C8 α,γ deficiency usually have undetectable C8 antigen with standard immunochemical techniques. As expected, patients with either form of the deficiency have a marked reduction in serum bactericidal activity.[66,67]

Clinical Expression

Like deficiencies of other components of the membrane attack complex, systemic neisserial infections have been the predominant clinical presentation of C8 deficiency.[4,5,65]

Molecular Genetic Basis

Deficiency of C8 β is more common among individuals of European descent and C8 α,γ deficiency is more common among individuals of African descent. Approximately 86% of C8 β−null alleles are the result of C-to-T transition in exon 9, which results in the generation of a premature stop codon.[68-70] Only a limited number of patients with C8 α,γ deficiency have been examined, and in most instances an intronic mutation alters the splicing of exons 6 and 7 of the C8A chain and creates an insertion that generates a premature stop codon.[71]

C9 Deficiency

Molecular Biology and Pathophysiology

The gene for C9 is located on the short arm of chromosome 5, approximately 2.5 Mb from the genes for C6 and C7.[1] The protein product has sequence homology to other members of the membrane attack complex.

Affected individuals have markedly reduced levels of both C9 antigen and functional activity. However, the hemolysis of antibody-sensitized erythrocytes can occur with the insertion of a membrane attack complex lacking C9 (i.e., C5b-8) and thus is not strictly dependent on C9. Therefore patients with C9 deficiency have some total hemolytic activity, although it is reduced to between one third and one half of the lower limit of normal.[72,73] Similarly, their sera possess some bactericidal activity, although the rate of killing is significantly reduced.[74]

Clinical Expression

Genetically determined C9 deficiency is uncommon among Asians but is relatively common among individuals of Japanese descent, with a frequency of 1:1000.[75] As with patients with deficiencies of the other components of the membrane attack complex, individuals with C9 deficiency have an increased susceptibility to systemic neisserial infections.[4,5,76]

Molecular Genetic Basis

The common mutation among individuals of Japanese descent is a nonsense mutation in exon 4.[75]

C1 Esterase Inhibitor Deficiency

Molecular Biology and Pathophysiology

Inherited C1 esterase inhibitor (C1-INH) is encoded by a gene on the long arm of chromosome 11.[1] C1-INH binds covalently to C1r and C1s, leading to dissociation of the C1 macromolecular complex and inhibition of the enzymatic actions of C1r and C1s.

Genetically determined C1 esterase inhibitor deficiency is inherited as an autosomal dominant trait. In the most common form (type I), accounting for approximately 85% of the patients, the sera of affected individuals are deficient in both C1-INH protein (5% to 30% of normal) and C1-INH function.[77-80] In the other less common form (type II), a dysfunctional protein is present in normal or elevated concentrations, but the functional activity of C1-INH is markedly reduced.[77-80] The dysfunctional C1-INH molecules from different families differ not only from normal C1-INH but from each other with respect to their electrophoretic mobility, ability to bind C1s, and ability to inhibit both synthetic and natural substrates.[81-83] In patients with type I C1-INH deficiency, the diagnosis can be established easily by demonstrating a decrease in serum C1-INH protein when assessed by immunochemical techniques. However, in patients with type II C1-INH deficiency, the diagnosis must rest on demonstrating a decrease in C1-INH functional activity. In either case, C4 levels are usually reduced below the lower limit of normal both during and between attacks[79] because of its uncontrolled cleavage by C1s.

The levels of normal C1-INH function in patients with either type of hereditary angioedema (HAE) are lower than what might be expected in a hemizygote: 5% to 30% of normal in type I C1-INH deficiency and little or none in type II C1-INH deficiency. In addition, the immunochemical levels of the dysfunctional protein in the type II disorder may be higher than normal, rather than the expected 50% of normal. It has been suggested that in the type I disorder, the markedly lower levels of C1-INH are the result of both decreased synthesis and increased catabolism consequent to the complexing of the normal C1-INH with the activated enzymes that it normally inhibits. Similarly, it has been suggested that the low levels of normal C1-INH and elevated levels of dysfunctional C1-INH protein in the type II disorder are the result of decreased synthesis and increased catabolism of the normal C1-INH and, at least in some cases, decreased catabolism of the dysfunctional C1-INH consequent to its inability to complex with C1.[84]

The pathophysiologic mechanisms by which the absence of C1-INH activity leads to the angioedema characteristic of the disorder are still incompletely understood. In addition to its role in inhibiting C1, C1-INH is the major inhibitor of kallikrein, and therefore diminished levels of C1-INH lead to unregulated activation of the classical pathway and kallikrein after exposure to a mild trigger.[85-88] Bradykinin and C2a appear to be the primary mediators of the angioedema.[86]

Clinical Expression

C1-INH deficiency is responsible for the clinical disorder HAE.[77] The clinical symptoms of HAE are the result of submucosal or subcutaneous noninflammatory edema.[89] The three most prominent areas of involvement are the skin, upper respiratory tract, and gastrointestinal tract.[78,79]

Attacks involving the skin may involve an extremity, the face, or genitalia. In some instances, there may be changes just preceding the edema such as subtle mottling, a transient serpiginous erythema, or frank erythema marginatum. The edema usually expands outward from a single site and may vary in size from a few centimeters to the involvement of a whole extremity. The lesions are pale rather than red, are not usually warm, and are characteristically nonpruritic. However, early in the development of the lesion, there may be a feeling of tightness in the skin because of the accumulation of subcutaneous fluid. Attacks usually progress for 1 to 2 days and resolve over an additional 2 to 3 days.

Attacks involving the upper respiratory tract represent a significant cause of morbidity, and occasionally death, in patients with HAE. In one series published in 1976, pharyngeal edema had occurred at least once in nearly two thirds of the patients.[79] The patient may initially experience a "tightness" in the throat; swelling of the tongue, buccal mucosa, and oropharynx follows. In some instances, laryngeal edema, accompanied by hoarseness and stridor, occurs and progresses to respiratory obstruction; this is a life-threatening emergency. In fact, in that same series, tracheotomies had been performed in 1 of every 6 patients with HAE.[79]

Symptoms in the gastrointestinal tract are related to edema of the bowel wall and may include anorexia, dull aching of the abdomen, vomiting, and, in some cases, crampy abdominal pain. Abdominal symptoms are often prominent in childhood and can occur in the absence of concurrent cutaneous or pharyngeal involvement. In some instances, abdominal symptoms may be the only ones the patient has ever had, leading to difficulty in diagnosis.

Although the onset of symptoms occurs in more than half of the patients before adolescence,[78,79] in some patients their first symptoms do not occur until they are well into adult life. However, in just over half of the patients, no specific events can be clearly identified as initiating attacks, anxiety, or stress, as is frequently cited.[78,79] Dental extractions and tonsillectomy can initiate edema of the upper airway, and cutaneous edema may follow trauma to an extremity. Some patients report attacks after the use of tight-fitting clothing or shoes, whereas others have related cold exposure to the onset of symptoms.

Molecular Genetic Defect

The division of C1-INH deficiency into two categories based on the presence or absence of a dysfunctional protein has no correlation with clinical phenotype and only limited correlation with genotype because there are some examples of C1-INH mutations in which a dysfunctional protein is produced but is degraded so rapidly that it is not detectable in the serum.

Alu-mediated deletions and duplications account for the most common C1-INH−null genotypes.[90,91] The *C1-INH* gene contains a total of 17 *Alu*-repetitive DNA elements, and these are responsible for most of the gene rearrangements leading to *C1-INH* deficiency. A variety of single-base changes and smaller deletions and duplications have also been identified.[90] Most patients with type II HAE deficiency have a mutation that interferes with the reactive center arginine residue. The other mutations identified in patients with a dysfunctional protein are usually found in the hinge region, thereby inactivating the *C1-INH*.[90]

Factor I Deficiency

Molecular Biology and Pathophysiology

The gene for factor I is located on the long arm of chromosome 4.[1] Factor I is a serine protease that cleaves C3b to produce iC3b, an inactive cleavage product that cannot function in the C3-cleaving enzyme of the alternative pathway.

Patients with factor I deficiency have uncontrolled activation of C3 via the alternative pathway.[92,93] There is normally a continuous low-grade generation of the alternative pathway C3-cleaving enzyme, C3b,Bb, which is inhibited by factor I. In the absence of factor I, there is no control imposed on the formation and expression of the alternative pathway C3-cleaving enzyme, and as a result there is the continued activation and cleavage and activation of C3.[90,92] Patients with factor I deficiency therefore have a secondary consumption of native C3 with markedly reduced levels of both antigenic and functional C3 in their sera and a corresponding decrease in serum opsonic, bactericidal, and chemotactic activity.[92,93]

Clinical Expression

The most common clinical expression of factor I deficiency has been an increased susceptibility to infection.[4,5,93] Like patients with C3 deficiency, factor I−deficient patients have infections caused by encapsulated pyogenic bacteria, such as *Streptococcus*, *Pneumococcus*, *Meningococcus*, and *H. influenzae*, organisms for which C3 is an important opsonic ligand. Also, like patients with C3 deficiency, some patients have had elevated levels of circulating immune complexes. In fact, there has been one report of a transient illness resembling serum sickness characterized by fever, rash, arthralgia, hematuria, and proteinuria.[94]

Molecular Genetic Defect

The molecular genetic basis for factor I deficiency has been identified in only a few patients and was found to be diverse.[95]

Properdin Deficiency

Molecular Biology and Pathophysiology

Properdin is the only gene of the complement system that is encoded on the X chromosome.[1] Properdin stabilizes the alternative pathway C3 and C5 convertases by extending the half-lives of the C3 and C5 converting enzymes.

Properdin deficiency is inherited as an X-linked recessive trait. It has been divided into three subtypes based on protein phenotypes. Type I properdin deficiency has no detectable properdin in the serum, type II deficiency has detectable but reduced levels of properdin, and type III deficiency, identified in a single family, is associated with normal serum levels of properdin protein but absent function. Patients with properdin deficiency have absent function of the alternative pathway. Similarly, serum bactericidal activity for some strains of meningococci is reduced in properdin-deficient serum.

Clinical Expression

Approximately 50% of the patients described with properdin deficiency have had systemic meningococcal disease.[4,5] Isolated cases of SLE and discoid lupus are also seen in properdin-deficient patients.

Molecular Genetic Basis

The mutations responsible for properdin deficiency are diverse. The patients who produce no detectable properdin typically have early stop codons,[96,97] whereas the patients who produce some properdin have missense mutations or splicing defects.[96,97] The single kindred with dysfunctional properdin had a single base-pair substitution, which affected binding to C3.[98]

MANAGEMENT OF GENETICALLY DETERMINED COMPLEMENT DEFICIENCIES

Prevention of Infectious Diseases

Two strategies have been attempted to reduce susceptibility to infections and/or modify the clinical course of the infections in patients with genetically determined deficiencies of complement.

One strategy is to immunize these patients against common bacterial pathogens such as *Pneumococcus, H. influenzae,* and *Meningococcus.* Unfortunately, because the complement system participates in the generation of a normal immune response,[99] complement-deficient patients may not respond as well as complement-sufficient hosts.[100] Another limitation to the use of immunization in complement-deficient patients is that the vaccines may not include all of the serotypes to which complement-deficient patients are susceptible. For example, the new pneumococcal conjugate vaccine is limited to seven serotypes, and the meningococcal vaccine contains only serotypes A, C, Y, and W.

A second strategy in the prevention of infection is the use of prophylactic antibiotics. Because patients with complement deficiencies have a high risk of recurrent episodes of blood-borne infections and because immunizations may not afford them complete protection, some patients have been placed on antibiotic prophylaxis. However, any recommendation for antibiotic prophylaxis must be viewed in the context of the emergence of antibiotic resistance among bacteria.

Management of Rheumatic Disorders

Regardless of the rheumatologic disorder, it is most often treated with the same immunosuppressive agents and antiinflammatory medications as one would use in a complement-sufficient patient.

Management of Angioedema

The treatment of C1-INH deficiency is different from that of other complement deficiencies in that there are specific measures available to ameliorate symptoms and to prevent recurrence. In some patients, their episodes of angioedema may be sufficiently frequent or difficult to manage to justify long-term prophylaxis. Attenuated androgens such as stanozolol or danazol are highly effective[101] and act by increasing transcription of the normal allele of *C1INH.*[102] However, because of their androgenic effects, their use in children is very limited. Another class of agents used for long-term prophylaxis is the antifibrinolytic agents.[103,104] Tranexamic acid and aminocaproic acid act by blocking plasmin generation. Although their efficacy is less than that of attenuated androgens, the incidence of side effects is also less than that of attenuated androgens. For this reason, these agents may be preferred in childhood.

In some instances, patients may require short-term prophylaxis for surgery or oral procedures. Attenuated andro-

gens, fibrinolytic agents, fresh frozen plasma, and C1 esterase concentrate have all been used successfully for short-term prophylaxis.[102]

C1 esterase inhibitor concentrate is the most effective agent for the treatment of acute attacks.[102,105] However, it is not yet approved for use in the United States, and its use is usually restricted to life-threatening situations. Epinephrine, antihistamines, and corticosteroids are of no proven benefit in C1-INH−deficient patients.

SECONDARY COMPLEMENT DEFICIENCIES

Secondary complement deficiencies are relatively common. Any pathologic process that results in activation of the complement cascade or interferes with the synthesis of complement components can result in a secondary complement deficiency.

The Newborn

In full-term infants, the levels of most components of either the classical or alternative pathways are 50% to 80% of adult levels.[106] However, both C8 and C9 seem to be more severely depressed, with levels in full-term newborn infants as low as 28% and 10%, respectively, of maternal levels.[107,108] The serum levels of individual components of complement in premature infants have also been studied. Significant levels of C4, C3, C7, C9, factor B, properdin, and C1 esterase inhibitor have been detected in fetal serum as early as the end of the first trimester or the beginning of the second trimester.[106-112] There is a general tendency for levels of these components to increase with age, and their levels in premature infants generally correlate with gestational age.[106-116]

Because many of the components of complement are reduced in neonatal sera, those serum activities that depend on the complement system, such as serum opsonic and chemotactic activities, are also reduced.[117-120] It has not always been possible to ascribe the deficient opsonizing or chemotactic activity found in the sera of newborn infants solely to a deficient complement system because deficiencies in other humoral factors, such as IgM, that are important in the generation of these activities may contribute as well.

Nephrotic Syndrome

Children with the idiopathic nephrotic syndrome have an increased susceptibility to pneumococcal peritonitis and sepsis. Although they are susceptible at any point in their illness, they are at greatest risk when they are in relapse and spilling large amounts of protein, such as factor B, in their urine. Their serum-opsonizing activity is reduced, and when factor B is added back to their sera, the defect is corrected,[121] suggesting that loss of factor B in the urine is responsible for their deficient opsonizing activity and thus may contribute to their increased susceptibility to infection.

Systemic Lupus Erythematosus and Other Rheumatologic Disorders

SLE is a systemic disorder in which immune complexes are generated and deposited in end organs, leading to the classical pathologic changes in lupus. The immune complexes may activate the complement cascade, especially the classical pathway, leading to consumption of individual components such as C3 and C4. The activation of the complement system typically precedes clinical flare, and the degree of hypocomplementemia, specifically levels of C3 and C4, generally reflects the degree of clinical activity.[122-124]

Although complement activation as a result of the circulating immune complexes is particularly characteristic of lupus, it has also been described in juvenile rheumatoid arthritis, Sjögren's syndrome, a variety of vasculitides, and mixed connective tissue disease. Hypocomplementemia as a result of immune complex formation is seen less frequently in inflammatory bowel disease, sarcoidosis, Behçet's syndrome, and myasthenia gravis.

Serum Sickness

Serum sickness is the consequence of immune complex formation in response to the administration of drugs (e.g., penicillin, cefaclor, and minocycline), foreign proteins (e.g., antithymocyte globulin, therapeutic monoclonal antibodies, or antivenoms), or, in some instances, infections.[125,126] Although rash, fever, and arthralgia/arthritis are the most common clinical findings, severe cases may progress to renal involvement.[127] Immune complexes are present in the circulation early in the process. Most cases have significant hypocomplementemia, and when it occurs it is characterized by low CH_{50}, C3, and C4 levels.[128]

Sepsis

Acute bacterial sepsis, specifically gram-negative sepsis, may be associated with transient hypocomplementemia. Generally, the hypocomplementemia reflects activation of both the alternative and classical pathways and is characterized by low levels of C3 and C4, as well as total hemolytic activity (CH_{50}) and the generation of the cleavage products, C3a and C5a.[129-131] The hypocomplementemia is most commonly found in patients who have some degree of cardiovascular compromise and is strongly correlated with the severity of the shock and morbidity.

Cirrhosis

Patients with cirrhosis have decreased serum concentrations of C3, C4, and total hemolytic activity.[132-134] The presence of decreased levels of C3 and C4 correlates with the degree of liver decompensation and levels of serum proteins synthesized in the liver, such as albumin and certain coagulation factors, suggesting that decreased hepatic synthesis is the basis for the decreased levels of C4 and C3. There is a correlation between the low levels of C3 and a predisposition to spontaneous bacterial peritonitis and mortality in cirrhosis.[135,136]

Cardiopulmonary Bypass, Extracorporeal Membrane Oxygenation, and Hemodialysis

A variety of therapeutic maneuvers, such as cardiopulmonary bypass, extracorporeal membrane oxygenation, and hemodialysis, bring the patient's blood in contact with artificial surfaces or membranes. As a result, there may be activation of the complement system with concurrent decreases of

BOX 11-1	**KEY CONCEPTS**
	Clinical Presentation of Complement Deficiencies

- Increased susceptibility to infection
- Rheumatic disorders
- Angioedema
- Specific illness depends on which complement component is involved

individual components, such as C3, and of total hemolytic complement.[137,138] As a consequence of the activation of the complement system, there also is generation of biologically active cleavage products, such as C3a and C5a. A number of studies have suggested that the generation of these anaphylatoxins is responsible for the generalized inflammatory response that follows cardiopulmonary bypass (postperfusion syndrome) and hemodialysis (pulmonary neutrophil sequestration).[137-139]

Malnutrition

Children with malnutrition, both kwashiorkor and marasmus, have decreased levels of serum total hemolytic complement activity as well as most of the individual components of complement, such as C3 and C5.[140] Dietary treatment of the malnutrition results in normalization of the complement levels. The degree of the decrease in complement components, such as C3, correlates strongly with serum albumin, suggesting that the decrease is the result of poor synthetic function in the liver.

CONCLUSIONS

Complement represents a bridge between innate and adaptive immunity. It is important for the phagocytosis of immune complexes, mainly through the fixation of C1-C4-C32-C3; for antibody-independent opsonization of bacteria via alternate pathway–mediated fixation and activation of C3; for lysis of bacteria via activation of the late complement components C5 to C9; for solubilizing immune complexes; and for elimination of apoptotic cells. Complement deficiencies manifest themselves either as susceptibility to recurrent infections or as susceptibility to autoimmune/immune complex–mediated diseases (Box 11-1). Deficiencies of early components of the classical complement cascade C1, C2, C4, and C3 are associated with both autoimmune/immune complex diseases and susceptibility to infections. Deficiencies of components of the alternate pathway (factor I and properdin) and of late components of the complement system C5 to C9 and of components of the alternate complement pathway are associated with only susceptibility to infections, primarily to neisserial infections in the case of deficiency of C5 through C9. The diagnosis of a complement component deficiency must be entertained in all cases with recurrent bacterial and viral infections that resemble in their presentations antibody deficiency syndromes, particularly in the face of elevated or upper-range levels of serum immunoglobulins and adequate antibody titers. The diagnosis of a deficiency in the early components of the classical complement cascade must be entertained in all cases of rheumatic diseases, particularly in cases presenting as SLE, discoid lupus, or vasculitis and if they are associated with increased incidence of infections. A diagnosis of deficiency of the complement regulatory protein C1 esterase inhibitor must be considered in cases of nonitching angioedema in the absence of urticaria, particularly in the presence of a similar family history and in cases precipitated by trauma.

REFERENCES

1. Sullivan KE, Winkelstein JA: Genetically determined deficiencies of complement. In Scriver CR, Beaudet AL, Sly WS, et al, eds: *Metabolic basis of inherited disease*, ed 8, New York, 2001, McGraw-Hill Book.
2. Winkelstein JA: Complement and natural immunity, *Clin Allergy Immunol* 3:421-428, 1983.
3. Singer L, Colten HR, Wetsel RA: Complement C3 deficiency: human, animal, and experimental models, *Pathobiology* 62:14-28, 1994.
4. Figueroa JE, Densen P: Infectious diseases associated with complement deficiencies, *Clin Microb Rev* 4:359-395, 1991.
5. Ross SC, Densen P: Complement deficiency states and infection: epidemiology, pathogenesis and consequences of neisserial and other infections in an immune deficiency, *Medicine* 63:243-273, 1984.
6. Ellison RT, Kohler PH, Curd JG, et al: Prevalence of congenital and acquired complement deficiency in patients with sporadic meningococcal disease, *N Engl J Med* 308:913-916, 1983.
7. Merino J, Rodriguez-Valverde V, Lamelas JA: Prevalence of deficits of complement components in patients with recurrent meningococcal infections, *J Infect Dis* 148:331-336, 1983.
8. Leggiadro RJ, Winkelstein JA: Prevalence of complement deficiencies in children with systemic meningococcal infections, *Pediatr Infect Dis* 6:75-79, 1987.
9. Fijen CA, Juijper EJ, Hannema AJ, et al: Complement deficiencies in patients over ten years old with meningococcal disease due to uncommon serogroups, *Lancet* 2:585-588, 1989.
10. Nielsen HE, Koch C, Magnussen P, et al: Complement deficiencies in selected groups of patients with meningococcal disease, *Scand J Infect Dis* 21:389-396, 1989.
11. Schifferli JA, Bartolotti SR, Peters DK: Inhibition of immune precipitation by complement, *Clin Exp Immunol* 42:387-394, 1980.
12. Schifferli JA, Steiger G, Hauptmann G, et al: Formation of soluble immune complexes by complement in sera of patients with various hypocomplementemic states, *J Clin Invest* 76:2127-2133, 1985.
13. Cornacoff JB, Hebert LA, Smead WL, et al: Primate erythrocyte-immune complex-clearing mechanism, *J Clin Invest* 71:236-247, 1983.
14. Botto M, Dell'Agnola C, Bygrave AE, et al: Homozygous C1q deficiency causes glomerulonephritis associated with multiple apoptotic bodies, *Nat Genet* 19:56-59, 1998.
15. Navratil JS, Ahearn JM: Apoptosis and autoimmunity: complement deficiency and systemic lupus erythematosus revisited, *Curr Rheumatol Rep* 2:32-38, 2000.
16. Provost TT, Arnett FC, Reichlin M: Homozygous C2 deficiency, lupus erythematosus, and anti-Ro (SSA) antibodies, *Arthritis Rheum* 26:1279-1282, 1983.
17. Meyer O, Hauptmann G, Tappeiner G, et al: Genetic deficiency of C4, C2 or C1q and lupus syndromes: association with anti-Ro (SS-A) antibodies, *Clin Exp Immunol* 62:678-684, 1985.
18. Bowness P, Davies KA, Norsworthy PJ, et al: Hereditary C1q deficiency and systemic lupus erythematosus, *Q J Med* 87:455-464, 1994.
19. Hauptmann G, Tappeiner G, Schifferli JA: Inherited deficiency of the fourth complement, *Immunodefic Rev* 1:3-22, 1988.
20. Sellar GC, Blake DJ, Reid KBM. Characterization and organization of the genes encoding the A-, B-, and C-chains of human complement subcomponent C1q, *Biochem J* 274:481-490, 1991.
21. Loos M, Heinz HP: Component deficiencies. 1. The first component: C1q, C1r, C1s, *Prog Allergy* 39:212-231, 1986.
22. Petry F: Molecular basis of hereditary C1q deficiency, *Immunobiology* 199:286-294, 1998.
23. Petry F, Berkel AI, Loos M: Repeated identification of a nonsense mutation in the C1qA-gene of deficient patients in South-East Europe, *Mol Immunol* 33(suppl 1):9, 1996.
24. Berkel AI, Birben E, Oner C, et al: Molecular, genetic and epidemiologic studies on selective complete C1q deficiency in Turkey, *Immunobiology* 201:347-355, 2000.
25. Petry F, Le DT, Kirschfink M, et al: Nonsense and missense mutations in the structural genes of complement component C1q A and C chains are linked with two different types of complete selective C1q deficiencies, *J Immunol* 155:4734-4738, 1995.
26. Awdeh ZL, Alper CA: Inherited structural polymorphism of the fourth component of human complement, *Proc Natl Acad Sci U S A* 77:3576-3580, 1978.
27. Clark RA, Klebanoff SJ: Role of the classical and alternative complement pathways in chemotaxis and opsonization: studies of human serum deficient in C4, *J Immunol* 120:1102-1108, 1978.
28. Mascart-Lemone F, Hauptmann G, Goetz J, et al: Genetic deficiency of C4 presenting with recurrent infections and a SLE-like disease, *Am J Med* 75:295-304, 1983.
29. Isenman DE, Young JR: The molecular basis for the difference in immune hemolysis activity of the Chido and Rogers isotypes of human complement component C4, *J Immunol* 132:3019-3027, 1984.
30. Christiansen FT, Dawkins RL, Uko G, et al: Complement allotyping in SLE: association with C4A null, *Aust N Z J Med* 13:483-488, 1983.
31. Fielder AHL, Walport MJ, Batchelor JR, et al: Family study of the major histocompatibility complex in patients with systemic lupus erythematosus: importance of null alleles of C4A and C4B in determining disease susceptibility, *Br Med J* 286:425-428, 1983.
32. Howard PF, Hochberg MC, Bias B, et al: Relationship between C4 null genes, HLA-D region antigens, and genetic susceptibility to systemic lupus erythematosus in Caucasian and Black Americans, *Am J Med* 81:187-192, 1986.
33. Petri M, Watson R, Winkelstein JA, et al: Clinical expression of systemic lupus erythematosus in patients with C4A deficiency, *Medicine* 72:236-244, 1993.
34. Welch TR, Brickman C, Bishof N, et al: The phenotype of SLE associated with complete deficiency of complement isotype C4A, *J Clin Immunol* 18:48-51, 1998.
35. Rowe PC, McLean RH, Wood RA, et al: Association of C4B deficiency with bacterial meningitis, *J Infect Dis* 160:448-451, 1989.
36. Biskof NA, Welch TR, Beischel LS: C4B deficiency: a risk factor for bacteremia with encapsulated organisms, *J Infect Dis* 162:248, 1990.
37. Kemp ME, Atkinson JP, Skanes VM, et al: Deletion of C4A genes in patients with systemic lupus erythematosus, *Arthritis Rheum* 30:1015-1022, 1987.
38. Barba G, Rittner C, Schneider PM: Genetic basis of human complement C4A deficiency, *J Clin Invest* 91:1681-1686, 1993.
39. Braun L, Schneider PM, Giles CM, et al: Null alleles of human complement C4. Evidence for pseudogenes at the C4A locus and gene conversion at the C4B locus, *J Exp Med* 171:129-140, 1990.
40. Ruddy S, Klemperer MR, Rosen FS, et al: Hereditary deficiency of the second component of complement in man: correlation of C2 hemolytic activity with immunochemical measurements of C2 protein, *Immunology* 18:943-954, 1970.
41. Friend P, Repine J, Kim Y, et al: Deficiency of the second component of complement (C2) with chronic vasculitis, *Ann Intern Med* 83:813-816, 1975.
42. Geibink GS, Verhoef J, Peterson PK, et al: Opsonic requirements for phagocytosis of *Streptococcus pneumoniae* types VI, XVIII, XXIII and XXV, *Infect Immun* 18:291-297, 1977.
43. Repine JE, Clawson CC, Friend PS: Influence of a deficiency of the second component of complement on the bactericidal activity of neutrophils in vitro, *J Clin Invest* 59:802-809, 1977.
44. Ruddy S: Component deficiencies: the second component, *Prog Allergy* 39:250-266, 1986.
45. Sullivan KE, Petri M, McLean R, et al: Prevalence of a mutation which causes C2 deficiency in a population of patients with SLE, *J Rheum* 21:1128-1133, 1994.
46. Gelfand EW, Clarkson JE, Minta JO: Selective deficiency of the second component of complement in a patient with anaphylactoid purpura, *Clin Immunol Immunopathol* 4:269-276, 1975.
47. Leddy JP, Griggs RC, Klemperer MR, et al: Hereditary complement (C2) deficiency with dermatomyositis, *Am J Med* 58:83-91, 1975.
48. Perlemuter G, Chassada S, Soubrane O, et al: Multifocal stenosing ulcerations of the small intestine revealing vasculitis associated with C2 deficiency, *Gastroenterology* 110:1628-1632, 1996.
49. Fasano MB, Hamosh A, Winkelstein JA: Recurrent systemic bacterial infections in homozygous C2 deficiency, *Pediatr Allergy Immunol* 1:46-49, 1990.
50. Johnson CA, Densen P, Hurford R, et al: Type I human complement C2 deficiency: a 28-base pair gene deletion causes skipping of exon 6 during RNA splicing, *J Biol Chem* 267:9347-9353, 1992.

51. Truedsson L, Alper CA, Awdeh ZL, et al: Characterization of type I complement C2 deficiency MHC haplotypes. Strong conservation of the complotype/HLA-B region and absence of disease association due to linked class II genes, *J Immunol* 151:5856-5863, 1993.

52. Wetsel RA, Kulics J, Lokki ML, et al: Type II human complement C2 deficiency. Allele-specific amino acid substitutions (Ser189-Phe; Gly444-Arg) cause impaired C2 secretion, *J Biol Chem* 271:5824-5831, 1996.

53. Wang X, Circolo A, Lokki ML, et al: Molecular heterogeneity in deficiency of complement protein C2 type I, *Immunology* 93:184-191, 1998.

54. Colten HR: Tissue specific regulation of inflammation, *J Appl Physiol* 72:1-7, 1992.

55. Botto M, Fong KY, So AK, et al: Homozygous hereditary C3 deficiency due to a partial gene deletion, *Proc Natl Acad Sci U S A* 89:4957-4961, 1992.

56. Botto M, Fong KY, So AK, et al: Molecular basis of hereditary C3 deficiency, *J Clin Invest* 86:1158-1163, 1990.

57. Wang X, Fleischer DT, Whitehead WT, et al: Inherited human complement C5 deficiency. Nonsense mutations in exons 1 (Gln1 to Stop) and 36 (Arg1458 to Stop) and compound heterozygosity in three African-American families, *J Immunol* 154:5464-5471, 1995.

58. Wurzner R, Hobart MJ, Fernie BA, et al: Molecular basis of subtotal complement C6 deficiency, *J Clin Invest* 95:1877-1883, 1995.

59. Zhu Z, Atkinson TP, Hovanky KT, et al: High prevalence of complement component C6 deficiency among African-Americans in the south-eastern USA, *Clin Exp Immunol* 119:305-310, 2000.

60. Hobart MJ, Fernie BA, Fijen KA, et al: The molecular basis of C6 deficiency in the western Cape, South Africa, *Hum Genet* 103:506-512, 1998.

61. Fernie BA, Orren A, Sheehan G, et al: Molecular bases of C7 deficiency. Three different defects, *J Immunol* 159:1019-1026, 1997.

62. Fernie BA, Hobart MJ: Complement C7 deficiency: seven further molecular defects and their associated marker haplotypes, *Hum Genet* 103:513-519. 1998.

63. Horiuchi T, Ferrer JM, Serra P, et al: A novel nonsense mutation at Glu-631 in a Spanish family with complement component 7 deficiency, *J Hum Genet* 44:215-218, 1999.

64. Nishizaka H, Horiuchi T, Zhu Z-B, et al: Genetic bases of human complement C7 deficiency, *J Immunol* 157:4239-4243, 1996.

65. Tedesco F: Component deficiencies. 8. The eighth component, *Prog Allergy* 39:295-306, 1986.

66. Jasin HE: Absence of the eighth component of complement in association with systemic lupus erythematosus-like disease, *J Clin Invest* 60:709-715, 1977.

67. Nicholson A, Lepow I: Host defense against *Neisseria meningitidis* requires a complement-dependent bactericidal activity, *Science* 205:298-299, 1979.

68. Kaufmann T, Hansch G, Rittner C, et al: Genetic basis of human complement C8 beta deficiency, *J Immunol* 150:4943-4947, 1993.

69. Saucedo L, Ackermann L, Platonov AE, et al: Delineation of additional genetic basis for C8β deficiency, *J Immunol* 155:5022-5028, 1995.

70. Kotnik V, Luznik-Bufon T, Schneider PM, et al: Molecular, genetic and functional analysis of homozygous C8 b-chain deficiency in two siblings, *Immunopharmacology* 38:215-221, 1997.

71. Densen P, Ackerman L: The genetic basis of C8α-γ deficiency, *Mol Immunol* S1:68, 1996.

72. Inai S, Kitamura H, Hiramatsu S, et al: Deficiency of the ninth component of complement in man, *J Clin Lab Immunol* 2:85-87, 1979.

73. Lint TF, Zeitz HJ, Gewurz H: Inherited deficiency of the ninth component of complement in man, *J Immunol* 125:2252-2257, 1980.

74. Harriman GR, Esser AF, Podack ER, et al: The role of C9 in complement-mediated killing of *Neisseria*, *J Immunol* 127:2386-2390, 1981.

75. Horiuchi T, Neshizaka H, Jojima T, et al: A nonsense mutation at Arg 95 is predominant in C9 deficiency in Japanese, *J Immunol* 160:1509-1513, 1998.

76. Lint TF, Gewurz H: Component deficiencies. 9. The ninth component, *Prog Allergy* 39:307-310, 1986.

77. Donaldson VH, Evans RR: A biochemical abnormality in hereditary angioneurotic edema. Absence of serum inhibitor of C1-esterase, *Am J Med* 35:37-43, 1963.

78. Cicardi M, Bergamaschini L, Marasini B, et al: Hereditary angioedema: an appraisal of 104 cases, *Am J Med Sci* 284:2-9, 1982.

79. Frank MM, Gelfand JA, Atkinson JP: Hereditary angioedema: the clinical syndrome and its management, *Ann Intern Med* 84:580-593, 1976.

80. Rosen FS, Charache P, Pensky J, et al: Hereditary angioneurotic edema: Two genetic variants, *Science* 148:957-965, 1965.

81. Rosen FS, Alper CA, Pensky J, et al: Genetically determined heterogeneity of the C1 esterase inhibitor in patients with hereditary angioneurotic edema, *J Clin Invest* 50:2143-2149, 1971.

82. Donaldson VH, Harrison RA, Rosen FS, et al: Variability in purified dysfunctional C1-inhibitor proteins from patients with hereditary angioneurotic edema. Functional and analytical gel studies, *J Clin Invest* 75:124-132, 1985.

83. Harpel PC, Hugli TE, Cooper NR: Studies on human plasma C1 inactivator-enzyme interactions, II: structural features of an abnormal C1 inactivator from a kindred with hereditary angioneurotic edema, *J Clin Invest* 55:605-611, 1975.

84. Lachmann PJ, Rosen FS: The catabolism of C1(−)inhibitor and the pathogenesis of hereditary angio-edema, *Acta Pathol Microbiol Immunol Scand* 92:35-39, 1984.

85. Klemperer MR, Donaldson VH, Rosen FS: Effect of C1 esterase on vascular permeability in man: studies in normal and complement-deficient individuals and in patients with hereditary angioneurotic edema, *J Clin Invest* 47:604-611, 1968.

86. Curd JG, Progais LJ Jr, Cochrane CG: Detection of active kallikrein in induced blister fluids of hereditary angioedema patients, *J Exp Med* 152:742-747, 1980.

87. Schapira M, Silver LD, Scott CF, et al: Prekallikrein activation and high-molecular-weight kininogen consumption in hereditary angioedema, *N Engl J Med* 308:1050-1053, 1983.

88. Schreiber AD, Kaplan AP, Austen KF: Inhibition by C1INH of Hageman factor fragment activation of coagulation, fibrinolysis, and kinin generation, *J Clin Invest* 52:1402-1409, 1973.

89. Sheffer AL, Craig JM, Willims-Kretschmer K, et al: Histopathological and ultrastructural observations on tissues from patients with hereditary angioneurotic edema, *J Allergy* 47:292-297, 1971.

90. Davis AE III, Bissler JJ, Cicardi M: Mutations in the C1 inhibitor gene that result in hereditary angioneurotic edema, *Behring Inst Mitt* 93:313-320, 1993.

91. Stoppa-Lyonnet D, Duponchel C, Meo T, et al: Recombinational biases in the rearranged C1-inhibitor genes of hereditary angioedema patients, *Am J Hum Genet* 49:1055-1062, 1991.

92. Abramson N, Alper CA, Lachmann PJ, et al: Deficiency of C3 inactivator in man, *J Immunol* 107:19-27, 1971.

93. Vyse TJ, Spath PJ, Davies KA, et al: Hereditary complement factor I deficiency, *Q J Med* 87:385-401, 1994.

94. Solal-Celigny P, Laviolette M, Hebert J, et al: C3b inactivator deficiency with immune complex manifestations, *Clin Exp Immunol* 47:197-205, 1982.

95. Vyse TJ, Morley BJ, Bartok I, et al: The molecular basis of hereditary complement factor I deficiency, *J Clin Invest* 97:925-933, 1996.

96. Westberg J, Nordin G, Fredrikson N, et al: Sequence-based analysis of properdin deficiency: identification of point mutations in two phenotypic forms of an X-linked immunodeficiency, *Genomics* 29:1-8, 1995.

97. Spath PJ, Sjoholm AG, Fredrikson GN, et al: Properdin deficiency in a large Swiss family: identification of a stop codon in the properdin gene, and association of meningococcal disease with lack of the IgG2 allotype marker G2m(n), *Clin Exp Immunol* 118:278-284, 1999.

98. Fredrikson GN, Westberg J, Kuijper EJ, et al: Molecular genetic characterization of properdin deficiency type III: dysfunction due to a single point mutation in exon 9 of the structural gene causing a tyrosine to aspartic acid interchange, *Mol Immunol* 33(suppl 1):1, 1996.

99. Carroll MC, Fisher MB: Complement and the immune response, *Curr Opin Immunol* 9:64, 1997.

100. Biselli R, Casapollo I, D'Amelio R, et al: Antibody response to meningococcal polysaccharides A and C in patients with complement defects, *Scand J Immunol* 37:644-650, 1993.

101. Gelfand JA, Sherins RJ, Alling DW, et al: Treatment of hereditary angioedema with danazol: reversal of clinical and biochemical abnormalities, *N Engl J Med* 295:1444-1448, 1976.

102. Agostoni A, Cicardi M, Cugno M, et al: Clinical problems in the C1-inhibitor deficient patient, *Behring Inst Mitt* 93:306-312, 1993.

103. Frank MM, Sergent JS, Kane MA, et al: Epsilon aminocaproic acid therapy of hereditary angioneurotic edema: a double blind study, *N Engl J Med* 286:808-812, 1972.

104. Sheffer AL, Austen KF, Rosen FS: Tranexamic acid therapy in hereditary angioneurotic edema, *N Engl J Med* 287:452-454, 1972.

105. Waytes AT, Rosen RS, Frank MM: Treatment of hereditary angioedema with vapor-heated C1 inhibitor concentrate, *N Engl J Med* 334:1630-1634, 1996.

106. Johnston RB Jr, Altenburger KM, Atkinson AW Jr, et al: Complement in the newborn infant, *Pediatrics* 64:S781-S786, 1979.

107. Ballow M, Fang F, Good RA, et al: Developmental aspects of complement components in the newborn, *Clin Exp Immunol* 18:257-266, 1974.

108. Adinolfi M, Beck SE: Human complement C7 and C9 in fetal and newborn sera, *Arch Dis Child* 50:562-564, 1975.
109. Adinolfi M: Levels of two components of complement (C4 and C3) in human fetal and newborn sera, *Dev Med Child Neurol* 12:306-308, 1970.
110. Adinolfi M: Human complement: onset and site of synthesis during fetal life, *Am J Dis Child* 131:1015-1023, 1977.
111. Adinolfi M, Gardner B: Synthesis of B1E and B1C components of complement in human foetuses, *Acta Paediatr Scand* 56:450-454, 1967.
112. Gitlin D, Biasucci A: Development of gamma G, gamma A, gamma M, beta-1-C/beta-1-A, C1 esterase inhibitor, ceruloplasmin, transferrin, hemopexin, haptoglobin, fibrinogen, plasminogen, alpha$_1$ antitrypsin, orosomucoid, beta-lipoprotein, alpha$_2$ macroglobulin and prealbumin in the human conceptus, *J Clin Invest* 48:1433-1436, 1969.
113. Fireman P, Zuchowski DA, Taylor PM: Development of human complement system, *J Immunol* 103:25-31, 1969.
114. Adamkin D, Stitzel A, Urmson J, et al: Activity of the alternative pathway of complement in the newborn infant, *J Pediatr* 93:604-608, 1978.
115. Sawyer MK, Forman ML, Kuplic LS, et al: Developmental aspects of the human complement system, *Biol Neonate* 19:148-162, 1971.
116. Strunk RC, Fenton LF, Gaines JA: Alternative pathway of complement activation in full term and premature infants, *Pediatr Res* 13:641-643, 1979.
117. Dossett JH, Williams RC Jr, Quie PG: Studies on interaction of bacteria, serum factors and polymorphonuclear leukocytes in others and newborns, *Pediatrics* 44:49-57, 1969.
118. Forman ML, Stiehm ER: Impaired opsonic activity but normal phagocytosis in low birth weight infants, *N Engl J Med* 281:926-931, 1969.
119. McCracken GH Jr, Eichenwald HF: Leukocyte function and the development of opsonic and complement activity in the neonate, *Am J Dis Child* 121:120-126, 1971.
120. Marodi L, Leijh PCJ, Braat A, et al: Opsonic activity of cord blood sera against various species of microorganisms, *Pediatr Res* 19:433-436, 1985.
121. McLean RH, Forsgren A, Bjorksten B, et al: Decreased serum factor B concentration associated with decreased opsonization of *Escherichia coli* in the idiopathic nephrotic syndrome, *Pediatr Res* 11:910-916, 1977.
122. Buyon JP, Tamerius J, Belmont HM, et al: Assessment of disease activity and impending flare in patients with systemic lupus erythematosus. Comparison of the use of complement split products and conventional measurements of complement, *Arthritis Rheum* 35:1028-1036, 1992.
123. Lloyd W, Schur PH: Immune complexes, complement, and anti-DNA in exacerbations of systemic lupus erythematosus (SLE), *Medicine* 60:208-217, 1981.
124. Swaak AJG, Groenwold J, Bronsveld W: Predictive value of complement profiles and anti-ds DNA in systemic lupus erythematosus, *Ann Rheum Dis* 45:359-366, 1986.
125. Heckbert SR, Stryker WS, Coltin KL, et al: Serum sickness in children after antibiotic exposure: estimates of occurrence and morbidity in a health maintenance organization population, *Am J Epidemiol* 132:336-342, 1990.
126. Parshuram CS, Phillips RJ: Retrospective review of antibiotic-associated serum sickness in children presenting to a paediatric emergency department, *Med J Aust* 169:116, 1998.
127. Border WA, Noble NA: From serum sickness to cytokines: advances in understanding the molecular pathogenesis of kidney disease [editorial], *Lab Invest* 68:125-128, 1993.
128. Bielory L, Eascon P, Lawley TD, et al: Serum sickness and hematopoietic recovery with antithymocyte globulin in bone marrow failure patients, *Br J Haematol* 63:729-736, 1986.
129. Fearon DT, Ruddy S, Schur PH, et al: Activation of the properdin pathway of complement in patients with gram-negative bacteremia, *N Engl J Med* 292:937-940, 1975.
130. Fust G, Petras GY, Ujhelyi E: Activation of the complement system during infections due to gram-negative bacteria, *Clin Immunol Immunopathol* 5:293-302, 1976.
131. Sprung CL, Schultz DR, Marcial E, et al: Complement activation in septic shock patients, *Crit Care Med* 14:525-528, 1986.
132. Ellison RT III, Horsburgh R Jr, Curd J: Complement levels in patients with hepatic dysfunction, *Dig Dis Sci* 35:231-235, 1990.
133. Potter BJ, Trueman AM, Kones EA: Serum complement in chronic liver disease, *Gut* 14:451-456, 1973.
134. Potter BJ, Elias E, Fayers PM, et al: Profiles of serum complement in patients with hepatobiliary diseases, *Digestion* 18:371-383, 1978.
135. Andreu M, Sola R, Sitges-Serra A, et al: Risk factors for spontaneous bacterial peritonitis in cirrhotic patients with ascites, *Gastroenterology* 104:1133-1138, 1993.
136. Homann C, Varming K, Hogasen K, et al: Acquired C3 deficiency in patients with alcoholic cirrhosis predisposes to infection and increased mortality, *Gut* 40:544-549, 1997.
137. Chenoweth DE, Cooper SW, Hugli TE, et al: Complement activation during cardiopulmonary bypass, *N Engl J Med* 304:497-503, 1981.
138. Jacob HS, Craddock PR, Hammerschmidt DE, et al: Complement-induced granulocyte aggregation, an unsuspected mechanism of disease, *N Engl J Med* 302:789-794, 1980.
139. Hosea SW, Brown E, Hammer C, et al: Role of complement activation in a model of adult respiratory distress syndrome, *J Clin Invest* 66:375-382, 1980.
140. Sirisina S, Suskind R, Edelman R, et al: Complement and C3-proactivator levels in children with protein-calorie malnutrition and effect of dietary treatment, *Lancet* 1:1016-1020, 1973.

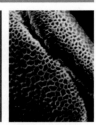

CHAPTER 12

White Blood Cell Defects

SERGIO D. ROSENZWEIG ■ STEVEN M. HOLLAND

White blood cells (WBCs) can be easily classified into lymphoid (T, B, and NK) and myeloid (neutrophils, eosinophils, basophils, and monocytes/macrophages) by virtue of their lineage-restricted progenitor origin. This chapter focuses especially on neutrophils and monocytes and the disorders that arise from their quantitative and functional defects.

Mature neutrophils develop in the bone marrow from a myeloid stem cell over about 14 days, during which time proliferation, differentiation, and maturation take place. Mature neutrophils, with their load of primary, secondary, and tertiary granules, are released into the bloodstream where they stay 6 to 10 hours before exiting by diapedesis to sites of inflammation. In the tissues they may work in ways that are primarily phagocytic, bactericidal or fungicidal or in the removal of damaged tissue.[1] Neutrophil disorders can be divided into quantitative disorders, marked typically by neutropenias, and functional disorders, marked by failures in specific metabolic or interactive pathways. Quantitative disorders include neutrophilia (> 7000 neutrophils per microliter in adult patients) and neutropenia (mild: < 1500 neutrophils per microliter, moderate: 1500 to 1000 neutrophils per microliter, severe: < 500 neutrophils per microliter). With very few exceptions (e.g., chronic idiopathic neutrophilia, leukocyte adhesion deficiencies, myeloproliferative diseases), neutrophilia is dependent on causes extrinsic to the neutrophils (e.g., acute or chronic infection, steroids, epinephrine). On the other hand, the causes of neutropenia are multiple and can be intrinsic or extrinsic to neutrophils or their progenitors (Table 12-1). Neutropenia usually falls into categories of decreased production or increased destruction or a combination of these two. Qualitative myeloid disorders include defects in motility (adhesion, chemotaxis), defects in phagocytosis, defects of granule synthesis and release, and defects in killing (see Table 12-1).

Neutropenia or a functional neutrophil disorder should be suspected in patients with recurrent, severe bacterial or fungal infections, especially those caused by unusual organisms (e.g., *Chromobacterium violaceum*) or in uncommon locations (e.g., liver abscess; Table 12-2). Viral and parasitic infections are not apparently increased in these patients, and should direct attention elsewhere. Initial laboratory evaluation for these patients should take into account the clinical presentation and a careful consideration of where the defect is likely to be. Some assays, such as repeated WBC counts with differentials or microscopic evaluation of neutrophils, are relatively simple and

can readily exclude certain disorders. Neutrophil or monocyte flow cytometric analysis requires a careful consideration of which markers to examine. Functional assays, such as oxidative burst testing, phagocytosis, or chemotaxis, are currently the most difficult because so few laboratories do them reliably or routinely (Table 12-3). Therefore careful consideration of the likely defect and mutation is crucial to guide intelligent and successful testing. We will consider some of the clinical, diagnostic, and management aspects of a few of the best characterized myeloid disorders.

Severe Congenital Neutropenia (Kostmann's Syndrome)

Severe congenital neutropenia (SCN), or Kostmann's syndrome, comprises a heterogeneous group of disorders with variable inheritance patterns that share the common characteristics of bone marrow granulocytic maturation arrest at the promyelocyte or myelocyte stage, severe chronic neutropenia (fewer than 200 neutrophils per microliter), and increased susceptibility to acute myeloid leukemia.

In 1956 Kostmann described a Swedish kindred with SCN inherited in an autosomal recessive pattern.[2]

Among patients with Kostmann's syndrome, single-allele mutations in the granulocyte colony-stimulating factor (G-CSF) receptor (G-CSFR, 1p35-p34.3) have been described and are associated with the development of acute myeloid leukemia.[3,4] However, not all patients with SCN/Kostmann's syndrome show mutations in the G-CSF receptor, which suggests that these mutations may be epiphenomena that occur in the setting of SCN but do not cause it.[5-7] More recently, Dale et al[8] found that 22 out of 25 patients with SCN had heterozygous mutations in the gene encoding neutrophil elastase (ELA2, 19p13.3). Interestingly, mutations in this same gene are also responsible for cyclic neutropenia.[9] The mutations in neutrophil elastase that cause cyclic neutropenia tend to be clustered around the catalytically active site of ELA2, whereas the mutations that are associated with SCN are located in a different part of the gene that winds up on a different side of the three-dimensional structure of the protein.[8]

The clinical manifestations of SCN appear promptly after birth: 50% of affected infants are symptomatic before the first month of life and 90% within the first 6 months; omphalitis, upper and lower respiratory tract infections, and skin and liver abscesses are the most frequent infections. Subcutaneous

TABLE 12-1 Neutrophil Disorders: Causes

Neutrophilia

- Usually dependent on causes *extrinsic* to the neutrophils (e.g., acute or chronic infection)

Neutropenia

- Caused by defects *intrinsic* to the neutrophils or their progenitors (severe congenital neutropenia, cyclic neutropenia, neutropenia associated with other well-defined syndromes [e.g., Schwachman syndrome, Fanconi syndrome, dyskeratosis congenita, Chédiak-Higashi syndrome, reticular dysgenesis, and warts, hypogammaglobulinemia, infections, and myelokathexis syndrome])
- Caused by defects *extrinsic* to the neutrophil or their progenitors (infections, drugs, immune-mediated metabolic diseases, nutritional deficiencies, bone marrow infiltration)

Motility Disorders

- Adhesion: Leukocyte adhesion deficiency type 1, 2, 3, or 4
- Chemotaxis: Leukocyte adhesion deficiency type 1, 2, or 4; localized juvenile periodontitis, neutrophil β-actin deficiency, secondary to extensive burns, secondary to alcohol consumption

Phagocytosis Disorders

- Leukocyte adhesion deficiency type 1 (complement mediated only); secondary to antibody deficiencies; complement deficiencies; mannose binding protein deficiency

Disorders of Granule Formation and Content

- Chédiak-Higashi syndrome; specific granule deficiency

Microbicidal Disorders

- Chronic granulomatous disease; myeloperoxidase deficiency; glucose-6-phosphate dehydrogenase deficiency, glutathione pathway deficiencies

---

TABLE 12-2 Infections and White Blood Cell Count Defects: Features Highly Suspicious of Phagocyte Disorders

Severe Infections		Recurrent Infections		Specific Infections		Unusually Located Infections	
Type of Infection	Diagnosis to Consider	Site of Infection	Diagnosis to Consider	Microorganisms	Diagnosis to Consider	Site of Infection	Diagnosis to Consider
Cellulitis	Neutropenia, LAD, CGD, HIES	Skin	Neutropenia, CGD, LAD, HIES	Staphylococci	Neutropenia, LAD, CGD, HIES	Umbilical stump	LAD
Colitis	Neutropenia, CGD	Gums	LAD, neutrophil motility disorders	*Serratia marcescens, Chromobacterium violaceum, Nocardia, Burkholderia cepacia*	CGD	Liver abscess	CGD
						Gums	LAD, neutrophil motility disorders
Osteomyelitis	CGD, IFN-γ/IL-12 pathway defects	Upper and lower respiratory tract	Neutropenia, CGD, HIES, functional neutrophil disorders	Aspergillus	Neutropenia, CGD, HIES		
		Gastrointestinal tract	CGD, IFN-γ/IL-12 pathway defects (salmonella)	Nontuberculous mycobacteria, bacille Calmette-Guérin	IFN-γ/IL-12 pathway defects, CGD, SCID		
		Lymph nodes	CGD, IFN-γ/IL-12 pathway defects (mycobacteria)	Candida	Neutropenia, CGD, myeloperoxidase deficiency		
		Osteomyelitis	CGD, IFN-γ/IL-12 pathway defects (mycobacteria)				

LAD, Leukocyte adhesion deficiency; *CGD,* chronic granulomatous disease; *HIES,* hyper-IgE syndrome; *SCID,* severe combined immunodeficiency syndrome.

TABLE 12-3 Laboratory Evaluation of Patient with Suspected Neutrophil Disorder*

Test	Normal Test Exclusions
White blood cell count and differential (repeated)	All forms of neutropenia
Neutrophil morphologic evaluation	Specific granule deficiency; Chédiak-Higashi syndrome
Flow cytometry	
CD18	Leukocyte adhesion deficiency type 1 (LAD-1) (complete)
CD15s (Sialyl-Lewis X)	LAD-2
Dihydrorhodamine (DHR) oxidation	Chronic granulomatous disease (CGD) (severe G6PD deficiencies and glutathione pathway deficiencies have abnormal DHR oxidation as well)
STAT-1 phosphorylation	IFN-γR1, IFN-γR2 deficiency
STAT-4 phosphorylation	IL-12Rβ1 deficiency
Bone marrow aspirate	
Neutrophil maturation	Severe congenital neutropenia; cyclic neutropenia
Neutrophil retention	Warts, hypogammaglobulinemia, infections, and myelokathexis syndrome
Nitroblue tetrazolium (NBT) reduction	CGD (severe G6PD deficiencies and glutathione pathway deficiencies have abnormal NBT reduction as well)

*Patients should be evaluated considering their family history, physical examination, and associated comorbid factors.

recombinant G-CSF (5 µg/kg/day; range from 1 to 120 µg/kg, depending on patient response) has dramatically changed the prognosis of these patients.[10] Since the advent of recombinant G-CSF, reductions in the number of infections and hospitalization days, and an increase in life expectancy have been described.[11-13]

Recently, Devriendt et al[14] described a family with an X-linked form of SCN (XLN) caused by mutations in the Wiskott-Aldrich syndrome protein (WASP). In contrast to the WASP mutations that produce classical Wiskott-Aldrich syndrome or X-linked thrombocytopenia, most of which are caused by mutations resulting in reduced WASP transcription or translation, the mutation causing XLN (L270P) disrupts a WASP autoinhibitory domain, thereby creating a constitutively active mutant protein.

Cyclic Neutropenia/Cyclic Hematopoiesis

Cyclic neutropenia/cyclic hematopoiesis is typically inherited as an autosomal dominant trait and is characterized by regular cyclic fluctuations in all hematopoietic lineages. However, clinical manifestations are almost exclusively associated with variations in neutrophils. Neutrophil counts cycle on an average of every 21 days (range 14 to 36 days), including periods of severe neutropenia ($> 200/\mu l$) that last from 3 to 10 days.[15,16] Different single-base heterozygous substitutions in ELA2 (neutrophil elastase 2, 19p13.3) have been identified in all pedigrees analyzed.[9] Most patients have clinical manifestations of neutropenia in early childhood. Oral ulcerations, gingivitis, lymphadenopathy, pharyngitis/tonsillitis, and skin lesions are the most frequently reported findings. Early loss of permanent teeth as a consequence of chronic gingivitis and periapical abscesses is a common feature.[17] Bone marrow aspirates obtained during periods of neutropenia show maturation arrest at the myelocyte stage or, less frequently, bone marrow hypoplasia.[18]

G-CSF dramatically improves peripheral neutrophil counts and decreases morbidity in cyclic neutropenic patients.[17,19] Interestingly, infections and hospitalizations appear to naturally lessen with age.[17]

Myelokathexis/Warts, Hypogammaglobulinemia, Infections, and Myelokathexis Syndrome

Myelokathexis (from the Greek for *retained in the bone marrow*) is a congenital disorder associated with severe chronic neutropenia, in which an autosomal dominant inheritance pattern appears the most likely.[20] A significant number of patients with myelokathexis have warts, hypogammaglobulinemia, and infections, with different degrees of severity. Therefore the acronym *WHIM* (warts, hypogammaglobulinemia, infections, and myelokathexis) has been proposed for this syndrome.[21] In these patients, unlike in other forms of congenital neutropenia, bone marrow aspirates show myeloid hypercellularity with increased numbers of granulocytes at all stages of differentiation. Recurrent sinopulmonary infections are frequent. During episodes of infection, neutrophil counts are typically increased compared with baseline levels. Steroids, subcutaneous epinephrine, and intravenous endotoxin, as well as G-CSF and granulocyte-macophage colony-stimulating factor (GM-CSF), have all been shown to mobilize mature neutrophils from the bone marrow.[22] Sustained therapy with G-CSF or GM-CSF has proved effective in rapidly increasing the number of neutrophils in the peripheral blood and decreasing the number of infections.[22] The presence of warts and hypogammaglobulinemia, although not severe, suggests a broader immunologic defect including that of the T and B cells. Interestingly, normalization of immunoglobulin levels has been observed during G-CSF and GM-CSF treatments.[21,22]

IMMUNE-MEDIATED NEUTROPENIAS
Alloimmune Neonatal Neutropenia

Alloimmune neonatal neutropenia (ANN) is a form of immune-mediated neutropenia first described by Lalezari and Bernard[23] in 1966. ANN is produced by the transplacental transfer of maternal antibodies against NA1 and NA2, two isotypes of the immunoglobulin receptor FcγRIIIb, causing immune destruction of neonatal neutrophils.[24] This problem typically arises in otherwise normal children of apparently normal, healthy mothers. Several of the healthy mothers did not express FcγRIIIb on their own neutrophils, leading to the elaboration of antibodies against FcγRIIIb expressed on fetal neutrophils following sensitization during pregnancy.[25-27] These complement-activating antineutrophil antibodies can be detected in 1 in 500 live births, making the potential incidence of ANN high. This disease should be considered in the evaluation of all infants with neutropenia, with or without infection. Antibody-coated neutrophils in ANN are phagocytosed in the reticuloendothelial system and removed from the circulation, leaving the neonate neutropenic and prone to infections. Omphalitis, cellulites, and pneumonia may be the presenting infections within the first 2 weeks of life. The diagnosis can be made by detection of neutrophil-specific alloantibodies in maternal serum. Parenteral antibiotics (even in the absence of other signs of sepsis) and G-CSF should be included in the initial management of ANN.[28,29] Intravenous gamma globulin may not be effective in reversing ANN.[29] As expected, ANN tends to spontaneously improve with the waning of maternal antibody levels, but this process may take months.

Primary and Secondary Autoimmune Neutropenia

Autoimmune neutropenia (AIN) is a rare disorder, caused by peripheral destruction of neutrophils and/or their precursors by autoantibodies present in patient serum or mediated by large granular lymphocytes (CD3+/CD8+/CD57+ T cells) in the bone marrow. Autoimmune neutropenia can be either primary or secondary. The neutropenia is an isolated clinical entity in primary AIN and associated with another disease in secondary AIN.

Primary Autoimmune Neutropenia

Primary AIN is the most common cause of chronic neutropenia (absolute neutrophil count < 1500/μl lasting at least 6 months) in infancy and childhood.[30,31] Primary AIN has a slight female predominance and has been reported in about 1:100,000 live births,[32] ten times more frequent than SCN. Antibodies directed against different neutrophil antigens can be detected in almost all patients. Approximately one third of these autoantibodies are anti-NA1 and -NA2, two of the glycosylated isoforms of FcγRIIIb (the same targets recognized in ANN). Almost 85% of these antibodies are of an IgG isotype. Other antigens toward which autoantibodies can be found are CD11b/CD18 (Mac-1), CD32 (FcγRII), and CD35 (C3b complement receptor).[33,34] The average age at diagnosis for primary AIN is 8 months. The majority of patients present with either skin or upper respiratory tract infections. Infrequently, some patients may suffer from severe infections such as pneumonia, meningitis, or sepsis.[34] The diagnosis may be incidental, as patients may remain asymptomatic despite low neutrophil counts. Monocytosis is also frequent. Neutrophil counts are usually below 1500/μl, with the majority of patients having more than 500 neutrophils/μl at diagnosis. The neutrophil count may transiently increase twofold to threefold during severe infections and return to neutropenic levels following resolution.[31,34] Bone marrow findings may be normal or hypercellular. The cause of this disease remains unknown, but it is not clearly associated with Parvovirus B19 infection.[34-36]

Detection of granulocyte-specific antibodies is key to the diagnosis of primary AIN and may require repeated testing.

Granulocyte immunofluorescence testing (GIFT) is a sensitive method for detection of antigranulocyte antibodies.[34]

The prognosis of primary AIN is very good because it is usually a self-limited disease. The neutropenia remits spontaneously within 7 to 24 months in 95% of patients, preceded by the disappearance of autoantibodies from the circulation. Symptomatic treatment with antibiotics for infections is usually sufficient. Prophylactic antibiotic treatment should be reserved for those with recurrent infections. Cotrimoxazole, ampicillin, and first-generation cephalosporins are the most commonly used prophylactic antibiotics. Treatment for severe infections or in the setting of emergency surgery often now includes G-CSF. High-dose IV immunoglobulin and corticosteroids have been used in the past.[34,37]

Secondary Autoimmune Neutropenia

Secondary AIN can be seen at any age but is more common in adults and has a more variable clinical course. Various systemic and autoimmune diseases such as systemic lupus erythematosus, Hodgkin's disease, large granular lymphocyte proliferation or leukemia, Epstein-Barr virus infection, cytomegalovirus infection,[38] HIV infection, and Parvovirus B19 infection[39] have been associated with secondary AIN. These patients are predisposed to the development of other autoimmune problems as well. Antineutrophil antibodies typically have pan-FcγRIII specificity rather than specificity to the FcγRIII subunits, making the resulting neutropenia more severe. Anti-CD18/11b antibodies have been detected in a subset of patients.[31] Secondary AIN responds best to therapy directed at the underlying cause.[40]

DEFECTS OF GRANULE FORMATION AND CONTENT

Chédiak-Higashi Syndrome

Chédiak-Higashi syndrome (CHS) is a rare and life-threatening autosomal recessive disease, clinically characterized by oculocutaneous albinism, frequent pyogenic infections, neurologic abnormalities, and a relatively late-onset lymphoma-like "accelerated phase." The disease is caused by mutations in the lysosomal trafficking regulator gene, LYST or CHS1 (1q42.1-q42.2).[41,42] The mechanism by which LYST works is still elusive,[43] and therefore so is the pathophysiology of CHS. A truncated LYST protein is the most frequent genetic defect found.[44] Affected patients show hypopigmentation of the skin, iris, and hair because of giant and aberrant melanosomes (macromelanosomes). Hair color is light brown to blonde, with a characteristic metallic silver-gray sheen. Under light microscopy, CHS hair shafts show small pathognomonic aggregates of clumped pigment (Figure 12-1).

Giant azurophil granules formed from the fusion of multiple primary granules are seen in neutrophils, eosinophils, and basophils. In fact, enlarged cytoplasmic granules are found in all granule-containing cells. Neutropenia is also frequently seen.[45,46] Normocellular to hypercellular bone marrow,[45] poor response to stimuli of bone marrow granulocyte release,[46] normal circulating granulocyte half-life, and elevated serum lysozyme levels suggest intramedullary destruction of neutrophils.

Monocyte and neutrophil chemotaxis is diminished.[47] Phagocytosis is normal or increased,[48,49] but bacterial killing is

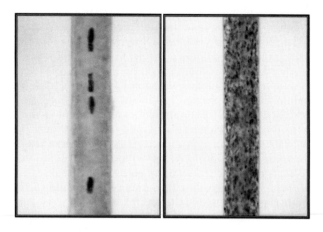

FIGURE 12-1 Pigment distribution in hair. Normal hair *(left)* shows pigment typically located in the cortex of the hair shaft. In Chédiak-Higashi syndrome *(right)*, small aggregates of clumped melanin are haphazardly distributed all along the hair shaft. (×20)

delayed, probably because of low levels of primary granule enzymes.[50,51] Natural killer (NK) cells show very low cytotoxicity,[52,53] but neutrophil and monocyte antibody–dependent cellular cytotoxicity is intact.[52] B cell function is usually unaffected.[52,54] Neurologic involvement of the peripheral and central nervous systems is common. Progressive neuropathy of the legs, cranial nerve palsies, seizures, mental retardation, and autonomic dysfunction are reported.[55-58]

The accelerated phase, one of the main causes of death in CHS, is clinically indistinguishable from other hemophagocytic syndromes, with fever, hepatosplenomegaly, lymphadenopathy, cytopenias, hypertriglyceridemia, hypofibrinogenemia, hemophagocytosis, and tissue lymphohistiocytic infiltration.[59] Defective surface expression of CTLA-4 probably contributes to the accelerated phase.[60] Etoposide (VP16), steroids, and intrathecal methotrexate (when the CNS is involved) have been effective treatments.[61] However, without successful bone marrow transplantation, the accelerated phase usually recurs.

Neutrophil-Specific Granule Deficiency

Neutrophil-specific granule deficiency is a rare, heterogeneous, autosomal recessive disease characterized by the profound reduction or absence of neutrophil-specific granules and their contents.[62,63] In several cases a homozygous, recessive mutation was found in C/EBP epsilon (14q11.2).[64] However, other cases do not have mutations in C/EBP epsilon, suggesting genetic heterogeneity. C/EBP epsilon is a member of the CCAAT/enhancer binding proteins, transcription factors that play critical roles in myelopoiesis and cellular differentiation.[65]

In neutrophil-specific granule deficiency there is a paucity or absence of neutrophil-specific granules, neutrophils with bilobed nuclei predominate (pseudo–Pelger-Huët anomaly), and increased susceptibility to pyogenic infections of the skin, ears, lungs, and lymph nodes are described.[62,66-68] Neutrophils have very low specific granule contents (e.g., lactoferrin) and low to absent defensins, a primary granule product. Electron microscopy shows absent peroxidase-negative granules in some patients and empty peroxidase-negative granules in

others. Superoxide production is normal. Staphylococcal activity may be reduced because of poor phagocytosis, but candidacidal activity is normal.[63] Hemostasis abnormalities, caused by reduced levels of platelet-associated, high-molecular-weight von Willebrand factor and platelet fibrinogen and fibronectin, have been reported.[69]

The diagnosis of specific granule deficiency is suggested by the peripheral smear and confirmed by electron microscopy and specific enzyme detection. Eosinophils may not be detectable on routine smears.[62] Management of these patients is complicated by their poor inflammatory responses. Grampositive cocci infections are common. Aggressive diagnosis of infection, prolonged and intensive therapy, and early use of surgical excision and débridement are necessary.

DEFECTS OF OXIDATIVE METABOLISM

Chronic Granulomatous Disease

Chronic granulomatous disease (CGD) is a genetically heterogeneous disease characterized by recurrent life-threatening infections caused by catalase-positive bacteria and fungi and exuberant granuloma formation. The disease is caused by defects in NADPH oxidase, the enzyme responsible for the phagocyte respiratory burst and the generation of superoxide. The NADPH oxidase exists as two groups of components: a heterodimeric, membrane-bound complex embedded in the walls of secondary granules and four distinct cytosolic proteins.[70] The structural components are referred to as *phox* proteins for *ph*agocyte *ox*idase. The secondary granule membrane

TABLE 12-4 Prevalence of Infection by Site in 368 Patients with Chronic Granulomatous Disease*

Type of Infection (Most Frequent Microorganisms Isolated)	Total Number (N = 368) (%)
Pneumonia (*Aspergillus* spp; *Staphylococcus* spp; *Burkholderia cepacia*; *Nocardia* spp; *Mycobacteria* spp)	290 (79%)
Abscess (*Staphylococcus* spp; *Serratia* spp; *Aspergillus* spp)	250 (68%)
Suppurative adenitis (*Staphylococcus* spp; *Serratia* spp; *Candida* spp)	194 (53%)
Osteomyelitis (*Serratia* spp; *Aspergillus* spp; *Paecilomyces* spp; *Staphylococcus* spp)	90 (25%)
Bacteremia/fungemia (*Salmonella* spp; *Burkholderia cepacia*; *Candida* spp; *Staphylococcus* spp; *Pseudomonas* spp)	65 (18%)
Cellulitis (*Chromobacterium violaceum* and *Serratia marsescens* were identified in one case each)	18 (5%)
Meningitis (*Candida* spp was identified in three cases)	15 (4%)
Other†	112 (30%)

Modified from Winkelstein JA, Marino MC, Johnston RB Jr, et al: *Medicine (Baltimore)* 79:155-169, 2000.

*These data include patients on variable prophylactic regimens, if any, and are meant to portray the natural history of disease over the last 20 years.

†Includes impetigo, sinusitis, otitis media, septic arthritis, urinary tract infection/pyelonephritis, gingivitis/periodontitis, chorioretinitis, gastroenteritis, paronychia, conjunctivitis, hepatitis, epididymitis, empyema, epiglottitis, cardiac empyema, mastoiditis, and suppurative phlebitis.

complex is cytochrome-b_{558}, composed of a 91-kd glycosylated β chain (gp91^{phox}) and a 22-kd nonglycosylated α chain (p22^{phox}), which binds heme and flavin. The cytosol contains the structural components p47^{phox} and p67^{phox} and the regulatory components p40^{phox} and rac. On cellular activation the cytosolic components p47^{phox} and p67^{phox} are phosphorylated and bind tightly together. In association with p40^{phox} and rac, these proteins combine with the cytochrome complex (gp91^{phox} and p22^{phox}) to form the intact NADPH oxidase. An electron is taken from NADPH and donated to molecular oxygen, leading to the formation of superoxide. In the presence of superoxide dismutase, this is converted to hydrogen peroxide, which, in the presence of myeloperoxidase and chlorine in the phagosome, is converted to bleach. Until recently, the metabolites of superoxide themselves were thought to be the critical mediators of bacterial killing. However, Reeves et al[71] have recently shown that phagocyte production of reactive oxygen species is most critical for microbial killing through the activation of certain primary granule proteins inside the phagocytic vacuole. This new paradigm for NADPH oxidase-mediated microbial killing suggests that the reactive oxidants are most critical as intracellular signaling molecules, leading to activation of other pathways rather than exerting a microbicidal effect per se.

Mutations in all of the four structural genes of the NADPH oxidase have been found to cause CGD. The most common genotype, accounting for nearly two thirds of the cases, involves mutations in gp91^{phox} and the remainder of cases are autosomal recessive; there are no autosomal dominant cases of CGD.[72] The frequency of CGD in the United States may be as high as 1:100,000. Clinically, CGD is quite variable but the majority of patients are diagnosed as toddlers and young children.[72] Infections and granulomatous lesions are the usual first manifestations. The lung, skin, lymph nodes, and liver are the most frequent sites of infection (Table 12-4). The overwhelming majority of infections in CGD are caused by only five organisms: *Staphylococcus aureus, Burkholderia cepacia, Serratia marcescens, Nocardia,* and *Aspergillus.* Trimethoprim/sulfamethoxazole prophylaxis has reduced the frequency of bacterial infections in general and staphylococcal infections in particular. On prophylaxis, staphylococcal infections are essentially confined to the liver and cervical lymph nodes.[72] Staphylococcal liver abscesses encountered in CGD are dense, caseous, and difficult to drain, requiring surgery in almost all cases.[73] With the great successes in antibacterial prophylaxis and therapy, fungal infections, typically caused by *Aspergillus* species, are now the leading cause of mortality in CGD.[72]

The gastrointestinal and genitourinary tracts are frequently affected (Figure 12-2). Esophageal, jejunal, ileal, cecal, rectal, and perirectal involvement with granulomata mimicking Crohn's disease has been described.[74-79] Gastric outlet obstruction is especially common and may be the initial presentation of CGD.[80-82] Walther et al[83] found that 38% of CGD patients had some kind of urologic event, including bladder granulomata, ureteral obstruction, and urinary tract infection. All patients with granulomata of the bladder or stricture of the ureter had defects of the membrane component of the NADPH oxidase (gp91^{phox} and p22^{phox}).

Steroid therapy is quite effective and surprisingly well tolerated when used for treatment of obstructive lesions. Prednisone given at about 1 mg/kg for a brief initial period and then tapered to a low dose on alternate days is quite successful.[84-87] Because the frequency of relapse/recurrence of gastrointestinal granulomatous disease is high, prolonged low-dose maintenance is often necessary. Other therapies for severe granulomatous complications include cyclosporine A[88] and colostomy for refractory rectal disease; several cases have been treated with infliximab (humanized monoclonal antibody against TNF-α). The latter therapy must still be viewed

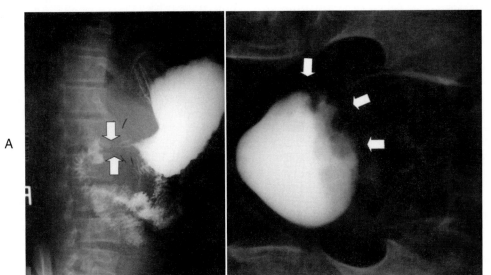

FIGURE 12-2 Gastrointestinal and genitourinary obstructive lesions in chronic granulomatous disease (CGD). **A,** High-grade obstruction of the gastric outlet in a 17-year-old boy with gp91^{phox}-deficient CGD *(arrows).* He had early satiety, weight loss, and intermittent vomiting for several weeks. He improved rapidly on steroid therapy. **B,** Extensive bladder granuloma formation in the superior aspect of the bladder in a 3-year-old boy with gp91^{phox}-deficient CGD *(arrows).* Note the mildly dilated ureter on the obstructed side. This child presented with dysuria and right hydronephrosis that responded promptly to steroids.

with caution, as infliximab increases the rates of infection in normal individuals.

The X-linked carriers of gp91^{phox} have two populations of phagocytes: one that produces superoxide and one that does not, giving carriers a characteristic mosaic pattern on oxidative testing. Discoid lupus erythematosus–like lesions, aphthous ulcers, and photosensitive rashes have been seen in gp91^{phox} carriers. Similarly, screening of patients with discoid lupus erythematosus detected a significant number of previously unsuspected CGD carriers.[89,90] Infections are not usually seen in these female carriers unless the normal neutrophils are below 5% to 10%, in which case these carriers are at risk for CGD-type infections.[72,91]

The diagnosis of CGD is usually made by direct measurement of superoxide production, ferricytochrome-c reduction, chemiluminescence, nitroblue tetrazolium (NBT) reduction, or dihydrorhodamine oxidation (DHR). Currently, we prefer the latter assay because of its relative ease of use, its ability to distinguish X-linked from autosomal patterns of CGD on flow cytometry, and its sensitivity to even very low numbers of functional neutrophils.[92,93]

Several other conditions affect the respiratory burst. Glucose-6-phosphate dehydrogenase deficiency may lead to a decreased respiratory burst and increased susceptibility to bacterial infections.[94] However, G6PD deficiency is most often associated with some degree of hemolytic anemia, whereas CGD is not. Diverse pathogens, including *Legionella pneumophila*, *Toxoplasma gondii*, *Chlamydia*, *Entamoeba histolytica*, and *Ehrlichia risticii*, have been shown to inhibit the respiratory burst *in vitro*. Recently, human granulocytic ehrlichiosis (*Anaplasma phagocytophila*) infection has been shown to suppress the respiratory burst by down-regulating gp91^{phox}.[95]

CGD should be considered because of severe or recurrent bacterial or fungal infections in children, especially those of the lung or liver. Infections with unusual organisms such as *B. cepacia*, *S. marcescens*, *C. violaceum*, *Nocardia*, or *Aspergillus* species should always initiate a search for CGD in patients of any age without other predisposing factors. Granulomatous events such as gastrointestinal or genitourinary obstruction are also suggestive. Immunoblot, flow cytometry, and molecular techniques can be used to determine the specific genotype. Molecular determination of specific mutations is available from various research and commercial laboratories and is necessary for prenatal diagnosis. Male sex, earlier age at presentation, and increased severity of disease suggest X-linked disease, but these are only rough guides. The precise gene defect should be determined in all cases because it is critical for genetic counseling and helps in prognosis. Autosomal recessive forms of CGD (mostly p47^{phox} deficient) have a significantly better prognosis than X-linked disease.[72]

Prophylactic trimethoprim/sulfamethoxazole (5 mg/kg/day based on trimethoprim) reduces the frequency of major infections from about once every year to once every 3.5 years.[96] It reduces staphylococcal and skin infections[97] without increasing the frequency of serious fungal infections in CGD.[98] A recent trial of itraconazole prophylaxis showed marked efficacy in prevention of fungal infection in CGD (100 mg daily for patients < 13 y or < 50 kg; 200 mg daily for those ≥ 13 y or ≥ 50 kg). Interferon gamma (IFN-γ) was shown in a large multinational, multicenter, placebo-controlled study to reduce the number and severity of infections in CGD by 70% compared with placebo. These benefits held true regardless of the inheritance pattern of CGD, sex, or use of prophylactic antibiotics. Interestingly, no significant difference could be detected in terms of *in vitro* superoxide generation, bactericidal activity, or cytochrome-b levels.[99] Systemic IFN-γ also augmented neutrophil activity against *Aspergillus* conidia *in vitro*.[100] Therefore our current recommendation is to use prophylaxis with trimethoprim/sulfamethoxazole, itraconazole, and IFN-γ (50 μg/m^2) in CGD.

The erythrocyte sedimentation rate is the most sensitive laboratory test of ongoing infection. Because the differential diagnosis for a given process in these patients includes bacteria, fungi, and granulomatous processes, a microbiologic diagnosis is critical. In severe infections, leukocyte transfusions are often used, although the efficacy is anecdotal. In CGD, irradiation of the granulocyte product is not necessary for prevention of graft versus host disease and it does inhibit the bactericidal activity of the cells.[101,102]

In a longitudinal analysis of 47 patients, Mouy et al[103] found an 8-year survival rate of 70.5% for children born before 1978 and a 92.9% survival rate for those born later. More recently, in a retrospective voluntary registry, Winkelstein et al[72] found mortality for the X-linked form of the disease to be about 5% per year and 2% per year for the autosomal recessive varieties.[72] The greatest cause of mortality for CGD in developed countries remains *Aspergillus* pneumonia.

Bone marrow transplantation leading to stable chimerism has been successfully performed in patients with CGD.[104] Ozsahin et al[105] performed successful bone marrow transplantation on a child with CGD and refractory *Aspergillus* infection. More recently, Horwitz et al[106] performed low-intensity, nonablative transplant from HLA-identical siblings into CGD patients. Success was greater in children than adults, but transplant-related toxicities, such as graft versus host disease, were problematic. Clinical trials of p47^{phox} gene therapy have shown marking of cells in the periphery for several months, but clinical benefit has not been shown, presumably because of the low numbers of corrected cells in the circulation (< 0.01%).[107]

Myeloperoxidase Deficiency

Myeloperoxidase (MPO) deficiency is an autosomal recessive trait with a variable range of expressivity. It is also the most common primary phagocyte disorder: 1/4000 individuals have complete MPO deficiency, and 1/2000 have a partial defect.[108-111] Myeloperoxidase (17q23) is synthesized in neutrophils and monocytes, packaged in the azurophilic granules, and released either into the phagosome or the extracellular space where it catalyzes the conversion of H_2O_2 to hypohalous acid (in neutrophils the halide is Cl$^-$ and the acid is bleach). Despite *in vitro* studies showing that MPO-deficient neutrophils are markedly less efficient than normal neutrophils in killing *C. albicans* and hyphal forms of *Aspergillus fumigatus*, infection in MPO deficiency is rare. Of the MPO-deficient patients who have had clinical findings, infections caused by different *Candida* strains were the most common: mucocutaneous, meningeal, and bone infections, as well as sepsis, have been described.[111-116] Diabetes mellitus appears to be a critical cofactor for *Candida* species infections in the context of MPO deficiency.[108,117,118] Definitive diagnosis is established by neutrophil/monocyte peroxidase histochemical staining or specific protein detection. There is no specific treatment for MPO deficiency; diabetes should be sought and controlled, and infections should be treated.

LEUKOCYTE ADHESION DEFICIENCIES

For over a century leukocyte movement from the bloodstream toward inflamed sites has been recognized as crucial in preventing and fighting infections. Leukocyte adhesion to the endothelium, to other leukocytes, and to bacteria is critical in the ability of leukocytes to travel, communicate, inflame, and fight infection. Different families of adhesion molecules mediate these processes, critical among which are the integrins and selectins.

Leukocyte Adhesion Deficiency Type 1

Leukocyte adhesion deficiency type 1 (LAD-1) is an autosomal recessive disorder produced by mutations in the common β2 chain (CD18) of the β2 integrin family (ITGB2, 21q22.3; Table 12-5). Each of the β2 integrins is a heterodimer composed of an α chain (CD11a, CD11b, or CD11c), noncovalently linked to a common β2 subunit (CD18). The α-β heterodimers of the β2 integrin family include CD11a/CD18 (lymphocyte function–associated antigen-1 (LFA-1), CD11b/CD18 (macrophage antigen-1, Mac-1 or complement receptor-3, CR3), and CD11c/CD18 (p150,95 or complement receptor-4, CR4).[119] CD18 is required for normal expression of the α-β heterodimers. Therefore mutations resulting in failure to produce a functional β2 subunit lead to either very low or no expression of CD11a, CD11b, or CD11c and thus cause LAD-1.[120-123]

The severe phenotype of LAD-1 is caused by less than 1% of normal expression of CD18 on neutrophils, whereas the moderate phenotype shows from 1% to 30% of normal expression.[124-126] Recently, patients with normal β2 integrin expression but without functional activity were described.[127,128] Therefore expression of CD18 alone is not sufficient to exclude the diagnosis of LAD-1: functional assays must be performed if the clinical suspicion is high.

Patients with the severe phenotype of LAD-1 characteristically have delayed umbilical stump separation and omphalitis,

persistent leukocytosis (> 15,000/μl) even in the absence of obvious active infection, and severe, destructive gingivitis and periodontitis with associated loss of dentition and alveolar bone. Recurrent infections of the skin, upper and lower airways, bowel, and perirectal area are common and usually caused by *S. aureus* or gram-negative bacilli. Infections tend to be necrotizing and may progress to ulceration (Figure 12-3). Typically, no pus is seen in these lesions and there is almost complete absence of neutrophil invasion on histopathology. Aggressive medical management with antibiotics, neutrophil transfusions, and prompt surgery, when indicated, are required. Impaired healing of infectious, traumatic, or surgical wounds is also characteristic of LAD-1 patients. Scars tend to acquire a dystrophic "cigarette-paper" appearance. Patients with the moderate phenotype tend to be diagnosed later in life, have normal umbilical separation, have fewer life-threatening infections, and live longer.[124,125] However, leukocytosis, periodontal disease, and delayed wound healing are still common.

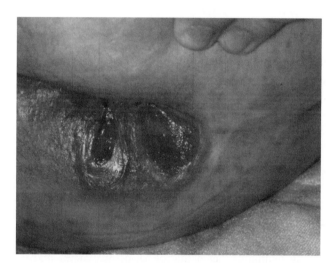

FIGURE 12-3 Ulcerative perirectal lesion in an 18-year-old boy with leukocyte adhesion deficiency type 1. No pus was seen and there was poor inflammation in the surrounding tissues.

TABLE 12-5 Leukocyte Adhesion Deficiency Syndromes

Leukocyte Adhesion Deficiency (LAD)	Type 1 (LAD-1)	Type 2 (LAD-2, or CDG-IIc)	Type 3 (LAD-3)	Type 4 (LAD-4)
OMIM	116920	266265; *605881	(E-selectin *131210)	602049
Inheritance pattern	Autosomal recessive	Autosomal recessive	Unknown	Autosomal dominant
Affected protein(s)	Integrin β2 common chain (CD18)	Glucosylated proteins (e.g., Sialyl-Lewis X, Le^x)	Endothelial E-selectin expression	Rac2
Neutrophil function affected	Chemotaxis, tight adherence	Rolling, tethering	Rolling, tethering	Chemotaxis, superoxide production
Delayed umbilical cord separation	Yes (severe phenotype only)	Yes	Yes	Yes
Leukocytosis/neutrophilia	Yes	Yes	No (mild neutropenia)	Yes

CDG-IIc, Congenital disorder of glycosylation type IIc; *OMIM,* Online Mendelian Inheritance in Man.

Flow cytometry analysis of LAD-1 blood samples shows significant reduction (moderate phenotype) or near absence (severe phenotype) of CD18 and its associated molecules CD11a, CD11b and CD11c on neutrophils and other leukocytes. LAD-1 patients show diminished neutrophil migration *in vivo* (Rebuck skin windows) and *in vitro*.[124,125] Adherence of affected granulocytes to glass, plastic, nylon, wool, and to other LAD neutrophils is greatly reduced and does not improve after stimulation.[124,125] Complement-mediated phagocytosis is severely impaired because of the absence of CD18/CD11b (CR3/Mac-1). Nevertheless, IgG-mediated phagocytosis is unaffected as is superoxide production, chemiluminescence, and primary and secondary granule release.[124,125] Antibody-dependent cell-mediated cytotoxicity (ADCC) is diminished in LAD-1 patients. Although viral infections are not a major problem in these patients in infancy, there have been deaths resulting from viral infections in affected young adults,[124] presumably reflecting some specific antibody synthesis impairment caused by poor cell-cell interaction.

At present, bone marrow transplantation is the only definitive treatment.[129-131] Preclinical gene-therapy studies have been performed in LAD-1,[132-134] but thus far there have been no clinical benefits in humans.

Leukocyte Adhesion Deficiency Type 2 (Congenital Disorder of Glycosylation Type IIc)

LAD-2, or congenital disorder of glycosylation type IIc (CDG-IIc), is very rare autosomal recessive inherited disease in which fucose metabolism is primarily affected because of mutations in the GDP-fucose transporter gene (11p11-q11)[135,136] (see Table 12-5). Lack of the GDP-fucose transporter leads to a lack of expression of Sialyl-Lewis X and other fucosylated proteins that function as ligands for the endothelial selectins, molecules that mediate the loose, rolling adhesion of neutrophils along postcapillary venules.[137,138] The clinical phenotype is not only characterized by infections of the skin, lung, and gums; leukocytosis; and poor pus formation, but includes mental retardation, short stature, distinctive facies, and the Bombay (hh) blood phenotype. However, unlike LAD-1 patients, the frequency and severity of infections tend to decline with time.[139] *In vitro* LAD-2 cells show impaired random and chemoattractant-directed neutrophil migration, as well as defective neutrophil homotypic aggregation.[140] Defective neutrophil adherence to IL-1β or TNF-α–stimulated endothelial cells have also been described.[141]

Marquardt et al[142] have reported a significant reduction in infectious episodes and neutrophil baseline counts, as well as improved psychomotor capabilities, in a LAD-2 patient after prolonged oral fucose treatment. Using a different therapeutic scheme and fucose dose, these results were not seen in the two patients reported and followed by Etzioni and Tonetti.[143]

Leukocyte Adhesion Deficiency Type 3

A female patient with deficient endothelial expression of E-selectin was described by DeLisser et al[144] (see Table 12-5). The patient had *Pseudomonas* omphalitis, recurrent ear and urinary tract infections, and severe soft tissue infections with impaired pus formation. She had a mild, chronic neutropenia with appropriate leukocyte increases in response to infections or GM-CSF. The patient has two normal half-sisters and had a full sibling who died *in utero* because of a staphylococcal infection, which leaves the inheritance pattern still unclear. No alterations in the E-selectin cDNA were detected, but circulating E-selectin levels were twice those of controls. So far, no specific neutrophil functional impairment has been found; altogether, these data suggest a defect in E-selectin tethering or secretion.

Leukocyte Adhesion Deficiency Type 4

Ambruso et al[145] and Williams et al[146] reported a male patient with an autosomal dominant mutation in the Rho GTP-ase Rac2 gene (Rac2, 22q12.13-q13.2; see Table 12-5). This molecule, comprising more than 96% of Rac in neutrophils, is a member of the Rho family of GTP-ases and is critical to the regulation of the actin cytoskeleton and superoxide production. The patient had delayed umbilical cord separation, perirectal abscesses, failure to heal surgical wounds, and absent pus in infected areas despite neutrophilia. Chemotaxis and superoxide production were impaired.[145,146] In addition, the patient's neutrophils showed defective azurophilic granule release[145] and impaired phagocytosis.[146] These defects are thought to reflect Rac interaction with the actin cytoskeleton (chemotaxis) and the NADPH oxidase (superoxide production). Four months after a matched related bone marrow transplantation, the patient was thriving, showing 100% donor cells in his bone marrow, and normalized superoxide production.[146]

IFN-γ/IL-12 Pathway Deficiencies (IFN-γ Receptor 1, IFN-γ Receptor 2, IL-12 Receptor β1, IL-12 p40, STAT-1)

The mononuclear phagocyte is crucial for protection against intracellular infections and for antigen presentation. It is also necessary for lymphocyte stimulation, lymphocyte proliferation, cytokine production, and response. Mycobacteria infect macrophages, leading to the production of interleukin 12 p70 (IL-12, a heterodimer of IL-12 p40 and IL-12 p35). IL-12 stimulates T cells and NK cells through its receptor (IL-12R, a heterodimer of IL-12Rβ1 and IL-12Rβ2) to produce IFN-γ. IFN-γ acts through its receptor (a heterodimer of IFN-γR1 and IFN-γR2) on macrophages (and on all nucleated cells) to up-regulate specific genes and activities. On phagocytes, IFN-γ increases production of tumor necrosis factor α (TNF-α) and further up-regulates IL-12. IFN-γ also causes mycobacterial killing through unknown mechanisms. IFN-γ binds to IFN-γR1, the ligand-binding chain, leading to its dimerization. Following this event, two IFN-γR2 chains—the signal-transducing chains—join the receptor complex. IFN-γR1 and IFN-γR2 are constitutively associated with their respective Janus kinases, Jak-1 and Jak-2. Mutual transphosphorylation of the Janus kinases leads to tyrosine phosphorylation of the intracellular domain of the IFN-γR1 at tyrosine (Y) 440. This tyrosine is the docking site for latent cytosolic signal transducer and activator of transcription-1 (STAT-1). Janus kinases mediate STAT-1 tyrosine 701 and serine 727 phosphorylation, leading to the homodimerization of two phospho–STAT-1 (STAT-1P) molecules, which then translocate to the nucleus and up-regulate the transcription of numerous IFN-γ–regulated genes[147] (Figure 12-4).

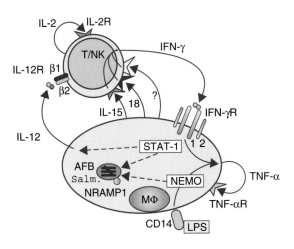

FIGURE 12-4 Schematic representation of the interferon gamma *(IFN-γ)/* interleukin-12 *(IL-12)* pathway. Ingested pathogens such as acid-fast bacilli *(AFB)* or salmonella (Salm.) stimulate IL-12 production by macrophages *(MΦ)*. Acting through its cognate IL-12 receptor, composed of the IL-12 receptor β1 chain (IL-12Rβ1) and the IL-12 receptor β2 chain (IL-12Rβ2), IL-12 stimulates T and NK cells to produce IFN-γ and IL-2. Homodimeric IFN-γ binds to the IFN-γ receptor complex *(IFN-γR)*. IFN-γ receptor 1 *(IFN-γR1)* is the binding chain, whereas IFN-γ receptor 2 *(IFN-γR2)* is necessary to transmit the signal intracellularly through the signal transduction and activator of transcription 1 *(STAT-1)*. The mechanisms by which IFN-γ stimulates intracellular microorganism killing are not fully understood but are likely to be numerous (e.g., up-regulation of MHC expression and IL-12 production, enhancement of antigen processing and reactive oxygen species production, reduction of the phagosomal pH). IFN-γ also stimulates tumor necrosis factor-α (TNF-α) production. TNF-α, acting through the TNF-α receptor *(TNF-αR)*, also shows effects against intracellular infections. Patients with mutations in the NFκB essential modulator *(NEMO)*, a protein critical in the TNF-α signaling pathway, have enhanced susceptibility to mycobacterial disease as well as other infections. IL-12 is not the only cytokine that stimulates IFN-γ production: IL-15, IL-18, and probably other factors have the same effect. Lipopolysaccharide *(LPS)* stimulation through the CD14/Toll-like receptor 2 complex can also stimulate IL-12 production.

Patients with defects in IFN-γR1 (6q23-q24), IFN-γR2 (21q22.1-q22.2), IL-12 receptor β1 (19p13.1), IL-12 p40 (5q31.1-33.1), and STAT-1 (2q32.2-q32.3) have been identified through their susceptibility to mycobacteria as well as to *Salmonella* infections.[148,149] Although these patients have a common infection susceptibility, there are phenotypic distinctions for the different genotypes.

Patients with autosomal recessive mutations leading to abolition of IFN-γR1 or IFN-γR2 expression have the most severe phenotypes. They present early in life, especially if they receive bacille Calmette-Guérin vaccination. These patients have poor or no granuloma formation in response to mycobacterial infections and typically develop repeated, disseminated, life-threatening infections caused by mycobacteria, salmonellae, and some viruses. In contrast, a common dominant mutation in IFN-γR1 is the result of 818del4, which leads to a truncation of the molecule that preserves the ligand-binding aspects but removes its recycling domain. Therefore the mutant IFN-γR1 protein remains stuck on the cell surface, where it binds IFN-γ but cannot signal appropriately. Patients with this autosomal dominant mutation in IFN-γR1 are less severely affected. They usually present before age 7 with pulmonary nontuberculous mycobacterial infection but then may go on to develop recurrent multifocal nontuberculous

osteomyelitis. Patients with IL-12 p40, IL-12 receptor β1, and STAT-1 mutations usually have a phenotype not as severe as complete IFN-γR1 and IFN-γR2 deficiency. Recent studies suggest that for IL-12 receptor β1 deficiency, the infection risk for nontuberculous mycobacteria is much higher in childhood but wanes after age 12.[150]

Defects in this pathway can be detected in several ways. Flow cytometry has proved to be very efficient for IFN-γR1 defects, as this protein is expressed on all nucleated cells all the time, to varying extents. In the case of the autosomal dominant form of IFN-γR1 deficiency, the protein is overabundant on the cell surface and therefore very easy to detect.[151] In contrast, direct detection of IFN-γR2 and IL-12Rβ1 requires cell culture and proliferation. Detection of intracellular phosphorylated STAT-1 after IFN-γ stimulation or phosphorylated STAT-4 after IL-12 stimulation is an indirect means of demonstrating functional integrity of the IFN-γ and IL-12 receptors, respectively.[152,153] Direct detection of IL-12 p40 or IL-12 p70 can be used for the diagnosis of patients who are deficient in IL-12 p40.[154] Defects in STAT-1 require research techniques.[155]

Treatment of infections in these patients poses special problems. For the patients with complete IFN-γR defects, there is no benefit to the use of subcutaneous IFN-γ to help in the clearance of mycobacterial disease. However, in patients with autosomal dominant IFN-γR1 deficiency, IL-12 defects, or IL-12R defects, IFN-γ is effective. Bone marrow transplantation for IFN-γR defects has been disappointing overall, for reasons that are still unclear. Currently, we recommend long-term prophylaxis against environmental mycobacterial infections with a macrolide such as azithromycin or clarithromycin.

Hyper-IgE and Recurrent Infection Syndrome

Hyper-IgE and recurrent infection syndrome (HIES, Job's syndrome) is a rare autosomal disorder characterized by recurrent infections, typically of the lower respiratory system and skin; eczema; extremely elevated levels of IgE; eosinophilia; and abnormalities of the connective tissue, skeleton, and dentition. The majority of patients have facial abnormalities including ocular hypertelorism; a prominent, protruding, triangular mandible; and a broad, somewhat bulbous nose[156] (Table 12-6). Failure of primary dental deciduousness, leading either to failure of secondary dentition erup-

TABLE 12-6 Characteristics of Hyper-IgE Recurrent Infection (Job's) Syndrome

Clinical Findings in Hyper-IgE Syndrome	Percentage
Eczema	100
Characteristic facies (> 16y)	100
Skin boils	87
Pneumonias	87
Mucocutaneous candidiasis	83
Lung cysts	77
Scoliosis (> 16y)	76
Delayed dental exfoliation	72
Pathologic fractures	57

Modified from Grimbacher B, Holland SM, Gallin JI, et al: *N Engl J Med* 340:692-702, 1999.

tion or retention of both sets of teeth, is common.[156] Many patients also have abnormalities of bone formation and metabolism, which may result in fractures, severe scoliosis, kyphosis, and craniosynostosis.[156] HIES occurs spontaneously in all racial and ethnic groups and in many cases is transmitted as an autosomal dominant trait.[156]

IgE is greatly elevated at some point in the life of all patients with HIES.[156-158] A few patients have been observed to drop their IgE levels below 2000 IU/ml as they get older and yet retain their susceptibility to infection.[156] Grimbacher et al[156] confirmed autosomal dominant transmission in seven families extending over several generations with variable expressivity. The rate of spontaneous occurrence is unknown, but sporadic cases account for at least half of those recognized so far. Several of the families described by Grimbacher et al[159] are linked to proximal 4q. However, several autosomal dominant families are not linked to 4q, suggesting that there are at least two genetically distinct types of autosomal dominant HIES. There may also be autosomal recessive forms of HIES, as suggested by several consanguineous kindred in which there are multiple affected members.[160] Therefore HIES is likely a complex autosomal disorder with both dominant and recessive forms.

The clinical manifestations of HIES are distinct. Patients usually present within the first days to months of life with severe eczema. Other early signs include mucocutaneous candidiasis and severe diaper rash. Sinus or pulmonary infections, predominantly with *S. aureus* or *Haemophilus influenzae,* are common. Postinflammatory pneumatoceles are often noted early in life; otitis media and externa are common. Infections occur less frequently in bones and joints and very infrequently in the liver, kidneys, and the gastrointestinal tract; documented sepsis is rare. Other pathogens that have been recovered include *Aspergillus* species, *Pseudomonas aeruginosa, Streptococcus pneumoniae,* group A streptococci, *Cryptococcus neoformans, Pneumocystis carinii,* and *C. albicans.* Cerebrovascular events (strokes, reversible ischemic neurologic deficits, unidentified bright objects/T2 hyperintensities on magnetic resonance imaging scans, carotid artery aneurysms) have been seen in an unusually high number of our patients (unpublished observations). Neoplasms, including Hodgkin's disease, histiocytic lymphoma of the brain in a 10-year-old girl, carcinoma of the tongue, nodular sclerosing Hodgkin's disease, and Barrett's esophagus, have also occurred in HIES patients.

Frequent bony abnormalities have been noted in HIES. Of the nine patients reported by Geha and Leung,[161] five had experienced at least one bone fracture. Of the six patients they tested by single-photon absorptiometry, all showed reduction in bone density. Likewise, the frequency of pathologic fractures in the population reported by Grimbacher et al[156] was 58%. Although the general mechanism for these abnormalities is unknown, Leung et al[162] demonstrated increased *in vitro* bone resorption by monocytes from patients with HIES.

Mucocutaneous candidiasis with involvement of the mouth, vagina, intertriginous areas, fingernails, and toenails affects about 50% of patients with HIES.[156,158] High-dose intravenous antibiotics for a prolonged course are required for eradication of infection and to prevent bronchopleural fistula formation and bronchiectasis. Empirical acute coverage should consider *S. aureus, H. influenzae,* and *S. pneumoniae.*

The former two organisms account for the majority of acute infections. Colonization of pneumatoceles and bronchiectatic lungs with *P. aeruginosa* and *Aspergillus* species can be especially problematic. Cases of esophageal and colonic cryptococcosis have been reported.[163]

The role of prophylactic antibiotics has not been rigorously investigated in this setting, but there is general consensus for their use. Most investigators direct coverage at *S. aureus* with a synthetic penicillin. A scoring system has been devised to aid in the formal diagnosis of HIES patients.[159]

CONCLUSIONS

Various defects of phagocytes have been painstakingly elucidated over the last several decades. Despite the fact that profound neutropenia predisposes patients to essentially all members of the bacterial and fungal kingdoms, metabolic defects in neutrophils and monocytes have relatively narrow spectra of infection. Some of these disorders have almost pathognomonic infection profiles (e.g., CGD, IFN-γ/IL-12 pathway defects). We have now put genetic faces to some of

---

BOX 12-1

KEY CONCEPTS

White Blood Cell Defects: Evaluation and Management

- Patients with white blood cell (WBC) defects usually present early in life with recurrent bacterial or fungal infections.
- Certain infections, such as *Burkholderia cepacia, Nocardia,* and nontuberculous mycobacteria, should always prompt an inquiry into the possibility of an underlying immune defect.
- Specific infection locations, such as omphalitis or osteomyelitis, should raise the suspicion of immune abnormalities.
- Abnormal aspects of host response, such as lack of fever, local inflammation, or pus, should immediately alert the clinician to the possibility of a WBC defect.
- It is better to perform the right test once than the entire battery of immune defect tests several times. Careful consideration of the clinical and microbiologic presentation usually indicates the right path to pursue.
- There is no substitute for the right drug, and that requires knowing the pathogen. Because the spectrum of infection in these diseases may range over several microbiologic kingdoms, empiric therapy is to be discouraged in favor of firm diagnoses.
- Prophylactic antibiotics, antifungal agents, and cytokines are highly successful in treating chronic granulomatous disease and appear to be useful in some other immunodeficiencies as well.
- A molecular diagnosis should be sought whenever possible. The expanding knowledge of genotype-phenotype relationships suggests that not all defects, even those within the same gene, are created equal.

the names of these puzzling diseases, like Kostmann's syndrome and cyclic neutropenia. It still comes as something of a surprise that these two distinct clinical entities are caused by mutations in the same gene. Also, the years of careful work on the genetic and biochemical defects in chronic granulomatous disease and myeloperoxidase deficiency still do not adequately explain the marked infection susceptibility in CGD on the one hand and the remarkable lack of infections in patients with MPO deficiency on the other. These observations remind us that the simple recognition of genes and pathways should not be confused with careful and complete understanding of the mechanism. The latter, despite all the complex diagrams, remains elusive (Boxes 12-1 and 12-2).

Although we have been very successful in identifying rare and flagrant defects affecting white cells that lead to severe infections, the more subtle defects that cause recurrent staphylococcal infections, mucocutaneous candidiasis, and hydradenitis, to name only a few of the vexing problems that frequently confront the clinical immunologist, remain to be determined. Careful study of the known pathways, assiduous following of the ramifications of those pathways to the points where they converge with new pathways, and conscientious characterization of clinical phenotypes will lead to the discovery of these elusive immune defects. In the process we will gain new insights into exactly how we remain so remarkably healthy in the face of so many daily microbial challenges.

In general, attenuated or inactivated viral vaccines are not contraindicated in individuals with primary phagocyte disorders, as antiviral cell-mediated immunity is intact.

Bacille Calmette-Guérin vaccination should be avoided in individuals with chronic granulomatous disease (CGD) or IFN-γ/IL-12 pathway defects, as well as in their newborn close relatives, until the defect is ruled out.

Mulching and gardening should be avoided by individuals with increased susceptibility to aspergillus infections, such as patients with CGD, hyper-IgE syndrome, and neutropenia.

Patients with white blood cell defects often fail to mount a normal inflammatory response, so clinicians and parents must keep a high index of suspicion for asymptomatic or hyposymptomatic infection.

Standard recommendations for duration of therapy of infections are based on assumptions in normal specimens. In the patient with a white cell defect, the host contribution to resolution of infection may be relatively small, leading to a need for longer or more intensive antibiotic or antifungal therapy.

When infections are necrotizing or poorly responsive to antibiotic therapy, surgery may be needed, even in situations in which it would not be needed in unaffected individuals (e.g., liver abscesses and lymphadenitis in CGD almost always need operative removal).

Obtain experienced, expert advice whenever possible.

Online Mendelian Inheritance in Man (OMIM) website (www.ncbi.nlm.nih.gov:80/entrez/query.fcgi?db=OMIM)

1. Conkrite EP, Vincent PV: Granulocytopoiesis in hemopoietic cellular proliferation. In Strohlman F, ed: *Hematopoietic cellular proliferation*, New York, 1970, Grune & Stratton.
2. Kostmann R: Infantile genetic agranulocytosis, *Acta Paediatr Scand [suppl]* 45:1-178, 1956.
3. Dong F, Brynes R, Tidow N, et al: Mutations in the gene for the granulocyte colony-stimulating-factor receptor in patients with acute myeloid leukemia preceded by severe congenital neutropenia, *N Engl J Med* 333:487-493, 1995.
4. Tidow N, Pilz C, Teichmann B, et al: Clinical relevance of point mutations in the cytoplasmic domain of the granulocyte-colony stimulating factor receptor gene in patients with severe congenital neutropenia, *Blood* 89:2369-2375, 1997.
5. Dong F, Hoefsloot L, Schelen A, et al: Identification of a nonsense mutation in the granulocyte-colony-stimulating factor receptor in severe congenital neutropenia, *Proc Natl Acad Sci U S A* 91:4480-4484, 1994.
6. Guba SC, Boxer LA, Emerson SG: G-CSF receptor transmembrane and intracytosolic structure in patients with congenital neutropenia, *Blood* 82:23a, 1993.
7. Sandoval C, Adams-Graves P, Parganas E, et al: The cytoplasmic portion of the G-CSF receptor is normal in patients with Kostmann syndrome, *Blood* 82:185a, 1993.
8. Dale DC, Person RE, Bolyard AA, et al: Mutations in the gene encoding neutrophil elastase in congenital and cyclic neutropenia, *Blood* 96:2317-2322, 2000.
9. Horwitz M, Benson KF, Person RE, et al: Mutations in ELA2, encoding neutrophil elastase, define a 21-day biological clock in cyclic haematopoiesis, *Nat Genet* 23:433-436, 1999.
10. Zeidler C, Boxer L, Dale DC, et al: Management of Kostmann syndrome in the G-CSF era, *Br J Haematol* 109:490-495, 2000.
11. Bonilla MA, Gillio AP, Ruggeiro M, et al: Effects of recombinant human granulocyte colony-stimulating factor on neutropenia in patients with congenital agranulocytosis, *N Engl J Med* 320:1574-1580, 1989.
12. Bonilla MA, Dale D, Zeidler C, et al: Long-term safety of treatment with recombinant human granulocyte colony-stimulating factor (r-metHug-CSF) in patients with severe congenital neutropenias, *Br J Haematol* 88:723-730, 1994.
13. Freedman MH: Safety of long-term administration of granulocyte colony-stimulating factor for severe chronic neutropenia, *Curr Opin Hematol* 4:217-224, 1997.
14. Devriendt K, Kim AS, Mathijs G, et al: Constitutively activating mutation in WASP causes X-linked severe congenital neutropenia, *Nat Genet* 27:313-317, 2001.
15. Wright DG, Dale DC, Fauci AS, et al: Human cyclic neutropenia: clinical review and long-term follow-up of patients, *Medicine (Baltimore)* 60:1-13, 1981.
16. Dale DC, Hammond WP: Cyclic neutropenia: a clinical review, *Blood Rev* 2:178-185, 1988.
17. Palmer SE, Stephens K, Dale DC: Genetics, phenotype, and natural history of autosomal dominant cyclic hematopoiesis, *Am J Med Genet* 66:413-422, 1996.
18. Souid AK: Congenital cyclic neutropenia, *Clin Pediatr (Phila)* 34:151-155, 1995.
19. Hammond WP IV, Price TH, Souza LM, et al: Treatment of cyclic neutropenia with granulocyte colony-stimulating factor, *N Engl J Med* 320:1306-1311, 1989.
20. Gorlin RJ, Gelg B, Diaz GA, et al: WHIM syndrome, an autosomal dominant disorder: clinical, hematological, and molecular studies, *Am J Med Genet* 91:368-376, 2000.
21. Wetzler M, Talpaz M, Kleinerman ES, et al: A new familial immunodeficiency disorder characterized by severe neutropenia, a defective marrow release mechanism and hypogammaglobulinemia, *Am J Med* 89:663-672, 1990.
22. Hord JD, Whitlock JA, Gay JC, et al: Clinical features of myelokathexis and treatment with hematopoietic cytokines: a case report of two patients and review of the literature, *J Pediatr Hematol Oncol* 19:443-448, 1997.

23. Lalezari P, Bernard GE: An isologous antigen-antibody reaction with human neutrophils, related to neonatal neutropenia, *J Clin Invest* 45:1741-1750, 1966.

24. Dale DC: Immune and idiopathic neutropenia, *Curr Opin Hematol* 5:33-36, 1998.

25. Huizinga TW, Kuijpers RW, Kleijer M, et al: Maternal genomic neutrophil FcRIII deficiency leading to neonatal isoimmune neutropenia, *Blood* 76:1927-1932, 1990.

26. Stroncek DF, Skubitz KM, Plachta LB, et al: Alloimmune neonatal neutropenia due to an antibody to the neutrophil Fc-gamma receptor III with maternal deficiency of CD16 antigen, *Blood* 77:1572-1580, 1991.

27. Fromont P, Bettaieb A, Skouri H, et al: Frequency of the polymorphonuclear Fc-gamma receptor III deficiency in the French population and its involvement in the development of neonatal alloimmune neutropenia, *Blood* 79:2131-2134, 1992.

28. Rodwell RL, Gray PH, Taylor KM, et al: Granulocyte colony stimulating factor treatment for alloimmune neonatal neutropenia, *Arch Dis Child Fetal Neonatal Ed* 75:F57-F58, 1996.

29. Gilmore M, Stroncek D, Korones D: Treatment of alloimmune neonatal neutropenia with granulocyte colony-stimulating factor, *J Pediatr* 125:948-951, 1994.

30. Bernini JC: Diagnosis and management of chronic neutropenia during childhood, *Pediatr Clin North Am* 43:773-792, 1996.

31. Bruin MC, von dem Borne AE, Tamminga RY, et al: Neutrophil antibody specificity in different types of childhood autoimmune neutropenia, *Blood* 94:1797-1802, 1999.

32. Lyall EG, Lucas GF, Eden OB: Autoimmune neutropenia of infancy, *J Clin Pathol* 45:431-434, 1992.

33. Hartman KR, Wright DG: Identification of autoantibodies specific for the neutrophil adhesion glycoproteins CD11b/CD18 in patients with autoimmune neutropenia, *Blood* 78:1096-1104, 1991.

34. Bux J, Behrens G, Jaeger G, et al: Diagnosis and clinical course of autoimmune neutropenia in infancy: analysis of 240 cases, *Blood* 91:181-186, 1998.

35. Murray JC, Morad AB: Childhood autoimmune neutropenia and human parvovirus B19 [letter], *Am J Hematol* 47:336, 1994.

36. Hartman KR, Brown KE, Green SW, et al: Lack of evidence for parvovirus B19 viraemia in children with chronic neutropenia [letter; comment], *Br J Haematol* 88:895-896, 1994.

37. Smith MA, Smith JG: The use of granulocyte colony-stimulating factor for treatment of autoimmune neutropenia, *Curr Opin Hematol* 8:165-169, 2001.

38. Soderberg C, Sumitran-Karuppan S, Ljungman P, et al: CD13-specific autoimmunity in cytomegalovirus-infected immunocompromised patients, *Transplantation* 61:594-600, 1996.

39. Gautier E, Bourhis JH, Bayle C, et al: Parvovirus B19 associated neutropenia: treatment with Rh G-CSF, *Hematol Cell Ther* 39:85-87, 1997.

40. Bussel JB, Abboud MR: Autoimmune neutropenia of childhood, *Crit Rev Oncol Hematol* 7:37-51, 1987.

41. Barbosa MD, Nguyen QA, Tchernev VT, et al: Identification of the homologous beige and Chédiak-Higashi syndrome genes, *Nature* 382:262-265, 1996.

42. Nagle DL, Karim MA, Woolf EA, et al: Identification and mutation analysis of the complete gene for Chédiak-Higashi syndrome, *Nat Genet* 14:307-311, 1996.

43. Introne W, Boissy RE, Gahl WA: Clinical, molecular, and cell biological aspects of Chédiak-Higashi syndrome, *Mol Genet Metab* 68:283-303, 1999.

44. Certain S, Barrat F, Pastural E, et al: Protein truncation test of LYST reveals heterogeneous mutations in patients with Chédiak-Higashi syndrome, *Blood* 95:979-983, 2000.

45. Blume RS, Wolff SM: The Chédiak-Higashi syndrome: studies in four patients and a review of the literature, *Medicine (Baltimore)* 51:247, 1972.

46. Blume RS, Bennet JM, Yankee RA, et al: Defective granulocyte regulation in the Chédiak-Higashi syndrome, *N Engl J Med* 279:1009, 1968.

47. Clawson CC, White JG, Repine JE: The Chédiak-Higashi syndrome: evidence that defective leukotaxis is primarily due to an impediment by giant granules, *Am J Pathol* 92:745, 1978.

48. Root RK, Rosenthal AS, Balestra DJ: Abnormal bactericidal, metabolic, and lysosomal functions of Chédiak-Higashi syndrome leukocytes, *J Clin Invest* 51:649-665, 1972.

49. Wolff SM, Dale DC, Clark RA, et al: The Chédiak-Higashi syndrome: studies of host defense, *Ann Intern Med* 76:293-306, 1972.

50. Gallin JI, Elin RJ, Hubert RT, et al: Efficacy of ascorbic acid in Chédiak-Higashi syndrome (CHS): studies in humans and mice, *Blood* 53:226-234, 1979.

51. Stossel TP, Root RK, Vaughan M: Phagocytosis in chronic granulomatous disease and Chédiak-Higashi syndrome, *N Engl J Med* 286:120-123, 1972.

52. Klein M, Roder J, Haliotis T, et al: Chédiak-Higashi gene in humans. II. The selectivity of the defect in natural killer and antibody-dependent cell-mediated cytotoxicity function, *J Exp Med* 151:1049-1058, 1980.

53. Haliotis T, Roder J, Klein M, et al: Chédiak Higashi gene in humans. I. Impairment of natural-killer function, *J Exp Med* 151:1039-1048, 1980.

54. Merino F, Klein GO, Henle W, et al: Elevated antibody titers to Epstein-Barr virus and low natural killer cell activity in patients with Chédiak-Higashi syndrome, *Clin Immunol Immunopathol* 27:326-339, 1983.

55. Sung JH, Meyers JP, Stadlan EM, et al: Neuropathological changes in Chédiak-Higashi syndrome, *J Neuropathol Exp Neurol* 28:86-118, 1969.

56. Lockman LA, Kennedy WR, White JG. The Chédiak-Higashi syndrome: electrophysiological and electron microscopic observations on the peripheral neuropathy, *J Pediatr* 70:942-951, 1967.

57. Misra VP, King RHM, Harding AE, et al: Peripheral neuropathy in the Chédiak-Higashi syndrome, *Acta Neuropathol* 81:354-358, 1991.

58. Uyama E, Hirano T, Ito K, et al: Chédiak-Higashi syndrome presenting as parkinsonism and dementia, *Acta Neurol Scand* 89:175-183, 1994.

59. Henter JI, Elinder G, Ost A, et al: Diagnostic guidelines for hemophagocytic lymphohistiocytosis, *Semin Oncol* 18:29-33, 1991.

60. Barrat FJ, Le Deist F, Benkerrou M, et al: Defective CTLA-4 cycling pathway in Chédiak-Higashi syndrome: a possible mechanism for deregulation of T lymphocyte activation, *Proc Natl Acad Sci U S A* 96:8645-8650, 1999.

61. Bejaoui M, Veber F, Girault D, et al: Phase acceleree de la maladie de Chédiak-Higashi, *Arch Fr Pediatr* 46:733, 1989.

62. Gallin JI, Fletcher MP, Seligmann BE, et al: Human neutrophil-specific granule deficiency: a model to assess the role of the neutrophil-specific granules in the evolution of the inflammatory response, *Blood* 59:1317-1329, 1982.

63. Strauss RG, Bove KE, Jones JF, et al: An anomaly of neutrophil morphology with impaired function, *N Engl J Med* 290:478-484, 1974.

64. Lekstrom-Himes JA, Dorman SE, Kopar P, et al: Neutrophil-specific granule deficiency results from a novel mutation with loss of function of the transcription factor CCAAT/enhancer binding protein epsilon, *J Exp Med* 189:1847-1852, 1999.

65. Lekstrom-Himes J, Xanthopoulos KG: Biological role of the CCAAT/enhancer-binding protein family of transcription factors, *J Biol Chem* 273:28545-28548, 1998.

66. Ambruso DR, Sasada M, Nishiyama H, et al: Defective bactericidal activity and absence of specific granules in neutrophils from a patient with recurrent bacterial infections, *J Clin Immunol* 4:23-30, 1984.

67. Breton-Gorius J, Mason DY, Buriot D, et al: Lactoferrin deficiency as a consequence of a lack of specific granules in neutrophils from a patient with recurrent infections, *Am J Pathol* 99:413-428, 1980.

68. Komiyama A, Morosawa H, Hanamura K, et al: Abnormal neutrophil maturation in a neutrophil defect with morphologic abnormality and impaired function, *J Pediatr* 94:19-25, 1979.

69. Parker RI, McKeown LP, Gallin JI, et al: Absence of the largest platelet-von Willebrand multimers in a patient with lactoferrin deficiency and a bleeding tendency, *Thromb Haemost* 67:320-324, 1992.

70. Segal BH, Leto TL, Gallin JI, et al: Genetic, biochemical, and clinical features of chronic granulomatous disease, *Medicine (Baltimore)* 79:170-200, 2000.

71. Reeves EP, Lu H, Jacobs HL, et al: Killing activity of neutrophils is mediated through activation of proteases by K+ flux, *Nature* 416:291-297, 2002.

72. Winkelstein JA, Marino MC, Johnston RB Jr, et al: Chronic granulomatous disease: report on a national registry of 368 patients, *Medicine (Baltimore)* 79:155-169, 2000.

73. Lublin M, Bartlett DL, Danforth DN, et al: Hepatic abscess in patients with chronic granulomatous disease, *Ann Surg* 235:383-391, 2002.

74. Harris BH, Boles ET: Intestinal lesions in chronic granulomatous disease of childhood, *J Pediatr Surg* 8:955-956, 1973.

75. Sty JR, Chusid MJ, Babbit DP, et al: Involvement of the colon in chronic granulomatous disease of childhood, *Radiology* 132:618, 1979.

76. Markowitz JF, Aranow E, Rausen AR, et al: Progressive esophageal dysfunction in chronic granulomatous disease, *J Pediatr Gastroenterol Nutr* 1:145-149, 1982.

77. Werlin SL, Chusid MJ, Caya J, et al: Colitis in chronic granulomatous disease, *Gastroenterology* 82:328-331, 1982.

78. Lindahl JA, Williams FH, Newman SL: Small bowel obstruction in chronic granulomatous disease, *J Pediatr Gastroenterol Nutr* 3:637-640, 1984.

79. Isaacs D, Wright VM, Shaw DG, et al: Chronic granulomatous disease mimicking Crohn's disease, *J Pediatr Gastroenterol Nutr* 4:498-501, 1985.

80. Griscom NT, Kirkpatrick JA, Girdany BR, et al: Gastric antral narrowing in chronic granulomatous disease of childhood, *Pediatrics* 54:456-460, 1974.

81. Johnson FE, Humbert JR, Kuzela DC, et al: Gastric outlet obstruction due to X-linked chronic granulomatous disease, *Surgery* 78:217-223, 1975.

82. Stopyrowa J, Fyderek K, Sikorska B, et al: Chronic granulomatous disease of childhood: gastric manifestation and response to salazosulfapyridine therapy, *Eur J Pediatr* 149:28-30, 1989.

83. Walther MM, Malech HL, Berman A, et al: The urologic manifestations of chronic granulomatous disease, *J Urol* 147:1314-1318, 1992.

84. Chin TW, Stiehm ER, Faloon J, et al: Corticosteroids in treatment of obstructive lesions of chronic granulomatous disease, *J Pediatr* 111:349-352, 1987.

85. Narita M, Shibata M, Togashi T, et al: Steroid therapy for bronchopneumonia in chronic granulomatous disease, *Acta Pediatr Jpn Overseas Ed* 33:181-185, 1991.

86. Quie PG, Belani KK: Corticosteroids for chronic granulomatous disease, *J Pediatr* 111:393-394, 1987.

87. Southwick FS, van der Meer JWM: Recurrent cystitis and bladder mass in two adults with chronic granulomatosis, *Ann Intern Med* 109:118-121, 1988.

88. Rosh JR, Tang HB, Mayer L, et al: Treatment of intractable gastrointestinal manifestations of chronic granulomatous disease with cyclosporine, *J Pediatr* 126:143-145, 1995.

89. Brandrup F, Koch C, Petri M, et al: Discoid lupus erythematosus-like lesions and stomatitis in female carriers of X-linked chronic granulomatous disease, *Br J Dermatol* 104:495-505, 1981.

90. Kragballe K, Borregaard N, Brandrup F, et al: Relation of monocyte and neutrophil oxidative metabolism to skin and oral lesions in carriers of chronic granulomatous disease, *Clin Exp Immunol* 43:390-398, 1981.

91. Bolscher BG, de Boer M, de Klein A, et al: Point mutations in the B-subunit of cytochrome b558 leading to X-linked chronic granulomatous disease, *Blood* 77:2482-2487, 1991.

92. Vowells SJ, Sekhsaria S, Malech HL, et al: Flow cytometric analysis of the granulocyte respiratory burst: a comparison study of fluorescent probes, *J Immunol Methods* 178:89-97, 1995.

93. Vowells SJ, Fleisher TA, Sekhsaria S, et al: Genotype-dependent variability in flow cytometric evaluation of reduced nicotinamide adenine dinucleotide phosphate oxidase function in patients with chronic granulomatous disease, *J Pediatr* 128:104-107, 1996.

94. Roos D, van Zwieten R, Wijnen JT, et al: Molecular basis and enzymatic properties of glucose 6-phosphate dehydrogenase volendam, leading to chronic nonspherocytic anemia, granulocyte dysfunction, and increased susceptibility to infections, *Blood* 94:2955-2962, 1999.

95. Banerjee R, Anguita J, Roos D, et al: Cutting edge: infection by the agent of human granulocytic ehrlichiosis prevents the respiratory burst by down-regulating gp91phox, *J Immunol* 164:3946-3949, 2000.

96. Gallin JI, Buescher ES, Seligmann BE, et al: NIH conference. Recent advances in chronic granulomatous disease, *Ann Intern Med* 99:657-674, 1983.

97. Forrest CB, Forehand JR, Axtell RA, et al: Clinical features and current management of chronic granulomatous disease, *Hematol Oncol Clin North Am* 2:253-266, 1988.

98. Margolis DM, Melnick DA, Alling DW, et al: Trimethoprim-sulfamethoxazole prophylaxis in the management of chronic granulomatous disease, *J Infect Dis* 162:723-726, 1990.

99. International Chronic Granulomatous Disease Cooperative Study Group: A controlled trial of interferon gamma to prevent infection in chronic granulomatous disease, *N Engl J Med* 324:509-516, 1991.

100. Rex JH, Bennett JE, Gallin JI, et al: Normal and deficient neutrophils can cooperate to damage *Aspergillus fumigatus* hyphae, *J Infect Dis* 162:523-528, 1990.

101. Buescher ES, Gallin JI: Radiation effects on cultured human monocytes and on monocyte-derived macrophages, *Blood* 63:1402-1407, 1984.

102. Buescher ES, Gallin JI: Effects of storage and radiation on human neutrophil function in vitro, *Inflammation* 11:401-416, 1987.

103. Mouy R, Fischer A, Vilmer E, et al: Incidence, severity, and prevention of infections in chronic granulomatous disease, *J Pediatr* 114:555-560, 1989.

104. Kamani N, August CS, Campbell DE, et al: Marrow transplantation in chronic granulomatous disease: an update with 6-year follow-up, *J Pediatr* 113:697-700, 1988.

105. Ozsahin H, von Planta M, Muller I, et al: Successful treatment of invasive aspergillosis in chronic granulomatous disease by bone marrow transplantation, granulocyte colony-stimulating factor-mobilized granulocytes, and liposomal amphotericin-B, *Blood* 92:2719-2724, 1998.

106. Horwitz ME, Barrett AJ, Brown MR, et al: Treatment of chronic granulomatous disease with nonmyeloablative conditioning and T-cell-depleted hematopoietic allograft, *N Engl J Med* 344:881-888, 2001.

107. Malech HL, Maples PB, Whiting-Theobald N, et al: Prolonged production of NADPH oxidase-corrected granulocytes after gene therapy of chronic granulomatous disease, *Proc Natl Acad Sci U S A* 94:12133-12138, 1997.

108. Parry MF, Root RK, Metcalf JA, et al: Myeloperoxidase deficiency: prevalence and clinical significance, *Ann Intern Med* 95:293,1981.

109. Kitahara M, Eyre HJ, Simonian Y, et al: Hereditary myeloperoxidase deficiency, *Blood* 57:888-893, 1981.

110. Nauseef WM, Root RK, Malech HL: Biochemical and immunologic analysis of hereditary myeloperoxidase deficiency, *J Clin Invest* 71:1297, 1983.

111. Nauseef WM: Myeloperoxidase deficiency, *Hematol Oncol Clin North Am* 2:135, 1988.

112. Okuda T, Yasuoka T, Oka N: Myeloperoxidase deficiency as a predisposing factor for deep mucocutaneous candidiasis: a case report, *J Oral Maxillofac Surg* 49:183-186, 1991.

113. Ludviksson BR, Thorarensen O, Gudnason T, et al: *Candida albicans* meningitis in a child with myeloperoxidase deficiency, *Pediatr Infect Dis J* 12:162-164, 1993.

114. Nguyen C, Katner HP: Myeloperoxidase deficiency manifesting as pustular candidal dermatitis, *Clin Infect Dis* 24:258-260, 1997.

115. Chiang AK, Chan GC, Ma SK, et al: Disseminated fungal infection associated with myeloperoxidase deficiency in a premature neonate, *Pediatr Infect Dis J* 19:1027-1029, 2000.

116. Lehrer RI, Cline MJ: Leukocyte myeloperoxidase deficiency and disseminated candidiasis: the role of myeloperoxidase in resistance to *Candida* infection, *J Clin Invest* 48:1478, 1969.

117. Cech P, Stalder H, Widmann JJ, et al: Leukocyte myeloperoxidase deficiency and diabetes mellitus associated with *Candida albicans* liver abscess, *Am J Med* 66:149-153, 1979.

118. Larrocha C, Fernandez de Castro M, Fontan G, et al: Hereditary myeloperoxidase deficiency: study of 12 cases, *Scand J Haematol* 29:389-397, 1982.

119. Repo H, Harlan JM: Mechanisms and consequences of phagocyte adhesion to endothelium, *Ann Med* 31:156-165, 1999.

120. Springer TA, Thompson NS, Miller LJ, et al: Inherited deficiency of the MAC-1, LFA-1, p150,95 glycoprotein family and its molecular basis, *J Exp Med* 160:1901-1918, 1984.

121. Kishimoto TK, Hollander N, Roberts TM, et al: Heterogeneous mutations of the beta subunit common to the LFA-1, Mac-1 and p150,95 glycoproteins cause leukocyte adhesion deficiency, *Cell* 50:193-201, 1987.

122. Kishimoto TK, O'Connor K, Springer TA: Leukocyte adhesion deficiency: aberrant splicing of a conserved integrin sequence causes a moderate deficiency phenotype, *J Biol Chem* 264:3588-3596, 1989.

123. Sligh JE, Hurwitz MY, Zhu C, et al: An initiation codon mutation in CD18 in association with the moderate phenotype of leukocyte adhesion deficiency, *J Biol Chem* 267:714-718, 1992.

124. Anderson DC, Schmalstieg FC, Finegold MJ, et al: The severe and moderate phenotypes of heritable Mac-1, LFA-1 deficiency: their quantitative definition and relation to leukocyte dysfunction and clinical features, *J Infect Dis* 152:668-689, 1985.

125. Anderson DC, Springer TA: Leukocyte adhesion deficiency: an inherited defect in the Mac-1, LFA-1, and P150,95 glycoprotein, *Annu Rev Med* 38:175, 1987.

126. Fischer A, Lisowska-Grospierre B, Anderson DC, et al: Leukocyte adhesion deficiency: molecular basis and functional consequences, *Immunodefic Rev* 1:39-54, 1988.

127. Kuijpers TW, van Lier RAW, Hamann D, et al: Leukocyte adhesion deficiency type 1 (LAD-1)/variant, *J Clin Invest* 100:1725-1733, 1997.

128. Hogg N, Stewart MP, Scarth SL, et al: A novel leukocyte adhesion deficiency caused by expressed but nonfunctional beta2 integrins Mac-1 and LFA-1, *J Clin Invest* 103:97-106, 1999.

129. LeDiest F, Blanche S, Keable H, et al: Successful HLA nonidentical bone marrow transplantation in three patients with leukocyte adhesion deficiency, *Blood* 74:512-518, 1989.

130. Fischer A, Landais P, Friedrich W: Bone marrow transplantation (BMT) in Europe for primary immunodeficiencies other than severe combined immunodeficiency, *Blood* 83:1149-1154, 1994.

131. Thomas C, Le Deist F, Cavazzana-Calvo M, et al: Results of allogeneic bone marrow transplantation in patients with leukocyte adhesion deficiency, *Blood* 86:1629-1635, 1995.

132. Hibbs ML, Wardlaw AJ, Stacker SA, et al: Transfection of cells from patients with leukocyte adhesion deficiency with an integrin beta subunit (CD18) restores lymphocyte function-associated antigen-1 expression and function, *J Clin Invest* 85:674-681, 1990.

133. Wilson JM, Ping AJ, Krauss JC, et al: Correction of CD18-deficient lymphocytes by retrovirus-mediated gene transfer, *Science* 248:1413-1416, 1990.

134. Bauer TR, Schwartz BR, Conrad Liles W, et al: Retroviral-mediated gene transfer of the leukocyte integrin CD18 into peripheral blood CD34+ cells derived from a patient with leukocyte adhesion deficiency type 1, *Blood* 91:1520-1526, 1998.

135. Lübke T, Marquardt T, Etzioni A, et al: Complementation cloning identifies CDG-IIc, a new type of congenital disorders of glycosylation, as a GDP-glucose transporter deficiency, *Nat Genet* 28:73-76, 2001.

136. Lühn K, Wild MK, Eckhardt M, et al: The gene defective in leukocyte adhesion deficiency II encodes a putative GDP-fucose transporter, *Nat Genet* 28:69-72, 2001.

137. Frydman M, Etzioni A, Eidlitz-Markus T, et al: Ramban-Hasharon syndrome of psychomotor retardation, short stature, defective neutrophil motility and Bombay phenotype, *Am J Med Genet* 44:297-302, 1992.

138. Etzioni A, Frydman M, Pollack S, et al: Brief report: recurrent severe infections caused by a novel leukocyte adhesion deficiency, *N Engl J Med* 327:1789-1792, 1992.

139. Etzioni A, Gershoni-Baruch R, Pollack S, et al: Leukocyte adhesion deficiency type II: long-term follow-up, *J Allergy Clin Immunol* 102:323-324, 1998.

140. Etzioni A: Adhesion molecule deficiencies and their clinical significance, *Cell Adhesion Comm* 2:257-260, 1994.

141. Phillips ML, Schwartz BR, Etzioni A, et al: Neutrophil adhesion deficiency syndrome type 2, *J Clin Invest* 96:2898-2906, 1995.

142. Marquardt T, Luhn K, Srikrishna G, et al: Correction of leukocyte adhesion deficiency type II with oral glucose, *Blood* 94:3976-3985, 1999.

143. Etzioni A, Tonetti M: Glucose supplementation in leukocyte adhesion deficiency type II (letter), *Blood* 95:3641-3642, 2000.

144. DeLisser HM, Christofidou-Solomidou M, Sun J, et al: Loss of endothelial surface expression of E-selectin in a patient with recurrent infections, *Blood* 94:884-894, 1999.

145. Ambruso DR, Knall C, Abell AN, et al: Human neutrophil immunodeficiency syndrome is associated with an inhibitory Rac2 mutation, *Proc Natl Acad Sci U S A* 97:4654-4659, 2000.

146. Williams DA, Tao W, Yang F, et al: Dominant negative mutation of the hematopoietic-specific Rho GTPase, Rac2, is associated with a human phagocyte immunodeficiency, *Blood* 96:1646-1654, 2000.

147. Bach EA, Aguet M, Schreiber RD: The IFN gamma receptor: a paradigm for cytokine receptor signaling, *Annu Rev Immunol* 15:563-591, 1997.

148. Dorman SE, Holland SM: Defects in the interferon gamma and IL-12 pathways, *Cytol Growth Factor Rev* 11:321-333, 2000.

149. Casanova JL, Abel L: Genetic dissection of immunity to mycobacteria: the human model, *Annu Rev Immunol* 20:581-620, 2002.

150. Fieschi C, Dupuis S, Catherinot E, et al: Low penetrance, broad resistance and favorable outcome of IL-12 receptor β1-deficiency: medical and immunological implications, *J Exp Med* (in press).

151. Jouanguy E, Lamhamedi-Cherradi S, Lammas D, et al: A human IFNGR1 small deletion hotspot associated with dominant susceptibility to mycobacterial infection, *Nat Genet* 21:370-378, 1999.

152. Fleisher AT, Dorman SE, Anderson JA, et al: Detection of intracellular phosphorylated STAT-1 by flow cytometry, *Clin Immunol* 90:425-430, 1999.

153. Uzel G, Frucht DM, Fleisher A, et al: Detection of intracellular phosphorylated STAT-4 by flow cytometry, *Clin Immunol* 100:270-276, 2001.

154. Altare F, Durandy A, Lammas D, et al: Impairment of mycobacterial immunity in human interleukin-12 receptor deficiency, *Science* 280:1432-1435, 1998.

155. Dupuis S, Dargemont C, Fieschi C, et al: Impairment of mycobacterial but not viral immunity by a germline human STAT1 mutation, *Science* 293:300-303, 2001.

156. Grimbacher B, Holland SM, Gallin JI, et al: Hyper-IgE syndrome with recurrent infections: an autosomal dominant multisystem disorder, *N Engl J Med* 340:692-702, 1999.

157. Buckley RH, Becker WG: Abnormalities in the regulation of human IgE synthesis, *Immunol Rev* 41:288, 1978.

158. Donabedian H, Gallin JI: The hyperimmunoglobulin E recurrent infection (Job's) syndrome: a review of the NIH experience and the literature, *Medicine (Baltimore)* 62:195, 1983.

159. Grimbacher B, Schaffer AA, Holland SM, et al: Genetic linkage of hyper-IgE syndrome to chromosome 4, *Am J Hum Genet* 65:735-744, 1999.

160. Renner ED, Holland SM, Schmitt M, et al: Autosomal recessive hyper-IgE syndrome: a distinct disease entity, *J Pediatr* (in press).

161. Geha RS, Leung DYM: Hyper immunoglobulin E syndrome, *Immunodeficiency Rev* 1:155, 1989.

162. Leung DY, Key L, Steinberg JJ, et al: Increased in vitro bone resorption by monocytes in the hyper-immunoglobulin E syndrome, *J Immunol* 140:84-88, 1988.

163. Hutto JO, Bryan CS, Greene FL, et al: Cryptococcosis of the colon resembling Crohn's disease in a patient with the hyperimmunoglobulinemia E-recurrent infection (Job's) syndrome, *Gastroenterology* 94:808, 1988.

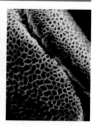

CHAPTER **13**

Rheumatic Diseases of Childhood: Therapeutic Principles

J. ROGER HOLLISTER

The rheumatic diseases of childhood encompass a wide spectrum of symptomatology. As a group, these illnesses are considered to be autoimmune disorders, implying that pathogenesis involves the host's immune system producing inflammation in the affected organs. Important disease differentials include those caused by a specific agent (e.g., septic arthritis, Lyme disease), malignancy (e.g., solid tumors or hematologic neoplasia), and allergic disorders (e.g., chronic sinusitis, chronic urticaria, or serum sickness). Table 13-1 lists the disease differential. Figure 13-1 is an algorithm for an approach to the evaluation of musculoskeletal pain in childhood.

JUVENILE RHEUMATOID ARTHRITIS

Juvenile rheumatoid arthritis (JRA) is the most common rheumatic disease of childhood.[1] It affects approximately one in a thousand children under the age of 16. There is a three to one female predominance except for the systemic-onset type, which is more gender neutral. The cause of JRA remains unknown. The most promising research suggests a multigene predisposition in combination with an unknown environmental agent. Diet, trauma, person-to-person transmission, and geographic locale have been eliminated as potential causes. The pathogenesis involves chronic inflammation of synovial tissue with infiltration of neutrophils and activated macrophages and lymphocytes. Many cytokines are locally active, and tumor necrosis factor (TNF) may play a central regulatory role.[2,3] There are three disease-onset patterns that have been recognized, and the natural history and complications are sufficiently unique to each type to merit the distinction.

Diagnosis

Pauciarticular JRA is the most common type. There are two peaks of onset: one between the ages of 1 and 5 years and the other between 12 and 16 years. Most patients present with a gradual onset of pain and swelling in one to five joints. The pattern is frequently asymmetric. The knee is most commonly affected, followed by the ankle, wrist, and elbow. The role of trauma as the triggering event for the chronic inflammatory process is difficult to analyze because children frequently experience mild extremity trauma as a result of their normal daily activities. Although there may be a history of such minor trauma, joint swelling lasting more than 24 hours is distinctly unusual from orthopedic causes. Similarly, internal mechanical derangements such as torn menisci are very uncommon in childhood.

The pain may range from being quite severe to extremely mild, where only the joint swelling is manifest. Morning stiffness or gelling during the day is very characteristic and suggests an inflammatory cause to the joint swelling. It is important to obtain a history with regard to limping or failure to use an upper extremity in judging the significance of joint pain,

---

TABLE 13-1 Differential Diagnosis of Musculoskeletal Pain

I. Autoimmune diseases
  A. Arthritides
    Juvenile rheumatoid arthritis
    Spondyloarthropathies
    Reactive, acute rheumatic fever
      Postdysentery
      Transient synovitis
  B. Collagen vascular disorders
    Systemic lupus erythematosus
    Juvenile dermatomyositis
    Vasculitis: Henoch-Schönlein purpura, polyarteritis nodosa, Kawasaki disease, Wegener's granulomatosis
II. Infections
  A. Bacterial septic arthritis
  B. Lyme disease
  C. Viral: Parvo B19
III. Malignancy
  A. Solid tumors
  B. Leukemia
  C. Neuroblastoma
IV. Orthopedic
  A. Trauma
  B. Aseptic necrosis (Legg-Calvé-Perthes disease)
  C. Slipped capital femoral epiphysis
  D. Stress fracture
  E. Spondylolysis and spondylolisthesis
  F. Osteochondroses (Osgood-Schlatter disease, Sever's disease)
V. Pain syndromes
  A. Growing pains
  B. Fibromyalgia
  C. Overuse syndrome
  D. Hypermobility syndrome
  E. Reflex sympathetic dystrophy

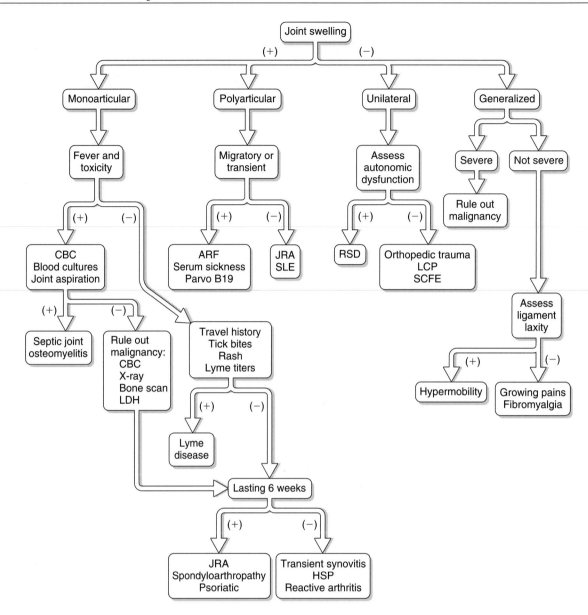

FIGURE 13-1 Algorithm for evaluation of musculoskeletal pain in childhood. *CBC,* Complete blood cell count; *ARF,* acute rheumatic fever; *JRA,* juvenile rheumatoid arthritis; *SLE,* systemic lupus erythematosus; *RSD,* reflex sympathetic dystrophy; *LCP,* Legg-Calvé-Perthes disease; *SCFE,* slipped capital femoral epiphysis; *LDH,* lactic dehydrogenase; *HSP,* Henoch-Schönlein purpura.

particularly in individuals whose joint swelling may not be apparent.

It is unusual for JRA to begin in a single hip, and such onset requires a wider differential diagnosis, particularly of orthopedic conditions within the hip. With onset below the age of 3 years, particularly with involvement of a single knee, there is the possibility of leg-length discrepancy over time and significant muscle atrophy.[4] There is suggestive evidence that a local steroid injection may prevent these sequelae.

The pauciarticular pattern of JRA onset defines a type of arthritis that is uniquely at risk for chronic, asymptomatic anterior uveitis. This may occur in up to 30% of such children if they are antinuclear antibody (ANA) positive. Detection of the uveitis is not possible with a routine ophthalmoscope, and therefore these children need to be in a screening program with an ophthalmologist for slit-lamp evaluation of the earl-

est signs of inflammation. Early detection of the uveitis is important in preventing sequelae, which may lead to decreased visual acuity or even blindness.[5]

Pauciarticular presentation in males over the age of 10, particularly with lower-extremity involvement, suggests the possibility of a spondyloarthropathy (see the section "Spondyloarthropathies").

POLYARTICULAR JUVENILE RHEUMATOID ARTHRITIS

Polyarticular JRA affects many joints, large and small, and frequently manifests a symmetric pattern. This type of JRA most resembles adult rheumatoid arthritis in its clinical presentation. It is important to obtain both a history and physical evidence of joint swelling in defining these individuals because there are other causes of only arthralgias (see Figure 13-1). It is this group of patients who may manifest rheumatoid nodules over areas of dermal trauma such as the elbows or feet. Systemic features are more common in this group of patients and include afternoon fatigue and anemia.

A subgroup of polyarticular JRA patients has positive tests for rheumatoid factor, most often in the older-age onset children. In long-term follow-up studies, the presence of rheumatoid factors in serum connotes more aggressive disease with a greater possibility of joint damage and disability.[1] Therefore seropositive children with polyarticular JRA should be treated early with second-level antiinflammatory or immunosuppressive medications.

The third type of JRA, *systemic-onset JRA (called Still's disease* in Europe), is the least common form. It presents to the physician as a fever of unknown origin (FUO). The fevers are prolonged, lasting from weeks to months. They are high-grade fevers reaching 104° to 105° F on a daily basis, often at the same time each day.[6] They have a quotidian or double quotidian pattern with normal or subnormal temperature levels in between. Sustained fevers throughout a 24-hour period are not characteristic. Patients may experience chills and toxicity with the fevers, which improve during afebrile intervals. Appetite is frequently decreased, and weight loss may occur.

A diagnostic rash occurs in 90% of patients with systemic-onset JRA[7] (Figure 13-2). The rash consists of an evanescent 3- to 5-mm erythematous macular or barely papular lesion occurring most commonly on the trunk and proximal extremities; however, the rash can involve the face and hands and feet as well. A rash located in a single area for more than 24 hours is incompatible with the diagnosis. The rash may be asymptomatic or occasionally pruritic and is frequently found during fever elevations. The rash may demonstrate the Koebner phenomenon of rash induction with dermal trauma. In patients with a diagnostic rash, extensive evaluation for other causes of an FUO may not be necessary.

Less specific symptoms or findings include lymphadenopathy, hepatospondomegaly, or serositis. Joint symptoms may be lacking in the first several weeks of the FUO in these patients. Arthralgia may be more prominent than arthritis.

Laboratory assessment of systemic-onset JRA shows striking evidence of inflammation. The white blood cell count is frequently elevated in the 20,000 to 30,0000 range with a left shift. Sedimentation rate is always elevated, usually between 60 to 80 mm/hr. A normal sedimentation rate excludes the diagnosis of systemic-onset JRA. Anemia may be significant, with hemoglobin as low as 7 g/dl but rarely lower. Platelet counts should be normal and are frequently significantly elevated. Thrombocytopenia is a worrisome finding and suggests an alternative diagnosis such as malignancy, lupus, or macrophage activation syndrome.

Laboratory Assessment

The laboratory assessment of JRA should include a complete blood cell count (CBC), sedimentation rate, ANA, and rheumatoid factor (the latter in older-age polyarticular presentation); the results may be nondiagnostic. Pauciarticular JRA with a single involved joint may demonstrate a normal sedimentation rate, which does not mitigate against the diagnosis in a patient who by history and physical examination demonstrates chronic synovitis. A positive ANA in a patient with pauciarticular disease increases the risk of uveitis from 10% to 30%. All ANA-positive pauciarticular patients need 3-month ophthalmologic screening, whereas ANA-negative patients can be screened every 6 months. The duration of the ophthalmologic screening should be for 4 years after the onset of the arthritis regardless of whether the disease enters remission. Systemic-onset JRA patients never have a positive ANA or rheumatoid factor. In older-age onset males with lower-extremity presentation, a human leukocyte antigen (HLA)-B27 test may be positive in support of the diagnosis of a spondyloarthopathy.

X-rays of involved joints show little more than soft tissue swelling. Bone scans in perplexing patients usually show tracer uptake on both sides of the joint, which is consistent with arthritis and not indicative of osteomyelitis. Magnetic resonance imaging (MRI) scans are rarely indicated but, when performed, show increased joint fluid with evidence of synovial inflammation. The use of tagged white blood cell scans in patients with FUO has not been critically studied for sensitivity and specificity.

Differential Diagnosis

Pain in a single extremity requires that infection and malignancy be excluded. With either of these conditions, the pain is usually progressive and severe. If a joint is not swollen, osteomyelitis, bone tumor, or hematologic malignancy is possible. An x-ray and blood count with sedimentation rate can help to distinguish these entities. In questionable cases, a bone scan can help differentiate osteomyelitis, and serum lactate dehydrogenase (LDH) can discriminate conditions with rapid cell turnover such as malignancy.[8]

If a joint is acutely swollen with progressive pain, fever, toxicity, and erythema over the joint, septic arthritis must be excluded by aspiration of the joint (see Figure 13-1). A septic hip will not, however, demonstrate joint swelling, but patients are usually systemically ill, the pain is rapidly progressive, and the white blood count and sedimentation rate are markedly elevated. *Staphylococcus* accounts for the vast majority of septic joints, and in acute situations, treatment with the appropriate antibiotic is reasonable until the results of the cultures are known. With monoarticular involvement and a preceding history of viral infection and only moderate pain, a reactive

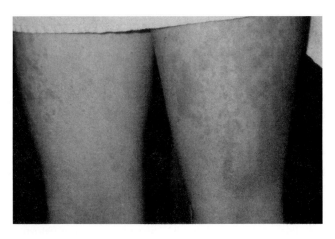

FIGURE 13-2 Skin eruption in systemic juvenile rheumatoid arthritis.

arthritis or transient synovitis may be the most likely explanation; blood work and sedimentation rates will be normal.

With polyarticular joint complaints and swelling, the differential diagnosis includes rheumatic fever, systemic lupus erythematosus (SLE), disseminated gonococcal infection, and in the adolescent population Parvo B19 viral arthritis. The arthritis of rheumatic fever is frequently migratory and quite painful. Evidence of rheumatic carditis should be carefully sought with auscultation for a regurgitant heart murmur. Markedly elevated sedimentation rates are the hallmark of rheumatic fever and poststreptococcal arthritis. Evidence of recent streptococcal infection with antibody titers is essential to the diagnosis. The polyarthralgia and polyarthritis of SLE is usually accompanied by other evidence of multi-organ involvement with that disease. Disseminated gonococcal infection with polyarthralgia and eventual monoarthritis is usually accompanied by embolic skin lesions, onset during menstruation, and a history of recent unprotected sex. Parvovirus B19 polyarthritis may be distinguished by exposure to children with fifth disease, skin rash, and low-grade fever.

Lyme arthritis resembles pauciarticular JRA; however, it occurs as discrete, recurrent episodes of arthritis lasting 2 to 6 weeks.[9] It appears primarily in five states, all of which are endemic for Lyme disease. A negative test for antibodies to *Borrelia burgdorferi* strongly argues against this diagnosis.

Treatment

The treatment principles for JRA are shown in Box 13-1. The treatment of JRA begins with nonsteroidal antiinflammatory drugs (NSAIDs). For younger children who require liquid medications, naprosyn (7.5 mg/kg twice daily) or ibuprofen (10 mg/kg two or three times daily) is available; newer agents are currently under development. For older children, naprosyn 250 to 375 mg twice daily, diclofenac 50 to 75 mg twice daily, or tolmetin (30 mg/kg/day) should provide symptomatic relief. Newer NSAIDs, including the COX2 inhibitors, are currently being tested in children; their advantages include less gastric irritation and no effect on platelet function.

BOX 13-1	**THERAPEUTIC PRINCIPLES** Juvenile Rheumatoid Arthritis

ANTIINFLAMMATORY MEDICATIONS

Nonsteroidal antiinflammatory drugs
COX2 inhibitors
Steroids
Analgesics

REHABILITATION TECHNIQUES

Physical therapy
Occupational therapy
Psychologic support
Exercise

ADVANCED THERAPIES

Immunosuppressants
Biologic agents

Temporary symptomatic relief from steroids such as prednisone 5 mg daily or twice daily should be done in consultation with a pediatric rheumatologist.

Second-line therapy of JRA begins with methotrexate in a low dose, administered on a weekly basis. Newer agents, including TNF inhibitors (etanercept and infliximab), are available for patients in whom methotrexate therapy fails.[10]

Prognosis

Overall, the prognosis for patients with JRA is markedly better than it was in the late 1990s. Treatment with second-line agents has reduced disability and the need for total joint replacement; 80% to 90% of children should have a favorable course and are able to maintain a largely normal lifestyle. Less favorable prognosis is associated with systemic-onset JRA that becomes chronic arthritis, chronic uveitis, and rheumatoid factor–positive polyarticular JRA.[1]

SPONDYLOARTHROPATHIES
Diagnosis

The spondyloarthropathies are a group of inflammatory disorders in childhood, which at disease onset and over the course of time are distinguishable from the more common JRA.[11] Several characteristics of these patients set them apart and with proper classification should suggest somewhat different treatments and follow-up protocols. As a group, these patients have an older age of onset (usually over the age of 9 years), males are much more affected than females, and pauciarticular lower-extremity synovitis is most typical. The history frequently reveals evidence of enthesitis (inflammation at the insertion of tendons and ligaments on bone), most often at the heel or at the knee over the tibial tuberosity; enthesitis is very uncommon in children with JRA. Furthermore, the history frequently reveals other members of the family in preceding generations with ankylosing spondylitis, psoriasis, inflammatory bowel disease, or Reiter's disease. These individuals, in particular those with a strong family history, may be HLA-B27 positive. Axial involvement (sacroiliitis or lumbosacral pain) may not be present at disease onset but may evolve over time, which allows better classification of these individuals.

Extraarticular manifestations include acute iritis (a hot, red, photophobic process markedly different from the silent, chronic uveitis seen in JRA patients). Psoriatic skin lesions, symptoms of inflammatory bowel disease, or the quite rare triad of Reiter's syndrome (conjunctivitis, urethritis, and arthritis) may be found.

As with other inflammatory arthritic conditions, the history may indicate morning stiffness and fatigue, which may be helpful in distinguishing these entities from osteochondroses (Osgood-Schlatter disease or Sever's disease).

Laboratory Assessment

Laboratory assessment may reveal an elevated sedimentation rate or C-reactive protein (CRP) indicative of inflammation as the source of the patient's symptoms as opposed to trauma or overuse. ANA is rarely positive and rheumatoid factors are absent. Positive tests for HLA-B27 provide supportive information but are not diagnostic.[12] The test is positive in approximately 80% to 90% of patients as opposed to 6% to 8% in the general Caucasian population. Therefore, a negative HLA-B27 does exclude the diagnosis if the clinical symptomatology is characteristic.

Radiologic techniques are not especially useful early in the disease course. Routine x-rays may show swelling of peripheral joints. MRI, which is expensive, may show the same inflammatory process at the enthesis or tendon sheath, which is evident on physical examination.

Differential diagnosis includes patients with JRA, overuse syndromes such as plantar fasciitis, and the osteochondroses.

Pathology

Pathologic specimens from affected areas reveal chronic inflammation indistinguishable from JRA. The pathogenesis of these diseases in patients who are HLA-B27 positive may relate to specific environmental triggers (see a fuller discussion in Chapter 14).

Treatment

Patients identified as having a spondyloarthopathy do not need to undergo long-term screening slit-lamp examinations as JRA patients would need to do because their eye symptoms are dramatic and lead to early referral to an ophthalmologist.

In patients with axial involvement of the lumbosacral spine or sacroiliac joints, physical therapy to maintain good posture is very important. Should a child's illness evolve into typical ankylosing spondylitis, fusion of axial joints is possible, and physical therapy should ensure that this be done in the most functional position possible. Orthotics may be of some benefit in managing the enthesitis in the foot.

Although no control trials in children have been conducted, naproxen (15 mg/kg/day), tolmetin (20 to 30 mg/kg/day), and indomethacin (2 to 4 mg/kg/day) are more effective than other nonsteroidal agents. Refractory cases may benefit from treatment with sulfasalazine.[13] Response to methotrexate is less impressive than it is in JRA patients. Treatment with the new anti-TNF agents appears effective in adult series and may well be applied to children with these disorders.

SYSTEMIC LUPUS ERYTHEMATOSUS

SLE is the prototypic autoimmune disease with the most diverse clinical presentation resulting from multiorgan disease.[14] Disease pathogenesis is related to the deposition in tissue of soluble immune complexes. The spectrum of manifestations is not caused by tissue-specific autoantibodies but rather by immune complex deposition with subsequent inflammatory events with neutrophils, lymphocytes, complement activation, and cytokine production. Initiation and perpetuation of the disease may be caused by autoreactive T lymphocytes that have escaped clonal deletion and poorly regulated B lymphocytes producing autoantibodies.[15]

SLE is not a common disease. Various estimates from several different series have concluded that the annual incidence is approximately 0.36 case per hundred thousand children under the age of 16; SLE under the age of 6 is rare. The female-to-male ratio is approximately 8:1, depending on the series. SLE appears to be both more common and more severe in the African-American and Hispanic populations.

Diagnosis

The diagnosis of SLE has benefited from criteria developed and validated by the American College of Rheumatology and are listed in Table 13-2. If 4 of the 11 criteria are fulfilled in an individual patient, there is a 90% probability that SLE is the correct diagnosis.

Musculoskeletal symptoms of joint pain and swelling are the most common organ system manifestations of SLE. They are present at onset or during disease evolution in more than 90% of patients.[16] If patients present with only constitutional symptoms such as fatigue, malaise, subjective weakness, or a weight loss, one should not seriously consider SLE or an ANA unless arthritic symptoms are part of the history. The pain of the arthritis, although it is a "nonerosive" process, may be more striking than the degree of inflammation in the individual joints found on physical examination.

Rashes in SLE may take many forms (Figure 13-3). Vasculitic rashes appear as 3- to 4-mm erythematous, nonblanching macular, or macular/papular, which may be seen on many parts of the body, including the palms and soles. Malar rashes across the cheeks and over the bridge of the nose, which gave the disease its name because it was felt to resemble the mask or bite of the wolf, are present in fewer than 50% of SLE patients. Besides erythema in that distribution, there should be evidence of scaling and follicular plugging. Photosensitive rashes may be seen in other parts of the body besides the malar distribution, where ultraviolet light exposure occurs. However, true photosensitivity occurs in only 30% of SLE patients. These individuals must protect the skin from ultraviolet exposure, as a flare of the skin disease may lead to a generalized autoimmune activation of the symptoms in many other organs. Urticaria as a skin manifestation is very uncommon in SLE. Evidence of other organ involvement should be sought in urticarial patients before ordering an ANA because there is a considerable false-positive ANA rate in chronic urticaria patients.

TABLE 13-2 American College of Rheumatology 1997 Criteria for Systemic Lupus Erythematosus

Malar (butterfly) rash
Discoid—lupus rash
Photosensitivity
Oral or nasal mucocutaneous ulceration
Nonerosive arthritis
Nephritis
    Proteinuria 0.5 g/day
    Cellular casts
Encephalopathy
    Seizures
    Psychosis
Pleuritis or pericarditis
Cytopenias
Positive immunoserology
    Antibodies to dsDNA
    Antibodies to Smith nuclear antigen
    Positive tests for antiphospholipid antibodies (lupus anticoagulant or anticardiolipin antibodies)
Positive antinuclear antibody

From Hochberg MC: *Arthritis Rheum* 40:1725, 1997.

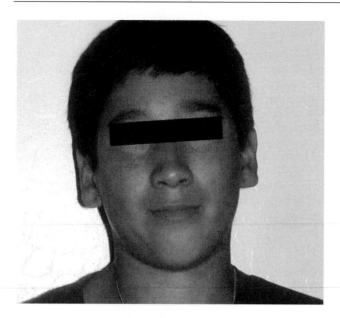

FIGURE 13-3 Rash in systemic lupus erythematosus.

Chest pain may suggest lung or heart involvement in SLE. Pleuritis is the most common lung manifestation in SLE. Pleuritic chest pain and shortness of breath are the usual symptoms. Physical examination may reveal diminished breath sounds indicating a pleural effusion, which can be documented by a chest x-ray. Pulmonary hemorrhage, a rare but potentially lethal manifestation of SLE, should be suspected in patients with cough, hypoxia, and rapid fall in hemoglobin. Hemoptysis may not be present. Costochondritis may mimic pleuritic chest pain, but on physical examination there are discrete tender areas at the costochondral junctions along the sternum.

Pericarditis is the most common cardiac manifestation of SLE. The chest pain is usually precordial and it is worse in the recumbent position. A chest x-ray will show cardiomegaly, and an echocardiogram can ascertain that this is caused by pericardial fluid as opposed to cardiac dilation. Electrocardiogram changes are a less sensitive way of detecting pericarditis. Liebman-Sachs endocarditis is an unusual finding in the pediatric population; when it occurs, it most often involves the mitral value with a new onset of a systolic regurgitant heart murmur.

Gastrointestinal involvement in SLE is uncommon; however, acute pancreatitis with severe left upper quadrant pain penetrating to the back can be an emergent situation. Liver involvement may produce mild elevation of hepatocellular enzymes but rarely causes symptoms.

Lupus nephritis produces no symptoms at disease onset. Microscopic hematuria, proteinuria, and cellular casts are indications of lupus nephritis. Hypertension, which requires treatment, is a frequent concomitant of lupus nephritis, especially when steroid therapy is initiated. In the past, lupus nephritis was a major cause of death, and in the modern era it is still capable of producing end-stage renal disease. Therefore aggressive therapy is indicated, although patients rarely experience symptoms directly attributable to the nephritis.

Anemia and thrombocytopenia reflect other aspects of this autoimmune diathesis. Autoimmune Coombs' positive hemolytic anemia is less common than an inflammatory anemia

of chronic disease with decreased red cell production. Teenagers with the new onset of idiopathic thrombocytopenic purpura should be screened for wider evidence of an autoimmune process.

Neuropsychologic involvement in SLE patients is rare as a presenting symptom with the exception of chorea. Seizures, stroke, and peripheral neuropathies are manifestations that are easy to discern. The more difficult issues arise with psychologic symptoms such as affective disorders, organic brain syndromes, and psychosis. Radiologic imaging is most helpful in patients with focal neurologic findings, but when the manifestations are primarily psychologic, computed tomography (CT) scans and MRIs are frequently normal.[17] Headaches are common in lupus patients and frequently have the characteristics of a vascular headache, but their occurrence does not necessarily parallel other manifestations of the disease and may exist when the rest of the patient's lupus is in excellent control.

Constitutional symptoms, which are not specific for lupus but nonetheless trouble the patient, include fever, weight loss, and fatigue. The organic fatigue of SLE tends to occur in the afternoon and evening, and it interferes with activities that patients enjoy doing. The fatigue may also be the last symptom to improve once therapy has been initiated.

Laboratory Assessment

A CBC will frequently show an anemia, leukopenia, or thrombocytopenia. Anemia is Coombs' positive in 15% of patients but it is often indicative of the anemia of chronic disease. The leukopenia most often shows a relative lymphopenia. Thrombocytopenia may manifest large platelets, suggesting autoimmune destruction.

The sedimentation rate is elevated in 90% of patients with SLE.[16] Although it is not specific, this test is very useful in discerning patients with inflammatory causes for their symptomatology. In many settings it may be worthwhile to measure the sedimentation rate before an ANA is ordered.

Because the ANA test is positive in more than 95% of SLE patients, a negative ANA effectively excludes the diagnosis of SLE. In SLE the titer of ANA is usually high (> 1:160). The fluorescent pattern reported on the ANA is not very helpful.

False-positive ANAs are seen more in the pediatric population. These are usually of low titer (> 1:320). In patients in whom the sedimentation rate is normal and the ANA is of low titer, further laboratory assessment is frequently not necessary. The reasons for the false-positive ANA incidence in pediatric patients may relate to frequent viral or streptococcal infections. Repetition of low titer–positive ANAs is not recommended because they are likely to remain positive.

In patients in whom there is a high titer–positive ANA, an ANA profile provides increased disease specificity if it is positive. Table 13-3 lists the elements of the ANA profile and their disease associations. Only 60% of patients fulfilling the diagnostic criteria for SLE will have elements positive on the ANA profile. Anti-DNA antibodies reflect disease activity; the other antibodies do not.

With successful treatment of SLE, the anti-DNA antibody levels should fall. Recrudescence of disease may be heralded by increases in anti-DNA levels.

In patients with lupus nephritis, the routine urinalysis is the most sensitive indicator of both disease activity and

TABLE 13-3 Antinuclear Antibody Profile

Test	Disease Association
Anti-DNA	Systemic lupus erythematosus (SLE) with nephritis
Anti-SM (Smith)	SLE
Anti-SSA/anti SSB	SLE with photosensitivity
	Sjögren's syndrome
	Neonatal SLE
Antiribonuclear protein	SLE and mixed connective tissue disease
Anticentromere or anti-SCL70	Scleroderma

response to therapy. Hematuria is usually microscopic. Cellular casts are helpful but depend on the freshness of the specimen. Proteinuria can be quantitated and followed with a spot, protein-to-creatinine ratio. Values less than 0.2 are normal, and values greater than 2.0 are indicative of nephrotic levels of proteinuria. Timed collections of urine to quantitate proteinuria are both tedious and frequently inaccurate. Similarly, serum creatinine levels provide accurate information; however, the glomerular filtration rate must be below 50% of normal before seeing an elevation in the serum creatinine. In questionable cases, timed creatinine clearances can provide additional information.

The serum C3 level is useful both for SLE diagnosis and monitoring disease activity.[18] Total hemolytic complement values correlate well in lupus patients with the C3 and are technically more difficult. However, in patients in whom a complement deficiency leading to SLE is a strong consideration, a single CH_{50} value can be obtained, and if the result is zero, individual complement factor levels can be measured to ascertain the complement deficiency. Measurements of complement split products (C3a, C5a, and others) have not been proven to improve the laboratory reflection of disease activity more than the C3 level itself. As with anti-DNA antibodies, C3 values that are low in untreated disease, indicating complement consumption, will improve with therapy and disease control. C3 levels that fall during therapy may herald a disease flare. However, some patients maintain low C3 levels, and therapy should be adjusted to the degree of patient symptomatology. C4 levels are not useful in the diagnosis or management of SLE. The frequency of various C4 null genes in the population is sufficiently frequent that this will result in persistently low C4 levels regardless of therapy and disease control.

In patients with SLE, measurements of antiphospholipid antibodies are important because these antibodies contribute to an increased risk of venous and arterial thromboses.[19] Anticardiolipin antibodies detect one type of prothrombotic antibody. The presence of a lupus anticoagulant (a different epitope) is most often detected with a prolonged partial tissue prothrombin time, which does not correct when mixed with fresh plasma. A Russell viper venom time should also be measured as a sensitive indicator of a lupus anticoagulant. Patients who have antiphospholipid antibodies should be treated with one baby aspirin per day (see treatment section). Unfortunately, these antibodies are relatively steroid resistant and are likely to exist for long periods of time regardless of disease therapy.

Treatment

Successful management of SLE begins with education of the patients and their families. SLE is a complicated disease, and it is to be anticipated that it will take two or three education sessions for them to feel comfortable with the information. It is important that all those involved realize that SLE is a lifelong condition. They also need to know that the possibility of a drug-free remission occurs in only a small percentage of patients; the remainder can be expected to do well but remain on medication. At disease onset, fatigue and decreased endurance occur in the majority of patients, and they should modify their schedules to include adequate amounts of rest. There is no proof that any specific diet is beneficial to the disease. Patients treated with steroids should take a diet adequate in calcium (1500 mg/day), and the diet should be a no-salt-added diet to reduce the cosmetic puffiness associated with salt and water retention.

In mild SLE nonsteroidal medications can provide significant benefit to the musculoskeletal symptomatology. In the absence of renal disease, most nonsteroidal medications are safe. In patients with renal disease, treatment with sulindac (150 or 200 mg twice daily) may have fewer renal side effects.

Antimalarial therapy has been a cornerstone for the management of certain aspects of SLE. These medications exert a significant antiinflammatory effect. Hydroxychloroquine is used in a dose of 5 to 7 mg/kg/day, with a maximum of 400 mg once a day, and has been shown to be beneficial for the skin disease, joint symptoms, and fatigue. However, it takes a good while for the benefits to be realized by the patient, so a trial of 8 to 12 weeks should be envisioned. The side effects include occasional nausea, rare skin pigment change, and the possibility of a retinopathy for which ophthalmologic supervision is necessary at 6-month intervals.

Steroid therapy is the cornerstone of acute management of SLE with major organ involvement or cytopenias. High-dose steroid therapy is necessary at disease onset at a dose of 2 mg/kg/day divided into doses every 12 hours. For seriously ill children, more rapid control of symptoms can be achieved with intravenous Solu-Medrol (30 mg/kg with a maximum dose of 1000 mg) given once a day for 3 days followed on the fourth day with prednisone at 2 mg/kg/day. The long-term goal in steroid therapy for the management of SLE is to reduce the dose to a nontoxic level.

With control of symptomatology and laboratory improvement (i.e., normal erythrocyte sedimentation rate, improved C3 levels, and clearing of urinary sediment), the dose of prednisone is reduced and condensed to a single daily dose. The legion of steroid side effects (see Chapter 41) mandates a dose reduction to the lowest level that will keep the patient well. In children, there are unique steroid side effects seen with very low levels of daily prednisone administration. Growth suppression and osteoporosis can occur with doses in the 3- to 5-mg range if taken on a daily basis. However, up to 15 mg of prednisone can be taken every other day without these side effects occurring,[20] so the goal of therapy is to get to every-other-day management.

Anticoagulation therapy is necessary in patients who have antiphospholipid antibodies (anticardiolipin antibodies or a lupus anticoagulant). In patients who have not had a thrombotic event, treatment with one baby aspirin per day is indicated. If a thrombotic event has occurred, anticoagulation over several years is necessary with warfarin or subcutaneous heparin. With warfarin an international normalized ratio should be maintained between 2 and 3.

In patients who fail to achieve the goal of every-other-day steroid management, addition of immunosuppressant medications is necessary. Azathioprine is most often the initial immunosuppressant at a dose of 2 to 3 mg/kg/day. Side effects include bone marrow suppression, opportunistic infections, nausea, and liver function abnormalities. Mycophenolate mofetil is a newer immunosuppressive agent that inhibits the enzyme inosine monophosphate dehydrogenase, leading to a reduced synthesis of guanosine nucleosides. The dose is 15 to 50 mg/kg/day divided twice daily with a maximum of 1 to 1.5 g twice a day. Side effects include bone marrow suppression, opportunistic infections, and diarrhea. Methotrexate administered once a week may be beneficial for the arthritic manifestations of SLE; however, it is not an effective agent to treat major organ involvement such as kidney disease. Patients who fail management with azathioprine or mycophenolate mofetil are candidates for treatment with cyclophosphamide with a monthly intravenous pulse protocol or daily basis. Consultation with a pediatric rheumatologist is indicated should that be the case.

Many biologic agents are currently under study to modify aspects of the immune response in patients with SLE; unfortunately, animal studies with anti-TNF medications, which have proven to be so successful in managing JRA, have suggested disease worsening with these agents in SLE patients.

Prognosis

The disease course with SLE is waxing and waning. The first year after diagnosis may be the most difficult because new organ system involvement is frequently seen. By the end of the second year, most patients will have set their individual disease manifestations and organ system involvement. For instance, new onset of renal disease or central nervous system disease is unusual if not seen in the first 2 years. In most patients, disease control can be achieved over the first year by lowering medications to nontoxic levels.

The prognosis for survival with SLE has improved markedly since the 1980s.[21] Most series have shown a 10-year survival of 85% to 90%. Over this same interval, the causes of death in SLE patients have changed. Although end-stage renal disease was previously the major cause of death, with modern management including dialysis and kidney transplant, renal deaths are now rare, and serious systemic infections now count for most of the mortality in lupus. These infections are caused by both the underlying disease and its immune disregulation and the effects of steroidal and immunosuppressive medications that are necessary for disease control. Immunization against pneumococcus and meningococcus is indicated in all patients. Pneumocystis prophylaxis should be used in patients on high-dose steroid and immunosuppressant therapy.

There is the second increase in mortality caused by accelerated arteriosclerosis in patients who have survived the acute autoimmune phase of the disease.[21]

KAWASAKI DISEASE

Kawasaki disease (formerly known as *mucocutaneous lymph node syndrome*) is an acute, dramatic type of vasculitis seen primarily in young children.[22] Although uncommon, it is the second most common form of vasculitis after Henoch-Schönlein purpura (HSP). The cause of the vasculitis is unknown, and morbidity and mortality were significant prior to treatment with intravenous immunoglobulin (IVIG). The disease description was published first in Japan in 1967 where the disease remains more common, but it is seen worldwide. It is most common in children less than 2 years of age, and the majority of cases occur in children less than 5 years of age. Many series suggest it is somewhat more common in males. In the United States it is estimated to have an annual incidence of 5.95 per 100,000 children in the Chicago area under the age of 5 years; familial occurrence is unusual, and concordance in twins is low.

Diagnosis

The criteria for the diagnosis have been created and validated and are summarized in Table 13-4. Three phases of the disease have been identified; in the acute febrile phase the children become abruptly ill with high-grade fever ($> 39°$ C) and an unusual degree of irritability. Over the next 3 or 4 days (but in no particular order) other manifestations develop, including red eyes, red and cracked lips, swollen lymph nodes, a pleomorphic rash, and redness and edema of the hands and feet. In the subacute phase, defined as that interval of 3 to 4 weeks (if untreated) when the fever resolves, peeling of the digits and perineum occurs and arthritis may be seen in some children, but most importantly this is the period that coronary artery aneurysms are most frequently found on echocardiography. Finally, in the convalescent phase the acute-phase reactants in the laboratory have normalized, and the children are basically asymptomatic.

Clinical characteristics of the illness at presentation may appear unique and classic; however, atypical cases are frequently seen. The fever is high grade and unresponsive to antibiotics. The conjunctivitis appears as nonpurulent erythema. Uveitis may be found on slit-lamp examination, contributing further to the diagnosis. The oral manifestations include red and cracked lips, mucosal erythema, and, frequently, a "strawberry tongue." Lymphadenopathy, although sometimes dramatic, in other cases is not greatly different from that in other viral causes of fever. The rash is erythematous, occurring primarily on the trunk and the perineum and progressing to the extremities. The rash is never vesicular or crusting. Changes in the extremities are primarily manifested by edema of the hands and feet, often with erythema of the

TABLE 13-4 Kawasaki Disease Criteria*

Criteria	Characteristics
Fever	$> 39°$ C for > 5 days
Conjunctivitis	Bilateral, nonsuppurative
Lymphadenopathy	Cervical, > 1.5 cm nonpurulent
Rash	Polymorphous
Changes in lips or oral mucosa	Red, cracked lips; "strawberry" tongue, erythematous oropharynx
Changes in extremities	Erythema and edema of palms and soles, desquamation of fingertips

From Centers for Disease Control: *MMWR* 34:33, 1985.
*Diagnosis requires five of six criteria or four criteria plus coronary aneurysm on echocardiography.

palms and soles. A tachycardia out of proportion to the fever or degree of anemia should raise concern about myocarditis in the acute phase of the illness.

Other manifestations seen in some patients include sterile pyuria, aseptic meningitis, and hydrops of the gallbladder.

Laboratory Assessment

Laboratory assessment shows evidence of significant inflammation in the first few days of the disease. The white blood count is frequently elevated and shifted to the left, often with toxic granulations; there may be a mild anemia. The platelet count is often elevated, but in atypical cases the evolution to a characteristic thrombocytosis with platelet counts greater than 700,000 may be delayed into the second or third week of the illness. Sedimentation rates and CRP values are elevated. The initial evaluation should also include an electrocardiogram and echocardiography. Coronary artery dilatations but not true aneurysms are found early on.

In the differential diagnosis of Kawasaki disease, scarlet fever mimics the disease most closely but the rash has a dry "sandpaper" texture, throat cultures are positive for streptococcus, and elevated antistreptolysin O titers are found. Adenoviral infection may also mimic Kawasaki disease. In doubtful cases, the response to IVIG and the evolution of symptoms over time may allow a more accurate diagnosis. Among other collagen vascular diseases, systemic-onset JRA also presents with dramatic fevers, but the rash is totally different. Infantile polyarteritis nodosa may present many of the same features and in autopsy series shares the same pathology as that found in Kawasaki disease.

Pathology

The pathology of Kawasaki disease is characterized by a narcotizing vasculitis of medium-sized arteries, with the coronary arteries being most often involved. In subacute and convalescent stages, aneurysms may develop as the inflammation diminishes. These aneurysms may regress over time, but they may also be the sites of future thrombosis causing myocardial ischemia.

The cause of Kawasaki disease is unknown. Although seasonality and clustering of new cases are observed, no person-to-person spread has been found. Many features of Kawasaki disease are seen in patients with toxic shock syndrome caused by *Streptococcus* or *Staphylococcus,* but proof of this mechanism has been difficult to reproduce. A recent multicenter study of Kawasaki patients found bacterial isolates of streptococci and staphylococci that produced certain exotoxins capable of producing a "superantigen" response in these children.[23] Genetic predisposition is inconclusive across various ethnic populations. Although IgA may be found in affected vessels, the responsible antigen has not been identified.

Treatment

The introduction of IVIG as a treatment for Kawasaki disease has dramatically changed the natural history and outcome of this condition. Patient response is often dramatic with defervescence of fever; reduction in irritability; and diminishment of rash, edema, and lymphadenopathy. The dose of IVIG is 2 g/kg administered over 10 to 12 hours.[24] With a conclusively favorable response, the patient can be discharged. If symptoms recur, a second dose of IVIG at 2 g/kg may produce a permanent cessation of acute symptoms. With the occasional failure of IVIG, treatment with steroids (2 mg/kg/day or pulse intravenous Solu-Medrol 30 mg/kg)[25,26] will frequently control the inflammation. In the rare patient, cyclophosphamide may be necessary.

In the acute inflammatory phase, salicylates (100 mg/kg/day in divided doses) are used for their antiinflammatory and anticoagulant effects. With the resolution of fever, the dose is changed to 5 mg/kg/day as an anticoagulant measure.

Follow-up echocardiography is a mandatory part of the treatment sequence. If no aneurysms are detected during this subacute phase, the prognosis should be very good and the salicylates can be discontinued. In patients with persistent aneurysm, long-term anticoagulation to prevent thrombosis is indicated.

Prognosis

Overall, the prognosis today for Kawasaki disease is largely favorable; however, there are patients in whom late morbidity and mortality are found because of progressive coronary artery disease.[27]

JUVENILE DERMATOMYOSITIS

Juvenile dermatomyositis (JDMS) is a unique autoimmune disease in childhood. It is characterized by a pathognomonic rash and proximal muscle weakness.[28] The disease has a remarkably stable incidence worldwide at approximately 0.4 case per 100,000 children of the age of 16; girls are more often affected than boys. The rash frequently begins before symptoms of muscle weakness. JDMS is considered a separate type of inflammatory myopathy based on the original classification by Bohan and Peters in the early 1970s. It is distinguished from adult dermatomyositis by the absence of associated malignancy, a unique vascular pathology, and a tendency to run a self-limited course.

Diagnosis

The muscle disease presents most often as the subacute onset of proximal muscle weakness. The hips are more affected than the shoulders, with symptoms of difficulty with stairs, getting out of a chair, and other lower-extremity functions. Shoulder girdle manifestations may include difficulty doing the hair or reaching for items over the head. Untreated, the weakness may progress to difficulty in getting off the floor, lifting the head off the bed, and inability to perform a sit-up. The weakness is usually out of proportion to degree of soreness or tenderness in the affected muscles. The distal muscles of the hands and feet are spared until very late in the course of the disease. In severely involved patients, there may be a history of difficulty swallowing or dysphonia (a new nasal quality to the voice). On physical examination, patients demonstrate weakness of the proximal muscles including the neck flexors, shoulder girdle, abdominal muscles, and hip muscles. In younger children, evidence of this may be gained by asking them to lift their heads off the examination table, perform a sit-up, and rise from the floor from a supine position. In this latter example, evidence of the Gower maneuver may be obtained as children appear to "climb up their legs" while using shoulder girdle musculature to substitute for weakness in the hip girdle. Deep tendon reflexes and other aspects of the neurologic examination should be normal.

In most patients the pathognomonic rash has a unique distribution on the body not seen with any other rash of childhood (Figure 13-4). The most commonly affected areas are the extensor surfaces of the knuckles, elbows, and knees. The rash begins initially as an erythematous, scaling eruption that may form papules known as *Gottron's papules.* The cheeks may also develop the rash, with a malar distribution similar to lupus; the upper chest may develop a rash in a "shawl" distribution; and lastly, the upper eyelids may manifest a rash that produces a faint purple discoloration referred to as *heliotrope,* so named for the purple flower. The rash may be photosensitive. Although the rash is necessary for diagnosis, its extent and severity may not parallel the course of the muscle weakness.

Other symptoms may include fever, weight loss, fatigue, and abdominal pain. If the abdominal pain is severe and cramping, vasculitis of the gastrointestinal tract may be present, which can be dangerous because it includes a risk of perforation.

The cause of JDMS is unknown. Familial cases are rare, but some studies have indicated a genetic predisposition to the disease with an increase carriage of HLA-B8 and DQA 1*0501.[29-31]

The diagnosis is established with five elements: proximal muscle weakness, characteristic rash, elevated muscle enzymes, myopathic electromyelogram, and occasionally a muscle biopsy. Most authorities would omit the latter two criteria if the other elements were met. Laboratory tests may include evidence of acute inflammation with an elevated sedimentation rate, anemia, and elevated acute-phase reactants. However, evidence of muscle injury with elevated muscle enzymes in the serum is the most useful test. In addition, these enzymes can be used to follow the response to treatment. At onset, a full panel of muscle enzyme profiles, including LDH, SGOT, SGPT, CPK, and aldolase, should be obtained. The last test has been most sensitive and useful. Aldolase values may be the last to normalize with treatment, indicating full disease control. The ANA may be positive but is nonspecific. Antimyositis-specific antibodies have not been useful in JDMS.

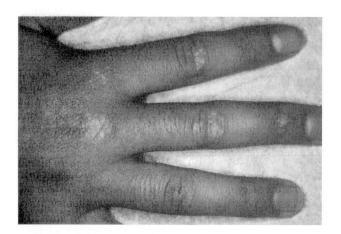

FIGURE 13-4 Rash in juvenile dermatomyositis.

Diagnosis

The differential diagnosis includes other rheumatic diseases such as SLE and mixed corrective tissue disease. Viral myositis demonstrates more muscle pain than does JDMS, although muscle enzymes may be very high in the acute phase. The calf musculature is always involved in viral myositis. Neuropathic causes such as weakness are important to rule out. In conditions such as Guillain-Barré syndrome, distal muscle weakness is found. In difficult cases, an electromyelogram is helpful in distinguishing a myopathy from a neuropathy.

MRI of the involved musculature has provided new and useful information, although it should be reserved for selected cases. In JDMS, abnormalities are demonstrated in a patchy distribution characteristic of the disease. If a muscle biopsy is necessary, involved areas can be selected (with MRI) and the chance of the sampling error giving a normal biopsy result can thereby be reduced. In addition, late in the course of JDMS when muscle enzymes may no longer reflect disease activity, an abnormal MRI indicates continuing disease activity.

Pathology

The pathology of the rash shows epidermal atrophy, hydropic degeneration of basal cells, and moderate dermal infiltrate with vascular dilation; immunofluorescence is negative. The muscle pathology shows evidence of vascular inflammation in the muscle with muscle fiber degeneration, necrosis, and regeneration. Perifascicular atrophy in the muscles is believed to be highly characteristic of JDMS even in the absence of inflammation in the particular biopsy sample.

The autoimmune pathogenesis of JDMS appears to involve both humoral and cell-mediated immunity. Although antibodies to muscle are not demonstrated in JDMS, the vasculature of the involved muscle demonstrates immunoglobulin and complement deposits. Cellular immune mechanisms have been suggested from studies showing that lymphocytes with JDMS are stimulated to blast formation on exposure to muscle antigens *in vitro.* Similarly, studies have indicated that patients' lymphocytes are capable of destroying cultured fetal muscle cells *in vitro.*

The cause of this autoimmune attack on skin and muscles is unknown. Because some series have shown seasonality at onset and there are viral models of myositis in experimental animals, there continues to be interest in trying to identify a viral cause of JDMS. However, a recent study examining muscle biopsy specimens with active disease prior to treatment was unsuccessful in identifying a viral cause.[32] This study used polymerase chain reaction technology with primers to more than 20 viruses and controls, which demonstrated that two or three DNA copies could be detected. Importantly, cancers that had been identified in adults with dermatomyositis have not been found in children with JDMS.

The disease course in JDMS may be quite heterogeneous.[28] Three distinct patterns have been identified. The first is monocyclic, in which the patient has the illness for approximately 2 years, requiring treatment during that interval, but thereafter has a return to normal health. In the polycyclic pattern there can be periods of disease activity that alternate with remission and the patient can be taken off all medications; remissions may be as long as 5 years in duration. The third course is described as chronic, where patients require therapy past the 2-year point. These patients may be detected at disease onset by capillary, nail-fold microscopy showing capillary dropout, dilatation, tortuosity, and telangiectasia.

Calcinosis is a postinflammatory sequela, which may be limited to one or two deposits in some patients or extensive debilitating deposits in rare cases. No effective preventive treatments have been developed. Surgical removal should be used only when the calcium deposits produce functional difficulties.

Although no control studies have been performed, the usual standard of therapy is with high-dose steroids. In severely weak patients, treatment may be initiated with pulse Solu-Medrol intravenously in a dose of 30 mg/kg/day for 3 days. Muscle enzyme levels should begin to fall with that therapy, and then prednisone (2 mg/kg/day in split dose) is given by mouth until disease control is achieved. Many authors have attributed treatment failures to underdosing with steroids or premature withdrawal of medication. Disease control is reflected in normalization of muscle enzymes and return of strength. With normalization of the muscle enzymes, a steroid taper is initiated with laboratory monitoring so that reductions in steroid dose cannot lead to return of disease activity. Elevations of muscle enzymes during steroid therapy may herald disease recurrence before a patient becomes clinically ill. In uncomplicated patients, alternate-day dosing of prednisone should be possible within 3 to 4 months. The dose of alternate-day steroids should be decreased to 10 mg every other day, which is essentially a nontoxic dose. Cushingoid side effects will regress, and linear growth will resume. This dose of steroid should be continued for 2 years. Calcium supplementation should be administered during steroid therapy, as steroid-induced osteoporosis is compounded by reduced physical activity.

Physical therapy modalities are employed to reverse contractures should they occur. Resistive exercises may be prescribed in children over the age of 8 years to aid in muscle strength recovery. Plaquenil and sunscreens may be used for treatment of the rash.

Immunosuppressant therapy may be necessary in patients who are not improving on prednisone or those in whom the steroid burden is too great. Again, control studies are lacking for this rare disease, but the current standard of care is to use steroid-sparing agents beginning with methotrexate at a dose of 1 mg/kg (maximum dose 50 mg) administered subcutaneously once a week.[33] Imuran has been shown to be beneficial in adult dermatomyositis in one controlled study.[34] The dose is 2 to 3 mg/kg/day. Cyclosporin A has provided additional benefit in patients who achieve inadequate disease control with steroids and methotrexate.[35]

IVIG has been reported to be beneficial in a small series of patients.[34] This adjunctive therapy may be used early in the treatment of the disease, when immunosuppressive medication is begun.

WEGENER'S GRANULOMATOSIS

Wegener's granulomatosis is a rare form of vasculitis that is lethal if untreated; it frequently presents with chronic upper respiratory symptoms suggestive of more benign entities.[36] Wegener's granulomatosis as a distant disease entity was first recognized in the German literature in the 1930s as a triad of upper and lower respiratory disease and glomerulonephritis.

The granulomatous inflammation affects medium-sized vessels. Left untreated, the disease may have a 90% mortality 5 years after disease onset; 3% of patients with Wegener's granulomatosis have disease onset at less than 20 years. The disease prevalence may approximate 0.1 per 100,000 individuals under the age of 16 years. The cause of Wegener's granulomatosis is unknown, but research continues to focus on the role of infection, given the unusual distribution of the vasculitic inflammation.

Upper respiratory involvement is characterized by inflammation of the nasal mucosa, sinuses, and middle ear. Sinusitis or otitis media unresponsive to aggressive antibiotic or surgical management should raise a suspicion of Wegener's granulomatosis, especially if there are constitutional symptoms such as fever and weight loss.

Lower respiratory symptoms include cough, dyspnea, hemoptysis, and stridor. Wegener's granulomatosis should be suspected in patients presenting with pulmonary hemorrhage characterized by hypoxia, pulmonary infiltrates, and rapid development of anemia. The stridor is caused by tracheal involvement with granulomas.

The renal disease of Wegener's granulomatosis is that of a glomerulonephritis with proteinuria, hematuria, and cast formation. Azotemia at disease diagnosis is an ominous sign because the glomerulonephritis is a necrotizing process with early, irreversible crescent formation, whereas other aspects of Wegener's granulomatosis may be fully reversible with treatment. The crescentic glomerulonephritis may be stabilized but not fully reversed.

Less common manifestations of Wegener's granulomatosis are purpuric skin lesions resembling those of HSP, arthralgias, and arthritis. Fever, weight loss, and fatigue, which are nonspecific symptoms, should nonetheless alert the physician that a more benign diagnosis may need further investigation.

Central nervous system lesions and involvement of the eye are late manifestations of disease activity.

Diagnosis

The differential diagnosis of Wegener's granulomatosis includes chronic, allergic upper respiratory disease. Patients presenting with pulmonary hemorrhage may have SLE, idiopathic pulmonary hemosiderosis, Goodpasture's syndrome, or Churg-Strauss syndrome, but the latter two entities are extremely rare in childhood. Lower-extremity purpura may be seen in HSP and SLE.

X-rays of the sinuses show chronic mucosal thickening. Chest x-ray demonstrates scattered pulmonary infiltrates that may be transient or segmental, suggestive of pulmonary hemorrhage. CT scans of the lungs frequently demonstrate the nodular inflammatory process indicative of Wegener's granulomatosis.

Laboratory Assessment

Initial laboratory tests are indicative of systemic inflammation. Anemia, leukocytosis, and thrombocytosis are nonspecific indicators of inflammation. Similarly, an elevated sedimentation rate and CRP are usually found. An elevated level of carbon monoxide diffusion in the lung is suggestive of pulmonary hemorrhage. The urinalysis demonstrates hematuria, proteinuria, and casts.

The development of the antineutrophilic cytoplasmic antibody (ANCA) test has provided greater than 90% sensitivity and greater than 90% specificity for Wegener's granulomatosis.[37] The usual antibody detected is the c-ANCA, which can be further elucidated by enzyme-linked immunosorbent assay (ELISA) techniques for antibody to the cytoplasmic PR3 antigen.[38] A p-ANCA antibody may occasionally be found but is also seen in patients with polyarteritis nodosum, crescentic glomerulonephritis, and inflammatory bowel disease. This antibody can be confirmed by an ELISA technique with myeloperoxidase as antigen. In patients with refractory otitis media, sinusitis, or lower-extremity purpura, a negative ANCA serves to eliminate diagnosis of this very serious disease.

Pathology

Pathologic specimens demonstrate a granulomatous vasculitis of vessel walls or the interstitium with collections of macrophages, neutrophils, and giant cells; however, obtaining diagnostic tissue is frequently difficult. Sinus tissue biopsies may only show chronic inflammation without the diagnostic findings. Similar sampling problems are found with transbronchial lung biopsies or needle kidney biopsies. The ANCA test has supplanted the necessity for aggressively pursuing pathologic tissue. The pathogenesis of Wegener's granulomatosis is incompletely understood. There is evidence to suggest that an ANCA antibody is capable of enhancing neutrophilic release of tissue-damaging enzymes.[37]

Treatment

Unless Wegener's granulomatosis is limited to the upper respiratory tract, treatment should be aggressive. High-dose steroid therapy (1 to 2 mg/kg/day) in a split dose or with initial pulse Solu-Medrol (30 mg/kg/day) in severely ill patients produces the most rapid improvement in symptoms. However, cyclophosphamide (2 mg/kg/day) should be started immediately because there is some lag time in its effect on the disease, and treatment with steroids alone has no effect on disease mortality.[37] The potential for sterility caused by cyclophosphamide, which must be given for 1 to 2 years, may be ameliorated by using testosterone in males and Lupron in females. Methotrexate may be considered in limited disease and as maintenance therapy in patients who have achieved excellent disease control with cyclophosphamide. However, relapses of patients on methotrexate are not uncommon and may lead to reinstitution of cyclophosphamide therapy.

The anti-TNF therapies (etanercept and infliximab) are showing early promise in the treatment of Wegener's granulomatosis, but long-term data are not available.

Prognosis

Wegener's granulomatosis is highly lethal if untreated. Drug-free remissions are rare, but with modern therapy many patients are able to lead a normal life. In children the incidence of subglottic stenosis is five times more common than in adults.[36] Chronic inflammation of the nasal mucosa may lead to cartilage collapse in the nose and a "saddle" deformity. The renal lesion of Wegener's granulomatosis is the most difficult to reverse, but patients can be maintained for many years with only mild renal insufficiency; some patients, however, may progress to end-stage renal disease.

HENOCH-SCHÖNLEIN PURPURA

HSP is the most common form of leukocytoclastic vasculitis in children.[39] It is uniquely mediated by IgA immune complex deposition. The annual incidence is 13.5 per 100,000 children under the age of 16. Boys are more commonly affected than girls (1.5:1). It is more common in winter and often is preceded by a viral upper respiratory infection. Beta-hemolytic streptococcal bacteria may be important in recurrent HSP but not population-based studies.[40]

Diagnosis

The clinical manifestations include lower extremity purpura, arthralgia, arthritis, abdominal pain, and hematuria, which may be grossly apparent.

The skin lesions begin as macular, papular, or urticarial lesions but progress to a nonblanching purpura. The majority of lesions are on the lower extremities and buttocks, although they may be scattered elsewhere. Arthralgias and arthritis are most commonly in the lower extremities and are often associated with edema of the hands and feet; in young children the edema may involve the scalp and scrotum.

Gastrointestinal involvement is suggested by abdominal pain that becomes colicky or cramping. Submucosal vasculitis and hemorrhage produce hematest-positive stools. Vasculitic involvement of the intestine may lead to intussusception (4.5% in some series) or, more rarely, to intestinal perforation.

Renal involvement is usually silent with microscopic hematuria and proteinuria; occasionally gross hematuria may be found. A nephritic presentation with hypertension and azotemia increases the risk of a persistent IgA nephropathy.

Laboratory Assessment

There is no diagnostic test for HSP. A CBC should not show a thrombocytopenia, which would indicate other important disease entities. The sedimentation rate is usually normal or only slightly elevated. Sedimentation rates greater than 40 mm/hr may suggest other disease entities, such as SLE or Wegener's granulomatosis, and appropriate tests for these entities should be ordered. The serum IgA level is elevated in 50% of patients during the acute phase. In doubtful cases or cases with prolonged disease activity (seen particularly in the adolescent population), a skin biopsy of a fresh lesion will demonstrate diagnostic IgA deposits.[41]

Prognosis

In the majority of young children the disease runs a self-limited course, lasting 2 to 4 weeks with full recovery. Older children (above 10 years) may have a more protracted course, but their outcome remains nonetheless good. Recurrences are not uncommon (15% to 40% in some series). They are most common within the first 2 years following the initial episode.

Treatment

In the majority of patients, the treatment is supportive. Nonsteroidal antiinflammatory agents can be helpful for the arthritic manifestations. Steroids are indicated (1 to 2 mg/kg/day in split

9. Szer IS, Taylor E, Steere AC: The long-term course of Lyme arthritis in children, *N Engl J Med* 325:159-163, 1991.
10. Lovell DJ, Giannini EH, Reiff A, et al: Efficacy and safety of etanercept (tumor necrosis factor receptor p75 Fc fusion protein; Enbrel) in children with polyarticular-course juvenile rheumatoid arthritis, *N Engl J Med* 342:1703-1710, 2000.
11. Cabral DA, Malleson PN, Petty RE: Spondyloarthropathies of childhood, *Pediatr Clin North Am* 42:1051-1070, 1995.
12. Petty RS, Cassidy JT: Juvenile ankylosing spondylitis. In Cassidy JT, Petty RE, eds: *Textbook of pediatric rheumatology,* ed 4, Philadelphia, 2001, WB Saunders.
13. Dougados M, Boumier P, Amor B: Sulphasalazine in ankylosing spondylitis: a double blind control study in 60 patients, *Br Med J* 293:911-914, 1986.
14. Lang BA: A clinical overview of systemic lupus erythematosus in childhood, *Pediatr Rev* 14:194-201, 1993.
15. Tsokos GC, Wong HK, Enyedy EJ, et al: Immune cell signaling in lupus, *Curr Opin Rheumatol* 12:355-363, 2000.
16. Iqbal S, Sher MR, Good RA, et al: Diversity in presenting manifestations of systemic lupus erythematosus in children, *J Pediatr* 135:500-505, 1999.
17. West SG: Lupus and the central nervous system, *Curr Opin Rheumatol* 8:408-414, 1996.
18. Singsen BH, Berstein BH, King KK, et al: Systemic lupus erythematosus in childhood: correlation between change in disease activity and serum complement levels, *J Pediatr* 89:358-364, 1976.
19. Petri M: Pathogenesis and treatment of the antiphospholipid syndrome, *Med Clin North Am* 81:151-177, 1997.
20. Auerbach HS, Williams M, Kirkpatrick JA, et al: Alternate-day prednisone reduces morbidity and improves pulmonary function in cystic fibrosis, *Lancet* 2:686-688, 1985.
21. Petri M: Long-term outcomes in lupus, *Am J Managed Care* 7:S480-S485, 2001.
22. Burns JC: Kawasaki disease, *Adv Pediatr* 48:157-177, 2001.
23. Leung DYM, Meissner H, Shulman ST, et al: Prevalence of superantigen-secreting bacteria in patients with Kawasaki disease, *J Pediatr* 140:742-746, 2002.
24. Newburger JW, Takahashi MT, Beiser AS, et al: A single intravenous infusion of gamma globulin as compared with four infusions in the treatment of acute Kawasaki syndrome, *N Engl J Med* 324:1633-1639, 1991.
25. Wright DA, Newburger JW, Baker A, et al: Treatment of immune globulin-resistant Kawasaki disease with pulsed doses of corticosteroids, *J Pediatr* 128:146-149, 1996.
26. Dale RC, Saleem MA, Daw S, et al: Treatment of severe complicated Kawasaki disease with oral prednisolone and aspirin, *J Pediatr* 137:723-726, 2000.
27. Fulton DR, Newburger JW: Long-term cardiac sequelae of Kawasaki disease, *Curr Rheum Reports* 2:324-329, 2000.
28. Pachman LM: Juvenile dermatomyositis: pathophysiology and disease expression, *Pediatr Clin North Am* 42:1071-1098, 1995.
29. Reed AM, Pachman LM, Hayford J, et al: Immunogenetic studies in families of children with juvenile dermatomyositis, *J Rheumatol* 25:1000-1002, 1998.
30. Pachman LM, Fedezyna TO, Lechman TS, et al: Juvenile dermatomyositis: the association of the TNF alpha-308A allele and disease chronicity, *Curr Rheumatol Reports* 3:379-386, 2001.
31. Tezak Z, Hoffman EP, Lutz JL, et al: Gene expression profiling in DQA1*0501+ children with untreated dermatomyositis: a novel model of pathogenesis, *J Immunol* 168:4154-4163, 2002.
32. Pachman LM, Litt DL, Rowley AH, et al: Lack of detection of enteroviral or bacterial DNA in magnetic resonance imaging-directed muscle biopsies from twenty children with active untreated juvenile dermatomyositis, *Arthritis Rheum* 38:1513-1518, 1995.
33. Miller LC, Sisson BA, Tucker LB, et al: Methotrexate treatment of recalcitrant childhood dermatomyositis, *Arthritis Rheum* 35:1143-1149, 1992.
34. Dalakas MC, Illa I, Dambrosia JM, et al: A controlled trial of high-dose intravenous immune globulin infusions as treatment for dermatomyositis, *N Engl J Med* 329:1993-2000, 1993.
35. Reiff A, Rawlings DJ, Shaham B, et al: Preliminary evidence for cyclosporin A as an alternative treatment of recalcitrant juvenile rheumatoid arthritis and juvenile dermatomyositis, *J Rheumatol* 24:2436-2443, 1997.
36. Rottem M, Fauci AS, Hallahan CW, et al: Wegener granulomatosis in children and adolescents: clinical presentation and outcome, *J Pediatr* 122:27-31, 1993.

BOX 13-2

KEY CONCEPTS

Diagnosis of Rheumatic Diseases of Childhood

- The diagnosis of the rheumatic diseases of childhood is based on history and physical examination.
- Laboratory tests add supportive information but seldom produce diagnoses not indicated by the history and physical examination.
- Most autoimmune diseases demonstrate evidence of inflammation in laboratory tests, which guides the clinician away from trauma, allergy, or emotions as possible causes.

dose) in patients who present with cramping abdominal pain in order to prevent the complications of intussusception or perforation.[42] Steroid therapy may be required for 2 to 3 weeks with a tapering schedule, depending on the recurrence of abdominal pain as the steroids are tapered. The treatment for a nephritic renal presentation remains controversial, although most authors use steroids and a combination of immunosuppressant agents. A fish-oil diet has been shown to be beneficial in adults with IgA nephropathy.[43] The proteinuria of persistent IgA nephropathy in HSP patients may also improve when treatment with angiotensin-converting enzyme inhibitors is instituted.

The vast majority of children make a full recovery from HSP. Long-term morbidity is caused by IgA nephropathy with progression to end-stage renal disease. Patients with a nephritic or nephritic-orthotic presentation should be referred to a renal specialist.

CONCLUSIONS

The panoply of illnesses included in the rheumatic diseases of childhood accounts for a major segment of chronic disease. Although proximate causes for these diseases are not known, increasing evidence indicates that genetic predisposition together with environmental influences will explain disease expression. Treatment advances since the 1990s have improved the outcome for the majority of patients (Box 13-2).

REFERENCES

1. Ilowite NT: Current treatment of juvenile rheumatoid arthritis, *Pediatrics* 109:109-115, 2002.
2. Jarvis JN: Pathogenesis and mechanisms of inflammation in the childhood rheumatic diseases, *Curr Opin Rheumatol* 10:459-467, 1998.
3. Glass DN, Giannini EH: JRA as a complex genetic trait, *Arthritis Rheum* 42:2261-2268, 1999.
4. Vostrejs M, Hollister JR: Muscle atrophy and leg length discrepancies in pauciarticular juvenile rheumatoid arthritis, *Am J Dis Child* 142:343-345, 1988.
5. Chylack TL Jr: The ocular manifestations of juvenile rheumatoid arthritis, *Arthritis Rheum* 20:217-223, 1977.
6. McMinn FJ, Bywaters EGL: Differences between the fever of Still's disease and that of rheumatic fever, *Ann Rheum Dis* 18:293, 1959.
7. Isdale IC, Bywaters EGL: The rash of rheumatoid arthritis and Still's disease, *Q J Med* 25:377-379, 1956.
8. Wallendahl M, Stork L, Hollister JR: The discriminating value of serum LDH values in children with malignancy presenting as joint pain, *Arch Pediatr Adolesc Med* 150:70-73, 1996.

37. Duna GF, Galperin C, Hoffman GS: Wegener's granulomatosis, *Rheum Dis Clin North Am* 21:949-986, 1995.

38. Jenne DE, Tschopp J: Wegener's autoantigen decoded, *Nature* 346, 1990.

39. Lanzkowsky S, Lanzkowsky L, Lanzkowsky P: Henoch-Schoenlein purpura, *Pediatr Rev* 13:130-137, 1992.

40. Nielsen HE: Epidemiology of Schonlein-Henoch purpura, *Acta Paediatr Scand* 77:125-131, 1988.

41. Faille-Kuyber EH, Kater L, Kooiker CJ, et al: IgA-deposits in cutaneous blood-vessel walls and mesangium in Henoch-Schonlein syndrome, *Lancet* 1:892-893, 1973.

42. Szer I: Henoch-Schonlein purpura: when and how to treat, *J Rheumatol* 23:1661-1665, 1996.

43. Donadio JV, Bergstalh EJ, Offord KP, et al: A controlled trial of fish oil in IgA nephropathy, *N Engl J Med* 331:1194-1199, 1994.

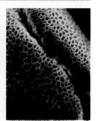

CHAPTER **14**

Autoimmune Diseases

STUART E. TURVEY ■ ROBERT P. SUNDEL

Horror autotoxicus was the evocative term coined by Paul Ehrlich at the turn of the twentieth century to describe the process of autoimmunity. Today we recognize that failure of the normal mechanisms involved in maintaining immunologic self-tolerance can result in such seemingly unrelated diseases as insulin-dependent diabetes mellitus (IDDM), rheumatoid arthritis (RA), rheumatic fever, and psoriasis. Autoimmune diseases are a fascinating but poorly understood group of conditions that involve all organ systems and affect approximately 5% of the population in Western countries.[1]

The definition of an *autoimmune disease* is somewhat vague but involves the demonstration of a destructive immune response, such as autoantibodies or autoreactive lymphocytes, directed against "self" tissues in the absence of infection or other discernible causes. Traditionally, autoimmune diseases have been characterized as either organ specific (e.g., IDDM) or systemic (e.g., systemic lupus erythematosus [SLE]) (Figure 14-1). Although clinically useful, this distinction does not correspond to causation. To understand autoimmunity, it is important to appreciate the range of self-tolerance mechanisms that prevent the generation of a damaging autoimmune response in the "normal" individual, as well the proposed infectious and environmental triggers that can initiate autoimmune disease in a genetically susceptible host.

In this chapter, we attempt to unify the current understanding of the factors involved in the initiation and progression of an autoimmune response and outline both current and novel therapeutic options available for physicians involved in the management of patients with autoimmune disease.

COMPONENTS OF THE IMMUNE RESPONSE: MAINTENANCE OF SELF-TOLERANCE

The extraordinary recognition capabilities of the mammalian immune system that have evolved to provide protection from the myriad of infectious agents result from random generation of antigen receptors on the surface of T and B cells. Theoretically, this lymphocyte repertoire allows for the discrimination of 10^9 through 10^{11} antigenic determinants.[2] Within this random pool of receptors, some will have high affinity for "self" antigens, and *tolerance* is the term used to describe the process that eliminates or neutralizes such autoreactive cells. Knowledge of the mechanisms involved in the maintenance of

self-tolerance is central to the understanding of the potential causes of autoimmune disease, as well as the development of strategies to reestablish tolerance in the face of ongoing autoimmunity.

T Cell Tolerance

The prevention of autoimmune destruction of healthy tissues is essential for well-being and survival. Accordingly, a range of mechanisms has evolved to prevent the development of autoimmunity. Both central (i.e., thymic) and peripheral mechanisms are involved in the establishment and maintenance of T cell tolerance (Figure 14-2).

Central T Cell Tolerance

The deletion of self-reactive T cells in the thymus is the central mechanism responsible for the maintenance of T cell tolerance. Immature T cells migrate from the bone marrow to the thymus; there they encounter peptides derived from endogenous proteins bound to major histocompatibility complex (MHC) molecules. T cells whose receptors have very low affinity for these self-peptide MHC complexes do not receive signals that prevent spontaneous apoptosis, and these cells therefore die "from neglect" in the thymus. T cells with high-affinity receptors for these complexes, and hence those that would be destined to be autoreactive, receive a signal to undergo apoptosis. This process is called *negative selection*. The remaining T cells, which have receptors with an intermediate affinity for self-peptide—MHC complexes, mature in the thymus and migrate to the periphery. This process, referred to as *positive selection*, involves the active rescue of MHC-restricted thymocytes from programmed cell death.

This rigorous selection process allows survival of T cells that are likely to be useful in host defense because their T cell receptors (TCRs) have the ability to recognize peptide presented in the context of self-MHC molecules. On the other hand, they do not have such high-affinity receptors that they will inevitably cause autoimmunity (these concepts are extensively reviewed[3-5]). Not all self-antigens are expressed in the thymus; therefore, a variety of peripheral mechanisms also participate in T cell tolerance.

Peripheral T Cell Tolerance

A range of mechanisms contributes to the maintenance of tolerance in the periphery.[6-10] Depending on the level of antigen

159

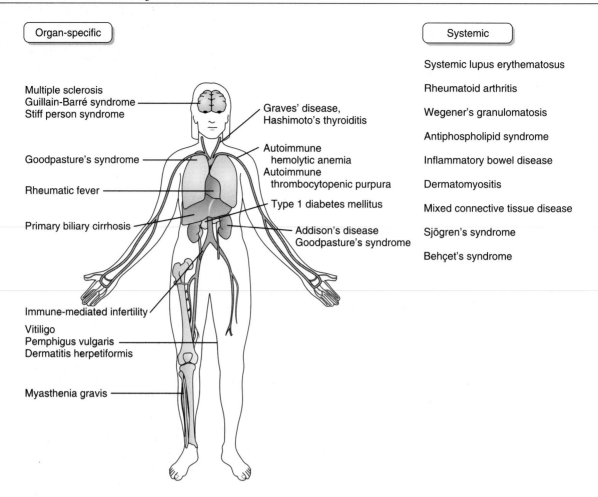

Organ-specific

Multiple sclerosis
Guillain-Barré syndrome
Stiff person syndrome

Goodpasture's syndrome

Rheumatic fever

Primary biliary cirrhosis

Immune-mediated infertility

Vitiligo
Pemphigus vulgaris
Dermatitis herpetiformis

Myasthenia gravis

Graves' disease,
Hashimoto's thyroiditis

Autoimmune
  hemolytic anemia
Autoimmune
  thrombocytopenic purpura

Type 1 diabetes mellitus

Addison's disease
Goodpasture's syndrome

Systemic

Systemic lupus erythematosus

Rheumatoid arthritis

Wegener's granulomatosis

Antiphospholipid syndrome

Inflammatory bowel disease

Dermatomyositis

Mixed connective tissue disease

Sjögren's syndrome

Behçet's syndrome

FIGURE 14-1 Some organ-specific and systemic autoimmune diseases.

expression and on whether the antigen is encountered in the presence or absence of inflammation, there are a number of possible outcomes for autoreactive T cells.

Ignorance. Under normal conditions, potentially autoreactive T cells may ignore their antigens, thereby maintaining self-tolerance. Such immunologic ignorance may be caused by expression of the antigen at a level below the threshold required to induce the activation of T cells or by the physical separation of the antigen from T cells (e.g., by the blood-brain barrier).

Anergy. T cells interacting with specific peptide-MHC complexes may become anergic if those interactions occur at a chronically low level or in the absence of co-stimulation. These cells do not produce IL-2 after antigen stimulation and have increased thresholds for activation. In this situation, tolerance is maintained by "re-tuning" the threshold for T cell activation to a level that favors lymphocyte nonreactivity.

Deletion. A series of deletional mechanisms is involved in "catching" self-reactive T cells that are exported from the thymus. The presentation of antigens in the absence of co-stimulation not only fails to prime T cells but also can result in deletion. Another mechanism of peripheral deletion results from the lack of growth factors for which all activated T cells compete. In addition, a pathway involving Fas (CD95) and its

ligand can mediate the death of autoreactive T cells. Engagement of the Fas receptor induces apoptosis in Fas-positive cells. The importance of this mechanism in maintaining tolerance is illustrated by the autoimmune lymphoproliferative syndrome (ALPS).[11] Patients with defects in Fas-mediated apoptosis develop cell- and autoantibody-mediated attacks on multiple organs, including the hematopoietic and gastrointestinal systems.

Regulation. The immune system has evolved multiple mechanisms to maintain protective immunity without the development of immune pathology. There is compelling evidence that CD4+ T cells specializing in the suppression of immune responses play a critical role in immune regulation. Inadequate generation or loss of this regulatory T cell population causes autoimmune disease in animal models.[9] The recent description of regulatory T cells in humans, enriched in the CD4+CD25+ population, is an exciting observation that opens the door for investigations into whether dysfunction of this population is involved in autoimmunity.[12]

B Cell Tolerance

Germline B cells producing polyreactive IgM autoantibodies and monospecific IgG autoantibodies produced by somatic point mutation are relatively common inhabitants of the B cell compartment. Several mechanisms are available to filter out

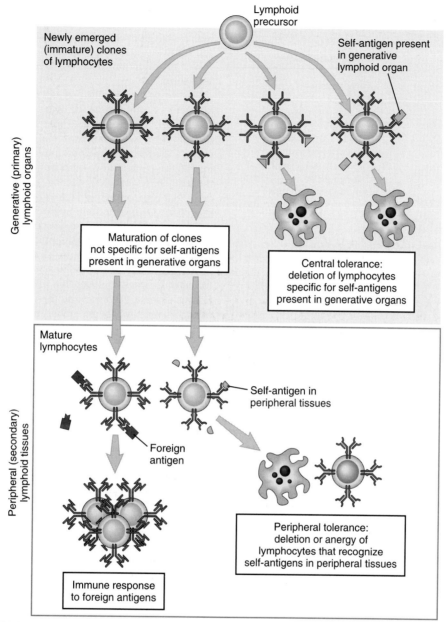

FIGURE 14-2 Central and peripheral mechanisms for self-tolerance. A range of mechanisms, occurring in both central and peripheral lymphoid tissues, act to minimize the chance of autoimmunity developing. (From Abbas A, Lichtman AL, Pober J: *Cellular and molecular immunology,* ed 4, Philadelphia, 2000, WB Saunders.)

autoreactive B cells from the B cell repertoire. Immature B cells are clonally deleted in the bone marrow, whereas autoreactive B cells are eliminated in the T cell zones of the spleen or lymph nodes. B lymphocytes that escape this surveillance may be functionally inactivated ("anergized"), or the specificity of the B cell receptor may be adjusted when an autoantigen is encountered ("receptor editing") (see reviews[4,6]). Nevertheless, B cell tolerance appears to depend predominantly on a lack of cognate B-T cell interactions: membrane immunoglobulin cross-linked in the absence of T cell help results in anergy or deletion of the autoreactive B cells. Accordingly, we focus on the dominant role of T cells in immune tolerance and autoimmunity.

Despite the fact that pathogenic autoantibodies do not appear to arise without a contribution of T cells, autoantibodies often mediate tissue damage and clinical manifestations of particular diseases. Thus anti-Ro antibodies have long been recognized to associate with congenital heart block in infants born to mothers with systemic lupus erythematosus. Recently, these antibodies were shown to block calcium channel current and to induce heart block in a perfused fetal heart model.[13] Thus determination of serum levels of autoantibodies may be helpful in confirming a diagnosis in a particular autoimmune condition. Some of the diseases marked by such specific autoantibodies are listed in Table 14-1.

TABLE 14-1 Autoantibodies Associated with the Development of Autoimmune Diseases

Autoantibody Target	Autoimmune Disease
Thyroid-stimulating hormone receptor	Graves' disease
Acetylcholine receptor	Myasthenia gravis
Basement membrane protein of glomeruli and alveoli	Goodpasture's syndrome
Neutrophil granule proteins	Antineutrophil cytoplasm antibody–associated vasculitides
Thyroid peroxidase	Hashimoto's thyroiditis
Phospholipids (especially phospholipid-β_2–glycoprotein I complex)	Antiphospholipid syndrome
Intrinsic factor	Pernicious anemia
Epidermal cell desmosome (especially desmoglein 3)	Pemphigus vulgaris
Platelet antigens (especially platelet glycoprotein IIb/IIIa)	Autoimmune thrombocytopenic purpura
Double-stranded DNA	Systemic lupus erythematosus
Immunogloubulin	Rheumatoid factor– associated rheumatoid arthritis
Erythrocyte antigens (especially Rh antigens, I antigen)	Autoimmune hemolytic anemia
Insulin and glutamic acid decarboxylase	Type 1 insulin-dependent diabetes mellitus

PRINCIPLES OF DISEASE MECHANISM

Pathogenesis of Autoimmune Disease Initiation

With all of these overlapping mechanisms working to prevent the immune system from attacking host tissues, how does autoimmune disease arise? Our current understanding is that the inheritance of an individual's set of genetic blueprints contributes susceptibility to the development of autoimmunity. Each person's unique genetic repertoire modulates susceptibility to autoimmunity in general and to any specific autoimmune disease in particular. Subtle variation in the genes controlling the development of the immune system and in the genes that activate, maintain, and regulate immune reactions leads to a wide spectrum of immune responsiveness. A given individual is more or less susceptible to autoreactivity, requiring more or less environmental disruption of the delicate balance between protection from infection and development of autoimmunity before *horror autotoxicus* actually develops.

Genetic Effects of Autoimmunity

Genetic factors are crucial for determining susceptibility to autoimmunity.[14] Nonetheless, because of the redundancies of the immune system, they are generally not sufficient by themselves to cause the development of autoimmune diseases. Thus autoimmunity due to mutation of a single gene is very rare, with only a few well-documented examples. Autoimmune polyglandular syndrome type I, also known as autoimmune polyendocrinopathy–candidiasis–ectodermal dystrophy, is an autosomal recessive disorder caused by mutations in the autoimmune regulator *(AIRE)* gene.[15] Another defect in regulatory genes causes the autosomal dominant condition ALPS, which is characterized by accumulation of T cells, as well as autoimmune phenomena.[11] As described earlier, this condition results from mutations in Fas, a key molecule involved in reduction in the size of T cell clones after immune activation.

The impact of genetic predisposition in the more common polygenic autoimmune disorders is most clearly demonstrated in the analysis of disease concordance rates between monozygotic twins. For example, in RA both identical twins express the disease in approximately 15% of cases,[16] whereas for IDDM, concordance rates from 23% to 53% have been reported.[17,18] Nevertheless, the lack of 100% concordance indicates that environmental factors contribute to overall disease expression. It has become apparent that susceptibility genes are frequently not disease specific but rather control the propensity for the development of any one of a number of clinically distinct autoimmune diseases. This is demonstrated in polyglandular autoimmune syndrome type II, in which affected individuals may develop primary adrenal insufficiency, Graves' disease, autoimmune thyroiditis, IDDM, primary hypogonadism, myasthenia gravis, and/or celiac disease. This is also seen in nonobese diabetic mice where a range of autoimmune phenomena develops in addition to the type 1 diabetes for which they are usually studied.[19]

The role of some susceptibility genes in increasing the risk of a range of autoimmune diseases is being studied at the molecular level. For example, cytotoxic T lymphocyte–associated protein 4 (CTLA-4, CD152) is expressed on the surface of activated T cells and is critical for down-regulation of immune responses. Allelic variants in the gene encoding CTLA-4 that result in a decrease in the inhibitory signal delivered by CTLA-4 have been associated with a number of autoimmune phenomena, including IDDM, primary biliary cirrhosis, and thyroid disease.[20-22]

The most potent genetic influence on susceptibility to autoimmunity appears to be MHC.[23] This was first shown to be important when HLA-B27 was identified as a potent risk factor for the development of ankylosing spondylitis more than 20 years ago. Approximately 90% of whites with the disease carry this allele, whereas its frequency in a control population is only approximately 9%. The disease therefore occurs 10 times as often among persons carrying the HLA-B27 allele as among persons without this allele.[24] Disease associations with MHC vary in strength, however, and in all the conditions that have been studied, several other genes in addition to those of the HLA region are likely to be involved. Thus African blacks develop ankylosing spondylitis despite the virtually complete absence of the HLA-B27 allele in this population.

The nature of the association with HLA markers has not been fully elucidated in any of the autoimmune diseases. The primary role of MHC molecules, antigen presentation of peptides to TCRs, is involved not only in T cell activation in the periphery but also in positive and negative selection in the thymus.[25] On this basis, it has been proposed that the MHC molecules associated with a predisposition to autoimmunity might be particularly good at presenting self-peptides. For example, HLA-DQ8 may be associated with the development of IDDM because of the ability of this MHC class II molecule to present peptides derived from insulin to T cells, and in this way the MHC allele contributes to the recognition and ultimate destruction of pancreatic islet cells. Nevertheless, on the basis of our understanding of the mechanisms responsible for maintenance of T cell tolerance in healthy individuals, there are a number of other ways in which a single MHC allele could contribute to autoimmunity. Thus certain MHC haplotypes might increase positive selection or decrease negative selection of autoreactive T cells in the thymus, or they might reduce intrathymic selection of regulatory T cells. Further complicating any theory is the fact that some HLA alleles confer protection against disease, such as *HLA-DQB1*0602* and type 1 diabetes.[26] Any explanation of the role of MHC alleles in disease susceptibility will thus have to account for the mechanisms responsible for this protection as well.

Gender and Autoimmunity

Although men and boys tend to contract infectious diseases more commonly than do women and girls, autoimmune diseases preferentially affect females, with the largest skewing seen in SLE and autoimmune thyroid disease.[27] Possible explanations for this gender bias include such factors as the modulatory effect of sex steroids on immune responsiveness and sex-linked genetic factors. It is likely that the basis for gender differences in autoimmune disease is multifactorial, with contributions being made by genetics, hormones, and the environment.

Pregnancy-associated changes in autoimmunity offer another window on disease differences between the genders. Multiple sclerosis and RA often improve during pregnancy (when estrogen and progesterone levels are highest) and then flare in the postpartum period as hormone levels plummet. This observation has particularly implicated hormonal effects on immune modulation and autoimmunity. In general, immune responses seem to be more robust in women, and the hormone estrogen appears to be immunostimulatory. Sex hormones have been shown to modulate a range of immune responses including antigen presentation and co-stimulation, lymphocyte activation, cytokine gene transcription, and adhesion molecule expression.[28,29] Nonetheless, many autoimmune diseases are more prevalent even in prepubertal girls and postmenopausal women, when sex hormone levels are not significantly different from those in males. Thus additional factors must explain the sex bias of autoimmune diseases.

Acquired Influences on the Development of Autoimmunity

The role for acquired or environmental factors in the development of autoimmunity is perhaps most vividly illustrated in the observation that the disease concordance rates between monozygotic twins do not nearly approach 100%. Microbial infections are the most heavily investigated of the environmental triggers, although noninfectious triggers have also been documented.

Infectious Triggers. Infections could trigger an autoimmune response by either antigen-specific or antigen-nonspecific mechanisms.[30,31]

1. *Antigen-specific (molecular mimicry).* Antigen-specific mechanisms responsible for triggering the development of autoimmunity depend on the concept of molecular mimicry. In this situation, a microbial antigenic determinant is structurally similar to a protein made by the host, such that the immune response appropriately generated against the invading microbe then inappropriately cross-reacts with host tissue, resulting in autoimmune destruction.[32]

   The best evidence for the role of molecular mimicry in autoimmune disease probably comes from antibiotic-resistant Lyme arthritis. Lyme disease, which is caused by the tick-borne spirochete *Borrelia burgdorferi,* is a multistage infection initially manifested as localized erythema migrans. This is followed within days or weeks by disseminated infection that principally affects the nervous system, heart, or joints.[33] In about 10% of patients, particularly those with *HLA-DRB1*0401* or related alleles, the arthritis persists for months or even years after appropriate antibiotic therapy even though all live spirochetes appear to have been eradicated. These patients tend to have high-titer IgG recognizing the outer surface protein A (OspA) of *B. burgdorferi.*

   A breakthrough in the understanding of the role of autoimmunity in the development of treatment-resistant Lyme arthritis occurred with recognition that the immunodominant peptide of OspA (OspA$_{165-173}$) presented by *HLA-DRB1*0401* is homologous to a peptide derived from the human protein leukocyte function–associated antigen 1 (hLFA-1$\alpha_{L332-340}$). hLFA-1 is an adhesion molecule that is highly expressed on T cells in synovium. In treatment-resistant Lyme arthritis, after dissemination of *B. burgdorferi* to multiple tissues, including joints, those individuals carrying *HLA-DRB1*0401* or related alleles mount an immune response that includes T cells reacting against the OspA$_{165-173}$ peptide. In the course of this immune response, which eventually eradicates the infecting spirochetes, a range of proinflammatory molecules is upregulated (including LFA-1α). As a result, there is enhanced presentation of self-peptides derived from LFA-1α augmenting and propagating the intraarticular inflammatory response even after the triggering infectious agent is completely cleared.[30]

   Other infections implicated in autoimmunity due to molecular mimicry include group A β-hemolytic streptococcal infections and rheumatic fever, *Trypanosoma cruzi* and Chagas' disease, *Campylobacter jejuni* and Guillain-Barré syndrome, and coxsackieviruses, cytomegalovirus or rubella, and IDDM[34] (Table 14-2). Nevertheless, these associations have not been fully characterized at the molecular level; therefore, many questions remain concerning the specificity of particular organisms and the susceptibility of particular individuals.

2. *Antigen-nonspecific (bystander activation).* In the antigen-nonspecific model, autoimmunity is thought to be the result of "bystander activation." In this situation, no particular microbial antigen is involved. Rather, infection results in tissue damage, releasing large quantities of normally sequestered self-antigens. Simultaneously, products of microorganisms, such as lipopolysaccharide and bacterial DNA, act as adjuvants and substantially improve immune responses to unrelated antigens. Specifically, inflammation resulting from infection induces expression of MHC classes I and II molecules and co-stimulatory molecules (e.g., CD40, CD40L, CD80, and CD86) on local antigen-presenting cells while also enhancing their antigen-processing machinery.

TABLE 14-2 Infections Associated with the Development of Autoimmune Disease

Autoimmune Disease	Infectious Agent
Rheumatic fever	Group A β-hemolytic streptococci
Guillain-Barré	*Campylobacter jejuni*, Epstein-Barr virus, cytomegalovirus, *Mycoplasma pneumoniae*
Antibiotic-resistant Lyme arthritis	*Borrelia burgdorferi*
Reactive arthritis	*Yersinia, Shigella, Salmonella, Chlamydia trachomatis*
Mixed cryoglobulinemia	Hepatitis C virus
Myocarditis	Coxsackieviruses
Human T cell lymphotrophic virus type 1—associated myelopathy/tropical spastic paraparesis	Human T cell–lymphotrophic virus type 1
Chagas' disease	*Trypanosoma cruzi*

Infecting organisms may also provoke polyclonal lymphocyte activation through the production of a mitogen or superantigen.[30,35] The potency of bystander activation in generating an immune response is clearly demonstrated in the success of routine vaccines in preventing common infections. Immunizations depend on bystander activation by administering the antigenic protein (e.g., tetanus toxoid) with an adjuvant known to cause nonspecific inflammation.

This cycle of microbial infection, cell death, inflammation, enhanced antigen presentation, and autoimmunity has not been demonstrated clearly in humans. Still, the hypothesis is supported by clinical observation that nonspecific infections (e.g., a urinary tract infection or viral upper respiratory illness) are often accompanied by a "flare" in underlying autoimmune diseases such as arthritis or inflammatory bowel disease. Nevertheless, it must be emphasized that autoimmunity is not an inevitable consequence of infection and tissue damage. The inherent mechanisms of self-tolerance are protective in all except a subset of individuals rendered susceptible because of genetic predisposition or immune imbalance from other insults.

Noninfectious Triggers. Noninfectious agents can also contribute to the development of autoimmunity. A range of drugs, including procainamide, penicillamine, and hydralazine, has been associated with the induction of antinuclear antibodies and a lupus-like syndrome.[36] Hemolytic anemia can develop after treatment with penicillin and cephalosporins, probably because the antibiotics bind to red cell membranes, creating a neoantigen that subsequently elicits the production of destructive autoantibodies.[37] Minocycline may cause an autoimmune vasculitis mediated by antineutrophil cytoplasm antibodies.[38] Chemotherapy or bone marrow transplantation may elicit a wide variety of autoantibodies and autoimmune phenomena, perhaps because of disruption of the normal balance between tolerogenic and immunogenic factors.

PATHOGENESIS OF AUTOIMMUNE DISEASE PROGRESSION

Mechanisms of Tissue Injury

No single mechanism is responsible for the variety of manifestations seen in autoimmune conditions. Once an autoimmune response is initiated, both autoreactive T cells and autoantibodies can contribute to tissue damage. For ease of understanding, autoimmune diseases are often classified as antibody-mediated or cell-mediated diseases based on the predominant immune mechanism involved in the disease (see Figure 14-1).

T cells can kill target tissues directly through the use of perforin and granzyme, as well as cause cellular dysfunction and death through the release of cytokines. T cell—mediated cytotoxicity alone seems to be essential for the development of IDDM, whereas the release of cytokines (including tumor necrosis factor [TNF]) plays a central role in the pathogenesis of RA.

Autoantibodies disrupt tissue function through a range of mechanisms, including the formation of immune complexes, opsonization and subsequent antibody-directed cellular cytotoxicity, and complement activation, as well as interference with normal cellular functioning.[35] Such interference with cellular physiology was first described in connection with blocking of the acetylcholine receptor, resulting in muscle weakness in myasthenia gravis. Autoantibodies can also activate receptors, such as the antibodies in Graves' disease that bind to receptors for thyroid-stimulating hormone. In addition, some autoantibodies seem to be markers for disease and have unclear pathogenic potential, such as the generation of antibodies against insulin and glutamic acid decarboxylase in patients with IDDM.[39] A range of autoantibodies and their associated autoimmune diseases are listed in Table 14-1.

Although T cell— or autoantibody-mediated mechanisms may predominate in any single autoimmune disease, this distinction is rather arbitrary and probably inappropriate. In established disease conditions, it is likely that both T cells and antibodies contribute to tissue damage. A further confounding feature is the fact that additional effector processes can supersede the mechanism initiating autoimmune-mediated tissue damage as the disease progresses. These complexities clearly have implications for the design of therapies to treat and prevent autoimmune disease.[35]

Epitope Spreading and Disease Progression

It has been suggested that all autoimmune diseases are initiated as a response to a single antigen.[40] Animal studies and limited human data demonstrate that as the disease progresses and becomes chronic, the immune response often broadens to include other parts (or epitopes) of the same molecule and even other molecules, a process called *epitope spreading*.[41] Epitope spreading describes the observed diversification of epitope specificity from an initial focused immune response to one directed against other antigenic targets. This epitope spreading can occur from one epitope to another in the same molecule (intramolecular epitope spreading) or to epitopes on a different molecule (intermolecular epitope spreading). Regardless of the initial antigenic stimulus, whether autoimmune or even infectious, the resulting inflammation and tissue damage prime a cascade of T cell responses with ever-expanding specificities. Epitope spreading is likely to enhance the efficiency of protective immune responses in clearing infections and tumors. Unfortunately, when the immune response is generated against the self instead, epitope spreading may cause the process to become more generalized and less responsive to treatment over time.[42] This may be one explanation for the observation that in many autoimmune conditions, most persuasively RA, treatment efficacy varies inversely with disease duration.[43]

The phenomenon of epitope spreading is one major barrier to the development of strategies to prevent autoimmunity in an antigen-specific manner. Current approaches to the management of autoimmune conditions such as SLE or multiple sclerosis rely on generalized suppression of the immune system. It is far more desirable to design autoantigen-specific forms of immune modulation that leave the immune system essentially intact to deal with infections and malignancies. Unfortunately, in an established autoimmune disease, the identity of the initiating antigen can usually no longer be determined and may not even be relevant once epitope spreading has occurred. In addition, the hierarchy of epitopes targeted by the developing autoimmune response is likely to vary between patients on the basis of the individual's HLA haplotype, further complicating treatment design.

THERAPEUTIC STRATEGIES

Given the pleomorphic manifestations of autoimmunity, rather than attempting to describe management options for individual disease, we provide an overview of currently available therapeutic strategies and outline novel approaches that are under investigation. As described in earlier sections, autoimmune diseases differ significantly in the immune mechanisms responsible for tissue destruction; the challenge for the future lies in determining the optimal therapeutic approach for each disorder.

Current Therapies

Until recently, therapy for autoimmune disease had been limited to two general strategies: global nonspecific suppression of the immune response (e.g., the use of corticosteroids for SLE) and supportive therapy for the organ dysfunction resulting from the destructive autoimmune process (e.g., insulin therapy or islet transplantation for those with IDDM).

Established therapeutic options for autoimmune disease are listed in Table 14-3.

An important clinical observation, which is supported by studies in experimental animal models, is that it is much easier to prevent autoimmune disease or at least obtain control early in the development of disease than it is to ameliorate established autoimmunity with tissue damage. On this basis, it is our clinical practice to attempt to achieve complete remission of autoimmune diseases using aggressive immunomodulatory therapy as soon as possible after diagnosis.[44] With this approach, it is possible to show a significant reduction in the number of patients with long-term disability from disease, as well as a significant decrease in the total duration of immunosuppressive therapy that is required.[45]

Novel and Experimental Therapies

Altered Peptide Ligands

Optimal therapy for autoimmune disease would involve silencing of only the pathogenic T cell clones responsible for disease activity. Unfortunately, it is rarely possible to identify or predict the autoantigens involved in human disease. Altered peptide ligands (APLs) have been used in multiple sclerosis in an attempt to treat disease in an antigen-specific fashion. APLs are analogues of peptide determinants, with one (or a few) substitution(s) at the amino acid positions essential for contact with the TCR, permitting them to compete for TCR binding and to interfere with the cascade of events necessary for full T cell activation.[46] Two clinical trials tested the effects of treating patients with multiple sclerosis with an APL derived from a peptide representing an immunodominant T cell epitope of myelin basic protein. Unfortunately, these studies were suspended due to significant toxicity, including immediate-type hypersensitivity reactions[47] and a higher incidence of multiple sclerosis exacerbation.[48] It is likely that further advances with APLs will depend on tailoring therapy for individual patients based on the antigen epitopes relevant for disease progression in the individual.

Co-Stimulation Blockade

Another approach to the treatment of autoimmune disease has been aimed at inhibiting T cell activation. Mounting an appropriate immune response depends on the careful regulation of lymphocyte activation, such that full T cell activation depends on the delivery of at least two signals. Cross-linking of the TCR, which occurs when it binds to peptide through MHC complexes on cell surfaces, provides signal 1. Lymphocytes activated by means of the antigen receptors alone, in the absence of co-stimulatory signals or signal 2, fail to produce cytokines, are unable to sustain proliferation, and often undergo apoptosis or become unresponsive to subsequent stimulation. The additional signals required for the activation of lymphocytes come from various co-stimulatory molecules on the surfaces of neighboring cells and soluble mediators such as cytokines. Some of the molecules on the surface of T cells that bind to co-stimulatory molecules on antigen-presenting cells include CD28, whose ligands are CD80 (B7-1) and CD86 (B7-2); CD154 (CD40 ligand), which binds to CD40; and inducible co-stimulator (ICOS) and ICOS ligand.[49,50]

Interference with these co-stimulatory interactions provides an attractive target for disrupting undesirable immune responses, such as those seen in autoimmunity or organ transplant rejection. A major benefit of this therapeutic approach is that it is not necessary to know the identity of the antigen involved in immune activation because co-stimulation blockade is antigen independent. A number of clinical trials have been undertaken to investigate the use of co-stimulation blockade in human autoimmune disease.

The role of the CD28/CD152 pathway in psoriasis was investigated in a study using CTLA4Ig, which is a soluble chimeric protein consisting of the extracellular domain of human CTLA-4 (CD152) and a fragment of the Fc portion of human IgG1. CTLA4Ig binds to B7-1 (CD80) and B7-2 (CD86) molecules on antigen-presenting cells (APCs) and thereby blocks the CD28-mediated co-stimulatory signal for T cell activation. CTLA4Ig administered to study patients with

TABLE 14-3 Common Current Therapeutic Options for Treating Autoimmune Disease

	Mechanism of Action	Diseases Treated	Dosage	Principal Toxicities	Monitoring and Precautions
Disease-modifying antirheumatic drugs					
Methotrexate	Blocks folate metabolism and purine synthesis Increases adenosine levels (anti-inflammatory mediator)	Arthritis (rheumatoid, psoriatic) Ankylosing spondylitis	10 mg/m^2 qwk PO/SQ/IV, escalate as tolerated	Hepatitis, nausea, oral ulcers, bone marrow suppression, pneumonitis (rare in children)	LFTs q4-8wks, periodic CBCs; folate can limit gastrointestinal and hematologic toxicity
Hydroxychloroquine	? Blocks lysosome antigen processing	SLE	≤ 7.0 mg/kg/d PO, maximum 400 mg/d, divided qd to bid	Retinopathy, nausea, rash, agranulocytosis	Ophthalmologic evaluation q6mos, CBCs, LFTs q3-6mos
Sulfasalazine	? Increases adenosine levels	Psoriatic arthritis Reactive arthritis Inflammatory bowel disease	Goal: 40-70 mg/kg/d PO divided bid/tid, maximum 3 g, start slowly	Rash, nausea, leukopenia, hepatitis, headache, photosensitivity, Stevens-Johnson syndrome	CBCs + LFTs qmo × 3-4 mos then periodically
Leflunomide	Blocks pyrimidine synthesis	Rheumatoid arthritis	Adult: 10-20 mg/d	Diarrhea, hepatitis, bone marrow suppression, alopecia/rash	LFTs qmo until stable, then q4-8wks
Biologic response modifiers					
Etanercept	Blocks TNF-α and lymphotoxin	Arthritis (rheumatoid, psoriatic) Ankylosing spondylitis	0.4 mg/kg SQ twice weekly, maximum 25 mg twice weekly	Injection site reactions, infections, cytopenias, ? multiple sclerosis	Sole biologic agent approved by the Food and Drug Administration for children
Infliximab	Blocks TNF-α	Arthritis (rheumatoid, psoriatic) Ankylosing spondylitis Crohn's disease Ulcerative colitis	3-5 mg/kg IV q6-8wks	Infections (especially reactivation tuberculosis)	None; use with low-dose methotrexate to inhibit development of antibodies against drug
Immunosuppressive agents					
Azathioprine	Active metabolite 6-MP, blocks purine synthesis	Rheumatoid arthritis SLE Dermatomyositis	1-3+ mg/kg/d PO	Bone marrow suppression, infection (especially zoster), nausea, hepatitis, rash	CBC, LFTs
Cyclosporine A	Blocks synthesis of IL-2 and other cytokines by inhibiting calcineurin	Arthritis (rheumatoid, psoriatic) Macrophage activation syndrome	5-10 mg/kg/d divided bid	Hypertension, nephrotoxicity, hyperlipidemia, diabetes, tremor, seizures, gingival hyperplasia, hirsutism, skin cancer, lymphoma	Blood pressure, UA, CBC, BUN/Cr, glucose, LFTs, K, Mg q2wks × 3 mos then q2-3mos; multiple drug interactions
Mycophenolate mofetil	Blocks purine synthesis	SLE	600 mg/m^2/dose bid, maximum 1 g bid	Bone marrow suppression, infections, nausea, diarrhea	CBC
Cyclophosphamide	Alkylate DNA, leading to strand breakage	Lupus nephritis Systemic vasculitis (e.g., Wegener's granulomatosis) Goodpasture's syndrome	Monthly IV: 500-1000 mg/m^2, maximum 1.2 g (with concurrent mesna) PO: 50-100 mg/m^2/d	Bone marrow suppression, nausea, alopecia, bladder toxicity, infertility, cardiotoxicity	Whole blood cell count; periodic UA, BUN/Cr; long-term monitoring for leukemia and bladder cancer; PCP prophylaxis if on steroids

LFTs, Liver function tests; *CBCs,* complete blood counts; *SLE,* systemic lupus erythematosus; *TNF,* tumor necrosis factor; *UA,* urinalysis; *BUN/Cr,* blood urea nitrogen/creatinine; *K,* serum potassium; *Mg,* serum magnesium; *PCP, Pneumocystis carinii* pneumonia.

stable plaque psoriasis was well tolerated and resulted in clinical improvement of the skin condition.[51]

Another target for co-stimulatory blockade has been the interaction between CD40 and CD154 (CD40 ligand). CD154 is expressed mainly on activated T cells and platelets, whereas its receptor (CD40) is found on endothelial cells and professional APCs, including dendritic cells and macrophages. CD40 ligation leads to APC secretion of a range of cytokines, as well as increases cell surface expression of MHC class II molecules, adhesion molecules, and the co-stimulatory ligands CD80 and CD86. In this case, clinical usefulness did not parallel laboratory predictions. Despite promising animal studies, trials of a monoclonal antibody directed against CD154 in patients with SLE were suspended because of an increased risk of thromboembolic complications.[52] Nevertheless, this approach remains attractive, and trials with other monoclonal antibodies are under way.

Modulation of the Cytokine Cascade

A very exciting new option for the management of autoimmune and inflammatory conditions has passed from development to the bedside. It is based on abrogating the effects of proinflammatory cytokines known to be involved in disease pathogenesis.

Two agents, etanercept (Enbrel) and infliximab (Remicade), are available for neutralizing the key inflammatory cytokine TNF-α. This strategy has a strong theoretical basis, with literature substantiating the central role of TNF in arthritis and other inflammatory conditions. TNF activates macrophages, endothelial cells, synoviocytes, and other cells and induces the production of additional proinflammatory cytokines and chemokines.[53,54] Etanercept is a genetically engineered, dimerized, fully humanized fusion protein composed of a TNF receptor and an IgG1:Fc portion that acts as a soluble "decoy receptor" binding both TNF-α and TNF-β. Infliximab is a chimeric (mouse/human) anti–TNF-α monoclonal antibody. Both drugs bind to TNF-α with high affinity, preventing its interaction with the TNF receptor and the consequent promotion of inflammation.

The efficacy of TNF neutralization has been demonstrated in patients with RA and other disorders, including juvenile rheumatoid arthritis, psoriatic arthritis, Crohn's disease, ankylosing spondylitis, and vasculitides such as Wegener's granulomatosis. Nevertheless, these medications are not without side effects. The reported association between treatment with infliximab and the development of tuberculosis[55] is a graphic reminder of the inevitable increase in infections whenever immunosuppression, however specific and focused, is undertaken. In addition, enhanced production of antinuclear, anti-DNA, and anticardiolipin antibodies and (rarely) progression to SLE have all been associated with anti-TNF therapy.[56] Interference with the finely tuned immune system must be done with caution and humility because all of the consequences of our manipulations are impossible to predict.

Ablation and Reconstitution of the Immune System

High-dose cytotoxic therapy followed by autologous stem cell transplantation has been proposed as a novel treatment for severe autoimmune disease on the basis that it may allow reestablishment of self-tolerance during the window of time free of memory–T cell influence.[57,58] However, in early studies, the underlying autoimmune disease was noted to progress or

relapse in a number of patients. The reasons for these treatment failures remain unclear, although possibilities include failure of high-dose therapy to eradicate autoaggressive lymphocytes, reinfusion of autoaggressive lymphocytes with the autograft, and renewed challenge from the autoantigen. To avoid the potential complication of reintroducing autoreactive lymphocytes, high-dose cyclophosphamide without stem cell rescue was performed in a small group of patients with a variety of severe autoimmune diseases. This approach is known to spare early hematopoietic stem cells, allowing bone marrow reconstitution over time. Treatment with high-dose cyclophosphamide resulted in several complete remissions in the small study population.[59] Prospective randomized studies should now determine the value and safety of immunoablation with or without stem cell transplantation compared with standard therapy for a range of autoimmune conditions.

The development of rituximab has potentially provided an elegant way to address autoimmune diseases that are predominantly antibody mediated, such as autoimmune cytopenias (e.g., idiopathic thrombocytopenic purpura) and SLE. Rituximab is a humanized monoclonal antibody against CD20, a cell surface molecule expressed on B cells from the pre−B cell stage to the early plasma cell stage of differentiation. Rituximab results in depletion of pre−B and mature B lymphocytes by both cell- and complement-mediated cytotoxicity. Rituximab was developed for the treatment of relapsed or refractory CD20-positive, B cell non–Hodgkin's lymphoma.[60] The use of rituximab to provide targeted immunotherapy for antibody-mediated autoimmune disease is an attractive notion. However, the relative risks and benefits of this therapy remain unknown, and adequate prophylactic measures will have to be considered to prevent opportunistic infections.[61]

Prevention of Autoimmune Disease

The luxury of developing strategies aimed at preventing autoimmunity is currently available only for type 1 diabetes mellitus. In this condition, the presence of autoantibodies against islet constituents can be used to accurately predict the risk of progression to overt diabetes before patients manifest any clinical or biochemical abnormalities. The largest prevention trial published to date involved subcutaneous administration of insulin in nondiabetic relatives of patients with diabetes who had a projected 5-year risk of diabetes of greater than 50%.[62] Despite encouraging results in animal models and pilot studies in humans, insulin in the dose and regimen used in this study neither delayed nor prevented the development of diabetes in this high-risk population. Although these results are disappointing, it is possible that the intervention was initiated too late in the cycle of disease progression to influence the outcome in these high-risk individuals. An ongoing trial examining the utility of oral insulin administration in relatives of patients who have a projected 5-year risk of 26% to 50% will assess the benefit of an intervention applied earlier in disease genesis.

A second preventative approach is to intervene at the time of diagnosis of diabetes when there is still some residual β cell function. Studies of immunosuppressive medications, including cyclosporine, azathioprine, prednisone, and antithymocyte globulin, have demonstrated some clinical benefit, although the benefits in a young and otherwise healthy population were not thought to warrant the risks of immune suppression. Recently, a humanized monoclonal antibody directed against the CD3 molecule (hOKT3χ1 [Ala-Ala]) was used in a small number of patients with new-onset type 1 diabetes mellitus.[63] T cells are thought to be predominantly responsible for β cell destruction in autoimmune diabetes, making the CD3 molecule that is expressed on the surface of all T cells an attractive target. In this study, treatment with the anti-CD3 monoclonal antibody mitigated the deterioration in insulin production and improved metabolic control during the first year in the majority of patients, although the long-term consequences of this therapy remain unknown.

CONCLUSIONS

Loss of self-tolerance results in the panoply of autoimmune phenomena physicians are asked to manage. Rather than viewing each autoimmune disease in isolation, it is now appreciated that a complex interaction among genetic predisposition, environmental influences, and immune regulation contributes to the development of autoimmunity (Box 14-1). Advances in understanding the cellular and molecular bases of normal and abnormal immune responses have fueled investigations into the development of novel approaches for treating autoimmune disease. We are entering an exciting era in which standard nonspecific immunosuppressive strategies are being replaced with therapies designed to specifically target the pathogenic mechanisms involved in each particular autoimmune disease. Approaches that scarcely can be imagined today are likely to become lynchpins of our therapeutic armamentarium of tomorrow.

Acknowledgment

This work was supported by the Samara Jan Turkel Center for Pediatric Autoimmune Disease.

REFERENCES

1. Jacobson DL, Gange SJ, Rose NR, et al: Epidemiology and estimated population burden of selected autoimmune diseases in the United States, *Clin Immunol Immunopathol* 84:223-243, 1997.
2. Delves PJ, Roitt IM: The immune system (first of two parts), *N Engl J Med* 343:37-49, 2000.
3. Mackay IR: Science, medicine, and the future: tolerance and autoimmunity, *Br Med J* 321:93-96, 2000.
4. Kamradt T, Mitchison NA: Tolerance and autoimmunity, *N Engl J Med* 344:655-664, 2001.
5. Sebzda E, Mariathasan S, Ohteki T, et al: Selection of the T cell repertoire, *Annu Rev Immunol* 17:829-874, 1999.
6. Goodnow CC: Pathways for self-tolerance and the treatment of autoimmune diseases, *Lancet* 357:2115-2121, 2001.
7. Schwartz RH: T cell clonal anergy, *Curr Opin Immunol* 9:351-357, 1997.
8. Miller JF, Basten A: Mechanisms of tolerance to self, *Curr Opin Immunol* 8:815-821, 1996.
9. Shevach EM: Regulatory T cells in autoimmunity, *Annu Rev Immunol* 18:423-449, 2000.
10. Walker LS, Abbas AK: The enemy within: keeping self-reactive T cells at bay in the periphery, *Nat Rev Immunol* 2:11-19, 2002.
11. Bleesing JJ, Straus SE, Fleisher TA: Autoimmune lymphoproliferative syndrome: a human disorder of abnormal lymphocyte survival, *Pediatr Clin North Am* 47:1291-1310, 2000.
12. Read S, Powrie F: CD4(+) regulatory T cells, *Curr Opin Immunol* 13:644-649, 2001.
13. Boutjdir M, Chen L, Zhang ZH, et al: Arrhythmogenicity of IgG and anti-52-kD SSA/Ro affinity-purified antibodies from mothers of children with congenital heart block, *Circ Res* 80:354-362, 1997.
14. Boyton RJ, Altmann DM: Transgenic models of autoimmune disease, *Clin Exp Immunol* 127:4-11, 2002.
15. Peterson P, Nagamine K, Scott H, et al: APECED: a monogenic autoimmune disease providing new clues to self-tolerance, *Immunol Today* 19:384-386, 1998.
16. Silman AJ, MacGregor AJ, Thomson W, et al: Twin concordance rates for rheumatoid arthritis: results from a nationwide study, *Br J Rheumatol* 32:903-907, 1993.
17. Kyvik KO, Green A, Beck-Nielsen H: Concordance rates of insulin dependent diabetes mellitus: a population based study of young Danish twins, *Br Med J* 311:913-917, 1995.
18. Kaprio J, Tuomilehto J, Koskenvuo M, et al: Concordance for type 1 (insulin-dependent) and type 2 (non-insulin-dependent) diabetes mellitus in a population-based cohort of twins in Finland, *Diabetologia* 35:1060-1067, 1992.
19. Silveira PA, Baxter AG: The NOD mouse as a model of SLE, *Autoimmunity* 34:53-64, 2001.
20. Kouki T, Sawai Y, Gardine CA, et al: CTLA-4 gene polymorphism at position 49 in exon 1 reduces the inhibitory function of CTLA-4 and contributes to the pathogenesis of Graves' disease, *J Immunol* 165:6606-6611, 2000.
21. Awata T, Kurihara S, Iitaka M, et al: Association of CTLA-4 gene A-G polymorphism (IDDM12 locus) with acute-onset and insulin-depleted IDDM as well as autoimmune thyroid disease (Graves' disease and Hashimoto's thyroiditis) in the Japanese population, *Diabetes* 47:128-129, 1998.
22. Agarwal K, Jones DE, Daly AK, et al: CTLA-4 gene polymorphism confers susceptibility to primary biliary cirrhosis, *J Hepatol* 32:538-541, 2000.
23. Vyse TJ, Todd JA: Genetic analysis of autoimmune disease, *Cell* 85:311-318, 1996.
24. Klein J, Sato A: The HLA system (first of two parts), *N Engl J Med* 343:702-709, 2000.
25. Klein J, Sato A: The HLA system (second of two parts), *N Engl J Med* 343:782-786, 2000.
26. Sanjeevi CB, Landin-Olsson M, Kockum I, et al: Effects of the second HLA-DQ haplotype on the association with childhood insulin-dependent diabetes mellitus, *Tiss Antigens* 45:148-152, 1995.
27. Beeson PB: Age and sex associations of 40 autoimmune diseases, *Am J Med* 96:457-462, 1994.
28. Whitacre CC, Reingold SC, O'Looney PA: A gender gap in autoimmunity, *Science* 283:1277-1278, 1999.
29. Whitacre CC: Sex differences in autoimmune disease, *Nat Immunol* 2:777-780, 2001.
30. Benoist C, Mathis D: Autoimmunity provoked by infection: how good is the case for T cell epitope mimicry? *Nat Immunol* 2:797-801, 2001.
31. Rose NR: Infection, mimics, and autoimmune disease, *J Clin Invest* 107:943-944, 2001.
32. Albert LJ, Inman RD: Molecular mimicry and autoimmunity, *N Engl J Med* 341:2068-2074, 1999.
33. Steere AC: Lyme disease, *N Engl J Med* 345:115-125, 2001.
34. Rose NR, Mackay IR: Molecular mimicry: a critical look at exemplary instances in human diseases, *Cell Mol Life Sci* 57:542-551, 2000.
35. Davidson A, Diamond B: Autoimmune diseases, *N Engl J Med* 345:340-350, 2001.
36. Price EJ, Venables PJ: Drug-induced lupus, *Drug Saf* 12:283-290, 1995.

37. Gehrs BC, Friedberg RC: Autoimmune hemolytic anemia, *Am J Hematol* 69:258-271, 2002.

38. Elkayam O, Yaron M, Caspi D: Minocycline-induced autoimmune syndromes: an overview, *Semin Arthritis Rheum* 28:392-397, 1999.

39. Atkinson MA, Eisenbarth GS: Type 1 diabetes: new perspectives on disease pathogenesis and treatment, *Lancet* 358:221-229, 2001.

40. Marrack P, Kappler J, Kotzin BL: Autoimmune disease: why and where it occurs, *Nat Med* 7:899-905, 2001.

41. Vanderlugt CL, Miller SD: Epitope spreading in immune-mediated diseases: implications for immunotherapy, *Nat Rev Immunol* 2:85-95, 2002.

42. Mottonen T, Hannonen P, Korpela M, et al: Delay to institution of therapy and induction of remission using single-drug or combination-disease-modifying antirheumatic drug therapy in early rheumatoid arthritis, *Arthritis Rheum* 46:894-898, 2002.

43. Lard LR, Boers M, Verhoeven A, et al: Early and aggressive treatment of rheumatoid arthritis patients affects the association of HLA class II antigens with progression of joint damage, *Arthritis Rheum* 46:899-905, 2002.

44. Landewe RB, Boers M, Verhoeven AC, et al: COBRA combination therapy in patients with early rheumatoid arthritis: long-term structural benefits of a brief intervention, *Arthritis Rheum* 46:347-356, 2002.

45. Fisler RE, Liang MG, Fuhlbrigge RC, et al: Aggressive management of juvenile dermatomyositis results in improved outcome and decreased incidence of calcinosis, *J Am Acad Dermatol* 47:505-511, 2002.

46. Sloan-Lancaster J, Allen PM: Altered peptide ligand-induced partial T cell activation: molecular mechanisms and role in T cell biology, *Annu Rev Immunol* 14:1-27, 1996.

47. Kappos L, Comi G, Panitch H, et al: Induction of a non-encephalitogenic type 2 T helper-cell autoimmune response in multiple sclerosis after administration of an altered peptide ligand in a placebo-controlled, randomized phase II trial. The Altered Peptide Ligand in Relapsing MS Study Group, *Nat Med* 6:1176-1182, 2000.

48. Bielekova B, Goodwin B, Richert N, et al: Encephalitogenic potential of the myelin basic protein peptide (amino acids 83-99) in multiple sclerosis: results of a phase II clinical trial with an altered peptide ligand, *Nat Med* 6:1167-1175, 2000.

49. Delves PJ, Roitt IM: The immune system (second of two parts), *N Engl J Med* 343:108-117, 2000.

50. Frauwirth KA, Thompson CB: Activation and inhibition of lymphocytes by costimulation, *J Clin Invest* 109:295-299, 2002.

51. Abrams JR, Lebwohl MG, Guzzo CA, et al: CTLA4Ig-mediated blockade of T-cell costimulation in patients with psoriasis vulgaris, *J Clin Invest* 103:1243-1252, 1999.

52. Kawai T, Andrews D, Colvin RB, et al: Thromboembolic complications after treatment with monoclonal antibody against CD40 ligand, *Nat Med* 6:114, 2000.

53. O'Shea JJ, Ma A, Lipsky P: Cytokines and autoimmunity, *Nat Rev Immunol* 2:37-45, 2002.

54. Choy EHS, Panayi GS: Cytokine pathways and joint inflammation in rheumatoid arthritis, *N Engl J Med* 344:907-916, 2001.

55. Keane J, Gershon S, Wise RP, et al: Tuberculosis associated with infliximab, a tumor necrosis factor alpha-neutralizing agent, *N Engl J Med* 345:1098-1104, 2001.

56. Charles PJ, Smeenk RJ, De Jong J, et al: Assessment of antibodies to double-stranded DNA induced in rheumatoid arthritis patients following treatment with infliximab, a monoclonal antibody to tumor necrosis factor alpha: findings in open-label and randomized placebo-controlled trials, *Arthritis Rheum* 43:2383-2390, 2000.

57. Traynor AE, Schroeder J, Rosa RM, et al: Treatment of severe systemic lupus erythematosus with high-dose chemotherapy and haemopoietic stem-cell transplantation: a phase I study, *Lancet* 356:701-707, 2000.

58. Brodsky RA, Petri M, Jones RJ: Hematopoietic stem cell transplantation for systemic lupus erythematosus, *Rheum Dis Clin North Am* 26:377-387, viii, 2000.

59. Brodsky RA, Petri M, Smith BD, et al: Immunoablative high-dose cyclophosphamide without stem-cell rescue for refractory, severe autoimmune disease, *Ann Intern Med* 129:1031-1035, 1998.

60. White CA, Weaver RL, Grillo-Lopez AJ: Antibody-targeted immunotherapy for treatment of malignancy, *Annu Rev Med* 52:125-145, 2001.

61. Cheson BD: Rituximab: clinical development and future directions, *Expert Opin Biol Ther* 2:97-110, 2002.

62. Diabetes Prevention Trial-Type 1 Diabetes Study Group: Effects of insulin in relatives of patients with type 1 diabetes mellitus, *N Engl J Med* 346:1685-1691, 2002.

63. Herold KC, Hagopian W, Auger JA, et al: Anti-CD3 monoclonal antibody in new-onset type 1 diabetes mellitus, *N Engl J Med* 346:1692-1698, 2002.

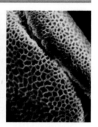

CHAPTER 15

Autoimmune Lymphoproliferative Syndrome

THOMAS A. FLEISHER

Down-regulation of the immune response has become a subject of increased focus as immunologists look for regulatory mechanisms that may play a role in the genesis of chronic inflammatory disorders. This emerging area of investigation complements the extensive work done in characterizing the differentiation and activation of immune cells. The primary lymphoid immune deficiency diseases have provided critical insights into many aspects of lymphocyte development, antigen recognition, and cell activation. In a similar fashion, a recently described prototypic human disorder that affects one pathway involved in the control of immune responses has provided important insights into mechanisms controlling the immune response via cell elimination. This disorder, the autoimmune lymphoproliferative syndrome (ALPS), has now been thoroughly characterized and represents the first human immune disorder that involves a congenital defect in lymphocyte-programmed cell death, or apoptosis. The active induction of apoptosis is mediated by several receptor-ligand pairs and provides one mechanism for controlling the extent of antigen-specific lymphocyte responses.[1,2] One apoptotic pathway that is particularly critical within the lymphocyte compartment depends on the interaction of the lymphocyte surface receptor Fas (CD95, Apo-1) and its specific ligand (FasL). Fas is up-regulated on T cells after cell activation and appears to be a critical signaling pathway for apoptosis in concert with T cell receptor (TCR) restimulation.[3] This provides a means to modulate T cell responses, particularly during chronic antigen stimulation, and to eliminate autoreactive cells and possibly malignant lymphoid cells.

A link between Fas-mediated lymphocyte apoptosis and autoimmune disease emerged from work in the *lpr* and *gld* murine models of systemic lupus erythematosus. Studies revealed that these autoimmune models were associated with defective lymphocyte apoptosis.[4] Ultimately this was demonstrated to be the product of mutations in the genes encoding either Fas or FasL in the *lpr* and *gld* mice, respectively.[5,6] The characteristics of these mice include the development of massive lymphadenopathy, antinuclear antibodies, circulating immune complexes with resultant glomerulonephritis, and a striking increase in circulating CD3+/CD4−/CD8− (double-negative) T cells. Homozygous mutations in either of these genes result in marked inhibition of lymphocyte apoptosis that normally is induced by the interaction between this receptor-ligand pair. Thus these murine models provided evidence for a critical role of the Fas

apoptotic pathway in the development of an autoimmune process. The pathogenic mechanism of disease in these mice is more complicated in that only certain strains of mice with either the *lpr* or the *gld* genetic defect develop autoimmune disease, whereas other strains with the same mutation do not. This is strong evidence that the genetic defect in either Fas or FasL is linked to an additional host factor or factors that either facilitate or protect against the development of autoimmunity.

EPIDEMIOLOGY

In 1967 Canale and Smith[7] described a group of patients who presented in early childhood with generalized lymphadenopathy and hepatosplenomegaly associated with autoimmune anemia/thrombocytopenia and increased gammaglobulins. A case report with similar findings followed, and the common feature in these patients was the chronic but nonmalignant nature of their symptoms. The underlying basis for disease in these patients remained unknown until 1992, when Sneller and colleagues[8] reported two patients with similar features and noted that there was a marked increase in circulating α/β-TCR−positive CD3+ T cells that did not express either CD4 or CD8. These T cells are referred to as α/β–double-negative T (DNT) cells and constitute less than 1% of peripheral blood lymphocytes in normal adults. The presence of autoimmunity, lymphadenopathy, and expansion of α/β-DNT cells in these patients led Sneller et al[8] to suggest that this could represent the human equivalent to the murine models of autoimmunity noted earlier (Table 15-1). Additional reports followed describing similar patients with childhood presentation of nonmalignant lymphoaccumulation and autoimmunity linked to an expansion of α/β-DNT cells. Sneller and colleagues[8] referred to this disorder as ALPS, a description that is now accepted by all groups who study these patients.

The apparent link between these patients and the *lpr/gld* autoimmunity models provided the rationale to study lymphocyte apoptosis in the patients; the results demonstrated a marked decrease in Fas-mediated *in vitro* lymphocyte apoptosis. These experiments involved activating lymphocytes *in vitro* to up-regulate Fas expression and then inducing the apoptotic signal by cross-linking Fas with a monoclonal antibody to this receptor and accessing the degree of cell death. The finding of a Fas-mediated apoptotic defect in these patients fueled the need to evaluate *TNFRSF6*, the gene that encodes Fas. These studies identified heterozygous mutations in

TABLE 15-1 Comparison of Features Found in Autoimmune Lymphoproliferative Syndrome and in the Murine Autoimmune *lpr/gld* Models

	Autoimmune Lymphoproliferative Syndrome	Mice
Lymphadenopathy	±	+
Splenomegaly	±	+
Hyper-IgG	±	+
Increased α/β–double-negative T cells	±	+
Immune cytopenia	±	−
Nephritis	±	+

many patients diagnosed with ALPS.[9] After the initial reports in 1995, an increasing number of patients with mutations in *TNFRSF6* have been identified worldwide, including some patients originally described by Canale and Smith.[10-12] In addition, a substantial number of patients with typical features of ALPS have now been found without mutations in *TNFRSF6*. Studies directed at the genes encoding FasL and intracellular proteins involved in the apoptotic pathway have identified patients with mutations in the FasL gene *(TNFSF6)* and the *cystinyl-asp*artate–requiring protein*ase* (caspase) 10 gene *(CASP10)*.[13,14] However, there remain ALPS patients with presently unknown genetic defects.

The typical clinical course in ALPS begins with nonmalignant peripheral lymphadenopathy that usually develops within the first 5 years of life.[15,16] Typically, this is associated with splenomegaly and hypersplenism that often necessitates splenectomy. There also may be hepatomegaly and peripheral lymphocytosis involving expansion of α/β-DNT cells, as well as B cells in some patients. The presence of B cell lymphocytosis is often accompanied by a polyclonal increase in serum immunoglobulins.

Autoimmunity most frequently presents as autoimmune hemolytic anemia either alone or with idiopathic thrombocytopenia purpura (ITP). This is associated with autoantibodies to the blood cells; typically, the direct Coombs' test is positive. Thrombocytopenia can be significant with platelet counts below 20,000/mm³; some ALPS patients may also develop neutropenia that appears to be immunologically mediated. Dermatologic findings are common in ALPS, with urticarial rashes representing the most frequent finding. Additional autoimmune disease that has been reported less frequently in ALPS patients includes glomerulonephritis and polyneuropathy. There also is a dramatically increased incidence of lymphoma in individuals with Fas mutations and other features of ALPS, with an increased relative risk of 51 for Hodgkin's disease and 14 for non–Hodgkin's lymphomas.[17]

The enlarged lymph nodes found in ALPS are characterized by follicular hyperplasia and marked paracortical expansion, with immunoblasts and plasma cells.[18] In addition, the paracortical areas demonstrate large numbers of infiltrating α/β-DNT cells. These findings resemble reactive lymph nodes associated with viral infection with the exception that histiocytes and apoptotic bodies are not found in the nodes of ALPS patients. The DNT cells in the lymph nodes and peripheral blood have the same immunophenotypic characteristics, including HLA-DR, CD57, and CD45RA expression.

GENETIC BASIS OF AUTOIMMUNE LYMPHOPROLIFERATIVE SYNDROME

As previously noted, the initial investigations in ALPS patients were directed at screening *TNFRSF6*, the gene encoding Fas. This gene consists of nine exons (Figure 15-1), the first five of which code for three cysteine-rich extracellular domains characteristic of the tumor necrosis factor receptor (TNFR) family.[19] The sixth exon codes for a transmembrane domain, and the last three (exons 7 through 9) code for the intracellular domain (see Figure 15-1). Within the intracellular domain is a critical region coded for by exon 9; this is referred to as the death domain, and this portion of the protein is directly involved in the apoptotic signaling pathway.

Five of the first seven ALPS patients seen at the National Institutes of Health demonstrated unique mutations in *TNFRSF6*.[7] After this report, patients with ALPS features were found by other investigators to have *TNFRSF6* mutations.[8-10] To date there have been 62 *TNFRSF6* mutations in ALPS patients from 69 different families reported to the ALPS on-line database maintained by the National Human Genome Research Institute at the National Institutes of Health (www. nhgri.nih.gov/DIR/GMBB/ALPS). These are most frequently missense or nonsense mutations and are found throughout the gene, although the majority (about 55%) are found in exon 9, which encodes the death domain.

These studies revealed that the majority of ALPS patients have a heterozygous mutation in *TNFRSF6*. This contrasts with the *lpr* model, which is an autosomal recessive disorder that requires mutations in both genes for autoimmunity to develop. There have been a small number of ALPS patients with homozygous or compound heterozygous defects in Fas, and these were associated with a more severe clinical phenotype presenting during the neonatal period that prompted bone marrow transplantation.[20,21]

A minority of ALPS patients, however, do not have mutations affecting *TNFRSF6*, and evaluation of the gene encoding FasL recently established that one patient with typical findings of ALPS has a heterozygous defect affecting FasL.[13,15,22] In addition, two patients with normal Fas and FasL have been demonstrated to have a defect in caspase 10, an intracellular proenzyme that is activated by a specific protein (Fas-associated death domain [FADD]) after its binding to the death domains of the trimerized Fas receptor.[14] Thus, although

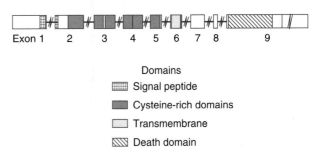

FIGURE 15-1 Gene organization of the *TNFRSF6* gene encoding the Fas protein.

the apoptotic defect in the majority of patients with ALPS results from a heterozygous defect in the gene encoding Fas, other molecular abnormalities in the Fas pathway can also lead to phenotypically similar diseases. These findings form the basis of the current classification scheme for ALPS.

- ALPS type Ia: mutation in the gene encoding Fas (*TNFRSF6*)
- ALPS type Ib: mutation in the gene encoding FasL (*TNFSF6*)
- ALPS type II: mutation in the gene encoding caspase 10 (*CASP10*)
- ALPS type III: no known mutation

The mutations in *TNFRSF6* found in ALPS patients were verified as causes of the apoptotic defect through the use of transfection experiments.[7] In these studies, murine thymoma cells were transfected with cDNA encoding either wild-type (normal) or mutant (patient) Fas. After the transfection of a murine cell line, human Fas expression could be demonstrated (Figure 15-2). The transfected cells were then exposed to anti-Fas antibody, and the level of cell death was evaluated. In these studies, only the cells transfected with normal Fas demonstrated significant levels of cell death after exposure to anti-Fas antibody. In contrast, despite human Fas expression by cells transfected with patient cDNA, the cells did not undergo apoptosis after cross-linking with the antibody.

As noted earlier, the majority of ALPS patients have heterozygous defects in *TNFRSF6,* and additional transfection experiments were designed to confirm that one defective copy of *TNFRSF6* was sufficient to induce a functional defect in Fas-mediated death. Using a series of cotransfection experiments with various ratios of normal and patient cDNA, it became clear that introduction of equal quantities of normal and patient cDNA into the murine cell line resulted in Fas surface expression at levels similar to that seen in the single cDNA transfection experiments (see Figure 15-2). However, despite the comparable surface Fas expression, the addition of anti-Fas antibody to the cotransfected murine cells did not induce a normal level of apoptosis (see Figure 15-2). These experiments demonstrate that heterozygous mutations in *TNFRSF6* seen in the majority of ALPS patients inhibit Fas function. In the case of mutations affecting the death domain, this appears to be a dominant negative inhibition based on the requirement of the receptor to homotrimerize to signal apoptosis.[23] Thus if the normal and mutant alleles in an ALPS patient produce equivalent amounts of protein, seven of eight Fas homotrimers would contain at least one mutant protein.[15] Further experiments were designed to examine the Fas apoptotic pathway in the setting of a heterozygous Fas mutation by evaluating the level of intracellular FADD binding to the Fas trimeric death domain.[24] These studies confirmed that FADD binding is diminished in the majority of ALPS patients with heterozygous mutations affecting the death domain. The decrease in FADD binding supports the hypothesis that Fas trimers containing one or more copies of the mutant protein are nonfunctional and explains the defective lymphocyte apoptosis observed in this group of ALPS patients (Figure 15-3). The mechanism responsible for the apoptotic defect in some ALPS patients with extracellular domain mutations has also been shown to be a dominant interfering defect and has helped to establish that the Fas homotrimer preassociates before the FasL encounter.[25] The cellular basis of many of the

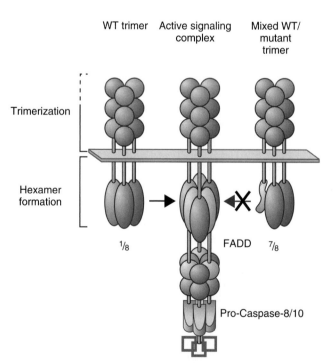

FIGURE 15-3 Schematic representation of the impact of a heterozygous mutation on trimeric Fas with the resultant block in signaling by the Fas homotrimer and inhibition of apoptosis. Normally homotrimeric FasL engages the trimeric Fas, resulting in the binding of three molecules of FADD protein (active signaling complex) with initiation of the intracellular cascade. The presence of one or more mutant Fas proteins (mixed WT/mutant) in the trimer inhibits the apoptotic cascade. *WT,* Wild type (nonmutant); *FADD,* Fas-associated death domain.

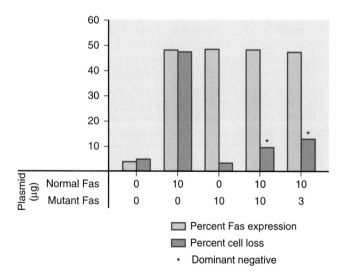

FIGURE 15-2 Transfection experiments using either normal (wild-type) or mutant (autoimmune lymphoproliferative syndrome) human cDNA. The target for the transfection is a murine thymoma cell line that does not express human Fas. After transfection, the cell line was tested for surface expression of human Fas by surface staining using flow cytometry and for induction of apoptosis using an antibody to human Fas to cross-link the surface protein, followed by assessment of the degree of cell death.

extracellular mutations has not been determined, although in some patients it may be linked to decreased levels of Fas expression.[26]

Extensive evaluation of family members of ALPS patients has identified multiple family members within individual pedigrees who have identical heterozygous mutations but who may have few, if any, features of ALPS.[27] Some have selected findings associated with ALPS, including increased DNT cells and a history of autoimmune cytopenia, whereas others are asymptomatic. A review of the clinical and genetic information in 16 ALPS pedigrees revealed that the site of the *TNFRSF6* mutation has a direct impact on the development of disease manifestation.[28] Specifically, in 11 families with mutations of exons 7 through 9, 38 of 43 (88%) individuals had at least one ALPS-associated feature and 19 (44%) of these family members had significant morbidity associated with these symptoms. In contrast, only 3 of 17 (18%) of the individuals in the five families with extracellular *TNFRSF6* mutations had any features of ALPS, and none had significant morbidity. Taken together, these findings establish that the site of the *TNFRSF6* mutation affects disease penetrance and severity.

IMMUNE FUNCTION IN AUTOIMMUNE LYMPHOPROLIFERATIVE SYNDROME

Immunologic evaluation of ALPS patients was initially directed at the DNT cells, and these were found to have limited *in vitro* functional activity. The CD4 T cells in ALPS appear to be skewed toward Th2 T cells based on the increased amounts of interleukin (IL)-4 and IL-5 secreted after *in vitro* activation.[29] In addition, T cells produce decreased levels of interferon gamma and IL-2 after *in vitro* activation, suggesting a concomitant decrease in Th1 T cell activity. There are markedly elevated serum levels of IL-10 in ALPS patients; this appears to be at least in part a product of the α/β-DNT cells and the circulating monocytes.[30] The increase in IL-10 production is likely contributing to the skewed T-helper pattern because IL-10 is a potent inhibitor of IL-12 and as a result also an inhibitor of Th1 development.

The immunologic data suggest that the overproduction of IL-10 is likely the reason for the increased production of IL-4 and IL-5. It also suggests that the skewing of the T cell compartment may contribute to the emergence of autoimmune B cells and the initiation of systemic autoimmune disease. This situation may be further enhanced by the lymphocyte apoptotic defect that could result in diminished elimination of autoreactive T cells and B cells (Box 15-1).

BOX 15-1

KEY CONCEPTS

Immunopathogenesis of Autoimmune Lymphoproliferative Syndrome

- Lymphadenopathy: persistence of lymphocytes that normally would die
- Autoimmunity: failure to eliminate autoreactive lymphocytes
- Lymphoma: inability to eliminate lymphocyte oncogenic mutations

---

BOX 15-2

KEY CONCEPTS

Autoimmune Lymphoproliferative Syndrome Differential Diagnosis

- Lymphoid malignancy
- Chronic viral infection
- Primary autoimmune hemolytic anemia
- Primary idiopathic thrombocytopenic purpura

DIFFERENTIAL DIAGNOSIS

The constellation of clinical and laboratory findings in ALPS patients is rather unique. However, the initial presentation of lymphadenopathy often raises the issue of lymphoid malignancy; this generally requires a biopsy to distinguish the changes associated with ALPS from those found in a malignant process. The initial findings can also be suggestive of a chronic viral infection such as Epstein-Barr virus, although there are no serologic studies or *in situ* hybridization data to support this. The autoimmunity seen in ALPS patients is most commonly directed against red blood cells and platelets. The laboratory findings associated with the autoimmunity do not distinguish patients with ALPS from those who do not have this disorder in that there is a broad range of autoantibody specificities observed among the patients. Finally, the increased risk for the development of lymphoma appears to be lifelong and careful vigilance is required to monitor for this complication in all family members known to have Fas mutations (Box 15-2).

EVALUATION AND TREATMENT

The diagnostic triad for ALPS is nonmalignant lymphoaccumulation, defective *in vitro* Fas-mediated lymphocyte apoptosis, and increased levels of α/β-DNT cells.[15,16,31] Clearly, after a history and physical examination, flow cytometric evaluation of peripheral blood lymphocytes is necessary to evaluate increased levels of α/β-DNT cells (Table 15-2). As noted previously, this is often accompanied by a B cell lymphocytosis,

---

TABLE 15-2   Laboratory Findings in Autoimmune Lymphoproliferative Syndrome

Immunologic
    Lymphocytes
        Increase: α/β–double-negative T cells, CD8 T cells, B cells
        Decrease: CD4/CD25 T cells, CD27+ B cells
    Immunoglobulins: increased IgG, IgA, and IgE
    Cytokines: increased levels of serum IL-10
    Autoantibodies: directed at blood cells
Hematologic
    Lymphocytosis
    Anemia
    Thrombocytopenia
    Neutropenia
    Eosinophilia
Chemistry
    Increased vitamin B_{12} level

the majority of which coexpress CD5, increased levels of CD8 T cells, and decreased levels of CD4/CD25 T cells.[32] The assessment of Fas-mediated lymphocyte apoptosis was described earlier and must be performed to establish this diagnosis. Once ALPS has been diagnosed, it is important to establish the site of the genetic defects. Because mutations in *TNFRSF6* represent the most common defects, we typically sequence this gene first. If these studies are unrevealing, we move to sequence the genes encoding FasL and caspase 10. As previously noted, there remain ALPS patients without defined genetic abnormalities, but studies are under way evaluating other members of the apoptotic intracellular signaling pathway.

ALPS patients with autoimmune disease typically have autoantibodies directed at the blood cells affected. However, there is no consistent pattern in terms of antigen specificity for the autoantibodies among the ALPS patients. In addition, there is only infrequent autoantibody reactivity to non−blood cell autoantigens, and when found, these tend to be of low titer and little clinical consequence. As previously noted, ALPS patients have increased serum IL-10 levels and often have increased levels of vitamin B12 and eosinophilia (see Table 15-2).

The lymphoid expansion typically diminishes with age; thus therapy directed at this feature of ALPS is generally not necessary in most ALPS patients. The splenomegaly is often associated with hypersplenism, and splenectomy is common among ALPS patients. The autoimmune cytopenias typically respond to corticosteroids; this therapy is also associated with a decrease in lymphadenopathy that rapidly reappears after discontinuation of the therapy. The ITP associated with ALPS often responds to corticosteroids, although exacerbations are not uncommon and these may become resistant to conventional therapy in some patients. ALPS thrombocytopenia often does not respond to intravenous immunoglobulin therapy in contrast to most childhood ITP cases. Preliminary data suggest that mycophenolate mofetil may be useful in the treatment of ALPS patients with ITP who are unresponsive to standard therapy. A recent report suggests that Fansidar (sulfadoxine-pyrimethamine) may improve autoimmune cytopenias and diminish lymphadenopathy in certain ALPS patients, but the usefulness of this approach remains to be confirmed in controlled studies.[33] The potential for lymphoma appears to be a lifelong risk, whereas the treatment of lymphomas in ALPS patients appears to follow standard response patterns.

CONCLUSIONS

ALPS represents a nonmalignant human lymphocyte disorder that results from defective lymphocyte apoptosis (Box 15-3). This disorder has many features in common with the *lpr* and *gld* murine models of autoimmunity, including defective Fas-induced lymphocyte apoptosis. The apoptotic abnormality appears to facilitate lymphoaccumulation and to alter the elimination of autoreactive lymphocytes contributing to the development of autoimmunity. ALPS patients without mutations in *TNFRSF6* have been identified that have mutations in either FasL or intracellular proteins involved in initiating apoptosis. A third group of ALPS patients has been identified; these patients have the same functional abnormality in Fas-mediated *in vitro* lymphocyte apoptosis but have as yet no defined genetic abnormality.

BOX 15-3

KEY CONCEPTS

Diagnostic Criteria for Autoimmune Lymphoproliferative Syndrome

Required
- Nonmalignant lymphadenopathy
- Increased percentage and/or numbers of α/β T cell receptor double negative T cells
- Defective *in vitro* lymphocyte apoptosis

Supportive
- Autoimmune disease
- Family history

Evaluation of extended family pedigrees has established that the development of clinical ALPS requires more than defective Fas-mediated lymphocyte apoptosis. Whether the additional requirements are genetic or environmental remains unknown, but these findings are consistent with the observation that only certain murine strains with either the *lpr* or *gld* mutations develop autoimmunity, whereas other strains do not. Preliminary data suggest that one possible contributing factor is alteration in lymphocyte immunoregulation mediated by CD25+CD4 T cells.[32]

The markedly increased risk of both Hodgkin's and non–Hodgkin's lymphoma in ALPS patients provides clear evidence that the Fas-mediated apoptosis also plays an important role in the elimination of lymphoid cells that have malignant potential. This risk appears to be lifelong because a number of patients have developed lymphoma in the fifth and sixth decades.

The lymphocyte response pattern in ALPS is characterized by Th2-type responses, with increased *in vitro* levels of IL-4 and IL-5 production accompanied by decreased interferon gamma production as well as elevated serum IL-10 levels. Interestingly, these changes are not accompanied by any obvious increased susceptibility to infection with intracellular pathogens or by an increased presence of atopic disease. This pattern of immunologic response combined with defective Fas-mediated lymphocyte apoptosis may allow selected autoreactive T cells and B cells to develop. The striking predominance of hematologic autoimmune disease suggests that the Fas apoptotic pathway, potentially in concert with other immunoregulatory changes, is particularly critical in controlling autoreactive lymphocytes directed at hematopoietic cells.

The results of these studies have established a genetic basis for the majority of ALPS patients and have provided the first direct evidence for a human autoimmune disease linked to a defect in lymphocyte apoptosis. ALPS may serve as a model human disease for defining the immunologic factors that lead to the development of selected humoral autoimmunity. In addition, ALPS could provide a clinical situation to investigate immunomodulatory therapy that potentially could control certain autoimmune diseases. Taken together, ALPS represents a new category of an "experiment of nature" involving lymphocyte apoptosis that provides important insights into the role of apoptosis in controlling lymphocyte development and homeostasis.

HELPFUL WEBSITE

National Human Genome Research Institute at the National Institutes of Health website (www.nhgri.nih.gov/DIR/GMBB/ALPS)

REFERENCES

1. Lenardo M, Chan FK-M, Hornung F, et al: Mature lymphocyte apoptosis: immune regulation in a dynamic and unpredictable antigenic environment, *Annu Rev Immunol* 17:221-253, 1999.
2. Siegel RM, Fleisher TA: The role of Fas and related death receptors in autoimmune and other disease states, *J Allergy Clin Immunol* 103:729-738, 1999.
3. Griffith TS, Brunner T, Fletcher SM, et al: Fas ligand-induced apoptosis as a mechanism of immune privilege, *Science* 270:1189-1192, 1995.
4. Kono DH, Theofilopoulos AN: Genetics of systemic autoimmunity in murine models of lupus, *Int Rev Immunol* 19:367-387, 2000.
5. Watanabe-Fukunaga R, Brannan CI, Copeland NG, et al: Lymphoproliferation disorder in mice explained by defects in Fas antigen that mediates apoptosis, *Nature* 356:314-317, 1992.
6. Takahashi T, Tanaka M, Brannan CI, et al: Generalized lymphoproliferative disease in mice, caused by a point mutation in the Fas ligand, *Cell* 76:969-976, 1994.
7. Canale VC, Smith CH: Chronic lymphadenopathy simulating malignant lymphoma, *J Pediatr* 70:891-899, 1967.
8. Sneller MC, Straus SE, Jaffe ES, et al: A novel lymphoproliferative/autoimmune syndrome resembling murine *lpr/gld* disease, *J Clin Invest* 90:334-341, 1992.
9. Fisher GH, Rosenberg FJ, Straus SE, et al: Dominant interfering Fas gene mutations impair apoptosis in a human autoimmune lymphoproliferative syndrome, *Cell* 81:935-946, 1995.
10. Rieux-Laucat F, Le Deist F, Hivbroz C, et al: Mutations in Fas associated with human lymphoproliferative syndrome and autoimmunity, *Science* 268:1347-1349, 1995.
11. Drappa J, Vaishnaw AK, Sullivan KE, et al: Fas gene mutations in the Canale-Smith syndrome, an inherited lymphoproliferative disorder associated with autoimmunity, *N Engl J Med* 335:1643-1649, 1996.
12. Bettinardi A, Brugnoni D, Quiròs-Roldan E, et al: Missense mutations in the Fas gene resulting in autoimmune lymphoproliferative syndrome: a molecular and immunological analysis, *Blood* 89:902-909, 1997.
13. Wang J, Zheng L, Lobito A, et al: Inherited human caspase 10 mutations underlie defective lymphocyte and dendritic cell apoptosis in autoimmune lymphoproliferative syndrome type II, *Cell* 98:47-58, 1999.
14. Pan TQ, Atkinson TP, Makris CM, et al: ALPS (autoimmune lymphoproliferative syndrome) associated with a mutation in Fas-ligand [abstract 48]. Presented at the 14th Annual Conference on Clinical Immunology and 5th International Symposium on Clinical Immunology, Washington, DC, April 15-17, 1999.
15. Bleesing JJH, Straus SE, Fleisher TA: Autoimmune lymphoproliferative syndrome: a human disorder of abnormal lymphocyte survival, *Pediatr Clin North Am* 47:1291-1310, 2000.
16. Sneller MC, Wang J, Dale JK, et al: Clinical, immunologic, and genetic features of an autoimmune lymphoproliferative syndrome associated with abnormal apoptosis, *Blood* 89:1341-1348, 1997.
17. Straus SE, Jaffe ES, Puck JM, et al: The development of lymphomas in families with autoimmune lymphoproliferative syndrome with germline Fas mutations and defective lymphocyte apoptosis, *Blood* 98:194-200, 2001.
18. Lim MS, Straus SE, Dale JK, et al: Pathological findings in human autoimmune lymphoproliferative syndrome, *Am J Pathol* 153:1541-1550, 1998.
19. Behrmann I, Walczak H, Krammer PH: Structure of the human APO-1 gene, *Eur J Immunol* 24:3057-3062, 1994.
20. Benkerrous M, LeDiest F, de Villartay JP, et al: Correction of Fas (CD95) deficiency by haploidentical bone marrow transplantation, *Eur J Immunol* 27:2043-2047, 1997.
21. Sleight BJ, Frederiksen JK, Zacharias DA, et al: Correction of autoimmune lymphoproliferative syndrome by bone marrow transplantation, *Bone Marrow Transplant* 22:375-380, 1998.
22. Dianzani U, Bragardo M, DiFranco D, et al: Deficiency of the Fas apoptosis pathway without Fas gene mutations in pediatric patients with autoimmune/lymphoproliferation, *Blood* 89:2871-2879, 1997.
23. Choi Y, Ramnath VR, Eaton AS, et al: Expression in transgenic mice of dominant interfering Fas mutations: a model of human autoimmune lymphoproliferative syndrome, *Clin Immunol* 93:34-45, 1999.
24. Martin DA, Sheng L, Siegel TM, et al: Defective CD95/APO-1 signal complex formation in human autoimmune syndrome type Ia, *Proc Natl Acad Sci U S A* 96:4552-4557, 1999.
25. Siegel RM, Frederiksen JK, Zacharias DA, et al: Fas preassociation required for apoptosis signaling and dominant inhibition by pathogenic mutations, *Science* 288:2354-2357, 2000.
26. Vaishnaw AK, Orlinck JR, Chu J-L, et al: The molecular basis for apoptotic defects in patients with CD95 (Fas/APO-1) mutations, *J Clin Invest* 103:355-363, 1999.
27. Infante AJ, Britton HA, DeNapoli T, et al: The clinical spectrum in a large kindred with autoimmune lymphoproliferative syndrome caused by a Fas mutation that impairs lymphocyte apoptosis, *J Pediatr* 133:629-633, 1998.
28. Jackson CE, Fischer RE, Hsu AP, et al: Autoimmune lymphoproliferative syndrome with defective Fas: genotype influences penetrance, *Am J Hum Genet* 64:1002-1014, 1999.
29. Fuss IJ, Strober W, Dale JK, et al: T helper 2 T cell cytokine abnormalities in autoimmune lymphoproliferative syndrome, a syndrome marked by defective apoptosis and humoral autoimmunity, *J Immunol* 158:1912-1918, 1997.
30. Lopatin U, Yao X, Williams RK, et al: Increases in circulating and lymphoid tissue IL-10 in autoimmune lymphoproliferative syndrome (ALPS) are associated with disease expression, *Blood* 97:3161-3170, 2001.
31. Rieux-Laucat F, Blanchère S, Danielan S, et al: Lymphoproliferative syndrome with autoimmunity: a possible genetic basis for dominant expression of the clinical manifestations, *Blood* 94:2575-2582, 1999.
32. Bleesing JJH, Brown MR, Straus SE, et al: Immunophenotypic profiles in families with the autoimmune lymphoproliferative syndrome, *Blood* 98:2466-2473, 2000.
33. van der Werff Ten Bosch J, Schotte P, Ferster A, et al: Reversion of autoimmune lymphoproliferative syndrome with an antimalarial drug: preliminary results of a clinical cohort study and molecular observations, *Br J Haematol* 117:176-188, 2002.

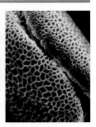

CHAPTER 16

Epstein-Barr Virus Infections

JAMES F. JONES

All viral illnesses are identified by the combination of their clinical components and specific laboratory parameters. The clinical components are dictated by the characteristics of the infectious agent, its predilection for binding to certain cell types, its mode of replication, and the types of host responses that are genetically controlled by the host. The laboratory parameters detect representations of the host response, isolate the infective agent, or identify its presence by protein or nucleic acid identification. Epstein-Barr virus (EBV) infections in particular must be understood by pediatricians and allergist-immunologists because of the cellular targets of the virus and the orchestrated immune responses required to control the infection. One of the three primary targets for infection is the B lymphocyte. Other primary targets are epithelial cells in a variety of anatomic sites. A recent study suggests that B lymphocytes are actually required in order for a person to become infected.[1] The previous hypothesis supported initial infection of oropharyngeal epithelial cells followed by spread to B cells with establishment of latent infection in both cell types. This study could not identify the virus in oropharyngeal cells obtained from patients who totally lack B cells (Bruton thymidine kinase deficiency). T lymphocytes are also a target, but little is known about either the process of such infections or the clinical consequences, except for the development of T cell lymphomas.[2]

The immunologic response is required to control active replication (production of new virions) and to control reactivation of an active infection once the typical herpesvirus latent state is achieved.[3] The immune response must also be tempered because the proliferation of noninfected lymphoid cells that accompanies the infection needs to be controlled. The immune response is then required to control infection of one or more of its constituent members and at the same time to prevent exaggerated host responses that could cause injury.[4,5]

As discussed further, the clinical expression of EBV infections is extraordinarily variable.[6,7] This variability is dictated by genetically controlled host responses that induce the clinical illness. It is also dependent on the presence or absence of appropriate "restraint" of the active response. Although multiple attempts have been made, no specific relationships between various viral genome structures and differing clinical states have been identified.

Antibodies to the virus are present in populations throughout the world. In the not too distant past it was found that a majority of younger children in developed countries are spe-cific antibody negative.[8] One can hypothesize that with the advent of a higher percentage of children below school age receiving care during the day outside of the home, exposure to the virus occurs at a younger age. Unfortunately, this question has not been formally addressed. It should be clear, however, that infectious mononucleosis (IM) is not the only clinical entity of importance in childhood and adolescence. Diagnosis requires recognition of symptoms, signs, and laboratory findings that constitute the spectrum of EBV infections, not just the IM syndrome. The nonspecific heterophile test should not be the procedure relied upon to diagnose all infections with this virus as it has been in the past.[9]

EPIDEMIOLOGY/ETIOLOGY

Epidemiology

The prevalence of EBV antibodies (demonstrating exposure to the virus with replication as evidence of infection) in children and adolescents does not correspond to the prevalence of EBV-associated illness. The incidence of IM as reported in 1972 in adolescents and young adults was 45 cases/100,000/year.[10] As recently as in the early 1980s the majority of children in the United States and other western countries remained free of specific anti-EBV antibodies until adolescence.[8] At that time if a child developed classic IM, a syndrome consisting of pharyngitis and cervical lymphadenopathy, hepatosplenomegaly, an increased lymphocyte count with a high percentage of atypical lymphoid cells, a positive heterophile test, and generalized malaise, there was an 85% chance that the infection was caused by EBV. This illness presentation was assumed to be the first exposure to the virus as acquired in adolescence. The determinants of the expression of EBV infection as IM in adolescents are unclear. It may be that there are indeed factors relating to adolescence per se that influence the presentation of classic IM. For example, familial factors may be as important in expression of illness as is the age of onset. Typically in a family of five susceptible persons, if one individual develops IM, only one of the remaining four susceptible persons will also demonstrate illness after the exposure. If the family member first presenting with IM is a child, however, the development of IM in other family members occurs at a higher rate.[11]

The prevalence of specific antibodies in young children throughout the world varies with socioeconomic status more than it does with identifiable illnesses. In countries, cities, and rural living sites that lack modern hygienic conditions, most children are seropositive for EBV by the age of 2 years; no clinical illness is common among these children. In the United States, children with illnesses such as nonspecific upper respiratory tract infections, pharyngitis, isolated hepatosplenomegaly, cough, vomiting, and diarrhea were found to have antibody patterns consistent with primary disease in a prospective study of acute hospitalizations.[12] A different approach was taken by Roberts et al,[13] who examined hospital records of children with EBV infections to determine the range of clinical illnesses. These researchers found that 16 of 41 patients ranging from 4 weeks to 13 years of age had "serious" problems, including pneumonia, chronic active hepatitis, gastrointestinal hemorrhage, prolonged intermittent fever, failure to thrive, and bone marrow failure; the remainder had typical IM. Clinical illnesses consistent with IM in younger children (under 15 years) vary in symptom patterns from those in adolescents according to Rehse and Helwig.[14] The younger children were more likely to display exudative pharyngitis, exanthems, and hepatosplenomegaly than were the adolescents, but the remaining syndromic components were similar.

It is interesting to note that virtually no new population-based epidemiologic studies have been published in the last 15 years. One recent study of 66 infants from China beginning at birth with samples every 4 months until 2 years of age found that all children were positive at birth, but 8 of them remained seropositive at 8 months of age.[15] However, 60% were positive by the end of the study. One factor influencing this observation is that EBV infections are not reportable diseases. Secondly, it is generally assumed that IM is the "only" infection with this virus and that it is a self-limited process with minor consequences. Unfortunately, the latter issue has not been formally studied. A third known factor that may influence epidemiologic studies is the fact that 90% of adults over 30 years of age are EBV seropositive, but only one third of them have had an illness identified as being caused by an EBV infection.

IM, however, is not the only illness associated with infection.[6,16] The initial illness may obviously be totally asymptomatic or it may include the following organ systems: central and peripheral nervous systems, hematologic system, eyes, skin, cardiovascular system, respiratory tract, gastrointestinal tract (including oral cavity and salivary glands), genitourinary tract, and breast tissue.[17] Severe infections that may be short-lived if responsive to treatment or prolonged if unresponsive to treatment or left untreated have also been described.[18] Table 16-1 lists some of the established clinical consequences associated with EBV infection.

Another category of EBV-associated diseases that deserves particular emphasis is cancer. Tumors that carry the virus include Burkitt's lymphoma (cell lines from this tumor were found to have the virus by electron microscopy); nasopharyngeal carcinoma; Hodgkin's and non–Hodgkin's lymphomas of B cell origin; NK and T cell lymphomas; leiomyomas in a variety of anatomic sites; and primarily B cell tumors that occur in patients with posttransplantation lymphoproliferative disorder (PTLD), human immunodeficiency virus (HIV), and other types of immunosuppression.[19] The most recent entry into the EBV-associated cancer arena is breast cancer, in which tumor cells were found by several independent investigators to contain the viral genome.[20]

More recently, old questions regarding a potential role for EBV in triggering autoimmune diseases have resurfaced; one such illness is systemic lupus erythematosus.[21]

Etiology

The reader is referred to a recent virology text for a detailed description of the virus and its replication.[22] For this discussion, it is important to review a few facts. The virus is a double-stranded DNA member of the herpesvirus family (herpesvirus 4). In its infectious and new virion production state the structure of the virion is linear. New virion production is associated with expression of a variety of replicative and structural proteins. Once infected, certain B cells somehow become the reservoir of the virus in its latent state (approximately 1 in 10^6 infected cells). These cells carry the viral DNA in closed, circular extrachromosomal episomes that replicate only with cell division and express a small number of latent proteins. The virus has been completely sequenced

---

TABLE 16-1 Clinical Illnesses Caused by Epstein-Barr Virus Infection

Nervous system	**Hematologic system**	**Immunologic system**
Meningitis	Anemia	X-linked lymphoproliferative syndrome (sphingolipid
Encephalitis	Thrombocytopenia	activator protein deficiency)
Acute hemoplagia	Neutropenia	Acquired hypogammaglobulinemia
Cerebellar ataxia	Aplastic anemia	
Alice-in-Wonderland syndrome	Leukopenia	**Oral cavity**
Psychoses	Hemophagocytic syndrome	Hairy leukoplakia
Guillain-Barré syndrome		Parotiditis
Acute transverse myelitis	**Skin**	
Sleep disorders	Chronic urticaria	**Opthalmologic system**
Peripheral neuropathies	Ampicillin-associated exanthem	Uveitis
	Gianotti-Crosti syndrome	Conjunctival lymphoid infiltrates
Pulmonary system		
Lymphoid interstitial pneumonia	**Gastrointestinal system**	**Genitourinary system**
Pulmonary lymphomatoid granulomatosis	Hepatitis	Vaginal ulcers
Pneumonia	Vanishing bile duct syndrome	Penile ulcers
Follicular bronchitis-bronchiolitis		Interstitial nephritis
	Congenital infection	

and contains approximately 100 open reading frames, but all the potential proteins have not been identified. Infection begins with binding of the virus to the CR2 or C3d complement receptors.

The production of symptoms in healthy persons requires levels of assumed normal immune function, as seen in Table 16-2.[23-25] A study by Svedmyr et al[26] attempting to evaluate the early immunologic events in IM in teenagers observed that symptoms coincided with the immune response. Perhaps surprisingly, there appeared to be little if any host response during the 4- to 6-week incubation period. Two general types of responses are required for control of the primary infection: cellular responses directed against the infected cells and humoral responses directed against free virions. These responses vary with active replication (new virion production) and the latent stage. The majority of the information describing these processes has thus far been generated from *in vitro* studies.[27]

Although antibody responses are the primary method of identifying infection, it is important to note that those antibodies are not functional in resolution of the illness; they are simply markers of the response, albeit important ones. The antibody responses identified in clinical laboratories identify responses to the viral capsid antigen (VCA), early antigen(s) (EA[s]), and the Epstein-Barr nuclear antigen (EBNA). Using assay systems that include the "gold standard" immunofluorescent antibody (IFA) technique or an enzyme-based recognition technique, IgM, IgA, and IgG isotype antibodies to the various proteins or protein complexes can be detected.[28] Antibodies that detect membrane antigen (gp 350/220) are associated with virus neutralization, but measurement of these antibodies is not standard clinical practice.

Cell-mediated responses include natural killer activity, lymphokine-activated cell cytotoxicity, and specific EBV protein–directed T cell cytotoxicity, appearing in that order as detected *in vitro*.[29] The last process is determined by the genetic makeup of the host.[30] Specific T cell receptor sequences (Vβ) bind to specific viral peptides expressed on the infected cells during both latent replication and new virion replication. One study suggests that IM is associated with selective Vβ utilization.[31]

The consequences of this recognition process then lead to a litany of inflammatory events producing the illness and controlling the infection.[25] Through Class I HLA restriction, certain individuals have selective patterns of viral peptide recognition that are in part associated with the two different stages of viral replication. Early evaluations of these processes concentrated on the genetics of T cell responses to proteins expressed during latent infection.[4] Similar work identified an important role for restrictions in recognition of proteins expressed in new virion replication.

Possible Role of Allergy in EBV Infections

Assignment of IM to an allergic origin was suggested in the 1940s by Randolph and Hettig[32] before EBV was identified as the causative agent of the classic syndrome in adults. The clinical symptoms allowing this assignation were fatigue, swollen lymph nodes, and a history of allergy.

Preliminary observations comparing the history of the presence or the absence of clinical IM in EBV-seropositive subjects with or without IgE allergy demonstrated a history of IM in 77% of patient with allergy but only in 25% of those

TABLE 16-2 Signs and Symptoms of EBV Infection and Possible Mechanisms

Signs/Symptoms	Possible Mechanisms

Nonspecific symptoms
  Malaise
  Headache
  Anorexia
  Myalgia
  Chills
  Arthralgia
  Nausea
	Mediators of inflammation:
	  IFN-α, IL-1, TNF-α, and
	  others

Lymphadenopathy	IFN-α, proliferation of infected
	  and noninfected lymphoid
	  cells

Fever	IL-1, TNF-α

Pharyngitis	Direct infection of epithelial
	  cells; mediators of inflamma-
	  tion: bradykinin; immune-cell
	  injury of infected cells

Splenomegaly	Cellular proliferation in re-
	  sponse to mediators; infected
	  lymphoid cells

Palatal exanthem	Lymphoid follicle infection; me- diators of inflammation
Jaundice	Unknown
Rash	Unknown

Encephalitis/meningitis (other
  neurologic problems)
	Mediators of inflammation; in-
	  filtrating lymphocytes

Pneumonia	Infected lymphoid cells
Hematologic	IFN-α; direct infection; viral transformation of B cells
Cardiac	Unknown; possibly IFN
Pancreas	Unknown
Vestibular, other otologic problems	Unknown
Ocular (including palpebral edema)	Unknown

Hairy leukoplakia	Direct infection of epithelial
	  cells in immunocompromised
	  patients

Tumors	Possible EBV-genome–induced alteration of cell growth

From Jones J, Katz B: Epstein-Barr virus infections in normal and immuno-suppressed patients. In Glaser R, Jones J, eds: *Herpesvirus infection*, Philadelphia, 1994, WB Saunders.
EBV, Epstein-Barr virus; *IFN*, interferon; *TNF*, tumor necrosis factor; *IL*, interleukin.

without allergy (Jones J, unpublished observations). Because the frequency of allergy in the general population is approximately 30%, it may be that the presence of allergy may then predispose the patient to the expression of the EBV IM that occurred in one third of individuals found to be seropositive.

Several studies from Sweden have shown that both children and adults with allergies have higher anti-VCA antibody titers than nonallergic individuals.[33,34] A general elevation in serum immunoglobulin levels is typically seen in acute IM as part of the proliferation, stimulation, and increased stimulation of B cells, but IgE levels are particularly increased to high levels.[35] In addition, although less frequent than IgM- and IgG-bearing B cells, IgE-expressing B cell clones can be established by infection with EBV.[36] Regardless of the surface isotype, some of these clones actually produce antibodies, including autoantibodies with specificity for endogenous hormones, particularly antithyroid antibodies.[37]

DIFFERENTIAL DIAGNOSIS

Although classic IM is frequently caused by EBV, similar conditions are perhaps too often incorrectly labeled EBV mononucleosis even though they are not causally related to an EBV infection. Typical examples include (1) patients with malaise with or without fever, a sore throat, and mildly enlarged cervical lymph nodes but no hematologic changes or hepatosplenomegaly and with a positive heterophile spot test; (2) patients with malaise and a positive spot test; and (3) patients with a compatible clinical illness whose spot tests are negative but whose specific antibody patterns are simply those of past infection and are interpreted by the performing laboratory or treating physician as being consistent with active infection. The use of tables that outline antibody patterns and are reported along with numerical values by the performing laboratory may lead to faulty interpretations of disease activity. These tables were originally described on the basis of IFA results and formulated based on long-term (at least 10-year) studies. Similar studies using the more sensitive but less quantitative enzyme-associated tests have been published. For example, anti-EA antibodies may persist in healthy patients and therefore do not always indicate an active or convalescent infection; thus some reevaluation of the usefulness of such tables is appropriate.

Since all systemic infections share the same basic symptoms, the differential diagnosis of EBV infections must start with a blank slate. Some infections are more likely than others to be considered "mono-like illnesses" and therefore can be mistaken for an EBV infection. These include cytomegalovirus, HHV-6/7, adenovirus, and HIV infections. All these infections share infection of cells associated with the immune system. An additional virus yielding overlapping symptoms is parvovirus B19. All these agents are capable of establishing prolonged or latent infections and, except for HIV, are all DNA viruses. A parasite, *Toxoplasmosis gondii,* also produces an infection with similar clinical components plus a positive heterophile test.[38] In each of these instances the proper diagnosis is achieved by virtue of specific laboratory testing. An EBV infection may be considered by the presence of problems that are common to clinical presentations that are not typically considered in the IM category; for example, a patient with chronic urticaria unresponsive to standard therapy with antithyroid antibodies[39] was subsequently found to have an active EBV infection. Another example is that of chronic thrombocytopenia and/or chronic neutropenia, each of which and their consequences may be the only heralds of an EBV infection. As mentioned in the introduction, the heterophile antibody test in one form or another, particularly those used in small laboratories, is often positive in clinical situations that are caused by EBV infections. Other infectious agents that may trigger the production of this antibody are malaria, rubella, and, not unusually, *T. gondii.* Heterophile antibodies that can be absorbed with sera from different species are also present in serum sickness.[9]

The question of complications of IM needs to be discussed. If one considers IM as the disease caused by EBV, conditions that are not always present in IM have been considered to be "complications"; such conditions could include hepatitis or meningitis.[40] But in the broader universe of EBV diseases, both these conditions can be direct components of the infection. On the other hand, a relatively common feature is neutropenia. A true complication would then be a bacterial infection, such as subcutaneous abscesses that would only occur in the presence of neutropenia. Peritonsillar abscesses and subcapsular splenic hematomas are considerations for other true complications, as is enlargement of the oral lymphoid mass, which creates airway obstruction and requires intervention.

EVALUATION AND MANAGEMENT

Diagnosis of any EBV infection in 2002 starts with a high level of suspicion for this agent as the cause of a very wide spectrum of clinical problems. Any patient even suspected of any of the clinical entities listed in Table 16-1 should be assumed to have an EBV infection unless there is a clear alternative explanation. The importance of identification of EBV-related diseases is not merely academic and there are several methods of approaching treatment of these problems. The first laboratory test is determination of the presence or absence of specific EBV antibodies. Depending on the results of such tests and the clinical status of the patient, testing for viral DNA or expressed RNA may be recommended.

The antibody pattern seen in acute primary infections as determined by both IFA and enzyme tests is positive IgM and IgG anti-VCA and positive anti-EA but negative anti-EBNA. The latter is thought only to appear once the active infection is under control and the virus has assumed its latent state, during which EBNA proteins are being produced. The magnitude of the response is not as important as the pattern, except when anti-VCA and anti-EA titers are more than 1:10,000 and 1:640, respectively, and anti-EBNA titers are 1:40 or lower. Comparable quantitative statements cannot be made about levels generated by the family of enzyme-linked assays.

How the host first "sees" EBNA proteins, however, remains unclear and there are variations on the antibody pattern when patients are first evaluated. Very early in the infection one may observe only anti-EA antibodies. The EA proteins are seen during the early stages of productive replication and may generate specific responses before the production of structural proteins identified by the anti-VCA antibodies. Perhaps the most useful finding to suggest an active infection, either a primary or reactivated state, is the absence of anti-EBNA.[6] Table 16-3 addresses the pattern and magnitude of antibody responses that are typically seen at various stages of clinical EBV infections and is based on IFA titers because there are no experimentally determined observations using the enzyme-linked systems.

The exception to reliance on antibodies for identification of EBV infection per se is a severe infection in infants. As with other infectious illnesses, overwhelming infections in these children may not be associated with specific antibody production. This situation is one indication for the use of nucleic acid or a viral protein presence in tissues, peripheral blood cells, or fluids such as serum, plasma, ascites, and effusions or transudates from a variety of sources.[41,42]

The presence of viral DNA in any of these specimens confirms an EBV infection, but does its presence support a cause-and-effect relationship for the clinical situation under evaluation? This question must be asked because of the presumed

TABLE 16-3 Diagnostic Levels of Anti-EBV Antibody Titers (Immunofluorescent Titers)

	Stage of Infection			
	Active Primary	*Reactivated*	*Severe*	*Past*
Anti-VCA				
IgM	1:10-1:40	Negative	Negative	Negative
IgG	1:20-1:5120	1:80-1:5120	≥ 1:10,000	1:80-1:5120
Anti-EA	1:20-1:320*	1:20-1:320	> 1:640	1:20-1:320
Anti-EBNA	Negative†	< 1:40	< 1:40	≥ 1:40
Heterophile Ab	Positive‡	N/A	N/A	Negative

EBV, Epstein-Barr virus; *VCA*, viral capsid antigen; *EA*, early antigen; *EBNA*, Epstein-Barr nuclear antigen; *N/A*, not applicable.
*May be only positive titer very early in infection.
†May remain positive for 12 months with resolution of illness and positive anti-EBNA.
‡85% positive in classic infectious mononucleosis; magnitude of response is not meaningful.

permanence of the latent state in B cells. It is possible that the viral genome as identified by the presence of DNA in lymph node cells is simply such a finding. If viral DNA, however, is found free in serum or plasma in an ill patient who has not mounted an anti-EBNA response, the likelihood of an ongoing active infection is very high (Box 16-1). In the normal course of a primary EBV infection typified by IM, free viral DNA is usually not found in serum or plasma after 2 weeks of illness.[43] The same can be said for the presence of viral DNA in tumor cells that have undergone genomic rearrangements.

Several methodologic issues need to be addressed at this time. If sufficient viral DNA can be found in tissue or saliva by Southern blotting, it suggests a high copy number and not simply the presence of virus at the lower limits of detection. But which components of the viral genome might be optimum targets for such an assay? There are a number of inherent repeat areas of the viral genome that have served as natural amplification factors. For instance, the BAM H1 W restriction fragment sequence may be repeated more than 10 times in a specific virus isolate but only a few times in others. Use of this fragment in identifying new EBV disease associations have been recorded.[2] This fragment was also useful when applied to *in situ* hybridization techniques in the same report.

More recently gene amplification techniques, such as polymerase chain reaction (PCR), have assumed prominence in identification of viral nucleic acids. The sensitivity of these procedures makes them naturally useful as diagnostic tools. The use of quantitative testing approaches some of the questions raised by the query of whether one is simply identifying latent infections. This issue has been particularly important in evaluation of PTLD states.[44] The sensitivity of PCR allows use of virtually any portion of the viral genome as long as the genomic sequence is known to be consistently present in all isolates.

The application of PCR for identification of messenger RNA (RT-PCR) as representative of viral genes undergoing active replication was an important advance.[45] In latent infections two small RNAs known as EBERs are abundantly expressed (over 10^5 copies), making such infections an excellent target for this technique and for *in situ* hybridization studies. The use of EBERs is ideal for the detection of latent infection; however, they are not present in situations where the tissue in question hosts an active infection associated with new virion production, such as hairy leukoplakia, or in T cell lymphomas where there might be incomplete replication but no detectable establishment of a latent infection.[46]

The use of identification of viral proteins in cells or tissues also commonly depends on the presence of latent stage proteins such as latent membrane protein (LMP). This protein is not expressed in cells in which the virus is actively replicating. Again, reliance on detection of this protein or other latent state proteins as the only approach or in conjunction with EBER identification may prevent detection of the virus and lead to faulty conclusions that may prevent therapeutic intervention.

Choice of the technique used for identification of the virus will be guided by the reason or reasons for needing to know of its presence. For instance, the number of copies of latent transcripts in lymphoid cells in patients with PTLD may be of prognostic value and indicators for therapy[44] (see Box 16-1).

TREATMENT

Treatment (Box 16-2) is based on the clinical circumstance and varies, whether the virus is actively producing new virions or is in the latent state, but cell proliferation is out of control. Treatment of IM is usually supportive and requires adequate rest, fluids, and the avoidance of contact sports if hepatosplenomegaly is significant. A circumstance that arbitrarily requires intervention is classic IM in a high school or college student at the time of final examinations where school

BOX 16-1	**KEY CONCEPTS**
	Evaluation and Management

- Consider Epstein-Barr virus (EBV) in patients with clinical features seen in spectrum of EBV-associated diseases.
- Specific EBV antibody testing is second step.
- Absence of anti–Epstein-Barr nuclear antigen antibodies supports an active infection, particularly accompanied by IgM antiviral capsid antigen and antiearly antigen antibodies.
- Viral DNA, RNA, and proteins in tissue support an EBV infection.
- Quantitative and semiquantitative assays assist in determination of reactivated infection in immunosuppressed patients.

absence would be costly. Oral steroid therapy has been described as helpful with lessening symptoms without adverse effect on the duration of the infection or inhibition of antibody production.[47] The use of intravenous and/or oral antiviral therapy with viral thymidine kinase inhibitors, such as acyclovir, in acute IM demonstrated a mild shortening of the acute illness and fever with no adverse effects.[48,49] The results, however, did not generate overwhelming enthusiasm for routine therapy with this group of compounds. Although there have been no formal studies, clinical experience with individuals in this age group who have prolonged (arbitrarily defined as > 2 weeks) of active disease with systemic complaints accompanied by pharyngitis preventing normal fluid intake, persistently elevated liver function test values, absence of anti-EBNA antibodies, and presence of viral DNA in serum or plasma by semiquantitative PCR demonstrated marked improvement over a few days with a combination of oral corticosteroids and oral acyclovir or related compounds (Jones, unpublished observations).

In the case of severe disease, defined by multisystem involvement, IgG anti-VCA antibody titers greater than 1:10,000, anti-EA titers greater than 1:640, and anti-EBNA titers ranging from 0 to less than 1:40, intravenous immunoglobulin (IVIG) has been given to provide neutralizing and ADCC antibodies along with corticosteroids and antiviral drugs (Jones J, unpublished observations). No trials of this combination have been performed because these patients are infrequently seen, but the responses have been dramatic when accompanied by standard or heroic supportive care. Monitoring of serum and plasma-free viral DNA and changes in the abnormal antibody titers along with clinical responses are required; however, one should not consider this approach without the nucleic acid data.

The standard initial therapy for PTLD is to decrease the amount of immunosuppressive therapy. This approach is usually effective when the proliferative response is polyclonal in nature or the copy number of latent viral genomes in the proliferating cells is not considered to be dangerously elevated. If the proliferating cell population is oligoclonal, more vigorous intervention is required and may include alteration of the type of immunosuppressive therapy and addition of antiviral agents. The presence of monoclonal cells indicates tumor development and requires cytotoxic therapy. A detailed discussion of the pathophysiology and treatment of PTLD is provided by Davis.[50]

A relatively recent approach to the more serious PTLD state is the use of cloned T cells derived *in vitro* and directed against patient B cell lines.[51] These clones may be derived from the patient or matched or even unmatched donors. The goal of therapy is cytotoxic T cell control of the proliferating B cells. This mode of therapy has recently been applied to patients with chronic active infections determined by persistent viral DNA in serum or plasma and abnormal antibody responses.[52]

A most intriguing concept of therapy reported by Slobod et al[53] is based upon laboratory observations made by Chodosh et al.[54] These researchers found that maintenance of the latent state in EBV-transformed cell lines could be inhibited *in vitro* in the presence of hydroxyurea. This chemical (drug) prevents the formation of new deoxynucleotides, among other actions. The chemical process by which linear EBV genomes become closed circles is not entirely clear, but based on this work, the production of new deoxynucleotides is required. Two AIDS patients had central nervous system B cell lymphomas known to carry the EBV genome in the latent state. The patients were treated with low-dose hydroxyurea and had marked clinical response, including shrinkage of the tumor mass. Perhaps this mode of therapy needs further evaluation because the persistence of the virus in its latent state is a major source of morbidity in EBV infections.

The best therapy in infectious disease practice is prevention. EBV immunization has been proposed for several years. Possible candidate vaccines include structural protein preparations and DNA vaccines. Because viral vaccines that undergo replication induce long-lasting immunity, development of an EBV vaccine that would undergo active partial replication but not establish latency would be worthy of consideration (see Box 16-2).

CONCLUSIONS

According to most practitioners, IM remains the primary illness associated with EBV infection; one of the aims of this chapter is to dispel this belief. The spectrum of illness is broad and it is deep in terms of potential disease severity. EBV infections in general cannot be reliably diagnosed by depending on the use of the heterophile antibody test in any of its forms. The only time that it is associated with EBV infection is in classic IM, and in that instance the syndrome per se with the typical WBC changes and increases in liver enzymes negates a need for the test. If heterophile antibodies are present, they are simply present; if they are not present, they are simply not present. There is no such thing as a false-positive or false-negative heterophile test, at least in terms of EBV infections. Specific antibody testing is the starting point for establishing an infection with this virus. Improvements are required in recommendations regarding interpretation of serologic test results. When in doubt about antibody test values in a patient, requesting that the tests be performed by the IFA method is often beneficial.

Another aim is to broaden the reader's understanding of diagnosis and treatment. EBV infections do not have to be considered "just a virus infection that will go away with time." In most cases, this statement is true but in situations in which resolution of the active process does not occur within the expected 1 to 2 weeks, steps can be taken to determine if therapy is required. The rite of passage through childhood no longer requires suffering through an EBV infection.

BOX 16-2   **KEY CONCEPTS**
Treatment

- Infectious mononucleosis: supportive; corticosteroids for airway obstruction (possibly combined with antiviral drugs)
- Severe infections: corticosteroids (or cyclosporin A), antiviral drugs, intravenous immunoglobulin, cytotoxic T cells
- Posttransplantation lymphoproliferative disorder: initial decrease in immunosuppression; same as for severe infections; antimetabolites
- Prevention: future immunizations

REFERENCES

1. Faulkner G, Burrows S, Khanna R, et al: X-linked agammaglobulinemia patients are not infected with Epstein-Barr virus: implications for the biology of the virus, *J Virol* 73:1555-1564, 1999.
2. Jones J, Shurin S, Abramowsky C, et al: T-cell lymphomas containing Epstein-Barr viral DNA in patients with chronic Epstein-Barr virus infections, *N Engl J Med* 318:733-741, 1988.
3. Rickinson A, Moss D: Human cytotoxic T lymphocyte responses to Epstein-Barr virus infection, *Ann Rev Immunol* 15:405-431, 1997.
4. Khanna R, Burrows SR, Moss DJ: Immune regulation in Epstein-Barr virus-associated diseases, *Microbiol Rev* 59:387-405, 1995.
5. Cohen J: The biology of Epstein-Barr virus: lessons learned from the virus and the host, *Curr Opin Immunol* 11:365-370, 1999.
6. Okano M: Epstein-Barr virus infection and its role in the expanding spectrum of human diseases, *Acta Paediatr* 87:11-18, 1998.
7. Schuster V, Kreth H: Epstein-Barr virus infection and associated diseases in children, *Eur J Pediatr* 1:718-725, 1992.
8. Henle W, Henle G: Epidemiologic aspects of Epstein-Barr virus (EBV)-associated diseases, *Ann N Y Acad Sci* 80:326-331, 1980.
9. Sumaya C, Ench Y: Epstein-Barr virus infectious mononucleosis in children: II. Heterophil antibody and viral-specific responses, *Pediatrics* 75:1011-1019, 1985.
10. Heath CJ, Brodsky A, Potodsky A: Infectious mononucleosis in a general population, *Am J Epidemiol* 95:46, 1972.
11. Sumaya C, Ench Y: Epstein-Barr virus infections in families: the role of children with infectious mononucleosis, *J Infect Dis* 154:842-850, 1986.
12. Fleisher G, Henle W: Primary Epstein-Barr virus infection in American infants, *J Infect Dis* 139:553-558, 1979.
13. Roberts W, Wotherspoon R, Herrod HG: Morbidity of Epstein-Barr virus infection in children. In Ablashi DV, Levine PH, Pagano JS, eds: *Epstein-Barr virus and human disease,* Clifton, NJ, 1987, Humana Press.
14. Rehse C, Helwig H: Das krankheitsbild der infektiosen mononucleose im kindesalter, *Monatsschr Kinderheilkd* 133:806-810, 1985.
15. Chan K, Tam S, Peiris JS, et al: Epstein-Barr virus (EBV) infection in infancy, *J Clin Virol* 21:57-62, 2001.
16. Kawa K: Epstein-Barr virus-associated diseases in humans, *Int J Hematol* 71:108-117, 2000.
17. Jones J, Katz B: Epstein-Barr virus infections in normal and immunosuppressed patients. In Glaser R, ed: *Herpesvirus infection,* Philadelphia, 1994, WB Saunders.
18. Kimura H, Hoshino Y, Kanegane H, et al: Clinical and virologic characteristics of chronic active Epstein-Barr virus infection, *Blood* 98:280-286, 2001.
19. Pagano J: Epstein-Barr virus: the first human tumor virus and its role in cancer, *Proc Assoc Am Physicians* 111:573-580, 1999.
20. Bonnet M, Guinebretiere J, Kremmer E, et al: Detection of Epstein-Barr virus in invasive breast cancers, *J Natl Cancer Inst* 91:1376-1381, 1999.
21. James J, Kaufman K, Farris A, et al: An increased prevalence of Epstein-Barr virus infection in young patients suggests a possible etiology for systemic lupus erythematosus, *J Clin Invest* 100:3019-3026, 1997.
22. Ascherio A, Munch M: Epstein-Barr virus and multiple sclerosis, *Epidemiology* 11:220-224, 2000.
23. Wright-Browne V, Schnee A, Jenkins M, et al: Serum cytokine levels in infectious mononucleosis at diagnosis and convalescence, *Leuk Lymphoma* 30:583-589, 1998.
24. Crawford DH: Biology and disease associations of Epstein-Barr virus, *Philos Trans R Soc Lond B Biol Sci* 356:461-473, 2001.
25. Andersson J: Clinical and immunological considerations in Epstein-Barr virus-associated diseases, *Scand Univ Press* 100:S72-S82, 1996.
26. Svedmyr E, Ermberg O, Seeley K: Virologic, immunologic, and clinical observations on a patient during the incubation, acute and convalescent phases of infectious mononucleosis, *Clin Immunol Immunopathol* 30:437-450, 1984.
27. Apolloni A, Moss D, Stumm R, et al: Sequence variation of cytotoxic T cell epitopes in different isolates of Epstein-Barr virus, *Eur J Immunol* 22:183-189, 1992.
28. Linde A: Diagnosis of Epstein-Barr virus-related diseases, *Scand J Infect Dis* 100:S83-S88, 1996.
29. Konttinen Y, Bluestein H, Zvaifler N: Regulation of the growth of Epstein-Barr virus-infected B cells: temporal profile of the *in vitro* development of three distinct cytotoxic cells, *Cell Immunol* 103:84-95, 1986.
30. Rickinson A, Wallace L, Epstein M: HLA-restricted T-cell recognition of Epstein-Barr virus-infected B cells, *Nature* 283:865-867, 1980.
31. Steven NM, Annels NE, Kumar A, et al: Immediate early and early lytic cycle proteins are frequent targets of the Epstein-Barr virus-induced cytotoxic T cell response, *J Exp Med* 185:1605-1617, 1997.
32. Randolph TG, Hettig RA: The coincidence of allergic disease, unexplained fatigue, and lymphadenopathy: possible diagnostic confusion with infectious mononucleosis, *Am J Med Sci* 306-314, 1945.
33. Rystedt I, Strannegard I, Strannegard O: Increased serum levels of antibodies to Epstein-Barr virus in adults with history of atopic dermatitis, *Int Arch Allergy Immunol* 75:179-183, 1984.
34. Strannegard I, Strannegard O: Epstein-Barr virus antibodies in children with atopic disease, *Int Arch Allergy Immunol* 64:314-319, 1981.
35. Bahna S, Heiner D, Horwitz C: Sequential changes of the five immunoglobulin classes and other responses in infectious mononucleosis, *Int Arch Allergy Immunol* 74:1-8, 1984.
36. Thyphronitis G, Max E, Finkelman FD: Generation and cloning of stable human IgE-secreting cells that have rearranged the C epsilon gene, *J Immunol* 146:1496-1502, 1991.
37. Robinson J, Stevens K: Production of autoantibodies to cellular antigens by human B cells transformed by Epstein-Barr virus, *Clin Immunol Immunopathol* 33:339-350, 1984.
38. Sayre M, Jehle D: Elevated toxoplasma IgG antibody in patients tested for infectious mononucleosis in an urban emergency department, *Ann Emerg Med* 84:383-386, 1988.
39. Dreyfus D, Schocket A, Milgrom H: Steroid-resistant chronic urticaria associated with anti-thyroid microsomal antibodies in a nine-year-old boy, *J Pediatr* 128:576-578, 1996.
40. Alpert G, Fleisher G: Complications of infection with Epstein-Barr virus during childhood: a study of children admitted to the hospital, *Pediatr Infect Dis* 3:304-306, 1984.
41. Ambinder RF, Mann RB: Detection and characterization of Epstein-Barr virus in clinical specimens, *Am J Pathol* 145:239-252, 1994.
42. Fan H, Gullery M: Epstein-Barr viral load measurement as a marker of EBV-related disease, *Molec Diag* 6:279-289, 2001.
43. Yamamoto M, Kimura H, Hironaka T, et al: Detection and quantification of virus DNA in plasma of patients with Epstein-Barr virus-associated diseases, *J Clin Microbiol* 33:1765-1768, 1995.
44. Rowe D, Qu L, Reyes J, et al: Use of quantitative competitive PCR to measure Epstein-Barr virus genome load in the peripheral blood of pediatric transplant patients with lymphoproliferative disorders, *J Clin Microbiol* 35:1612-1615, 1997.
45. Gulley M: Molecular diagnosis of Epstein-Barr virus-related diseases, *J Molec Diag* 3:1-10, 2001.
46. Raab-Traub N, Webster-Cyriaque J: Epstein-Barr virus infection and expression in oral lesions, *Oral Dis* 3:S164-S170, 1997.
47. Brandfonbrener A, Epstein A, Wu S: Corticosteroid therapy in Epstein-Barr virus infection: effect on lymphocyte class, subset, and response to early antigen, *Arch Intern Med* 146:337-339, 1986.
48. Andersson J, Britton S, Ernberg I, et al: Effect of acyclovir on infectious mononucleosis: a double-blind, placebo-controlled study, *J Infect Dis* 153:283-290, 1986.
49. Yao Q, Ogan P, Rowe M, et al: The Epstein-Barr virus: host balance in acute infectious mononucleosis patients receiving acyclovir anti-viral therapy, *Int J Can* 43:61-66, 1989.
50. Davis C: The antiviral prophylaxis of post-transplant lymphoproliferative disorder, *Springer Semin Immunopathol* 20:437-453, 1998.
51. Liu Z, Savoldo B, Huls H, et al: Epstein-Barr virus (EBV)-specific cytotoxic T lymphocytes for the prevention and treatment of EBV-associated post-transplant lymphomas, *Recent Results Cancer Res* 159:123-133, 2002.
52. Savoldo B, Huls M, Liu Z, et al: Autologous Epstein-Barr virus (EBV)-specific cytotoxic T cells for the treatment of persistent active EBV infection, *Blood* 100:4059-4066, 2002.
53. Slobod K, Taylor G, Sandlund J, et al: Epstein-Barr virus-targeted therapy for AIDS-related primary lymphoma of the central nervous system, *Lancet* 356:1493-1494, 2000.
54. Chodosh J, Holder VP, Gan Y, et al: Eradication of latent Epstein-Barr virus by hydroxyurea alters the growth-transformed cell phenotype, *J Infect Dis* 177:1194-1201, 1998.

SECTION C

IMMUNE-DIRECTED THERAPIES

RAIF S. GEHA

CHAPTER **17**

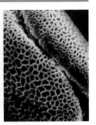

Intravenous Immune Serum Globulin Therapy

MARK BALLOW

At the beginning of World War II, Cohn and colleagues[1] from Harvard University developed an ethanol fractionation method to separate plasma proteins into stable fractions. Fraction II was an antibody-rich fraction that could be administered in small amounts intramuscularly and had a protective effect against measles and hepatitis A. In 1952 Bruton[2] described the first case of agammaglobulinemia and showed that replacement with Cohn's fraction II immunoglobulin was effective in the treatment of these patients. However, this replacement could be done only intramuscularly because administration intravascularly caused serious side effects. In the early 1960s the Swiss Red Cross Laboratories developed methods to adapt the Cohn fraction II immunoglobulin for intravenous use, and in 1981 the first commercial intravenous immunoglobulin (IVIG) became available in the United States.

IMMUNOGLOBULIN REPLACEMENT THERAPY IN PRIMARY IMMUNODEFICIENCY

The goal of immunoglobulin replacement therapy in patients with primary immunodeficiency is to provide adequate antibodies to prevent infections and long-term complications, especially pulmonary disease. Any patient with profound hypogammaglobulinemia and/or defective antibody production may be a candidate for IVIG[3] (Table 17-1). Transient hypogammaglobulinemia of infancy is not an indication for immunoglobulin replacement.[4] Most of these children are able to produce adequate antibodies in response to immunization despite low serum concentration of immunoglobulins and usually resolve their hypogammaglobulinemia between the age of 3 and 5 years. The administration of exogenous immunoglobulin may inhibit antibody production in these patients. It is very important to evaluate the ability of the patient to produce specific antibodies to polysaccharide or protein antigens. Immunoglobulin replacement therapy should be considered only in patients with deficiencies in antibody

formation but not necessarily in patients with low levels of immunoglobulin or IgG subclasses. The approved and potential uses for IVIG as replacement or adjunct therapy in patients with infection or inflammatory disorders are shown in Table 17-2.

Preparation of IVIG

Most of the IVIG preparations are derived from plasma by Cohn's ethanol fractionation method or its Cohn-Oncley modification.[5] This fractionation process obtains four fractions. Fraction II is the immunoglobulin-rich fraction containing 95% to 99% IgG. There are small varying amounts of IgM, IgA, IgD, IgE, and other proteins.[6] Cohn fraction II can only be given intramuscularly. The side effects of Cohn fraction II when given intravenously are thought to result from aggregation of the IgG molecules and their anticomplementary activity, which can produce an anaphylactoid reaction. Several methods have been used to eliminate IgG aggregates, including treatment with trace amounts of proteolytic enzymes such as pepsin, ultracentrifugation, reduction of sulfhydryl bonds followed by alkylation at low pH, or polyethylene glycol and DEAE-Sephadex (Table 17-3). Other additions such as sugars, amino acids, or albumin stabilize the IgG molecules from reaggregation and also protect it during lyophilization. Treatment with solvent and detergent or with pasteurization is also used as a final step for viral inactivation, especially for enveloped viruses.

IVIG is made from pooled plasma from at least 10,000 donors, but each pool may contain up to 60,000 donors and contains a broad spectrum of antibodies with biologic activities, especially for infectious pathogens. It contains at least 90% intact monomeric IgG with a normal ratio of subclasses and is free of aggregates. The biologic activity of the IgG is maintained especially for Fc-mediated function; it contains no infectious agents or other potentially harmful contaminants. Although there is no standardization for the titer of

TABLE 17-1 Intravenous Immunoglobulin Replacement Therapy in Patients with Primary Immune Deficiency

Patients with a B cell immune deficiency
  Bruton's agammaglobulinemia (infantile X-linked agammaglobulinemia)
  Abnormalities in pre–B cell receptor complex
    Igα defects
    Surrogate light chain defects
    B cell linker protein defect
    μ Heavy chain defects
  Autosomal recessive hyper-IgM
  NFκB essential modulator
  Common variable immunodeficiency
  Selective antibody deficiency
Patients with combined or T cell immunodeficiency
  Severe combined immunodeficiency syndrome, all types
  Wiskott-Aldrich syndrome
  Ataxia-telangiectasia
  DiGeorge syndrome/complete type
  X-linked hyper-IgM syndrome (CD40 ligand deficiency)

TABLE 17-2 Uses of Intravenous Immunoglobulin in Patients with Immunodeficiency Disorders and in Patients with an Infectious or Inflammatory Process

Food and Drug Administration approved
  Patients with primary immunodeficiency
  Children with human immunodeficiency virus/acquired immunodeficiency syndrome
  Chronic lymphocytic leukemia with recurrent infections and humoral immunodeficiency
  Kawasaki disease
  Following bone marrow transplantation
Potential uses
  Anemia associated with chronic human parvovirus B19 infection
  Staphylococcal and streptococcal (superantigen-induced) toxic shock syndromes
  Prevention of infection in low-birth-weight infants
  Neonatal and adult sepsis

antibodies against common organisms such as *Streptococcus pneumoniae* and *Haemophilus influenzae,* each lot must contain adequate levels of antibody to certain microbial agents. These products may vary slightly from each manufacturer and from lot to lot but they are generally comparable. Some products containing very low amounts of IgA may be beneficial in some immune deficiency patients with complete IgA deficiency because they minimize the risk of IgA sensitization and possible anaphylactic reactions[7] (Box 17-1).

All current preparations are essentially equivalent, and are selected on the basis of cost, availability, convenience, and the amount of IgA if used for IgG immune deficient patients with complete IgA deficiency. There are two forms of IVIG preparations: a lyophilized form and a liquid form. The liquid form may be more convenient because no reconstitution is required but this form generally needs to be kept refrigerated. The characteristics of IVIG preparations available in the United States are shown in Table 17-3.

BOX 17-1 **KEY CONCEPTS**
Intravenous Immune Serum Globulin

- Cold ethanol fractionation (Cohn fraction II)
- > 95% IgG; > 90% monomeric IgG
- Traces of other immunoglobulins, e.g., IgA and IgM, and serum proteins
- Addition of sugar, amino acids or albumin stabilizes IgG from aggregation
- Intact Fc receptor biologic function
    Opsonization and phagocytosis
    Complement activation
- Normal half-life for serum IgG
- Normal proportion of IgG subclasses
- Broad spectrum of antibodies to bacterial and viral agents

The half-life of antibodies varies. It depends on the isotype and the subclass of the antibody. Total IgG has a half-life of approximately 17 to 30 days,[8,9] but the half-life of IgG3 is much shorter (7.5 to 9 days)[9,10] compared with IgG1 and IgG2, which have half-lives of approximately 27 to 30 days. Generally, it should take about 3 months after beginning monthly IVIG infusions or a dosage change to reach equilibration (steady state).[6] Infusing increased amounts of IVIG results in a more rapid catabolic rate because the catabolism of IgG is concentration dependent.[10] This process is mediated by the Fc receptors on phagocytic cells.[11]

Dosage

The recommended dose for IVIG as replacement therapy is generally 400 to 600 mg/kg/mo given every 4 weeks in patients with primary immune deficiency. A higher dose of immunoglobulin can lead to higher peak and trough levels of serum IgG.[12] On average, peak serum IgG levels increase approximately 250 mg/dl,[12] and trough levels increase 100 mg/dl[13] for each 100 mg/kg of IVIG infused. Several trials had been conducted to compare the efficacy of immunoglobulin given intramuscularly versus intravenously and low doses (> 200 mg/kg) versus high doses (> 250 mg/kg). In 1987 Bernatowska et al[14] compared 150 mg/kg with 500 mg/kg and showed that the higher dose decreased the number of days of fever and the number of days on antibiotics and improved pulmonary function. The benefits of the higher dose of IVIG were more significant in children who had severe clinical symptoms. In a randomized crossover study, Roifman et al[15] administered either 200 mg/kg or 600 mg/kg of IVIG to 12 patients with antibody deficiency and chronic lung disease; pulmonary function improved in patients on the higher doses of IVIG therapy. In 1992 Liese et al[16] reported that 29 patients with X-linked agammaglobulinemia (XLA) who received immunoglobulin replacement therapy between 1965 and 1990 showed a significant decrease in the incidence of pneumonia and the number of hospitalized days in patients receiving 350

TABLE 17-3 Commercial Intravenous Immunoglobulin Preparations

Brand (Manufacturer)	Manufacturing Process	pH	Additives	Parenteral Form and Final Concentrations	IgA Content (µg/ml)
Gammagard S/D (Baxter Healthcare Corp, Hyland Immuno)	Cohn-Oncley cold ethanol fractionation, followed by ultrafiltration and ion exchange chromatography; solvent detergent treated	6.8	5% solution: 0.3% albumin, 2.25% glycine, 2% glucose	Lyophilized powder 5%, 10%	< 3.7 (5% solution)
Gamimune N (Bayer Corp Pharmaceutical)	Cold ethanol fractionation, diafiltration and ultrafiltration; solvent detergent treated	4-4.5	5% solution: 9%-11% maltose; 10% solution: 0.16-0.24 M glycine	Sterile solution 5%, 10%	270
Gammar-P.I.V. (Aventis Behring)	Cohn-Oncley cold ethanol Heat-treated pasteurization	6.8	5% solution: 5% sucrose, 3% albumin, 0.5% NaCl	Lyophilized powder 5%	25
Iveegam EN (Baxter Healthcare Corp, Hyland Immuno)	Modified Cohn-Oncley process; ion exchange gel; PEG precipitation	7	5% solution: 5% glucose, 0.3% NaCl	Lyophilized powder 5%	< 10
Polygam S/D (Baxter Healthcare Corp, Hyland Immuno for the American Red Cross)	Cohn-Oncley cold ethanol fractionation, followed by ultrafiltration and ion exchange chromatography; solvent detergent treated	6.8	5% solution: 0.3% albumin, 2.25% glycine, 2% glucose	Lyophilized powder 5%, 10%	< 1.6 (5% solution)
Panglobulin (Swiss Red Cross for the American Red Cross)	Cold alcohol fractionation, filtration	6.6	Per gram of IgG: 1.67 g sucrose, < 20 mg NaCl	Lyophilized powder 3%, 6%, 9%, 12%	720
Sandoglobulin (ZLB Bioplasma Inc.)	Cold alcohol fractionation, filtration	6.6	Per gram of IgG: 1.67 g sucrose, < 20 mg NaCl	Lyophilized powder 3%, 6%, 9%, 12%	720
Venoglobulin-S (Alpha Therapeutics)	Cohn-Oncley cold ethanol fractionation, followed by PEG fractionation and ion exchange chromatography; solvent detergent treated	5.2-5.8	5% solution: 5% sorbitol, 0.13% albumin 10% solution; 5% sorbitol, 0.26% albumin	Sterile solution 5%, 10%	11-14

Data from Manufacturers' literature; www.E-Medicine.com; Thampakkul S, Ballow M: *Allergy Immunol Clin North Am* 21:165, 2001; Schwartz SA: *Pediatr Clin North Am* 47:1355-1369, 2000.

to 600 mg/kg IVIG every 3 weeks compared with patients receiving less than 200 mg/kg IVIG every 3 weeks or 100 mg/kg of IM gamma globulin every 3 weeks. The improvements were more evident when the high-dose IVIG was initiated before the age of 5 years. Eijkhout et al[17] studied the effects of two different doses of IVIG on the incidence of recurrent infections in patients with primary immune deficiency in a randomized, double-blind, multicenter crossover study. Standard doses of IVIG included 300 mg/kg every 4 weeks for adults, and 400 mg/kg every 4 weeks for children. The administration of high IVIG doses (adults: 600 mg/kg, children: 800 mg/kg) significantly reduced the number (3.5 vs. 2.5 per patient) and duration (median, 33 days vs. 21 days) of infections. Trough levels also increased during high-dose therapy. Importantly, the incidence and type of side effects did not differ between the standard and high-dose therapies.

In 1999 Kainulainen et al[18] published data on 22 patients with primary hypogammaglobulinemia and pulmonary abnormalities who were treated with IVIG. Despite adequate trough serum IgG levels (> 500 mg/dl), silent and asymptomatic pulmonary changes occurred. Quartier et al[19] performed a retrospective study of the clinical features and outcomes of 31 patients with XLA receiving replacement IVIG

therapy between 1982 and 1997. IVIG was given at doses of greater than 250 mg/kg every 3 weeks with a mean serum trough level between 500 and 1140 mg/dl (median: 700 mg/dl). The incidence of bacterial infections requiring hospitalization fell from 0.4 to 0.06 per patient per year; however, enteroviral meningoencephalitis still developed in three patients. Of 23 patients evaluated by pulmonary function tests and chest computed tomography scans, 3 had obstructive disease, 6 had bronchiectasis, and 20 had chronic sinusitis. The authors concluded that although early treatment with IVIG and achieving a trough serum IgG level of more than 500 mg/dl were effective in preventing severe, acute bacterial infections, these levels may not prevent pulmonary disease and sinusitis. The authors suggest that more intensive therapy to maintain a higher serum IgG level (e.g., > 800 mg/dl) may improve pulmonary outcome in patients with XLA. As these studies demonstrate, pulmonary abnormalities are the most important factors associated with morbidity and mortality in patients with primary immunodeficiencies. The number of infections, days missed from school or work, and hospitalized days may not be sufficient indicators of adequate treatment, so the improvement or maintenance of pulmonary function is an important measure of the success of therapy.

Administration

In patients with primary immune deficiency the replacement dose of IVIG is generally 400 to 600 mg/kg. All brands of IVIG are probably equivalent as replacement therapy, although there are differences in viral inactivation processes, for example, solvent detergent versus pasteurization and liquid versus lyophilized. The choice of brands may be dependent on the hospital or home care formulary and the local availability and cost. The dose, manufacturer, and lot number should be recorded for each infusion in order to perform look-back procedures in case of adverse events or other consequences. It is crucial to record all side effects that occur during the infusion. Liver and renal function should also be monitored periodically, approximately every 6 months. Antigen detection for hepatitis B and polymerase chain reaction (PCR) for hepatitis C should be performed if clinically indicated.

Intravenous Administration

The recommended rates of IVIG infusion were determined in early studies using reduced and alkylated IgG.[20] Such preparations led to rate-related side effects in 50% of patients. Newer preparations are more tolerable but manufacturers still recommend rates (3 to 4 mg/kg/min) from the early studies. With some preparations much higher rates can be tolerated in selected patients who have had no adverse reactions with conventional rates.[21] The Food and Drug Administration (FDA) recommends that for patients at risk for renal failure, for example, those with preexisting renal insufficiency, diabetes, age greater than 65, volume depletion, sepsis, and paraproteinemia and those who use nephrotoxic drugs, recommended doses should not be exceeded and that infusion rates and concentrations should be the minimum levels that are practical. The maximum suggested infusion rate for sucrose-containing IVIGs is 3 mg sucrose/kg/min (2 mg/kg/min for Sandoglobulin; 1 mg/kg/min for Gammar-P IV).[22]

The initial treatment should be administered in the hospital or a blood product infusion center and should be closely supervised by experienced personnel. The risk of developing adverse reactions during the initial treatment is much higher and is generally associated with the presence of infections and formation of immune complexes. In patients with active infection, the dose should be halved, that is, 200 to 300 mg/kg, and repeated 2 weeks later to achieve a full dose. Thereafter, adverse reactions are uncommon unless patients have active infection.

To minimize cost and inconvenience, self-administration and home treatment have been studied and used successfully.[23,24] For home therapy, patients need to be selected carefully. Patients must have several uneventful treatments in the hospital and be trained under close supervision to ensure correct techniques and should be able to recognize and treat side effects. Infusions should be done only in the presence of a responsible adult who is knowledgeable and ready to respond to an adverse event. Patients receiving home treatment should be seen regularly to monitor clinical status, liver function, renal function, and trough serum IgG levels.[25]

Subcutaneous Administration

Berger et al[26] were the first to describe the use of the subcutaneous route for immunoglobulin replacement therapy in 1980. It was reported as safe, well tolerated, and effective in achieving adequate serum IgG levels. Although used successfully in several studies,[27,28] it was not very popular because it was time-consuming as a result of the slow rate of infusion (1 to 2 ml/hr). Home treatment with rapid subcutaneous infusion was studied more extensively in the 1990s. Studies by Waniewski et al[29] showed that subcutaneous infusions of gamma globulin (100 mg/kg) reach a steady state after 6 months if given weekly or in a week in patients given daily infusions for 5 days and thereafter weekly. A multicenter study by Gardulf et al[30] of 165 patients with primary hypogammaglobulinemia or IgG-subclass deficiency receiving 33,168 subcutaneous infusions (27,030 at home) showed significant reductions in adverse systemic reactions compared with those who received intramuscular or intravenous administration. Anaphylactoid reactions did not occur. Patients achieved significant increases in serum IgG after 6 months of initiating immunoglobulin therapy. The use of subcutaneous instead of intravenous infusions resulted in yearly cost reductions of approximately $10,000.[30] Local tissue reactions include swelling, soreness, redness, induration, local heat, itching, and bruising and are often transient. Each subcutaneous infusion requires a small portable syringe pump together with a 10-ml syringe and an infusion set with a 0.4-mm butterfly needle. The needle should be bent at a 60- to 90-degree angle before insertion, although special subcutaneous needles are available for use in diabetic patients. The length of the needle should be adjusted to the thickness of the subcutaneous tissue of each patient. Before infusion, the line needs to be checked to ensure that there is no blood return. Infusions need to be given weekly at two to six sites. Infusion sites are usually on the abdominal wall and thigh. The rate of infusion on the pump is set initially at 10 ml/hr of 16.5% mercury-free immunoglobulin and may be increased 1 ml/hr every month up to15 ml/hr if no adverse reactions occur. In the United States, where 16.5% intramuscular immunoglobulin contains mercury, 10% or 12% IVIG may be used. Before home treatment, patients need to be carefully taught the correct technique for self-administration and how to recognize possible side effects. Rapid subcutaneous immunoglobulin infusion is safer, less expensive, better tolerated, and preferred by some patients. It should be considered an alternative in selected patients, especially those with frequent adverse reactions by the intravenous route.

Side Effects

Nonanaphylactic Reactions

Most adverse reactions of IVIG are related to the administration of IVIG and are rate related. Common adverse events include tachycardia, chest tightness, back pain, arthralgia, myalgia, hypertension or hypotension, headache, pruritus, rash, and low-grade fever (Table 17-4). More serious reactions include dyspnea, nausea, vomiting, circulatory collapse, and loss of consciousness. Patients with more profound immunodeficiency or patients with active infections have more severe reactions. The reactions are related to the anticomplementary activity of IgG aggregates in the IVIG.[31] In addition, the formation of oligomeric or polymeric IgG complexes can interact with Fc receptors and trigger the release of inflammatory mediators.[32] These adverse reactions have occurred with less frequency (10% to 15%) and with less severity in the more recent preparations of IVIG. Fatigue, myalgia, and headache may be delayed and may last several hours after the infusion. Slowing the infusion rate or discontinuing therapy until symptoms subside may diminish the reaction. Pretreatment with nonsteroidal antiinflammatory agents such as ibuprofen (10 mg/kg/dose), acetaminophen (15 mg/kg/dose), diphenhydramine (1 mg/kg/dose) and/or hydrocortisone (6 mg/kg/dose, maximum 100 mg)[13,31,33] 1 hour before the infusion may prevent the adverse reactions.

Aseptic meningitis can occur with large doses and rapid infusions and in the treatment of patients with autoimmune or inflammatory diseases.[34-37] Interestingly, this adverse reaction rarely occurs in immunodeficient subjects.[35] Symptoms, including headache, stiff neck, and photophobia, usually develop within 24 hours after completion of the infusion and may last 3 to 5 days. Spinal fluid pleocytosis occurs in most patients.[34,35,37] Long-term complications are minimal.[37] The cause of aseptic meningitis is unclear, but migraine has been reported as a risk factor and may be associated with recurrence despite the use of different IVIG preparations and slower rates of infusion.[34]

TABLE 17-4 Adverse Effects of Intravenous Immunoglobulin Administration

Common
  Chills
  Headache
  Backache
  Myalgia
  Malaise, fatigue
  Fever
  Pruritis
  Rash, flushing
  Nausea, vomiting
  Tingling
  Hypotension or hypertension
  Fluid overload
Uncommon (multiple reports)
  Chest pain or tightness
  Dyspnea
  Severe headaches
  Aseptic meningitis
  Renal failure
Rare (isolated reports)
  Anaphylaxis
  Arthritis
  Hyperviscosity
    Thrombosis/cerebral infarction
    Myocardial infarction
    Acute encephalopathy
  Cardiac rhythm abnormalities
  Coagulopathy
  Hemolysis: alloantibodies to blood type A/B
  Cryoglobulinemia
  Neutropenia
  Alopecia
  Uveitis
  Noninfectious hepatitis
  Hypothermia
  Lymphocytic pleural effusion
Potential (no reports)
  Creutzfeldt-Jakob disease
  Human immunodeficiency virus infections
  Parvovirus B19

Acute renal failure is a rare but significant complication of IVIG treatment. Histopathologic findings of acute tubular necrosis, vacuolar degeneration, and osmotic nephrosis are suggestive of osmotic injury to the proximal renal tubules; 55% of the cases were patients treated for idiopathic thrombocytopenic purpura (ITP), and less than 5% involved patients with primary immunodeficiency.[22] This complication may relate to the higher doses of IVIG used in ITP. The majority of cases were treated successfully with conservative treatment, but 17 patients who had serious underlying conditions died. Preliminary reports suggest that IVIG products using sucrose as a stabilizer may have a greater risk for this renal complication (see Table 17-3). The infusion rate for sucrose-containing IVIG should not exceed a sucrose level of 3 mg/kg/min. Risk factors for this adverse reaction include preexisting renal insufficiency, diabetes mellitus, dehydration, age greater than 65, sepsis, paraproteinemia, and concomitant use of nephrotoxic agents. For patients at increased risk, monitoring blood urea nitrogen and creatinine before starting the treatment and periodically thereafter is necessary. If renal function deteriorates, the product should be changed to an IVIG that does not contain sucrose.

More uncommon or rare complications of IVIG treatment are provided in Table 17-4. Because IVIG preparations are prepared from a large number of donors, antibodies against A/B blood-group antigens are present. Nonagglutinating antibodies in the IVIG may cause hemolytic reactions, especially if large amounts are infused.[38] Patients receiving large doses of IVIG may also develop fluid overload or hyperviscosity that can compromise cardiac function.

Anaphylactic Reactions

IgE antibodies to IgA have been reported to cause severe transfusion reactions in IgA-deficient patients.[7,39] There are few reports of true anaphylaxis in patients with selective IgA deficiency and common variable immunodeficiency who developed IgE antibodies to IgA after treatment with IVIG.[7] The symptoms are typical of an IgE-mediated anaphylactic reaction. The severity ranges from mild reactions to death. The serum levels of IgE antibody against IgA were found to correlate with anaphylaxis.[7] However, several patients with antibodies against IgA did not have anaphylactic reactions when treated with IVIG preparations containing very low concentrations of contaminating IgA (see Table 17-3).[7,40] Thus if replacement of immunoglobulin is needed in these patients, IVIG products containing minimal amounts of IgA should be used.

Infectious Complications

Hepatitis C infection in patients receiving IVIG products was initially reported in experimental lots in Europe and the United States. Hepatitis C infection usually occurred in clusters associated with contaminated lots[41,42] and specific manufacturing procedures. Bjoro et al[41] reported a group of patients infected with hepatitis C who had primary hypogammaglobulinemia and who received contaminated IVIG; 17 of 20 patients were positive for hepatitis C virus (HCV) RNA, and all had abnormal liver tests and liver biopsies. The course of HCV infection in these patients was rapidly progressive and the responses to treatment with interferon-α2b were poor, especially in patients infected with multiple HCV serotypes. The clinical course of HCV infection in patients with immune deficiency is not well defined. Bresee et al[43] reported that only 11% of children with primary immune deficiency receiving contaminated IVIG became infected with HCV and developed hepatitis. More long-term follow-up studies will be necessary to determine the outcome and consequences of HCV infection in patients with primary immune deficiency. Routine screening of plasma donors for hepatitis C RNA by reverse transcriptase–PCR and the addition of a viral inactivation process in the final manufacturing step, for example, treatment with solvent/detergent or pasteurization, has significantly reduced the risk of transmission of HCV and other viruses. There have been no reports of transmission of human immunodeficiency virus and Cruetzfeldt-Jakob disease in patients receiving IVIG therapy thus far.

IVIG AS AN IMMUNE-MODULATING AGENT

Since the first report by Imbach et al[44] on the use of IVIG in childhood ITP, IVIG has been used for the treatment of a variety of inflammatory and autoimmune disorders (Table 17-5). A number of mechanisms have been postulated for the immunomodulatory effects of IVIG (Table 17-6).[45] Platelet counts rise rapidly in children with ITP following the administration of 1 to 2 g/kg IVIG.[46] Fehr et al[47] and Bussel[48] suggested that the rapid responses following IVIG treatment in ITP were caused by a blockade of the reticuloendothelial system (RES). Clarkson et al[49] demonstrated a marked increase in platelet count using a monoclonal antibody directed against the low affinity Fcγ receptor found on neutrophils, NK cells, and macrophages, suggesting that this effect might be related to specific blockade of low-affinity Fcγ receptors on macrophages in the spleen and in other parts of the RES system. Debre et al[50] reported that children with acute ITP treated with intravenous Fcγ fragments from a preparation of IVIG showed a rapid increase in platelet counts. These studies using the Fcγ fragment as therapy strengthens the hypothesis that Fcγ receptor blockade is responsible for the rapid increase in platelet counts as the main mechanism of action of IVIG in ITP, although other immune regulatory mechanisms could be involved.

As in childhood ITP, Kawasaki disease (KD) is an FDA-approved therapeutic indication for IVIG administration.[51] The disease is an acute multisystem disease of unknown etiology that primarily affects young children. Although the acute illness is generally self-limited, coronary artery abnormalities related to a generalized inflammation and immune activation of small and medium-sized blood vessels develop in up to 25% of untreated patients. Geographic clustering, epidemics, and even pandemics in Japan and seasonal variations (for example, late winter and spring), suggest an infectious etiology. The observation that children less than 6 months or more than 8 years of age are rarely affected suggests that the lack of a protective antibody against the putative KD agent may be an important risk factor for development of the disease. Finally, in support of its infectious etiology, the acute onset of disease has clinical features that are suggestive of infection. Leung et al[52,53] have proposed that enterotoxins producing *Staphylococcus* and *Streptococcus* acting as superantigens are responsible for the inflammatory and immunologic changes seen in patients with KD. IVIG has been shown to contain high titers of specific antibodies that inhibit the activation of T cells by

TABLE 17-5 Treatment of Patients with Autoimmune and Inflammatory Diseases

Proven Efficacy by Controlled Studies

Idiopathic thrombocytopenic purpura
Autoimmune neutropenia
Kawasaki syndrome
Guillain-Barré syndrome
Chronic inflammatory demyelinating polyradiculoneuropathy
Multifocal motor neuropathy
Dermatomyositis (adult)
Lambert-Eaton myasthenic syndrome

Probable Treatment Efficacy*

Myasthenia gravis
Toxic shock syndrome
Toxic epidermal necrolysis
Asthma (subset of patients requiring high-dose oral corticosteroids)

Possible Treatment Efficacy†

Autoimmune hemolytic anemia
Autoimmune coagulopathies
Multiple sclerosis
Obsessive-compulsive and tic disorders (pediatric autoimmune neuropsychiatric disorders associated with streptococcus)
Polymyositis
Recurrent spontaneous abortion
Rheumatoid arthritis (adult)
Systemic vasculitis (antineutrophil cytoplasm antibody positive or related to parvovirus B19 disease)
Demyelinating peripheral neuropathy with IgM monoclonal paraproteins
Rasmussen's aneurysm
Postinfectious or vaccine-related childhood seizure disorders (West's syndrome; Lennox-Gastaut syndrome)
Chronic urticaria with autoantibodies to FcεRI

Little or No Treatment Efficacy

Inclusion-body myositis
Paraneoplastic neurologic syndrome
Systemic lupus erythematosus
Atopic dermatitis

From Sacher RA: *J Allergy Clin Immunol* 108:S139-S146, 2001.
*Few placebo-controlled trials or supported by strong open-label clinical trials.
†Supported by open-label studies and anecdotal reports.

staphylococcal and streptococcal superantigens.[54] These findings may account for the observation that treatment of acute KD with IVIG results in a marked reduction of macrophage and T cell activation.[55,56] The efficacy of IVIG in suppressing the immune activation associated with KD, and more importantly, its ability to prevent the development of coronary artery aneurysms may relate to the neutralizing antibody activity in IVIG against these bacterial enterotoxins.[52] The findings that a threshold dose of IVIG is needed to decrease signs of acute inflammation in KD[57] and that some patients require retreatment[58] suggest that IVIG contains variable antitoxin titers.[59] Toxin neutralization is probably not the only beneficial effect of IVIG in KD.

TABLE 17-6 Mechanisms of Action of Intravenous Immunoglobulin

1. Neutralization of autoimmune antibodies by antiidiotypic antibodies in the intravenous immunoglobulin (IVIG)
2. Induction of antiinflammatory cytokines (interleukin 1 receptor antagonist)
3. Inhibition of complement uptake on target tissues and attenuation of complement-mediated tissue damage
4. Neutralization of staphylococcal and streptococcal exotoxins
5. Inhibition of Fas-mediated cell death by Fas-blocking antibodies in the IVIG
6. Enhancement of glucocorticoid receptors binding affinity
7. Inhibition of B cell function and modulation of cytokine production by monocytes and T cells through the FcγRIIB receptor
8. Neutralization of antibodies to cytokines (IL-1, TNF-α, IFN-α, IFN-γ, and IL-6)
9. Fc receptor blockade of reticuloendothelial system
10. Solubilization of immune complexes

Other potential mechanisms of IVIG in KD include immunomodulation of cytokine production or cytokine effects and inhibition of vascular endothelial cell activation. Others have also demonstrated that IVIG inhibits the production of IL-1, TNF-α, TNF-β, and IFN-γ from peripheral blood mononuclear cells stimulated with bacterial superantigens or lipopolysaccharide.[60] Furthermore, Xu et al,[61] using human umbilical vein endothelial cells, recently demonstrated that IVIG inhibited endothelial cell proliferation and down-regulated the mRNA expression of adhesion molecules (ICAM-1, VCAM-1), chemokines (MCP-1), growth factors (M-CSF and GM-CSF), and proinflammatory cytokines (TNF-α, IL-1α, IL-6). Thus IVIG may exert its antiinflammatory effects in KD by interrupting or modifying a number of different steps in the inflammatory cascade starting with the inhibition of effector cell function and cytokine-induced endothelial cell activation.

Several diseases and animal models have been reported to show that IVIG might also work by inhibiting complement uptake on target cells. Basta et al,[62] using an animal model of Forssman shock, demonstrated that high-dose IVIG prevented the death of guinea pigs. The inflammatory process in this guinea pig model is mediated by complement uptake and activation on endothelial cells that result in tissue damage. These investigators postulated that very high levels of serum IgG from IVIG therapy prevent active C3 and C4 fragments from binding to target cells, resulting in the modulation of acute complement-dependent tissue injury. Basta et al[63] showed that IVIG not only inhibited the uptake of C3 fragments onto antibody-sensitized cells but also C4, an early complement component.

Dermatomyositis (DM) is a disease characterized by the subacute onset of muscle weakness, affecting predominantly the proximal muscle groups, and is often accompanied or preceded by a typical skin rash. Although its cause is unknown, DM is considered to be an autoimmune disease based on the perivascular and interfascicular inflammatory infiltrates and circulating autoantibodies to endothelial cells and histidyl-tRNA synthetase (Jo-1).[64, 65] A humoral immune process directed against the intramuscular capillaries characterizes the immunopathogenesis of DM. This process leads to a complement-mediated endomysial microangiography with deposition of the membrane attack complex (MAC) consisting of activated complement components C5b-9 on the intramuscular capillaries.[65] The endomysial capillary damage as a result of MAC deposition leads to microinfarcts within the muscle fascicles, muscle ischemia, inflammation, and eventually perifascicular atrophy.[66] The expression of ICAM-1 is increased on the endomysial blood vessels and muscle cells, which further facilitates the infiltration of inflammatory cells, mainly CD4+ T cells and some B cells.[66,67] The efficacy of IVIG treatment in adult DM has been demonstrated in a double-blind, placebo-controlled study by Dalakas et al.[65,66] In one research project, although composed largely of case reports and small, uncontrolled studies, IVIG has also been shown to be effective in juvenile DM.[68,69] Basta and Dalakas[70] showed that in DM patients treated with high-dose IVIG, the sera showed a significant inhibitory activity for the uptake of activated C3 fragments (C3b) onto sensitized human erythrocytes. The reduction in C3b uptake paralleled the magnitude of clinical improvement. The maximum inhibition of C3 uptake occurred within hours after IVIG infusion, started to rebound 2 days after IVIG treatment, and reached baseline levels after 30 days. Muscle biopsies of patients improving after IVIG showed disappearance of the MAC deposits from the endomysial capillaries.[65,70] In addition, Dalakas et al[65] demonstrated that IVIG markedly decreased ICAM-1 expression in muscle tissues after IVIG treatment.

The pathophysiology of a number of autoimmune diseases may be related to pertubations of the idiotype network.[71] Several groups have postulated that IVIG contains antiidiotypic antibodies that down-regulate the immune response.[72,73] A number of diseases may serve as models for this mechanism of IVIG, including patients with circulating autoantibody inhibitors to Factor VIII coagulant activity, systemic lupus erythematosus, and antineutrophil cytoplasm antibody (ANCA)–associated vasculitis. The presence of antiidiotypic antibodies in IVIG was first suggested by the response to IVIG therapy of a patient with autoimmunity to Factor VIII.[74] The treatment of two patients with high-titer autoantibodies to Factor VIII coagulant activity with high-dose IVIG resulted in a rapid and prolonged suppression of this autoantibody.[75] Sultan et al[74] showed that IVIG could also inhibit this Factor VIII autoantibody inhibitor activity *in vitro* and that the inhibitory effect resided with the F(ab′)$_2$ fragment.

Dietrich and Kazatchkine[73] extended these observations to other disease-associated autoimmune diseases. Using commercial sources of IVIG these investigators prepared F(ab′)$_2$ fragments that could neutralize or bind to known autoantibodies, such as anti-Factor VIII, antithyroglobulin, anti-DNA, antiintrinsic factor, and ANCA. ANCA-associated vasculitis may be a good example of the possible therapeutic effects of antiidiotypic antibody in IVIG on a disease caused by autoantibodies. IVIG contains antibodies with idiotypic specificities that can bind and neutralize potentially pathogenic autoantibodies such as antibodies to GM1 ganglioside (anti-GM1 antibodies) in patients with Guillain-Barré syndrome (GBS) and chronic inflammatory demyelinating polyradiculoneuropathy (CIDP) and antiacetylcholine receptor (AChR) antibodies in myasthenia gravis (MG).[76-79] Malik et al[80] showed that antiidiotypic antibodies in the IVIG directed against idiotypes located on the anti-GM1 immunoglobulin molecule blocked the binding of the anti-GM1 antibodies to its target antigen. These studies suggest that an idiotype/antiidiotype interaction is a possible mechanism by which IVIG could modulate the immune-mediated disease process and contribute to the remyelination in patients with GBS and CIDP. Support for a similar mechanism in MG comes from the fact that IgG or F(ab′)$_2$ fragments in the IVIG preparations are capable of binding to AChR antibodies *in vitro*.[81] Vassilev et al[82] showed that normal human IVIG could suppress experimental MG in mice with severe combined immunodeficiency syndrome. Further studies are necessary to determine the significance of these antiidiotypic antibodies in IVIG as immune modulators in the pathogenesis of these autoimmune neurologic diseases.

In ITP patients treated with IVIG several studies have shown a decrease in antiplatelet antibody production.[48,83] Changes in the immunoregulatory function of T cells and B cells have been proposed as a mechanism for this decrease in antiplatelet antibodies following IVIG therapy. IVIG may have other immune-modulating effects in addition to blockade of the Fcγ receptor. Studies have shown that the addition of IVIG *in vitro* suppresses lymphocyte proliferative responses to a variety of T cell mitogens.[84,85] This suppressive activity was dependent on the Fc portion of IVIG in that the F(ab′)$_2$ fragments had no effect. Other studies have suggested that the target cell for inhibition of antibody production was the B lymphocyte rather than the T cell.[86,87] In severely ill asthmatic children dependent on oral steroids and treated with high-dose IVIG, Mazer and Gelfand[88] demonstrated a decrease in total serum IgE and allergen-specific IgE antibodies. Sigman et al[89] showed that IVIG *in vitro* could modulate IgE production. High concentrations of IVIG, in a dose-dependent manner, inhibited IgE production of anti-CD40/IL-4–stimulated B cells. This effect was not caused by a blocking antibody in the IVIG but by impairment of IgE synthesis. The inhibitory effect on IgE production was associated with a decrease in Cε mRNA transcripts.

B cells and a subpopulation of T cells express a low-affinity Fcγ receptor (FcγRIIB).[90,91] This receptor provides an inhibitory signal to cells through a pathway mediated by an immunoregulatory tyrosine-based inhibition motif (e.g., ITIM). Similar inhibitory Fcγ receptors are present on basophils and mast cells. Samuelsson et al[92] investigated a murine model of immune thrombocytopenia and found that the protective effects of IVIG required the inhibitory Fcγ receptor (e.g., FcγRIIB) because either disruption of the receptor or blocking with a monoclonal antibody reversed the therapeutic effects. This immune modulatory action of IVIG may work in concert with the antiidiotypic antibodies in IVIG discussed previously. Co-ligation of the B cell receptor by an antiidiotypic antibody and binding of this antibody via the Fc moiety to the FcγRIIB receptor could induce a specific negative regulatory signal to the B cell, leading to inhibition of B cell activation and subsequently antibody production. The observations on the effects of IVIG in patients with steroid-dependent asthma[88,93] may be related to similar FcγRIIB regulatory receptors on basophils and mast cells.

Another mechanism of action of IVIG related to specific antibodies in the IVIG is its effect on apoptosis. Viard et al[94] reported that IVIG could inhibit the apoptotic process, for example, program cell death in patients with toxic epidermal necrolysis (TEN, or Lyell's syndrome), which is a severe drug-induced bullous skin reaction. In *in vitro* studies IVIG was demonstrated to protect the keratinocytes from apoptosis by blocking the effects of Fas L on the Fas receptor. These investigators also determined that the depletion of anti-Fas antibodies from IVIG abrogated the ability of IVIG to inhibit Fas L–mediated apoptosis. In an open, uncontrolled trial of IVIG (0.2 to 0.75 g/kg/day for 4 consecutive days) in 10 TEN patients, skin progression was halted within 1 to 2 days and was followed by rapid skin healing and a favorable outcome. These immune-modulating effects of IVIG in patients with TEN represent another unique mechanism by which IVIG can modify the disease process and may prove to be useful in other Fas-mediated inflammatory or autoimmune diseases.

CONCLUSIONS

Immunoglobulin replacement is the mainstay of treatment for patients with primary humoral immune deficiency. The goal of the treatment is to provide a broad spectrum of antibodies to prevent infections and chronic long-term complications. The usual dose is 400 to 600 mg/kg/mo but may vary, and some individuals may actually require higher doses during active infection. A serum trough level above 500 mg/dl has been shown to be effective in the prevention of infections; however, recent studies have suggested that even higher doses and those that achieve IgG trough levels above 700 mg/dl may

---

BOX 17-2

THERAPEUTIC PRINCIPLES
Principles of intravenous immunoglobulin treatment

PATIENTS WITH PRIMARY IMMUNE DEFICIENCY

Initial dosage: 300-400 mg/kg every 4 weeks for replacement therapy
Increase to 400-600 mg/kg to gain clinical improvement
Maintain a serum trough level of > 500 mg/dl
May adjust the dose and/or dosing interval depending on clinical response
Record manufacturer, lot number, and dose with each infusion
Equilibration takes several months even when dosage changes made
Check trough levels if patient continues to have infections or before any dose change
Monitor
Liver and renal function tests every 6 months
Hepatitis C nucleotide testing by reverse transcriptase–polymerase chain reaction when indicated
Pulmonary function

PATIENTS WITH AUTOIMMUNE DISORDERS

Dosage: 1-2 g/kg over 1-2 days or 400 mg/kg for 4-5 days
Careful monitoring during infusion for side effects
Caution in patients at risk for adverse reactions (e.g., age over 65 years), conditions such as underlying renal or cardiovascular disease, hypercoagulable state, diabetes, volume depletion, or paraproteinemia
Caution with hyperosmolar intravenous immunoglobulin preparations

be desirable. Immunoglobulin can be given intramuscularly, intravenously, or subcutaneously. Generally, IVIG replacement therapy is considered safe in the majority of patients; side effects are usually mild and treatable by premedication. Improvements in good manufacturing practices, closer screening of plasma donors, testing of the source plasma with sensitive nucleic acid assays (e.g., PCR), and additional viral inactivation steps have made IVIG a better and safer plasma-derived product. The majority of the application of IVIG therapy is in patients with autoimmune disorders. The use of IVIG in these patient groups has not only led to a new treatment modality but has enhanced our understanding of the disease pathogenesis and the mechanisms by which IVIG may modulate the immune and inflammatory processes (Box 17-2).

REFERENCES

1. Cohn EJ, Luetscher JA Jr, Oncley JL, et al: Preparation and properties of serum and plasma proteins. III. Size and charge of proteins separating upon equilibration across membranes with ethanol-water mixtures of controlled pH, ionic strength and temperature, *J Am Chem Soc* 62: 3396-3400, 1940.
2. Bruton OC: Agammaglobulinemia, *Pediatrics* 9:722-728, 1952.
3. Ballow M: Primary immunodeficiency disorders: antibody deficiency, *J Allergy Clin Immunol* 109:581-591, 2002.
4. Tiller TL Jr, Buckley RH: Transient hypogammaglobulinemia of infancy: review of the literature, clinical and immunologic features of 11 new cases and long-term follow-up, *J Pediatr* 92:347-353, 1978.
5. Cohn EJ: The history of plasma fractionation. In Andrus EC, Bronk DW, Carden GA Jr, et al, eds: *Advances in military medicine*, vol 1, Boston, 1948, Little, Brown.
6. Eibl MM, Wedgwood RJ: Intravenous immunoglobulin: a review, *Immunodef Rev* 1:1-42, 1989.
7. Burks AW, Sampson HA, Buckley RH: Anaphylactic reactions after gamma globulin administration in patients with hypogammaglobulinemia: detection of IgE antibodies to IgA, *N Engl J Med* 314:560-564, 1986.
8. Fischer SH, Ochs HD, Wedgwood RJ, et al: Survival of antigen-specific antibody following administration of intravenous immunoglobulin in patients with primary immunodeficiency diseases, *Monogr Allergy* 23:225-235, 1988.
9. Mankarious S, Lee M, Fischer S, et al: The half-lives of IgG subclasses and specific antibodies in patients with primary immunodeficiency who are receiving intravenously administered immunoglobulin, *J Lab Clin Med* 112:634-640, 1988.
10. Waldmann TA, Strober W: Metabolism of immunoglobulins, *Prog Allergy* 13:1-110, 1969.
11. Yu Z, Lennon VA: Mechanism of intravenous immune globulin therapy in antibody-mediated autoimmune diseases, *N Engl J Med* 340:227-228, 1999.
12. Ochs HD, Fischer SH, Wedgewood RJ, et al: Comparison of high-dose and low-dose intravenous immunoglobulin therapy in patients with primary immunodeficiency diseases, *Am J Med* 76:78-82, 1984.
13. Stiehm ER: Immunodeficiency disorders: general conditions. In Stiehm ER, ed: *Immunologic disorders in infants and children,* ed 4, Philadelphia, 1996, WB Saunders.
14. Bernatowska E, Madalinski K, Janowicz W, et al: Results of a prospective controlled two-dose crossover study with intravenous immunoglobulin and comparison (retrospective) with plasma treatment, *Clin Immunol Immunopathol* 43:153-162, 1987.
15. Roifman CM, Schaffer FM, Wachsmuth SE, et al: Reversal of chronic polymyositis following intravenous immune serum globulin therapy, *JAMA* 258:513-515, 1987.
16. Liese JG, Wintergerst U, Tympner KD, et al: High- vs low-dose immunoglobulin therapy in the long-term treatment of X-linked agammaglobulinemia, *Am J Dis Child* 146:335-339, 1992.
17. Eijkhout HW, van der Meer JWM, Kallenberg CGM, et al: The effect of two different dosages of intravenous immunoglobulin on the incidence of recurrent infections in patients with primary hypogammaglobulinemia: a randomized, double-blind, multicenter crossover trial, *Ann Intern Med* 135:165-174, 2001.
18. Kainulainen L, Varpula M, Liippo K, et al: Pulmonary abnormalities in patients with primary hypogammaglobulinemia, *J Allergy Clin Immunol* 104:1031-1036, 1999.
19. Quartier P, Debre M, DeBlie J, et al: Early and prolonged intravenous immunoglobulin replacement therapy in childhood agammaglobulinemia: a retrospective survey of 31 patients, *J Pediatrics* 134:589-596, 1999.
20. Ammann AJ, Ashman RF, Buckley RH, et al: Use of intravenous gammaglobulin in antibody immunodeficiency: results of a multicenter controlled trial, *Clin Immunol Immunopathol* 22:60-67, 1982.
21. Schiff RI: Individualizing the dose of intravenous immune serum globulin for therapy of patients with primary humoral immunodeficiency, *Vox Sanguinis* 49:15-24, 1985.
22. Centers for Disease Control and Prevention: Renal insufficiency and failure associated with immune globulin intravenous therapy—United States, 1986-1998, *MMWR Morb Mortal Wkly Rep* 48:518-521, 1999.
23. Kobayashi RH, Kobayashi AD, Lee N, et al: Home self-administration of intravenous immunoglobulin therapy in children, *Pediatrics* 85:705-709, 1990.
24. Daly PB, Evans JH, Kobayashi RH, et al: Home-based immunoglobulin infusion therapy: quality of life and patient health perceptions, *Ann Allergy* 67:504-510, 1991.
25. Schiff RI: Transmission of viral infections through intravenous immune globulin, *N Engl J Med* 331:1649-1650, 1991.
26. Berger M, Cupps TR, Fauci AS: Immunoglobulin replacement therapy by slow subcutaneous infusion, *Ann Intern Med* 93:55-66, 1980.
27. Bayston K, Leahy MF, McCreanor JD, et al: Subcutaneous gammaglobulin: effective management of hypogammaglobulinaemia, *N Z Med J* 98:652, 1985.
28. Leahy MF: Subcutaneous immunoglobulin home treatment in hypogammaglobulinaemia, *Lancet* 2:48, 1986.
29. Waniewski J, Gardulf A, Hammarstrom L: Bioavailability of gammaglobulin after subcutaneous infusions in patients with common variable immunodeficiency, *J Clin Immunol* 14:90-97, 1994.
30. Gardulf A, Andersen V, Bjorkander J, et al: Subcutaneous immunoglobulin replacement in patients with primary antibody deficiencies: safety and costs, *Lancet* 345:365-369, 1995.
31. Lederman H, Roifman T, Lavi S, et al: Corticosteroids for prevention of adverse reactions to intravenous immune serum globulin infusions in hypogammaglobulinemic patients, *Am J Med* 81:443-446, 1986.
32. Camussi G, Aglietta M, Coda R, et al: Release of platelet activating factor (PAF) and histamine. II. The cellular origin of human PAF monocytes, polymorphonuclear neutrophils and basophils, *Immunology* 42:191-199, 1981.
33. Roberton DM, Hosking CS: Use of methylprednisolone as prophylaxis for immediate adverse infusion reactions in hypogammaglobulinaemic patients receiving intravenous immunoglobulin: a controlled trial, *Aust Paediatr J* 24:174-177, 1988.
34. Sekul EA, Cupler EJ, Dalakas MC: Aseptic meningitis associated with high-dose intravenous immunoglobulin therapy: frequency and risk factors, *Ann Intern Med* 121:259-262, 1994.
35. Scribner CL, Kapit RM, Phillips ET, et al: Aseptic meningitis and intravenous immunoglobulin therapy, *Ann Intern Med* 121:305-306, 1994.
36. Kats E, Shindo S, Eto Y, et al: Administration of immune globulin associated with aseptic meningitis, *JAMA* 259:3269-3270, 1988.
37. Brannagan TH, Nagle KJ, Lange DJ, et al: Complications of intravenous immune globulin treatment in neurologic disease, *Neurology* 47:674-677, 1996.
38. Robertson VM, Dickson LG, Romond EH, et al: Positive antiglobulin tests due to intravenous immunoglobulin in patients who received bone marrow transplant, *Transfusion* 27:28-31, 1987.
39. Cunningham-Rundles C: Intravenous immune serum globulin in immunodeficiency, *Vox Sanguinis* 49:8-14, 1985.
40. Apfelzweig R, Piszkiewicz D, Hooper JS: Immunoglobulin A concentrations in commercial immune globulins, *J Clin Immunol* 7:46-50, 1987.
41. Bjoro K, Froland SS, Yun Z, et al: Hepatitis C infection in patients with primary hypogammaglobulinemia after treatment with contaminated immune globulin, *N Engl J Med* 331:1607-1611, 1994.
42. Yap PL, McOmish F, Webster ADB, et al: Hepatitis C virus transmission by intravenous immunoglobulin, *J Hepatol* 21:455-460, 1994.
43. Bresee JS, Mast EE, Coleman PJ, et al: Hepatitis C virus infection associated with administration of intravenous immune globulin, *JAMA* 276:1563-1567, 1996.
44. Imbach P, Barandun S, d'Apuzzo V, et al: High-dose intravenous gammaglobulin for idiopathic thrombocytopenic purpura in childhood, *Lancet* 1:1228-1231, 1981.

45. Ballow M: Mechanisms of action of intravenous immune serum globulin in autoimmune and inflammatory diseases, *J Allergy Clin Immunol* 100:151-157, 1997.

46. Blanchette VS, Luke B, Andrew M, et al: A prospective, randomized trial of high-dose intravenous immune globulin G therapy, oral prednisone therapy, and no therapy in childhood acute immune thrombocytopenic purpura [see comments], *J Pediatr* 123:989-995, 1993.

47. Fehr J, Hofmann V, Kappeler U: Transient reversal of thrombocytopenia in idiopathic thrombocytopenic purpura by high-dose intravenous gamma globulin, *N Engl J Med* 306:1254-1258, 1982.

48. Bussel J: Modulation of Fc receptor clearance and antiplatelet antibodies as a consequence of intravenous immune globulin infusion in patients with immune thrombocytopenic purpura, *J Allergy Clin Immunol* 84:566-578, 1989.

49. Clarkson SB, Bussel JB, Kimberly RP, et al: Treatment of refractory immune thrombocytopenic purpura with an anti-Fc gamma receptor antibody, *N Engl J Med* 314:1236-1239, 1986.

50. Debre M, Bonnet MC, Fridman WH, et al: Infusion of Fc gamma fragments for treatment of children with acute immune thrombocytopenic purpura, *Lancet* 342:945-949, 1993.

51. Newburger JW, Takahashi M, Burns JC, et al: The treatment of Kawasaki syndrome with intravenous gamma globulin, *N Engl J Med* 315:341-347, 1986.

52. Leung DY: Kawasaki syndrome: immunomodulatory benefit and potential toxin neutralization by intravenous immune globulin, *Clin Exp Immunol* 104:49-54, 1996.

53. Leung DY, Schlievert PM, Meissner HC: The immunopathogenesis and management of Kawasaki syndrome, *Arthritis Rheum* 41:1538-1547, 1998.

54. Takei S, Arora YK, Walker SM: Intravenous immunoglobulin contains specific antibodies inhibitory to activation of T cells by staphylococcal toxin superantigens, *J Clin Invest* 91:602-607, 1993.

55. Leung DYM, Burns J, Newburger J, et al: Reversal of lymphocyte activation *in vivo* in the Kawasaki syndrome by intravenous gammaglobulin, *J Clin Invest* 79:468-472, 1987.

56. Leung DYM, Cotran RS, Kurt-Jones EZ, et al: Endothelial cell activation and increased interleukin 1 secretion in the pathogenesis of acute Kawasaki disease, *Lancet* 2:1298-1302, 1989.

57. Newburger JW, Takahashi M, Beiser AS, et al: A single intravenous infusion of gamma globulin as compared with four infusions in the treatment of acute Kawasaki syndrome, *N Engl J Med* 324:1633-1639, 1991.

58. Burns JC, Capparelli EV, Brown JA, et al: Intravenous gamma-globulin treatment and retreatment in Kawasaki disease. US/Canadian Kawasaki Syndrome Study Group, *Pediatr Infect Dis J* 17:1144-1148, 1998.

59. Norrby-Teglund A, Basma H, Andersson J, et al: Varying titers of neutralizing antibodies to streptococcal superantigens in different preparations of normal polyspecific immunoglobulin G: implications for therapeutic efficacy, *Clin Infect Dis* 26:631-638, 1998.

60. Gupta M, Noel GJ, Schaefer M, et al: Cytokine modulation with immune gamma-globulin in peripheral blood of normal children and its implications in Kawasaki disease treatment, *J Clin Immunol* 21:193-199, 2001.

61. Xu C, Poirier B, Van Huyen JPD, et al: Modulation of endothelial cell function by normal polyspecific human intravenous immunoglobulins, *Am J Pathol* 153:1257-1266, 1998.

62. Basta M, Kirshbom P, Frank MM, et al: Mechanism of therapeutic effect of high-dose intravenous immunoglobulin: attenuation of acute, complement-dependent immune damage in a guinea pig model, *J Clin Invest* 84:1974-1981, 1989.

63. Basta M, Fries LF, Frank MM: High doses of intravenous Ig inhibit in vitro uptake of C4 fragments onto sensitized erythrocytes, *Blood* 77:376-380, 1991.

64. Dalakas MC: Polymyositis, dermatomyositis, and inclusion-body myositis, *New Engl J Med* 325:1487-1498, 1991.

65. Dalakas MC, Illa I, D'Ambrosia JM, et al: A controlled trial of high-dose immune globulin infusions as treatment for dermatomyositis, *New Engl J Med* 329:1993-2000, 1993.

66. Dalakas MC: Clinical relevance of IVIG in the modulation of the complement-mediated tissue damage: implications in dermatomyositis, Guillain Barré syndrome and myasthenia gravis. In Kazatchkine MA, Morell A, eds: *Intravenous immunoglobulin: research and therapy*, London, 1996, Parthenon.

67. Soueidan SA, Dalakas MC: Treatment of autoimmune neuromuscular diseases with high-dose intravenous immune globulin, *Pediatr Res* 33:S95-S100, 1993.

68. Lang BA, Laxer RM, Murphy G, et al: Treatment of dermatomyositis with intravenous gammaglobulin, *Am J Med* 91:169-172, 1991.

69. Sansome A, Dubowitz V: Intravenous immunoglobulin in juvenile dermatomyositis: four-year review of nine cases, *Arch Dis Child* 72:25-28, 1995.

70. Basta M, Dalakas MC: High-dose intravenous immunoglobulin exerts its beneficial effect in patients with dermatomyositis by blocking endomysial deposition of activated complement fragments, *J Clin Invest* 94:1729-1735, 1994.

71. Shoenfeld Y: Idiotypic induction of autoimmunity: a new aspect of the idiotypic network, *FASEB J* 8:1296-1301, 1994.

72. Rossi F, Kazatchkine MD: Antiidiotypes against autoantibodies in pooled normal human polyspecific IgG, *J Immunol* 143:4104-4109, 1989.

73. Dietrich G, Kazatchkine MD: Normal immunoglobulin G (IgG) for therapeutic use (intravenous Ig) contain antiidiotypic specificities against an immunodominant, disease-associated, cross-reactive idiotype of human anti-thyroglobulin autoantibodies, *J Clin Invest* 85:620-625, 1990.

74. Sultan Y, Rossi F, Kazatchkine MD: Recovery from anti-VIIIc (antihemophilic factor) autoimmune disease is dependent on generation of antiidiotypes against anti VIIIc autoantibodies, *Proc Natl Acad Sci U S A* 84:828-831, 1987.

75. Sultan Y, Kazatchkine MD, Maisonneuve P, et al: Anti-idiotypic suppression of autoantibodies to factor VIII (antihaemophilic factor) by high-dose intravenous gammaglobulin, *Lancet* 2:765-768, 1984.

76. Dalakas MC: Mechanism of action of intravenous immunoglobulin and therapeutic considerations in the treatment of autoimmune neurologic diseases, *Neurology* 51:S2-S8, 1998.

77. Van Der Meché FGA: The Guillain-Barré syndrome: pathogenesis and treatment, *Rev Neurol (Paris)* 152:355-358, 1996.

78. Van der Meché FGA, Visser LH, Jacobs BC, et al: Guillain-Barré syndrome: multifactorial mechanisms versus defined subgroups, *J Infect Dis* 176:S99-S102, 1997.

79. Yuki N, Miyagi F: Possible mechanism of intravenous immunoglobulin treatment on anti-GM1 antibody-mediated neuropathies, *J Neurol Sci* 139:160-162, 1996.

80. Malik U, Oleksowicz L, Latov N, et al: Intravenous gamma-globulin inhibits binding of anti-GM1 to its target antigen, *Ann Neurol* 39:136-139, 1996.

81. Liblau R, Gajdos PH, Bustarret A, et al: Intravenous gamma-globulin in myasthenia gravis: interaction with anti-acetylcholine receptor autoantibodies, *J Clin Immunol* 11:128-131, 1991.

82. Vassilev T, Yamamoto M, Aissaoui A, et al: Normal human immunoglobulin suppresses experimental myasthenia gravis in SCID mice, *Eur J Immunol* 29:2436-2442, 1999.

83. Bussel J, Pahwa S, Porges A, et al: Correlation of *in vitro* antibody synthesis with the outcome of intravenous gamma-globulin treatment of chronic idiopathic thrombocytopenic purpura, *J Clin Immunol* 6:50-56, 1986.

84. Antel J, Medof M, Oger J, et al: Generation of suppressor cells by aggregated human globulin, *Clin Exp Immunol* 43:351-356, 1981.

85. Hashimoto F, Sakiyama Y, Matsumoto S: The suppressive effect of gamma globulin preparations on in vitro pokeweed mitogen-induced immunoglobulin production, *Clin Exp Immunol* 65:409, 1986.

86. Kondo N, Ozawa T, Mushiake K, et al: Suppression of immunoglobulin production of lymphocytes by intravenous immunoglobulin, *J Clin Immunol* 11:152-158, 1991.

87. Stohl W: Cellular mechanisms in the in vitro inhibition of pokeweed mitogen induced B cell differentiation by immunoglobulin for intravenous use, *J Immunol* 136:1407-1413, 1986.

88. Mazer BD, Gelfand EW: An open-label study of high-dose intravenous immunoglobulin in severe childhood asthma, *J Allergy Clin Immunol* 87:976-983, 1991.

89. Sigman K, Ghibu F, Sommerville W, et al: Intravenous immunoglobulin inhibits IgE production in human B lymphocytes, *J Allergy Clin Immunol* 102:421-427, 1998.

90. Daeron M: Fc receptor biology, *Ann Rev Immunol* 15:203-234, 1997.

91. Kimberly RP, Salmon JE, Edberg JC: Receptors for immunoglobulin G, *Arthritis Rheum* 38:306-314, 1995.

92. Samuelsson A, Towers TL, Ravetch JV: Anti-inflammatory activity of IVIG mediated through the inhibitory Fc receptor, *Science* 291:484-486, 2001.

93. Salmun LM, Barlan I, Wolf H, et al: Effects of intravenous immunoglobulin on steroid consumption in patients with severe asthma: a double-blind, placebo-controlled, randomized trial, *J Allergy Clin Immunol* 103:810-815, 1999.

94. Viard I, Wehrli P, Bullanim R, et al: Inhibition of toxic epidermal necrolysis by blockade of CD95 with human intravenous immunoglobulin, *Science* 282:490-493, 1998.

CHAPTER 18

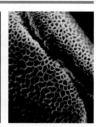

Bone Marrow Transplantation

REBECCA H. BUCKLEY

Even though bone marrow transplantation was first attempted in humans a half-century ago, it was unsuccessful except in identical twins until after the major histocompatibility complex (MHC) was discovered in 1968.[1,2] In that same year, immune function was corrected in two children with very different but invariably fatal genetically determined immunodeficiency diseases, Wiskott-Aldrich syndrome and X-linked severe combined immunodeficiency (SCID), by transplanting into them unfractionated human leukocyte antigen (HLA)–identical sibling bone marrow cells.[3,4] The correction of these, and later many other types of primary immunodeficiency diseases by bone marrow transplantation, has taught us that the defects in most such diseases are intrinsic to cells of one or more hematopoietic lineages and not the result of failure of the microenvironment to support the growth and development of those cells. Bone marrow transplantation has also been used successfully in the treatment of many other conditions, including malignancies, radiation injury, bone marrow aplasia, hemoglobinopathies, osteopetrosis, storage diseases, and other inborn errors of metabolism. This chapter focuses only on its use in the treatment of genetically determined immunodeficiency diseases.

The objective of bone marrow transplantation for primary immunodeficiency diseases is to restore immunocompetence by engrafting normal stem cells that can develop into immunocompetent cells (Box 18-1). Normal bone marrow and peripheral blood both contain self-replicating cells that can give rise to erythrocytes, granulocytes, cells of the monocyte-macrophage lineage, megakaryocytes, and immunocompetent T and B cells.[5] Until recently, the only adequate therapy available for patients with severe primary cellular immunodeficiencies was successful transplantation of allogeneic immunocompetent tissue. However, impressive success in achieving immune reconstitution through the administration of autologous gene-corrected stem cells into infants with X-linked SCID[6,7] offers the hope that this approach will someday replace the need for allogeneic stem cell transplantation for many of these disorders.

HUMAN LEUKOCYTE ANTIGEN AND THE ROLE OF THE IMMUNE SYSTEM IN BONE MARROW TRANSPLANTATION

Unlike solid organ transplantation, where the primary obstacle to overcome is potential rejection of the transplanted organ by the recipient, the immune response is a major problem in both directions in bone marrow transplantation

---

BOX 18-1

KEY CONCEPTS

Importance of Major Histocompatibility Complex in Bone Marrow Transplantation

- Allogeneic T cells recognize foreign tissues as a consequence of disparity in major histocompatibility complex antigens, particularly class II antigens.
- Human severe combined immunodeficiency (SCID) results from an absence of T cells (and in some cases also B and/or natural killer cells). The purpose of bone marrow transplantation in SCID is to engraft a normal hematopoietic stem cell that can differentiate into T cells and other immune cells.
- Until 2 decades ago, bone marrow transplantation was possible only when there was a human leukocyte antigen—identical related donor.
- This problem has since been circumvented by rigorous depletion of postthymic T cells from the donor marrow. Thus even half-matched (parental) stem cells can be used successfully for immune reconstitution. The stem cells are matured in the infant's thymus, where positive and negative selection occurs, and the T cells that emerge do not cause graft-versus-host disease.

Modified from Buckley RH: Bone marrow reconstitution in primary immunodeficiency. In Rich RR, Fleisher TT, Shearer WT, et al, eds: *Clinical immunology: principles and practice*, ed 2, St Louis, 2001, Mosby.

(Box 18-2). Not only can recipients of a bone marrow transplant reject the transplanted marrow, but also there is the problem that the transplanted bone marrow cells can reject the recipient: graft-versus-host disease (GVHD). Also in contrast to solid organ transplantation, where successful grafts have been attained without HLA matching through the use of cyclosporine and other immunosuppressive agents, it has long been known that HLA disparity is a major problem for bone marrow transplantation (see Box 18-1). HLA class II antigen disparity is more of a problem than class I differences because successful transplantation of unfractionated marrow has been accomplished despite HLA class I incompatibility[4] but not usually when there is class II incompatibility.[8] This is because recipient class II HLA antigens stimulate genetically different donor T cells to proliferate and become cytotoxic, causing GVHD. The reverse problem is also possible for the same reason in those recipients who have residual immunocompe-

KEY CONCEPTS

Host-versus-Graft and Graft-versus-Host Reactions in Bone Marrow and Cord Blood Transplantation

■ If the host has any T cell function, the allogeneic marrow graft will probably be rejected regardless of the degree of human leukocyte antigen (HLA) compatibility (except in the case of identical twins); therefore engraftment will fail unless pretransplantation chemotherapy is administered.

■ Preconditioning the immunodeficient host who has any degree of T cell function is done with agents designed to eliminate that function.

■ If host T cell function is absent (because of either the underlying defect or pretransplantation chemotherapy), the T cells in the graft may attack the host tissues, principally the skin, liver, and intestine (graft-versus-host disease [GVHD]).

■ GVHD risk factors include unrelated donor, HLA-mismatched donor, pretransplantation conditioning (GVHD occurs even in HLA-identical transplants), older age of the recipient, and previous viral infections.

■ Treatment of acute or chronic GVHD is imperfect, and the drugs used to treat it make the immunodeficient host even more immunodeficient and susceptible to infections for which there is no effective treatment.

■ The best approach to GVHD is prevention.

Modified from Buckley RH: Bone marrow reconstitution in primary immunodeficiency. In Rich RR, Fleisher TT, Shearer WT, et al, eds: *Clinical immunology: principles and practice*, ed 2, St Louis, 2001, Mosby.

tence; that is, host T cells recognize donor marrow HLA class II antigens and effect marrow rejection. In addition, it is known that effective immune responses require the sharing of genetically identical class II HLA antigens by interacting T, B, and antigen-presenting cells. However, this sharing is still possible if only one of the two HLA haplotypes is identical between donor and recipient,[9] as was repeatedly shown over the past two decades in the case of T cell–depleted, half-matched bone marrow stem cell transplants into infants with SCID.[10,11]

The two early successes in immune reconstitution of primary immunodeficiency diseases in 1968 were followed over the next 15 years by many disappointments because of the rare availability of HLA-matched sibling donors for patients with lethal primary T cell defects. In the first report of the outcomes of bone marrow transplantation for SCID in 1977, only 14 of 69 patients with SCID who received marrow or fetal tissue transplants worldwide were surviving with functional grafts.[8] Until 1980, only HLA-identical unfractionated bone marrow could be used for bone marrow transplantation because of the lethal GVHD that ensued if mismatched donors were used.[8]

In the late 1970s, studies in rats[12] and mice[13] showed that removal of all (or nearly all) postthymic T cells from MHC nonidentical donor marrow or spleen cell suspensions enabled successful rescue of lethally irradiated animals without causing fatal GVHD. This was accomplished in rats by treating donor marrow or spleen cells with anti–T cell antisera[12] and in mice by agglutinating the unwanted cells with plant lectins.[13] The remaining immature marrow or splenic non–T

cells restored lymphohematopoietic function in the ablated MHC-disparate animals.

Following the leads from their work in mice,[13] Reisner et al[14] demonstrated in the early 1980s that removal of most mature T cells from half-matched parental marrow allowed successful immune reconstitution of human infants with SCID by the remaining cells without subsequent GVHD. Since that time, this approach has been successfully applied numerous times to the treatment of SCID.[10,11,15-19] Moreover, the resulting chimeras have proved extremely useful in the study of human thymic educative T and B cell ontogeny (Figure 18-1),[15,18-21] tolerance induction,[22] and mechanisms of MHC restriction for antigen presentation.[9]

GRAFT-VERSUS-HOST DISEASE

GVHD remains the major barrier to widespread successful application of bone marrow transplantation for the correction of many different diseases.[23-25] Acute GVHD begins 6 or more days after transplantation (or posttransfusion in the case of nonirradiated blood products) with high unrelenting fever, a morbilliform maculopapular erythematous rash, and severe diarrhea.[24] The rash becomes progressively confluent and may involve the entire body surface; it is both pruritic and painful and eventually leads to marked exfoliation. Eosinophilia and lymphocytosis develop, followed shortly by hepatosplenomegaly, abnormal liver function tests, and hyperbilirubinemia. The diarrhea is watery and voluminous and may become bloody as the disease progresses. Nausea, vomiting, and severe, cramping abdominal pain occur as a consequence of the gastrointestinal involvement, which is also accompanied by a protein-losing enteropathy. The latter contributes to marked generalized edema ("third spacing") seen in more severe, acute GVHD. The most severe forms of acute GVHD are also characterized by bone marrow aplasia, marked susceptibility to infection, and death in a high proportion of cases.

Staging

Staging of GVHD is based on the severity and number of organ systems involved.[24] The four categories generally defined are grade 1, 1+ to 2+ skin rash without gut involvement and with no more than 1+ liver involvement; grade 2, 1+ to 3+ skin rash with either 1+ to 2+ gastrointestinal involvement or 1+ to 2+ liver involvement or both; grade 3, 2+ to 4+ skin rash with 2+ to 4+ gastrointestinal involvement with or without 2+ to 4+ liver involvement (a decrease in performance status and fever also characterize grades 2 and 3, with increasing severity per stage); and grade 4, pattern and severity of GVHD similar to those in grade 3, with extreme constitutional symptoms.

If the patient does not die and acute GVHD persists, it is termed *chronic* after 100 days. Chronic GVHD may evolve from acute GVHD or may develop in the absence of or after resolution of acute GVHD. It occurs in 45% to 70% of conditioned patients receiving HLA-matched bone marrow transplants.[26] Skin lesions of chronic GVHD resemble scleroderma, with hyperkeratosis, reticular hyperpigmentation, atrophy with ulceration, and fibrosis and limitation of joint movement. Other manifestations include the sicca syndrome, disordered immunoregulation as evidenced by autoantibody and immune complex formation and polyclonal and monoclonal

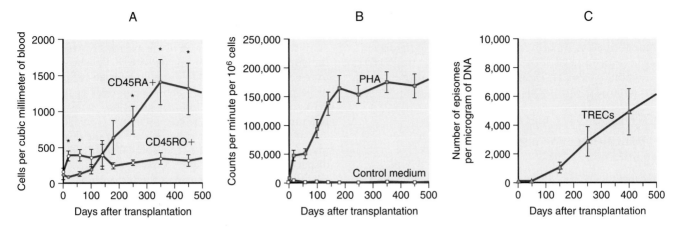

FIGURE 18-1 Memory (CD45RO+) versus naive (CD45RA+) T cells (**A**), T cell proliferation in response to PHA (**B**), and T cell receptor excision circles (TRECs) (**C**) after bone marrow transplantation with T cell–depleted human leukocyte antigen–identical ($N = 7$) or –haploidentical ($N = 71$) related bone marrow stem cells into infants with severe combined immunodeficiency (SCID) without pretransplant chemoablation or posttransplant graft-versus-host disease prophylaxis. The findings indicate that thymic processing is crucial for the development of new T cells from normal allogeneic stem cells in these infants with SCID. (From Patel DD, Gooding ME, Parrott RE, et al: *N Engl J Med* 342: 1325-1332, 2000.)

hyperimmunoglobulinemia, idiopathic interstitial pneumonitis, and frequent infections.[27]

Etiology and Pathogenesis

The principal cause of GVHD is that the recipient with absent T cell function (or one made equally T cell deficient by irradiation or chemotherapy) cannot reject bone marrow, matched or mismatched.[23] By contrast, engrafted, genetically different immunocompetent donor T cells recognize foreign HLA antigens on the recipient's cells and respond to them.[23-25,27] In the case of HLA-identical bone marrow transplants, GVHD is likely the result of responses by donor T cells[28,29] to recipient minor locus histocompatibility or Y chromosome–associated transplantation antigens because a significantly higher incidence of GVHD occurs in male patients who receive MHC-matched female marrow than in patients receiving MHC and sex-matched marrow.[8,23,27] In the case of unfractionated marrow transplants from HLA class II–mismatched donors, this reaction of the donor T lymphocytes against the recipient is almost invariably fatal. The severity of GVHD increases with the recipient's age, gender mismatch, prior herpesvirus infections,[23] the use of HLA-matched unrelated donors (MUDs), and, if a related donor is not HLA identical, the degree of genetic disparity and/or the rigor with which T cells are depleted from the marrow. GVHD is usually mild and self-limited in SCID hosts not administered pretransplantation immunosuppression who receive unfractionated HLA-identical marrow. However, in 60% of recipients who receive pretransplantation irradiation or immunosuppressive drugs, GVHD is moderate to severe and fatal in 15% to 20% despite HLA identity.[24,25]

Diagnosis

Although the diagnosis is strongly suspected when the earlier constellation of clinical manifestations is fully developed, histologic diagnosis is often necessary at earlier stages to exclude other causes of rash (e.g., drug-related rashes), hepatitis (e.g., infections with herpesviruses), or diarrhea (e.g., caused by in-

fectious agents). Skin biopsies in acute GVHD reveal basal vacuolar degeneration or necrosis, spongiosis, single cell dyskeratosis, eosinophilic necrosis of epidermal cells, and a dermal perivascular round cell infiltration.[25] Similar necrotic changes occur in the liver and intestinal tract and eventually in most other tissues. However, in the early stages of GVHD, the histology can resemble that of drug reactions or some forms of hepatitis, in which case the only definitive means of establishing a diagnosis is by identifying donor-derived cells in the blood or target organ. This has been facilitated greatly by the use of polymerase chain reaction to amplify DNA polymorphisms associated with variations in the length of dinucleotide or trinucleotide microsatellite repeats.[30]

Treatment

Many regimens have been used to mitigate GVHD in both MHC-incompatible and -compatible bone marrow transplants. For all unfractionated HLA-identical related or unrelated bone marrow or cord blood transplants into patients for whom pretransplantation chemotherapy is administered to prevent rejection, it is necessary to use GVHD prophylaxis. Such patients are usually administered cyclosporine daily for 6 to 9 months or methotrexate (15 mg/M² on the first day posttransplantation and 10 mg/M² on the third, sixth, and eleventh days and weekly thereafter until day 100) or both, in which case a shorter course of methotrexate is used.[31] For unfractionated HLA-identical sibling bone marrow transplants or rigorously T cell–depleted haploidentical (half-matched) bone marrow transplants into infants with SCID, it is usually unnecessary to give immunosuppressive agents to prevent GVHD. However, when GVHD does occur in the latter situations, steroids (or even cyclosporine) are occasionally needed to treat more severe forms of the condition.

The previously mentioned immunosuppressive agents have not prevented GVHD entirely; moreover, they can adversely affect the immune cells one is trying to engraft. Once severe GVHD has become established, it is extremely difficult to treat. Antithymocyte serum, steroids, cyclosporine, and murine monoclonal antibodies to human T cell surface antigens have ameliorated many, but the course has been inexorably fatal in others similarly treated.[25] Anticytokine and anticytokine receptor antibodies are being evaluated for their potential efficacy in mitigating GVHD.[32] The best approach to GVHD is prevention (see Box 18-2). By far the best preventive approach is the removal of postthymic T cells from the donor marrow.

METHODS OF T CELL DEPLETION

Soybean Lectin and Sheep Erythrocyte Agglutination

This method of T cell depletion involves agglutination of most mature marrow cells with soybean lectin, followed by sedimentation of clumped cells and subsequent removal of T cells from the unagglutinated marrow by sheep erythrocyte rosetting and density-gradient centrifugation.[14,33] For an adequate yield of stem cells, it is necessary to collect approximately 1 L of bone marrow from the donor. This is usually not a problem because a parent is usually chosen as the donor, and the donations are made under general anesthesia. Paradoxically, although soy lectin is very effective in removing most mature marrow cells, it does not bind to human T cells. Thus after soy lectin agglutination, there are still numerous T cells in the unagglutinated fraction.[33] To remove the T cells, two steps of sheep erythrocyte rosette depletion are required. The final cell preparation contains few, if any, lymphocytes; is phytohemagglutinin (PHA) and mixed leukocyte culture nonresponsive; consists of immature myeloid, stem, and dendritic cells; and represents less than 5% to 10% of the initial number of nucleated marrow cells.[33] There is abundant evidence that such preparations contain stem cells because they have immunologically reconstituted numerous infants with SCID.

Other Methods of T Cell Depletion

Another method of depleting postthymic T cells from donor marrow is incubation with monoclonal antibodies to human T cells plus a source of complement.[34,35] T cell depletion is not as effective with monoclonal antibody treatment as with the soy lectin, sheep red blood cell (SRBC) rosette-depletion method, possibly as a result of modulation of T cell antigens from the surface of the T cells without destroying them. As a consequence, somewhat more frequent and severe GVHD has been observed. Recently, better (but not complete) T cell depletion has been achieved by using solid-phase anti-CD34 monoclonal antibodies for positive selection of stem cells, followed by purging with a monoclonal antibody to CD2.[36] The more recent version of the Isolex 300i anti-CD34 (Baxter Scientific, Irvine, CA) product has resulted in less T cell contamination. However, the efficiency in selecting CD34+ cells has varied greatly among the different commercially available solid-phase devices, with the CliniMACs (Miltenyi Biotec, Auburn, CA) product generally giving higher yields of CD34+ cells. These devices also enable closed system handling of the marrow cells.

PREVENTION OF REJECTION

Immunosuppressive agents commonly used to ensure the acceptance of solid-organ grafts or the prevention of GVHD have deleterious effects on the very cells one is trying to engraft in patients with genetically determined immunodefi-

ciency. Therefore, immunosuppressive and myeloablative agents used to prevent bone marrow graft rejection must be administered before infusion of the marrow to avoid injury to the donor cells. Except in infants with SCID who are unable to reject allografts, all other immunodeficient recipients have to be preconditioned with chemotherapeutic agents to prevent graft rejection. In those transplant recipients with some potential to reject grafts, factors influencing the likelihood of engraftment of donor marrow cells are (1) the degree of immunoincompetence of the recipient, (2) the degree of MHC disparity between donor and recipient, (3) the degree of presensitization of the recipient to the histocompatibility antigens of the donor, (4) the number of marrow cells administered, (5) the type of conditioning regimen given the recipient, and (6) whether T cell–depletion techniques are used. Conditioning agents used most widely have included procarbazine, cyclophosphamide, busulfan, melphalan, and antithymocyte globulin. A combination of 2 or 4 mg/kg busulfan daily for 4 days followed by 50 mg/kg cyclophosphamide daily for 4 days has been commonly used.[37] In patients with primary immunodeficiency who do require conditioning, preparation of the recipient need only be directed at immunosuppression and myeloablation (see Box 18-2). Thus total body irradiation (TBI), required to eradicate malignant cells, is not usually necessary. Because of the toxicity of high-dose conditioning regimens, however, there has been considerable recent interest in using a minimally myelosuppressive-conditioning regimen based on low-dose TBI or fludarabine alone or in combination with other drugs, followed by a short course of immunosuppression and postgrafting cyclosporine and methotrexate or mycophenolate mofetil.[38-40]

SOURCES OF STEM CELLS FOR TRANSPLANTATION

The various potential sources of stem cells are listed in Box 18-3; these include bone marrow and peripheral blood (including cord blood) from related or unrelated,[10] HLA-

---

BOX 18-3

THERAPEUTIC PRINCIPLES
Sources of Stem Cells for the Treatment of Primary Immunodeficiency

HLA-identical sibling (or other relative) bone marrow

HLA-identical sibling cord blood

Haploidentical (half-matched) related (parental) bone marrow

    T cell depleted by soy lectin/SRBC

    T cell depleted by monoclonal antibodies

MUD bone marrow

    Unfractionated

    T cell depleted by monoclonal antibodies

    MUD cord blood

Modified from Buckley RH: Bone marrow reconstitution in primary immunodeficiency. In Rich RR, Fleisher TT, Shearer WT, et al, eds: *Clinical immunology: principles and practice,* ed 2, St Louis, 2001, Mosby. *HLA,* Human leukocyte antigen; *SRBC,* sheep red blood cell; *MUD,* matched unrelated donor.

matched or -mismatched donors. HLA-identical related bone marrow (unfractionated or T cell depleted) and HLA-identical sibling cord blood are still considered the treatments of choice for all patients in need of a transplant. Even those sources do not guarantee graft acceptance or freedom from GVHD because of minor locus histocompatibility antigenic differences. However, HLA-identical sibling cord blood appears to have less GVHD potential than does HLA-identical sibling bone marrow.[41] If a patient with a severe cellular immunodeficiency or other type of invariably fatal primary immunodeficiency is fortunate enough to have an HLA-identical sibling, unfractionated bone marrow cells can be given. Such marrow cell suspensions contain, in addition to stem cells, mature T and B cells. In most cases both T cell and B cell immunity have been fully constituted by such matched transplants, with evidence of function detected as early as 2 weeks after transplantation when no pretransplantation conditioning and no posttransplantation GVHD prophylaxis are required. Adoptive transfer of mature T cells is the explanation for the very rapid onset of immune function after matched unfractionated bone marrow or cord blood transplantation.[11] Despite the availability of molecular typing, unfractionated MUD bone marrow or cord blood transplants cause significantly more GVHD than do related matched transplants because of incompatibility for HLA antigens not typed for (e.g., class I*c* locus and class II DQ and DP antigens) or to minor locus histocompatibility differences.[42] These disparities result in a much greater need for long-term use of immunosuppressive agents to prevent or mitigate GVHD in MUD transplants, which is self-defeating when the goal is immunoreconstitution. Rigorous T cell depletion permits administration of HLA-mismatched related donor bone marrow or MUD bone marrow or cord blood. However, in actual practice, rigorous T cell depletion is rarely applied to MUD bone marrow or cord blood transplantation. By contrast, the ability to use rigorously T cell–depleted haploidentical (half-matched) related parental bone marrow stem cells has been a major advance in the treatment of primary immunodeficiency diseases. It not only is effective in causing immune reconstitution but also has permitted the omission of immunosuppressive drugs for GVHD prophylaxis. When T cell–depleted marrow is given, the stem cells must go to the host thymus for maturation, a process that takes 90 to 120 days before T cells enter the circulation.[10,11,15,21]

Bone Marrow Transplantation Procedure

Bone marrow transplantation is the simplest of all transplantation procedures, offering little risk to the donor because it involves removal of a tissue that is readily regenerated. The bone marrow cells are usually obtained via aspiration with a 14- or 16-gauge needle from multiple sites along both iliac crests while the donor is under general anesthesia.[43] An alternate site in adults is the sternum or, in children, the upper third of the tibia. The aspirate is placed in heparinized tissue culture medium and passed through metal screens with diminishing apertures to remove bone spicules, and the nucleated marrow cells are enumerated. In the case of unfractionated HLA-identical bone marrow or cord blood, the cells are then given to the recipient intravenously in a manner similar to a blood transfusion. In the case of T cell–depleted marrow, the final fraction is given this same way.

Indications for Bone Marrow Transplantation

Except for infants with complete DiGeorge syndrome, who have no HLA-identical donors and who therefore require a cultured allogeneic thymic transplant, all infants and children with genetic defects in immune function that lead to death at an early age are potential candidates for allogeneic bone marrow or blood stem cell transplantation. Patients with many different types of immune defects have received such transplants, with varying degrees of success. These defects include SCID, Wiskott-Aldrich syndrome, combined immunodeficiency (CID), Omenn's syndrome, leukocyte adhesion deficiency (LAD), MHC antigen deficiency, Chédiak-Higashi syndrome, chronic granulomatous disease (CGD), DiGeorge's syndrome, purine nucleoside phosphorylase (PNP) deficiency, cartilage hair hypoplasia, hyper-IgM syndrome, interleukin (IL)-2 deficiency, and X-linked lymphoproliferative disease.

Problems after Bone Marrow Transplantation

Multiple problems occur during the posttransplantation period, particularly in patients given pretransplantation conditioning. Thus marrow transplantation should be carried out only by experienced teams. The dominant problems are GVHD, as noted earlier, and infections. In addition, multiple transfusions of blood products are usually necessary for chemoablated patients during the 7 to 20 days before erythroid and myeloid engraftment occurs. The availability of granulocyte colony-stimulating factor (G-CSF) has shortened the time to development of neutrophils after transplantation. All transfusions that contain immunocompetent cells should be irradiated with 1500 to 3000 rad to prevent GVHD and, if the recipient is cytomegalovirus (CMV) seronegative, the transfusions should be from CMV-seronegative donors. Family members can be used as blood donors during this period.

Infections

Because patients with primary cellular immunodeficiency are highly susceptible to opportunistic viral, fungal, and facultative intracellular microorganisms, they frequently develop an untreatable infection before their defects are diagnosed and before transplantation.[27] In addition, the immunodeficiency that occurs in the posttransplantation period for patients who have had conditioning regimens and who are receiving GVHD prophylactic drugs adds to the high incidence of infections in those patients, regardless of whether GVHD is present.[27] Another contributing factor is the profound granulocytopenia that occurs in conditioned patients; however, the use of G-CSF has reduced the severity of this problem. The advent of GVHD prolongs the impaired immunity and further heightens the susceptibility to infection. Protective isolation is necessary. The most problematic infectious agents include *Candida albicans, Aspergillus* spp., *Pneumocystis carinii*, CMV, herpes simplex virus, varicella-zoster virus, Epstein-Barr virus (EBV), parainfluenza, enteroviruses, and adenoviruses.[27] Bacterial infections with high-grade pathogens also occur but, if identified in time, can usually be treated effectively with antibiotics. Intravenous gamma globulin therapy has also helped reduce the frequency and severity of infections with common bacterial and viral agents. The use of trimethoprim-sulfamethoxazole or intravenous pentamidine has vastly reduced the mortality rate from *P. carinii* pneumonia. Trimethoprim-sulfamethoxazole and intravenous pentamidine are effective prophylactic agents for this infection. Intravenous ribavirin is somewhat effective against adenovirus and parainfluenza infections. Acyclovir is highly effective in treating varicella-zoster and herpes simplex infections and may have some prophylactic effect for EBV infections, and ganciclovir and CytoGam are helpful in controlling CMV infections. Nevertheless, little other than the development of normal host T cell function will attenuate ongoing infections with CMV, EBV, enteroviruses, parainfluenza 3, and adenoviruses. Infections frequently lead to death before T cell function develops; this is particularly true if severe GVHD occurs.

Identification of Engraftment

Four types of markers are used to identify donor cells in marrow recipients: chromosomal differences,[44] erythrocyte and leukocyte antigens, serum allotypes, and DNA sequence polymorphisms. If donor and recipient are of the opposite sex, karyotypic markers can be detected as early as 2 weeks after grafting. Serum immunoglobulin allotypic markers are useful in documenting the chimerism of B cells.

Effectiveness of Bone Marrow Transplantation for the Treatment of Primary Immunodeficiency Diseases

Although precise figures are not available, more than 1200 patients worldwide with many different forms of genetically determined immunodeficiency have received bone marrow transplants over the past 34 years in attempts to correct their underlying immune defects (Box 18-4). Possibly because of both earlier diagnosis before the development of untreatable opportunistic infections and the availability of better antimicrobial agents to treat infections, the results of bone marrow transplantation have improved considerably during the past 17 years.[10,11,15,18,45-47] A worldwide survey conducted by the author from 1994 through 1997, with, subsequent additions of published cases from the literature, revealed that 239 of 302 (79%) patients with primary immunodeficiency transplanted with HLA-identical marrow during a period of 29 years survived.

Most encouraging, however, were the results of T cell–depleted haploidentical (half-matched) marrow transplants in patients with primary immunodeficiency. From the same survey, it was ascertained that 646 such transplants had been performed and that 363 (56%) of the patients survived. The significance is even more impressive when it is realized that most of the 646 recipients would have died had not T cell–depletion techniques been developed.

Severe Combined Immunodeficiency

Bone marrow transplantation has been more widely applied and more successful in infants with SCID than in those with any other primary immunodeficiency. Because infants with SCID lack T cells, there is no need to administer pretransplantation chemotherapy (Box 18-5). In the same survey and literature review, only 126 infants with SCID were reported as having received HLA-identical marrow, and 106 (84%) survived. By contrast, 477 infants with SCID had received haploidentical marrow, and 301 (63%) survived worldwide; how-

<table>
<tr><td>BOX
18-4</td><td>KEY CONCEPTS
Bone Marrow Transplantation in Immunodeficiency</td></tr>
</table>

- Approximately 79% of all immunodeficient patients transplanted with HLA-identical sibling bone marrow or cord blood survive. There is evidence for engraftment of both adoptively transferred mature donor T cells and donor stems that develop into new T cells in the patient's thymus. These new T cells have undergone both positive and negative selection in the host thymus.

- Approximately 56% of all immunodeficient patients transplanted with T cell–depleted, HLA-haploidentical bone marrow survive. Immune reconstitution in this type of transplant depends on engraftment of donor stems that develop into new T cells in the patient's thymus, where they undergo both positive and negative selection.

- The time required for stem cells to be processed by the patient's thymus is a minimum of 90 to 120 days. Even the vestigeal thymus of infants with severe combined immunodeficiency syndrome is able to process donor stem cells to become mature and functioning T cells.

- The difference in time to development of T cell function (14 days for unfractionated HLA-identical marrow or cord blood versus 90 to 120 days for T cell–depleted HLA-identical or haploidentical bone marrow transplants) is because of the adoptive transfer of mature donor T and B cells.

- The use of MUD bone marrow or cord blood donors at this time offers no clear advantage over the use of HLA-haploidentical related donors. Major problems of either type of MUD transplant are a long delay in identifying a donor; the need for heavy and prolonged GVHD prophylaxis with cyclosporine, methotrexate, and/or steroids; a substantial rate of serious GVHD despite the use of the latter; and resultant prolongation of the immunodeficiency causing further susceptibility to opportunistic infections.

Modified from Buckley RH: Bone marrow reconstitution in primary immunodeficiency. In Rich RR, Fleisher TT, Shearer WT et al, eds: *Clinical immunology: principles and practice*, ed 2, St Louis, 2001, Mosby.
HLA, Human leukocyte antigen; *MUD,* matched unrelated donor; *GVHD,* graft-versus-host disease.

ever, the haploidentical transplants were not T cell depleted until after 1980. Nevertheless, this is a major accomplishment because SCID is 100% fatal without marrow transplantation or, in the case of infants who are adenosine deaminase (ADA) deficient, enzyme-replacement therapy. The latter is helpful for only a small percentage of infants with SCID because ADA deficiency accounts for only approximately 15% of cases of SCID.[10,47,48] Only 17 infants with SCID were reported as having received MUD transplants, and 12 (71%) survived. Six infants with SCID were reported as having received related or unrelated cord blood transplants, and five survived. The percentages of infants with SCID who received either HLA-identical or haploidentical marrow and who were found to be surviving in the author's survey were roughly similar to those in reviews of the European experience with unfractionated HLA-identical and T cell–depleted, haploidentical (or

KEY CONCEPTS

*Bone Marrow Transplantation in Patients
with Severe Combined Immunodeficiency*

- Infants with severe combined immunodeficiency (SCID) have no T cell function; therefore they cannot reject marrow grafts or T cells. They are at a high risk for fatal graft-versus-host disease (GVHD) from blood products that contain mature T cells.

- Because they cannot reject grafts, there is no need for chemotherapeutic or antilymphocyte conditioning before they receive marrow or blood stem cell grafts. Because they will continue to have their own neutrophils, platelets, and red blood cells, they will not require many transfusions and will not be as susceptible to fungal or bacterial infections.

- The kinetics of stem cell education by the SCID thymus is identical regardless of whether patients are given pretransplantation chemotherapy. In addition, the use of pretransplantation chemotherapy does not ensure that B cell function will develop.

- Because they do not need pretransplantation conditioning, this helps reduce the likelihood of GVHD if they are given unfractionated human leukocyte antigen (HLA)–identical or T cell–depleted, HLA-haploidentical related marrow or blood stem cell grafts. Thus GVHD prophylaxis with cyclosporine and/or methotrexate can be omitted, and immune function can develop without being impeded by these immunosuppressive drugs.

Modified from Buckley RH: Bone marrow reconstitution in primary immunodeficiency. In Rich RR, Fleisher TT, Shearer WT, et al, eds: *Clinical immunology: principles and practice*, ed 2, St Louis, 2001, Mosby.

More important, our studies have shown that such transplants can provide normal numbers of T cells and normalize T cell function in all molecular types of SCID (Figure 18-2). Despite the fact that all infants with SCID have vestigial thymuses, we recently demonstrated that the T cells that emerge after transplantation in these chimeras are thymically derived.[11,21] They are CD45RA+ and they contain extrachromosomal DNA circles formed during intrathymic T cell development (T cell receptor recombination excision circles [TRECs]). Before transplantation, neither the few host T cells that are present nor any transplacentally transferred maternal T cells contain TRECs and they are CD45RO+. However, after transplantation there is the gradual emergence of both CD45RA+ and TREC-containing T cells, coinciding with the development of T cell function (see Figure 18-1). Most impressive is the fact that 34 of 35 (97%) infants we have transplanted in the first 3.5 months of life currently survive[11,54] (Figure 18-3). Thus there appears to be no advantage in per-

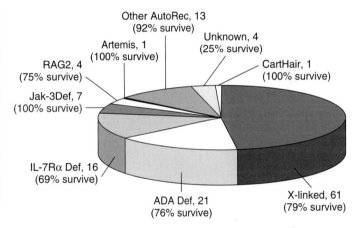

FIGURE 18-2 Survival rates for bone marrow transplants given 128 infants with different types of severe combined immunodeficiency syndrome, showing that bone marrow transplantation is effective for all known genetic types.

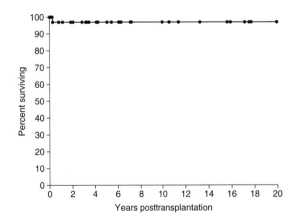

FIGURE 18-3 Kaplan-Meier survival curve for 35 consecutive infants with severe combined immunodeficiency syndrome who received bone marrow transplants at the author's institution from human leukocyte antigen–identical (N = 2) or –haploidentical (N = 31) donors before they were 3.5 months of age without pretransplantation chemoablation or posttransplantation graft-versus-host disease prophylaxis. Thirty-four (97%) infants survived for periods of 2 months to 20.4 years after transplantation. The one death occurred from a cytomegalovirus infection.

non–T cell–depleted) bone marrow transplants in SCID.[49-51] The SCID survival rates in Europe were 76% in the HLA-identical group and ranged from 35% to 60% in the half-matched transplants. A further retrospective analysis of the influence of the SCID phenotype on the outcome of haploidentical marrow transplants by the European Group for Bone Marrow Transplantation and the European Society for Immunodeficiency found the disease-free survival to be significantly better for patients with B+ SCID (60%) than for those with B− SCID (35%) (P = 0.002).[52] However, 12 of 16 (75%) infants with the B− Athabascan form of SCID caused by Artemis deficiency were reported as surviving after bone marrow transplantation in this country.[53]

During the past 20 years, the author and associates have transplanted 128 infants with SCID, and 98 of these (78%) are currently surviving from 1 month to 20.4 years after transplantation. No pretransplantation conditioning was given except to three infants who also received cord blood transplants. Only 15 had HLA-identical donors; all of the 15 survive with functioning grafts. One hundred thirteen infants with SCID received half-matched related donor stem cells prepared by the soy lectin, SRBC-rosetting T cell–depletion technique,[14] and 85 (75%) of these patients survive. Survival rates were similar whether the patients were ADA normal (78%) or ADA deficient (75%), and there was no significant difference in disease-free survival for B+ versus B− SCID.

forming such transplants *in utero* as opposed to performing them soon after birth.[55,56] *In utero* transplants also carry the risks associated with injecting the fetus and the inability to detect GVHD during gestation.

Wiskott-Aldrich Syndrome

The second largest group of immunodeficiency patients who have received bone marrow transplants since 1968 are those with Wiskott-Aldrich syndrome.[57-64] In a recent report from the International Bone Marrow Transplant Registry,[62] 170 patients with Wiskott-Aldrich syndrome had been transplanted, and the 5-year probability of survival for all patients was 70% (95% confidence interval, 63% to 77%). Probabilities differed by donor type: 87% (74% to 93%) with HLA-identical sibling donors, 52% (37% to 65%) with other related donors, and 71% (58% to 80%) with unrelated donors ($P = 0.0006$). Boys who had received an unrelated donor transplant before age 5 had survival similar to those receiving HLA-identical sibling transplants. The facts that all such patients require myeloablation and cytoreduction to prevent graft rejection; that they have been multiply transfused with allogeneic platelets before transplantation, resulting in resistance to engraftment; that they may have developed chronic herpesvirus infections before transplantation; and that they are prone to develop malignancy are all likely factors contributing to their failure to survive the 3 to 4 months required for stem cells to mature to functioning T cells from a T cell—depleted marrow graft. Many of the deaths were from EBV-associated B-lymphocyte lymphoproliferative disorders.[45]

Combined Immunodeficiency

Patients with CIDs characterized by less severe T cell defects than in SCID constituted the third largest group of patients who received bone marrow transplants since 1968.[46] Thirty-three (51%) of 65 patients so treated were reported as surviving. HLA-identical marrow transplants were clearly more successful (13 of 17, or 76%) than T cell—depleted, haploidentical (15 of 38, or 39%)[51] or MUD adult marrow (0 of 2) transplants, but 5 of 7 recipients of cord blood transplants were surviving.[65]

Omenn's Syndrome

Forty-five patients with Omenn's syndrome were reported in the literature[45,51,66,67] or to the author as having received marrow transplants since 1968, and 23 (51%) were alive at the time. As with the other non-SCID defects, however, the greatest success was with HLA-identical sibling transplants: 9 of 12 (75%) were surviving, whereas only 11 of 27 (41%) haploidentical marrow and 3 of 6 (50%) MUD marrow recipients were alive.

Leukocyte Adhesion Deficiency

Twenty-five (76%) of 33 patients with leukocyte adhesion deficiency type 1 (LAD-1) were alive after bone marrow transplantation at the time of the survey and review.[45,51,68,69] All types of marrow transplantation were successful in this condition: 6 of 8 (75%) HLA-identical sibling transplants, 15 of 21 (71%) T cell—depleted haploidentical marrow transplants,

2 of 2 (100%) MUD adult marrow transplants, and 2 of 3 cord blood transplants.

Major Histocompatibility Complex Antigen Deficiency Syndromes

Fourteen (5%) of 26 patients with the bare lymphocyte syndrome were reported alive after having received marrow transplants.[70,71] These included 4 (44%) of 9 who received HLA-identical sibling marrow but only 7 (35%) of 20 who received T cell—depleted, haploidentical marrow; 2 (100%) of 2 who received MUD marrow and 1 (100%) of 1 who received a related cord blood transplant.[45,50,70-72]

Chédiak-Higashi Syndrome

Eighteen (78%) of 23 patients with Chédiak-Higashi syndrome who received bone marrow transplants were reported to be alive.[45,57,73,74] These included 10 (83%) of 12 who received HLA-identical sibling marrow, 1 (20%) of 5 who received haploidentical marrow, and 6 (100%) of 6 who received MUD marrow.

Chronic Granulomatous Disease

Twenty (71%) of 28 patients with CGD who had received bone marrow transplants were reported as surviving, and a majority of these were chimeric.[75-80] The overall survival figures include 18 (72%) of 25 HLA-identical sibling marrow recipients and 2 (67%) of 3 recipients of MUD marrow.[81] Very recently, success has been reported in treating CGD patients with the "mini-transplant" approach using HLA-identical sibling donors.[38,79]

DiGeorge Syndrome

Eleven patients with the complete DiGeorge syndrome were reported to the author as undergoing marrow transplantation, whereas an additional four underwent fetal thymus or cultured mature thymic tissue transplantation.[82,83] The only survivors were two of the three who received unfractionated HLA-identical sibling marrow and two of the two who were recipients of explants of cultured thymic epithelium. Twenty-six additional patients were identified from the literature in the report by Goldsobel et al[82] in 1987 as having undergone fetal thymus or cultured thymic epithelial transplantation, and at the time of their review only eight were alive and well. However, more recently, 16 additional infants with complete DiGeorge syndrome were transplanted with cultured thymic tissue, and 10 of these are surviving.[83]

Other Primary Immunodeficiencies

Other disorders treated successfully by bone marrow transplantation include X-linked hyper-IgM (13 of 21 surviving),[84-89] reticular dysgenesis (9 of 11 surviving),[90] PNP deficiency (3 of 8 surviving),[91,92] cartilage hair hypoplasia (4 of 7 surviving), X-linked lymphoproliferative syndrome (6 of 9 surviving),[89,93-95] pigmentary dilution (Griscelli) syndrome (3 of 7 surviving),[96] IL-2 deficiency (2 of 2 surviving),[46] common variable immunodeficiency (CVID) (0 of 4 surviving), chronic mucocutaneous candidiasis (0 of 1 surviving), ataxia-

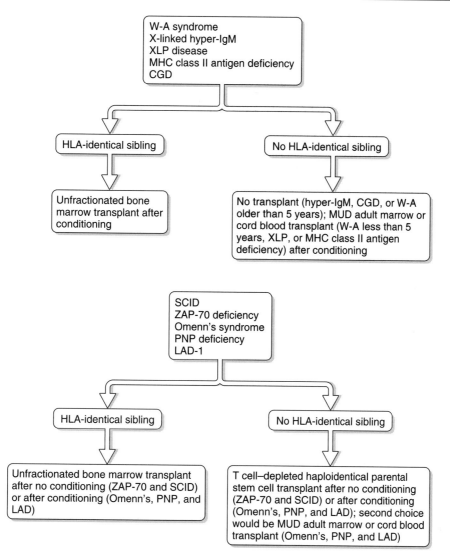

FIGURE 18-4 Algorithm showing decision points about transplantation for patients with primary immunodeficiency. *W-A,* Wiskott-Aldrich; *XLP,* X-linked lymphoproliferative; *MHC,* major histocompatibility complex; *CGD,* chronic granulomatous disease; *HLA,* human leukocyte antigen; *MUD,* matched unrelated donor; *SCID,* severe combined immunodeficiency; *PNP,* purine nucleoside phosphorylase; *LAD,* leukocyte adhesion deficiency.

telangiectasia (0 of 4 surviving), and Fas (CD95) deficiency (1 of 1 surviving).[97] The author and associates have also performed transplants on 51 patients with non-SCID immunodeficiency, with the following survival rates: 11 (42%) of 26 with CID, 5 (71%) of 7 with LAD, 2 (100%) of 2 with Chédiak-Higashi syndrome, 2 (100%) of 2 with CGD, 1 (100%) of 1 with ZAP-70 deficiency, 2 (40%) of 5 with Omenn's syndrome, 1 (33%) of 3 with PNP deficiency, 1 (50%) of 2 with Wiskott-Aldrich syndrome, 1 (100%) of 1 with X-linked hyper-IgM, and 1 each with Griscelli syndrome and IFN-γR2 deficiency, neither of whom survived.

CONCLUSIONS

Figure 18-4 contains a clinical algorithm concerning decision making for bone marrow transplantation in the primary immunodeficiency diseases for which this has been done most often. It is likely that this algorithm will change in the near future as gene therapy becomes available for these defects.

HELPFUL WEBSITES

The Severe Combined Immunodeficiency website (www.scid.net)
The Immune Deficiency Foundation website (www.primaryimmune.org.)

REFERENCES

1. Pillow RP, Epstein RB, Buckner CD, et al: Treatment of bone marrow failure by isogeneic marrow infusion, *N Engl J Med* 275:94-97, 1966.
2. Amos DB, Bach FH: Phenotypic expressions of the major histocompatibility locus in man (HL-A): leukocyte antigens and mixed leukocyte culture reactivity, *J Exp Med* 128:623-637, 1968.
3. Bach FH, Albertini RJ, Joo P, et al: Bone marrow transplantation in a patient with the Wiskott-Aldrich syndrome, *Lancet* 2:1364-1366, 1968.
4. Gatti RA, Meuwissen HJ, Allen HD, et al: Immunological reconstitution of sex-linked lymphopenic immunological deficiency, *Lancet* 2:1366-1369, 1968.
5. Wu AM, Till JE, Siminovitch L, et al: Cytological evidence for a relationship between normal hematopoietic colony-forming cells and cells of the lymphoid system, *J Exp Med* 127:455-464, 1968.

6. Cavazzana-Calvo M, Hacein-Bey S, deSaint Basile G, et al: Gene therapy of human severe combined immunodeficiency (SCID)-X1 disease, *Science* 288:669-672, 2000.

7. Hacein-Bey-Abina S, Le Deist F, Carlier F, et al: Sustained correction of X-linked severe combined immunodeficiency by *ex vivo* gene therapy, *N Engl J Med* 346:1185-1193, 2002.

8. Bortin MM, Rimm AA: Severe combined immunodeficiency disease. Characterization of the disease and results of transplantation, *JAMA* 238:591-600, 1977.

9. Roberts JL, Volkman DJ, Buckley RH: Modified MHC restriction of donor-origin T cells in humans with severe combined immunodeficiency transplanted with haploidentical bone marrow stem cells, *J Immunol* 143:1575-1579, 1989.

10. Buckley RH, Schiff SE, Schiff RI, et al: Hematopoietic stem cell transplantation for the treatment of severe combined immunodeficiency, *N Engl J Med* 340:508-516, 1999.

11. Myers LA, Patel DD, Puck JM, et al: Hematopoietic stem cell transplantation for severe combined immunodeficiency in the neonatal period leads to superior thymic output and improved survival, *Blood* 99:872-878, 2002.

12. Muller-Ruchholtz W, Wottge HU, Muller-Hermelink HK: Bone marrow transplantation in rats across strong histocompatibility barriers by selective elimination of lymphoid cells in donor marrow, *Transplant Proc* 8:537-541, 1976.

13. Reisner Y, Itzicovitch L, Meshorer A, et al: Hematopoietic stem cell transplantation using mouse bone marrow and spleen cells fractionated by lectins, *Proc Natl Acad Sci U S A* 75:2933-2936, 1978.

14. Reisner Y, Kapoor N, Kirkpatrick D, et al: Transplantation for severe combined immunodeficiency with HLA-A, B, D, DR incompatible parental marrow cells fractionated by soybean agglutinin and sheep red blood cells, *Blood* 61:341-348, 1983.

15. Buckley RH, Schiff SE, Sampson HA, et al: Development of immunity in human severe primary T cell deficiency following haploidentical bone marrow stem cell transplantation, *J Immunol* 136:2398-2407, 1986.

16. O'Reilly RJ, Keever CA, Small TN, et al: The use of HLA-non-identical T cell depleted marrow transplants for correction of severe combined immunodeficiency disease, *Immunodef Rev* 1:273-309, 1989.

17. Dror Y, Gallagher R, Wara DW, et al: Immune reconstitution in severe combined immunodeficiency disease after lectin-treated, T cell depleted haplocompatible bone marrow transplantation, *Blood* 81:2021-2030, 1993.

18. Giri N, Vowels M, Ziegler JB, et al: HLA non-identical T cell depleted bone marrow transplantation for primary immunodeficiency diseases, *Aust N Z J Med* 24:26-30, 1994.

19. Wijnaendts L, LeDeist F, Griscelli C, et al: Development of immunologic functions after bone marrow transplantation in 33 patients with severe combined immunodeficiency, *Blood* 74:2212-2219, 1989.

20. Moen RC, Horowitz SD, Sondel PM, et al: Immunologic reconstitution after haploidentical bone marrow transplantation for immune deficiency disorders: treatment of bone marrow cells with monoclonal antibody CT-2 and complement, *Blood* 70:664-669, 1987.

21. Patel DD, Gooding ME, Parrott RE, et al: Thymic function after hematopoietic stem-cell transplantation for the treatment of severe combined immunodeficiency, *N Engl J Med* 342:1325-1332, 2000.

22. Schiff SE, Buckley RH: Modified responses to recipient and donor B cells by genetically donor T cells from human haploidentical bone marrow chimeras, *J Immunol* 138:2088-2094, 1987.

23. Ferrara JL, Deeg HJ: Graft-versus-host disease, *N Engl J Med* 324:667-674, 1991.

24. Glucksberg H, Storb R, Fefer A, et al: Clinical manifestations of graft-versus-host disease in human recipients of marrow from HLA-matched sibling donors, *Transplantation* 18:295-304, 1974.

25. Deeg HJ, Henslee-Downey PJ: Management of acute graft-versus-host disease, *Bone Marrow Transplant* 6:1-8, 1990.

26. Weisdorf D, Haake R, Blazar B, et al: Treatment of moderate/severe acute graft-versus-host disease after allogeneic bone marrow transplantation: an analysis of clinical risk features and outcome, *Blood* 75:1024-1030, 1990.

27. Skinner J, Finlay JL, Sondel PM, et al: Infectious complications in pediatric patients undergoing transplantation with T lymphocyte-depleted bone marrow, *Pediatr Infect Dis* 5:319-324, 1986.

28. Theobald M, Nierle T, Bunjes D, et al: Host-specific interleukin-2-secreting donor T-cell precursors as predictors of acute graft-versus-host disease in bone marrow transplantation between HLA-identical siblings, *N Engl J Med* 327:1613-1617, 1992.

29. Schwarer AP, Jiang YZ, Brookes PA, et al: Frequency of anti-recipient alloreactive helper T-cell precursors in donor blood and graft-versus-host disease after HLA-identical sibling bone marrow transplantation, *Lancet* 341:203-205, 1993.

30. Wang L, Juji T, Tokunaga K, et al: Polymorphic microsatellite markers for the diagnosis of graft-versus-host disease, *N Engl J Med* 330:398-401, 1994.

31. Storb R, Deeg HJ, Whitehead J, et al: Methotrexate and cyclosporine compared with cyclosporine alone for prophylaxis of acute graft versus host disease after marrow transplantation for leukemia, *N Engl J Med* 314:729-735, 1986.

32. Ozsahin H, Tuchschmid P, Lauener R, et al: Blockade of acute grade IV skin and eye graft-versus-host disease by anti-interleukin-2 receptor monoclonal antibody in genoidentical bone marrow transplantation setting, *Turk J Pediatr* 40:231-235, 1998.

33. Schiff SE, Kurtzberg J, Buckley RH: Studies of human bone marrow treated with soybean lectin and sheep erythrocytes: stepwise analysis of cell morphology, phenotype and function, *Clin Exp Immunol* 68:685-693, 1987.

34. Reinherz EL, Geha R, Rappeport JM, et al: Reconstitution after transplantation with T-lymphocyte-depleted HLA haplotype-mismatched bone marrow for severe combined immunodeficiency, *Proc Natl Acad Sci U S A* 79:6047-6051, 1982.

35. Hale G, Waldmann H: Control of graft-versus-host disease and graft rejection by T cell depletion of donor and recipient with Campath-1 antibodies. Results of matched sibling transplants for malignant diseases, *Bone Marrow Transplant* 13:597-611, 1994.

36. Martin-Hernandez MP, Arrieta R, Martinez A, et al: Haploidentical peripheral blood cell transplantation with a combination of CD34 selection and T cell depletion as graft-versus-host disease prophylaxis in a patient with severe combined immunodeficiency, *Bone Marrow Transplant* 20:797-799, 1997.

37. Blazar BR, Ramsay NKC, Kersey JH, et al: Pretransplant conditioning with busulfan (Myleran) and cyclophosphamide for nonmalignant diseases. Assessment of engraftment following histocompatible allogeneic bone marrow transplantation, *Transplantation* 39:597, 1985.

38. Nagler A, Ackerstein A, Kapelushnik J, et al: Donor lymphocyte infusion post-non-myeloablative allogeneic peripheral blood stem cell transplantation for chronic granulomatous disease, *Bone Marrow Transplant* 24:339-342, 1999.

39. Carella AM, Giralt S, Slavin S: Low intensity regimens with allogeneic hematopoietic stem cell transplantation as treatment of hematologic neoplasia, *Haematologica* 85:304-313, 2000.

40. Carella AM, Champlin R, Slavin S, et al: Mini-allografts: ongoing trials in humans, *Bone Marrow Transplant* 25:345-350, 2000.

41. Rocha V, Wagner JE Jr, Sobocinski KA, et al: Graft-versus-host disease in children who have received a cord-blood or bone marrow transplant from an HLA-identical sibling. Eurocord and International Bone Marrow Transplant Registry Working Committee on Alternative Donor and Stem Cell Sources, *N Engl J Med* 342:1846-1854, 2000.

42. Barker JN, Davies SM, DeFor T, et al: Survival after transplantation of unrelated donor umbilical cord blood is comparable to that of human leukocyte antigen-matched unrelated donor bone marrow: results of a matched-pair analysis, *Blood* 97:2957-2961, 2001.

43. Thomas ED, Storb R, Clift RA, et al: Bone marrow transplantation, *N Engl J Med* 292:823-843, 1975.

44. Van Den Berg H, Vossen JM, van den Bergh RL, et al: Detection of Y chromosome by *in situ* hybridization in combination with membrane antigens by two-color immunofluorescence, *Lab Invest* 64:623-628, 1994.

45. Fischer A, Landais P, Friedrich W, et al: Bone marrow transplantation (BMT) in Europe for primary immunodeficiencies other than severe combined immunodeficiency: a report from the European Group for BMT and the European Group for Immunodeficiency, *Blood* 83:1149-1154, 1994.

46. Berthet F, Le Deist F, Duliege AM, et al: Clinical consequences and treatment of primary immunodeficiency syndromes characterized by functional T and B lymphocyte anomalies (combined immune deficiency), *Pediatrics* 93:265-270, 1994.

47. Stephan JL, Vlekova V, Le Deist F, et al: Severe combined immunodeficiency: a retrospective single-center study of clinical presentation and outcome in 117 cases, *J Pediatr* 123:564-572, 1993.

48. Buckley RH, Schiff RI, Schiff SE, et al: Human severe combined immunodeficiency (SCID): genetic, phenotypic and functional diversity in 108 infants, *J Pediatr* 130:378-387, 1997.

49. Haddad E, Landais P, Friedrich W, et al: Long-term immune reconstitution and outcome after HLA-nonidentical T-cell-depleted bone marrow transplantation for severe combined immunodeficiency: a European retrospective study of 116 patients, *Blood* 91:3646-3653, 1998.

50. Fischer A, Landais P, Friedrich W, et al: European experience of bone marrow transplantation for severe combined immunodeficiency, *Lancet* 336:850-854, 1990.

51. Lanfranchi A, Verardi R, Tettoni K, et al: Haploidentical peripheral blood and marrow stem cell transplantation in nine cases of primary immunodeficiency, *Haematologica* 85:41-46, 2000.

52. Bertrand Y, Landais P, Friedrich W, et al: Influence of severe combined immunodeficiency phenotype on the outcome of HLA non-identical T cell-depleted bone marrow transplantation, *J Pediatr* 134:740-748, 1999.

53. O'Marcaigh AS, DeSantes K, Hu D, et al: Bone marrow transplantation for T-B- severe combined immunodeficiency disease in Athabascan-speaking native Americans, *Bone Marrow Transplant* 27:703-709, 2001.

54. Kane L, Gennery AR, Crooks BN, et al: Neonatal bone marrow transplantation for severe combined immunodeficiency, *Arch Dis Child Fetal Neonatal Ed* 85:F110-F113, 2001.

55. Wengler GS, Lanfranchi A, Frusca T, et al: *In-utero* transplantation of parental CD34 haematopoietic progenitor cells in a patient with X-linked severe combined immunodeficiency (SCIDX1), *Lancet* 348:1484-1487, 1996.

56. Flake AW, Roncarolo MG, Puck JM, et al: Treatment of X-linked severe combined immunodeficiency by *in utero* transplantation of paternal bone marrow, *N Engl J Med* 335:1806-1810, 1996.

57. Parkman R, Rappeport J, Geha R, et al: Complete correction of the Wiskott-Aldrich syndrome by allogenic bone-marrow transplantation, *N Engl J Med* 298:921-927, 1978.

58. Brochstein JA, Gillio AP, Ruggiero M, et al: Marrow transplantation from human leukocyte antigen-identical or haploidentical donors for correction of Wiskott-Aldrich syndrome, *J Pediatr* 119:907-912, 1991.

59. Rumelhart SL, Trigg ME, Horowitz SD, et al: Monoclonal antibody T cell depleted HLA-haploidentical bone marrow transplantation for Wiskott-Aldrich syndrome, *Blood* 75:1031-1035, 1990.

60. Mullen CA, Anderson KD, Blaese RM: Splenectomy and/or bone marrow transplantation in the management of the Wiskott-Aldrich syndrome: long-term follow-up of 62 cases, *Blood* 82:2961-2966, 1993.

61. Lenarsky C, Weinberg K, Kohn DB, et al: Unrelated donor bone marrow transplantation for Wiskott-Aldrich syndrome, *Bone Marrow Transplant* 12:145-147, 1993.

62. Filipovich AH, Stone JV, Tomany SC, et al: Impact of donor type on outcome of bone marrow transplantation for Wiskott-Aldrich syndrome: collaborative study of the International Bone Marrow Transplant Registry and the National Marrow Donor Program, *Blood* 97:1598-1603, 2001.

63. Miano M, Porta F, Locatelli F, et al: Unrelated donor marrow transplantation for inborn errors, *Bone Marrow Transplant* 21:S37-S41, 1998.

64. Ozsahin H, Le Deist F, Benkerrou M, et al: Bone marrow transplantation in 26 patients with Wiskott-Aldrich syndrome from a single center, *J Pediatr* 129:238-244, 1996.

65. Knutsen AP, Wall DA: Kinetics of T-cell development of umbilical cord blood transplantation in severe T-cell immunodeficiency disorders, *J Allergy Clin Immunol* 103:823-832, 1999.

66. Gomez L, Le Deist F, Blanche S, et al: Treatment of Omenn syndrome by bone marrow transplantation, *J Pediatr* 127:76-81, 1995.

67. Loechelt BJ, Shapiro RS, Jyonouchi H, et al: Mismatched bone marrow transplantation for Omenn syndrome: a variant of severe combined immunodeficiency, *Bone Marrow Transplant* 16:381-385, 1995.

68. Le Deist F, Blanche S, Keable H: Successful HLA nonidentical bone marrow transplantation in three patients with the leukocyte adhesion deficiency, *Blood* 74:512, 1989.

69. Thomas C, LeDeist F, Cavazzana-Calvo M, et al: Results of allogeneic bone marrow transplantation in patients with leukocyte adhesion deficiency, *Blood* 86:1629-1635, 1995.

70. Canioni D, Patey N, Cuenod B, et al: Major histocompatibility complex class II deficiency needs an early diagnosis: report of a case, *Pediatr Pathol Lab Med* 17:645-651, 1997.

71. Klein C, Cavazzana-Calvo M, Le Deist F, et al: Bone marrow transplantation in major histocompatibility complex class II deficiency: a single center study of 19 patients, *Blood* 85:580-587, 1995.

72. Bonduel M, Pozo A, Zelazko M, et al: Successful related umbilical cord blood transplantation for graft failure following T cell-depleted non-identical bone marrow transplantation in a child with major histocompatibility complex class II deficiency, *Bone Marrow Transplant* 24:437-440, 1999.

73. Haddad E, Le Deist F, Blanche S, et al: Treatment of Chédiak-Higashi syndrome by allogenic bone marrow transplantation: report of 10 cases, *Blood* 85:3328-3333, 1995.

74. Liang JS, Lu MY, Tsai MJ, et al: Bone marrow transplantation from an HLA-matched unrelated donor for treatment of Chédiak-Higashi syndrome, *J Formos Med Assoc* 99:499-502, 2000.

75. Hobbs JR, Monteil M, McCluskey DR, et al: Chronic granulomatous disease 100% corrected by displacement bone marrow transplantation from a volunteer unrelated donor, *Eur J Pediatr* 151:806-810, 1992.

76. Kamani N, August CS, Campbell DE, et al: Marrow transplantation in chronic granulomatous disease: an update, with 6-year follow up, *J Pediatr* 113:697-700, 1988.

77. di Bartolomeo P, Girolamo G, Angrilli P, et al: Reconstitution of normal neutrophil function in chronic granulomatous disease by bone marrow transplantation, *Bone Marrow Transplant* 4:695-700, 1989.

78. Rappeport JM, Newburger PE, Goldblum RM, et al: Allogeneic transplantation for chronic granulomatous disease, *J Pediatr* 101:952-955, 1982.

79. Horwitz ME, Barrett AJ, Brown MR, et al: Treatment of chronic granulomatous disease with nonmyeloablative conditioning and a T-cell-depleted hematopoietic allograft, *N Engl J Med* 344:881-888, 2001.

80. Ozsahin H, von Planta M, Muller I, et al: Successful treatment of invasive aspergillosis in chronic granulomatous disease by bone marrow transplantation, granulocyte colony-stimulating factor-mobilized granulocytes, and liposomal amphotericin-B, *Blood* 92:2719-2724, 1998.

81. Seger RA, Ezekowitz RAB: Treatment of chronic granulomatous disease, *Immunodeficiency* 5:113-130, 1994.

82. Goldsobel AB, Haas A, Stiehm ER: Bone marrow transplantation in DiGeorge syndrome, *J Pediatr* 111:40-44, 1987.

83. Markert ML, Boeck A, Hale LP, et al: Thymus transplantation in complete DiGeorge syndrome, *N Engl J Med* 341:1180-1189, 1999.

84. Thomas C, de Saint Basile G, Le Deist F, et al: Brief report: correction of X-linked hyper-IgM syndrome by allogeneic bone marrow transplantation, *N Engl J Med* 333:426-429, 1995.

85. Scholl PR, O'Gorman MR, Pachman LM, et al: Correction of neutropenia and hypogammaglobulinemia in X-linked hyper-IgM syndrome by allogeneic bone marrow transplantation, *Bone Marrow Transplant* 22:1215-1218, 1998.

86. Fasth A: Bone marrow transplantation for hyper-IgM syndrome, *Immunodeficiency* 4:323, 1993.

87. Duplantier JE, Seyama K, Day NK, et al: Immunologic reconstitution following bone marrow transplantation for X-linked hyper IgM syndrome, *Clin Immunol* 98:313-318, 2001.

88. Khawaja K, Gennery AR, Flood TJ, et al: Bone marrow transplantation for CD40 ligand deficiency: a single centre experience, *Arch Dis Child* 84: 508-511, 2001.

89. Ziegner UH, Ochs HD, Schanen C, et al: Unrelated umbilical cord stem cell transplantation for X-linked immunodeficiencies, *J Pediatr* 138: 570-573, 2001.

90. De Santes KB, Lai SS, Cowan MJ: Haploidentical bone marrow transplants for two patients with reticular dysgenesis, *Bone Marrow Transplant* 17:1171-1173, 1996.

91. Broome CB, Graham ML, Saulsbury FT, et al: Correction of purine nucleoside phosphorylase deficiency by transplantation of allogeneic bone marrow from a sibling, *J Pediatr* 128:373-376, 1996.

92. Carpenter PA, Ziegler JB, Vowels MR: Late diagnosis and correction of purine nucleoside phosphorylase deficiency with allogeneic bone marrow transplantation, *Bone Marrow Transplant* 17:121-124, 1996.

93. Williams LL, Rooney CM, Conley ME, et al: Correction of Duncan's syndrome by allogeneic bone marrow transplantation, *Lancet* 342:587-588, 1993.

94. Gross TG, Filipovich AH, Conley ME, et al: Cure of X-linked lymphoproliferative disease (XLP) with allogeneic hematopoietic stem cell transplantation (HSCT): report from the XLP registry, *Bone Marrow Transplant* 17:741-744, 1996.

95. Pracher E, Panzer-Grumayer ER, Zoubek A, et al: Successful bone marrow transplantation in a boy with X-linked lymphoproliferative syndrome and acute severe infectious mononucleosis, *Bone Marrow Transplant* 13:655-658, 1994.

96. Schneider LC, Berman RS, Shea CR, et al: Bone marrow transplantation (BMT) for the syndrome of pigmentary dilution and lymphohistiocytosis (Griscelli's syndrome), *J Clin Immunol* 10:146-153, 1990.

97. Benkerrou M, Le Deist F, De Villartay JP, et al: Correction of Fas (CD95) deficiency by haploidentical bone marrow transplantation, *Eur J Immunol* 27:2043-2047, 1997.

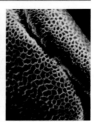

CHAPTER 19

Immunizations

EDINA H. MOYLETT ■ IMELDA CELINE HANSON

The science of vaccinology began in 1796 when Dr. Edward Jenner used material from cowpox lesions to "vaccinate" an 8-year-old boy.[1] The impact of immunization on a global health scale was significantly altered by the work of Salk and Salk[1] and Sabin[2] on inactive and live attenuated polio vaccines, respectively. Universal polio immunization ultimately resulted in the eradication of naturally occurring disease in the United States by 1979 and in the entire western hemisphere by 1991. For many infections (e.g., polio, measles), global disease eradication is now scientifically attainable. In fact, these goals are more dependent on global maintenance of health care delivery system infrastructure and development of mechanisms to limit the use of many infectious diseases in bioterrorism events. For certain important childhood illnesses, adverse events have hampered vaccine development and implementation. An example includes the recent report of intussusception with the Rotavirus quadrivalent vaccine licensed in 1998.[3] Rotavirus continues to be the most common cause of severe gastroenteritis among children worldwide.

In May 1980, the World Health Assembly certified that the world was free of naturally occurring smallpox.[4] Controversy existed regarding the maintenance of laboratory strains of smallpox, and recent political events, most notably U.S. anthrax infection after bioterrorism events,[5] have prompted the possibility of reintroducing routine immunization against smallpox and revisiting current recommendations for anthrax vaccine delivery.[6] The current U.S. childhood immunization schedule recommends that children receive vaccinations against up to 13 different infectious agents from birth to teenage years; the adult schedule recommends additional dosing throughout adult life (dT) and, for special populations, periodic influenza and pneumococcal vaccines.[7] The number of infectious agents to be added to such schedules will depend on scientific advancement and availability of resources for their distribution.

COMPONENTS OF THE IMMUNE RESPONSE

Passive Immunization

Protection against microbial infection may be acquired via passive or active immunization. Examples of passive immunization include the administration of pooled human plasma rich in antibodies directed against a multitude of pathogens. Such products have been formulated and licensed globally for intramuscular immunoglobulin (IG) or intravenous immunoglobulin (IVIG) administration; in addition, product manufacturing may target a specific pathogen, hyperimmune globulin. Historically, IG was used for protection after measles or hepatitis A infection. Intravenous or intramuscular formulations with high titers against certain infections, such as RSV-IVIG (RespiGam), varicella zoster immunoglobulin (VZIG), hepatitis B immunoglobulin (HBIG), and cytomegalovirus-IVIG (CytoGam), have also been used as either preexposure prophylaxis (RespiGam, CytoGam) or after specific infection exposure (HBIG, VZIG, tetanus-IG, and rabies-IG). Passive immunization offers an advantage of immediate acquisition of humoral immunity in the recipient. The disadvantage is that no immune memory is evoked and therefore long-lasting protection is not provided. Additional disadvantages include the potential risk for transmission of blood-borne pathogens, considering the origin of these products. Although modern sterilizing techniques and additional virucidal steps make this unlikely, infectious transmission has been reported often before routine accessibility of serologic testing for a specific pathogen.[8]

In addition to preexposure or postexposure therapy, IG or, more frequently, IVIG has been used to provide humoral immunity to patients with underlying defects in antibody production or infection, such as severe combined immunodeficiency, common variable immunodeficiency, or specific antibody deficiency states. Higher doses of IVIG (2 g/kg) have been reported as efficacious when used as immune-modulating therapy for patients with certain autoimmune or inflammatory conditions.[9]

Passive immunization has also been used as antitoxin therapy of equine or human origin to treat diphtheria, tetanus, and botulinum infection. Antitoxins immediately neutralize circulating toxins, allowing the adaptive arm of the immune system a chance to provide antigen-specific neutralizing antibodies. Stringent guidelines are linked to the administration of equine antiserum therapy to minimize the risk of associated serum sickness.

Active Immunization

Active immunization depends on an antigenic vaccine and an intact immune system in the recipient for optimal efficacy. Box 19-1 outlines those requirements that are necessary for optimal vaccine development. Many different antigenic vaccine components exist; each is discussed here.

KEY CONCEPTS

Features of an Effective Vaccine

Safety
- Does not cause infection in the recipient

Protective
- Must protect against illness resulting from exposure to the live pathogen
- Protection should be long-lasting or preferably lifelong

Induction of an immune response
- Neutralizing antibody should be generated to defend the vaccine recipient against invading pathogens
- Cellular response should be produced if defense is required against intracellular or viral pathogens

Practical considerations
- Acceptable side effect profile
- Low cost of production
- Ease of storage
- Ability to produce large quantities
- Ease of administration

Vaccine Types

Table 19-1 outlines vaccines that are suggested by the Advisory Committee for Immunization Practices and the American Academy of Family Physicians for routine delivery to children and adults in the United States.[7,10] Many more vaccines, providing protection to 25 organisms, are licensed in the United States and are recommended in specific clinical settings. Vaccine types vary and include attenuated live viral or bacterial vaccines, killed (subunit, toxoid, or conjugate) vaccines, and recombinant, DNA, or vector vaccines. Each of these uses varying methods of promoting an immune response.

Killed or Inactivated Vaccines. A killed or inactivated vaccine consists of an inactive preparation of the pathogen eliminating the chance of reversion to the "infectious" wild type. Traditionally, chemicals such as formalin used in the deactivation process do not alter determinants of antigenicity, permitting an immune response to develop. Pathogens have been adapted using various methods, including whole-organism inactivation (e.g., cholera and pertussis vaccine), exotoxin detoxification (e.g., diphtheria and tetanus toxoid vaccines), use of soluble capsular material either alone (e.g., pneumococcal polysaccharide vaccine) or covalently linked to carrier proteins (e.g., *Haemophilus influenzae* type B conjugate vaccines), and use of purified extracts of components of the organism (e.g., subunit influenza and acellular pertussis vaccines). Immunity occurring after the administration of inactivated vaccines is typically humoral, and efficacy is measured by postimmunization neutralizing antibody levels. Neutralizing antibodies (IgG) produced on reexposure to the immunizing antigen result from the rapid expansion of memory B cells and provide infection control. Inability of a killed vaccine component to replicate in the host minimizes triggering the arm of the immune system responsible for eliciting cytotoxic cellular responses, thus limiting development of a cellular response. In addition, the absence of replication limits

mucosal surface secretory IgA production. This limits the efficacy of a killed or inactivated vaccine against pathogens whose transmission occurs across mucosal barriers where IgA plays a significant role in host defense. Increased safety is an obvious feature of killed vaccines. However, lifelong protection is not inferred after inactivated vaccine administration, necessitating repeat or "booster" doses.

Conjugate Vaccines. Many polysaccharide-encapsulated bacteria, including *Haemophilus* spp. and *Streptococcus pneumoniae,* are of particular pathogenic importance in children younger than 2 years. The most effective defense against these microorganisms is opsonization of the polysaccharide coat with antibody. The most effective vaccine would elicit antibodies against the polysaccharide capsule of the bacteria. Polysaccharide antigens mount a T cell–independent immune response, resulting in low-affinity, high-avidity IgM production. The response to polysaccharide antigens is most inefficient in infants, who have high morbidity from such pathogens because of the immaturity of their immune system. To augment this suboptimal infant immune response, *Haemophilus* spp. and *S. pneumoniae* antigens have successfully been conjugated to carrier proteins to which the immune system has already been exposed (e.g., tetanus and diphtheria toxoids). The subsequent immune response is T cell dependent and invokes generation of immunologic memory. Conjugated *H. influenzae* B vaccines, licensed since 1987, have resulted in a dramatic reduction in severe pediatric morbidity due to this organism.[11] A heptavalent pneumococcal conjugate vaccine, licensed for use in 2000, has also impacted disease prevalence of acute otitis media in children.[12]

Subunit Vaccines. Subunit vaccines often involve the use of recombinant DNA technology to augment immunogenicity. As an example, the currently available subunit hepatitis B vaccine clones the hepatitis B surface antigen (HBsAg) gene into yeast, yielding synthesis of HBsAg within the yeast cell.[13] Similar recombinant DNA technology has been applied in the commercially available Lyme vaccine.[14] The immunogenicity of peptide vaccines may also be augmented through the formation of aggregates such as immunostimulating complexes, virus-like particles, antigen-coated beads, and lipid-encapsulating antigen.

Live-Attenuated Vaccines. Live-attenuated vaccines meet the criteria for eliciting a complete immune response because they induce limited viral replication of adequate amplitude to elicit a protective immune response without resulting in significant clinical infection. The majority of antiviral vaccines currently licensed for use in the United States are live-attenuated vaccines. Attenuation is usually achieved by viral passage in nonhuman cell lines. Virus strains selected for use in attenuated vaccines are chosen for their instability or growth limitations in human cells. Attenuation may also be achieved by passage of a virus through conditions (temperature, pH, etc.) not favorable for replication in normal human hosts. An example is the not yet licensed intranasal cold-adapted influenza virus vaccine[15] that has been documented as safe and efficacious in clinical trials to date.[16] Because live-attenuated vaccines mimic natural infection, the immune response achieved is usually lifelong, eliminating the need for booster series. Moreover, mucosal immunity and cellular

TABLE 19-1 Recommended and Minimum Ages and Intervals between Vaccine Doses for Children[a]

Vaccine	Recommended Age for This Dose	Minimum Interval to Next Dose
Hepatitis B1[b]	Birth to 2 mo	4 wk
Hepatitis B2	1-4 mo	8 wk
Hepatitis B3[c]	6-18 mo	—
Diphtheria and tetanus toxoids and acellular pertussis (DTaP)1	2 mo	4 wk
DTaP2	4 mo	4 wk
DTaP3	6 mo	6 mo[d,e]
DTaP4	15-18 mo	6 mo[d]
DTaP5	4-6 yr	—
Haemophilus influenzae type b (Hib)1[f]	2 mo	4 wk
Hib2	4 mo	4 wk
Hib3[g]	6 mo	8 wk
Hib4	12-15 mo	—
Inactivated poliovirus vaccine (IPV)1	2 mo	4 wk
IPV2	4 mo	4 wk
IPV3	6-18 mo	4 wk
IPV4	4-6 yr	—
Pneumococcal conjugate vaccine (PCV)1[h]	2 mo	4 wk
PCV2	4 mo	4 wk
PCV3	6 mo	8 wk
PCV4	12-15 mo	—
Measles, mumps, and rubella (MMR)1	12-15 mo[i]	4 wk
MMR2	4-6 yr	—
Varicella[j]	12-15 mo	4 wk[j]
Hepatitis A1	≥ 2 yr	6 mo[d]
Hepatitis A2	≥ 30 mo	—
Influenza[k]	—	4 wk
Pneumococcal polysaccharide (PPV)	—	5 yr
PPV2	—	—

Modified from Atkinson WL, Pickering LK, Schwartz B, et al: *MMWR CDC Surveill Summ* 51:1-35, 2002.

[a]Combination vaccines are available. The use of licensed combination vaccines is preferred to separate injections of their equivalent component vaccines. When administering combination vaccines, the minimum age for administration is the oldest age for any of the individual components; the minimum interval between doses is equal to the greatest interval of any of the individual antigens. (From Centers for Disease Control and Prevention: *MMWR Morb Mortal Wkly Rep* 48:5, 1999.)

[b]A combination hepatitis B–Hib vaccine is available (Comvax, manufactured by Merck Vaccine Division). This vaccine should not be administered to infants younger than 6 weeks because of the Hib component.

[c]Hepatitis B3 should be administered ≥ 8 weeks after hepatitis B2 and 16 weeks after hepatitis B1, and it should not be administered before age 6 months.

[d]Calendar months.

[e]The minimum interval between DTaP3 and DTaP4 is recommended to be ≥ 6 months. However, DTaP4 does not need to be repeated if administered ≥ 4 months after DTaP3.

[f]Second doses of PPV are recommended for persons at highest risk for serious pneumococcal infection and those who are likely to have a rapid decline in pneumococcal antibody concentration. Revaccination 3 years after the previous dose can be considered for children at highest risk for severe pneumococcal infection who would be younger than 10 years at the time of revaccination. (See Centers for Disease Control and Prevention: *MMWR Morb Mortal Wkly Rep* 46:1-24, 1997.)

[g]For a regimen of only polyribosylribitol phosphate-meningococcal outer membrane protein (PRP-OMP, PedvaxHib, manufactured by Merck), a dose administered at age 6 months is not required.

[h]For Hib and PCV, children receiving the first dose of vaccine at age ≥ 7 months require fewer doses to complete the series. (See Centers for Disease Control and Prevention: *MMWR Morb Mortal Wkly Rep* 40:1-7, 1991 and Centers for Disease Control and Prevention: *MMWR Morb Mortal Wkly Rep* 49:1-35, 2000.)

[i]During a measles outbreak, if cases are occurring among infants younger than 12 months, measles vaccination of infants aged ≥ 6 months can be undertaken as an outbreak control measure. However, doses administered at younger than 12 months should not be counted as part of the series. (From Centers for Disease Control and Prevention: *MMWR Morb Mortal Wkly Rep* 47:1-57, 1998.)

[j]Children aged 12 months to 13 years require only one dose of varicella vaccine. Persons aged ≥ 13 years should receive two doses separated by ≥ 4 weeks.

[k]Two doses of inactivated influenza vaccine, separated by 4 weeks, are recommended for children aged 6 months to 9 years who are receiving the vaccine for the first time. Children aged 6 months to 9 years who have previously received influenza vaccine and persons aged ≥ 9 years require only one dose per influenza season.

responses can be achieved, improving immunity against natural infection.

Live-attenuated vaccines may pose risks for immunocompromised hosts, in whom they may behave as virulent opportunistic pathogens. An example includes virus-associated paralytic poliomyelitis (VAPP), which occurs when the live-attenuated oral poliovirus vaccine (OPV) is administered to an immunocompromised patient or to a contact of an immunocompromised patient.[17] In VAPP, vaccine virus strains replicate in the gut unchecked and may revert to the wild type

with disastrous consequences. All live-attenuated vaccines are associated with a risk for reversion to the wild type and ensuing dissemination, especially in the immunocompromised setting.

DNA Vaccines. DNA-based vaccination uses a novel technique to efficiently stimulate humoral and cellular immune responses to protein antigens. DNA that encodes foreign antigens may be incorporated into plasmids or vectors.[18] In animal models, plasmid-coated beads have been blasted across the skin by means of a gene gun and are then taken up by dendritic cells with a strong resultant T-helper cell response and subsequent antibody production. Attenuated viruses or bacteria may be used as vectors containing DNA-encoding antigen from another infectious agent. The DNA contained in the vector codes for important T and B cell epitopes with resultant cellular and humoral immune responses. Leading candidate virus vectors include poxviruses (e.g., vaccinia, fowlpox, and canarypox) that have the ability to replicate but not infect human cells. Possible adverse events subsequent to DNA vaccination include the formation of anti-DNA antibodies, unexpected consequences of persistent expression of foreign antigen, and the potential for a transformational event.

Peptide Vaccines. Peptides representing part of an antigen may be used as a vaccine. The advantages of such peptides are that the product is chemically defined, stable, and safe and contains only important B and T cell epitopes. However, it is difficult to replicate exact immunogenic epitopes. Also, peptides are subject to proteolysis and poorly elicit both humoral and cellular responses. *In vivo* processing through natural antigen-processing pathways may be achieved by conjugating peptides with protein carriers or viral vectors. In addition, adjuvants such as lipid carriers load peptides into the host cell cytoplasm, allowing major histocompatibility complex class I restricted T cell responses to occur. Peptide vaccines have revolutionized the field of tumor immunogenetics.[19]

Adjuvants. A vaccine is only as successful as the quality of the immune response it stimulates. Certain antigens, namely peptides and polysaccharides, are poorly immunogenic. In addition, host factors such as extremes of age and poor nutritional status reduce immunogenicity for all, and specifically peptide and polysaccharide antigen, vaccines. Substances that improve the immunogenicity of antigens mixed with it have been defined as adjuvants. The use of adjuvants to enhance vaccine immunogenicity was introduced in the 1920s.[20] Despite extensive research, to date only aluminum-containing compounds (e.g., alum, aluminum hydroxide, and aluminum phosphate) are approved for use in humans. Adjuvants alter the immune response to antigen in a myriad of ways.[21-23] Of the proposed activities of adjuvants, two of the more important immune-modulating functions include (1) conversion of soluble proteins into particulate matter that is more easily ingested by antigen-presenting cells and (2) signal induction by microbial constituents of macrophages or dendritic cells to become more efficient at antigen presentation.

PRINCIPLES OF DISEASE MECHANISM

Both adult and childhood schedules for the delivery of developed immunizations exist to minimize morbidity of pathogens to differing age groups. Caveats for vaccine delivery are outlined for those at greatest risk of adverse events or for those for whom safety data do not adequately exist, such as pregnant women.

Childhood Schedules

The childhood vaccination schedule is published annually by the Advisory Committee on Immunization Practices, the American Academy of Family Physicians, and the American Academy of Pediatrics. The schedule includes delivery of the first doses of a single antigen (hepatitis B) at birth to 2 months, six vaccine antigens (diphtheria, tetanus, pertussis, *H. influenzae* type B, polio, and seven serotypes of *S. pneumoniae*) at 2 months, and four vaccine antigens (measles, mumps, rubella, and varicella) at 12 to 15 months of age. Initial vaccination for each of these antigens requires subsequent booster doses (see Table 19-1) to provide optimal production of neutralizing antibody in the recipient. Hepatitis A vaccine is recommended for children older than 2 years living in endemic areas of the United States; influenza vaccine is currently recommended for children 6 months of age and older with chronic diseases, such as chronic lung disease. In the future, recommendations for childhood delivery of influenza vaccine, like guidelines for adults, will be suggested for children 6 to 35 months old, who are reported in the literature to have the highest morbidity from influenza disease.[24,25] Strategies to enhance delivery of all recommended dosing includes taking advantage of all missed opportunities and offering an accelerated schedule for infants and children who could not meet the outlined dosing schedules. Table 19-1 provides minimal dosing intervals for each vaccine.

Multiple manufacturers provide varying formulations (antigen quantity and processing/preparation methodology) of the vaccines outlined in the U.S. childhood schedule. Interchangeability of vaccines has been documented for some but not all vaccine antigens. Data support the interchangeability of *H. influenzae* type B, hepatitis A, and hepatitis B vaccines.[26] In contrast, the literature does not completely support interchangeability of vaccines containing acellular pertussis antigen.

Adult Schedule

Certain vaccines should be kept updated in the adult population. Persons aged 65 years or older and all adults with underlying medical conditions that place them at increased risk for pneumococcal infection should receive at least one dose of the 23-valent pneumococcal vaccine. Similarly, all persons 50 years old or older should receive an annual influenza immunization, as should all adults with underlying medical conditions that place them at an increased risk for severe influenza infection.[27] Booster immunizations with tetanus and diphtheria toxoids (Tds) should be administered every 10 years after completion of the primary series. All adults born after 1956 should have received at least one dose of the measles, mumps, and rubella (MMR) vaccine or have other evidence of immunity. All other adults born after 1956 at increased risk for measles transmission (e.g., health care employees, college students, and those traveling to endemic areas) should have documentation of receipt of two doses of MMR on or after their first birthday or other evidence of immunity. Immunization against hepatitis A and B, as well as the recently licensed Lyme disease vaccine,[28] is recommended for those adults at increased risk for disease transmission or acquisition.

Special Populations/Conditions

Immunocompromised
Live-attenuated vaccines (viral and bacterial) are generally not administered to individuals with primary immunodeficiency syndromes who may have specific risks[29,30] or have acquired or

secondary immunodeficiencies. However, as with every rule in medicine, caveats exist. All live viral vaccines are contraindicated for patients with severely impaired cellular immunity, but individuals with hypogammaglobulinemia or dysgammaglobulinemia may receive varicella vaccine[31] and measles vaccine. In contrast, OPV should not be administered to any patient with impaired humoral immunity. Inactivated vaccines may be administered without adverse effects to patients with impaired immunity, although response may be suboptimal.

Recommendations for live-attenuated vaccine delivery to human immunodeficiency virus (HIV)–infected individuals vary according to the antigen considered. Given the severity of natural measles or varicella disease among HIV-infected patients, both live-attenuated vaccines are recommended for HIV-infected patients without evidence of immunocompromise (Centers for Disease Control and Prevention [CDC] class N1 or A1, age-specific CD4+ lymphocyte is 25%).[32,33]

Despite recent advances in immune reconstitution of patients with severe inherited immune defects, insufficient data exist regarding general recommendations for administration of live-attenuated vaccines to these immune-restored individuals. No vaccine contraindications exist for primary complement deficiencies; patients with phagocyte defects should not receive live bacterial vaccines.

Pregnancy

Vaccine delivery during pregnancy is generally considered a contraindication, or precautions are suggested for some vaccines. In general, live-attenuated vaccines are contraindicated during pregnancy because of a theoretical risk to the fetus. The potential for risk is not always realized; a recent report evaluated inadvertent administration of varicella virus vaccine to 58 women during the first and second trimesters of pregnancy with no reports of congenital varicella in 56 live births.[34] Although limited by number, this report identifies that theoretical risk in pregnancy is not always substantiated in the literature. Accidental administration of MMR or varicella virus vaccine during pregnancy should not be considered as an indication for termination. In contrast, indications for delivery of the live-attenuated yellow fever vaccine should be balanced against the infectious risk to the fetus for pregnant women traveling to a yellow fever–endemic area. Risk to the fetus or mother after immunization with inactivated viral or bacterial vaccines, or toxoids is not described in the literature; administration of these vaccines is often indicated (Td, influenza vaccine after 14 weeks' gestation for pregnancies during influenza season, etc.).[35]

Health Care Workers

Health care workers may have an increased risk for acquisition and transmission of infectious agents, especially blood-borne pathogens. Vaccine-preventable infections of special concern to those involved in health care delivery and especially pediatric practice include measles, mumps, rubella, hepatitis B, and varicella. Immunity to the latter infections should be documented before initiating employment in the health care setting and is often mandated. Annual influenza immunization should be offered to all health care workers. In certain settings, health care workers may be a source for or exposed to *Mycobacterium tuberculosis* and should therefore be tested annually.

Travel

For entry into certain countries, vaccinations may be recommended for foreign visitors, depending on the travel destination, exposure risk during travel, and length of travel. Information about international infectious disease outbreaks, vaccinations, and precautions for special populations can be found at the CDC National Center for Infectious Diseases Traveler's Health website (www.cdc.gov/travel).

Recent bioterrorism events have prompted review of the current recommendations for delivery of vaccines (anthrax, variola virus, *Yersiniae pestis*) whose distributions have been linked to specific indications. Infectious agents with potential for mass destruction include *Bacillus anthracis*, *Y. pestis*, *Francisella tularensis*, botulinum toxin, hemorrhagic fever viruses, and multidrug-resistant *M. tuberculosis*. CDC guidelines address the release of smallpox vaccine in the event of bioterrorism[36]; updated recommendations are available at the Infectious Disease Society of America (IDSA) website (www.idsociety.org). Current CDC recommendations (October 2002) suggest that in the absence of naturally occurring smallpox, the general public should not be vaccinated before an attack. However, because of imminent licensure of smallpox vaccine and vaccination of military personnel in the United States, pre-event immunization vaccination is suggested for public health outbreak investigation teams and health care workers (an estimated 500,000 individuals), who are likely to provide emergency services to postevent smallpox patients. Preexposure immunization with anthrax vaccine is licensed for individuals aged 18 to 65 years who have a high likelihood of contact with *B. anthracis* (e.g., laboratory personnel and abattoir workers); complete immunization guidelines are available from the CDC.[6]

ADVERSE EVENTS

The administration of any vaccine is associated with a risk for an adverse event. Common adverse events include erythema or pain at injection sites or generalized nonspecific symptoms such as malaise, irritability, and temperature elevation. Other specific adverse events causally linked to specific immunizations include anaphylaxis to vaccine components or stabilizing agents. Examples of such reactions include tetanus toxoid anaphylaxis, gelatin anaphylaxis in MMR,[37] and anaphylaxis to antibiotics (neomycin, streptomycin, polymyxin B, and others) used in specific vaccines.[38] Previously held theories that egg sensitivity predicted anaphylaxis to egg-containing vaccines like MMR, influenza, and yellow fever vaccine have been challenged by the reported observation that early sensitization may occur with gelatin-containing vaccines commonly delivered in the U.S. childhood vaccine schedule, such as acellular diphtheria-tetanus-pertussis (DTaP) vaccines.[39] Current vaccine delivery practice does not include avoidance of MMR for egg-sensitive individuals.[40]

Other possible causal associations for adverse events (multiple sclerosis from hepatitis B vaccine, inflammatory bowel disease and pervasive developmental disorder/autism from measles vaccine) have been purported after vaccine delivery but are refuted by careful, separate epidemiologic review including Institute of Medicine evaluations.[41-43] The U.S. Food and Drug Administration (FDA) licensed the first vaccine against Rotavirus in 1998, and 14 months later the vaccine was withdrawn after an association with intussusception was described.[44] Retrospective studies have failed to highlight a link between natural rotavirus infection and a risk for intussusception,[45] implicating the possibility of animal components used in the rotavirus vaccine as a cause for such complications.

Theoretical risks related to vaccine delivery have also been raised. Thimerosal, a mercury-containing preservative, has long been used as an additive in biologics and vaccines because of its ability to prevent bacterial and fungal contamination, particularly in multidose containers. Thimerosal is used as a preservative in the Hib, DTaP, and hepatitis B childhood vaccines. The Committee on Environmental Health of the American Academy of Pediatrics has outlined the forms of mercury that cause exposure to humans, the impact of that exposure on the fetus and young infants, environmental sources, potential for toxicity, and treatment options after exposure.[46] Anxiety among parents and caregivers concerning the risk of administering multiple mercury-containing vaccines prompted the development of thimerosal-free vaccines.[47]

Reporting of vaccine-related adverse events is encouraged through a passive surveillance system that is intended to capture rare reactions, delayed reactions, or reactions not detected in stringent pre- or post-FDA licensing studies. The Vaccine Adverse Event Reporting System (VAERS) is a spontaneous reporting system that addresses postlicensure vaccine safety. VAERS, jointly administered by the CDC and FDA, was created in 1990 to provide a standardized national method for the collection of all reports of clinically significant adverse events. The National Childhood Vaccine Injury Act of 1996 mandates that health care workers who administer vaccines and manufacturers of vaccines report certain adverse health effects that are linked to receipt of a vaccine to the VAERS system (1-800-822-7967).

CONCLUSIONS

Novel vaccine approaches (DNA and peptide vaccines) promise the potential for global reduction in infectious disease morbidity and/or sequelae in the twenty-first century. Continued developmental direction for vaccinology includes improving immunogenicity, thus limiting the necessity for booster doses, and improving safety, thus limiting adverse events. In addition to a scientific challenge for safe/immunogenic vaccine development, novel approaches will be necessary to adequately deliver these newer vaccines to populations at highest risk and thus the greatest need.

HELPFUL WEBSITES

Advisory Committee on Immunization Practices website (www.cdc.bov/nip/acip)
American Academy of Pediatrics website (www.aap.org)
American Academy of Family Physicians website (www.aafp.org)

REFERENCES

1. Salk J, Salk D: Control of influenza and poliomyelitis with killed virus vaccines, *Science* 195:834-847, 1977.
2. Sabin AB: Oral poliovirus vaccine. History of its development and prospects for eradication of poliomyelitis, *JAMA* 194:872-876, 1965.
3. Centers for Disease Control and Prevention: Intussusception among recipients of Rotavirus vaccine—United States, 1998-1999, *JAMA* 282:520-521, 1999.
4. World Health Organization: Declaration of global eradication of smallpox, *Wkly Epidemiol Rec* 55:145-152, 1980.
5. Centers for Disease Control and Prevention: Recognition of illness associated with the intentional release of a biologic agent, *MMWR Morb Mortal Wkly Rep* 50:893-897, 2001.
6. Centers for Disease Control and Prevention: Use of anthrax vaccine in the United States: recommendations of the Advisory Committee on Immunization Practices, *MMWR Morb Mortal Wkly Rep* 40:1-20, 2000.
7. Atkinson WL, Pickering LK, Schwartz B, et al: General recommendations on immunization. Recommendations of the Advisory Committee on Immunization Practices (ACIP) and the American Academy of Family Physicians (AAFP), *MMWR CDC Surveill Summ* 51:1-35, 2002.
8. Christie JM, Healey CJ, Watson J, et al: Clinical outcome of hypogammaglobulinemia patients following outbreak of acute hepatitis C: 2 yr follow-up, *Clin Exp Immunol* 110:4-8, 1997.
9. Tse SM, Silverman ED, McCrindle BW, et al: Early treatment with intravenous immunoglobulin in patients with Kawasaki disease, *J Pediatr* 140:450-455, 2002.
10. Ada G: Vaccines and vaccination, *N Engl J Med* 345:1042-1053, 2001.
11. Adams WG, Deaver KA, Cochi SL, et al: Decline of childhood *Haemophilus influenzae* type b (Hib) disease in the Hib vaccine era, *JAMA* 269:221-226, 1993.
12. Eskola J, Kilpi T, Palmu A, et al: Finnish Otitis Media Study Group. Efficacy of a pneumococcal conjugate vaccine against acute otitis media, *N Engl J Med* 344:403-409, 2001.
13. Wampler DE, Lehman ED, Boger J, et al: Multiple chemical forms of hepatitis B surface antigen produced in yeast, *Proc Natl Acad Sci U S A* 82:6830-6834, 1985.
14. Sikand VK, Halsey N, Krause PJ, et al: Pediatric Lyme Vaccine Study Group. Safety and immunogenicity of a recombinant *Borrelia burgdorferi* outer surface protein A vaccine against Lyme disease in healthy children and adolescents: a randomized controlled trial, *Pediatrics* 108:123-128, 2001.
15. Herlocher ML, Maassab HF, Webster RG: Molecular and biological changes in the cold-adapted "master strain" A/AA/6/60 (H2N2) influenza virus, *Proc Natl Acad Sci U S A* 90:6032-6036, 1993.
16. Belshe RB, Mendelman PM, Treanor J, et al: The efficacy of live attenuated, cold-adapted, trivalent, intranasal influenza virus vaccine in children, *N Engl J Med* 338:1405-1412, 1998.
17. Centers for Disease Control and Prevention: Prolonged poliovirus excretion in an immunodeficient person with vaccine-associated paralytic poliomyelitis, *MMWR Morb Mortal Wkly Rep* 46:641-643, 1997.
18. Gregersen JP: DNA vaccines, *Naturwissenschaften* 88:504-513, 2001.
19. Watanabe T, Watanabe S, Neumann G, et al: Immunogenicity and protective efficacy of replication-incompetent influenza virus-like particles, *J Virol* 76:767-773, 2002.
20. Weber J: Peptide vaccines for cancer, *Naturwissenschaften* 88:504-513, 2001.
21. Glenny AT, Pope CG, Waddington H, et al: Immunological notes, *J Pathol Bacteriol* 29:31, 1926.
22. Hem SL, White JL: Structure and properties of aluminum-containing adjuvants, *Pharm Biotechnol* 6:249-279, 1995.
23. Sun S, Kishimoto H, Sprent J: DNA as an adjuvant: capacity of insect DNA and synthetic oligodeoxynucleotides to augment T cell responses to specific antigen, *J Exp Med* 187:1145-1150, 1998.
24. Izurieta HS, Thompson WW, Dramarz P, et al: Influenza and the rates of hospitalization for respiratory disease among infants and young children, *N Engl J Med* 342:232-239, 2000.
25. Neuzil KM, Zhu Y, Griffin MR, et al: Burden of interpandemic influenza in children younger than 4 years: a 25-year prospective study, *J Infect Dis* 185:147-152, 2002.
26. Anderson EL, Decker MD, Englund JA, et al: Interchangeability of conjugated *Haemophilus influenzae* type B vaccines in infants, *JAMA* 273:849-853, 1995.
27. Bridges CB, Fukuda K, Uyeki TM, et al: Centers for Disease Control and Prevention, Advisory Committee on Immunization Practices. Prevention and control of influenza. Recommendations of the Advisory Committee on Immunization Practices (ACIP), *MMWR Recomm Rep* 51:1-31, 2002.
28. Steere AC, Sikand VK, Meurice F, et al: Vaccination against Lyme disease with recombinant *Borrelia burgdorferi* outer-surface lipoprotein A with adjuvant. Lyme Disease Vaccine Study Group, *N Engl J Med* 339:209-215, 1998.

29. Pohl KR, Farley JD, Jan JE, et al: Ataxia-telangiectasia in a child with vaccine-associated paralytic poliomyelitis, *J Pediatr* 121:405-407, 1992.

30. Inaba H, Hori H, Ito M, et al: Polio vaccine virus-associated meningoencephalitis in an infant with transient hypogammaglobulinemia, *Scand J Infect Dis* 33:630-631, 2001.

31. Centers for Disease Control and Prevention: Prevention of varicella. Updated Recommendations of the Advisory Committee on Immunization Practices (ACIP), *MMWR Morb Mortal Wkly Rep* 48:1-5, 1999.

32. American Academy of Pediatrics Committee on Infectious Diseases: Varicella vaccine update, *Pediatrics* 105:136-141, 2000.

33. Levin MJ, Gershon AA, Weinberg A, et al: AIDS Clinical Trials Group 265 team: immunization of HIV-infected children with varicella vaccine, *J Pediatr* 139:305-310, 2001.

34. Shields KE, Galil K, Seward J, et al: Varicella vaccine exposure during pregnancy: data from the first 5 years of the pregnancy registry, *Obstet Gynecol* 98:14-19, 2001.

35. Glezen WP: Maternal vaccines, *Prim Care* 28:791-806, 2001.

36. Centers for Disease Control and Prevention: Vaccinia (smallpox) vaccine recommendations of the Advisory Committee on Immunization Practices (ACIP), 2001, *MMWR Recomm Rep* 50:1-25, 2001.

37. Patja A, Makinen-Kiljunen S, Davidkin I, et al: Allergic reactions to measles-mumps-rubella vaccination, *Pediatrics* 107:E27, 2001.

38. Georgitis JW, Fasano MB: Allergenic components of vaccines and avoidance of vaccination-related adverse events, *Curr Allergy Rep* 1:11-17, 2001.

39. Nakayama T, Aizawa C, Kuno-Sakai H: A clinical analysis of gelatin allergy and determination of its causal relationship to the previous administration of gelatin-containing acellular pertussis vaccine combined with diphtheria and tetanus toxoids, *J Allergy Clin Immunol* 103:200-202, 1999.

40. James JM, Burks AW, Roberson PH, et al: Safe administration of the measles vaccine to children allergic to eggs, *N Engl J Med* 332:1262-1266, 1995.

41. Marwick C: US report finds no link between MMR and autism, *Br Med J* 322:1083, 2001.

42. Farrington CP, Miller E, Taylor B: MMR and autism: further evidence against a causal association, *Vaccine* 19:3632-3635, 2001.

43. Ascherio A, Zhang SM, Hernan MA, et al: Hepatitis B vaccination and the risk of multiple sclerosis, *N Engl J Med* 344:327-332, 2002.

44. Centers for Disease Control and Prevention: Withdrawal of Rotavirus vaccine recommendation, *MMWR Morb Mortal Wkly Rep* 48:1007, 1999.

45. Chang EJ, Zangwill KM, Lee H, et al: Lack of association between Rotavirus infection and intussusception: implications for use of attenuated Rotavirus vaccines, *Pediatr Infect Dis* 21:97-102, 2002.

46. Goldman LR, Shannon MW, American Academy of Pediatrics Committee on Environmental Health: Technical report: mercury in the environment: implications for pediatricians, *Pediatrics* 108:197-205, 2001.

47. Centers for Disease Control and Prevention: Recommendations regarding the use of vaccines that contain thimerosal as a preservative, *MMWR Recomm Rep* 48:996-998, 1999.

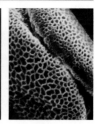

CHAPTER **20**

Gene Therapy and Allergy

CATHERINE M. BOLLARD ■ MALCOLM K. BRENNER

When investigators first considered using gene therapy to treat human disease, it was assumed that monogenic disorders would be the target, with the intent of restoring a functional gene to a defective cell. Moreover, because of the unknown risks of this novel therapeutic approach, these disorders had to be both immediately life-threatening and lacking in safe, effective alternative treatments. Allergic disorders do not meet these guidelines. Although a strong genetic component is doubtlessly present, allergic diseases are a complex, heterogeneous group of maladies with an equally complex and heterogeneous polygenic basis. Also, although allergic responses certainly can be fatal, the great majority of patients live with, rather than die from, their conditions, and it has been difficult to identify subgroups who might justifiably be exposed to the unknown risks of gene therapy. Gradually, however, these requirements have become less rigid. It has become appreciated that gene therapy may be of considerable value even for the treatment of complex genetic disorders. Cancer, for example, is a complex (albeit acquired) genetic disorder and yet represents by far the most common clinical setting for trials of gene transfer. In terms of safety, investigators have become reassured that gene therapy generally carries no untoward or unforeseen risks beyond those to be considered for any new therapy. Although there has been one well-publicized death attributed to administration of an adenoviral vector and a second patient has developed leukemia associated with retrovirus-mediated gene transfer for correction of immunodeficiency, it is important to appreciate that several thousand other patients have received treatment with gene transfer vectors or gene modified cells, apparently without associated severe toxicity or mortality.

For these reasons, serious consideration of gene therapy approaches to the treatment of allergic disorders is now justified. Because this proposed application represents an embryonic usage for a field that is itself in a highly rudimentary stage of development, the major purpose of this chapter is to explain the principles of gene therapy and to illustrate what it can and cannot do. We will show how it may be possible to use gene transfer either directly as therapy for allergic disorders or as a tool to validate target molecules and pathways whose function may later be modified by more conventional therapies. The examples and suggestions made here will be backed, where possible, by published experimental data. However, because this chapter is intended to be provocative and not just didactic, some unsupported speculation remains.

VECTORS

A prerequisite for any gene therapy approach is the ability to transduce the desired target cell. Several viral and nonviral gene transfer systems have entered or are about to enter clinical practice, and they are summarized in Box 20-1 and discussed later in more detail.[1-5] Each of these systems has its advantages and disadvantages, but none yet possess the generally desirable characteristics of high transduction efficiency, specific cell targeting, and high levels of gene expression. For many gene therapy approaches, including those intended to modulate the immune response to allergens, it would also be useful to control the transgene product. Although several different regulatory systems have been described and tested successfully in animal models,[6,7] none have yet been established to be safe and effective in humans.

Because no available vector systems yet come close to meeting the requirements for a truly effective agent, the choice has to be based on the "least bad" or best available alternative for the specific application proposed.

Viral Vectors

Murine Retroviral Based

Murine retroviruses, particularly the Moloney murine leukemia virus (MoMuLV), are vectors that are capable of integrating into host cell DNA. This capacity has lead to their extensive use in clinical settings where the target cell will undergo extensive division because a copy of the transgene will appear in every daughter cell. These clinical applications have included gene marking studies and the correction of severe combined immunodeficiency (SCID) syndromes.[8-11] MoMuLVs are single-stranded, enveloped RNA viruses that are transcribed by reverse transcriptase into double-stranded DNA. In a clinical vector the packaging signal and long terminal repeats (LTRs) are retained, whereas the structural and replicative genes (*gag, pol,* and *env*) of the wild type retrovirus are replaced by one or more genes of interest, driven either by the retroviral promoter in the 5 LTR or by an internal promoter. The retroviral constructs are made in cell lines in which the missing retrovirus genes are present *in trans* and thus reproduce and package a vector that is not replication competent. After production of viral particles and infection of target cells, the vector is uncoated in the cytosol and the RNA is transcribed via reverse transcriptase into DNA, which

KEY CONCEPTS

Advantages and Disadvantages of Vector Systems

Vector	Advantages	Disadvantages	Current uses
■ Murine retrovirus	■ Stable integration into dividing cells ■ Minimal immunogenicity ■ Stable packaging system	■ Low titer ■ Only integrates in dividing cells ■ Limited insertion size ■ Risk of silencing ■ Risk of insertional mutagenesis	■ Marker studies ■ Gene therapy approaches using hemopoietic stem cells or T cells (e.g., to treat immunodeficiency syndromes) ■ Transduction tumor cell lines
■ Lentivirus	■ Integrates into dividing cells ■ Expressed in nondividing cells ■ Larger insertion size than murine retroviruses	■ No stable packaging system ■ Complex safety issues	■ No approved trials as yet
■ Self-inactivating lentiviral vectors (SIN-Lenti)	■ Incapable of replication post-transfection → ? ■ Increased safety ■ Stable packaging system	■ ? Safety concerns remain	■ No approved trials as yet
■ Adenovirus	■ Infects wide range of cell types ■ Infects nondividing cells ■ High titers ■ High level of expression ■ Accepts 12-15 kb DNA inserts	■ Highly immunogenic ■ Nonintegrating	■ Direct *in vivo* applications ■ Transduction tumor cells
■ Adeno-associated virus (AAV)	■ Integrates into dividing cells ■ Infects wide range of cell types	■ No stable packaging cell line ■ Very limited insertion size	■ Replacement gene therapy approaches targeting muscle, liver, and brain cells
■ Herpesvirus	■ High titers ■ Transduces some target cells at high efficiency ■ Accepts large DNA inserts	■ No packaging cell lines ■ Nonintegrating ■ May be cytotoxic to target cells	■ Transduction tumor cells ■ Neurologic disorders
■ Liposomes and other physical methods using plasmid DNA	■ Easy to prepare in quantity ■ Virtually unlimited size ■ Limited immunogenicity	■ Inefficient entry into target cells ■ Nonintegrating	■ Topical applications ■ Transduction tumor cells

integrates into the host genome (Figure 20-1). The host range of MoMuLV viruses is determined by the gp70 envelope protein, which interacts with the target cells' receptors.[12] The envelope also affects the sensitivity of the vector to primate complement and hence determines the feasibility of using the virus for *in vivo* as well as *ex vivo* transduction of target cells. It is possible to modify the target cell range and to increase the physical stability and complement resistance of MoMuLV particles simply by growing the vector in packaging cell lines that supply a different envelope *in trans*. For example, retroviruses with the gibbon ape leukemia virus (GALV) envelope more efficiently transduce T lymphocytes than the same retrovirus expressing an amphotropic envelope.[13] Similarly, viruses with the feline leukemia virus envelope may have an enhanced capacity to transduce human hematopoietic stem cells.[14]

Unfortunately, modifying the viral envelope cannot overcome one of the main limitations of Moloney-based vectors, which is that the preintegration complex cannot penetrate the small pores in the nuclear membrane of resting cells. Because this preintegration complex is also unstable, Moloney vectors can only effectively transduce actively dividing cells in marked distinction to the lentiviral vectors described below.[15] This requirement for cell division has been a major limitation when human hematopoietic stem cells are the targets because few of these cells are in cycle at any one time, and efforts to increase the cycling fraction with growth factors may lead to differentiation and loss of stem cell activity.[16] More recently, the combination of MoMuLV with improved mixtures of cytokines (such as Flt 3 ligand, interleukin-3 [IL-3], and stem cell factor) and physical entrapment techniques (such as fibronectin) that bring vector and target cell into apposition has produced more satisfactory levels of transduction of human stem cells.[17]

Lentiviral Vectors

Because of the limitations of murine retroviruses, human and feline lentiviral vectors have attracted increasing attention as gene delivery systems.[4,18] Lentiviral vectors have been reported to readily transduce hemopoietic progenitor cells.[19] Because they form a more stable preintegration complex than MoMuLV, they are also able to infect quiescent subsets of primitive hemopoietic stem cells, such as the CD34+, CD38−, or CD38− lineage-negative population, where they persist and integrate once these cells enter the cycle.[20] The

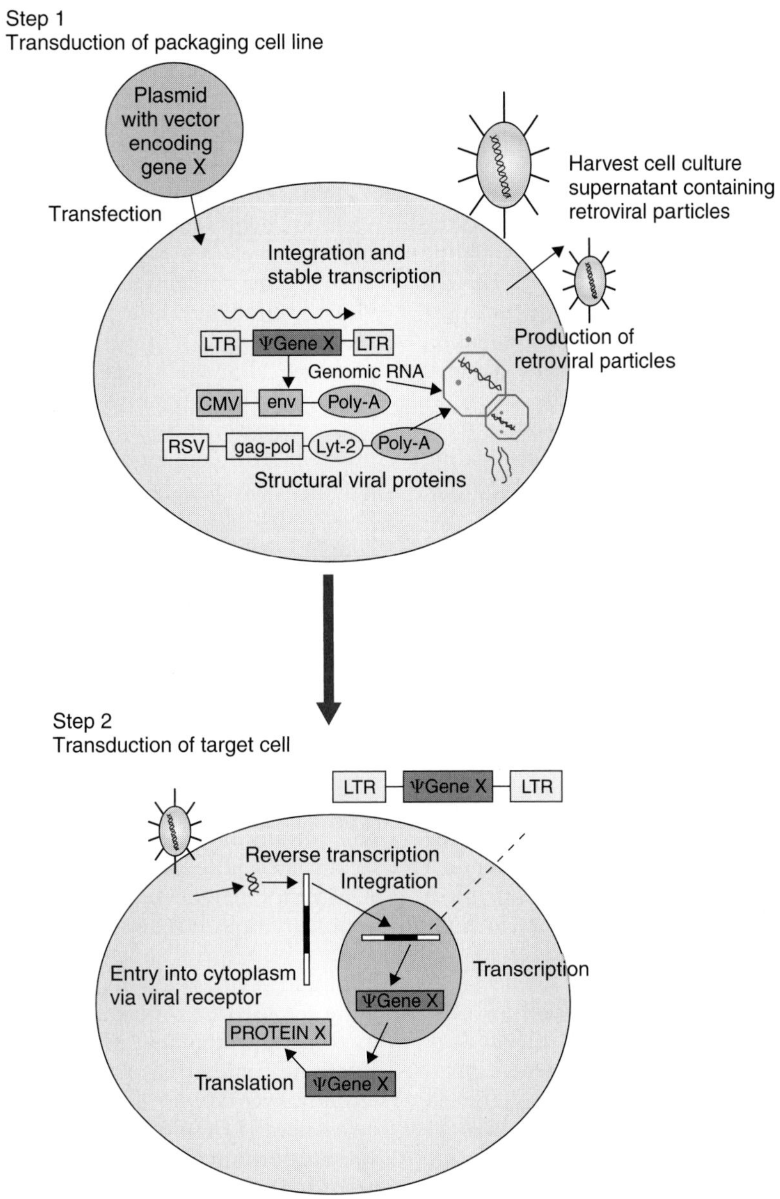

Step 1
Transduction of packaging cell line

FIGURE 20-1 Production of infectious retroviral particle and transduction of target cell. Production of an infectious retroviral particle from a bacterial plasmid that encodes a retroviral genome requires the introduction of the bacterial plasmid into mammalian cells *(Step 1)*. In the example shown, a replication-incompetent vector encoding the gene of interest is introduced (e.g., by CaPO$_4$-mediated transfection) into a packaging cell line. The packaging cell line is usually a mouse cell line that encodes the viral structural proteins *(gag, pol,* and *env)* necessary for the production of viral particles. In this example the bacterial plasmid is then stably transcribed from integrated plasmid molecules. The viral transcript is initiated at the 5' long terminal repeat *(LTR)* and terminated at the 3' LTR and is thus a full-length viral transcript. It contains the packaging sequence ψ, which is recognized by the structural proteins and allows it to be packaged into viral particles. A fully infectious but replication-incompetent viral particle containing the vector genome then buds from the packaging cell. The culture supernatant is removed from these cells and used to transduce target cells *(Step 2)*. The retrovirus interacts with a host cell receptor, enters the cell, reverse transcribes, and integrates. A full-length viral transcript can also be initiated in the 5' LTR and in the 3' LTR but the viral transcript only encodes the gene of interest and not any of the proteins required to make a viral capsid. Cells infected with this replication-incompetent vector cannot make more viral particles and there is no spread of the viral genome from an infected cell to other cells. However, the viral genome containing the gene of interest passes to all progeny cells, resulting in stable expression.

human immunodeficiency virus (HIV) can also efficiently infect terminally differentiated cells such as neurons,[21] and in both cell types, high levels of gene expression have been reported.

Although lentiviral vectors have clear advantages over murine retroviruses, substantial technical and safety problems remain before they can enter general clinical usage. At the technical level, the toxicity of some HIV proteins has made generation of stable packaging cells difficult.[4] More troubling perhaps, there is the public health concern that HIV-derived vector systems will recombine in vivo to form mutant infectious HIV particles, such as those formed by recombination with lentiviral sequences embedded in the human genome. Such concerns have prevented approval of any clinical protocols.[4,22] In an effort to further minimize this already remote possibility, third- and fourth-generation self-inactivating (SIN-L) lentiviral vectors have been generated in which the parental HIV-1 enhancer and promoter sequences from the lentivirus 3 LTR have been deleted.[23] When the SIN vector infects its target cells, it is incapable of transcribing vector-length RNA, reducing the likelihood of recombination to generate replication-competent retroviruses. Accumulating evidence from preclinical studies suggests that SIN vectors will be safe, and it is likely that they or their derivatives will soon be approved for clinical use.[24,25]

Adenoviral Vectors

Adenoviral vectors infect a wide range of cell types inside and outside the immune system and therefore do not carry the risk of insertional mutagenesis that is an unavoidable concern with current retroviral vectors. Unlike retroviruses, these vectors are nonintegrating and express their genes in nondividing cells. The vectors can be used to transduce cells ex vivo but are also stable in vivo and so can be used to infect cells in situ. Adenoviruses are a suitable delivery system for gene therapy approaches to treat allergic disorders if the strategy chosen requires high-level but short-term transgene expression by the target cell and if an immune response directed against the adenovector or its infected target cell is unlikely to be problematic.

First-generation adenoviral vectors are E1 (early protein) or E3 deletion mutants and are therefore replication incompetent. These viruses have been used for transfer of immunostimulatory genes into cancer cells to enhance the immune response, for transfer of prodrug metabolizing enzymes in an effort to sensitize normal or malignant cells to killing, and in gene correction studies, for example, in cystic fibrosis and hemophilia.[26,27]

Adenoviral vectors have many limitations. Because they are nonintegrating, the gene products are expressed from episomal DNA, and are lost after cell division; indeed, they can be inactivated even in nondividing cells.[28] Adenoviral vectors are therefore unsuited for any application that requires long-term expression in a rapidly turning over cell population. The vectors themselves also induce an acute inflammatory response, with release of cytokines including tumor necrosis factor-alpha (TNF-α), and interleukins such as IL-6 and IL-8. Indeed, the acute-phase response to injected adenoviral vectors has been fatal in humans.[29] Subsequent to this acute-phase response, adenoviral vectors also induce antibodies that can neutralize subsequent vectors administered to the patient, and

T cell responses directed to adenoviral and transgenic proteins. This cell-mediated immunity recognizes and eliminates cells expressing the low level of adenoviral proteins that are still present despite the removal of the early adenoviral genes responsible for facilitating viral DNA replication and structural protein synthesis.

In an effort to reduce the immunogenicity of adenoviral vectors, a helper-dependent vector system has been developed in which one virus (helper) contains all viral replication genes and the other contains only the therapeutic gene sequence, the viral inverted terminal repeats (ITRs), and the packaging recognition signal.[30] In principle, only the therapeutic virus is packaged, although a small number of helper particles do in fact contaminate the final product. The process is currently labor intensive, difficult to scale up, and there is a continued problem with contaminating helper virus even though the amounts have now been reduced to less than 0.1%.[31] Nevertheless, these helper-dependent vectors may be less likely to trigger a cellular response against the transduced target cell, allowing for more persistent transgene expression. They are now entering clinical trials.[26]

Adeno-Associated Viral Vectors

Adeno-associated viruses (AAVs) are integrating parvoviruses that normally depend on a helper virus (adenovirus or herpesvirus) for productive infection.[32] They can, however, exist as a latent provirus in the absence of the helper virus. Vectors based on AAV have been developed as gene transfer vehicles able to transduce a wide variety of cells including nondividing cells.[33] There is no known disease associated with AAV, and the AAV vector genome lacks viral coding sequences. Hence, the vector itself has not been associated with toxicity or inflammatory responses. Nonetheless, neutralizing antibodies are produced in vivo so that repeat administration of AAV may require the use of a different serotype. AAV vectors have been used in various animal models of genetic and acquired diseases, and clinical trials are under way using muscle and, more recently, liver delivery of the vector to patients with factor IX deficiency.[34-36] Despite the advantages of low toxicity and persistence, introduction of AAV vectors into clinical practice has been delayed by the labor-intensive nature of the large-scale production required for clinical trials and by the limited size of the transgene the parvovirus can package. Not only does this preclude their use for large structural genes, it will also hamper future efforts to include regulatory systems that can control the quantity of transgene product.

Herpesviruses

Herpesviruses have been proposed as high-efficiency vectors for many cell types. Although they usually do not integrate in the host cell, they have the potential to persist after primary infection in a latent state.[37,38] Deletion of the five immediate early (IE) genes allows herpes simplex virus (HSV) vectors to be grown in high titers in complementing cell lines without the production of replication-competent virus.[39] In fact, up to half the HSV genes are nonessential for virus replication in culture and can be removed. This allows insertion of a large payload, which may be multiple structural genes or structural and regulatory elements in combination.[40]

HSV vectors have now been used in numerous animal models including those in which peripheral[41] or central nervous system disorders are targeted,[42] and in cancer as well.[43,44] Clinical experience with these vectors is beginning to accrue, and it is likely that they will have wider application in human disease over the next few years, especially in disorders of the nervous system.

Nonviral Vectors

Because of the complexities associated with the manufacture of viral vectors and concerns over their immunogenicity, insertional mutagenesis, and toxicity, increasing attention has been paid to the nonviral vector system. Until recently these systems were profoundly limited for clinical applications because of their extreme inefficiency and lack of targeting to specific cell types. More recent developments have begun to show how these limitations can be overcome. Of particular interest is the increasing ability to combine nonviral and physical methods of gene transfer, for example, the use of plasmids coupled with local electroporation of target tissues *in situ* to favor gene uptake.

Most clinical experience with nonviral gene transfer has used plasmids injected primarily as DNA vaccines (see the section on producing a soluble protein). The efficiency of these plasmids has been increased by incorporating synthetic promoters, which may enhance the amount of transgene produced.[45] Plasmids are also administered following incorporation into liposomal complexes.[46,47] Cationic liposome/DNA complexes are the most widely used of these and fuse with the cell membrane and enter the endosomal uptake pathway. DNA released from these endosomes may then pass through the nuclear membrane and be expressed. Liposomal delivery of plasmid DNA is more efficient than direct injection, and because liposomes are relatively nontoxic they can be given repeatedly. Although levels of gene expression comparable to viral vectors have been obtained in some cellular targets, the DNA transferred by liposomes does not integrate the genome. Moreover, the ability to target these vectors is still relatively limited despite the incorporation of a variety of ligands into the liposome-DNA complex.[47]

Plasmids may also be successfully coupled with other physical methods of gene transfer. For example, successful gene transfer *in vivo* has been reported with the use of a bioballistic ("gene gun") technique in which DNA coated onto colloidal gold particles is driven at high velocity by gas pressure into the cell.[48] Alternatively, increased cellular uptake of plasmid may be obtained locally by application of an electrical charge (electroporation)[47,48] that induces reversible holes in the cell membrane. Laser light and ultrasonic transducers (optoporation and sonoporation, respectively) may have identical effects. Electroporation techniques have been successfully used to transfer the cytotoxic drug bleomycin into human tumors *in situ*, and the first clinical protocols using this approach for plasmid gene transfer are now under consideration by regulatory bodies.

Finally, a nonviral strategy termed *transkaryotic implantation* was recently employed in a clinical trial for the treatment of patients with severe hemophilia A. Somatic cells are isolated from a patient and transfected with a therapeutic gene using physical means, and then a rare transduced clone is isolated, expanded *ex vivo*, and reimplanted *in vivo*. An early study of this approach has shown some promise, but it remains cumbersome.[49]

Nonviral gene delivery would be more attractive if the transgene were able to integrate with higher efficiency in the host cell genome, and transposon technology may afford such an opportunity.[50] If a plasmid encoding a therapeutic gene (factor IX) and portions of a transposon is co-injected with a second plasmid encoding an enzyme that activates those transposon elements, there is chromosomal integration and transposition that lead to long-term expression (> 5 months) of factor IX at levels that were therapeutic in a mouse model of hemophilia B. It is not yet clear whether this type of approach would also improve the duration of plasmid-dependent gene expression in large animals or humans. In summary, advances in the technology of the components of nonviral vector systems will likely lead to a progressive increase in their effectiveness and a corresponding increase in their use in human gene therapy studies.

VECTOR SAFETY CONCERN

Adverse publicity has sensitized both investigators and the public to the potential dangers of gene transfer vectors. Every new therapeutic agent must of course be carefully monitored for adverse effects, and gene transfer vectors are no different. Beyond these general concerns, however, there are more specific issues that must be considered. We have already alluded to concerns about recombinational events following administration of retroviral vectors, but insertional mutagenesis is a potential consequence of any integration event, regardless of the vector used.[51] This risk is likely to be small: for example, gene marking studies have been performed with murine retroviruses in more than 100 patients, some of whom have more than 10 years of follow-up. Although no adverse effects attributable to retroviral gene transfer have been reported,[52] vigilance remains important. A recent article reported that murine marrow stem cells transduced with a murine retroviral vector encoding a marker gene called *truncated nerve growth factor receptor* (NGFR) used in some human studies[53] could cause leukemia after serial transplantation of transduced stem cells in mice.[54] More recently, a patient with severe combined immunodeficiency caused by common γ chain deficiency developed a T cell leukemia associated with integration of the retroviral vector used for correction. Hence, all recipients of gene transfer vectors now require a minimum of 15 years of follow-up, including genetic analysis of any tumors that may appear.

The major safety concern with nonintegrating viral vectors relates to their immunogenicity, a characteristic that may be particularly unwelcome in the allergic host. Immunity to adenoviral vectors is perhaps the best studied and illustrates the complex innate and immune host defense mechanisms that viral vectors may trigger. Inflammatory and immune responses are generated against the vector proteins themselves, while T cell responses appear against the low levels of adenoviral proteins expressed even when cells are transduced by defective viruses.[2,55] It is unlikely that it will ever be possible to safely ablate the multiplicity of immune defenses to viruses and viral vectors that have been developed. The ultimate need will be to develop synthetic vectors that combine the efficiency and targeting ability of viruses with the more benign physical characteristics of current plasmids.

EFFECTOR CELLS AND EFFECTOR MOLECULES

To devise successful gene therapy interventions for allergic responses, an understanding of the cellular and molecular mechanisms involved in generating and regulating these phenomena is required. A detailed description of all that is known about this subject is beyond the scope of this chapter; however, a basic overview of the effector cells and molecules of the immune system is provided in Figure 20-2 and in the section that follows, which are offered as a basis for explaining how components of the allergic response could in principle become targets for genetic manipulation.

Antigen-Presenting Cells

The nature of the immunogen and how it is presented in part determines what type of immune response will result. For an antigen to stimulate a T cell response, it requires presentation on antigen-presenting cells (APCs) such as dendritic cells (DCs). APCs take up antigen, process it to peptides, and present it in association with Class I and Class II molecules of the major histocompatibility complex (MHC). If these cells encounter T lymphocytes expressing an appropriate specific CD3 receptor for the MHC-peptide complex they are presenting, CD80 and CD86 surface molecules on the APCs engage the CD28 molecule on T cells and provide signals crucial for T cell survival and cytokine secretion.[56] The T cell's interaction with peptide and antigen-presenting cells helps determine whether a CD8 (recognizes antigen and class I MHC molecules) or a CD4 (recognizes antigen and class II MHC molecules) response is generated and whether a CD4 response is predominantly T helper cell type 1 (Th1), Th2, or Th regulatory (Tr). The population of T cells recruited in turn modifies the immunoglobulin (Ig) class of the antibody response made by antigen-specific B cells, and the class of Ig determines which downstream effector mechanisms are recruited. For example, activation of Th2 cells favors recruitment of IgE-producing B cells, with subsequent arming of basophils and mast cells for an acute hypersensitivity response.[57,58]

T Cells and T Helper Response

As described previously, Th cells are recruited when CD4+ T cells recognize the appropriate peptide presented in a complex associated with HLA Class II antigens on antigen-presenting cells. Three functional classes of T cells may result: Th1, Th2, or Tr. Th1 cells favor induction of cytotoxic/antiviral effector cells and produce cytokines such as IL-12 and interferon gamma (IFN-γ), which tend to antagonize the allergic response. Th2 cells favor induction of inflammatory and antibody responses, producing cytokines such as IL-4, IL-5, IL-6, IL-10, IL-13, and granulocyte-macrophage colony-stimulating factor. By promoting B cell synthesis of IgE, recruitment of Th2 cells can effectively arm basophils, mast cells, and eosinophils, which are also capable of releasing Th2-like proinflammatory cytokines in response to antigen.

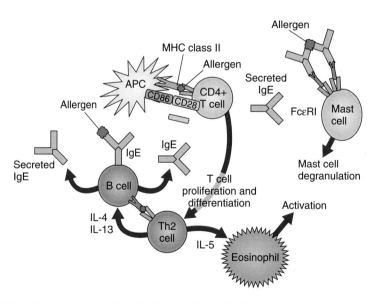

FIGURE 20-2 Effector response in allergy. In this figure CD4+ T cells recognize the allergen presented on the antigen-presenting cell *(APC)* by class II major histocompatibility complex *(MHC)* molecules. There is engagement of the costimulatory molecule CD28 on the T cell with CD86 or CD80 on the APC. If there is binding of a low-affinity antigen to the MHC class II molecule and engagement of CD86 with CD28, this biases toward T helper cell type 2 *(Th2)* development. This is in contrast to high-affinity antigen binding and engagement of CD80 with CD28, which biases toward *Th1* development. Th2 cells then secrete interleukins *(ILs)*, including IL-5, which stimulates eosinophilic activation, and IL-4 and IL-13, which help the B cells secrete IgE. Secreted IgE then binds to mast cells or basophils through high-affinity Fcε receptors *(FcεRI)*. Cross-linking of this receptor with exposure to the allergen results in mast cell degranulation. Both activation of eosinophils and mast cell degranulation trigger the release of inflammatory mediators including histamine, leukotrienes, prostaglandins, and cytokines, resulting in the clinical and pathologic manifestations of the allergic response.

Immune Tolerance

Besides promoting the immune response, CD4 T lymphocytes can also provide a regulatory function (in the form of Tr cells) and become involved in the phenomenon of immune tolerance. Antigen-specific tolerance had predominantly been considered to be a passive process involving inactivation or death of clones of antigen-specific cells following exposure to the specific antigen. These mechanisms probably do underlie tolerance to self-antigens, a fundamental property of the immune system (Figure 20-3). Immature or developing lymphocytes are more susceptible to tolerance induction than mature, competent cells, and during their development all lymphocytes go through a stage during which self-antigen recognition leads to their death or inactivation. Failure of this mechanism may lead to autoimmune disease. Elimination takes place in the generative lymphoid organs and is known as *central tolerance*. Of greater relevance to control of the allergic response is the phenomenon of *peripheral tolerance*, which affects mature lymphocytes. Such tolerance may result from passive unresponsiveness, or anergy, but it is now increasingly accepted that it may also be a more active process, in which antigen-specific Tr cells produce inhibitory signals that down-regulate the activity of antigen-specific T helper cells that would otherwise induce an inflammatory or cytotoxic T cell response.

Anergy can be induced if the APCs presenting the antigen lack or have had blocked one or more of the critical co-stimulatory molecules involved during antigen activation of T cells. Lacking appropriate co-stimulation, T cells are rendered incapable of responding to the antigen even if the antigen is later presented by competent APCs. Peripheral tolerance may also be induced by activation-induced cell death, in which repeated stimulation of T lymphocytes by antigens induces IL-2 release and up-regulates *Fas* ligand, increasing the sensitivity of the T cells to *Fas*-mediated apoptosis. The physiologic importance of this "clonal exhaustion" mechanism is unclear.

For many years there has been controversy about whether or not T cells also actively contribute to the induction and maintenance of tolerance to foreign and self-antigens (immune suppression), but this concept is gaining increasing acceptance and there is now convincing evidence that unresponsiveness of CD4+ T cells to systemic or mucosally delivered antigen can occur only after a transient period of T cell activation and can then be adoptively transferred to a naive animal.[59,60] The development of Tr cells takes approximately 2 weeks *in vivo* and their long-term persistence is antigen dependent.[61] Tr cells exhibit a cell-surface phenotype of CD4+, CD45RB[lo], CD25+, and CD38+ and express high levels of CTLA-4.[62]

A number of factors seem to favor the generation of Tr cells. The first is antigen activation in the presence of cytokines such as transforming growth factor-beta (TGF-β) and IL-10.[63,64] The second is the route of antigen administration. Studies using the autoantigen myelin basic protein have identified a unique subset of regulatory CD4 cells termed *Th3* that can be recruited by oral feeding of the antigen and that display a restricted pattern of cytokine expression including IL-4, IL-10, and TGF-β.[65] The third factor favoring Tr generation is activation of the Notch pathway when the T cell reaches its decision point for becoming a Th or a Tr cell. Vertebrates express multiple Notch receptors (Notches 1-4) and Notch ligands (jagged or serrate 1-2 and delta-like 1,3,4) and these pathways play an important role in determining cell fate. In the immune system, whether a lymphocyte will become a T cell or a B cell, a CD4+ or a CD8+ T cell, or a Tr or a Th cell appears to be determined largely by whether or not the Notch pathway is activated when each decision point is reached[66-70] (Figure 20-4). Hence, stimulation of the Notch pathway in the presence of a given antigen generates Tr cells that can actively diminish even a preexisting immune response to that antigen.[71]

B Lymphocytes and IgE

A subset of B cells releases immunoglobulin E (IgE), and elevated amounts of this immunoglobulin class are often present in the sera of patients with allergic disease. The Fc region of the IgE molecule binds at its C-3 domain with receptors such as CD23 and with the high-affinity receptor FcεRI, present on tissue mast cells, basophils, B cells, and other APCs, including DCs. When the host is exposed to the specific antigen, cross-linking of cell-bound IgE occurs and produces mast cell degranulation and release of inflammatory mediators such as histamine, prostaglandin D2, thromboxane A2, the leukotrienes C4 and B4, and Th2 cytokines. The biologic effects of these mast cell mediators and cytokines result in the clinical allergic response.

IL-4, produced by Th2 cells, is one important cytokine that favors IgE synthesis from B cells,[72,73] but IL-13 release plays an additional role.[74] Engagement of the C40 antigen on B cells by T cells or APCs expressing the CD40 ligand (CD154) also promotes IgE class switching.[75]

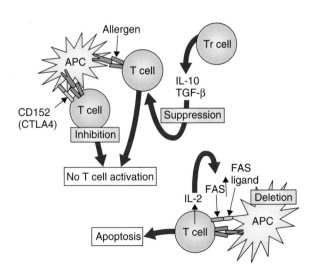

FIGURE 20-3 Mechanisms of peripheral tolerance. This figure shows three mechanisms by which T cell tolerance can be induced. Under the influence of interleukin-2 *(IL-2)*, activated T cells up-regulate the expression of the Fas (CD95) molecule on their surfaces. These cells can then receive their signals from cells that express Fas ligand and undergo apoptosis, a process known as deletion. T cells may also be inhibited by the interaction of the CD152 molecule expressed on some T cells with CD80 on antigen-presenting cells *(APCs)*. Finally, T regulatory *(Tr)* cells can suppress other T cells most likely through the production of inhibitory cytokines such as IL-10 and transforming growth factor-beta *(TGF-β)*.

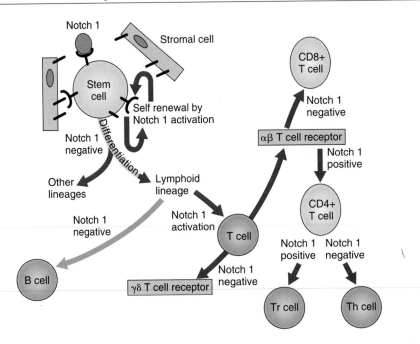

FIGURE 20-4 The Notch pathway. This figure highlights the influence of Notch activation on the lymphoid developmental pathway. If the Notch 1 pathway is triggered by binding of the Notch 1 receptor to its ligand, then stem cell proliferation and self-renewal are favored, whereas differentiation is inhibited. If the Notch pathway is inactive, stem cell differentiation is more likely to occur. In this example there is differentiation to the lymphoid lineage, where Notch 1 activation of lymphoid precursors induces them to become T rather than B lymphocytes. Once a cell has committed to the T lineage, Notch 1 activation induces expression of αβ versus γδ T cell receptors and differentiation toward CD8+ cytotoxic T cells rather than CD4+ T cells. Finally, Notch 1 activation of CD4+ T cells induces the development of T regulatory (*Tr*) cells over T helper (*Th*) cells.

WHAT CAN GENE THERAPY DO FOR THE ALLERGIC PATIENT?

Based on the cellular and molecular mechanisms underlying the immune response outlined in this chapter, it is possible to define several types of gene transfer interventions that could modify the nature of the allergic response. These are summarized in Box 20-2, and examples are illustrated below.

Correcting a Genetic Defect to Restore Cellular Function

If there are any specific underlying genetic defects involved in the predisposition to allergy, they are poorly understood. For this reason, it is premature to suggest specific gene replacement targets for the treatment of allergic diseases. Immune deficiency disorders, however, provide an excellent model of the way such gene replacement therapies might work and illustrate the limitations of the approach very clearly. Because the principles learned from these immunodeficiency studies will undoubtedly ultimately apply to gene correction efforts for allergic disorders, we will briefly describe the outcomes in human trials to date.

Severe combined immunodeficiency diseases (SCIDs) caused by common γ chain deficiency or due to adenosine deaminase (ADA) deficiency were among the first disorders treated by gene therapy. These disorders were chosen not just because they were life-threatening diseases in which the relevant genes were well characterized but also because studies of carriers showed that even a low level of correction could be beneficial and/or that gene-corrected cells had proliferative and survival advantages over the uncorrected population.

Common γ Chain Deficiency

This defect accounts for 50% to 60% of all cases of SCID. The defect is in the common cytokine receptor chain (γc), which is shared by the receptors for IL-2, IL-4, IL-7, IL-9, and IL-15. The result is a deficiency of mature T and natural killer (NK) lymphocytes and an increased number of B cells. In preclinical studies, γc-transduced CD34+ cells from SCID patients matured into T cells and NK cells *ex vivo*. These preclinical results led to a successful therapeutic study in France in 1999.[8] The first two patients treated had missense mutations resulting in loss of the transmembrane region of the γc. Autologous CD34+ stem cells derived from bone marrow were transduced with a γc retroviral vector with a transduction efficiency of 20% to 40%. Between 75 to 90 days after infusion of the transduced CD34+ cells, lymphocyte counts rose in both patients, and the T cells were shown to express the γc transgene and were polyclonal. The T cells were also functionally normal with normal proliferation in response to mitogenic stimuli, IL-2, and antigens after immunization. Both the patients remained well, and over the past 2 years nine additional patients have been treated in France, as have patients in Australia and the United Kingdom, all with similar benefits.[76] However, the development of leukemia in one of these patients is a cause for concern.

BOX 20-2	KEY CONCEPTS
	What Gene Therapy Can Do

What gene therapy can do	General examples	Examples of gene therapy for allergic diseases
■ Restore cell function/correcting cell deficits	■ Transduction of target cells with deficient gene as in SCID common γ chain deficiency; HSCs transduced with γc retroviral vector	■ No example yet in view of the polygenic nature of the allergic diseases
■ Change the function of the cell	■ Transduction of antigen-presenting cells with Notch 1 ligands to induce T cell anergy	■ In an asthma mouse model, dendritic cells transduced with Jagged-1 and pulsed with *Der p 1* → inhibition of proliferative T cell responses
■ Produce a protein	■ Transduction of protein gene into target cells	■ Adenoviral transfer of allergen gene to sensitize subjects → state of tolerance
		■ Mucosal transfer of IL-12 and IFN-γ to reduce Th2 cytokine expression
		■ Transfer of glucocorticoid receptor to epithelial cells
■ Produce an altered protein	■ Transduction of a mutant protein into cells to modify function of target cells	■ Administration of mutated versions of native allergen to induce anergy in T cells specific for native allergen
■ Remove a protein	■ Administration of ribozymes, intracellular antibodies (intrabodies), or intrakines	■ The use of anticytokine antibodies such as IL-4 to inhibit the Th2 response
		■ The use of antibodies targeted against the mediators of inflammation such as the leukotrienes
■ Provide insights into cell biology	■ Gene modification and/or marking of cells critical in cellular pathways to track function	■ Potentially could simulate activation or blockade of specific molecular pathways in specific cell types as a means to analyze constituents of the allergic response

Adenosine Deaminase Deficiency

ADA deficiency was the first disease to be treated by gene therapy using autologous T cells transduced with a retrovirus incorporating the ADA gene. These were administered to two patients over an 18- to 23-month period.[77] The study was partially successful as determined by immune function studies, and both children remained well at 3 years. However, the ADA enzyme replacement therapy could not be completely withdrawn. Other clinical trials followed, including the transduction of neonatal bone marrow cells and autologous cord blood cells with an ADA-encoding retrovirus in the presence of hemopoietic growth factors.[78] In one study, multilineage engraftment of the gene-modified cells and the generation of ADA-expressing T lymphocytes were observed after the transduced cord blood cells were infused back into patients.[79] However, as the dose of ADA enzyme was reduced, the proportion of the ADA-expressing mature T lymphocytes did not increase and was considered too low to be of clinical benefit: full-dose enzyme replacement therapy was therefore restarted.[80,81] More recently, an improved marrow stem cell transduction technique coupled with the use of cytotoxic drugs to reduce residual non-transduced stem cells in the patients has been associated with complete immune reconstitution in two patients and withdrawal of ADA replacement therapy in one.[82,83] These clinical results indicate that although human hemopoietic stem cells can be transduced with murine retrovirus-based vectors, the level of transduction and transgene expression is such that it may be necessary

to promote engraftment of the modified cells by using cytoreductive drugs against endogenous uncorrected cells.

Changing the Effector Function of the Cell

One of the best examples of this approach in allergy is the modification of antigen-presenting cells so that they induce a tolerogenic rather than an activating immune response. House dust mites (*Dermatophagoides pteronyssinus*) are well known to produce allergens strongly associated with childhood asthma.[84] A major component of the allergen is the enzymatically active protease *Der p 1*. In a murine model this protease has been shown to selectively cleave surface CD23 from B cells and interrupt the negative regulator of IgE production.[85,86] One means by which negative regulation could be restored would be by genetically modifying APCs. If they expressed high levels of Notch ligands as well as the allergen, any naive allergen-specific T cell they encountered would have Notch activation and would be switched to the Tr pathway (see Figure 20-4). These Notch-activated T cells could potentially down-regulate any preexisting response to the allergen. Transduction of murine splenic APCs with the Notch ligand Jagged-1, followed by pulsing with *Der p 1*, will indeed produce T cells capable of inhibiting the proliferative responses of primed lymph node T cells. Moreover, when Jagged-transduced DCs are injected into naive syngeneic mice, recognition of the antigen on these DCs leads to the development of long-lived, antigen-specific tolerance.[87] Similar experiments have been performed in humans, albeit not yet with conventional allergens. For example, it is possible to transduce human APCs with an adenoviral vector encoding the Notch ligand Jagged-1. When these APCs are cocultured with naive (CD45RA+) allogeneic T cells, the latter differentiate into Tr cells capable of specifically inhibiting T helper and T cytotoxic responses to fresh allogeneic APCs while sparing the response to third-party allogeneic APCs and other unrelated antigens.[88]

These results illustrate one of the important principles of gene transfer into immune system cells. Modification of the behavior of even a small percentage of cells of a single subpopulation may influence not just the behavior of that cell or the subpopulation to which it belongs but may also affect the entire immune system and produce distant actions on unmodified and apparently unrelated components. The amplification attributable to this network effect may help to overcome the limited efficiency of current vectors.

More limited and more direct genetic modification of cellular behavior is also feasible. Transfer of the glucocorticoid receptor to epithelial cells is one such possibility. NFκB is a transcription factor that is constitutively present within the cytoplasm bound to IκB molecules, which retain NFκB in an inactive state. Proinflammatory stimuli induce phosphorylation of the IκB molecules, leading to their degradation and transfer of NFκB to the nucleus, where it is activated and induces transcription of components that induce synthesis of the cytokine cascade. When corticosteroids bind their cytoplasmic receptor, the complex inhibits NFκB release. *In vitro* overexpression of the glucocorticoid receptor on epithelial cell line A549 leads to repression of transcription factor–mediated cytokine gene transcription, an effect that might be of value in the treatment of resistant asthma.[89] Unlike the induction of Tr cells, however, this type of approach is likely to require a high proportion of cells to be gene corrected *in situ* if clinical benefit were to result. It is not yet clear how this could be accomplished with our current vector systems.

Producing a Soluble Protein with Immunomodulating Activity

DNA plasmid–mediated gene transfer may be used to vaccinate patients with allergen genes in a modified form of specific immunotherapy (SIT).[90,91] Conventional SIT using gradually increasing doses of standardized allergen extracts has been effective for many antigens but is sometimes a high-risk approach when potent allergens (e.g., latex) are used.[92] In addition, SIT requires inconveniently frequent injections over a prolonged period of time. In animal models DNA vaccination appears to offer an alternative. Allergen-encoding vectors consisting of either naked plasmid DNA or of recombinant mycoplasma[93-96] have been successfully used for the prophylaxis of atopic responses, reduction of IgE titers, and a shift of the immune response from Th2 to Th1. These actions lead to a decrease in airway hyperresponsiveness and anaphylactic hypersensitivity. Because this approach is less effective at modifying a preexisting IgE response, efforts were made to boost its potency by substituting an adenoviral vector as the gene delivery system. For example, adenoviral vectors expressing the β-galactosidase enzyme can be given to mice intraperitoneally and the animals subsequently inoculated with β-galactosidase itself, using a route and schedule that normally induces a high level of IgE Ab and anaphylaxis. In the Adβgal-treated mice,

the development of specific IgE antibodies is blocked and the immune response shifted from a Th2 to a Th1 phenotype. Although it is unknown whether or not this approach would be significantly more effective at modulating a preexisting IgE response than a simple plasmid, the approach is being investigated using several different allergenic protein genes.[97] Even if this immunization method can be effectively implemented for preexisting immune responses, the approach has the fundamental limitation that it can be effective only when a small number of well-defined protein antigens are the cause of the allergic response. This criterion is met by some but by no means all of the atopy-inducing allergens.

Plasmids have also been explored for use in food allergies, where SIT is considered to be excessively risky.[98] In the AKR/J mouse the main peanut allergen is *Arah2*. Anaphylaxis can be induced by combined oral and intraperitoneal sensitization with peanut extracts, followed by intraperitoneal challenge with recombinant *Arah2*. Chitosan, a natural polysaccharide found in crustacean shells, is nontoxic and biodegradable. It can be complexed with plasmid DNA to form stable nanoparticles that can be endocytosed by gastrointestinal epithelial cells. If an *Arah2* plasmid is complexed with chitosan and fed to the AKR/J mice, there is an increase in serum IgG2a titers and a decrease in IgE titers compared with control mice. When the mice are sensitized and challenged, there is substantial blunting of response in the plasmid/chitosan group versus the controls.[99] Again, it remains unclear whether or not this strategy would work safely in individuals who are already hypersensitive.

Distinct from the vaccination approach, transgenic production of soluble proteins may also be used to modify patterns of cytokine expression in an effort to favor a less inflammatory immune response. This can be achieved either by increasing expression of the cytokines themselves or by changing expression of their receptors. For example, in a mouse model of asthma, mucosal transfer of IL-12 and IFN-γ genes significantly reduced Th2 cytokine expression and bronchial hyperresponsiveness.[100,101]

Finally, it has been shown that a lactose-intolerant rat can be rendered lactose tolerant following oral administration of an adeno-associated viral vector encoding the beta-galactosidase (βgal) transgene, which is expressed in both gut epithelial and lamina propria cells.[102] One highly speculative possibility is that it might be possible to use gene transfer of an appropriate metabolizing enzyme so that potential allergens can simply be destroyed before they have a chance to induce an immune response.

Express a Novel Engineered Protein

Until now we have focused on transfer of "naturally occurring" genes, but it is also possible to transfer genes that have been bioengineered to have specific properties lacking in their natural counterparts. The availability of such genes affords a number of therapeutic opportunities. For example, the balance between a desirable and undesirable immune response in an allergic patient is determined in part by the pattern of cytokines produced. We briefly outlined above how transgenic cytokines or cytokine receptors could be used to alter the prevailing balance between antiinflammatory and proinflammatory cytokines. A related alternative is to render cells more or less sensitive to a given cytokine by introducing genes for mutant receptors that have higher or lower affinity than the native receptor and that ideally have a dominant phenotype. Presently there are no examples where this application has been used in allergy, but there are several cancer applications that are conceptually relevant. When patients with relapsed Epstein-Barr virus (EBV)–positive Hodgkin's disease are treated with EBV-specific cytotoxic T lymphocytes (CTLs), the activity of these cells is diminished by the high level of TGF-β that the Hodgkin's tumor cells produce.[103] To overcome this problem, CTLs that can first be transduced with a retrovirus vector expressing a mutant dominant-negative TGF-β type II receptor (DNR) that blocks TGF-β signal transduction and renders the CTLs resistant to the anticytolytic and antiproliferative effects of TGF-β.[104] If related effects were obtained following transduction of T cells from atopic patients with mutant IL-4 or IL-10 receptors, it is likely that generation of a Th2 response would now be less favored.

Removing a Function

Although gene transfer can add or modify a pre-existing function in the immune system, it can also be used to remove an activity. One example given above is the transfer of mutant cytokine receptors that are dominant-negative inhibitors of the response. Much broader classes of "function-removing agents" exist, of which the best studied for clinical application are ribozymes, intrabodies, and intrakines.

Ribozymes represent a unique class of RNA molecules that can catalytically cleave specific target mRNA, thereby leading to its degradation.[105] Intrabodies are single-chain antibodies with Golgi retention signals incorporated into their sequence that can trap intracellular proteins before they reach their place of intracellular activity or are secreted by the cell.[106] Intrakines are chemokine fragments, also with Golgi retention signals, that trap cellular chemokine receptors before they appear on the cell surface. Sequences encoding all these agents have been successfully transferred and expressed in a variety of cell targets. To date, these "loss of function" molecules have been explored primarily in infectious and malignant diseases, where they can be used to prevent expression of HIV receptors on the target cell surface or to disrupt or trap oncogenic fusion transcripts/proteins created by gene translocations in tumor cells.[107-109] However, these "loss of function" molecules could also be used to prevent or treat allergic disorders. Ribozymes could destroy the transcripts for cytokines or cytokine receptors, and intrabodies could trap the equivalent proteins. Expression of intrakine genes would down-regulate chemokine receptors on T cells and reduce their ability to migrate in response to inflammatory or atopy-inducing signals. However, in allergy, as in most other projected applications, effectiveness would require not just the targeting of the appropriate cell type but also a high efficiency of transduction and high levels of gene expression; as we have already discussed, we are far from achieving these desirable ends.

Insights into Cell Biology and Target Validation for Small Molecules

Gene transfer ultimately may have much to offer in the treatment of the allergic disorders, but it is probable that for the next several years its most important role will be to help identify the cellular and molecular mechanisms underlying the allergic response and to help validate particular molecular targets for other therapeutic interventions. The ability to simulate activation or blockade of specific molecular pathways in specific cell types represents a powerful tool for analyzing the constituents of the allergic response, and knowledge of the molecular and cellular bases of allergic diseases will improve over time. An improvement in the technology for efficiently transferring genes in a targeted, safe, and controlled manner can also be anticipated. As our knowledge and practical capabilities increase, we can expect to see gene transfer making a significant contribution to the alleviation and cure of allergic diseases.

CONCLUSIONS

It is too early to assign a role to gene therapy for the treatment of allergic diseases, and we have outlined instead the potential strengths and current weaknesses of this technology (see Boxes 20-2 and 20-3). We have offered potential examples of how gene transfer can be applied to the allergic disorders. We predict that the transfer of antiinflammatory/immunomodulatory genes will provide a convenient way of controlling the allergic response and that exploitation of effective oral gene therapy in combination with the mucosal route of antigen presentation will be valuable for induction of antigenic tolerance.

HELPFUL WEBSITES

The American Society for Gene Therapy website (www.ASGT.edu)
The Center for Cell and Gene Therapy website (www.CAGT.org)

REFERENCES

1. Kay MA, Glorioso JC, Naldini L: Viral vectors for gene therapy: the art of turning infectious agents into vehicles of therapeutics, *Nat Med* 7:33-40, 2001.
2. Hitt MM, Graham FL: Adenovirus vectors for human gene therapy, *Adv Virus Res* 55:479-505, 2000.
3. High KA: Gene therapy: a 2001 perspective, *Haemophilia* 7(suppl 1):23-27, 2001.
4. Buchschacher GL Jr, Wong-Staal F: Development of lentiviral vectors for gene therapy for human diseases, *Blood* 95:2499-2504, 2000.
5. Xu K, Ma H, McCown TJ, et al: Generation of a stable cell line producing high-titer self-inactivating lentiviral vectors, *Mol Ther* 3:97-104, 2001.
6. Rossi FM, Blau HM: Recent advances in inducible gene expression systems, *Curr Opin Biotechnol* 9:451-456, 1998.
7. Wang Y, O'Malley BWJ, Tsai SY, et al: A regulatory system for use in gene transfer, *Proc Natl Acad Sci U S A* 91:8180-8184, 1994.
8. Hacein-Bey-Abina S, Le Deist F, Carlier F, et al: Sustained correction of X-linked severe combined immunodeficiency by *ex vivo* gene therapy, *N Engl J Med* 346:1185-1193, 2002.

BOX 20-3

KEY CONCEPTS
What Gene Therapy Cannot Do

- Produce a functional change in every cell
- Correct a deficit in every cell
- Produce tightly regulated transgenes
- Produce very high levels of products

9. Brenner MK: Gene marking, *Gene Therapy* 3:278-279, 1996.

10. Bollard CM, Heslop HE, Brenner MK: Gene-marking studies of hematopoietic cells, *Int J Hematol* 73:14-22, 2001.

11. Wivel NA, Wilson JM: Methods of gene delivery, *Hematol Oncol Clin North Am* 12:483-501, 1998.

12. Miller AD: Cell-surface receptors for retroviruses and implications for gene transfer, *Proc Natl Acad Sci USA* 93:11407-11413, 1996.

13. Lam JS, Reeves ME, Cowherd R, et al: Improved gene transfer into human lymphocytes using retroviruses with the gibbon ape leukemia virus envelope, *Hum Gene Ther* 7:1415-1422, 1996.

14. Kelly PF, Vandergriff J, Nathwani A, et al: Highly efficient gene transfer into cord blood nonobese diabetic/severe combined immunodeficiency repopulating cells with oncoretroviral vector particles pseudotyped with the feline endogenous retrovirus (RD114) envelope protein, *Blood* 96:1206-1214, 2000.

15. Miller DG, Adam MA, Miller AD: Gene transfer by retrovirus vectors occurs only in cells that are actively replicating at the time of infection, *Mol Cell Biol* 10:4239-4242, 1990.

16. Tisdale JF, Hanazono Y, Sellers SE, et al: *Ex vivo* expansion of genetically marked rhesus peripheral blood progenitor cells results in diminished long-term repopulating ability, *Blood* 92:1131-1141, 1998.

17. Pollok KE, Hanenberg H, Noblitt TW, et al: High-efficiency gene transfer into normal and adenosine deaminase-deficient T lymphocytes is mediated by transduction on recombinant fibronectin fragments, *J Virol* 72:4882-4892, 1998.

18. Amado RG, Chen IS: Lentiviral vectors—the promise of gene therapy within reach? *Science* 285:674-676, 1999.

19. Sutton RE, Wu HT, Rigg R, et al: Human immunodeficiency virus type 1 vectors efficiently transduce human hematopoietic stem cells, *J Virol* 72:5781-5788, 1998.

20. Case SS, Price MA, Jordan CT, et al: Stable transduction of quiescent CD34(+)CD38(−) human hematopoietic cells by HIV-1-based lentiviral vectors, *Proc Natl Acad Sci U S A* 96:2988-2993, 1999.

21. Naldini L, Blomer U, Gallay P, et al: *In vivo* gene delivery and stable transduction of nondividing cells by a lentiviral vector, *Science* 272:263-267, 1996.

22. Naldini L: Lentiviruses as gene transfer agents for delivery to non-dividing cells, *Curr Opin Biotechnol* 9:457-463, 1998.

23. Yu SF, Von Ruden T, Kantoff PW, et al: Self-inactivating retroviral vectors designed for transfer of whole genes into mammalian cells, *Proc Natl Acad Sci U S A* 83:3194-3198, 1986.

24. Xu K, Ma H, McCown TJ, et al: Generation of a stable cell line producing high-titer self-inactivating lentiviral vectors, *Mol Ther* 3:97-104, 2001.

25. Salmon P, Kindler V, Ducrey O, et al: High-level transgene expression in human hematopoietic progenitors and differentiated blood lineages after transduction with improved lentiviral vectors, *Blood* 96:3392-3398, 2000.

26. Alton E, Kitson C: Gene therapy for cystic fibrosis, *Expert Opin Investig Drugs* 9:1523-1535, 2000.

27. Balague C, Zhou J, Dai Y, et al: Stained high-level expression of full-length human factor VIII and restoration of clotting activity in hemophilic mice using a minimal adenovirus vector, *Blood* 95:820-828, 2000.

28. Michou AI, Santoro L, Christ M, et al: Adenovirus-mediated gene transfer: influence of transgene, mouse strain and type of immune response on persistence of transgene expression, *Gene Ther* 4:473-482, 1997.

29. Ferber D: Gene therapy. Safer and virus-free? *Science* 294:1638-1642, 2001.

30. Morsy MA, Caskey CT: Expanded-capacity adenoviral vectors—the helper-dependent vectors, *Mol Med Today* 5:18-24, 1999.

31. Morral N, O'Neal W, Rice K, et al: Administration of helper-dependent adenoviral vectors and sequential delivery of different vector serotype for long-term liver-directed gene transfer in baboons, *Proc Natl Acad Sci U S A* 96:12816-12821, 1999.

32. Inoue N, Russell DW: Packaging cells based on inducible gene amplification for the production of adeno-associated virus vectors, *J Virol* 72:7024-7031, 1998.

33. Miao CH, Nakai H, Thompson AR, et al: Nonrandom transduction of recombinant adeno-associated virus vectors in mouse hepatocytes *in vivo*: cell cycling does not influence hepatocyte transduction, *J Virol* 74:3793-3803, 2000.

34. Kay MA, Manno CS, Ragni MV, et al: Evidence for gene transfer and expression of factor IX in hemophilia B patients treated with an AAV vector, *Nat Genet* 24:257-261, 2000.

35. Russell DW, Kay MA: Adeno-associated virus vectors and hematology, *Blood* 94:864-874, 1999.

36. Stedman H, Wilson JM, Finke R, et al: Phase I clinical trial utilizing gene therapy for limb girdle muscular dystrophy: alpha-, beta-, gamma-, or delta-sarcoglycan gene delivered with intramuscular instillations of adeno-associated vectors, *Hum Gene Ther* 11:777-790, 2000.

37. Wolfe D, Goins WF, Kaplan TJ, et al: Herpesvirus-mediated systemic delivery of nerve growth factor, *Mol Ther* 3:61-69, 2001.

38. Burton EA, Wechuck JB, Wendell SK, et al: Multiple applications for replication-defective herpes simplex virus vectors, *Stem Cells* 19:358-377, 2001.

39. Samaniego LA, Neiderhiser L, DeLuca NA: Persistence and expression of the herpes simplex virus genome in the absence of immediate-early proteins, *J Virol* 72:3307-3320, 1998.

40. Krisky DM, Marconi PC, Oligino TJ, et al: Development of herpes simplex virus replication-defective multigene vectors for combination gene therapy applications, *Gene Ther* 5:1517-1530, 1998.

41. Chancellor MB, Yoshimura N, Pruchnic R, et al: Gene therapy strategies for urological dysfunction, *Trends Mol Med* 7:301-306, 2001.

42. Martino G, Poliani PL, Marconi PC, et al: Cytokine gene therapy of autoimmune demyelination revisited using herpes simplex virus type-1-derived vectors, *Gene Ther* 7:1087-1093, 2000.

43. Burton EA, Glorioso JC: Multi-modal combination gene therapy for malignant glioma using replication-defective HSV vectors, *Drug Discov Today* 6:347-356, 2001.

44. Dilloo D, Rill D, Entwistle C, et al: A novel herpes vector for the high-efficiency transduction of normal and malignant human hemopoietic cells, *Blood* 89:119-127, 1997.

45. Li X, Eastman EM, Schwartz RJ, et al: Synthetic muscle promoters: activities exceeding naturally occurring regulatory sequences, *Nature Biotechnol* 17:241-245, 1999.

46. Nabel GJ, Nabel EG, Yang ZY, et al: Direct gene transfer with DNA-liposome complexes in melanoma: expression, biologic activity, and lack of toxicity in humans, *Proc Natl Acad Sci U S A* 90:11307-11311, 1993.

47. Templeton NS, Lasic DD: New directions in liposome gene delivery, *Mol Biotechnol* 11:175-180, 1999.

48. Seemann S, Hauff P, Schultze-Mosgau M, et al: Pharmaceutical evaluation of gas-filled microparticles as gene delivery system, *Pharm Res* 19:250-257, 2002.

49. Roth DA, Tawa NE Jr, O'Brien JM, et al: Nonviral transfer of the gene encoding coagulation factor VIII in patients with severe hemophilia A, *N Engl J Med* 344:1735-1742, 2001.

50. Yant SR, Meuse L, Chiu W, et al: Somatic integration and long-term transgene expression in normal and haemophilic mice using a DNA transposon system, *Nat Genet* 25:35-41, 2000.

51. Donahue RE, Kessler SW, Bodine D, et al: Helper virus induced T cell lymphoma in nonhuman primates after retroviral mediated gene transfer, *J Exp Med* 176:1125-1135, 1992.

52. Heslop HE, Rill DR, Horwitz EM, et al: Gene marking to assess tumor contamination in stem cell grafts for acute myeloid leukemia. In Dicke KA, Keating A, eds: *Autologous blood and marrow transplantation*, Charlottesville, Va, 1999, Carden Jennings.

53. Bonini C, Ferrari G, Verzeletti S, et al: HSV-TK gene transfer into donor lymphocytes for control of allogeneic graft versus leukemia, *Science* 276:1719-1724, 1997.

54. Li Z, Dullmann J, Schiedlmeier B, et al: Murine leukemia induced by retroviral gene marking, *Science* 296:497, 2002.

55. Brenner M: Gene transfer by adenovectors, *Blood* 94:3965-3967, 1999.

56. Schwartz RH: Costimulation of T lymphocytes: the role of CD28, CTLA-4, and B7/BB1 in interleukin-2 production and immunotherapy, *Cell* 71:1065-1068, 1992.

57. Keane-Myers AM, Gause WC, Finkelman FD, et al: Development of murine allergic asthma is dependent upon B7-2 costimulation, *J Immunol* 160:1036-1043, 1998.

58. Kuchroo VK, Das MP, Brown JA, et al: B7-1 and B7-2 costimulatory molecules activate differentially the Th1/Th2 developmental pathways: application to autoimmune disease therapy, *Cell* 80:707-718, 1995.

59. Webb S, Morris C, Sprent J: Extrathymic tolerance of mature T cells: clonal elimination as a consequence of immunity, *Cell* 63:1249-1256, 1990.

60. Rocha B, von Boehmer H: Peripheral selection of the T cell repertoire, *Science* 251:1225-1228, 1991.

61. Metzler B, Wraith DC: Inhibition of T-cell responsiveness by nasal peptide administration: influence of the thymus and differential recovery of T-cell-dependent functions, *Immunology* 97:257-263, 1999.

62. Mason D, Powrie F: Control of immune pathology by regulatory T cells, *Curr Opin Immunol* 10:649-655, 1998.

63. Powrie F, Carlino J, Leach MW, et al: A critical role for transforming growth factor-beta but not interleukin 4 in the suppression of T helper type 1-mediated colitis by CD45RB (low) CD4+ T cells, *J Exp Med* 183:2669-2674, 1996.

64. Asseman C, Mauze S, Leach MW, et al: An essential role for interleukin 10 in the function of regulatory T cells that inhibit intestinal inflammation, *J Exp Med* 190:995-1004, 1999.

65. Chen Y, Kuchroo VK, Inobe J, et al: Regulatory T cell clones induced by oral tolerance: suppression of autoimmune encephalomyelitis, *Science* 265:1237-1240, 1994.

66. Robey E, Chang D, Itano A, et al: An activated form of Notch influences the choice between CD4 and CD8 T cell lineages, *Cell* 87:483-492, 1996.

67. Deftos ML, He YW, Ojala EW, et al: Correlating notch signaling with thymocyte maturation, *Immunity* 9:777-786, 1998.

68. Izon DJ, Punt JA, Xu L, et al: Notch 1 regulates maturation of CD4+ and CD8+ thymocytes by modulating TCR signal strength, *Immunity* 14:253-264, 2001.

69. Radtke F, Wilson A, Stark G, et al: Deficient T cell fate specification in mice with an induced inactivation of Notch 1, *Immunity* 10:547-558, 1999.

70. Pear WS, Aster JC, Scott ML, et al: Exclusive development of T cell neoplasms in mice transplanted with bone marrow expressing activated Notch alleles, *J Exp Med* 183:2283-2291, 1996.

71. Brenner M: To be or notch to be, *Nat Med* 6:1210-1211, 2000.

72. Coffman RL, Carty J: A T cell activity that enhances polyclonal IgE production and its inhibition by interferon-gamma, *J Immunol* 136:949-954, 1986.

73. Finkelman FD, Katona IM, Urban JF Jr, et al: IL-4 is required to generate and sustain *in vivo* IgE responses, *J Immunol* 141:2335-2341, 1988.

74. Minty A, Chalon P, Derocq JM, et al: Interleukin-13 is a new human lymphokine regulating inflammatory and immune responses, *Nature* 362:248-250, 1993.

75. Kawabe T, Naka T, Yoshida K, et al: The immune responses in CD40-deficient mice: impaired immunoglobulin class switching and germinal center formation, *Immunity* 1:167-178, 1994.

76. Dyer O: "Bubble baby" lives a normal life after gene therapy, *Br Med J* 324:872, 2002.

77. Blaese RM, Culver KW, Miller AD, et al: T lymphocyte-directed gene therapy for ADA-SCID: initial trial results after 4 years, *Science* 270:475-480, 1995.

78. Parkman R, Weinberg K, Crooks G, et al: Gene therapy for adenosine deaminase deficiency, *Annu Rev Med* 51:33-47, 2000.

79. Kohn DB, Weinberg KI, Nolta JA, et al: Engraftment of gene-modified umbilical cord blood cells in neonates with adenosine deaminase deficiency, *Nat Med* 1:1017-1023, 1995.

80. Kohn DB, Hershfield MS, Carbonaro D, et al: T lymphocytes with a normal ADA gene accumulate after transplantation of transduced autologous umbilical cord blood CD34+ cells in ADA-deficient SCID neonates, *Nat Med* 4:775-780, 1998.

81. Wimperis JZ, Brenner MK, Prentice HG, et al: Transfer of a functioning humoral immune system in transplantation of T- lymphocyte-depleted bone marrow, *Lancet* 1:339-343, 1986.

82. Aiuti A, Vai S, Mortellaro A, et al: Immune reconstitution in ADA-SCID after PBL gene therapy and discontinuation of enzyme replacement, *Nat Med* 8:423-425, 2002.

83. Kohn DB: Adenosine deaminase gene therapy protocol revisited, *Mol Ther* 5:96-97, 2002.

84. Sporik R, Holgate ST, Platts-Mills TA, et al: Exposure to house-dust mite allergen (Der p I) and the development of asthma in childhood: a prospective study, *N Engl J Med* 323:502-507, 1990.

85. Hewitt CR, Brown AP, Hart BJ, et al: A major house dust mite allergen disrupts the immunoglobulin E network by selectively cleaving CD23: innate protection by antiproteases, *J Exp Med* 182:1537-1544, 1995.

86. Herbert CA, King CM, Ring PC, et al: Augmentation of permeability in the bronchial epithelium by the house dust mite allergen Der p1, *Am J Respir Cell Mol Biol* 12:369-378, 1995.

87. Hoyne GF, Le Roux I, Corsin-Jimenez M, et al: Serrate 1-induced notch signalling regulates the decision between immunity and tolerance made by peripheral CD4(+) T cells, *Int Immunol* 12:177-185, 2000.

88. Yvon ES, Vigouroux S, Rousseau RF, et al: Non-professional APC overexpressing Jagged-1 induce naive peripheral T cells to become alloantigen-specific regulatory cells (abstract), *Cytotherapy* 4:125, 2002.

89. Mathieu M, Gougat C, Jaffuel D, et al: The glucocorticoid receptor gene as a candidate for gene therapy in asthma, *Gene Ther* 6:245-252, 1999.

90. Durham SR, Walker SM, Varga EM, et al: Long-term clinical efficacy of grass-pollen immunotherapy, *N Engl J Med* 341:468-475, 1999.

91. Bousquet J, Michel FB: Specific immunotherapy in asthma: is it effective? *J Allergy Clin Immunol* 94:1-11, 1994.

92. Leynadier F, Herman D, Vervloet D, et al: Specific immunotherapy with a standardized latex extract versus placebo in allergic healthcare workers, *J Allergy Clin Immunol* 106:585-590, 2000.

93. Janssen R, Kruisselbrink A, Hoogteijling L, et al: Analysis of recombinant mycobacteria as T helper type 1 vaccines in an allergy challenge model, *Immunology* 102:441-449, 2001.

94. Raz E, Tighe H, Sato Y, et al: Preferential induction of a Th1 immune response and inhibition of specific IgE antibody formation by plasmid DNA immunization, *Proc Natl Acad Sci U S A* 93:5141-5145, 1996.

95. Hsu CH, Chua KY, Tao MH, et al: Immunoprophylaxis of allergen-induced immunoglobulin E synthesis and airway hyperresponsiveness *in vivo* by genetic immunization, *Nat Med* 2:540-544, 1996.

96. Horner AA, Nguyen MD, Ronaghy A, et al: DNA-based vaccination reduces the risk of lethal anaphylactic hypersensitivity in mice, *J Allergy Clin Immunol* 106:349-356, 2000.

97. Sudowe S, Montermann E, Steitz J, et al: Efficacy of recombinant adenovirus as vector for allergen gene therapy in a mouse model of type I allergy, *Gene Ther* 9:147-156, 2002.

98. Moffatt MF, Cookson WO: Gene therapy for peanut allergy, *Nat Med* 5:380-381, 1999.

99. Roy K, Mao HQ, Huang SK, et al: Oral gene delivery with chitosan—DNA nanoparticles generates immunologic protection in a murine model of peanut allergy, *Nat Med* 5:387-391, 1999.

100. Hogan SP, Foster PS, Tan X, et al: Mucosal IL-12 gene delivery inhibits allergic airways disease and restores local antiviral immunity, *Eur J Immunol* 28:413-423, 1998.

101. Dow SW, Schwarze J, Heath TD, et al: Systemic and local interferon gamma gene delivery to the lungs for treatment of allergen-induced airway hyperresponsiveness in mice, *Hum Gene Ther* 10:1905-1914, 1999.

102. During MJ, Xu R, Young D, et al: Perioral gene therapy of lactose intolerance using an adeno-associated virus vector, *Nat Med* 4:1131-1135, 1998.

103. Poppema S, Potters M, Visser L, et al: Immune escape mechanisms in Hodgkin's disease, *Ann Oncol* 9(suppl)5:S21-S24, 1998.

104. Bollard CM, Rossig C, Calogne MJ, et al: Adapting a transforming growth factor beta-related tumor protection strategy to enhance antitumor immunity, *Blood* 99:3179-3187, 2002.

105. Lewin AS, Hauswirth WW: Ribozyme gene therapy: applications for molecular medicine, *Trends Mol Med* 7:221-228, 2001.

106. Marasco WA, Dana JS: Antibodies for targeted gene therapy: extracellular gene targeting and intracellular expression, *Adv Drug Deliv Rev* 31:153-170, 1998.

107. Marasco WA, LaVecchio J, Winkler A: Human anti-HIV-1 tat sFv intrabodies for gene therapy of advanced HIV-1 infection and AIDS, *J Immunol Methods* 231:223-238, 1999.

108. Mhashilkar AM, Biswas DK, LaVecchio J, et al: Inhibition of human immunodeficiency virus type 1 replication *in vitro* by a novel combination of anti-Tat single-chain intrabodies and NF- kappa B antagonists, *J Virol* 71:6486-6494, 1997.

109. Richardson JH, Sodroski JG, Waldmann TA, et al: Phenotypic knockout of the high-affinity human interleukin 2 receptor by intracellular single-chain antibodies against the alpha subunit of the receptor, *Proc Natl Acad Sci U S A* 92:3137-3141, 1995.

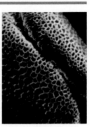

CHAPTER 21

Stem Cell Therapeutics: An Overview

MARISHA A. STANISLAUS ■ ALAN M. GEWIRTZ

Stem cells are the ultimate source of all body tissues. They are characterized biologically by two essential features. The first is that, until appropriately cued by environmental signals, they exist *in vivo* in a quiescent, undifferentiated state; the second is that they have the ability to self-renew. They are characterized initially as being totipotent, pluripotent, or monopotent. During normal embryogenesis, the "totipotent" (from the Latin word *totus,* meaning "entire") zygote, or fertilized egg, divides and differentiates into all the cells and specialized tissues (e.g., blood, neural, liver) that compose the human body. "Pluripotent" (from the Latin word *pluris,* meaning "several" or "many") stem cells are derived from the early human embryo or from fetal tissue that was destined to be a part of the gonads. These cells have the potential to develop into any of the cells that are ultimately derived from the three embryonic germ (EG) cell layers, that is, the endoderm, mesoderm, and ectoderm (Figure 21-1). Monopotent cells exist within the specialized tissue and, at least until recently, were thought to give rise only to cell types belonging to that tissue.

Stem cells can be of embryonic or adult origin. Embryonic stem (ES) cells are derived from the inner cell mass of the blastocyst, which forms in the early stages (4 to 5 days after fertilization) of embryonic development, before implantation in the uterine wall. These cells can self-renew and are pluripotent.[1] Adult stem cells may be found in many specialized tissues of the body, including the brain, bone marrow, liver, skin, gastrointestinal tract, cornea and retina of the eye, and even the dental pulp of the tooth. In the adult, all of these tissues are in a perpetual state of flux and, even in the absence of injury, are continuously giving rise to new cells to replace those that have worn out.[2] It was suggested earlier that adult stem cells are monopotent, but a number of recent investigations have suggested that they may be more "plastic" than previously thought. For example, adult stem cells derived from the bone marrow, apart from differentiating into blood and immune cells, can also develop into cells of nonhematopoietic lineages such as skeletal muscle,[3,4] microglia and astroglia in the brain,[5,6] and hepatocytes of the liver.[7] These observations have given rise to the notion that adult stem cells may be as programmable as ES cells, suggesting that they may be very useful in clinical medicine. Whether adult stem cells are truly pluripotent or able to replicate indefinitely in culture remains to be established.

EMBRYONIC STEM CELLS

Beginning in 1998, scientists discovered that ES cells could be isolated from early human embryos, grown in culture for long periods of time while maintaining a normal karyotype, and made to differentiate into a wide array of tissues and organs derived from all three EG layers.[8-12] These long-term cultures of ES cells have active telomerase and maintain long telomeres, which are markers of proliferating cells.[8,10,13,14] ES cells have also been successfully isolated from the primordial germ cells of the gonadal ridge of the 5- to 10-week fetus and are referred to as EG cells.[9,15] With continued development, the gonadal ridge develops into the testes or ovaries, and the primordial germ cells develop into the eggs or sperm. ES and EG cells differ in the conditions required for their isolation, culture, life span *in vitro,* and differentiation ability. ES cells can proliferate for up to 300 population doublings and can be passaged for more than 1 year in culture, whereas EG cells can proliferate for up to only 80 population doublings.[8,10,12,16] Most diploid somatic cells do not express high levels of telomerase and enter replicative senescence after a finite life span of 50 to 80 population doublings in tissue culture.[16] Thus properties of the cells of the early embryo, such as normal karyotype and high telomerase activity, are sustained in human ES cells in culture for extended periods of time.

Stem cell lines have been developed from both ES and EG cells. They are capable of self-renewal over long periods and can give rise to many differentiated cell types.[8,9,17,18] This discovery led to ES and EG cells being widely investigated for their potential to cure diseases by repairing or replacing damaged cells and tissues. One of the current perceived advantages of using ES cells over adult stem cells is that ES cells have the ability to proliferate for long periods of time *in vitro* and can be directed to differentiate into a broad range of cell types.[9,19] ES cells, when removed from feeder layers and transferred to suspension cultures, begin to differentiate into three-dimensional, multicellular aggregates of differentiated and undifferentiated cells termed "embryoid bodies." Embryoid bodies are composed of a haphazard collection of precursor and more fully differentiated cells from a wide variety of lineages and resemble early postimplantation embryos.[19] Frequently, within 7 to 14 days of transfer, these embryoid bodies progress through a series of stages that begin as a simple, morula-like ball of cells, eventually forming cavitated and cystic embryoid

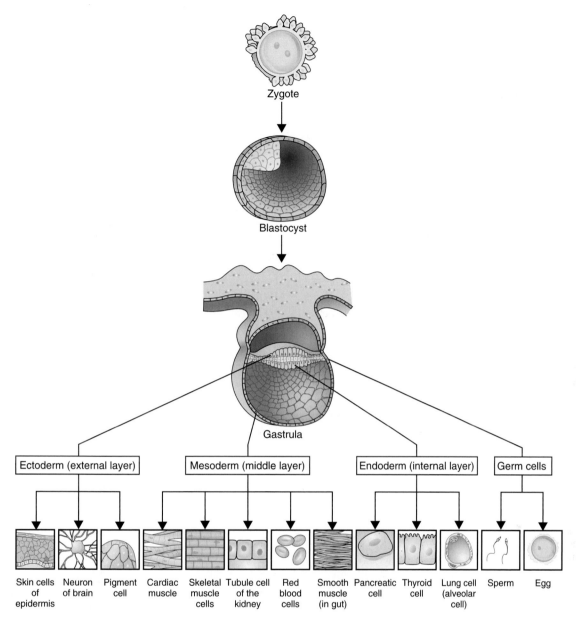

Zygote

Blastocyst

Gastrula

| Ectoderm (external layer) | Mesoderm (middle layer) | Endoderm (internal layer) | Germ cells |

Skin cells of epidermis · Neuron of brain · Pigment cell · Cardiac muscle · Skeletal muscle cells · Tubule cell of the kidney · Red blood cells · Smooth muscle (in gut) · Pancreatic cell · Thyroid cell · Lung cell (alveolar cell) · Sperm · Egg

FIGURE 21-1 Embryonic origin and developmental potential of specialized tissues within the human body. Note in particular the gastrula's three main germ cell layers, which develop from the blastocyst (from whose inner cell layer embryonic stem cells are derived). Of additional interest, the mesoderm ultimately gives rise to all formed elements of the blood (myeloid and erythroid) as well as the cells of the immune system. (Modified from Terese Winslow, Medical Illustrator, 2001.)

bodies.[11] *In vitro* differentiation experiments have shown that plated cultures of embryoid bodies show a variety of different morphologies, including rhythmically contracting cardiomyocytes, pigmented and nonpigmented epithelial cells, neural cells having outgrowths of axons and dendrites, and mesenchymal cells.[16] Recent studies have also demonstrated that embryoid bodies derived from the human ES cell line H9 express genes specific for each of the three EG layers, including α-fetoprotein, neurofilament 68-kDa subunit, gammaglobulin, and α−cardiac actin marking primitive endoderm, neuroectoderm, and mesoderm derivatives.[11,12,20]

The full developmental potential of ES cells is unveiled when these cells are studied in an *in vivo* environment, such as injection into a host blastocyst.[8,21] Human ES cells injected into mice with severe combined immunodeficiency (SCID) form benign teratomas, with advanced differentiated tissues representing all three EG layers.[8] These tissues include highly specialized derivatives of ectoderm, such as neural epithelium; of mesoderm, such as bone, cartilage, striated muscle, fetal glomeruli, and renal tubules; and of endoderm, such as the gut.[8] The formation of organized tissues during normal embryogenesis is controlled by many inductive events and complex epithelial-mesenchymal interactions. These events and interactions are seen to occur in teratomas but are less clear in *in vitro* differentiation.[16] Because we have yet to fully understand the precise inductive elements that regulate embryonic pattern formation and reproduce it *in vitro,* it would be very useful to explore methods of extracting cells/tissues of interest from the heterogeneous teratomas or to direct differentiation *in vivo* toward a particular lineage. Feasible methods to achieve this include (1) adding certain specific combinations of growth factors or chemical morphogens, (2) co-culturing/transplanting ES cells with inducer tissues or cells, (3) implanting ES cells into specific organs or regions, (4) overexpressing transcription factors associated with the development of specific tissues, (5) selecting cells that activate a particular lineage-specific program of gene expression, and (6) isolating cells of interest based on fluorescence-activated cell sorting.[16,20,22-30] Some of these methods have been used to enrich ES cell cultures for a particular cell type of interest *in vitro;* however, much remains to be done *in vivo.*[16]

POTENTIAL CLINICAL USES

Stem cells have been proposed to have a number of uses, but the most obvious, and potentially of greatest use, is to restore or replace tissue that has been damaged by disease or injury. Studies in animal models have shown that transplantation of fetal, ES, or pluripotent stem cell derivatives can successfully treat many chronic diseases or conditions such as Parkinson's disease, diabetes, injury of the spinal cord, Purkinje cell degeneration, Duchenne's muscular dystrophy, liver or heart failure, and osteogenesis imperfecta.[22,31-39] In this review, we highlight recent developments for three of these diseases—(diabetes, Parkinson's disease, and congestive heart failure (CHF)—which will serve as examples for the use of stem cells as therapeutic agents.

DIABETES

The ability to culture insulin-producing pancreatic islet cells from ES cells holds great promise for the cure of type 1 diabetes. In theory, a line of ES cells that could be cultivated into producing islet cells on demand could be made available. These cells could also be genetically engineered to avoid immune rejection.[16] On a more practical level, it is very difficult to induce ES cells to differentiate into a specific lineage. Purification of a single cell type from the initial mixed population is also difficult. Percentages of differentiated cells expressing a single phenotype in this mixture are very small, ranging typically from 0.1% to 0.5%.[40] Only rarely have specific culture conditions or growth factors led to the establishment of cultures containing only a single cell type.[19,20] Even in these cases, the human pluripotent cell lines retain a broad array of multilineage gene expression profiles despite the addition of specific growth factors.[19,20] Methods to circumvent the problem of purification of a single cell type include engineering the cells to use a tissue-specific promoter to drive the expression of either a selectable marker such as an antibiotic resistance gene[22,26,28] or a gene encoding the green fluorescence protein.[41,42] For the isolation of cells containing insulin,[22,40] transfected mouse ES cells with a chimeric construct containing the regulatory region of the insulin gene coupled to the

gene encoding neomycin resistance followed by isolating cells that were neomycin resistant. These cells, when cloned and cultured under low concentrations of glucose, underwent differentiation and were able to respond to changes in glucose concentration by up to a sevenfold increase in insulin secretion. When these cells were implanted into the spleens of streptozotocin-induced diabetic mice, the researchers were able to reverse the symptoms of diabetes and restore blood glucose concentrations to normal levels. These results showed that diabetes could be among the first applications of stem cell therapy.

In 2000, Schuldiner et al[20] reported that they were able to successfully culture human ES cells to form embryoid bodies, which spontaneously expressed *PDX-1,* a gene that controls the transcription of insulin. Assady et al[43] reported that these embryoid bodies contained 1% to 3% beta islet insulin-producing cells. They also found that the embryoid bodies express *glut-2* and islet-specific glucokinase genes, both of which are important for beta cell function and insulin secretion. When the cells were cultured with glucose, they were found to secrete insulin. The investigators were hopeful that refining the culture conditions could lead to the differentiation of pancreatic islets.

Research efforts have also been directed toward culturing islet cells from adult pancreatic tissue. Differentiated beta cells are difficult to proliferate in culture. However, one group has been able to engineer islet cells derived from human cadavers by adding DNA-encoding genes that stimulate cell proliferation to drive growth in culture. The cells were also engineered to stimulate the expression of the insulin gene because the establishment of this sort of cell line in culture causes the cells to lose the production of insulin. When the cells were transplanted into immune-deficient mice, they produced insulin in response to glucose. Investigations into whether these cells will reverse diabetes in diabetic mice are ongoing.[44,45] The cells that line pancreatic ducts have been shown to be a potential source of islet progenitor cells, and some studies have shown that when these ductal cells are cultured, they can be induced to differentiate into clusters containing both ductal and islet endocrine cells, which are found to secrete insulin when given glucose.[23]

DISEASES OF THE NERVOUS SYSTEM

Stem cells have tremendous therapeutic potential as a cell-based therapy to rebuild damaged neurons in diseases of the nervous system such as Parkinson's disease, amyotrophic lateral sclerosis (Lou Gehrig's disease), Alzheimer's disease, and others. Parkinson's disease is a neurodegenerative disease that progresses with age; it usually strikes after the age of 50 years. It affects neurons in the brain that secrete the neurotransmitter dopamine. As the neurons die, levels of dopamine being produced decrease, and this leads to the movement disorders characteristic of Parkinson's disease. Levodopa, which is converted to dopamine in the brain, is the mainstay of treatment for this disease, but most patients develop tachyphylaxis to its effects over time. In contrast to diabetes, in which the transplantation of islet cells is a therapeutic option, the implantation of fully differentiated dopamine-releasing neurons into the brain is not presently possible. Dopaminergic neurons do not survive transplantation, and it is very difficult to establish the appropriate connections with their normal target neurons in the striatum.[46]

It was previously thought that nerve cells in the brain do not divide. In recent years, however, many investigators have shown that stem cells that self-renew and differentiate appropriately into the three major neuronal lineages, neurons, astrocytes, and oligodendrocytes, do occur in the adult mammalian brain.[47-53] Fetal tissue is a very rich source of neuronal stem cells.[48] Human trials using fetal neuronal tissue from electively aborted fetuses have been conducted, and it was initially reported that they were able to achieve a clear reduction in the severity of the symptoms of patients with Parkinson's disease.[54-57] Using positron emission tomography (PET) scanning, scientists were able to measure an increase in dopamine neuron function in the striatum of the patients.[57] However, these trials were done on an "open-label" basis, meaning that both the investigator and patient knew which patient was the recipient of the transplanted tissue. In 2001, Freed et al[58] reported the results of the first double-blind placebo-controlled neural transplantation trial for Parkinson's disease. These results were not as encouraging as the initial reports. Patients receiving the transplants showed no significant benefit in a subjective assessment of the patient's quality of life, which was the primary end point of the study.[1,58,59] However, PET scans revealed that the transplanted dopamine neurons survived and grew, giving hope that the procedure might be made more effective by some modification in technique. Another double-blind trial is currently being conducted, and the results are anxiously awaited.[1]

Even if these trials prove to be successful, the use of cell implantation has a number of drawbacks, including the lack of sufficient amounts of well-characterized and standardized cell material. Furthermore, widespread application will likely be limited as long as access to embryonic donor tissue is required.[59] For these reasons, the development of alternative sources of cells for therapeutic purposes is the object of intense investigation. Candidate cells would form a renewable, unlimited source of cells capable of differentiating into functional dopamine neurons. Recently, Zhang et al[60] and Reubinoff et al[61] reported a potential alternative to the use of fetal tissue transplantation through the development of methods of inducing human ES cells to differentiate into neural stem cells, which differentiated in vitro into the three neural lineages. When these neural stem cells were transplanted into the brains of neonate rodents, they incorporated into the host brain, demonstrated widespread distribution, and differentiated into all three neural lineages. The transplanted cells migrated along established tracks and differentiated in a region-specific manner, which showed their capability to respond to local cues and participate in the processes of host brain development. Both groups also reported that they observed no evidence of teratoma or non-neural tissue formations in the brains of transplant recipients. Further studies are required to show the functionality of the newly generated neurons. Recent studies reported by Bjorklund et al[62] showed that undifferentiated mouse ES cells transplanted into the rat striatum spontaneously differentiated into dopaminergic neurons that restored cerebral function in the animal. Kawasaki et al[63] identified a stromal cell—derived inducing activity that promoted the in vitro differentiation of neural primate ES cells. When these dopamine-producing cells were transplanted into

the brains of mice with SCID, they were observed to give rise to dopaminergic neurite formation in the target tissue within 2 weeks. Kim et al[39] also reported successful results after infecting murine ES cells with a Nurr1 expression construct that allowed increased survival and neuronal differentiation of the transplanted ES cells.

It should be noted that there is much debate over how many populations of central nervous system stem cells exist, how they are related, and how they function in vivo. There are currently no identifiable markers that exist for identifying the neuronal stem cells in vivo, and the only way to test whether a certain population of central nervous system cells contains stem cells is to manipulate them in vitro.[50] Many of the transplantation studies that used nonselected ES cells as transplants resulted in spheroid-like aggregates containing differentiated neurons.[64] A selection procedure has been established that allows for the enrichment of nestin-expressing neural precursor cells, which have been shown to differentiate and participate in the normal rat brain.[63,65-67] The transplantation of selected neural precursor cells has shown better integration into the host tissue.[68,69] Recently, Andressen et al[69] genetically engineered murine ES cells to express the enhanced green fluorescent protein (EGFP) under the control of a thymidine kinase promoter/nestin second intron and were able to specifically detect EGFP in nestin-immunoreactive neural precursor cells. On transplantation into rat brains, these cells were observed to integrate into the host tissue and served as a pool for successive neuronal and glial differentiation. Thus a combination of a specific selection protocol for neural precursor cells with the specific expression of EGFP in these cells may offer a valuable opportunity to gain a pure neural precursor cell population for in vitro maintenance and expansion, followed by in vivo transplantation. Also, the use of fluorescence-activated cell sorting to purify EGFP-labeled neural precursor cells will be useful for the standardization of a donor cell population for cell replacement therapies.[69]

Another promising area in stem cell therapy of the nervous system that is briefly mentioned here involves the "repair mechanism." It was found that on brain injury, stem cells in two specific areas of the brain, the subventricular zone and the dentate gyrus of the hippocampus, proliferated and migrated toward the site of damage.[70] Fallon et al[71] have shown that transforming growth factor-α, a peptide involved in tissue repair and present in the earliest embryos, induces a "wave of migration" of stem cells when injected into damaged areas of the brain. Of equal interest, these stem cells subsequently differentiated into dopamine neurons. Also, it is important to note that treated rats did not show any of the behavioral abnormalities associated with the loss of the neurons. Further investigations of the beneficial effects on parkinsonian symptoms are ongoing.

The study of stem cell therapeutics for curing Parkinson's disease is a good model for nervous system disorders because it is a relatively easy target involving the replacement of only one particular cell type in a single area of the brain. However, therapies for other disorders, such as an injury of the spinal cord, where many cell types are destroyed, face much larger hurdles. Clearly, more research needs to be done, but the use of stem cells for treating nervous system disorders is rapidly advancing, and this approach appears to hold great promise for the future.

REPAIRING A DAMAGED HEART

CHF afflicts millions of people around the world, with 400,000 new cases being reported in the United States itself every year. CHF may result from many causes, including hypertension, infection, and coronary artery disease. Although many medical and surgical treatments for CHF are available, the long-term prognosis of these patients remains guarded, with an average life expectancy of about 5 years after diagnosis.[1] Using stem cells to repair damaged myocardium holds promise equal to that for the treatment of myocardial disease. Transplanting autologous stem cells would have clear-cut advantages over transplanting the whole organ because it would obviate the need for a donor and for the requisite immunosuppression needed to suppress rejection of the transplanted heart. It is now known that by using highly specific culture conditions, stem cells can be driven toward differentiating into cardiomyocytes, vascular endothelial cells that form the inner lining of new blood vessels, and smooth muscle cells that form the wall of blood vessels.[72,73] Of particular importance are the preclinical studies in rodent models in which heart failure is induced by myocardial infarction caused by selective ligation of the coronary arteries. Recently, Orlic and colleagues[74] showed that by injecting adult bone marrow−derived hematopoietic stem cells (HSCs) into the heart of a mouse that had been induced to have a heart attack, they were able to form new cardiomyocytes, vascular endothelium, and smooth muscle cells. Within 9 days after injection, the newly generated myocardium, including coronary arteries and capillaries, occupied up to 68% of the damaged portion of the ventricle. Mice that received the transplanted cells survived in much greater numbers than the control mice. These results suggested that the HSCs were able to respond to internal signals within the heart, migrate toward the injured ventricle, and give rise to specialized, differentiated heart cells. Jackson et al[75] performed a similar study using adult stem cells derived from mouse bone marrow and delivered these into the model mice via bone marrow transplantation. They found that after 2 to 4 weeks, the survival rate was 26%, with the damaged heart tissue showing the presence of donor-derived cardiomyocytes and endothelial cells. This study provided yet another alternative for the delivery and therapeutic strategy of stem cells for the repair/growth of cardiac tissue. Kocher et al[76] took this one step further and showed that human bone marrow−derived adult stem cells, when injected into rats, were able to give rise to vascular endothelial cells, forming new blood vessels.

Human ES cells are also showing much promise for cell-based cardiac therapy. In 2000, Itskovitz-Eldor et al[11] showed that human ES cells could reproducibly differentiate in culture into cells that exhibited cellular markers and the physical appearance of heart cells. Kehat et al[73] have also shown that human ES cells can also differentiate into myocytes that portray cardiomyocytic structural and functional properties. The next step in this research is to see whether these ES cells can repair and replace damaged heart cells in an animal model.

There is no doubt that adult and ES cells are proving to be very useful in stem cell therapy for replacing damaged heart tissue. However, many questions still remain to be answered. For instance, how many cells would be required to repair one human heart? How long will the replacement cells continue to function? Do the results from the animal models accurately reflect human heart conditions and transplantation responses? Would it be feasible for "at-risk" patients to donate their stem cells in advance so that no time is lost between having a heart attack and receiving the stem cell transplantation? The answers to these questions are being pursued by many investigators and, when received, will provide a much better idea of how useful stem cell therapy of damaged myocardium will turn out to be.

CLINICAL APPLICATIONS OF HEMATOPOIETIC STEM CELLS

It is probably fair to say that stem cell research began with the hematology community and the many scientists who were engaged in studies of hematopoiesis, the process of blood formation. The pioneering work of Till and McCullough[77] in the 1960s on hematopoietic cells helped define the two hallmark characteristics of all stem cells, namely their ability to self-renew and to differentiate into all the formed elements of the blood. Much research has been done to identify and characterize HSCs. This task has, however, proved difficult because the cells are rare and morphologically indistinguishable from other primitive cells. Thus one has to rely on cell surface proteins as markers for the isolation of HSCs. Much of the initial research on establishing such markers was done with mice, which laid the groundwork for human analyses.[78] For human HSCs, some of these markers are CD34+, lineage (lin)−, Thy1+, c-*kit*−/low, and CD38−/low.[79]

After destroying the patient's own hematopoietic cells using radiation and/or chemotherapy, HSCs collected from the blood or bone marrow of the donor are transfused into the recipient. An adult typically requires 7 to 10 million "stem" cells per kilogram of body weight for transplantation, and these are enriched in the CD34+ population of cells. CD34+ cells obtained from peripheral blood have been reported to engraft quicker but likely at the expense of causing more graft-versus-host disease (GVHD) than bone marrow−derived cells.[80] HSCs present in umbilical cord blood units are the least likely to incite GVHD but are difficult to use for adult transplantation because it is an infrequent occurrence that a sufficient number can be obtained from a single cord to transplant into a patient.[81] There are many complications of HSC transplantation in addition to GVHD, and these include prolonged immunosuppression and secondary malignancies (see also Chapter 18).

Adult HSC transplantation is by now a common procedure for the treatment of a variety of hematologic diseases, both "benign," such as aplastic anemia, beta-thalassemia, and globoid cell leukodystrophy, and inborn errors of metabolism such as Hunter's syndrome and Lesch-Nyhan syndrome.[1] Transplants are also widely used for the treatment of malignant hematologic diseases such as leukemia, lymphoma, and myeloma and, more recently, autoimmune diseases such as systemic lupus erythematosus.[82] Finally, the GVHD engendered by the transplant of competent donor immune cells is also finding use in the treatment of other solid tumor malignancies.[83]

STEM CELLS AND GENE THERAPY

A final area in which stem cells will undoubtedly influence clinical medicine is gene therapy. Gene therapy uses genetic engineering to alter, supplement, or replace the activity of an abnormal gene by introducing a normal copy of the gene or providing a gene that adds new functions. The initial clinical trials using gene therapy focused on replacing a defective gene with a normal copy of that gene in patients with single-gene disorders such as cystic fibrosis[84] and Duchenne muscular dystrophy.[85] Now, efforts are increasingly being directed toward complex, chronic diseases that involve more than one gene, including heart disease, arthritis, and Alzheimer's disease.

Two major strategies are used for delivering therapeutic transgenes to patients. The first is to use a "direct delivery" system whereby the therapeutic transgene is packaged into a delivery vehicle such as a disarmed virus and injected into the patient's target organ. This delivery method is limited to specific types of human cells that the viral vehicle can infect, composed largely of dividing cells. This limits their usefulness in treating diseases of organs such as the heart or brain, which are composed of mainly nondividing cells. The second strategy is to use "cell-based delivery" whereby the therapeutic transgene is packaged into a delivery vehicle such as a disarmed virus and introduced into a delivery cell such as a stem cell that is derived from the patient. These genetically modified cells are then multiplied in the laboratory and infused back into the patient. This method is more advantageous than direct gene transfer because it allows researchers more control over selection of genetically modified cells when they are manipulated outside the body and because investigators can control the level and rate of production of the therapeutic agent in the cells.[86]

Stem cells are of great benefit to cell-based gene therapy because they are self-renewing and thus may reduce or eliminate the repeated administrations of the gene therapy. Of the approximately 450 gene therapy clinical trials conducted in the United States so far, 40% have been cell based, of which 30% have used HSCs as the means of delivering transgenes into patients. These cells are the first choice for several reasons, including the facts that they can be readily isolated from the circulating blood or bone marrow of adults or the cord blood of newborns and that redelivering them into the patient is relatively easy via injection.

HSCs differentiate into a number of lineages in which the therapeutic transgene will reside. Apart from "homing" to the bone marrow, these stem cells are also capable of migrating to many different areas of the body, including the bone marrow, liver, spleen, and lymph nodes, which would be very useful in the treatment of diseases other than just those of the blood, such as liver metabolic disorders and Gaucher's disease.[1] So far HSCs have been the only kind of adult stem cell used in human trials. However, several other adult stem cells are being studied as vehicle candidates for gene therapy, including muscle-forming stem cells, or myoblasts[87,88]; bone-forming stem cells, or osteoblasts;[89] and neural stem cells.[90]

ES cells possess qualities such as pluripotency and unlimited proliferative capacity, which make them very attractive for use in cell-based gene therapy. At this stage, however, such ES cell therapy is still highly hypothetical and experimental because research is limited to only a few laboratories that have access to human ES cells. As time progresses and more advances are made, it will be necessary to identify optimal stages of differentiation for transplant and to prove that the transplanted ES cells are able to integrate, function, and survive in the recipient. There are some drawbacks to and concerns regarding the use of ES cells in therapy. Human ES cells used for

transplantation have the propensity to induce the formation of teratomas.[91,92] These teratomas are, however, typically benign. It has been found it is the undifferentiated ES cells that induce teratomas. Therefore this tumor formation might be avoided if a method was devised to remove the undifferentiated cells before transplantation. Researchers are now considering the possibility of genetically modifying ES cells, differentiating them in culture, and then isolating large, pure populations of differentiated cells for transplant. They could also be used as laboratory models for differentiation allowing the evaluation of vectors for gene delivery and translation within the patient.[1]

The immunologic status of human ES cells has not been studied in great detail, and the question of whether these cells would trigger immune rejection in the recipient remains to be answered. It is also important to understand the mechanisms by which ES cells can proliferate, yet remain undifferentiated in culture. The choice between self-renewal and differentiation is highly regulated by intrinsic signals and the external microenviroment.[93] To realize the true therapeutic potential of ES and EG cells, it is first important to understand the molecular and genetic bases by which these cells continue to replicate for prolonged periods of time. Second, to perform successful transplantations in patients, it is important to have a sufficient number of cells that can be manipulated to differentiate into the desired cell type. Achieving clinical success with ES cells looks promising and may provide solutions for many of the technical hurdles faced by therapeutic gene transfer today.

SCIENTIFIC AND ETHICAL ISSUES

Stem cells hold great promise to cure many diseases that were earlier thought to be incurable. However, their potential use in clinical therapy has raised many concerns, both scientific and ethical in nature. From the purely scientific perspective, as discussed earlier, many questions remain to be answered before they are considered safe for clinical applications. Of equal importance, however, are logistical and ethical issues associated with the use of material of fetal origin. Regarding the former issue, there is sufficient concern about the origin and identification of cells to warrant the existence of a "safety net" composed of a set of safeguards for human stem cells to be used in clinical applications. These include the following:

1. Donor sources of stem cells should be carefully screened for pedigree evaluation/genetic testing and infectious diseases.
2. Because most stem cells are maintained and expanded in culture before transplantation, it is imperative that controlled, standardized practices and procedures be followed to maintain the integrity, uniformity, and reliability of the human stem cell preparations.
3. Stem cells, and those of an embryonic origin in particular, are highly pluripotent and have the capacity to differentiate into all cell types. It is therefore imperative to gauge the purity of a cellular preparation through the rigorous and quantitative identification of cell types within a heterogeneous population of differentiating human cells.
4. Before transplantation, human stem cell preparations must be shown to possess relevant biologic activity. For

example, pancreatic islet-like cells must release insulin, cells intended for liver tissue regeneration must be capable of storing glycogen, and cardiomyocytes intended for heart transplantation must be shown to contract synchronously.

5. "Proof of concept" must be clearly established in an animal model to demonstrate the validity, efficacy, and safety of the intended therapy.[1]

The use of human ES cells in medical research has drawn much attention from the public, and many ethical issues have been raised that concern their use solely for the purpose of medical benefit. Many consider this research to be immoral, illegal, and unnecessary.[94] The fact that experiments using ES cells, as performed currently, result in the death of an embryo cannot be ignored. Stem cell research must not lead to an underground black market of "spare" embryos.[95] In principle, because pluripotent cells proliferate indefinitely, it should be possible for medical research to be conducted on the directed differentiation of stem cells using the relatively few human pluripotent stem cell lines that have been derived so far. This is the basis for the policy proposed by President George W. Bush, who limited funding of human ES cell research to the 64 human cell lines already established before August 9, 2001. This ruling is causing unrest among members of the scientific community, who claim that not all 64 lines can be used for research and distribution of the cell lines is restricted by patenting, commercial secrecy, and restrictive national and international material transfer agreements.[96] These ethical issues are not relevant to adult stem cell research in which cells are isolated from the adult, such as the harvesting of HSCs for bone marrow transplantation. However, this approach is somewhat problematic because adult stem cells are thought not to be as "plastic" as ES cells. Contrary to this view, the most recent experiment to address this issue suggests that a population of multipotent mesenchymal stem cells with all the developmental potential of ES cells may reside in human marrow.[97] If these observations are confirmed and the cells can be prospectively identified and isolated from marrow in sufficient numbers, one very difficult issue for stem cell therapy will have been solved.

CONCLUSIONS

As discussed in detail earlier and summarized in Box 21-1, stem cells can be found in embryonic as well as adult tissues, and their potential for treating a wide variety of common and uncommon diseases is almost as limitless as their ability to undergo cell divisions. Nonetheless, this therapeutic potential will be fulfilled only if stem cells can be isolated and purified in sufficient numbers to truly affect organ function. This would mean that the cells are present not only in sufficient numbers but also that they function as efficiently as the cell population they are designed to replace. If the present pace of research continues unabated, however, we will soon learn more about the differences and similarities of embryonic and adult stem cells and their ability to survive, proliferate, and function after transplantation. Accordingly, although it is difficult to predict the ultimate usefulness of stem cell-based therapy at this time, it is not difficult to conclude that this is an enormously important area of scientific research and one that has great potential monetary rewards. For these reasons,

| BOX 21-1 | **KEY CONCEPTS** *Stem Cell Therapeutics* |

- Stem cells are the source of all specialized cells of the body.
- These cells are defined by two essential characteristics: the ability to self-renew and the ability to differentiate into multiple different tissue types.
- There are two main types, depending on origin: embryonic and adult.

    Embryonic cells, derived from the inner layer of blastocysts, have the greatest ability to proliferate and differentiate into virtually any specialized tissue.

    Adult cells, derived from the differentiated tissues of developed organs, compared with embryonic cells, appear to have more limited ability to proliferate and differentiate.

- The potential for treating disease that results from damaged tissue is great, but the usefulness is not yet proved.
- Ethical, religious, and political issues associated with the derivation and use of embryonic cells have not been fully resolved and remain stumbling blocks that impede scientific investigation in this area.

Modified from Kirschstein R, Skirboll LR: Stem cells: scientific progress and future research directions. 2001, National Institute of Health publication http://www.nih.gov/news/stemcell/scireport.htm.

on a worldwide basis, attempts to regulate stem cell research will likely prove difficult. In countries like the United States, one must hope for thoughtful legislative action on this front or the whole endeavor may be driven underground and away from these shores. Open discussions between political bodies and the various interest groups in the scientific, medical, and religious communities need to take place to address the concerns of each and to ultimately provide a solution for what is clearly in the interest of all mankind.

REFERENCES

1. Kirschstein R, Skirboll LR: Stem cells: scientific progress and future research directions. 2001, National Institute of Health publication http://www.nih.gov/news/stemcell/scireport.htm.
2. Fuchs E, Segre JA: Stem cells: a new lease on life, *Cell* 100:143-155, 2000.
3. Ferrari G, Cusella-DeAngelis G, Coletta M, et al: Muscle regeneration by bone marrow-derived myogenic progenitors (published erratum appears in *Science* 281:293, 1998), *Science* 279:1528-1530, 1998.
4. Gussoni E, Soneoka Y, Strickland CD, et al: Dystrophin expression in the mdx mouse restored by stem cell transplantation, *Nature* 401:390-394, 1999.
5. Eglitis MA, Mezey E: Hematopoietic cells differentiate into both microglia and macroglia in the brains of adult mice, *Proc Natl Acad Sci U S A* 94:4080-4085, 1997.
6. Kopen GC, Prockop DJ, Phinney DG: Marrow stromal cells migrate throughout forebrain and cerebellum, and they differentiate into astrocytes after injection into neonatal mouse brains, *Proc Natl Acad Sci U S A* 96:10711-10716, 1999.
7. Petersen PE, Bowen WC, Patrene KD, et al: Bone marrow as a potential source of hepatic oval cells, *Science* 284:1168-1170, 1999.
8. Thomson JA, Itskovitz-Eldor J, Shapiro SS, et al: Embryonic stem cell lines derived from human blastocysts, *Science* 282:1145-1147, 1998.
9. Shamblott MJ, Axelman J, Wang S, et al: Derivation of pluripotent stem cells from cultured human primordial germ cells, *Proc Natl Acad Sci U S A* 95:13726-13731, 1998.

10. Amit M, Carpenter MK, Inokuma MS, et al: Clonally derived human embryonic stem cell lines maintain pluripotency and proliferative potential for prolonged periods of culture, *Dev Biol* 227:271-278, 2000.

11. Itskovitz-Eldor J, Schulding M, Karsenti D, et al: Differentiation of human embryonic stem cells into embryoid bodies comprising the three embryonic germ layers, *Mol Med* 6:88-95, 2000.

12. Reubinoff BE, Pera MF, Fong CY, et al: Embryonic stem cell lines from human blastocysts: somatic differentiation *in vitro* (published erratum appears in *Nat Biotechnol* 18:559, 2000), *Nat Biotechnol* 18:399-404, 2000.

13. Betts DH, King WA: Telomerase activity and telomere detection during early bovine development, *Dev Genet* 25:397-403, 1999.

14. Brenner CA, Wolny YM, Adler RR, et al: Alternative splicing of the telomerase catalytic subunit in human oocytes and embryos, *Mol Hum Reprod* 5:845-850, 1999.

15. Matsui Y, Zsebo K, Hogan BL: Derivation of pluripotential embryonic germ cells from murine primordial germ cells in culture, *Cell* 70:841-847, 1992.

16. Odorico JS, Kaufman DS, Thomson JA: Multilineage differentiation from human embryonic stem cell lines, *Stem Cells* 19:193-204, 2001.

17. Bongso A, Fong CY, Ng SC, et al: Isolation and culture of inner cell mass cells from human blastocysts, *Hum Reprod* 9:2110-2117, 1994.

18. Andrews PW, Damjanov I, Simon D, et al: Pluripotent embryonal carcinoma clones derived from the human teratocarcinoma cell line Tera-2. Differentiation *in vivo* and *in vitro*, *Lab Invest* 50:147-162, 1984.

19. Shamblott MJ, Axelman J, Littlefield JW, et al: Human embryonic germ cell derivatives express a broad range of developmentally distinct markers and proliferate extensively *in vitro*, *Proc Natl Acad Sci U S A* 98: 113-118, 2001.

20. Schuldiner M, Yanuka O, Itskovitz-Eldor J, et al: Effects of eight growth factors on the differentiation of cells derived from human embryonic stem cells, *Proc Natl Acad Sci U S A* 97:11307-11312, 2000.

21. Bradley A, Evans M, Kaufman MH, et al: Formation of germline chimeras from embryo-derived teratocarcinoma cell lines, *Nature* 309:255-256, 1984.

22. Soria B, Roche E, Berna G, et al: Insulin-secreting cells derived from embryonic stem cells normalize glycemia in streptozotocin-induced diabetic mice, *Diabetes* 49:157-162, 2000.

23. Bonner-Weir S, Taneja M, Weir GC, et al: In vitro cultivation of human islets from expanded ductal tissue, *Proc Natl Acad Sci U S A* 97:7999-8004, 2000.

24. Levinson-Dushnik M, Benvenisty N: Involvement of hepatocyte nuclear factor 3 in endoderm differentiation of embryonic stem cells, *Mol Cell Biol* 17:3817-3822, 1997.

25. Ferber S, Halkin A, Cohen H, et al: Pancreatic and duodenal homeobox gene 1 induces expression of insulin genes in liver and ameliorates streptozotocin-induced hyperglycemia, *Nat Med* 6:568-572, 2000.

26. Klug MG, Soonpaa MH, Koh GY, et al: Genetically selected cardiomyocytes from differentiating embryonic stem cells form stable intracardiac grafts, *J Clin Invest* 98:216-224, 1996.

27. Li A, Simmons PJ, Kaur P, et al: Identification and isolation of candidate human keratinocyte stem cells based on cell surface phenotype, *Proc Natl Acad Sci U S A* 95:3902-3907, 1998.

28. Li M, Pevny L, Lovell-Badge R, et al: Generation of purified neural precursors from embryonic stem cells by lineage selection, *Curr Biol* 8: 971-974, 1998.

29. Weissman IL: Stem cells: units of development, units of regeneration, and units in evolution, *Cell* 100:157-168, 2000.

30. Saitou M, Baton SC, Surani MA: A molecular programme for the specification of germ cell fate in mice, *Nature* 418:293-300, 2002.

31. Zhang W, Lee WH, Triarhou LC: Grafted cerebellar cells in a mouse model of hereditary ataxia express IGF-I system genes and partially restore behavioral function, *Nat Med* 2:65-71, 1996.

32. Lilja H, Arkadopoulos N, Blanc P, et al: Fetal rat hepatocytes: isolation, characterization, and transplantation in the Ngase analbuminemic rats, *Transplantation* 64:1240-1248, 1997.

33. Brustle O, Choudhary K, Karram K, et al: Chimeric brains generated by intraventricular transplantation of fetal human brain cells into embryonic rats, *Nat Biotechnol* 16:1040-1044, 1998.

34. Studer L, Tabar V, McKay RDG: Transplantation of expanded mesencephalic precursors leads to recovery in parkinsonian rats, *Nat Neurosci* 1:290-295, 1998.

35. McDonald JW, Liu XZ, Qu Y, et al: Transplanted and therapeutic effects of bone-marrow derived mesenchymal cells in children with osteogenesis imperfecta, *Nat Med* 5:309-313, 1999.

36. Horwitz EM, Prockop DJ, Fitzpatrick LA, et al: Transplantability embryonic stem cells survive, differentiate and promote recovery in injured rat spinal cord, *Nat Med* 5:1410-1412, 1999.

37. Kobayashi N, Miyazaki M, Fukaya K, et al: Transplantation of highly differentiated immortalized human hepatocytes to treat acute liver failure, *Transplantation* 69:202-207, 2000.

38. Li RK, Weisel RD, Mickle DA, et al: Autologous porcine heart cell transplantation improved heart function after a myocardial infarction, *J Thorac Cardiovasc Surg* 119:62-68, 2000.

39. Kim J-H, Auerbach JM, Rodriguez-Gomez JA, et al: Dopamine neurons derived from embryonic stem cells function in an animal model of Parkinson's disease, *Nature* 418:50-56, 2002.

40. Soria B, Skoudy A, Martin F: From stem cells to beta cells: new strategies in cell therapy of diabetes mellitus, *Diabetologia* 44:407-415, 2001.

41. Kolossov E, Fleischmann BK, Liu Q, et al: Functional characteristics of embryonic stem cell-derived cardiac precursor cells identified by tissue-specific expression of the green fluorescent protein, *J Cell Biol* 143: 2045-2056, 1998.

42. Hadjantonakis AK, Nagy A: FACS for the isolation of individual cells from transgenic mice harboring a fluorescent protein reporter, *Genesis* 27:95-98, 2000.

43. Assady S, Maor G, Amit M, et al: Insulin production by human embryonic stem cells, *Diabetes* 50:1691-1697, 2001.

44. Dufayet de la Tour D, Halvorsen T, Demeterco C, et al: B-cell differentiation from a human pancreatic cell line *in vitro* and *in vivo*, *Mol Endocrinol* 15:476-483, 2001.

45. Itkin-Ansari P, Demeterco C, Bossie S, et al: PDX-1 and cell-cell contact act in synergy to promote d-cell development in a human pancreatic endocrine precursor cell line, *Mol Endocrinol* 14:814-822, 2001.

46. Quinn NP: The clinical application of cell grafting techniques in patients with Parkinson's disease, *Prog Brain Res* 82:619-625, 1990.

47. Gage FH, Coates PW, Palmer TD, et al: Survival and differentiation of adult neuronal progenitor cells transplanted to the adult brain, *Proc Natl Acad Sci U S A* 92:11879-11883, 1995.

48. Johe KK, Hazel TG, Muller T, et al: Single factors direct the differentiation of stem cells from the fetal and adult central nervous system, *Genes Dev* 10:3129-3140, 1996.

49. McKay R: Stem cells in the central nervous system, *Science* 276:66-71, 1997.

50. Morrison SJ, White PM, Zock C, et al: Prospective identification, isolation by flow cytometry, and *in vivo* self-renewal of multipotent mammalian neural crest stem cells, *Cell* 96:737-749, 1999.

51. Weiss S, van der Kooy D: CNS stem cells: where's the biology (a.k.a. beef)? *J Neurobiol* 36:307-314, 1998.

52. Shihabuddin LS, Palmer TD, Gage FH: The search for neural progenitor cells: prospects for the therapy of neurodegenerative disease, *Mol Med Today* 5:474-480, 1999.

53. Temple S, Alvarez-Buylla A: Stem cells in the adult mammalian central nervous system, *Curr Opin Neurobiol* 9:135-141, 1999.

54. Madrazo I, Leon V, Torres C, et al: Transplantation of fetal substantia nigra and adrenal medulla to the caudate nucleus in two patients with Parkinson's disease, *N Engl J Med* 318:51, 1988.

55. Lindvall O, Rehncrona S, Gustavii B, et al: Fetal dopamine-rich mesencephalic grafts in Parkinson's disease, *Lancet* 2:1483-1484, 1988.

56. Lindvall O, Rehncrona S, Brundin P, et al: Human fetal dopamine neurons grafted into the striatum in 2 patients with severe Parkinson's disease: a detailed account of methodology and a 6-month follow-up, *Arch Neurol* 46:615-631, 1989.

57. Lindvall O, Brundin P, Widner H, et al: Grafts of fetal dopamine neurons survive and improve motor function in Parkinson's disease, *Science* 247:574-577, 1990.

58. Freed CR, Greene PE, Breeze RE, et al: Transplantation of embryonic dopamine neurons for severe Parkinson's disease, *N Engl J Med* 344: 710-719, 2001.

59. Dunnett SB, Bjorklund A, Lindvall O: Cell therapy in Parkinson's disease: stop or go? *Nat Rev Neurosci* 2:365-369, 2001.

60. Zhang SC, Wernig M, Duncan ID, et al: In vitro differentiation of transplantable neural precursors from human embryonic stem cells, *Nat Biotechnol* 19:1129-1133, 2001.

61. Reubinoff BE, Itsykson P, Turetsky T, et al: Neural progenitors from human embryonic stem cells, *Nat Biotechnol* 19:1134-1140, 2001.

62. Bjorklund LM, Sanchez-Pernaute R, Chung S, et al: Embryonic stem cells develop into functional dopaminergic neurons after transplantation in a Parkinson rat model, *Proc Natl Acad Sci U S A* 99:2344-2349, 2002.

63. Kawasaki H, Suemori H, Mizuseki K, et al: Generation of dopaminergic neurons and pigmented epithelia from primate ES cells by stromal cell-derived inducing activity, *Proc Natl Acad Sci U S A* 99:1580-1585, 2002.

64. Deacon T, Dinsmore J, Costantini LC, et al: Blastula-stage stem cells can differentiate into dopaminergic and serotonergic neurons after transplantation, *Exp Neurol* 149:28-41, 1998.

65. Okabe S, Forsberg-Nilsson K, Spiro AC, et al: Development of neuronal precursor cells and functional postmitotic neurons from embryonic stem cells *in vitro*, *Mech Dev* 59:89-102, 1996.

66. Brustle O, Spiro AC, Karram K, et al: In-vitro generated neural precursors participate in mammalian brain development, *Proc Natl Acad Sci U S A* 94:14809-14814, 1997.

67. Brustle O, Jones KN, Learish RD, et al: Embryonic stem cell-derived glial precursors: a source of myelinating transplants, *Science* 285:754-756, 1999.

68. Arnhold S, Lenartz D, Kruttwig K, et al: Differentiation of green-fluorescent protein-labeled embryonic stem cell-derived neural precursor cells into Thy-1 positive neurons and glia after transplantation into adult rat striatum, *J Neurosurg* 93:1026-1032, 2000.

69. Andressen C, Stocker E, Klinz FJ, et al: Nestin-specific green fluorescent protein expression in embryonic stem cell-derived neural precursor cells used for transplantation, *Stem Cells* 19:419-424, 2001.

70. Bjorklund A, Lindvall O: Self-repair in the brain, *Nature* 405:892-895, 2000.

71. Fallon J, Reid S, Kinyamu R, et al: *In vivo* induction of massive proliferation, directed migration, and differentiation of neural cells in the adult mammalian brain, *Proc Natl Acad Sci U S A* 97:14686-14691, 2000.

72. Pittenger MF, Mackay AM, Beck SM, et al: Multilineage potential of adult human mesenchymal stem cells, *Science* 284:143-147, 1999.

73. Kehat I, Kenyagin-Karsenti D, Druckman M, et al: Human embryonic stem cells can differentiate into myocytes portraying cardiomyocytic structural and functional properties, *J Clin Invest* 108:407-414, 2001.

74. Orlic D, Kajstura J, Chimenti S, et al: Bone marrow cells regenerate infarcted myocardium, *Nature* 410:701-705, 2001.

75. Jackson KA, Majka SM, Wang H, et al: Regeneration of ischemic cardiac muscle and vascular endothelium by adult stem cells, *J Clin Invest* 107:1-8, 2001.

76. Kocher AA, Schuster MD, Szabolcs MJ, et al: Neovascularization of ischemic myocardium by human bone-marrow-derived angioblasts prevents cardiomyocyte apoptosis, reduces remodeling and improves cardiac function, *Nat Med* 7:430-436, 2001.

77. Till JE, McCullough EA: A direct measurement of the radiation sensitivity of normal mouse bone marrow cells, *Radiat Res* 14:213-222, 1961.

78. Sprangrude GJ, Heimfeld S, Weissman IL: Purification and characterization of mouse hematopoietic stem cells, *Science* 214:58-62, 1988.

79. Baum CM, Weissman IL, Tsukamoto AS, et al: Isolation of a candidate human hematopoietic stem-cell population, *Proc Natl Acad Sci U S A* 89:2804-2808, 1992.

80. Cutler C, Giri S, Jeyapalan S, et al: Acute and chronic graft-versus-host disease after allogeneic peripheral blood stem-cell and bone marrow transplantation: a meta-analysis, *J Clin Oncol* 19:3685-3691, 2001.

81. Laughlin MJ: Umbilical cord blood for allogeneic transplantation in children and adults, *Bone Marrow Transplant* 27:1-6, 2001.

82. Traynor AE, Schroeder J, Rosa RM, et al: Treatment of severe systemic lupus erythematosus with high-dose chemotherapy and hematopoietic stem-cell transplantation: a phase 1 study, *Lancet* 356:701-707, 2000.

83. Childs R, Chernoff A, Contentin N, et al: Regression of metastatic renal-cell carcinoma after nonmyeloablative allogeneic peripheral-blood stem-cell transplantation, *N Engl J Med* 343:750-758, 2000.

84. Knowles MR, Hohneker KW, Zhou Z, et al: A controlled study of adeno-viral-vector-mediated gene transfer in the nasal epithelium of patients with cystic fibrosis, *N Engl J Med* 333:823-831, 1995.

85. Morgan JE: Cell and gene therapy in Duchenne muscular dystrophy, *Hum Gene Ther* 5:165-173, 1994.

86. Kaji EH, Leiden JM: Gene and stem cell therapies, *JAMA* 285:545-550, 2001.

87. Mohajeri MH, Figlewicz DA, Bohn MC: Intramuscular grafts of myoblasts genetically modified to secrete glial cell line-derived neurotrophic factor prevent motor neuron loss and disease progression in a mouse model of familial amyotrophic lateral sclerosis, *Hum Gene Ther* 10:1853-1866, 1999.

88. Ozawa CR, Springer ML, Blau HM: A novel means of drug delivery: myoblast-mediated gene therapy and regulatable retroviral vectors, *Annu Rev Pharmacol Toxicol* 40:295-317, 2000.

89. Laurencin CT, Attawia MA, Lu LQ, et al: Poly(actide-co-glycolide)/hydroxyapatite delivery of BMP-2 producing cells: a regional gene therapy approach to bone regeneration, *Biomaterials* 22:1271-1277, 2001.

90. Aboody KS, Brown A, Rainov NG, et al: Neural stem cells display extensive tropism for pathology in adult brain: evidence from intracranial gliomas, *Proc Natl Acad Sci U S A* 97:12846-12851, 2000.

91. Kleinsmith LJ, Pierce GB Jr: Multipotentiality of single embryonal carcinoma cells, *Cancer Res* 24:1544-1551, 1964.

92. Martin GR: Teratocarcinomas and mammalian embryogenesis, *Science* 209:768-776, 1980.

93. Watt FM, Hogan BL: Out of Eden: stem cells and their niches, *Science* 287:1427-1430, 2000.

94. Young FE: A time for restraint, *Science* 287:1424, 2000.

95. Perry D: Patients' voices: the powerful sound in the stem cell debate, *Science* 287:1423, 2000.

96. McLaren A: Ethical and social considerations of stem cell research, *Nature* 414:129-131, 2001.

97. Jiang Y, Jahagirdar BN, Reinhardt RL, et al: Pluripotency of mesenchymal stem cells derived from adult marrow, *Nature* 418:41-49, 2002.

DIAGNOSIS AND TREATMENT OF ALLERGIC DISEASE

DONALD Y.M. LEUNG

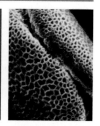

CHAPTER **22**

Laboratory *(In Vitro)* Analyses

ROBERT G. HAMILTON

The diagnostic immunology laboratory performs serologic and environmental analyses that supplement the clinical history and *in vivo* tests in the diagnosis and management of children with suspected type 1 hypersensitivity. This chapter discusses three groups of analytes that are measured in the laboratory: those that serve as *diagnostic confirmatory tests* when there is high suspicion of allergic disease based on a clinical history, those that permit *allergen exposure assessment and more effective management* of patients diagnosed with allergic disease, and those that are of *research interest* and have remained primarily in academic laboratories and are thus not offered by clinical immunology laboratories.

TYPE 1 HYPERSENSITIVITY RESPONSE IN HUMANS

Prausnitz and Kustner were the first to describe the mechanism of the type 1 hypersensitivity allergic reaction using an *in vivo* test when serum from Kustner, who was allergic to fish, was injected into the skin of Prausnitz. An immediate wheal-and-flare reaction in the skin was then induced when fish antigen was injected into the same skin site. A serum factor or atopic reagin in the sera of allergic subjects was suggested by their experiment and later shown by Ishizaka and Ishizaka[1] and Johansson and Benich[2] to be a novel immunoglobulin that was given the name *IgE*.

Table 22-1 summarizes the principal immune system components (italicized) that are involved in the induction of IgE antibody and elicitation of the effector mechanisms of Type 1 hypersensitivity. Inhalation, skin, or parenteral exposure to environmental *allergens* is the initiating event, during which these foreign molecules are exposed to antigen-presenting cells on mucosal surfaces. The antigen-presenting cells process the antigen and present antigenic epitopes to *T helper cells* that secrete *cytokines* (IL4, IL-10, IL-13), which induce *B cell* lymphocyte proliferation. Allergen-specific IgE antibody is produced as a part of the B cell immune response. IgE antibody circulates in the blood and binds to FcεR1 receptors on the

surfaces of *mast cells* and *basophils*. Upon re-exposure, some allergen cross-links IgE antibody on the mast cell surface, causing an influx in calcium, which in turn triggers the release of preformed *mediators* (*histamine, proteases*) and newly synthesized mediators (*leukotrienes, prostaglandins*). The pharmacologic effects of the mediators on blood vessels and airways as well as the induction of cell infiltration and accumulation produce a spectrum of clinical symptoms including hay fever, asthma, eczema, and anaphylaxis. *Cytokines* (IL-4, IL-5, IL-6) are reportedly released from degranulating mast cells and they serve to enhance the inflammatory and IgE responses.

Although there are a number of potential analytes that could be monitored in the laboratory to evaluate an individual for Type 1 hypersensitivity (see Table 22-1), allergen-specific IgE antibody is the most frequently measured analyte for diagnosis. IgE production is, however, under the control of T cells and the cytokines that they generate. The release of IL-4 and IL-13 causes T helper cell type 2 (Th2) to proliferate and B cells to switch to IgE antibody production. Alternatively, the generation of interferon (IFN)-γ, IL-2, and IL-12 favors Th1 cellular responses and suppression of the Th2 response. The mast cell is considered the most important effector cell. Mast cell enzymes such as tryptase that are released following the cross-linking of IgE antibody are clinically used as a marker for mast cell activation. Antigen-presenting cells, Th1 and Th2, cytokines, mast cells, basophils, and mediators are all important components of the Type 1 hypersensitivity response, but they have remained research analytes. See Chapters 4 and 5 for a more extensive discussion of the cellular, cytokine, and mediator components of the Type 1 hypersensitivity response.

ALLERGENS

Allergen preparations are typically mixtures of glycoproteins, lipoproteins, or proteins with conjugated chemical and drug haptens that have been solubilized from a well-defined

Antigen presentation
Allergen (exposure, entry at mucosal surfaces or local lymph nodes)
Antigen-presenting cells (processing and presentation)
Th2 lymphocytes
   Cytokines (promotors of IgE production: IL-4, IL-10, IL-13) (inhibitors of IgE production: IFN-γ)
B cell lymphocytes

IgE production and sensitization
IgE (allergen-specific IgE antibody)
Connective tissue fixed and mucosal mast cells with FcϵRI receptors
Circulating basophils with FcϵRI receptors

Mast cell activation and mediator release
Reexposure to *allergen* induces calcium ion influx into mast cells
Mast cell releases preformed and newly synthesized mediators
   Release of *tryptase*
   Exocytosis of preformed *histamine*
   Synthesis of newly formed lipid mediators from arachidonic acid
      Prostaglandin D$_2$
      Leukotriene B$_4$, C$_4$, D$_4$

Humoral immune responses
Chronic antigenic challenge (inadvertent or intentional [immunotherapy]) induces antigen-specific IgG and IgA antibodies in blood and secretions

*Analytes in italics are routinely measured in the clinical diagnostic allergy laboratory and thus are discussed in the text. Analytes that are underlined are considered research analytes and are not routinely measured in the clinical laboratory.

(usually biologic) source. Allergenic proteins elicit the formation of IgE antibody when introduced into an immunocompetent and genetically predisposed host. The concentration of all the allergenic epitopes together produces a defined, measurable biologic response in allergic individuals. More than 200 allergens of clinical importance have been identified among weeds, grasses, trees, animal danders, molds, house dust mites, parasites, insect venoms, occupational allergens, drugs, and foods. To illustrate the complex nature of one of these allergen groups (grass), an estimated 9000 species of grasses cover approximately 20% of the world's surface. Important cereals and forage plants reside in this family as well as grass mixtures for lawns. The grass plant flowers open for only a few hours, during which pollination can occur. There is a high degree of immunologic cross-reactivity within the grass genus *Festuca* (cocksfoot, meadow fescue, rye, meadow/Kentucky, blue/June, and timothy grasses). In contrast, Bermuda grass (*Cynodon dactylon*) shows moderate cross-reactivity to Johnson and Bahia grass but not to the other distantly related grasses. A comprehensive compendium of the known clinically important allergens, together with their scientific names, purified major allergen components, and working codes, are presented elsewhere.[3]

Natural rubber latex (see Chapter 58) is another important allergen group that is used in this chapter for illustrative purposes. Children who undergo multiple surgeries early in life are at an increased risk for becoming sensitized to natural rubber latex allergens. Frequent urologic, orthopedic, and

TABLE 22-2 Natural Rubber Latex (*Hevea brasiliensis*) Allergens

Name	Description	Allergen Group	MW (kDa)	Cross-reactions*
Hev b 1	Rubber elongation factor	14.6	Hev b 3-rp	1
Hev b 2	Beta 1/3 gluconase	34-36	Pan	2
Hev b 3	Prenyltransferase	24-27	Hev b 1-rp	1
Hev b 4	Microhelix	110/50		4
Hev b 5	Acidic protein	16-24		4
Hev b 6.02	Hevein protein	4.7	Foods	2, 3
Hev b 7	Patatin homologue	43-35		2, 3
Hev b 8	Profilin	14	Pan	4
Hev b 9	Enolase	51	Molds	4
Hev b 10	Superoxide dismutase	26	Pan-molds	4
Hev b 11	Chitinase	NA	Pan-foods	2

*Allergen cross-reaction groups: *1*, biosynthesis of polyisoprene polymer; *2*, pathogenesis-related proteins; *3*, latex coagulation-related proteins; *4*, structural proteins and housekeeping enzymes.

neurologic surgeries result in repeated exposures to natural rubber latex gloves as well as rubber bladder catheters and nonsterile powdered examination gloves that are used for removal of fecal impactions. Several potent latex allergens have been identified in these products (Table 22-2): *Hevea brasiliensis* (Hev b) 1 and 3 are proteins that facilitate biosynthesis of the polyisoprene polymer. Hev b 1 and 3 envelop rubber particles and promote rubber chain formation. They are attached to rubber particles except when they are solubilized into the fluid phase of the rubber sap. A second group (Hev b 2, 6, 7, and 11 and Hevamine) are pathogenesis-related (PR) proteins. These proteins are found in the central (C) serum or aqueous phase and they serve to protect the plant against pathogenic microorganisms. Hev b 2 (PR2) degrades fungal cell walls, Hev b 11 (PR3) degrades the chitin exoskeleton of insects, and Hev b 6 (PR4) is involved in plant wood repair. Hev b 6 and 7 constitute a separate group of allergens that are involved in modifying the latex coagulation process. Hevein, or Hev b 6.02, is a lectin-like protein that aids in latex coagulation by interacting with the n-acetyl d glucosamine and 22 kD glycoprotein receptor on the surface of the rubber particle. Hev b 7 inhibits coagulation. Hev b 4, 5, 8, 9, and 10 are structural proteins and housekeeping enzymes.

DIAGNOSIS

The most common diagnostic algorithm for human allergic disease begins with a thorough clinical history and physical examination. These are sequentially followed by *in vivo* skin testing, *in vitro* studies with serologic assays, and controlled provocation challenge tests as confirmatory measurements for the detection of IgE antibodies (Figure 22-1). The interrelationship among all of these components of the diagnostic plan is illustrated in this chapter using natural rubber latex as a model allergen system.

Latex allergy diagnosis begins with a comprehensive clinical history.[4] A child may present with complaints of allergic symptoms (hives, rhinoconjunctivitis, asthma, anaphylaxis)

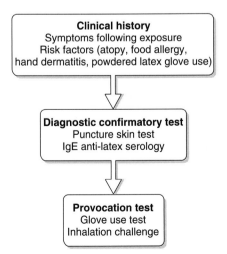

FIGURE 22-1 Diagnostic algorithm for latex allergy. If the clinical history is suggestive of latex allergy, a puncture skin test or IgE antibody serology that is performed to document the presence of IgE anti-latex. As a last resort, provocation tests can be performed to adjudicate discordant history and IgE anti-latex confirmatory test results.

that are temporally associated with exposure to a natural rubber product. The allergist probes the child's atopic history and specific latex allergy history using questions designed to identify predisposing risk factors, such as an atopic state (seasonal rhinitis, early-onset asthma, eczema, food allergy); the frequency, consistency, and magnitude of latex allergen exposure; and the presence of concomitant food allergy and hand dermatitis. The rubber-containing product type (dipped or molded) associated with the reported reactions provides clues that can strengthen the clinical suspicion of latex allergy. For instance, the rapid-onset allergic symptoms around latex toy balloons or other dipped rubber products (medical gloves, natural rubber toys) would be supportive. In contrast, respiratory or upper-airway symptoms, when the child has been around latex paint that does not contain natural rubber, diminish the probability of latex allergy. The type of exposure and time of onset, duration, and severity of the symptoms can help differentiate between Type 1 (protein-allergen–induced, immediate-type) and Type 4 (rubber chemical–induced, delayed-type) hypersensitivity. Other risk factors for IgE antibody production include a genetic predisposition for atopic disease or parental history of allergy, chronic infectious or acute viral illness, relative contributions of Th1/Th2 cells to the immune response, and the nutritional status of the individual.[4]

DIAGNOSTIC LABORATORY METHODS

Total serum IgE was initially used as a diagnostic marker for allergic disease.[5] However, because of the wide overlap in the total serum IgE levels between atopic and non-atopic populations,[6] allergen-specific IgE has superceded it as the single most important laboratory analyte in the diagnostic work-up for allergic disease. The radioallergosorbent test (RAST) was the first assay developed for the detection of IgE antibodies in human serum with defined allergen specificities.[7] The RAST is a noncompetitive, heterogeneous (separation step included), solid-phase immunoradiometric (radiolabeled antibody) assay (Figure 22-2) in which the allergen of interest was covalently coupled to cellulose (paper) discs. In a first RAST incubation human serum is incubated with the allergosorbent, during which time antibodies of all human isotypes (typically IgE and IgG, if present) bind to insolubilized antigens. Following a buffer wash, bound IgE is detected with ^{125}I-labeled antihuman IgE Fc. After a second buffer wash to remove unbound radiolabeled anti-human IgE, bound radioactivity is measured in a gamma counter and is proportional to the amount of allergen-specific IgE in the initial serum specimen. The early Phadebas RAST (Pharmacia, Uppsala, Sweden) was calibrated in arbitrary Phadebas RAST Units (PRU) per ml of IgE antibirch using a multipoint IgE antibirch reference serum curve bound to a birch pollen allergosorbent.

The basic RAST chemistry has remained essentially unchanged over more than 35 years. The number and quality of allergen extracts used in preparing allergosorbents have increased as a result of extensive research in new methods of extraction and quality control. New matrix materials such as the cellulose sponge have enhanced the binding capacity and reduced the nonspecific binding properties of allergosorbents. Various polyclonal and monoclonal anti-IgE detection antibody combinations ensure maximal assay sensitivity and specificity for human IgE. Automation has improved assay

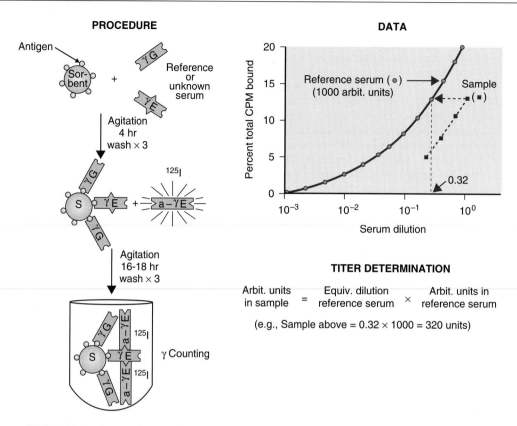

PROCEDURE

DATA

TITER DETERMINATION

$$\text{Arbit. units in sample} = \text{Equiv. dilution reference serum} \times \text{Arbit. units in reference serum}$$

(e.g., Sample above = 0.32 × 1000 = 320 units)

FIGURE 22-2 Schematic diagram of the radioallergosorbent test. In the first incubation, allergen-specific antibody of many human isotypes (primarily IgE and IgG) is bound from human serum to an allergosorbent. Following buffer washes to remove unbound serum proteins, bound IgE antibody is detected with ^{125}I-labeled rabbit anti-human IgE antibody. The CPM bound to the allergosorbent after a final buffer wash are proportional to the amount of specific IgE antibody in the original serum. Multiple dilutions of a reference (assigned 1000 arbitrary [arbit.] units) and the test sera are analyzed and their dose-response curves should dilute out in parallel. When the arbitrary units for the dilution of the test sample are determined by interpolation from the reference curve, the final titer or antibody estimates should be equivalent to each other when each dilution is corrected for its respective dilution factor. (From Middleton E Jr: *Allergies: principles and practice*, ed 4, vol 2, St Louis, 1983, Mosby.)

precision and reproducibility to the level where some IgE antibody assays on autoanalyzers require only single measurements to ensure accurate results. Nonisotopic labels have increased the shelf lives of reagents and have made the assays more user-friendly. Calibration systems used in current commercial assays employ a common strategy[8] in which a heterologous total serum IgE curve is used to convert allergen-specific IgE assay response data into quantitative dose estimates of IgE antibody. All these modifications have resulted in a "second-generation" of RAST-type assays that display superior analytical sensitivity and specificity and are more quantitative, reproducible, and automated than their earlier counterparts. These improvements have made the serologic assay for IgE antibody more diagnostically competitive with its *in vivo* puncture skin test counterpart. The intradermal skin test still appears to possess an inherent advantage in terms of analytical sensitivity and disadvantage of a loss of diagnostic specificity.[9]

Despite convergence toward improved performance and common calibration schemes, the specific IgE antibody levels that are measured in different commercial assays cannot be considered interchangeable or equivalent. Marked differences remain in the specificity of the allergen used in the allergen-containing reagents of different assays. Allergen preparations are almost always mixtures of proteins that vary in their composition (molecular weight, charge [isoelectric point], relative content) and immunogenicity or allergenic potency between manufacturers. The composition of an allergen reagent used in present-day serologic assays for IgE antibody quantitation should be expected to vary as a function of a number of factors. These are the season in which the raw material is collected, the degree of difficulty in identifying a pure source of material, the presence of morphologically similar raw materials that may cross-contaminate, and differences in the extraction process during allergen-reagent production by assay manufacturers. Allergen extracts selected for use in allergosorbents undergo extensive quality control using isoelectrofocusing, Sodium dodecyl sulfate-polyacrylamide gel electrophoresis, crossed-immunoelectrophoresis, and immunoblotting methods. There are also issues of stability during storage, heterogeneity of the human IgE antibody–containing sera used for quality control, and different criteria for acceptance of the finished allergen-containing reagent by different manufacturers. Thus allergosorbents from different manufacturers should be expected to detect different populations of IgE antibodies for any given allergen specificity.

IgE Antibody Assay Performance

Currently there is no Food and Drug Administration (FDA)–licensed natural rubber latex skin testing reagent available for use in skin testing in the United States.[4] Some allergists prepare their own skin testing extracts from latex gloves; however, these extracts are difficult to validate in terms of their potency, specificity, and stability. The clinician must therefore rely upon laboratory-based serologic assays as the only validated means for the detection of latex-specific IgE antibody in individuals with a suggestive clinical history of latex allergy. The strengths and weaknesses of today's commercial allergen-specific IgE antibody assay technology can be illustrated by examining the evolution in latex-specific IgE antibody assay performance.

The earliest RAST assays for latex-specific IgE antibody were reported at a 1992 international conference on sensitivity to latex products in medical devices.[10] These assays used latex allergens from gloves and centrifuged ammoniated and nonammoniated *Hevea brasiliensis* latex that were coupled to microtiter plates and agarose and cellulose particles. Direct comparison of RAST assay performance with matched glove, ammoniated and nonammoniated latex from common clone 600 of a *Hevea brasiliensis* tree led to the observation that all three sources of latex on the allergosorbent produced highly concordant numbers of positive latex-specific IgE antibody results.[11] Because nonammoniated latex was more uniform between batches, it was selected as the allergen source of choice.

In 1995 the FDA cleared the first commercial assay for latex-specific IgE antibody (Diagnostic Products Corporation [DPC] tube-based enzyme immunoassay). Subsequently a number of other assays were approved by the FDA, including the DPC Alastat Microplate in 1995 and DPC Immulite Assay and Pharmacia CAP System fluorescent enzyme immunoassay (FEIA) in 1996. The diagnostic performances of the three most widely used FDA-approved latex-specific IgE assays were directly compared in two independent studies.[12,13] When puncture skin testing with an investigational reagent from Greer Laboratories was used as the reference method, the Pharmacia CAP System and DPC Alastat Microplate displayed 76% and 73% diagnostic sensitivity, respectively, whereas their diagnostic specificity in comparison with the skin test was 97%. These data indicated that both the CAP and Alastat misclassified approximately 25% of latex-sensitized cases as being falsely negative for IgE antibody. The Hycor HyTECH, in contrast, displayed a diagnostic specificity of 73%, producing 27% false-positive results when compared with puncture skin testing. The low diagnostic sensitivity in the CAP System and Alastat was believed to be related to poorly represented and/or denatured allergens such as Hev b 2, 5, 6, and 7 in the allergen-containing reagents used in these assays.[14,15] This work has led to the development of an improved recombinant Hev b 5–enriched FEIA CAP allergosorbent that is currently being clinically evaluated for improved diagnostic sensitivity.

A second concern has focused on significant imprecision of the commercial latex–specific IgE antibody assays at levels close to their positive cutoffs (0.35 to 0.45 kIUa/L).[16] In fact, 35% of sera with latex-specific IgE antibody levels in this low-positive range produced discordant positive or negative mismatched discrepancies upon repeat testing. This has caused some investigators to routinely repeat latex-specific IgE antibody results between 0.3 and 0.4 kIU/L in duplicate. Others have concluded that latex-specific IgE results from the Alastat assay in the 0.35 to 0.7 kIU/L range should be considered equivocal or weakly positive.[17] Biagini et al[16] have, however, confirmed, using receiver-operator characteristic analysis, that the manufacturer-established positive cutoff of less than 0.35 kIU/L produces the best performance achievable for at least the CAP System and Alastat Microplate.

Comparison of IgE Antibody Serology with Other Measures of Allergic Disease

Second-generation IgE antibody assays have the ability to generate quantitative IgE antibody measurements in mass per volume units that are traceable to the World Health Organization International Reference Preparation for human IgE. In terms of conversion factors, Lindqvist et al[18] have shown that 1 allergen-specific IgE antibody unit (kUa/L) as measured in the CAP System is equivalent to 1 international unit (kU/L, or 2.4 µg/L) of IgE protein.

In 1997 Sampson and Ho[19] retrospectively investigated sera from 196 children and adolescents (mean age 5.2 years, 60% male) with atopic dermatitis who the researchers evaluated for food allergy over a 10-year period. Levels of IgE antibodies specific for cow's milk, chicken egg, peanut, wheat, soy, and fish were correlated with a diagnosis of food allergy as defined by positive double-blind, placebo-controlled food challenges or a convincing history of food-induced anaphylaxis. They were able to identify IgE antibody levels using the Pharmacia FEIA CAP System that could predict clinical reactivity (positive food challenges) with more than 95% certainty for egg (6 kUa/L), milk (32 kUa/L), peanut (15 kUa/L), and fish (20 kUa/L). The significance of this report rests in the potential for eliminating double-blind, placebo-controlled food challenges in children suspected of having IgE-mediated food allergy. In a 2001 report Sampson[20] extended his observations with a prospective study of 100 children and adolescents (mean age 3.8 years, 62% male) that had been referred for evaluation of food allergy. This prospective study verified the retrospective study–based 95% predictive decision points for egg, milk, peanut, and fish allergy. The study also confirmed that use of the positive criteria correctly diagnosed food allergy in more than 95% of children using the serum IgE antibody level. The study showed that quantitative food-specific IgE antibody measurements are useful for diagnosing symptomatic allergies to egg, milk, peanut, and fish in the pediatric population. The important conclusion of these studies is that the serologic IgE antibody test results eliminate the need for double-blind, placebo-controlled food challenges in a significant number of children.

For inhalant allergies, Wood et al[9] have shown that quantitative cat allergen–specific IgE antibodies are equivalent to puncture skin tests and superior in performance to intradermal skin tests in the diagnosis of clinical reactivity to cat allergen. When compared with a positive cat inhalation challenge outcome, the Pharmacia FEIA CAP System measurement displayed a diagnostic sensitivity of 69%, specificity of 100%, positive predictive value of 100%, and negative predictive value of 73%. In the house dust mite system De Lovinfosse et al[21] reported a significant correlation between the concentration of IgE specific to dust mite and the concentration of sensitizing mite allergen in the individual's mattress dust ($P = 0.001$). They reported a 77% probability of being exposed to high dust mite allergen (> 10 μg per gram of dust) when the serum IgE antimite levels were greater than 2 kUa/L and vice versa. These data showed that quantitative serum IgE antibody measurements can identify individuals who are not only sensitized to mites but also who are most in need of avoidance through environmental control measures. Other illustrations of the importance of quantitative allergen-specific IgE to respiratory allergy are reviewed elsewhere.[22] As a general rule for inhalant allergen specificities, the skin test and quantitative IgE antibody immunoassay can be viewed as interchangeable. One exception is in the monitoring of patients on immunotherapy, where a decrease in the positivity of the puncture skin test titration alone has been shown to predict continued remission after cessation of allergen immunotherapy.[23]

Multiallergen IgE Antibody Screening Assays

When a patient provides an equivocal history for allergic disease, it can be difficult to pinpoint with reasonable certainty the appropriate IgE antibody specificities for further diagnostic investigation. A multiallergen screen is a single RAST-type test that has the highest negative predictive value for atopic disease of any laboratory test currently available. The pediatric Phadiatop is Pharmacia's version of the multiallergen screen for evaluating children. It is a qualitative test that measures the presence of IgE antibody specific for a group of indoor, outdoor, and food aeroallergens that induce most of pediatric respiratory and food-related allergic disease. A negative multiallergen screen reduces the probability that allergic disease is the cause of the child's clinical problems. Multiallergen screen results are particularly useful in the diagnosis of pediatric allergic diseases where there is a need to detect allergen-specific IgE antibody in serum as a marker for sensitization.

In a 2001 study 143 children and adolescents were assigned an allergy status (103 positive, 40 negative) based on a combined history, skin prick test, and specific IgE antibody (UniCAP, Pharmacia) to seven common inhalants (mite, oak, ragweed, grass, dog, cat, and *Alternaria*).[24] The multiallergen screen (Phadiatop, Pharmacia) run on these same sera correctly identified the allergy status of all subjects, verifying the diagnostic sensitivity and specificity of the Phadiatop in differentiating sensitized individuals from those who are not sensitized to common inhalant allergens.

Mast Cell Tryptase

Serum levels of tryptase can be useful as a marker of mast cell activation in making the definitive diagnosis of anaphylaxis. Tryptase is a 134,000 Da serine esterase with four subunits, each containing an enzymatically active site.[25] When tryptase becomes dissociated from heparin, it spontaneously degrades into enzymatically inactive monomeric subunits. It is released from activated mast cells in parallel with prestored histamine and other newly generated vasoactive mediators. The α-tryptase concentration in blood is considered a measure of the mast cell number and it is estimated by subtracting the β-tryptase from the total tryptase concentration; in contrast, β-tryptase levels in blood are considered a measure of mast cell activation.

A noncompetitive fluorescent enzyme immunoassay (CAP System, Pharmacia, Uppsala, Sweden) is available to measure tryptase in human serum. It uses a capture monoclonal antibody that binds both α-protryptase and β-tryptase.[26] β-Tryptase is measured with a solid-phase noncompetitive immunoassay that uses a β-tryptase–specific capture monoclonal antibody. Before analysis both the α and β forms of tryptase are converted into an enzymatically inactive form. Total serum tryptase concentrations in healthy (nondiseased) individuals range from 1 to 10 ng/ml (average 5 ng/ml). If baseline total serum tryptase levels exceed 20 ng/ml, systemic mastocytosis should be suspected. β-Tryptase levels less than 1 ng/ml are observed in nondiseased individuals, and β-tryptase levels more than 1 ng/ml indicate mast cell activation. For optimal results, blood samples should be collected from 0.5 to 4 hours following the initiation of a suspected systemic reaction mediated by mast cells.[27] A peak β-tryptase level more than 10 ng/ml in a postmortem serum suggests systemic anaphylaxis as one probable cause of death. Systemic anaphylaxis induced by an insect sting can produce β-tryptase levels that peak at more than 5 ng/ml by 30 to 60 minutes after the sting and then decline, with a biologic half-life of approximately 2 hours.[28]

Serum Markers of Hypersensitivity Pneumonitis

Extrinsic allergic alveolitis, or hypersensitivity pneumonitis, is an inflammatory reaction involving the lung interstitium and terminal bronchioles.[29] A heavy exposure to antigenic organic dust (e.g., molds, bird droppings) can induce chills, fever, malaise, cough, and shortness of breath within hours of exposure. Although histology of the lung lesions indicates that a cell-mediated pathology is involved in hypersensitivity pneumonitis, most individuals have high levels of IgG antibody to the offending antigen in their sera that is used as a marker of the disease. Precipitating IgG antibody specific for antigens in organic dust has been measured in human serum to support the differential diagnosis of this condition. The classic double diffusion (Ouchterlony) technique has been routinely performed to detect precipitating antibodies in the diagnosis of this disease. In this assay, crude antigen extract and antibody (control or patient's serum) are delivered into closely spaced wells in a porous agarose gel. Visible white precipitin lines confirmed by lines of identity with known human antibody controls represent a positive test. Precipitating antibodies or precipitins are detected in the sera of nearly all ill patients in one study but also in the sera of 50% of asymptomatic individuals exposed to the relevant organic dust.[30] More recently, enzyme immunoassays for IgG antibody to selected organic dust antigens have been reported.[31] In many cases, however, the enzyme immunoassay appears to be too analytically sensitive and diagnostically nonspecific. For this reason the classic precipitin assays continue to be widely used for detecting IgG precipitins to antigens in pigeon serum, *Aureobasidium pullulans,* thermophilic *Actinomyces, Aspergillus fumigatus,* and extractable proteins from fecal material produced by parakeets and a variety of exotic household birds, such as Amazon, cockatiel, and blue front parrots.

MANAGEMENT

The management of individuals with allergic disease involves the combined use of pharmacotherapy, immunotherapy, and avoidance therapy. The clinical laboratory provides a number of analytical measurements that aid the clinician in optimizing venom immunotherapy and monitoring the humoral (IgG antibody) immune responses in patients on venom immunotherapy. Moreover, indoor aeroallergen levels are measured in the settled dust of home, workplace, and school environments both before and after remediation to document the need for allergen-avoidance measures and to verify that the environment has been cleared of allergen sources.

Optimizing Venom Immunotherapy

When considering the medically important *Hymenoptera*, it has been long known that cross-reactivity exists between the vespid venoms (yellow jacket, white-faced hornet, and yellow hornet) and Polistes wasp venom (PWV) proteins. Results from a competitive inhibition format of the IgE RAST specific for PWV have allowed allergists to more effectively select the venom specificities and to minimize the number of venoms that must be administered during immunotherapy. This targeted venom therapy is especially important for children in whom unnecessary administration of PWV may lead to *de novo* sensitization to Polistes allergens. In this assay the patient's serum (0.1 ml), containing IgE anti-PWV and IgE anti-yellow jacket venom (YJV), is incubated with 100 μg of soluble YJV. The serum-allergen mixture is then analyzed in a RAST-type assay for IgE anti-PWV. If greater than 95% of the IgE anti-PWV binding to PWV-allergosorbent is inhibited by preincubation with YJV, this indicates that the IgE anti-PWV is essentially completely cross-reactive with YJV. Moreover, this indicates that the individual can be treated with yellow jacket or mixed vespid venom alone and inclusion of PWV is unnecessary. In a study of 412 patients with a positive skin test to YJV and PWV, 36% of the patients' sera contained IgE anti-PWV that was inhibited more than 95% by soluble YJV.[32] The degree of IgE anti-PWV inhibition was independent of the IgE antibody level. Cost analysis of the RAST venom inhibition test and a conventional 5-year *Hymenoptera* venom immunotherapy program has shown that this serologic evaluation is cost-effective.

Monitoring Venom Immunotherapy

Allergen-specific IgG antibodies are not routinely measured in the clinical immunology laboratory because there is no general clinical indication for their measurement, except in the research monitoring of immunotherapy-induced humoral immune responses. The one exception is *Hymenoptera* venom-related allergy.[33] Some investigators believe that venom-specific IgG antibody measurements are useful in assessing the clinical and immunologic efficacy of venom immunotherapy, particularly in the early maintenance phase (3 to 6 months). Their measurement has also been used by some clinicians to periodically determine the efficacy of maintenance therapy doses and the frequency of injections and to evaluate adverse reactions and the relative need for increased venom immunotherapy doses.

Golden et al[34] studied serum from 109 subjects who had a positive history of insect sting–induced systemic allergic reactions and positive intradermal skin tests with *Hymenoptera* venoms. They set a prospective discriminator of 3 μg/ml of IgG antivenom to define two groups who had been on similar maintenance venom immunotherapy for a minimum of 2 years and were balanced in terms of age, gender, and skin test reactivity. A total of 87 challenge stings were performed in 46 patients in the low venom–specific IgG group (≤ 3 μg/ml) and 124 stings in 63 patients in the high group (venom-specific IgG > 3 μg/ml). Systemic symptoms occurred in 1.6% of subjects in the greater than 3 μg/ml group, in 16% of those with less than 3 μg/ml, and in 26% of subjects with low venom IgG who received less than 4 years of treatment. The venom-specific IgG level had no predictive value for subjects who received more than 4 years of therapy. The authors concluded that low venom–specific IgG levels are associated with an elevated risk of treatment failure during the first 4 years of immunotherapy with yellow jacket or mixed vespid venoms.

Facilitating Avoidance Therapy with Aeroallergen Measurements of Indoor Environments

Dust mite (*Dermatophagoides pteronyssinus, D. farinae*), cat epithelium/dander (*Felis domesticus*), dog epithelium/dander (*Canis familariasis*), cockroach (*Blatella germanica*), and mouse (*Mus musculus*) are known sources of potent indoor aeroallergens.[35] Single proteins from each of these biosources are being used as "indicator" allergens because their relative levels in surface dust allow their associated complex allergen sources to be tracked by room throughout a home, workplace, or school. The most widely used indicator allergens are listed in Table 22-3. Der f 1 and Der p 1 are 25 kDa allergenic proteins released into surface dust from dust mite fecal particles; Fel d 1 is a 35 kDa allergen excreted by the sweat glands of the domestic cat; Can f 1 is a 25 kDa allergen produced by the sweat glands of the dog; Bla g 1 is an allergen produced by the German cockroach; and MUP (mouse urinary protein) is a 19 kDa allergen excreted into urine by the mouse.

Assessment of an environment is accomplished by collecting a surface dust specimen from air ducts, floors, or other horizontal surfaces (bed, upholstered furniture) using an inexpensive dust collector attached to a standard household vacuum cleaner. The crude dust is sent to a clinical immunology laboratory, where it is processed by passing it through a sieve and mixing it with a protein containing physiologic buffer (1:20 weight per volume) to extract the soluble proteins. The extracted allergens are then quantified using noncompetitive (two-site) monoclonal antibody–based immunoenzymetric assays. Presently, there is a commercial source of assay reagents and standards and an interlaboratory proficiency survey conducted by the College of American Pathologists that has confirmed good laboratory performance of these aeroallergen measurements in selected laboratories.

A high level of one or more of the indoor aeroallergens identifies an allergen source in the home, workplace, or school that can sensitize or induce an allergic reaction in a sensitized individual. Levels of Der p 1 or Der f 1 allergen greater than 2000 ng/g of fine dust have been associated with an increased risk for allergic symptoms in sensitized individuals, whereas

TABLE 22-3 Analytes Measured in the Clinical Immunology Laboratory

Diagnosis
Allergen-specific IgE
  Multiallergen-specific IgE screen (adult and pediatric forms)
  Individual allergen specificities
Total serum IgE*
Precipitating antibodies specific for proteins in organic dust
Tryptase (α, β; mast cell protease and used as a marker for mast cell mediated anaphylaxis)
Other tests: complete blood count (CBC), sputum examination for eosinophils and neutrophils

Management
Allergen-specific IgG (*Hymenoptera*)
Indoor aeroallergen quantitation in surface dust
  Der p 1/Der f 1 (dust mite, *Dermatophagoides*)
  Fel d 1 (cat, *Felis domesticus*)
  Can f 1 (dog, *Canis familaris*)
  Bla g 1/Bla g 2 (cockroach, *Blattela germanica*)
  MUP (mouse, *Mus musculus* urinary protein)
Cotinine (metabolite of nicotine measured in serum, urine, and sputum and used as a marker of smoke exposure)

Research analytes
IgE specific autoantibodies
Eosinophil cationic protein
Mediators†,‡
  Preformed biogenic amine: histamine
  Newly formed leukotriene C_4 (LTC$_4$), prostaglandin D_2 (PGD$_2$)
Proteoglycans†
  Heparin
  Chondroitin sulfate E
Proteases†
  Mast cell chymase
  Mast cell carboxypeptidase cathepsin G
Fibroblast growth factor (bFGF)†
Cytokines
  Tumor necrosis factor-alpha
  Interleukin-4, -5, -6, -13‡

*Total serum IgE is the only one of these tests listed that is regulated under the CLIA 88.
†Primarily released from mast cells.
‡Primarily released from basophils.

an increased risk for sensitization has been associated with mite levels greater than 10,000 ng/g. In contrast, cat allergen levels greater than 8000 ng/g of Fel d 1 in fine dust have been suggested as threshold for sensitization. Comparable risk targets have also been used for dog (Can f 1) allergen levels in indoor environments. For cockroach and mouse urinary allergen, any detectable allergen in the indoor environment places a cockroach- or mouse-allergic individual at risk for symptoms and further sensitization.[36]

Mold/Fungus Evaluation in Indoor Environments

Accurate quantitation of the mold content of an environment is a challenge for any clinical laboratory. Four molds (*Alternaria, Aspergillus, Cladosporium,* and *Penicillium*) constitute the majority of indoor molds.[35] Fungal spores can be both viable and nonviable. The laboratory methods used for quantifying viable and nonviable spores are different. The total spore counts (nonviable and viable) can be determined by collecting particulate from the air impactor or suction device and then assessing the spore's morphology for the purpose of speciating the mold. Viable fungal spores that grow when environmental conditions are favorable are considered by some allergists to be more clinically important because they can colonize indoor environments and, in some cases, the respiratory tract. In one clinical laboratory a qualitative, viable mold spore analysis is performed on 5 mg of fine dust that is distributed over a microbiologic culture plate containing Sabouraud's dextrose agar. Visual inspection of the plate at 24 and 48 hours allows the total number of mold colonies to be quantified. The colony count at 24 hours can be viewed as an estimate of the mold burden of the environment. Repetitive subculturing and morphologic identification allow the species of the predominant molds to be determined; however, this is infrequently performed. Rather, once a mold contamination has been identified, remediation by cleaning with bleach and reducing humidity is generally instituted.

Individual mold "indicator" allergens have been detected by two-site immunoassays. Alt a 1, for instance, is a 28 kD protein from *Alternaria alternata/tenuis* that has been measured by an immunoenzymetric assay. However, the utility of the immunoassay for assessing mold content has been questioned because molds that inhabit indoor environments do not always produce the same repertoire of proteins. Mold growth depends on the specific environmental conditions present on any given day (e.g., nutrients, temperature, humidity). Moreover, their performance characteristics in most cases have not been validated. Thus, although immunoassays for selected mold allergens are available in research laboratories, they are not generally used as clinical tests to monitor environments for the quantity of mold growth.

There are no established mold spore contamination ranges that can be considered safe, partly because mold is ever present, different individuals have different relative sensitivities, and the target airborne mold allergens are difficult to sample and verify. Thus, it is not presently possible to identify an environment that will place a mold-allergic person at risk for symptoms. Multiple variables associated with mold spore heterogeneity, differential growth based on nutrients and environmental conditions, the degree of aerosolization, and variable specificity of the patient's IgE antibody complicate the interpretation of a mold spore measurement when attempting to predict a clinical outcome from any environmental exposure. Sometimes the indoor mold levels are compared with the outdoor mold levels collected at the same time. These are used to determine if airborne mold spores are significantly higher and thus play a more significant role in the allergy and asthma symptoms experienced indoors. Mold spore levels above 25,000 colonies per gram of fine dust have been identified in one study as a level that places a home in the 75th percentile for random homes monitored across the United States. When this proposed threshold level is exceeded, allergic individuals are encouraged to remediate their environments; this often involves replacing air duct filters, removing plants, and decreasing indoor humidity. A detailed overview of corrective strategies for remediation of indoor environments is beyond the scope of this chapter but can be found elsewhere in this book (see Chapter 26).

KEY CONCEPTS
Diagnosis

- Allergen-specific IgE antibody is the most important analyte measured in the clinical immunology laboratory for diagnosis of allergic disease. It is performed as a confirmatory test to support a clinical history that strongly suggests an allergic disorder.
- The radioallergosorbent test, or RAST, is a two-stage noncompetitive radioimmunoassay in which allergen-specific antibodies are bound to an allergosorbent and bound IgE antibodies are detected with radioiodinated antihuman IgE. A calibration curve analysis is performed in each assay to allow interpolation of response data into dose estimates of allergen-specific IgE.
- Clinically used, FDA-cleared, "second-generation" allergen-specific IgE antibody immunoassays are patterned after the RAST but they are more quantitative, reproducible, standardized, allergen specific, rapid, automated, and safer (nonisotopic). Quantitative IgE antibody results are reported in kIU/L, traceable to the World Health Organization IgE Standard (1 IU = 2.4 ng of IgE).
- The multiallergen screen is a qualitative RAST-type assay that measures allergen-specific IgE antibody to a panel of aeroallergens and, in a pediatric version, additional food allergens in a single test. The multiallergen screening assay produces qualitative (positive or negative) results that lead to subsequent investigation of the patient's serum or skin for IgE antibodies specific for individual clinically-defined allergen specificities.
- Competitive inhibition format of the RAST-type immunoassay is used to determine the relative potency of allergen extracts used in skin testing, to identify the extent of cross-reactivity of human IgE antibody for structurally similar allergens (e.g., Vespid versus Polistes wasp venom allergens) and in *Hymenoptera* venom allergy, to select appropriate venoms for immunotherapy.
- Quantitative IgE antibody levels to selected foods (milk, egg, fish, and peanut) if above a predefined IgE antibody threshold may eliminate the need for tedious and expensive double-blind, placebo-controlled food challenges (DBPCFCs). However, food antigen–specific IgG and IgG4 antibody levels do not correlate with the diagnostic results of DBPCFCs.

KEY CONCEPTS
Management

- Clinically successful aeroallergen immunotherapy is almost always accompanied by high (micrograms per milliliter) levels of allergen-specific IgG antibody in serum.
- Quantitative venom-specific IgG antibody levels can be useful in individualizing venom doses and injection frequencies for patients on maintenance venom immunotherapy for up to 4 years.
- Mast cell tryptase is a serine esterase that is used as a marker of mast cell activation during anaphylaxis. Immunoreactive tryptase levels in sera of healthy adults are typically less than 5 μg/L. Elevated levels (> 10 μg/L) are detectable 1 to 4 hours after the onset of systemic anaphylaxis with hypotension.
- Indoor allergens from dust mites, animal epidermis (cat, dog, mouse, rat), cockroaches, and a limited number of molds are quantified in processed house dust to investigate individual risk of allergic symptoms or sensitization and to monitor effects of environmental control.

RESEARCH ANALYTES

There are a number of immune system components involved in the induction of IgE antibody and effector mechanisms of Type 1 hypersensitivity (see Table 22-1) that are studied in the allergy research laboratory rather than in the clinical immunology laboratory. These include antigen-presenting cells that process and present allergens to lymphocytes, the Th1/Th2 lymphocyte axis and its associated cytokines that promote (IL-4, IL-10, IL-13) and inhibit (interferon-γ) IgE antibody production, B cell lymphocytes, the FcϵR1 receptors on basophils and connective tissue fixed and mucosal mast cells, histamine in serum and its release from mast cells and basophils, and lipid mediators (prostaglandin D_2 and leukotriene B_4, C_4, D_4) synthesized from arachidonic acid. In addition, IgE-specific autoantibodies and antihuman IgE autoantibodies, eosinophil cationic protein, proteoglycans (heparin and chondroitin sulfate E), fibroblast growth factors, and cathepsin G are all analytes that are measured in the research laboratory. Study of these components may better elucidate the mechanisms involved in the Type 1 hypersensitivity response.

CONCLUSIONS

The goal of the clinical immunology laboratory is to provide serologic testing that supports the clinician in the diagnosis and management of patients suspected of Type 1 hypersensitivity reactions (Boxes 22-1 and 22-2). To this end, the most important analyte measured in the clinical laboratory is allergen-specific IgE antibody. Selection of the laboratory and the IgE antibody assay methods and standards that it employs to ensure quality are the ultimate responsibility of the referring physician.[37] Performance on national diagnostic allergy proficiency surveys conducted by the College of American Pathologists and a successful inspection leading to federal licensure under the Clinical Laboratory Improvement Act of 1988 are both benchmarks that can be used by the physician to ensure that the clinical laboratory provides quality testing.

REFERENCES

1. Ishizaka K, Ishizaka T: Physiochemical properties of reaginic antibody. I. Association of reaginic activity with an immunoglobulin other than gamma A or gamma G globulin, *J Allergy* 37:169-172, 1967.
2. Johansson SGO, Benich H: Immunological studies of an atypical (myeloma) immunoglobulin, *Immunology* 13:381-394, 1967.

3. Matsson P, Hamilton RG, Adkinson NF Jr, et al: *Evaluation methods and analytical performance characteristics of immunological assays for human immunoglobulin E (IgE) antibodies of defined allergen specificities,* Wayne, Penn, 1997, National Committee on Clinical Laboratory Standards (NCCLS).

4. Hamilton RG, Peterson EL, Ownby DR: Clinical and laboratory-based methods in the diagnosis of natural rubber latex allergy, *J Allergy Clin Immunol* 110:S47-S56, 2002.

5. Barbee RA, Halomen M, Lebowitz M, et al: Distribution of IgE in a community population sample: correlations with age, sex and allergen skin test reactivity, *J Allergy Clin Immunol* 68:106-114, 1981.

6. Hamilton RG: Human immunoglobulins. In Leffell MS, Rose N, eds: *Handbook of human immunology,* Boca Raton, Fla, 1998, CRC Press.

7. Wide L, Bennich H, Johansson SGO: Diagnosis by an *in vitro* test for allergen specific IgE antibodies, *Lancet* 2:1105-1109, 1967.

8. Butler JE, Hamilton RG: Quantitation of specific antibodies: methods of expression, standards, solid phase considerations and specific applications. In Butler JE, ed: *Immunochemistry of solid phase immunoassays,* Boca Raton, Fla, 1991, CRC Press.

9. Wood RA, Phipatanakul W, Hamilton RG, et al: A comparison of skin prick tests, intradermal skin tests and RASTs in the diagnosis of cat allergy, *J Allergy Clin Immunol* 102:773-779, 1999.

10. Hamilton RG, Charous BL, Yunginger JW: End-product (glove) extracts useful in the laboratory assessment of IgE mediated latex hypersensitivity. In Proceedings of the International Latex Conference: Sensitivity of Latex in Medical Devices, Baltimore, November 5-7, 1992.

11. Hamilton RG, Charous BL, Adkinson NF Jr, et al: Serological methods in the laboratory diagnosis of latex rubber allergy: study of nonammoniated, ammoniated and glove extracts as allergen reagent sources, *J Lab Clin Med* 123:594-604, 1994.

12. Hamilton RG, Biagini RE, Krieg EF: Diagnostic performance of FDA-cleared serological assays for natural rubber latex specific IgE antibody, *J Allergy Clin Immunol* 103:925-930, 1999.

13. Ownby DR, Magera B, Williams PB: A blinded multi-center evaluation of two commercial *in vitro* tests for latex-specific IgE antibodies, *Ann Allergy Asthma Immunol* 84:193-196, 2000.

14. Chen Z, Rihs HP, Slater JE, et al: The absence of Hev b 5 antigen may cause false-negative results in serologic assays for latex-specific IgE antibodies, *J Allergy Clin Immunol* 106:S83, 2000.

15. Hamilton RG, Biagini R, MacKenzie B, et al: FDA-cleared immunoassays for latex-specific IgE are missing allergenic epitopes from multiple Hev b allergens, *J Allergy Clin Immunol* 109:S259, 2002.

16. Biagini RE, Krieg EF, Pinkerton LE, et al: Receiver operating characteristics analyses of Food and Drug Administration cleared serological assays for natural rubber latex specific immunoglobulin E antibody, *Clin Diagn Lab Immunol* 8:1145-1149, 2001.

17. Saxon A, Ownby D, Huard T, et al: Prevalence of IgE to natural rubber latex in unselected blood donors and performance characteristics of AlaSTAT testing, *Ann Allergy Asthma Immunol* 84:199-206, 2000.

18. Lindqvist A, Maaninen E, Zimmerman K, et al: Quantitative measurement of allergen-specific IgE antibodies applied in a new immunoassay system, UniCAP. In Basomba A, Hernandez F, DeRojas MD, eds: *Proceedings of the XVI European Congress of Allergology and Clinical Immunology ECACI 95,* Bologna, 1995, Monduzzi Editore.

19. Sampson HA, Ho DG: Relationship between food-specific IgE concentrations and the risk of positive food challenges in children and adolescents, *J Allergy Clin Immunol* 100:444-451, 1997.

20. Sampson HA: Utility of food-specific IgE concentrations in predicting food allergy, *J Allergy Clin Immunol* 107:891-896, 2001.

21. De Lovinfosse S, Charpin D, Dornelas A, et al: Can mite-specific IgE be used as a surrogate marker for mite exposure? *Allergy* 49:64-69, 1994.

22. Yunginger JW, Ahlstedt S, Eggleston PA, et al: Quantitative IgE antibody assays in allergic diseases (rostrum), *J Allergy Clin Immunol* 105:1077-1084, 2000.

23. Des Roches A, Paradis L, Knani J, et al: Immunotherapy with a standardized *Dermatophagoides pteronyssinus* extract. V. Duration of the efficacy of immunotherapy after its cessation, *Allergy* 51:430-433, 1996.

24. Williams PB, Siegel C, Portnoy J: Efficacy of a single diagnostic test for sensitization to common inhalant allergens, *Ann Allergy Asthma Immunol* 86:196-202, 2001.

25. Schwartz LB, Bradford TR: Regulation of tryptase from human lung mast cells by heparin: stabilization of the active tetramer, *J Biol Chem* 261:7372-7379, 1986.

26. Enander I, Matsson P, Andesson AS, et al: A radioimmunoassay for human serum tryptase released during mast cell activation, *J Allergy Clin Immunol* 85:154-159, 1990.

27. Schwartz LB, Yunginger JW, Miller J, et al: Time course of the appearance and disappearance of human mast cell tryptase in the circulation after anaphylaxis, *J Clin Invest* 83:1551-1557, 1989.

28. Van der Linden PW, Hack CE, Poortman J, et al: Insect sting challenge in 138 patients: relation between clinical severity of anaphylaxis and mast cell activation, *J Allergy Clin Immunol* 90:110-118, 1992.

29. Zacharisen MC, Schuleter DP, Kurup VP, et al: The long-term outcome in acute, subacute and chronic forms of pigeon breeder's disease hypersensitivity pneumonitis, *Ann Allergy Asthma Immunol* 88:175-182, 2002.

30. Fan LL: Hypersensitivity pneumonitis in children, *Curr Opin Pediatr* 14:323-326, 2002.

31. Mizobe T, Adachi S, Hamaoka A, et al: Evaluation of the enzyme-linked immunosorbent assay system for serodiagnosis of summer-type hypersensitivity pneumonitis, *Arerugi* 51:20-23, 2002.

32. Hamilton RG, Wisenauer JA, Golden DB, et al: Selection of *Hymenoptera* venoms for immunotherapy based on patient's IgE antibody cross-reactivity, *J Allergy Clin Immunol* 92:651-659, 1993.

33. Hamilton RG, Adkinson NF: Immunological tests for diagnosis and management of human allergic disease: total and allergen-specific IgE and allergen-specific IgG. In Rose NR, Conway de Macario E, Folds JD, et al, eds: *Manual of clinical laboratory immunology,* Washington, DC, 1997, American Society for Microbiology.

34. Golden DBK, Lawrence ID, Hamilton RG, et al: Clinical correlation of the venom-specific IgG antibody level during maintenance venom immunotherapy, *J Allergy Clin Immunol* 90:386-393, 1992.

35. Hamilton RG, Chapman MD, Platts-Mills TAE, et al: House dust aeroallergen measurements in clinical practice: a guide to allergen-free home and work environments, *Immunol Allergy Practice* 14:96-112, 1992.

36. Hamilton RG, Eggleston PA: Environmental allergen analyses, *Methods* 13:53-60, 1997.

37. Hamilton RG: Responsibility for quality IgE antibody results rests ultimately with the referring physician (invited editorial), *Ann Allergy Asthma Immunol* 86:353-355, 2001.

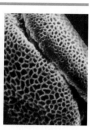

CHAPTER 23

In Vivo Testing for Immunoglobulin E–Mediated Sensitivity

HAROLD S. NELSON

In the United States, *in vivo* testing for the diagnosis of allergy is virtually synonymous with skin testing. Direct application of allergen to the mucous membranes of the eyes, nose, and bronchi is very rarely performed for clinical diagnosis in the United States. It is perhaps used more often in Europe, but there, too, it is less common than it was several decades ago. The preference for skin testing over allergen challenges to the conjunctiva, nose, or lungs is attributable to skin testing being less time consuming and more comfortable for the patient. It provides an objective end point rather than the subjective end points typical with conjunctival and nasal challenges. Finally, many allergens can be tested for in a single session compared with the limitation to a single allergen with mucosal challenges. There is little to suggest that the information gained from mucosal testing is different from that obtained by skin testing. Results of nasal challenges have been shown to correlate closely with skin tests,[1] as do the results of bronchial challenges, when the additional factor of nonspecific airway responsiveness to histamine is included.[2]

PREVALENCE OF POSITIVE SKIN TESTS

Reaction of the skin to extracts of environmental allergens is common, but not invariable, in patients with the so-called atopic diseases: perennial and seasonal rhinitis, bronchial asthma, and atopic eczema. Of 656 asthmatic patients referred for an allergy evaluation in London, 544 (84%) had at least one positive immediate reaction to prick skin testing with 22 common allergens.[3] Skin test reactivity was more common in those with onset of asthma before the age of 10, whereas those with onset after the age of 30 more commonly had a negative skin test. A similar percentage with positive skin tests has been reported in patients evaluated for rhinitis[4] and eczema.[5]

Positive reactions on skin testing are also common in studies of unselected residents in westernized societies. In an epidemiologic study in Tucson, Arizona, 34% of the subjects older than 2 years had at least one reaction to a battery of five or more allergens or mixes.[6] A study was conducted in 200 young and middle-aged adults with a battery of 13 extracts (10 pollen, 2 mite, and 1 cat).[7] Three groups were recruited for prick skin testing. In those with a personal history of rhinitis or asthma, 90% had at least one positive prick skin test. In those with no personal history of rhinitis or asthma but a close relative with one of these conditions, 46% had at least one positive prick skin test. Even in those who denied rhinitis or asthma personally or in close relatives, 29% had at least one positive prick skin test.

FACTORS AFFECTING THE SIZE AND PREVALENCE OF POSITIVE SKIN TESTS

Age

Epidemiologic studies in Tucson demonstrate the varying prevalences of positive immediate prick skin test reactions with age in their population.[6] When tested with a battery of five allergens or mixes, only 22% of those 3 or 4 years old had at least one positive test. The peak prevalence of reactivity was seen in the first half of the third decade, when 52% reacted to at least one test. The prevalence of a positive skin test then declined slowly until age 50, after which there was a more rapid falloff, reaching a low of 16% in the subjects older than 75 years. Further studies in this population related the presence of prick skin test reactivity to the reactivity of the skin to histamine and to the serum total IgE levels.[8] In dividing the study population into four age groups, they found that total IgE was highest in those 9 to 19 years old and declined progressively in the other three groups (20 to 34, 35 to 50, and >50 years old). Histamine reactivity was lowest in the 9- to 19-year-old group, however, and was higher in the three older groups. The prevalence of positive skin tests, presumably reflecting in part the interaction of specific IgE and reactivity of the skin to histamine, was highest in the 20- to 34-year-old group.

Supporting data for the above observations come from separate studies of levels of specific IgE and cutaneous reactivity to histamine by age.[9,10] A retrospective review was conducted of results in 326 patients whose sera were analyzed for total and specific IgE.[9] The peak levels for total IgE were in the second and third decades, whereas the highest levels for grass- and house dust mite–specific IgE were observed in those 10 to 15 years old. A prospective study of cutaneous reactivity to histamine was conducted in 365 subjects aged 1 to 85 years.[10] The size of the prick skin test to histamine increased progressively, peaking in those 21 to 38 years old. There was then very little difference until age 50. After this, there was a further decline in the mean reaction size. Representative values with the 27 mg/ml concentration of histamine were 3.8 mm for ages 0 to 3 years; 6.2 mm, ages 21 to 30 years; and 4.5 mm, ages 61 to 70 years.

Reactivity of the skin to histamine and codeine was examined in children from infancy to age 2.[11] Prick skin tests with both histamine and codeine (a nonimmunologic mast cell−degranulating agent) were particularly small up to age 6 months, although after 1 month of age there was usually some reactivity to both reagents. Due to the reduced reactivity to histamine in children younger than 2 years, adjustment of the interpretation for the size of the positive control is important.

Varying reactivity to histamine can have a significant effect on skin test reactions, even in adults.[12] In an epidemiologic study, 893 adults were prick skin tested with 14 allergens and tenfold dilutions of histamine, ranging from 1 to 0.001 mg/ml. In those positive only to the highest concentration of histamine, 56% had all negative skin tests to allergens and only 15% had six or more positive skin tests. By comparison, of those responding to 0.01 and 0.001 mg/ml histamine concentrations, only 11% had all negative skin tests to allergens and 60% had six or more positive tests.

Physiologic Factors

The size of the reaction of the skin has been reported to vary with the time of day, season of the year, menstrual cycle, subject's handedness, and part of the body used for testing. Although it had been reported that there was a circadian pattern to skin reactivity, a study in 20 children and 20 adults did not find any significant variation during the normal clinic hours.[13] Subjects were tested in duplicate with serial dilutions of short ragweed and histamine at 8 AM and 4 PM. No significant differences between the two sessions were observed at any dilution of either test material. The size of the skin reactions to histamine and allergens was examined over the course of 1 year.[14] It was found that reactions to both allergens and histamine were greater in October and February than in July and August.

Fifteen allergic women with seasonal rhinitis and/or asthma and 15 nonallergic female controls were skin tested three times during their menstrual cycle.[15] There were significantly greater reactions to histamine and morphine in both allergic and nonallergic women and to Parietaria extract in allergic women on days 12 to 16 of the cycle, corresponding to ovulation and peak estrogen levels. The size of the reaction to histamine on the forearms was compared with handedness in 176 subjects.[16] Significant differences between the size of the wheal and flare on the two forearms were observed. Subjects who were right handed with only right-handed relatives had significantly larger reactions on the left arm. Subjects who were either left handed or ambidextrous had significantly larger reactions on the right arm. Subjects who were right handed but had non−right-handed relatives had no difference in reaction between the two arms.

Reactivity of the Skin in Different Areas of the Body

The back is commonly used for percutaneous testing because it provides a large surface that can accommodate many tests. Although it may be acceptable to consider the back as homogenous for clinical purposes, there is a significant gradient of reactivity with the upper back being less reactive than the middle, which in turn is less reactive than the lower third. The wheal diameter was 30% less with allergens and 19% less with histamine on the upper compared with the lower back.[17] Often the forearm is used as an alternative site for percutaneous testing because there is no need for the patient to disrobe, and testing may be done with the patient sitting in a chair rather than lying down. It has been long recognized that the forearm is not as reactive as the back. In one study, the allergen-induced wheal diameter was 27% smaller and the flare diameter was 14% smaller.[18] Although the difference is not great, it is estimated that 2.3% of tests positive on the back would be negative if performed on the forearm.

Medication

Because histamine is a major mediator of the immediate skin test, drugs that have antihistamine properties suppress skin test reactions. Studies have been directed toward assessing the duration of this suppression after the medication is discontinued because this is often an important consideration for diagnostic allergy skin testing. Persistent suppression after multiple doses of first-generation antihistamines was studied.[19] The mean time for skin reactivity to return to normal after stopping the drug was 3 days for chlorpheniramine and tripelennamine and 5 days for hydroxyzine. However, some patients remained suppressed for 6 to 8 days. After multiple doses of the second-generation antihistamine fexofenadine, skin reactivity returned to normal 2 days later.[20] Single 25-mg doses of the tricyclic antidepressants desipramine and doxepin produced suppression that lasted an average of 2 and 6 days, respectively.[21] It was recommended that doxepin be withheld at least 7 days before skin testing. Multiple dosing of the H_2 antagonist ranitidine produced significant suppression of both the wheal and flare of the histamine skin test.[22] Suppression was only 18% of the mean diameter; therefore withholding the drug on the day of testing should be adequate.

There is no consensus regarding the effect of corticosteroids on allergy skin tests. In a prospective study, the topical application of corticosteroids for 4 weeks reduced the area of the allergen-induced wheal by 72% and the flare by 62%.[23] The reduction could at least in part be explained by an 85% reduction in the number of detectable mast cells in the treated skin. A prospective study of 1 week of oral corticosteroids, 24 mg/day methylprednisolone, found no effect on reactivity to ragweed.[24] A retrospective analysis of 25 patients who had been on oral steroids for longer, but varying, periods suggested that they had diminished skin reactivity to codeine, a nonimmunologic mast cell−degranulating agent.[25] However, a prospective study of 33 patients who received oral steroids for at least 1 year (median dosage, 20 mg/day prednisone; median duration, 2 years) revealed no suppression of skin reactions to either codeine or allergen.[26]

Allergy immunotherapy has been observed to reduce the immediate reaction to allergen skin testing.[27] The reductions in the immediate skin test are accompanied by reductions in nasal and conjunctival sensitivity.[27] Allergen immunotherapy reduces the late cutaneous reaction even more than the immediate reaction.[28]

Quantity and Quality of Extracts

The size of the reaction is a function of the patient's sensitivity and the amount of the relevant reagent injected. The relationship between dose and response is best expressed as a log/log relationship.[29] (The slope is steeper when the size of the reaction is expressed as the log of the area, as opposed to the log of the diameter.) When log-linear dose responses are calculated, the resulting curve is S shaped but linear in the midrange.[30] A tenfold increase in the concentration of allergen or histamine will produce an approximately 1.5-fold increase in mean diameter,[29] or a doubling of the area of the wheal.[29]

In the United States, standardized extracts are available for several grasses, ragweed, *Dermatophagoides pteronyssinus* and *farinae*, and cat. In general, other pollen extracts, although not standardized, are of good potency. Most extracts of dog dander[31] and probably most or all fungi[32] are relatively weak. In the cases of fungi and cockroach, proteases within the extracts may degrade susceptible proteins within the extract.[33]

A unique problem appears to exist with extracts of some foods. Many patients with documented food sensitivity will fail to react to commercial extracts or *in vitro* tests prepared from these extracts (but will react to testing with fresh extracts of the foods).[34,35] Reactions to fresh foods, but not commercial food extracts, have been reported with fruits and celery,[35,36] with shellfish and fish,[35,37] and even with peanuts and walnuts.[35] This report not withstanding, peanut extracts have been reported to be reliable in other studies.[36,38] In 76 children aged 5 months to 15 years, there were 31 positive blinded food challenges of 96 foods that yielded positive prick skin tests.[38] All of the positive challenges were to peanuts, eggs, milk, or soy. There were no positive open feeding challenges to foods that had not been positive on prick skin testing.

METHODS OF SKIN TESTING

Prick versus Intradermal Testing

There are two approaches to allergen skin testing. One is to introduce the allergen through a break in the skin. This may be percutaneous, via pricking, puncturing, or scratching.[33] In the latter, a linear scratch is made without drawing blood. Either this may be performed first, with the extract then dropped on the abraded skin, or the scratch may be made through a drop of extract. The scratch test has now in large part been abandoned because of greater discomfort, poorer reproducibility, and the possibility of leaving multiple liner depigmented areas for some time afterward.[39] The prick test is performed by introducing the tip of the device into the epidermis at an approximately 45-degree angle through a drop of extract; the tip is then lifted, creating a small, transient break in the epidermis. Prick testing can be performed with either solid needles or hollow hypodermic needles. Puncture testing is performed by pressing the tip of the device at a 90-degree angle to the skin. Usually the device that is used has a sharp point approximately 1 mm long, with a widening above to limit penetration into the skin.

The alternative to percutaneous testing is intracutaneous testing. A hypodermic syringe and needle are used. The needle is threaded into the dermis, where typically 0.01 to 0.02 ml of extract is injected. Intradermal testing is more sensitive than prick/puncture. For equivalency at threshold reactions, the extract for prick/puncture testing must be 1000-fold more concentrated.[40] Also, direct comparisons indicate that intradermal testing is more reproducible than percutaneous testing.[40] Nevertheless, there are many arguments in favor of the percutaneous test as the routine for allergy testing (Table 23-1). These include economy of time and patient comfort and safety. They apply to percutaneous versus intracutaneous

TABLE 23-1 Advantages of Percutaneous versus Intracutaneous Skin Testing

Percutaneous: Prick or Puncture	Intracutaneous
Safer	More sensitive (1:1000 at threshold)
Technically less demanding	More reproducible
Less painful	Requires less concentrated extracts
More rapidly performed	
Many tests in one session	
Positive and negative more easily distinguished (only true for low-trauma devices)	
Positive correlates better with clinical allergy	
Steeper dose-response curve (valuable for titrated testing)	
Extracts more stable (50% glycerin)	

testing no matter what the relative concentrations of extract employed. If, in addition, the intradermal test is performed with a concentration greater than 1:1000 that of the percutaneous test, in order to increase its sensitivity, additional considerations arise as to whether this increased sensitivity is clinically necessary or useful.

Diagnostic Usefulness of the Percutaneous Test

The prick skin test has served well in epidemiologic studies. Prick skin test reactivity to indoor allergens, but not pollens, has been shown to be a risk factor for asthma in children[41,42] and in adolescents and adults.[43] Prick skin test reactivity in asymptomatic freshmen in college carried an increased risk for the development of allergic rhinitis.[44,45] Three-year follow-up revealed that 18.2% of those with positive prick skin tests had developed allergic rhinitis compared with 1.8% of those with negative prick skin tests.[44] At 7-year follow-up, 31.9% of those with positive prick skin tests and 7.7% of those with negative prick skin tests had developed allergic rhinitis.[45] The larger the prick skin test as a freshman, the more likely the development of allergic rhinitis. Furthermore, after 7 years, new-onset asthma had developed in 5% of the prick skin test–positive group versus 1.5% in the prick skin test–negative group.[45]

Diagnostic Usefulness of the Intracutaneous Test

Although the intracutaneous test, at the strength customarily performed, is more sensitive, it may be questioned whether this increased sensitivity is clinically necessary. The prick skin test, performed with good-quality extracts, is positive in many subjects who do not have a personal or even a family history of allergy.[7] A number of studies have addressed the clinical usefulness of intracutaneous testing. In the Tucson epidemiologic study, 311 subjects representing a sample of the more than 3800 participants had prick skin testing followed, if negative, by intracutaneous testing with 1:1000 wt/v extract to 14 common allergens.[46] Subjects were divided by history into allergic and nonallergic groups. Prick test reactivity correlated with the presence of allergy symptoms. Conversely, positive reactions to intracutaneous testing, which followed a negative prick test for that allergen, showed no correlation with either the patient's clinical allergic status or the level of total serum IgE. Studies in smaller groups of patients have supported this epidemiologic data. Thirty-four subjects with perennial rhinitis who were prick skin test negative but intracutaneous test positive were compared with 19 subjects who had positive prick skin tests and to 13 healthy controls.[47] Although in the 19 prick skin test–positive subjects the radioallergosorbent test (RAST) was positive in 12 and leukocyte histamine release and nasal challenge were positive in 17 each, among the intracutaneous only–positive group, there were no positive RASTs or leukocyte histamine release tests and only 1 of 34 had a positive nasal challenge.

Two studies examined the intracutaneous test as a predictor of symptoms with natural exposure to the allergen.[48,49] In a study of the clinical usefulness of intradermal skin tests to grass, four groups were compared: three of the groups had a history of seasonal allergic rhinitis, one with positive prick skin tests to Timothy grass, one with a negative prick but a positive intradermal test to Timothy grass, and one with both negative prick and intracutaneous tests to Timothy grass. The fourth group comprised nonallergic control groups.[48] On the basis of nasal challenge with Timothy grass pollen, allergic reactions were present in 68% of those with positive prick skin tests to Timothy grass and in none of the nonallergic controls. In both the group with positive and those with negative intracutaneous tests to Timothy grass, 11% were positive. Subjects were then followed though the grass pollen season. Their symptom scores, recorded in a diary, were examined for a correlation with grass pollen counts. A positive correlation was present in 64% of those with positive prick skin tests and in none of the nonallergic controls. A positive correlation of symptoms with pollen count was present in 22% of those with a positive intracutaneous test and 21% of those with a negative intracutaneous test to Timothy grass. Both criteria for al-

lergy to Timothy grass, a positive nasal challenge, and a correlation between symptoms and grass pollen counts were met in 46% of those with positive prick skin tests but in none in the other three groups. Thus under the conditions of this study, the presence of a positive intradermal skin test response to Timothy grass in the presence of a negative skin prick test response to Timothy grass did not indicate the presence of clinically significant sensitivity to Timothy grass.[48]

In the second study, patients were challenged with cat exposure for 1 hour.[49] Both positive prick skin tests and RASTs to cats were highly predictive of development of symptoms on exposure to the cat room. Subjects with a negative skin prick test were just as likely to have a positive-challenge result if they had a negative (31%) as if they had a positive (24%) intracutaneous skin test. The authors concluded that, at least with regard to cat allergy, these results strongly suggest that major therapeutic decisions, such as environmental control or immunotherapy, should never be based on a positive intracutaneous skin test result alone.[49]

Expressing the Results of Skin Testing

The results of both percutaneous and intracutaneous skin tests are often reported in only semiquantitative terms. Results may be recorded only as positive or negative or in terms of 0 to 4+ without any indication of what size reactions these numbers represent.[50] At the very least, a record of skin testing should indicate certain information that will allow another physician to interpret the results. In addition to the concentration of extract used, the form should indicate whether the tests are percutaneous or intracutaneous and, if the former, which device was used for testing, whether testing was performed on the back or the arm, and the size of the positive and negative reactions. Finally, if an arbitrary grading system is used, the range of reaction for each grade should be clearly indicated on the form (Table 23-2).

TABLE 23-2 Semiquantitative Reporting of Skin Test Results

Criteria to read prick/puncture skin tests

0	No reaction or no difference from control
+	Erythema less than a nickel in diameter
++	Erythema greater than a nickel in diameter
+++	Wheal with surrounding erythema
++++	Wheal with pseudopods and surrounding erythema

Criteria to read intracutaneous tests when control ≥ 2 mm

0	No difference from control
+	Wheal 1½ to 2 times that of control or definite erythema greater than a nickel in diameter
++	Wheal 2 to 3 times that of control
+++	Wheal > 3 times that of control
++++	Wheal with pseudopods

Criteria to read intracutaneous tests when control < 2 mm

0	No difference from control
+	3- to 4-mm wheal with erythema or erythema greater than a nickel in diameter
++	4- to 8-mm wheal without pseudopods
+++	> 8-mm wheal without pseudopods
++++	Wheal with pseudopods and erythema

From Vanselow NA: Skin testing and other diagnostic procedures. In Sheldon JM, Lovell RG, Mathews KP, eds: *A manual of clinical allergy,* ed 2, Philadelphia, 1967, WB Saunders.

A superior method of expressing results is to measure the reaction and then enter the measurement on the form. This need not be excessively time consuming. Although area of the wheal and erythema is the most accurate, measurements of the product of the orthogonal diameters, the sum of the orthogonal diameters, and even the longest diameter correlate very well with area, with *r* values greater than 0.9.[51]

The Scandinavian Society of Allergology recommended that skin test results be standardized in relation to the size of the reaction to histamine, using 0.1 mg/ml of histamine for intradermal testing and 1 mg/ml of histamine for prick skin testing.[52] The suggested method was to calculate the mean diameter. If the reaction to allergen was the same size as the histamine reaction, the grade was 3+; if half that size, 2+; and if twice as large, 4+. Subsequent study suggested that the histamine control should be 10 mg/ml because of the small reactions with a high coefficient of variation with the 1 mg/ml histamine prick skin test.[53] Even the 20% to 30% coefficient of variation for reactions to 10 mg/ml raises questions regarding the desirability of standardizing to a histamine control, which if used for this purpose should be performed at least in duplicate.[54]

The reliability of different means of expressing the results of prick skin testing was compared in patients sensitive to dogs.[55] A determination of sensitivity to dogs was made in 202 children based on a composite score from history, RAST, and bronchial or conjunctival allergen challenges. The results of three common means of expressing results are shown in Table 23-3.

Although the overall efficacy of the histamine reference was greatest, in this study most allergists would prefer to have the maximum sensitivity to not miss any truly sensitive patients. Other methods, or clinical judgment, should then be used to distinguish between those who are only sensitized and those who are clinically allergic.[54]

Devices for Percutaneous Skin Testing

Intracutaneous skin tests are performed using a hypodermic syringe and needle. Percutaneous tests are performed with an ever-increasing variety of devices.[17,56] These devices differ in whether they are used to prick or puncture (some are used both ways). Some have a single stylus with a single or several points and are used to either prick or puncture through a drop of extract or to carry a drop of extract from the extract bottle; the application of extract and the puncture occur in one step.

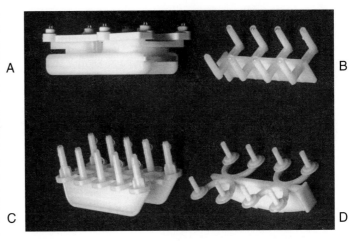

FIGURE 23-1 Four devices for performing multiple-puncture skin testing: **A,** Greertrack (Greer Labs, Lenoir, NC); **B,** MultiTest II (Lincoln Diagnostics, Decatur, IL); **C,** Polypik (Dermapik II Skin Test System, Biomedex Inc., Spokane, WA); and **D,** QuickTest (Quantities System, Planate Inc., Placentia, CA). All four devices are designed to be dipped into the extract wells and to carry a drop of extract on each head to be introduced into the skin by the puncture method.

Increasingly, devices are being introduced that have multiple heads so that up to eight tests can be accomplished with one application (Figure 23-1). In general, the multiheaded skin test devices are designed to first be dipped into the extract bottles and then applied to the skin in one step. The devices for percutaneous testing vary in the degree of trauma that they impart to the skin; therefore they vary in the size of positive reactions and in the likelihood of producing a reaction at the site of the negative control. These require different criteria for what constitutes a positive reaction (Table 23-4).

Allergy skin testing has come under the scrutiny of the U.S. Department of Labor Occupational Safety and Health Administration (OSHA). In 1995 they alerted their field personnel to the possible safety and health risks that may arise with the practice of using one device per person and wiping the device between tests. OSHA considered this practice to have the potential for a blood-borne pathogen exposure incident should the technician accidentally prick himself or herself with the device wiping it. The implications of this notice have led many allergists to abandon the use of solid-bore needles for percutaneous testing, leading to greater use of the newer devices, which are disposed of after each application of each test.

Placement of Adjacent Tests

There are two reports, both describing intracutaneous testing with Hymenoptera venom, which indicate that false-positive tests can result from an adjacent positive histamine control.[57,58] The influence of large, positive reactions to histamine or to allergen on adjacent prick skin tests was prospectively studied.[18] There was no evidence of falsely positive prick skin tests attributable to the large adjacent reactions, even when the test sites were separated only by 2 cm. Thus it appears that the augmentation that has been observed may be limited to intracutaneous testing and perhaps also to the active constituents in the Hymenoptera venom.

TABLE 23-3 Comparison of Criteria for a Positive Prick Skin Test to Dogs

Criteria	Sensitivity (%)	Specificity (%)	Overall Efficacy (%)
≥ 3-mm wheal diameter	98	82	89
≥ 5-mm wheal diameter	66	98	84
3+ histamine reference	92	93	93

From Vanto T: *Ann Allergy* 49:340-344, 1982.

TABLE 23-4 Size of Wheals that Are Larger than 99% of the Wheals with Saline Using the Same Device by the Same Operator

Devices for Which a 3-mm Wheal Would Be Significant		Devices for Which a >3-mm Wheal Should Be Used as Significant	
Device	99th Quantile of Reactions at the Negative Control Sites (mm)	Device	99th Quantile of Reactions at the Negative Control Sites (mm)
Quintest (HS) puncture	0	DermaPIK (Greer) prick	3.25
Smallpox needle (HS) prick	0	DuoTip (Lincoln) twist	3.5
DuoTip (Lincoln) prick	1.5	Bifurcated needle (ALO) prick	4.0
Lancet (HS) puncture	2.0	MultiTest (Lincoln) puncture	4.0
Lancet (ALK) puncture	3.0	Bifurcated needle (ALO) puncture	4.5
		DermaPIK (Greer) twist	5.0

From Nelson HS, Rosloniec DM, McCall LL, et al: *J Allergy Clin Immunol* 92:750-756, 1993; Nelson HS, Lahr J, Buchmeier BA, et al: *J Allergy Clin Immunol* 101: 153-156, 1998.
ALK, ALK America; *ALO,* Allergy Laboratories of Ohio; *Greer,* Greer Laboratories; *HS,* Hollister Steir; *Lincoln,* Lincoln Diagnostics.

SPECIAL CONSIDERATIONS

Safety of Skin Testing

Deaths have been reported with skin testing.[59] For the most part these were reactions to testing with horse serum or other potent allergens and, almost without exception, they were associated with intradermal testing.[59] Severe reactions can occur, however, even with prick skin testing in very sensitive patients treated with undiluted commercial or fresh food extracts.[60] In a private practice, 10,400 patients were skin tested first by prick and then followed, if negative, by intradermal testing.[61] Two systemic reactions occurred, both with intradermal testing: one occurred in a patient who had had a negative prick skin test, and the other occurred in a patient who did not have preliminary prick skin testing. The experience with allergy skin testing at the Mayo Clinic between 1992 and 1997 was reviewed.[59] Puncture skin testing was performed in 16,505 patients, whereas 1806 received puncture followed by intracutaneous skin testing for selected allergens (Hymenoptera venom, penicillin, and other drugs). Five patients experienced systemic reactions after puncture tests, whereas one patient experienced a systemic reaction to an intracutaneous test after a negative puncture test. Two of the five patients who experienced systemic reactions to puncture testing had positive reactions to latex. One patient reacted to both latex and aeroallergens, whereas two reacted only to aeroallergens. Thus for prick/puncture testing to aeroallergens, systemic reactions, none life threatening, occurred with an incidence of about 15 to 23 per 100,000 tests.

Local Allergy

Patients sometimes present with what sounds like a convincing clinical history of an allergic respiratory condition, but they have negative skin tests to the suspected, and sometimes to all, allergens. There are several studies that suggest that patients may be sensitive to an allergen and have IgE antibodies to that allergen in their nasal secretions, even though prick skin tests and *in vitro* tests for that same allergen are negative. A group of patients with perennial rhinitis was reported to have positive nasal challenges to house dust mite extract and a positive RAST for house dust mites performed on their nasal secretions, even though prick skin tests and RAST on peripheral blood were negative.[62] Two patients with positive nasal challenges and positive RASTs on nasal secretions, in whom prick skin tests and serum RASTs were negative, were reported among 17 patients who presented with conflicting histories and assessments of sensitivity.[63] Four additional patients with positive RAST on nasal secretions, with negative prick skin tests and serum RAST, were encountered among 53 consecutive patients with perennial rhinitis.[64] In the latter study, some of these nasal secretion RASTs were to pollens in patients without corresponding seasonal symptoms, and thus they were not clinically relevant.[64] Nine children of a mean age of 2 years and 5 months with rhinitis or asthma had both negative prick skin tests and serum RASTs for house dust mites. Mast cells from the nasal secretions from 7 of 9 children bound house dust mite allergen on their surface.[65] The investigators were able to block the binding by anti-IgE, indicating the mast cells were sensitized with house dust mite−specific IgE.

Delayed Reactions to Skin Tests

Immediate skin reactions to histamine typically peak at 8 minutes, whereas those to allergen peak at 15 minutes. Large allergen-induced immediate skin tests in a large test reaction area are followed by a late cutaneous reaction. Progressive erythema and induration occur at the site of the immediate reaction, peaking at 4 to 6 hours. These reactions can be triggered by mast cell mediators released by a variety of mechanisms, including allergens, anti-IgE, and nonimmunologic mast cell−degranulating agents, but not by histamine alone.[66] There appears to be a threshold size of the immediate reaction below which the late-phase reaction does not occur. Beyond that size, there is a rough correlation between the size of the immediate reaction and the size of the resulting late-phase reaction in the same individual[66] and in unselected patients.[67] The IgE-mediated late cutaneous reaction has not been described in the absence of an immediate reaction. The late-phase cutaneous reaction is not suppressed by antihistamines but is reduced by corticosteroids. Furthermore, it is markedly reduced by allergen immunotherapy, more so than the immediate reactions.[28]

Isolated, delayed reactions to allergy skin testing have been described.[68-70] Furthermore, when looked for, they appear to fairly commonly follow intracutaneous testing.[68,69] Two hundred ninety-two adult patients who had received a total of 2700 intracutaneous tests were examined after 20 minutes for immediate reactions and again after 48 hours for evidence of delayed reactions.[68] Immediate reactions were observed in 17% of the skin tests in allergic patients and 5% of the skin tests in nonallergic patients. At 48 hours, delayed reactions were present at 7% of the skin test sites in the allergic patients and 5% in the nonallergic patients. Delayed reactions were more than twice as common at sites of positive immediate as negative immediate skin reactions. Those occurring at the site of negative immediate skin tests had the histology of a delayed-type hypersensitive reaction. Positive reactions at 6 hours at sites that did not have an immediate reaction were sought in 50 children.[69] Eighteen children were reported to have 40 isolated late cutaneous reactions. All followed intracutaneous testing. None occurred after negative prick tests. The most common cause was the cockroach, but weeds, trees, cats, and ragweed were also common causes. In both of these studies, there was no suggestion that the late or delayed cutaneous reactions had clinical relevance. A single patient was described with seasonal rhinoconjunctivitis who had all negative prick skin tests and RASTs but developed positive reactions beginning several hours after the prick skin tests to pollen, which peaked after 20 to 40 hours.[70] The author speculated that these late skin tests could represent clinically relevant delayed-type hypersensitivity to pollen that was responsible for the patient's seasonal allergic rhinoconjunctivitis.

Relation of Skin Tests to *In Vitro* Measurements of Specific IgE

For most aeroallergens, the RASTs and enzyme-using variations are somewhat less sensitive than percutaneous tests, and both are much less sensitive than intracutaneous tests at the concentrations of allergen extract tests that are commonly used. Even though less sensitive than intracutaneous, the prick/puncture tests and RASTs are still often positive in patients without clinical symptoms. This has led to attempts to increase the diagnostic precision of these tests by defining cutoffs that enhance specificity without too great a loss in sensitivity. An ambitious study recruited 267 patients who were prick skin test positive and had a clear history of respiratory symptoms in relation to the allergen producing the positive skin test.[71] They were compared with 232 subjects with similar positive prick skin tests but negative histories of respiratory symptoms caused by the aeroallergens producing the positive prick skin tests. Finally, there were 243 nonallergic controls. Patients also had RASTs for the allergens that produced the positive prick skin tests. The investigators constructed receiver operating characteristic curves for sensitivity versus specificity for both RASTs and prick skin tests. They found maximum diagnostic accuracy at cutoffs of 11.7 kU/L in the Pharmacia CAP system (where the threshold for sensitivity is 0.35 kU/L). The cutoff for prick skin testing was a wheal of 32.2 mm (~6-mm diameter). They also reported that the diagnostic accuracy of the RAST exceeded that of the prick skin test. This conclusion may have been biased, however, by the inclusion criteria that all subjects have positive prick skin tests.

Despite similar sensitivity and performances by the *in vitro* and percutaneous tests, the quantitative relationship between them in individuals is relatively weak. Reactivity on intracutaneous skin testing and RAST was measured in 43 patients with rhinitis and/or asthma using five purified major allergens.[72] The overall correlation for skin testing versus serum IgE was only 0.68. For the same level of specific IgE, the amount of the allergen required in different subjects for a positive skin test varied by as much as 100-fold. Skin reactivity was adversely affected by total IgE. Skin testing correlated better than RAST with histamine release, suggesting that "releasability" might account for part of the residual variation in the correlation between skin test results and levels of IgE antibodies.

An additional factor may be the affinity for IgE-allergen binding.[73] Reactions on prick skin testing to ragweed and *Dermatophagoides pteronyssinus* were compared with Amb a 1– and Der p 1–specific IgE levels in 165 members from families with histories of clinical atopy. The donors with positive prick skin test reactions tended to have higher concentrations of specific IgE than those with negative prick skin tests. However, there was considerable overlap between the prick skin test–positive and prick skin test–negative groups, without a clear demarcation between them. Comparison of mean values between prick skin test–positive and prick skin test–negative groups was not statistically significant. Donors with positive prick skin test reactions had, on average, higher binding affinities than those with negative prick skin test results. These values differed significantly for the two groups ($P < 0.001$). The product of affinity and concentration, termed the *antibody capacity,* provided a much clearer demarcation between donors who were prick skin test positive and those who were prick skin test negative.

Relation of Skin Tests to Nasal Allergen Challenge and *In Vitro* Assessment of Specific IgE

Nasal allergen challenges with threefold increasing numbers of grass pollen grains, prick skin tests with threefold increasing concentrations of grass pollen extract, and RASTs using the same grass pollen extract were compared in 44 subjects with rhinitis during the grass pollen season and 10 nonallergic controls.[1] The nasal challenge method, which uses a total symptom score of 5 as an end point, has been validated by demonstration of the release of prostaglandin D_2 into nasal secretions at the end point and by correlation of threshold scores with symptoms on seasonal exposure to grass pollen. Nasal challenges were positive in 41 of 43 patients and 0 of 10 controls. There was a significant correlation ($R_s = 0.54$, $P < 0.005$) between the threshold for nasal challenge and that for prick skin testing. There was no significant correlation between nasal thresholds and levels of specific IgE, suggesting that releasability of mast cells and basophils may be an important parameter in determining symptoms.

Relation of Skin Tests to Bronchial Allergen Challenge

There is a relatively poor correlation between the results of allergen skin testing and bronchial allergen challenge. The reason is the presence of a second variable, nonspecific bronchial hyperresponsiveness, as measured by histamine or methacholine inhalation challenge. It was observed that positive bronchial allergen challenges occurred almost exclusively in subjects with positive prick skin tests[74] but that the correlation

KEY CONCEPTS
Skin Testing

- Skin testing with allergenic extracts is the favored method of *in vivo* testing for IgE-mediated sensitivity.
- The preferred method of skin testing is percutaneous (prick or puncture), with intracutaneous (intradermal) testing generally reserved for weak allergenic extracts, such as Hymenoptera venom or agents used for testing for drug allergy.
- Advantages of percutaneous (prick or puncture) over intracutaneous (intradermal) testing include the following:

  They are safer, less technically demanding, less painful, and more rapidly performed, and many tests can be performed in one session.

  The extracts are more stable and positive, and negative reactions are more easily differentiated.

  Most important, positive reactions correlate better with clinical sensitivity than is the case of intracutaneous tests.
- Advantages of the intracutaneous tests are a somewhat better reproducibility and greater sensitivity. The latter, however, has not been found to be useful for detecting clinically relevant sensitivity in several studies.
- The results of skin testing correlate only weakly with those from *in vitro* studies with the same allergen in the same patient. The size of the skin test reactions depends, in addition to the amount of specific IgE, on the binding affinity of the IgE antibody, the releasability of the patient's mast cells, and the reactivity of their skin to histamine.
- In a particular individual, the size of the skin test will also depend on the area of the body used for testing, with the back being more reactive than the arm.

between skin testing and bronchial allergen challenge could be improved considerably by incorporating the threshold of nonspecific bronchial responsiveness.[75,76] A prospective study confirmed these retrospective observations.[2] The early bronchoconstrictor response to allergen challenge could be predicted within an eightfold range by a formula using skin test reactivity and bronchial sensitivity to histamine. It was pointed out that this degree of prediction was better than the reproducibility of bronchial allergen challenge achieved by some investigators.

CONCLUSIONS

In the United States, *in vivo* testing for the diagnosis of allergy is virtually synonymous with skin testing. In comparison with allergen challenges to the conjunctiva, nose, and lungs, skin testing is less time consuming and more comfortable for the patient. It provides an objective end point rather than the subjective end points typical with conjunctival and nasal challenges, and, finally, many allergens can be tested for in a single session, compared with the limitation to a single allergen with mucosal challenges (Box 23-1).

Percutaneous prick or puncture skin testing is the most efficient method of diagnosing IgE-mediated sensitivity. It is rapidly accomplished and involves little discomfort to the patient, and the results correlate better than those of intracutaneous testing, with the presence of symptoms caused by the allergen. In addition to economy, it appears to have advantages over *in vitro* tests of IgE sensitivity in that it reflects not only the level of specific IgE sensitivity but also antigen-binding affinity of the IgE, mast cell releasability, and reactivity to the skin to histamine. It is important, however, in conducting percutaneous skin tests to pay attention to the quality of extracts and the characteristics of the device used and to express the results in a quantitative manner that can be interpreted by other practitioners.

REFERENCES

1. Bousquet J, Lebel B, Dhlvert H, et al: Nasal challenge with pollen grains, skin-prick tests and specific IgE in patients with grass pollen allergy, *Clin Allergy* 17:529-536, 1987.
2. Cockcroft DW, Murdock KY, Kirby J, et al: Prediction of airway responsiveness to histamine, *Am Rev Respir Dis* 135:264-267, 1987.
3. Hendrick DJ, Davies RJ, D'Souza MF, et al: An analysis of skin prick test reactions in 656 asthmatic patients, *Thorax* 30:2-8, 1975.
4. Viner AS, Jackman N: Retrospective study of 1271 patients diagnosed as perennial rhinitis, *Clin Allergy* 6:251-259,1976.
5. Rajka G: Prurigo Besnier (atopic dermatitis) with special reference to the role of allergy factors. II. The evaluation of the results of skin reactions, *Acta Derm Venereol* 41:1-39, 1961.
6. Barbee RA, Lebowitz MD, Thompson HC, et al: Immediate skin test reactivity in a general population sample, *Ann Intern Med* 84:129-133, 1976.
7. Adinoff AD, Rosloniec DM, McCall LL, et al: Immediate skin test reactivity to Food and Drug Administration-approved standardized extracts, *J Allergy Clin Immunol* 86:766-774, 1990.
8. Barbee RA, Brown WG, Kaltenborn W, et al: Allergen skin-test reactivity in a community population sample: correlation with age, histamine skin reactions, and total serum immunoglobulin E, *J Allergy Clin Immunol* 68:15-19, 1981.
9. Hanneuse Y, Delespesse G, Hudson D, et al: Influence of ageing on IgE-mediated reactions in allergic patients, *Clin Allergy* 8:165-174, 1978.
10. Skassa-Brociek W, Manderscheid J-C, Michel F-B, et al: Skin test reactivity to histamine from infancy to old age, *J Allergy Clin Immunol* 80: 711-716, 1987.
11. Menardo JL, Bousquet J, Rodiere M, et al: Skin test reactivity in infancy, *J Allergy Clin Immunol* 75:646-651, 1985.
12. Stuckey MS, Witt CS, Schmitt LH, et al: Histamine sensitivity influences reactivity to allergens, *J Allergy Clin Immunol* 75:373-376, 1985.
13. Vichyanond P, Nelson HS: Circadian variation of skin reactivity and allergy skin tests, *J Allergy Clin Immunol* 83:1101-1106, 1989.
14. Oppenheimer JJ, Nelson HS: Seasonal variation in immediate skin test reactions, *Ann Allergy* 71:227-229, 1993.
15. Kalogeromitros D, Katsarou A, Armenaka M, et al: Influence of the menstrual cycle on skin-prick test reactions to histamine, morphine and allergen, *Clin Exp Allergy* 25:461-466, 1995.
16. Wise SL, Meador KJ, Thompson WO, et al: Cerebral lateralization and histamine skin test asymmetries in humans, *Ann Allergy* 70:328-332, 1993.
17. Nelson HS, Rosloniec DM, McCall LL, et al: Comparative performance of five commercial skin test devices, *J Allergy Clin Immunol* 92:750-756, 1993.
18. Nelson HS, Knoetzer J, Bucher B: Effect of distance between sites and region of the body on results of skin prick tests, *J Allergy Clin Immunol* 97:596-601, 1996.
19. Cook TJ, MacQueen DM, Wittig HJ, et al: Degree and duration of skin test suppression and side effects with antihistamines, *J Allergy Clin Immunol* 51:71-77, 1973.
20. Dockhorn RJ, Hill EK, Hafner KB, et al: The duration of inhibition of skin prick test reactions after bid administration to steady-state of the non-sedating antihistamine Allegra (abst), *J Allergy Clin Immunol* 99 (1 Part 2):S446, 1997.
21. Rao KS, Menon PK, Hillman BC, et al: Duration of the suppressive effect of tricyclic antidepressants on histamine-induced wheal-and-flare reactions in human skin, *J Allergy Clin Immunol* 82:752-757, 1988.
22. Miller J, Nelson HS: Suppression of immediate skin tests by ranitidine, *J Allergy Clin Immunol* 84:895-899, 1989.

23. Pipkorn U, Hammarlund A, Enerback L: Prolonged treatment with topical glucocorticoids results in an inhibition of the allergen-induced wheal-and-flare response and a reduction in skin mast cell numbers and histamine content, *Clin Exp Allergy* 19:19-25, 1989.

24. Slott RI, Zweiman B: A controlled study of the effect of corticosteroids on immediate skin test reactivity, *J Allergy Clin Immunol* 554:229-234, 1974.

25. Olson R, Karpink MH, Shelanski S, et al: Skin reactivity to codeine and histamine during prolonged corticosteroid therapy, *J Allergy Clin Immunol* 86:153-159, 1990.

26. Des Roches A, Paradis L, Bougeard Y-H, et al: Long-term oral corticosteroid therapy does not alter the results of immediate allergy skin prick tests, *J Allergy Clin Immunol* 98:522-527, 1996.

27. Dantzler BS, Tipton WR, Nelson HS, et al: Tissue threshold changes during the first months of immunotherapy, *Ann Allergy* 45:213-216, 1980.

28. Nish WA, Charlesworth EN, Davis TL, et al: The effect of immunotherapy on the cutaneous late phase reaction to allergen, *J Allergy Clin Immunol* 93:484-493,1994.

29. Dreborg S, Holgersson M, Nilsson G, et al: The dose response relationship of allergen, histamine, and histamine releasers in skin prick test and the precision of the skin prick test method, *Allergy* 42:117-125, 1987.

30. Harris RI, Stern MA, Watson HK: Dose response curve of allergen and histamine in skin prick tests, *Allergy* 43:565-572, 1989.

31. Meiser JP, Nelson HS: Comparing conventional and acetone-precipitated dog allergen extract skin testing, *J Allergy Clin Immunol* 107:744-745, 2001.

32. Yuninger JW, Jones RI, Gleich GJ: Studies on Alternaria allergens, *J Allergy Clin Immunol* 58:405-413, 1976.

33. Esch RG: Role of proteases on the stability of allergic extracts. In Klein R, ed: *Regulatory control and standardization of allergic extracts,* Stuttgart, Germany, 1990, Gustav Fischer Verlag.

34. Dreborg S, Foucard T: Allergy to apple, carrot and potato in children with birch pollen allergy, *Allergy* 38:167-172, 1983.

35. Rosen JP, Selcow JE, Mendelson ML, et al: Skin testing with natural foods in patients suspected of having food allergies: is it a necessity? *J Allergy Clin Immunol* 93:1068-1070, 1994.

36. Ortolani C, Ispano M, Pastorello EA, et al: Comparison of results of skin prick tests (with fresh foods and commercial food extracts) and RAST in 100 patients with oral allergy syndrome, *J Allergy Clin Immunol* 83:683-690, 1989.

37. Ancona GR, Schumacher IC: The use of raw foods as skin testing material in allergic disorders, *Calif Med* 73:473-475, 1950.

38. Bock SA, Lee W-Y, Remigio L, et al: An appraisal of skin tests with food extracts for diagnosis of food hypersensitivity, *Clin Allergy* 8:559-564, 1978.

39. Vanselow NA: Skin testing and other diagnostic procedures. In Sheldon JM, Lovell RG, Mathews KP, eds: *A manual of clinical allergy,* ed 2, Philadelphia, 1967, WB Saunders.

40. Indrajana T, Spieksma FTM, Voorhorst R: Comparative study of the intracutaneous, scratch and prick tests in allergy, *Ann Allergy* 29:639-650, 1971.

41. Sears MR, Herbison GP, Holdaway MD, et al: The relative risks of sensitivity to grass pollen, house dust mite and cat dander in the development of childhood asthma, *Clin Exp Allergy* 19:419-424, 1989.

42. Henderson FW, Stewart PW, Burchinal MR, et al: Respiratory allergy and the relationship between early childhood lower respiratory illness and subsequent lung function, *Am Rev Respir Dis* 145:283-290, 1992.

43. Gergen PJ, Turkeltaub PC: The association of individual allergen reactivity with respiratory disease in a national sample: data from the second National Health and Nutrition Examination Survey, 1976-80 (NHANES II), *J Allergy Clin Immunol* 90:579-588, 1992.

44. Hagy GW, Settipane GA: Prognosis of positive allergy skin tests in an asymptomatic population. A three year followup of college students, *J Allergy* 48:200-211, 1971.

45. Hagy GW, Settipane GA: Risk factors for developing asthma and allergic rhinitis. A 7-year follow-up of college students, *J Allergy Clin Immunol* 58:330-336, 1976.

46. Brown WG, Halonen MJ, Kaltenborn WT, et al: The relationship of respiratory allergy, skin test reactivity, and serum IgE in a community population sample, *J Allergy Clin Immunol* 63:328-335, 1979.

47. Reddy PM, Nagaya H, Pascual HC, et al: Reappraisal of intracutaneous tests in the diagnosis of reaginic allergy, *J Allergy Clin Immunol* 61:36-41, 1978.

48. Nelson HS, Oppenheimer JJ, Buchmeier A, et al: An assessment of the role of intradermal skin testing in the diagnosis of clinically relevant allergy to timothy grass, *J Allergy Clin Immunol* 97:1193-1201, 1996.

49. Wood RA, Phipatanakul W, Hamilton RG, et al: A comparison of skin prick tests, intradermal skin tests, and RASTs in the diagnosis of cat allergy, *J Allergy Clin Immunol* 103:773-779, 1999.

50. Holbrich M, Nelson HS: Skin test recording techniques among allergists (abst), *J Allergy Clin Immunol* 101:S249, 1998.

51. Ownby DR: Computerized measurement of allergen-induced skin reactions, *J Allergy Clin Immunol* 69:536-538, 1982.

52. Scandinavian Society of Allergology: Standardization of diagnostic work in allergy, *Acta Allergol* 29:239-240, 1974.

53. Taudorf E, Malling H-J, Laursen LC, et al: Reproducibility of histamine skin prick test, *Allergy* 40:344-349, 1985.

54. Dreborg S: Skin testing. The safety of skin tests and information obtained from using different methods and concentrations of allergens, *Allergy* 48:473-478, 1993.

55. Vanto T: Efficacy of different skin prick testing methods in the diagnosis of allergy to dog, *Ann Allergy* 49:340-344, 1982.

56. Nelson HS, Lahr J, Buchmeier BA, et al: Evaluation of devices for prick skin testing, *J Allergy Clin Immunol* 101:153-156, 1998.

57. Tipton WR: Influence of histamine controls on skin tests with hymenoptera venom, *Ann Allergy* 44:204-205, 1980.

58. Koller DY, Pirker C, Jarisch R, et al: Influence of the histamine control on skin reactivity in skin testing, *Allergy* 47:58-59, 1992.

59. Valyaseui MA, Maddox DE, Li JTC: Systemic reactions to allergy skin tests, *Ann Allergy* 83:132-136, 1999.

60. Novembre E, Bernardini R, Bertini G, et al: Skin-prick test-induced anaphylaxis, *Allergy* 50:511-513, 1995.

61. Lin MS, Tanner E, Lynn J, et al: Non-fatal systemic allergic reactions induced by skin testing and immunotherapy, *Ann Allergy* 71:557-562, 1993.

62. Huggins KG, Brostoff J: Local production of specific IgE antibodies in allergic rhinitis patients with negative skin tests, *Lancet* 2:148-150, 1975.

63. Miadonna A, Leggieri E, Tedeschi A, et al: Clinical significance of specific IgE determination on nasal secretions, *Clin Allergy* 13:155-164, 1983.

64. Small P, Barrett D, Frenkiel S, et al: Measurement of antigen-specific IgE in nasal secretions of patients with perennial rhinitis, *Ann Allergy* 55:68-71, 1985.

65. Shimojo N, Hirano K, Saito K, et al: Detection of house dust mite (HDM)-specific IgE antibodies on nasal mast cells from asthmatic patients whose skin prick test and RAST are negative for HDM, *Int Arch Allergy Immunol* 98:135-139, 1992.

66. DeShazo RD, Levinson AI, Dvorak HF, et al: The late phase skin reaction: evidence for activation of the coagulation system in an IgE-dependent reaction in man, *J Immunol* 122:692-698, 1979.

67. Agarwal K, Zetterstrom O: Diagnostic significance of late cutaneous allergic responses and their correlation with radioallergosorbent test, *Clin Allergy* 12:489-497, 1982.

68. Green GR, Zweiman B, Beerman H, et al: Delayed skin reactions to inhalant antigens, *J Allergy* 40:224-236, 1967.

69. Liesl MB: Isolated late cutaneous reactions to allergen skin testing in children, *Ann Allergy* 84:294-298, 2000.

70. Lin RY: Delayed hypersensitivity to pollen skin prick tests and seasonal rhinitis, *J Allergy Clin Immunol* 95:911-912, 1995.

71. Pastorello EA, Incorvaia C, Ortolani C, et al: Studies on the relationship between the level of specific IgE antibodies and the clinical expression of allergy. I. Definition of levels distinguishing patients with symptomatic from patients with asymptomatic allergy to common aeroallergens, *J Allergy Clin Immunol* 96:580-587, 1995.

72. Witteman AM, Stapel SSO, Perdok GJ, et al: The relationship between RAST and skin test results in patients with asthma or rhinitis: a quantitative study with purified major allergens, *J Allergy Clin Immunol* 97:16-25, 1996.

73. Pierson-Mullany LK, Jackola DR, Blumenthal MN, et al: Evidence of an affinity threshold for IgE-allergen binding in the percutaneous skin test reaction, *Clin Exp Allergy* 32:107-116, 2002.

74. Bryant DH, Burns MW, Lazarus L: The correlation between skin tests, bronchial provocation tests and the serum level of IgE specific for common allergens in patients with asthma, *Clin Allergy* 5:145-157, 1975.

75. Killian D, Cockcroft DW, Hargreave FE, et al: Factors in allergen-induced asthma: relevance of the intensity of the airways allergen reaction and nonspecific bronchial reactivity, *Clin Allergy* 6:219-225, 1976.

76. Bryant DH, Burns WM: Bronchial histamine reactivity: Its relationship to the reactivity of the bronchi to allergens, *Clin Allergy* 6:523-532, 1976.

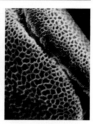

CHAPTER 24

Outdoor Allergens

JOHN W. YUNGINGER

Allergens are substances, usually proteins or glycoproteins, capable of inducing IgE-antibody responses (sensitization) in genetically predisposed individuals. Subsequent exposures to allergens can trigger immediate hypersensitivity responses such as rhinitis, conjunctivitis, or asthma in previously sensitized persons. The number of proteins from any given allergenic source will vary, but sensitized persons producing IgE antibodies to a source will often recognize more than one allergen. This chapter will review the nomenclature, biology, source, distribution, and quantitation of the most common outdoor allergens.

ALLERGEN NOMENCLATURE

Many clinically important allergens have been isolated and sequenced, and their structures have been defined.[1] The Allergen Nomenclature Committee of the International Union of Immunological Societies (IUIS) has devised a unified nomenclature system for purified allergens.[2] Allergens are phenotypically designated by the first three letters of the genus, followed by a space, then the first letter of the species, another space, and finally an Arabic number; occasionally, an additional letter must be added to either the genus or species designation. Allergens are genotypically designated with italics; for example, the two genes encoding the two polypeptide chains of the major cat (*Felis domesticus*) allergen Fel d 1 are designated *Fel d 1A* and *Fel d 1B*. Isoallergens are members of an allergen group that have 67% or greater amino acid sequence identity. Isoallergens and their variants that belong to the same allergen group are designated by suffixes of a period followed by four Arabic numerals. For example, two isoallergens from Timothy grass pollen (*Phleum pratense*), known originally as Phl p Va and Phl p Vb, are now designated as Phl p 5.0102 and Phl p 5.0201, respectively, whereas the two clones of the latter are designated as *Phl p 5.0201* and *Phl p 5.0202*. A contemporary Internet-based listing of purified allergens is maintained by the IUIS.[3]

OUTDOOR AEROALLERGEN SAMPLING

The major sources of outdoor allergens are plants and fungi. Traditional atmospheric surveys rely on capture and morphologic identification of pollen and spore unit structures. The various air-sampling devices (Table 24-1) have been described in detail by Muilenberg[4] and Solomon and Platts-Mills.[5] The simplest device is the Durham shelter, in which airborne particulates passively settle onto an adhesive-coated microscope slide. Entrapped pollen grains are stained with a basic fuchsin solution (Calberla stain) and identified by comparison with specimens in published atlases.[6] Data are reported as particles per square centimeter of slide area. More efficient air samplers include the intermittent rotating arm impactor (Rotorod sampler) and the intermittent suction trap (Kramer-Collins sampler), in which airborne particulates are deposited onto Lucite rods or adhesive strips for subsequent identification; these data are reported as particles per cubic meter. However, samplers that operate intermittently may miss sudden showers of pollens or fungal spores. Continuously operating samplers include the Burkard spore trap, in which particulates are deposited onto a slowly moving adhesive tape, and the Andersen sequential sieve impinger, in which viable fungal spores are separated into various aerodynamic sizes onto culture plates for subsequent incubation and identification. Culture methods identify only viable fungal particles, however, and many airborne spores do not grow on available culture media.

POLLENS

Biology

Pollen grains are the male gametes produced in pollen sacs (microsporangia) of the anthers of flowering plants (angiosperms) and conifers (gymnosperms). Wind-pollinated (anemophilous) plants are more allergenic than insect-pollinated (entomophilous) plants; outdoor pollen loads are derived overwhelmingly from the former. The lining cell layer of the anther sac cavity is the tapetum, which secretes tapetal fluid and also contains "pollen mother" cells, from which the protoplast of the pollen grain is derived (Figure 24-1).[7] Mature pollen grains contain a hard outer wall (exine) comprised of sporopollenin, a polyterpene derived from the tapetum.[8] A softer inner wall (intine) comprises pectin and cellulose and encloses pollen mother cell-derived cytoplasmic proteins, starches, sugars, lipids, carotenoids, and ascorbic acid.[8] The biochemistry of plant pollination and fertilization has recently been reviewed.[7]

Exposure

Exposure to pollen aeroallergens is dependent on the types of plants growing in a particular location, as well as pollen-specific characteristics such as buoyant density, ease of dispersion, and profusion. Approximately 20 to 100 pollen

TABLE 24-1 Outdoor Aeroallergen Samplers

Apparatus	Description	Advantages	Disadvantages
Durham sampler	Passive deposition of airborne particles on adhesive-coated microscope slide	Simplicity, low cost, durability	Cannot provide volumetric data
Rotorod sampler	Intermittent rotating arm impactor that captures airborne particles onto adhesive-coated Lucite rods	Provides volumetric data; unaffected by wind speed or direction	Loss of efficiency with particle overloading; episodic showers of airborne particulates may be missed
Andersen sampler	Suction sampler containing sequential sieves to deposit viable particles onto culture plates	High efficiency; identifies smaller fungal spores that are difficult to identify visually	Expense; requires wind orientation
Burkard trap	Suction sampler with small intake orifice that continuously deposits particles onto a slowly moving tape	High efficiency; provides volumetric data; no particle overloading	Expense
Kramer-Collins trap	Suction sampler that intermittently deposits particles onto rotating drum	High efficiency; provides volumetric data; moderate cost; wind-oriented	Episodic showers of airborne particulates may be missed

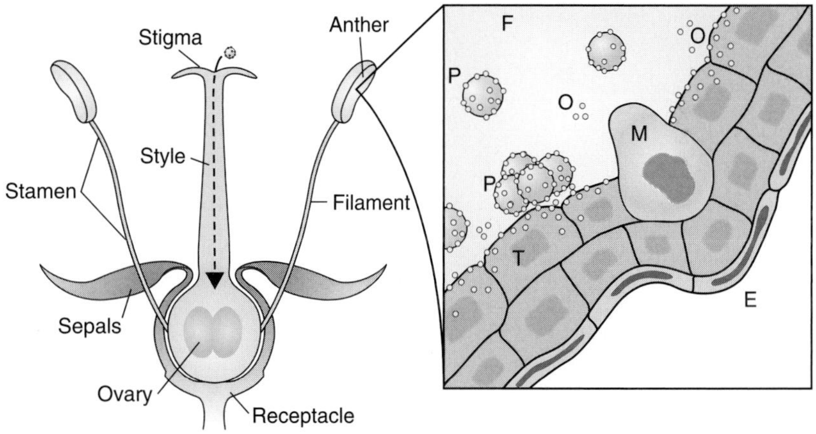

FIGURE 24-1 Schematic diagram of a segment of an anther sac wall and cavity. Pollen grains *(P)* are shown as tetrads and monads. *T,* Secretory tapetum; *M,* pollen mother (progenitor) cell; *F,* tapetal fluid; *O,* orbicules of sporopollenin; *E,* epidermis. Orbicules derive from the tapetal endoplasmic reticulum and occupy cell surface sites until released. (From Solomon WR: *J Allergy Clin Immunol* 109:895-900, 2002.)

grains/m^3 is sufficient to provoke symptoms in sensitized individuals. Pollen grains range from 10 to 100 μm in diameter, and most inhaled grains lodge in the nasal cavity or nasopharynx. However, allergens are also present on submicronic pollen-derived vectors such as starch grains (amyloplasts, approximately 700 per pollen grain, each approximately 3 μm in diameter) and exine fragments (0.3 to 2 μm in diameter) known variously as *orbicules, Übish bodies,*[7] or *P-particles* (polysaccharide-containing wall-precursor bodies).[9] These allergenic particles, when inhaled by sensitized individuals, are small enough to reach the lower respiratory tract and trigger asthma. In particular, starch granules from Timothy or rye grass pollen contain Phl p 5 and Lol p 5, respectively[10]; airborne concentrations of these amyloplasts increase tenfold during convective disturbances and can induce epidemics of thunderstorm-induced asthma.[11,12]

Allergenic Pollens in the United States

Selected examples of common pollens are shown in Figure 24-2. Residents of the United States are exposed to sequential pollen showers from trees (late winter to spring), grasses (spring to summer), and weeds (late summer to fall). Detailed listings of the pollens present in various floristic zones[5] or specific geographic regions of the United States[13-15] have been published. Contemporary pollen counts from throughout the United States are available from the website of the American Academy of Allergy, Asthma and Immunology.[16]

Trees
Selected examples of allergenic trees and shrubs are listed in Table 24-2, along with their distribution in the United States. Conifers shed large quantities of pollen, particularly in the southeastern United States, Rocky Mountains, and Pacific northwest. However, only that from mountain cedar is regarded as highly allergenic, producing seasonal rhinoconjunctivitis symptoms during December, January, and February in Oklahoma and Texas. Other species of cedar produce symptoms in more limited areas of the Pacific northwest. Among the angiosperms, ash, poplar, birch, maple, and oak species, as well as pecan, may be important in specific locales. White mulberry (*Morus alba*), an Asian species introduced as a boulevard tree in Arizona, is a potent sensitizer whose further planting is now prohibited by law.

Tree pollen production tends to be shorter and more intense than pollen production from grasses or weeds. In northern and eastern areas of the United States, elm and cedar pollens are the first to appear, followed in order by maple/box elder, birch, oak, and hickory/walnut. In southern California, ash and alder begin pollination in January, followed by juniper, cedar, and sycamore in February and willow, poplar, mulberry, oak, and olive in March and April.[15] Red elms

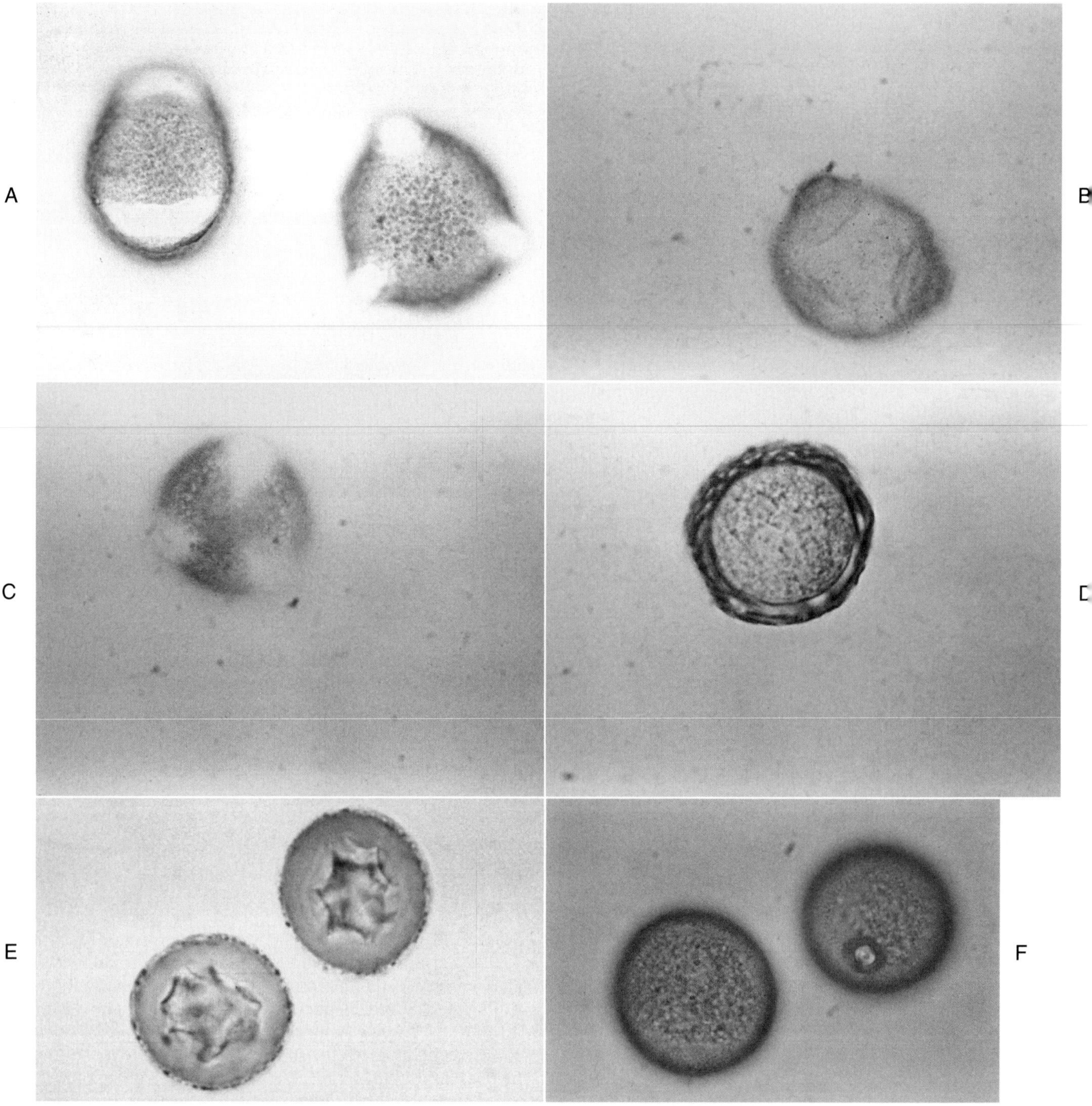

FIGURE 24-2 Selected examples of common pollen grains and fungal spores (Calberla stain). **A,** White oak (*Quercus alba*). **B,** White birch (*Betula populifolia*). **C,** Box elder (*Acer negundo*). **D,** American elm (*Ulmus americana*). **E,** Red cedar (*Juniperus virginiana*). **F,** Orchard grass (*Dactylis glomerata*).

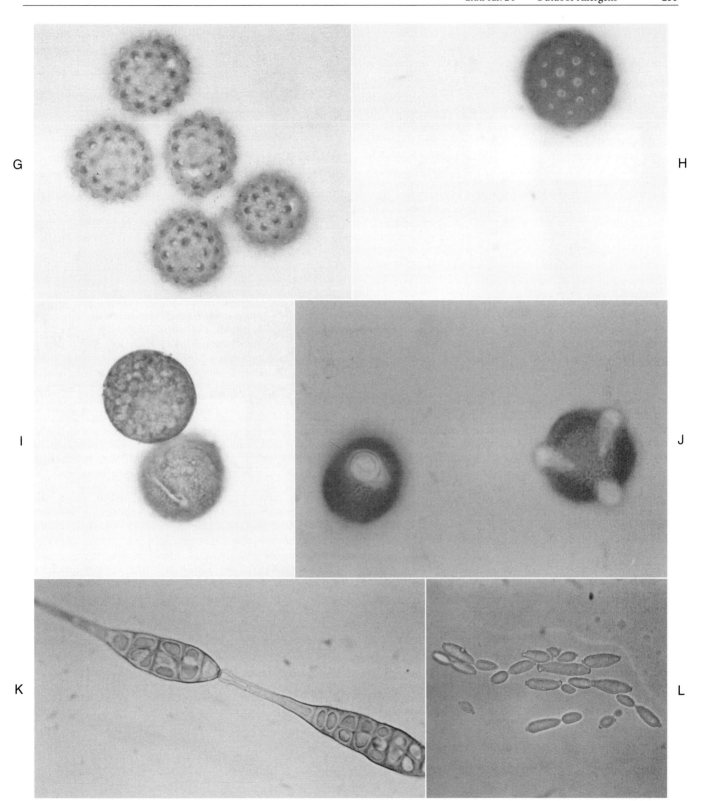

FIGURE 24-2, cont'd G, Giant ragweed (*Ambrosia trifida*). **H,** Lamb's quarters (*Chenopodium album*). **I,** Sheep sorrel (*Rumex acetosella*). **J,** Common sagebrush (*Artemisia tridentata*). **K,** *Alternaria.* **L,** *Cladosporium.*

TABLE 24-2 Selected Trees and Shrubs of Major Allergenic Importance in the United States

Botanical Family	Major Allergenic Genera	Distribution
Gymnosperms (conifers)		
Cupressaceae (cypress family)	*Juniperus ashei* (mountain cedar)	Central Texas, Oklahoma, Arkansas
	Juniperus virginiana (eastern red cedar)	Midwestern and eastern U.S.
	Juniperus scopulorum (Rocky Mountain juniper)	Rocky Mountains
Angiosperms (flowering plants)		
Aceraceae (maple family)	*Acer negundo* (box elder)	Great plains and mid-Atlantic states
	Acer rubrum (red maple)	Eastern U.S.; partially insect-pollinated
Betulaceae (birch family)	*Alnus incana* (white alder)	Northern U.S., Rocky Mountains
	Betula lutea (gray birch)	Northeastern U.S. and Allegheny Mountains
	Ostrya virginiana (American hop hornbeam)	Eastern and midwestern U.S.
Casuarinaceae (Australian pine family)	*Casuarina equisetifolia* (Australian pine)	California and Florida
Fabaceae (legume family)	*Prosopis glandulosa* (glandular mesquite)	Texas, Oklahoma, and southwestern U.S.
Fagaceae (beech family)	*Fagus grandifolia* (American beech)	Eastern and midwestern U.S.
	Quercus alba (white oak)	Eastern and midwestern U.S.
	Quercus rubra (red oak)	Eastern and midwestern U.S.
	Quercus virginiana (live oak)	Texas, Gulf coast, Florida
Juglandaceae (walnut family)	*Carya cordiformis* (bitternut hickory)	Midwestern and eastern U.S.
	Juglans nigra (black walnut)	Great plains; southwestern and southeastern U.S.
Moraceae (mulberry family)	*Morus rubra* (red mulberry)	Central and eastern U.S.
Oleaceae (olive family)	*Fraxinus pennsylvanica* (green ash)	Eastern two thirds of U.S.
	Olea europaea (common olive)	Introduced to California and southwestern U.S.
Platanaceae (plane tree family)	*Platanus occidentalis* (American sycamore)	Central and eastern U.S.
Salicaceae (willow family)	*Populus deltoides* (eastern cottonwood)	Eastern Rocky Mountains and Great Plains
Tiliaceae (linden family)	*Tilia americana* (American basswood or linden)	Northeastern and north central U.S.
Ulmaceae (elm family)	*Celtis occidentalis* (hackberry)	Great Plains and mid-Atlantic states
	Ulmus americana (American elm)	Eastern and midwestern U.S.

(southern Appalachian Mountains and Arkansas) and Chinese elms (southern California) pollinate in the fall from August to October. Although trees share many cross-reacting allergens within genera, there is generally little cross-reactivity between genera.

Grasses

Selected examples of allergenic grasses are listed in Table 24-3. Grass pollens are an important cause of allergic rhinoconjunctivitis in the United States, ranking second only to ragweed pollen. Most of the various grass pollen grains are indistinguishable morphologically. In the northern United States peak grass pollination occurs during May and June, whereas in southern California, Texas, and Florida the grass pollen season may extend from February through November. There is extensive cross-allergenicity among the northern grass species (June, orchard, Timothy, and red top),[17] whereas Bermuda grass allergens are more distinct. Although Bermuda grass pollen is dominant in the southern portions of the United States, Johnson grass, Bahia grass,

TABLE 24-3 Selected Grasses of Major Allergenic Importance in the United States

Botanical Family	Major Allergenic Genera	Distribution
Poaceae (grass family)		
Chloridoideae subfamily	*Cynodon dactylon* (Bermuda grass)	Southern half of U.S.
Panicoideae subfamily	*Paspalum notatum* (Bahia grass)	Southeastern U.S.
	Sorghum halepense (Johnson grass)	Southern half of U.S.
Pooideae subfamily		
Poeae tribe	*Dactylis glomerata* (orchard grass)	Northern three-quarters of U.S.
	Festuca elatior (meadow fescue)	Entire U.S. except Arizona and southern Florida
	Lolium perenne (perennial rye grass)	Entire U.S. except south Texas and south Florida
	Poa pratensis (June or Kentucky blue grass)	Entire U.S. except south Texas and south Florida
Aveneae tribe	*Anthoxanthum odoratum* (sweet vernal grass)	Eastern third of U.S. and Pacific coast
	Holcus lanatus (velvet grass)	Eastern half of U.S. and Pacific coast
Agrostideae tribe	*Agrostis alba* (red top grass)	Entire U.S. except Florida and southern California
	Phleum pratense (Timothy grass)	Entire U.S.
Bromeae tribe	*Bromus inermus* (smooth brome)	Northern half of U.S.

and Sudan grass (*Holcus sudanensis*) are also found in the southeastern coastal plains and in Florida. Salt grass (*Distichlis spicata*) and Canary grass (*Phalaris minor*) may be found in the arid southwestern region of the United States. Grass seed is an important field crop in the Willamette Valley of Oregon, with peak pollen levels reached in early summer. Pollens from other grass family members, such as cereal grains (corn, rye, oat, wheat), sedges, and rushes, do not commonly produce symptoms.

Weeds

Selected examples of allergenic weeds are listed in Table 24-4. In addition to the ragweed species listed, other species of ragweed are of local importance in southern and western areas of the United States. Hemp (*Cannabis sativa*) was cultivated in Illinois, Iowa, and eastern Nebraska during World War II for production of rope and may still be found in pastures and hedgerows; hemp pollen is modestly allergenic. Chenopod and amaranth pollens are present nearly perennially in southern Florida. Weed pollen levels diminish in mountainous regions at elevations above 5000 feet and most of the Pacific northwestern area remains ragweed-free. Pollens from entomophilous members of the composite family, such as dandelions, daisies, asters, marigolds, and chrysanthemums, do not commonly produce rhinitis.

Allergenic Pollens Outside the United States

Grasses are the most common cause of pollen allergy outside the United States, including both the temperate grasses and Bermuda grass. Birch and alder pollens are major causes of spring hay fever in the Scandinavian countries whereas Japanese red cedar ("sugi," *Cryptomeria japonica*) pollen is a major offender in Japan. Short ragweed can be found in eastern France and the Balkans, although mugwort is a more widespread weed allergen in Europe. Russian thistle pollen is a major weed allergen in the Middle East. Wall pellitory (*Parietaria officinalis*) pollen is an important aeroallergen in the Mediterranean basin. Listings of allergenic pollens present in Europe[18] and elsewhere in the world[19] have been published.

FUNGI
Biology

Fungi are eukaryotic organisms with rigid cell walls and require exogenous carbohydrates for nutrition. Fungi can be unicellular (yeasts) or multicellular. Biochemically, fungi are composed of chitin, a polymer of β-1,4-N-acetylglucosamine, or cellulose, a polymer of β-1,4-glucose.[20] Fungi are traditionally considered to be allergenic if extracts thereof produce positive immediate wheal-and-flare skin tests in atopic individuals, and selected examples are listed in Table 24-5. Fungal taxonomy is imprecise, and characterization of single fungal allergens has been hampered by the tendency of fungi to undergo spontaneous biochemical changes during repeated subculture.[21] Members of the Ascomycete and Basidiomycete families produce sexual (haploid) spores, but many ascomycetes and basidiomycetes also reproduce asexually via diploid spores (imperfect fungi, or Deuteromycetes) that are classified into form genera with completely different names. Although the most commonly recognized allergenic fungi arise from microscopic sources, macroscopic basidiomycetes (mushrooms, puffballs, and bracket fungi) are also allergenic. In most mushrooms studied to date, allergens have been found in spores, caps, and stalks.[22]

Exposure

Fungi are widespread throughout the United States, particularly in the central part of the country, where field crops support massive quantities of fungi.[23] The true prevalence of fungal allergy is unknown; estimates range from 3% to 91% depending on the population studied, the extracts used, and the species tested.[24] Fungal extracts used for diagnostic skin testing are unstandardized, making comparative studies difficult. In addition, diagnostic extracts are not available for many of the basidiomycetes, many of which do not sporulate in culture.[22] In the northern United States, outdoor fungal spore levels are virtually absent during winter months, rise during spring and summer, and peak during fall harvest season. In the southern part of the country fungal spores are abundant throughout the year. Viable fungi can even be

TABLE 24-4 Selected Weeds and Herbs of Major Allergenic Importance in the United States

Botanical Family	Major Allergenic Genera	Distribution
Asteraceae (composite family)	*Ambrosia artemisaefolia* (short ragweed)	Entire U.S. except southwest desert and California
	Ambrosia trifida (giant ragweed)	Eastern two thirds of U.S. except Florida
	Iva annua (rough marsh elder)	Atlantic coast and central Great Plains
	Artemisia vulgaris (common mugwort)	Northeastern and central U.S. and Rocky Mountains
	Artemisia tridentata (common sagebrush)	Rocky Mountains and Pacific coast
Chenopodiaceae (goosefoot family)	*Kochia scoparia* (burning bush)	Great plains and Rocky Mountains
	Salsola kali (Russian thistle)	Great plains and Rocky Mountains
	Chenopodium album (lamb's quarters)	Eastern and central U.S.
	Atriplex argenta (saltbush)	Rocky mountains and southwestern U.S.
Amaranthaceae (amaranth family)	*Amaranthus retroflexus* (rough pigweed)	Eastern and central U.S.
	Amaranthus tamariscinus (western water hemp)	Great Plains south through Texas
Plantaginaceae (plantain family)	*Plantago lanceolata* (English plantain)	Entire U.S.
Polygonaceae (buckwheat family)	*Rumex acetosella* (sheep sorrel)	Entire U.S.
Urticaceae (nettle family)	*Urtica dioica* (nettle)	Entire U.S. except southeast coast

TABLE 24-5 Selected Fungi of Allergenic Importance

Class	Representative Examples	Comments
Ascomycetes (asexual stage)	*Alternaria alternata*	Infects grasses and grains
	Aspergillus flavus	Saprophyte; found both indoors and outdoors
	Cladosporium herbarum	Parasite of spinach, bananas, and tomatoes
	Epicoccum purpurascens	Infects grasses and grains
	Fusarium roseum	Saprophyte and plant pathogen
	Helminthosporium solani	Parasite of potatoes and grains
	Penicillium spp.	Saprophyte; found both indoors and outdoors
	Stemphylium botryosum	Imperfect form of *Pleospora herbarum*
Basidiomycetes (asexual stage)	*Ganoderma lucidum*	Wood-rotting fungus
	Coprinus comatus	Shaggy or inky cap mushroom
	Pleurotus ostreatus	Oyster mushroom
	Malassezia furfur	Opportunistic cutaneous yeast
Zygomycetes	*Mucor* spp.	Found indoors or on composting vegetation
	Rhizopus nigricans	Found indoors or on composting vegetation

cultured from the air in desert environments.[25] Seasonal fungal spore release patterns are less well defined than those for pollens; in addition, the microscopic sources of most fungi make exposure assessments more difficult than is the case with pollens. Basidiomycete counts are highest in autumn and spring. Airborne spores of *Alternaria, Cladosporium, Helminthosporium, Stemphylium,* and *Drechslera* are more common during dry, windy weather whereas spores of *Phoma, Fusarium,* and *Cephalosporium* are more common during damp or foggy weather. Clinically, most fungus-sensitive persons are sensitized to multiple fungal species.

Specific Allergenic Fungi

Alternaria

Alternaria allergens are among the most clinically important fungal allergens, commonly causing late summer and fall asthma in agricultural areas (see Figure 24-2). Alternaria sensitivity has been associated with sudden, severe asthma episodes in children and young adults.[26] Alt a 1 is a major Alternaria allergen whose exact function is unknown. Several other individual Alternaria allergens have been isolated, including a heat shock protein, ribosomal proteins, and several enzymes.[27]

Aspergillus

Asp f 1, a major Aspergillus allergen, is a ribonuclease that shows extensive homology to mitogillin, a cytotoxin produced by *Aspergillus restrictus*.[24] Other *Aspergillus* allergens include a peroxisomal membrane protein, proteases, ribosomal proteins, and manganese superoxide dismutase.[27]

Cladosporium

Spores of *Cladosporium* (see Figure 24-2) are the most prevalent outdoor fungal type; at least eight individual allergens have been characterized, including an aldehyde dehydrogenase, an enolase, a ribosomal protein, and a heat shock protein.[27]

Penicillium

Spores of *Penicillium* can occur outdoors but are more important indoor fungal contaminants. Individual *Penicillium* allergens include two serine proteases and an acetylglucosaminidase.[27]

CLINICAL UTILITY OF POLLEN AND MOLD SPORE COUNTS

Quantitative or semiquantitative (high, medium, low) prevalence data for pollens and spores are commonly reported on Internet websites, in newspapers, or in televised weather reports. These measurements may be useful in estimating the onset, peak, and end of pollen seasons. However, given the time lag between sampling and publication of results, the lumping of several genera under one heading (e.g., "trees," "weeds"), the short-term fluctuations in pollen and spore levels, and the variance in levels between sampling locations, these data cannot be correlated reliably with individual patient symptoms.

AMORPHOUS OUTDOOR ALLERGENS

There is increasing recognition that allergens may exist on airborne particles other than intact pollen grains and fungal spores. These aeroallergens cannot be identified morphologically but can be measured immunochemically. Airborne particles $> 0.3\ \mu$ in diameter may be captured on filter papers using high-volume air samplers. The filters are then extracted into small volumes of buffer, and the allergen contents are measured by inhibition immunoassays using pooled IgE-containing sera from sensitized individuals.[28] In the case of individual aeroallergens that have been purified, characterized, and cloned, monoclonal antibody–based immunoassays can be used for their quantitation.

Insects

Several aquatic insects can produce widespread inhalant allergies. The larvae of caddis flies (order *Trichoptera*) develop in inland freshwater lakes and streams and later rise to the surface, where mature adults emerge and fly ashore.[29] Hairs shed from the wings and bodies of adult insects are allergenic, provoking conjunctivitis, rhinitis, or asthma in nearby sensitized residents. Mayflies (order *Ephemeroptera*) have a similar but shorter life cycle, and airborne pellicles shed from adult insects can elicit symptoms in sensitized persons.[29] Lake fly larvae (order *Diptera*) also mature in lakes and rivers before pupation and emergence of adult midges; in this case, the midge hemoglobin is the inciting allergen.[30]

Scales from moths (order *Lepidoptera*) can be primary skin irritants or can elicit IgE antibody formation. The tussock moth (*Hemerocampa pseudotsugata*) infests Douglas fir trees in the Pacific northwest and can sensitize forest workers or nearby residents.[31] Human sensitization to *Pseudaletia unipuncta* moth allergens has been documented in midwestern U.S. residents with fall hay fever.[32] Sensitization to moths and butterflies has also been reported in Japan.[33]

Grain Dust

During the 1980s soybean dust particles were responsible for multiple epidemics of asthma in Barcelona, Spain during the unloading of container ships.[34] The allergen responsible was subsequently identified as a glycoprotein derived from the soybean hull.[35] Similar epidemics of asthma had occurred in New Orleans several decades earlier,[36] but attempts to establish their exact etiology had been unsuccessful. However, a review of historical data on vessel cargo, prevailing wind direction, and hospital records revealed a strong correlation (odds ratio = 6.7, 95% CI 1.5 to 46.7) between emergency room visits for asthma and the presence of soy cargo in the harbor.[37]

OUTDOOR AIR POLLUTION

Allergic disorders, especially asthma, are characterized not only by increased reactivity to allergens but also increased nonspecific reactivity to a number of air pollutants. The U.S. Environmental Protection Agency oversees monitoring of several pollutants, including carbon monoxide, lead, nitrogen dioxide, and particulate matter < 10 μm (PM10) and < 2.5 μm (PM2.5) in diameter.

Sulfur Dioxide

Sulfur dioxide is generated by coal-burning industrial plants, power plants, and other fixed sources. In asthmatic persons sulfur dioxide induces bronchospasm at ambient concentrations of 0.5 ppm; this bronchospastic effect is magnified during exercise or exposure to cold, dry air.[38] Increased ambient exposure to sulfur dioxide has been linked to an increased number of emergency room visits for respiratory problems and increased hospitalization rates.[39] Sulfur dioxide may also contribute to acid aerosol (H_2SO_4) formation.

Ozone

Ozone is a by-product of atmospheric reactions that require nitrogen oxides, sunlight, and volatile organic compounds. Ozone levels > 0.11 ppm are associated with increased emergency room visits for asthma in school children.[40] Controlled ozone exposure induces an immediate decline in FEV_1 and a more gradual bronchial inflammatory reaction[41]; these effects are magnified by exercise.

Particulate Matter

Active agents in airborne particulate matter include silica, metals, acid aerosols, endotoxin, and polyaromatic hydrocarbons. Increased airborne PM10 levels are associated with

---

BOX 24-1

KEY CONCEPTS

Diagnostic Evaluation of Childhood Allergies

- Using the resources listed, ascertain the outdoor allergens present in the child's environment.
- Obtain an allergy history that includes the patient's home, day care, and/or school environment.
- By allergy skin testing or by immunoassays for specific IgE antibodies, determine whether the child is sensitized to environmental allergens.
- Correlate results of sensitization studies with the clinical history.

episodes of asthma exacerbation in children.[42] In nasal provocation studies involving ragweed-sensitive volunteers, challenge with ragweed allergen in the presence of diesel exhaust particles produced enhanced ragweed-specific IgE and IgG responses, increased Th2 cytokine expression, and decreased expression of interferon-γ, compared with challenge with ragweed allergen alone.[43] *In vitro* studies show that purified Lol p 1 grass allergen can bind to aggregated diesel exhaust carbon particles (1 to 2 μm in diameter).[44] Collectively, these studies suggest a mechanism whereby outdoor pollen allergens may interact with environmental pollutants to induce and perpetuate a Th2 inflammatory response in the lower airways of allergic individuals.

CONCLUSIONS

Optimal assessment of the allergic child requires the physician to be familiar with allergens in the child's outdoor and indoor environments (Box 24-1). Outdoor allergens are common triggers of childhood rhinoconjunctivitis and asthma. In addition to morphologically identifiable pollen grains and fungal spores, allergens may be present in smaller airborne particulates capable of penetrating the lower respiratory tract. Amorphous outdoor allergens may be quantitated by immunoassays utilizing monoclonal antibodies or pooled IgE antibody–containing sera from sensitized persons. Immune responses to outdoor allergens may be potentiated by simultaneous exposure to pollutants such as diesel exhaust particles.

HELPFUL WEBSITES

The Allergy Web website (www.allergyweb.com)
The National Allergy Bureau website (www.aaaai.org/nab)
The American Academy of Allergy, Asthma and Immunology website (www.aaaai.org/)
The American College of Allergy, Asthma and Immunology website (www.acaai.org/)

REFERENCES

1. Aalberse RC: Structural biology of allergens, *J Allergy Clin Immunol* 106:228-238, 2000.
2. King TP, Hoffman D, Lowenstein H, et al: Allergen nomenclature, *J Allergy Clin Immunol* 96:5-14, 1995.
3. Anonymous: Allergen nomenclature, International Union of Immunological Societies Allergen Nomenclature Sub-Committee, http://www.allergen.org/List.htm, 2002.

4. Muilenberg ML: Allergen assessment by microscopy and culture, *Immunol Allergy Clin North Am* 9:245-268, 1989.

5. Solomon WR, Platts-Mills TAE: Aerobiology and inhalant allergens. In Middleton E, Reed CE, Ellis EF et al, eds: *Allergy: principles and practice,* ed 5, St Louis, 1998, Mosby.

6. Lewis WH, Vinay P, Zenger VE, eds: *Airborne and allergenic pollen of North America,* Baltimore, 1983, The Johns Hopkins University Press.

7. Solomon WR: Airborne pollen: a brief life, *J Allergy Clin Immunol* 109:895-900, 2002.

8. Leuschner RM: Human biometeorology: pollen, *Experientia* 49:931-942, 1993.

9. Vrtala S, Fischer S, Grote M, et al: Molecular, immunological, and structural characterization of Phl p 6, a major allergen and P-particle-associated protein from Timothy grass (*Phleum pratense*) pollen, *J Immunol* 163:5489-5496, 1999.

10. Schäppi GF, Taylor PE, Pain MCF, et al: Concentrations of major grass group 5 allergens in pollen grains and atmospheric particles: implications for hay fever and allergic asthma sufferers sensitized to grass pollen allergens, *Clin Exp Allergy* 29:633-641, 1999.

11. Venables KM, Allitt U, Collier CG, et al: Thunderstorm-related asthma—the epidemic of 24/25 June 1994, *Clin Exp Allergy* 27:725-736, 1998.

12. Suphioglu C: Thunderstorm asthma due to grass pollen, *Int Arch Allergy Immunol* 116:253-260, 1998.

13. Samter M, Durham OC: *Regional allergy of the United States, Canada, Mexico, and Cuba,* Springfield, Ill, 1995, Charles C. Thomas.

14. Jelks ML: Aeroallergens of Florida, *Immunol Allergy Clin North Am* 9:381-397, 1989.

15. Ellis MH, Gallup J: Aeroallergens of Southern California, *Immunol Allergy Clin North Am* 9:365-380, 1989.

16. American Academy of Allergy, Asthma and Immunology: http://www.aaaai.org.

17. Leiferman KM, Gleich GJ: The cross-reactivity of IgE antibodies with pollen allergens. I. Analysis of various species of grass pollens, *J Allergy Clin Immunol* 58:129-139, 1976.

18. D'Amato G, Spieksma F, Liccardi G, et al: Pollen-related allergy in Europe, *Allergy* 53:567-578, 1998.

19. Roth A: *Allergy in the world,* Honolulu, 1978, University Press of Hawaii.

20. Burge HA: Airborne allergenic fungi, *Immunol Allergy Clin North Am* 9:307-319, 1989.

21. Schumacher MJ, Jeffrey SE: Variability of *Alternaria alternata:* biochemical and immunological characteristics of culture filtrates from seven isolates, *J Allergy Clin Immunol* 58:263-277, 1976.

22. Horner WE, Helbling A, Lehrer SB: Basidiomycete allergens, *Allergy* 53:1114-1121, 1998.

23. Burge HA, Rogers CA: Outdoor allergens, *Environ Health Perspect* 108:653-659, 2000.

24. Horner WE, Helbling A, Salvaggio JE: Fungal allergens, *Clin Microbiol Rev* 8:161-179, 1995.

25. Zhan ZU, Zhan MA, Chandy R, et al: Aspergillus and other moulds in the air of Kuwait, *Mycopathologia* 146:25-32, 1999.

26. O'Hollaren MT, Yunginger JW, Offord KP, et al: Exposure to an aeroallergen as a possible precipitating factor in respiratory arrest in young patients with asthma, *N Engl J Med* 324:359-363, 1991.

27. Stewart GA, Robinson C: The structure and function of allergens. In Adkinson NF Jr, Yunginger JW, Busse WW, et al, eds: *Middleton's allergy: principles and practice,* ed 6, St Louis, 2003, Mosby (in press).

28. Yunginger JW, Adolphson CR, Swanson MC: Quantitation and standardization of allergens. In Rose NR, Hamilton RG, Detrick B, eds: *Manual of clinical laboratory immunology,* ed 6, Washington, DC, 2002, ASM Press.

29. Mathews KP: Inhalant insect-derived allergens, *Immunol Allergy Clin North Am* 9:321-338, 1989.

30. Baur X, Dewair M, Haegele K: Common antigenic determinants of haemoglobin as basis of immunological cross-reactivity between chironomid species (Diptera, Chironomidae): studies with human and animal sera, *Clin Exp Immunol* 54:599-607, 1983.

31. Perlman F, Press E, Googins JA, et al: Tussockosis: reactions to Douglas fir tussock moth, *Ann Allergy* 36:302-307, 1976.

32. Wynn SR, Swanson MC, Reed CE, et al: Immunochemical quantitation, size distribution, and cross-reactivity of lepidoptera (moth) aeroallergens in southeastern Minnesota, *J Allergy Clin Immunol* 82:47-54, 1988.

33. Kino T, Chihara J, Fukuda K, et al: Allergy to insects in Japan. III. High frequency of IgE antibody responses to insects (moth, butterfly, caddis fly, and chironomid) in patients with bronchial asthma and immunochemical quantitation of the insect-related airborne particles smaller than 10 microns in diameter, *J Allergy Clin Immunol* 79:857-866, 1987.

34. Anto JM, Sunyer J, Rodriguez-Roisin R, et al: Community outbreaks of asthma associated with inhalation of soybean dust, *N Engl J Med* 320:1097-1102, 1989.

35. Swanson MC, Li JY, Wentz-Murtha PE, et al: Source of the aeroallergen of soybean dust: a low molecular mass glycoprotein from the soybean tela, *J Allergy Clin Immunol* 87:783-788, 1991.

36. Salvaggio J, Seabury J, Schoenhardt FA: New Orleans asthma. V. Relationship between Charity Hospital asthma admission rates, semiquantitative pollen and fungal spore counts, and total particulate aerometric sampling data, *J Allergy Clin Immunol* 48:96-114, 1971.

37. White MC, Etzel RA, Olson DR, et al: Reexamination of epidemic asthma in New Orleans, Louisiana, in relation to the presence of soy at the harbor, *Am J Epidemiol* 145:432-438, 1997.

38. Pierson WE, Koenig J: Respiratory effects of air pollution on allergic disease, *J Allergy Clin Immunol* 90:557-566, 1992.

39. Committee of the Environmental and Occupational Health Assembly of the American Thoracic Society: Health effects of outdoor air pollution, *Am J Respir Crit Care Med* 153:3-50, 1996.

40. White MC, Etzel RA, Wilcox WD, et al: Exacerbations of childhood asthma and ozone pollution in Atlanta, *Environ Res* 65:56-68, 1994.

41. Peden DB: Indoor and outdoor air pollution. In Adkinson NF Jr, Yunginger JW, Busse WW, et al, eds: *Middleton's allergy: principles and practice,* ed 6, St Louis, 2003, Mosby.

42. Anonymous: Children at risk from ozone air pollution—United States, 1991-1993, *MMWR Morb Mortal Wkly Rep* 44:309-312, 1995.

43. Diaz-Sanchez D, Tsien A, Fleming J, et al: Combined diesel exhaust particulate and ragweed allergen challenge markedly enhances human in vivo nasal ragweed-specific IgE and skews cytokine production to a T helper cell 2-type pattern, *J Immunol* 158:2406-2413, 1997.

44. Knox RB, Suphioglu C, Taylor P, et al: Major grass pollen allergen Lol p 1 binds to diesel exhaust particles: implications for asthma and air pollution, *Clin Exp Allergy* 27:246-251, 1997.

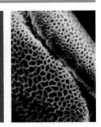

CHAPTER 25

Indoor Allergens

MARTIN D. CHAPMAN

House dust allergens have been associated with asthma since the 1920s, when Kern[1] and Cooke[2] independently reported a high prevalence of immediate skin tests to house dust extracts among patients with asthma. At the same time, Van Leeuven[3] showed that asthma patients who were admitted to a modified hospital room free of "climate allergens" (which he believed to be bacteria and molds) showed clinical improvement: some of the first experiments using allergen avoidance for asthma management. In the mid twentieth century, allergists sought to explain how such a heterogenous material as house dust could contain a potent allergen that appeared to be ubiquitous in dust extracts. The prevailing theory was that a chemical reaction occurred in dust resulting in the synthesis of the "house dust allergen." Researchers extracted house dust with phenol and other solvents to identify allergenically active compounds.[4] The puzzle was finally resolved in the 1960s, when Voorhorst and Spieksma[5] showed that the origin of house dust allergen was biologic rather than chemical. The allergenic potency of Dutch house dust extracts correlated with the numbers of house dust mites in the samples and extracts of pure mite cultures (Acari, Pyroglyphidae: *Dermatophagoides pteronyssinus* and *D. farinae*) gave positive skin tests at dilutions of 10^{-6} or greater.[5] Voorhorst and Spieksma[5] also showed a correlation of asthma symptoms with seasonal variation in mite numbers, providing the first evidence for exposure thresholds: exposure to 100 mites per gram of dust was associated with sensitization, and 500 mites per gram was associated with symptom exacerbation.

The prevalence of asthma has increased during the past 40 years, and current data suggest that approximately 10% of U.S. children have asthma. Sensitization and exposure to indoor allergens, principally dust mites, animal danders, cockroach (CR), and fungi, are among the most important risk factors for asthma.[6-9] The two principal mite species, *D. pteronyssinus* and *D. farinae*, account for more than 90% of the mite fauna in U.S. house dust samples. Other allergenic mites include *Euroglyphus maynei* and *Blomia tropicalis* (found in subtropical regions such as Florida, southern California, Texas, and Puerto Rico). Storage mites, such as *Lepidoglyphus destructor, Tyrophagus putrescentiae,* and *Acarus siro,* may cause occupational asthma among farmers, farm workers and their families, and grain handlers. The relationship among exposure, allergen sensitization, and asthma has been most thoroughly explored for dust mite allergens. Epidemiologic studies in many parts of the world have established that

exposure to 2 μg/g mite group 1 allergen in the dust results in allergic sensitization and that there is a dose-response relationship between exposure and the numbers of atopic individuals who become sensitized.[6-9] There is further evidence that asthma severity is related to mite allergen exposure.[10,11]

Childhood asthma is also strongly associated with sensitization to animal allergens, CR, and, to a lesser extent, mold allergens. Cat allergen (Fel d 1) has a ubiquitous distribution in the environment and can be found at clinically significant levels in houses that do not contain cats (similarly for dog allergen).[12-14] Rodent urinary proteins have long been associated with occupational asthma among laboratory animal handlers; recently a high prevalence of sensitization and exposure to mouse allergen was reported among inner-city children with asthma.[15] These children are also at the greatest risk of developing CR allergy. CR infestation of housing results in the accumulation of potent allergens that are associated with increased asthma mortality and morbidity among U.S. children, particularly African-American and Hispanic children, living in inner cities.[16,17] CR allergens appear to be particularly potent. Atopic individuals develop IgE responses after exposure to tenfold to a hundredfold lower levels of CR allergens than to dust mite or cat allergens.[18] Asthma is the most common disease associated with CR and occurs in CR-infested housing in inner cities, as well as in suburbs and rural areas.

Investigation of the role of indoor allergens in asthma has involved the identification of the most important allergens and the development of techniques to accurately monitor allergen exposure. This chapter reviews the structure and biologic function of indoor allergens and current allergen detection systems that are used to assess exposure in the laboratory and, increasingly, by patients themselves. The interpretation of exposure results and clinical significance of allergen exposure assessments is also discussed.

ALLERGEN STRUCTURE AND FUNCTION

Allergens are proteins or glycoproteins of 10 to 50 kDa that are readily soluble and able to penetrate the nasal and respiratory mucosae. Molecular cloning has determined the primary amino acid sequences of more than 500 allergens (see http://www.allergen.org), and 20 to 25 three-dimensional structures of indoor allergens have been resolved.[19] Structural analyses have not revealed any common features or motifs that are associated with the induction of IgE responses

KEY CONCEPTS
Indoor Allergens: Structure and Function

- Allergens are soluble proteins or glycoproteins of molecular weights of 10 to 50 kDa.
- Most major allergens have been cloned, sequenced, and expressed.
- More than 500 allergen sequences are deposited in protein databases (GenBank, PDB), and about 20 tertiary structures have been resolved by x-ray crystallography.
- Allergens have diverse biologic functions and may be enzymes, enzyme inhibitors, lipocalins, or regulatory or structural proteins.
- Allergens promote T cells to differentiate along the Th2 pathway to produce IL-4 and IL-13 and to initiate isotype switching to IgE.

(reviewed in Chapman et al[19] and Aalberse[20]). Allergens belong to several families of proteins and have diverse biologic functions: they may be enzymes, enzyme inhibitors, ligand-binding proteins, or structural or regulatory proteins (Box 25-1). A systematic allergen nomenclature has been developed by the International Union of Immunological Societies' (IUIS) Allergen Nomenclature Subcommittee: the first three letters of the source genus followed by a single letter for the species and a number denoting the chronologic order of allergen identification. Thus the abbreviated nomenclature for *Dermatophagoides pteronyssinus* allergen 1 is Der p 1. To be included in the IUIS nomenclature, the allergen must have been purified to homogeneity and/or cloned, and the prevalence of IgE antibody (ab) must have been established in an appropriate allergic population by skin testing or *in vitro* IgE ab assays.

Most dust mite allergens are digestive enzymes excreted with the feces, such as Der p 1 (cysteine protease), Der p 3 (serine protease), and Der p 6 (chymotrypsin). With the

exception of cat allergen Fel d 1, most animal allergens are ligand-binding proteins (lipocalins) or albumins. Lipocalins are 20- to 25-kDa proteins with a conserved, eight-stranded, antiparallel β-barrel structure; they serve to bind and transport small hydrophobic chemicals[21] (Figure 25-1). As a group, lipocalins have a variety of ligand-binding functions, but the rat and mouse urinary allergens are pheromone- or odorant-binding proteins, and it is likely that the other lipocalin animal allergens have similar functions. The CR allergen Bla g 4 is also a lipocalin. Other important CR allergens include Bla g 2, an inactive aspartic proteinase, Bla g 5 (glutathione transferase family), and Per a 7 (tropomyosin).[17] Fungal allergens have been cloned from *Alternaria, Aspergillus, Cladosporium, Penicillium,* and *Trichophyton* spp., and several of these allergens are proteolytic enzymes, heat shock proteins, or ribonucleases.[22] There is conflicting evidence as to whether biologic function influences allergenicity. Some researchers have proposed that the enzymatic activity of mite allergens promotes IgE synthesis and local inflammatory responses via cleavage of CD23 and CD25 receptors on B cells and by causing the release of pro-inflammatory cytokines (interleukin [IL]-8, IL-6, monocyte chemotactic protein-1 [MCP-1], and granulocyte-monocyte colony-stimulating factor [GM-CSF]) from bronchial epithelial cells. Mite protease allergens cause detachment of bronchial epithelial cells *in vitro* and disrupt intercellular tight junctions.[23,24] On the other hand, several potent allergens, including Der p 2, Fel d 1, Bla g 1, and Bla g 2, have no enzymatic activity, and some animal allergens (Can f 1 and Fel d 3) are cysteine protease inhibitors.[21]

Recombinant allergens have been produced in high-level expression systems in bacteria (*Escherichia coli*), yeast (*Pichia pastoris*), and baculovirus. In general, the allergenic activity of the recombinant allergens, assessed by skin testing and *in vitro* IgE antibody assays, is comparable to that of the natural allergens. The advantages of recombinant allergens are that they can be precisely manipulated, targeted, and engineered and they can be formulated at defined concentrations and potency.[19] Cocktails of two to four major allergens can be used

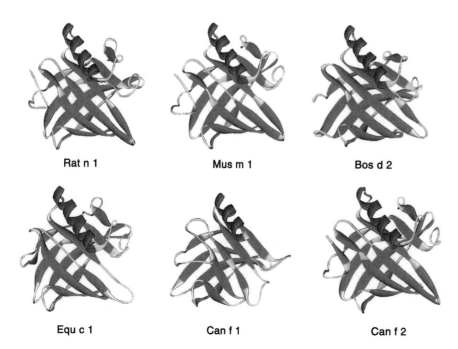

Rat n 1   **Mus m 1**   **Bos d 2**

Equ c 1   **Can f 1**   **Can f 2**

FIGURE 25-1 Molecular structures of the lipocalin allergens. Each lipocalin comprises eight antiparallel β sheets and an N-terminal α helix. (From Pomés A, Smith AM, Grégoire C, et al: *Allergy Clin Immunol Int* 13:162-169, 2001.)

for diagnostic purposes with the same specificity and sensitivity as natural allergen extracts. Recombinant allergens are being used to develop new generations of diagnostic tests, including microarrays and lateral flow devices, that could ultimately replace skin tests for allergy diagnosis.[25] They are also being used to develop new therapeutic strategies and vaccines for the treatment of allergic disease.

EVALUATION OF ALLERGEN EXPOSURE

Allergen Detection Systems

Biologists and pest management companies have counted dust mites in dust samples and trapped CR to assess infestation and allergen exposure. Although these methods are useful in studying population dynamics, seasonal variation, and the effect of physical and chemical methods for reducing mite and CR populations, they are time consuming and unsuitable for routine measurements of allergen exposure. Moreover, allergen levels may remain high when mite or CR levels have been reduced, and simply enumerating mite/CR may not be a reliable indicator of allergen exposure. Since the mid-1980s, quantitative assessments of allergen exposure have been made by measuring major allergens in reservoir dust samples (bed, carpet, soft furnishings) using monoclonal antibody (mAb)–based enzyme-linked immunosorbent assays (ELISAs). The advantages of these assays are high sensitivity (~1 ng/ml), high throughput (hundreds of samples per day), accurate quantification, and defined specificity. The ELISAs for indoor allergens use either

pairs of mAbs directed against nonoverlapping epitopes on the allergen molecule or capture mAb and polyclonal rabbit antibody for detection. Table 25-1 lists the antibody combinations and allergen standards for 17 ELISA systems for indoor allergens.[26] Critical elements in the development of ELISA tests are the use of high-affinity mAb of defined specificity and standards with known allergen content. A few national and international standards have been produced for the calibration of Der p 1, Can f 1, and Fel d 1 assays, and other standards are commercially available (Table 25-1). In most cases, these standards are allergen extracts that were calibrated to contain a known amount of allergen, but they are not purified allergens. Standards are important because they enable allergen measurements made by different laboratories to be directly compared. The World Health Organization (WHO)/IUIS Allergen Standardization Committee has initiated a multicenter project, involving researchers from academia, industry, and regulatory agencies, to develop international standards for purified allergens. This program is being coordinated through the European Union Certified Reference Materials for Allergenic Products (CREATE) project. The aim is to develop recombinant allergen standards for mite group 1 and group 2 allergens, as well as birch, rye grass, and olive pollen allergens. The purified allergens will be assessed for protein content and allergenic activity and will serve as primary standards for immunoassays.

Indoor allergen measurement by ELISA is the gold standard for exposure assessment; a growing number of academic and commercial reference laboratories across the United States

---

TABLE 25-1 Immunoassays for Indoor Allergens*

Allergen	Capture Monoclonal Antibody	Second Antibody	Allergen Standards
Mite			
Der p 1	5H8	4C1[B]	NIBSC 82/518
	10B9	5H8[B]	NIBSC 82/518
	PIA03	P1A01[B]	92-Dp
Der f 1	6A8	4C1[B]	UVA 93/02
	F1B01	F1A05	92-Df
Group 2	1D8	7A1[B]	UVA 97/01
Group 7	WH9	HD19[B]	NA
Blo t 5	4G9	4D9[B]	rBlo t 5
Lep d 2	Le5B5	RaαLep d 2	rLep d 2
Mammal			
Cat Fel d 1	6F9	3E4[B]	CBER Cat E10
Dog Can f 1	6E9	RaαCan f 1	NIBSC 84/685
Rat Rat n 1	RUP-6	RUP-1[B]	Affinity-purified Rat n 1
Mouse Mus m 1	RaαMus m 1	RaαMus m 1	JHU
Cow Bos d 2	mAb³	mAb¹[B]	nBos d 2
Horse Equ c 4	103	14G4[B]	NA
Cockroach			
Bla g 1	10A6	RaαBla g 1	UVA 97/02
Bla g 2	8F4	RaαBla g 2	UVA 97/02
Per a 3	A-2	E-4[AP]	Purified Per a 3
Fungi			
Asp f 1	4A6	RaαAsp f 1	Affinity-purified Asp f 1
Alt a 1	121G	121G[B]	rAlt a 1
	Mab-1	Mab-2	Affinity-purified nAlt a 1

Modified from Chapman MD, Tsay A, Vailes LD: *Allergy* 56:604-610, 2001.

NA, Not available.

*Two-site enzyme-linked immunosorbent assay (ELISA) using capture monoclonal antibodies to coat ELISA plates and biotinylated ([B]) of alkaline phosphatase ([AP]) monoclonal antibody for detection of rabbit polyclonal antibody.

offer ELISA testing services. Simple qualitative or semiquantitative tests that can be used in allergy clinics or physicians' offices or by consumers have recently been developed. The aim of these "point of care" tests is to provide patients with tests that can be used to monitor allergen levels in their homes and to reinforce education about the role of allergens in causing asthma. The first such test was Acarex (Werner and Mertz, Mainz, Germany), a dipstick that measures guanine in house dust (a surrogate for dust mites), followed by DUSTSCREEN (CMG-HESKA, Freibourg, Switzerland), an mAb-based test that measures multiple allergens on a nitrocellulose strip and is designed for use in allergy clinics.[26] Recently, lateral flow technology has been used to develop rapid tests that can measure specific allergens in 10 minutes (INDOOR Biotechnologies, Charlottesville, VA). These tests are analogous to pregnancy or human immunodeficiency virus tests and are designed for use by patients and other consumers. The mite allergen test uses the same mAb as the mite group 2 ELISA and can detect both *D. pteronyssinus* and *D. farinae*. The test includes a simple dust collection and extraction device (MITEST dust collector) that allows dust to be collected and extracted within 2 minutes[27] (Figure 25-2). The rapid test has indicator lines that provide patients with estimates of high, medium, and low allergen levels; these lines have been shown to correlate with group 2 levels determined by ELISA.[27] A "wipe test" (Bio-Check [DRAGER, Lubeck, Germany]) that uses similar lateral flow technology has also been produced in Europe.[28] In principle, lateral flow tests can be applied to other allergens, and prototypes for Fel d 1 and peanut allergens have been developed.

Allergen Sampling in Dust and Air

Allergens are typically measured on dust samples that are collected by vacuuming an area of 1 m² for 2 minutes and extracting 100 mg of fine dust in 2 ml of buffer.[6] Samples are usually collected from three or four sites in the home, including mattresses, bedding, bedroom or living room carpet, soft furnishings, or kitchen floors. The results are expressed as nanograms or micrograms of allergen per gram of dust. Measurements of group 1 allergens in bedding provide the best index of mite exposure and show a good correlation between results expressed as micrograms of allergen per gram of dust or per unit area (μg/m²).[29] Cat and dog allergens are widely distributed throughout the house and accumulate at clinically significant levels in houses that do not contain pets. Not surprisingly, the highest concentrations of CR allergens are usually found in kitchens, although in heavily infested homes allergen accumulates on flooring and in bedding.

Measurement of allergen levels in dust provides a valid index of exposure but cannot be used to monitor personal exposure. The aerodynamic properties of mite, cat, dog, and CR allergens have been studied using particle-sizing devices such as the Cascade impactor and Andersen sampler.[13,30-32] Mite and CR allergens occur on large particles of 10 to 40 μm in diameter and cannot be detected in rooms under undisturbed conditions. After a disturbance, such as using a vacuum cleaner without a filter, these particles remain airborne for about 20 to 40 minutes. In contrast, cat and dog allergens can be easily detected in air samples under undisturbed conditions and persist in the air for several hours. Animal dander particles (skin flakes) are less dense than mite feces, and approximately 25% of animal allergen occurs on smaller particles, 5 μm in diameter, that remain airborne. A novel personal sampling device (HALOGEN [Inhalix, Sydney, Australia]) has recently been developed that enables inhaled allergen particles to be visualized on antibody-coated slides. Silicone air samplers are worn in the nostrils for 4 to 8 hours during normal domestic activity, and inhaled particles are deposited onto the antibody-coated slides and detected by immunochemical staining. A "halo" forms on the slide around the allergen-

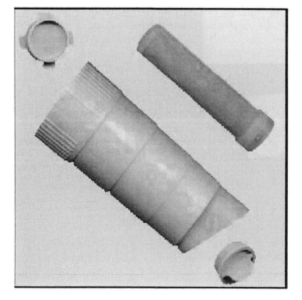

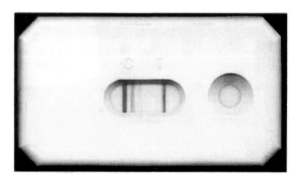

FIGURE 25-2 Rapid test for dust mite group 2 allergens. Dust samples are collected using the MITEST dust collection and extraction device *(left)*. The nylon filter is inserted into the collector and attached to the wand of a vacuum cleaner. Dust is sampled for 2 minutes and extracted in the tube. The extract is then applied to the well of the rapid test cassette *(right)*. The test shows a strong red line, and the intensity of the line can be compared with the high, medium, and low indicator lines to the left of the test line. (From Tsay A, Williams L, Mitchell EB, et al: *Clin Exp Allergy* 32:1596-1601, 2002.)

bearing particles that can be counted or the allergen can be measured using sensitive amplified ELISA systems. The HALOGEN assay has been used to monitor personal exposure to mite, cat, pollen, and fungus allergens (reviewed in O'Meara and Tovey[33]). Another new device for monitoring airborne allergen in homes is the Ionic Breeze Quadra (IBQ [Sharper Image, San Francisco, CA]), a commercial air filtration product. The IBQ is an electrostatic device that has three stainless steel blades that collect particles. The allergen can be measured by wiping the blades with filter paper and assaying the eluted allergen by ELISA. The IBQ has been shown to collect 0.5 to 8 μg Fel d 1 or Can f 1 over 24 hours and to detect mite allergens after disturbance.[34] The advantage of using the IBQ for air sampling is that it is silent and unobtrusive and can be operated in a room for several days without affecting the household or workplace.

Exposure Thresholds

Epidemiologic studies carried out in the United States, Europe, Australasia, and Japan have shown that sensitization to indoor allergens is the most significant risk factor for childhood asthma. Evidence from population surveys, case-control studies, prospective studies, and studies carried out at high altitudes or in hospital emergency departments were reviewed at the Third International Workshop in 1997.[6] The workshop confirmed that exposure to 2 μg/g mite group 1 allergens was a risk for sensitization to dust mites and that there was a dose-response relationship between the level of allergen exposure and sensitization. Adjusted odds ratios (ORs) for sensitization and exposure to 2 μg/g mite group 1 range from 3 to 6, and in many parts of the world sensitization to mites is the strongest independent risk factor for asthma. Recent studies have confirmed and extended these findings. A survey of 1054 middle school children in Virginia showed that dust mite sensitization was independently associated with asthma (OR 6.6, $P < 0.0001$) and that dust from 81% of homes contained more than 2 μg/g mite group 1 allergen.[35] A prospective study of 939 German schoolchildren followed up to age 7 showed a sevenfold difference in sensitization to mite between children exposed to less than 0.03 μg/g mite group 1 (first quartile) with those exposed to 1 to 240 μg (fourth quartile).[36]

Although the exposure data have been most thoroughly investigated for mite allergens, similar relationships between exposure and sensitization have been observed for other indoor allergens (Table 25-2). Most houses that contain cats or dogs have Fel d 1 or Can f 1 levels of greater than 10 μg/g, whereas homes that do not contain these pets may contain 1 to 10 μg/g animal allergen.[12-14] What distinguishes animal allergen exposure from other indoor allergens is the wide range of exposure levels (from < 0.5 to > 3000 μg/g) and the ubiquitous allergen distribution. Cat and dog allergens occur in schools, offices, workplaces, and public buildings, where they are passively transported by their owners, and they can cause both sensitization and symptoms in these environments.[37,38] An atopic child who lives at home without a cat can become sensitized by visiting homes or attending schools where cat allergen is present. A recent Swedish study showed a ninefold increased risk of asthma exacerbations at school among 6- to 12-year-old children who attended classes with other children who kept cats compared with those in classes with fewer than 18% cat owners.[39] Thus passive exposure of school children to animal allergens can exacerbate asthma, even among children who are being treated with asthma medications. Experimental challenge studies carried out in a room containing cats have shown that airborne Fel d 1 levels of 10 to 100 ng/m³ induced respiratory symptoms and caused changes in pulmonary function.[40,41] Similar airborne allergen levels are typically found in homes that contain cats. Somewhat paradoxically, two recent studies have shown that high-level exposure to Fel d 1 (> 20 μg/g) gives rise to a form of tolerance that results in a lower prevalence of IgE antibody responses.[42,43] This modified Th2 response is associated with production of high levels of Fel d 1–specific IgG4 antibody without IgE antibody.[42] In both studies, low-dose exposure to Fel d 1 (1 to 8 μg/g) was most strongly associated with the development of IgE antibody. The dose-response studies may explain why, in population surveys, sensitization to cats is often lower than that to dust mites. In countries such as New Zealand, where 78% of the population owns cats and high levels of allergen occur in houses, the prevalence of sensitization to cats is only 10% and cats is not as important a cause of asthma as dust mites.[44]

CR allergen exposure has been assessed by measuring Bla g 1 and Bla g 2, which cause sensitization on 30% to 50% and 60% to 80% of CR-allergic patients, respectively.[17] Most dust samples from CR-infested homes contain both allergens, although there is only a modest quantitative correlation between levels of the two allergens. Analysis of Bla g 1 and Bla g 2 levels in the homes of asthma patients admitted to the emergency departments in Atlanta, Georgia, and Wilmington, Delaware, showed that homes with visible evidence of CR contained more than 8 U/g Bla g 1 and more than 2 U/g (approximately 0.1 μg/g) Bla g 2.[45,46] In inner-city Baltimore, the proportion of asthmatic children (aged 4 to 9 years) with positive skin tests to CR increased from 32% among children exposed to 1 to 2 U/g Bla g 1 to 45% among children exposed to more than 4 U/g.[7] Multicenter case-control studies carried out

TABLE 25-2 Allergen Exposure Thresholds for Sensitization

	Allergen Level in Dust Sample				
Risk for Sensitization*	Mite Group 1 (μg/g)	Fel d 1 (μg/g)	Can f 1 (μg/g)	Bla g 1 (U/g)	Bla g 2 (μg/g)
High	> 10	1-8	1-8	> 8	> 1
Medium	2-10	8-20	8-20	1-8	0.08-0.4
Low	< 0.3†	< 0.5	< 0.5	< 0.6	<< 0.08
		> 20	> 20?		

*For atopic children.
†Levels found in "allergen-free" hospital rooms or in houses/apartments maintained for at least 6 months are less than 45% relative humidity.

among 12- to 13-year-old school children in Charlottesville, Virginia, and Los Alamos, New Mexico, showed that a four-fold increase in Bla g 2 exposure (from 0.08 to 0.33 μg/g) was associated with highly significant increases in wheal size of CR skin tests.[18] These studies provide evidence for a dose-response relationship between CR allergen exposure and sensitization. The reported CR allergen levels are severalfold lower than those for either mite or animal allergens, suggesting that CR may be more potent in stimulating IgE responses. The National Cooperative Inner City Asthma Study (NCICAS) showed that sensitization and exposure to CR (> 8 U/g Bla g 1) were associated with increased asthma morbidity. Among inner-city children from eight U.S. cities enrolled in the study, 37% were allergic to CR, and hospitalizations, unscheduled medical visits, and days lost from school due to wheezing or asthma were strongly associated with CR allergen exposure.[7,16] In the United States, high CR allergen levels are associated with lower socioeconomic status, living in inner cities, and race (African-American or Hispanic). However, CR allergy is not an entirely urban problem. Suburban and rural homes, including trailer homes, that harbor high levels of CR cause sensitization and respiratory disease in these populations. Moreover, asthma is the most important public health problem caused by CR infestation of homes.

The measurement of exposure to fungal allergens has proved more difficult than for other indoor allergens. Numerous fungal allergens have been cloned, and sensitive and specific assays for major allergens, such as Alt a 1 and Asp f 1, have been developed (see Box 25-1). The problems with measuring these allergens are related to the biology of fungal growth in houses. Unless houses are heavily contaminated, most *Aspergillus* occurs as spores and the Asp f 1 allergen is produced only when the spores germinate. Similarly, although the Alt a 1 assay is quite sensitive and the allergen can be eluted from spores, laboratory experiments indicate that unless the spore counts are very high (>100,000/ml), they are unlikely to be detected in the assay.[47,48] Success in using polyclonal antibody–based ELISA for "total" fungal allergens has been reported.[48] However, the limitations of these assays are that they measure both allergens and nonallergenic fungal proteins and that they cannot be used to provide quantitative assessments of allergen exposure. Other markers of fungal growth in houses include β(1-3) glucans, ergosterol, extracellular polysaccharides, and volatile organic compounds.[22] Until more clearly defined and validated allergen tests become available, it seems likely that volumetric air sampling and measurement of spore counts and fungi cultured from air/dust samples will remain the standard approaches to assess fungal exposure.

For mite, animal, and CR allergens, there are clear data on exposure thresholds that result in sensitization. However, an association between allergen exposure and asthma symptoms is less clear, and for mite and CR allergens, there is a poor relationship between current exposure and symptoms. A seminal 12-year prospective study by Sporik et al[49] of children born to atopic patients showed that the development of asthma at age 11 was strongly associated with high levels of dust mite exposure (>10 μg/g) in the first year of life. A mite allergen level of 10 μg/g has been regarded as a risk level for symptoms based on this study and earlier seasonal variation and hospital emergency department admission studies.[6] However, the German MAS study found no association between mite allergen

exposure and asthma in the prospective cohort followed through age 7.[36] The MAS study has several limitations: the reported mite allergen levels were very low compared with other countries and did not include a wide range of exposure (reviewed in an article by Sporik and Platts-Mills[44]). It has also been argued that the concept that there should be a direct relationship between allergen exposure and asthma is flawed because any association is entirely dependent on sensitization. Thus in Atlanta, there is no association between CR allergen exposure and asthma, unless the degree of sensitization is taken into account.[44]

Monitoring Allergen Exposure as Part of Asthma Management

Expert guidelines for asthma management, produced by the National Heart, Lung, and Blood Institute (NHLBI) and the American Academy of Allergy, Asthma and Immunology (AAAAI), recommend allergen avoidance as a primary goal of asthma management.[50,51] The guidelines recommend using patient histories and allergic sensitization as evidence of allergen exposure but do not include any environmental assessment. There are several flaws with this approach. Allergen levels in homes vary widely across the United States, depending on climate, geographic location, housing type and condition, and socioeconomic status. The National Allergen Survey reported that 22% of U.S. homes contain more than 10 μg/g mite allergen and illustrate that high mite allergen levels are a potential problem in many homes.[52] Conversely, many U.S. homes have low or undetectable allergen levels. For example, Der f 1 levels in Boston, Massachusetts, were 10-fold to 100-fold higher in single-family homes than in centrally heated apartments.[53] Thus marked variations in allergen exposure were demonstrated in a single U.S. city. Other observations show that inner-city homes located on the East Coast have lower mite allergen levels than those reported in the urban South.[7,17,45,54,55] Clinically relevant levels of cat allergen are found in homes that do not contain cats and in some schools. Finally, CR allergen is found in about 20% of homes that have no visible evidence of CR infestation.[46] The significance of these studies is that allergen exposure should not be assumed and that knowledge of allergen levels in the home is needed to provide objective advice about exposure and avoidance.

A detailed discussion of environmental control measures for reducing allergen levels is given in Chapter 22. Allergen measurements have been used to validate the efficacy of a variety of physical and chemical control methods, procedures, and devices, including mattress encasings, vacuum cleaner filters, acaricides, protein denaturants, detergents and carpet cleaners, and steam cleaning, humidity control, and air filtration systems. For example, the quality of mattress and pillow encasings was greatly improved by using microfine cotton fabrics, and the precise pore size of these fabrics for allergen exclusion was established by airflow experiments and allergen analysis by ELISA.[56] It is important that products and devices be tested for their effects on specific allergens so that allergists can make objective recommendations based on scientific and technical data and allergic patients and other consumers can verify claims made by manufacturers.

The availability of new rapid screening tests for indoor allergens will educate patients about the role of allergens in causing allergic disease. The importance of educating patients so that they can play a leading role in controlling their disease has recently been emphasized.[26,57] The objectives of making exposure measurements are to show that in addition to having IgE reactivity to an allergen, the patient may be exposed to the relevant allergen at home. This information is expected to reinforce the link among allergen sensitization, exposure, and disease activity; enable informed decisions to be made about treatment options; and encourage implementation and compliance with intervention procedures (Box 25-2). Support for this concept comes from recent European studies involving 360 asthma/rhinitis patients, which showed that the use of an "indoor environmental technician" to visit homes resulted in greater compliance with avoidance measures and greater reductions in allergen levels.[58] In well-designed clinical studies in the United States, it was reported that only 20% to 30% of patients adhere to avoidance recommendations.[51] Adherence improved to about 50% with intensive clinic-based education. These studies emphasize the need for improving compliance if allergen avoidance is to be effective. The hypothesis that knowledge of allergen exposure can be used as an educational tool that will encourage compliance needs to be tested in outreach studies. If these studies are successful, they could form the basis of simple environmental monitoring and control procedures to treat asthma, with significant cost savings and benefits for public health.

CONCLUSIONS

Children and adults in Western countries have adopted sedentary lifestyles and spend 90% of their time indoors, where they may be exposed to high levels of environmental allergens. Modern housing has low air exchange rates and results in high airborne allergen levels, especially animal allergens. Although these observations do not explain the increase in asthma prevalence that has occurred during the past 40 years, they may contribute to the increase in allergen sensitization seen in children. Epidemiologic studies worldwide have proved an association between allergen exposure and IgE-mediated sensitization and have consistently shown a strong association between allergen sensitization and asthma.[44] Allergen exposure can be accurately measured by ELISA for major allergens, which have been reported in more than 250 peer-reviewed publications. The gap in the repertoire is that there are few tests for fungal allergens; this has limited studies on the role of fungal allergen exposure in causing allergic disease and other respiratory conditions. Currently, measurement of allergen in reservoir dust samples provides the best index of allergen exposure in the home. An increasing array of semiquantitative tests is being developed for use in physicians' offices and by allergic patients. These tests should empower patients to monitor allergen levels in the home and to implement suitable avoidance procedures in consultation with allergists and allergy clinic staff. The next generation of allergy tests will enable multiple allergens to be tested on a dust or air sample at the same time and within 10 minutes, thus making allergen detection systems widely available for the consumer. Home allergen assessments will enable allergists to provide objective information about allergen exposure and will educate patients about allergic disease. This approach should encourage compliance with allergen avoidance and the implementation of procedures to reduce allergen levels. Environmental control is an integral part of asthma management and should be considered for children with atopic dermatitis. Prospective controlled trials are under way to establish whether the primary avoidance of allergens in infancy will reduce allergen sensitization and the prevalence of asthma. Preliminary results of a large cohort studied at 3 years show a reduced prevalence of wheeze among children on avoidance compared with control children.[59] The combination of improved allergen-monitoring techniques and validated allergen-avoidance procedures should enable low allergen conditions to be established in homes. This strategy should improve asthma management and reduce the public health problems associated with sensitization to indoor allergens.

BOX 25-2

THERAPEUTIC PRINCIPLES
Allergen Exposure Measurements in Clinical Practice

Provide objective assessments of current allergen exposure.

Educate patients about sensitization, exposure, and allergic disease.

Allow allergists or pediatricians to provide clear information about the efficacy of avoidance procedures or devices.

Reinforce advice about immunotherapy or avoidance.

Encourage compliance with avoidance procedures.

HELPFUL WEBSITES

The WHO/IUIS Allergen Nomenclature Sub-committee website (www.allergen.org)
The National Institute for Environmental Health Sciences website (www.niehs.nih.gov)
The American Academy of Allergy Asthma and Immunology website (www.aaaai.org)
The American College of Allergy Asthma and Immunology website (www.acaai.org)
The Environmental Protection Agency website (www.epa. gov)
The National Institute for Allergy and Infectious Diseases website (www.niaid.nih.gov/research/dait.htm)
The Allergy Report website (www.theallergyreport.org/main.html)

REFERENCES

1. Kern RA: Dust sensitization in bronchial asthma, *Med Clin North Am* 5:751-758, 1921.
2. Cooke RA: Studies in specific hypersensitiveness, IV: new aetiologic factors in bronchial asthma, *J Immunol* 7:147-162, 1922.
3. Van Leeuwen S: Asthma and tuberculosis in relation to "climate allergens," *Br Med J* 2:344-347, 1927.
4. Berrens L, Young E: Preparation and properties of purified house dust allergen, *Nature* 190:536-537, 1961.
5. Voorhorst R, Spieksma FthM, Varekamp H, et al: The house dust mite (*Dermatophagoides pteronyssins*) and the allergens it produces, *J Allergy* 39:325-339, 1967.
6. Platts-Mills TAE, Vervloet D, Thomas WR, et al: Indoor allergens and asthma: report of the Third International Workshop, *J Allergy Clin Immunol* 100:S1-S24, 1997.
7. Eggleston PA, Rosenstreich D, Lynn H, et al: Relationship of indoor allergen exposure to skin test sensitivity in inner-city children with asthma, *J Allergy Clin Immunol* 102:563-570, 1998.
8. Bush RK, Eggleston PA, eds: Guidelines for control of indoor allergen exposure, *J Allergy Clin Immunol* 107:S403-S440, 2001.
9. Peat JK: Can asthma be prevented? Evidence from epidemiological studies of children in Australia and New Zealand in the last decade, *Clin Exp Allergy* 28:261-265, 1997.

10. Custovic A, Taggart SCO, Francis HC, et al: Exposure to house dust mite allergens and the clinical activity of asthma, *J Allergy Clin Immunol* 98:64-72, 1995.

11. Chan-Yeung M, Manfreda J, Dimich-Ward H, et al: Mite and cat allergen levels in homes and severity of asthma, *Am J Respir Crit Care Med* 152:1805-1811, 1995.

12. Bollinger ME, Eggleston PA, Flanagan E, et al: Cat antigen in homes with and without cats may induce allergic symptoms, *J Allergy Clin Immunol* 97:907-914, 1996.

13. Custovic A, Green R, Fletcher A, et al: Aerodynamic properties of the major dog allergen Can f 1: distribution in homes, concentration, and particle size of allergen in the air, *Am J Resp Crit Care Med* 155:94-98, 1997.

14. Ingram JM, Sporik R, Rose G, et al: Quantitative assessment of exposure to dog (Can f 1) and cat (Fel d 1) allergens: relationship to sensitization and asthma among children living in Los Alamos, New Mexico, *J Allergy Clin Immunol* 96:449-456, 1995.

15. Phipatanakul W, Eggleston PA, Wright EC, et al: Mouse allergen, II: the relationship of mouse allergen exposure to mouse sensitization and asthma morbidity in inner-city children with asthma, *J Allergy Clin Immunol* 106:1075-1080, 2000.

16. Rosenstreich DL, Eggleston P, Kattan M, et al: The role of cockroach allergy and exposure to cockroach allergen in causing morbidity among inner-city children with asthma, *N Engl J Med* 336:1356-1363, 1997.

17. Arruda LK, Vailes LD, Ferriani VP, et al: Cockroach allergens and asthma, *J Allergy Clin Immunol* 107:419-428, 2001.

18. Sporik R, Squillace SP, Ingram JM, et al: Mite, cat, and cockroach exposure, allergen sensitisation, and asthma in children: a case-control study of three schools, *Thorax* 54:675-680, 1999.

19. Chapman MD, Smith AM, Vailes LD, et al: Recombinant allergens for diagnosis and therapy of allergic disease, *J Allergy Clin Immunol* 106:409-418, 2000.

20. Aalberse RC: Structural biology of allergens, *J Allergy Clin Immunol* 106:228-238, 2000.

21. Pomes A, Chapman MD, Vailes LD, et al: Cockroach allergen Bla g 2: structure, function, and implications for allergic sensitization, *Am J Respir Crit Care Med* 165:391-397, 2002.

22. Bush RK, Portnoy JM: The role and abatement of fungal allergens in allergic diseases, *J Allergy Clin Immunol* 107:S430-S440, 2001.

23. Shakib F, Schulz O, Sewell H: A mite subversive: cleavage of CD23 and CD25 by Der p 1 enhances allergenicity, *Immunol Today* 19:313-316, 1998.

24. Wan H, Winton HL, Soeller C, et al: Der p 1 facilitates transepithelial allergen delivery by disruption of tight junctions, *J Clin Invest* 104:123-133, 1999.

25. Hiller R, Laffer S, Harwanegg C, et al: Microarrayed allergen molecules: diagnostic gatekeepers for allergy treatment, *FASEB J* 16:414-416, 2002.

26. Chapman MD, Tsay A, Vailes LD: Home allergen monitoring and control: improving clinical practice and patient benefits, *Allergy* 56:604-610, 2001.

27. Tsay A, Williams L, Mitchell EB, et al: A rapid test for detection of mite allergens in homes, *Clin Exp Allergy* 32:1596-1601, 2002.

28. Polzius R, Wuske T, Mahn J: Wipe test for the detection of indoor allergens, *Allergy* 57:143-145, 2002.

29. Custovic A, Taggart SCO, Niven RM, et al: Evaluating exposure to mite allergens, *J Allergy Clin Immunol* 96:134-135, 1995.

30. Luczynska CM, Li Y, Chapman MD, et al: Airborne concentrations and particle size distribution of allergen derived from domestic cats (*Felis domesticus*). Measurements using cascade impactor, liquid impinger, and a two-site monoclonal antibody assay for Fel d I, *Am Rev Respir Dis* 141:361-367, 1990.

31. Ehnert B, Lau-Schadendorf S, Weber A, et al: Reducing domestic exposure to dust mite allergen reduces bronchial hyperreactivity in sensitive children with asthma, *J Allergy Clin Immunol* 90:135-138, 1992.

32. de Blay F, Sanchez J, Hedelin G, et al: Dust and airborne exposure to allergens derived from cockroach (Blattella germanica) in low-cost public housing in Strasbourg (France), *J Allergy Clin Immunol* 99:107-112, 1997.

33. O'Meara T, Tovey ER: Monitoring personal allergen exposure, *Clin Rev Allergy Immunol* 18:341-395, 2000.

34. Custis N, Woodfolk JA, Vaughan JW, et al: Use of a novel air cleaner to monitor airborne allergen, *J Allergy Clin Immunol* 109:S53, 2002.

35. Squillace SP, Sporik RB, Rakes G, et al: Sensitization to dust mites as a dominant risk factor for asthma among adolescents living in central Virginia. Multiple regression analysis of a population-based study, *Am J Respir Crit Care Med* 156:1760-1764, 1997.

36. Lau S, Illi S, Sommerfeld C, et al: Early exposure to house-dust mite and cat allergens and development of childhood asthma: a cohort study. Multicentre Allergy Study Group, *Lancet* 356:1392-1397, 2000.

37. Custovic A, Green R, Taggart SC, et al: Domestic allergens in public places, II: dog (Can f 1) and cockroach (Bla g 2) allergens in dust and mite, cat, dog and cockroach allergens in the air in public buildings, *Clin Exp Allergy* 26:1246-1252, 1996.

38. Patchett K, Lewis S, Crane J, et al: Cat allergen (Fel d 1) levels on school children's clothing and in primary school classrooms in Wellington, New Zealand, *J Allergy Clin Immunol* 100:755-759, 1997.

39. Almqvist C, Wickman M, Perfetti L, et al: Worsening of asthma in children allergic to cats, after indirect exposure to cat at school, *Am J Respir Crit Care Med* 163:694-698, 2001.

40. Wood RA, Eggleston PA. Environmental challenges to animal allergens. In Spector S, ed: *Provocation testing in clinical practice*, New York, 1994, Marcel Dekker.

41. Wood RA, Eggleston PA: The effects of intranasal steroids on nasal and pulmonary responses to cat exposure, *Am J Respir Crit Care Med* 151:315-320, 1995.

42. Platts-Mills T, Vaughan J, Squillace S, et al: Sensitisation, asthma, and a modified Th2 response in children exposed to cat allergen: a population-based cross-sectional study, *Lancet* 357:752-756, 2001.

43. Custovic A, Hallam CL, Simpson BM, et al: Decreased prevalence of sensitization to cats with high exposure to cat allergen, *J Allergy Clin Immunol* 108:537-539, 2001.

44. Sporik R, Platts-Mills TAE: Allergen exposure and the development of asthma, *Thorax* 56(suppl II):II58-II63, 2001.

45. Call RS, Smith TF, Morris E, et al: Risk factors for asthma in inner city children, *J Pediatr* 121:862-866, 1992.

46. Gelber LE, Seltzer LH, Bouzoukis JK, et al: Sensitization and exposure to indoor allergens as risk factors for asthma among patients presenting to hospital, *Am Rev Respir Dis* 147:573-578, 1993.

47. Vailes LD, Sridhara S, Cromwell O, et al: Quantitation of the major fungal allergens, Alt a 1 and Asp f 1 in commercial allergenic products, *J Allergy Clin Immunol* 107:641-646, 2001.

48. Barnes C, Tuck J, Simon S: Allergenic materials in the house dust of allergy clinic patients, *Ann Allergy Asthma Immunol* 86:517-523, 2001.

49. Sporik R, Holgate ST, Platts-Mills TA: Exposure to house-dust mite allergen (Der p I) and the development of asthma in childhood: a prospective study, *N Engl J Med* 323:502-507, 1990.

50. National Asthma Education and Prevention Program, Expert Panel Report 2. *Guidelines for the diagnosis and management of asthma*, Bethesda, MD, 1997, National Institutes of Health, National Heart, Lung, and Blood Institute. NIH Pub No. 97-4051.

51. American Academy of Allergy, Asthma and Immunology: Position statement. Environmental allergen avoidance in allergic asthma, *J Allergy Clin Immunol* 103:203-205, 1999.

52. Vojta PJ, Friedman W, Marker DA, et al: First National Survey of Lead and Allergens in Housing: survey design and methods for the allergen and endotoxin components, *Environ Health Perspect* 110:527-532, 2002.

53. Chew GL, Higgins KM, Gold DR, et al: Monthly measurements of indoor allergens and the influence of housing type in a northeastern US city, *Allergy* 54:1058-1066, 1999.

54. Miller RL, Chew GL, Bell CA, et al: Prenatal exposure, maternal sensitization, and sensitization *in utero* to indoor allergens in an inner-city cohort, *Am J Resp Crit Care Med* 164:995-1001, 2001.

55. Nelson RP Jr, DiNicolo R, Fernandez-Caldas E, et al: Allergen-specific IgE levels and mite allergen exposure in children with acute asthma first seen in an emergency department and in non asthmatic control subjects, *J Allergy Clin Immunol* 98:258-263, 2001.

56. Vaughan JW, McLaughlin TE, Perzanowski MS, et al: Evaluation of materials used for bedding encasement: effect of pore size in blocking cat and dust mite allergen, *J Allergy Clin Immunol* 103:227-231, 1999.

57. Platts-Mills TA, Vaughan JW, Carter MC, et al: The role of intervention in established allergy avoidance of indoor allergens in the treatment of chronic allergic disease, *J Allergy Clin Immunol* 106:787-804, 2000.

58. deBlay F, Fourgaut G, Lieutier-Colas F, et al: Mite allergen reduction: role of an indoor technician in patients' compliance and allergen exposure, *J Allergy Clin Immunol* 107:S218, 2001.

59. Custovic A, Simpson BM, Simpson A: Effect of environmental manipulation in pregnancy and early life on respiratory symptoms and atopy during first year of life: a randomised trial, *Lancet* 358:188-193, 2001.

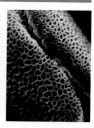

CHAPTER 26

Environmental Control

ROBERT A. WOOD

There is no doubt that aeroallergens play a major role in the pathogenesis of allergic disease, including asthma, allergic rhinitis, and atopic dermatitis. Among these, the indoor allergens are of particular importance. These principally include the allergens of house dust mites, domestic pets, cockroaches, and molds. The relative importance of these different allergens varies in different parts of the world depending on a variety of geographic and climatic factors. All studies agree, however, that children with asthma will have a high likelihood of becoming sensitized to whichever of these allergens are prominent in their local environments. This chapter focuses on the importance of allergen avoidance in the management of allergic disease.

DUST MITES

Dust mites are arachnids that live in the dust that accumulates in most homes, particularly the dust contained within fabrics. Favorite habitats include carpets, upholstered furniture, mattresses, pillows, and bedding materials. Their major food source is shed human skin scales, which are present in high numbers in most of these items. The major dust mite species known to be associated with allergic disease are *Dermatophagoides pteronyssinus* and *Dermatophagoides farinae*.[1-3] Other mites, including *Euroglyphus maynei* and *Blomia tropicalis* are also important in some areas, although their distribution is considerably more limited. Dust mites grow optimally in areas that are both warm and humid, and they grow very poorly when the relative humidity remains below 40%.[4] Dust mites grow from eggs to adults over the course of about 4 weeks and adult dust mites live for about 6 weeks, during which time females produce 40 to 80 eggs.[5]

Assessment of dust mite exposure has been accomplished largely through the analysis of settled dust samples. Although some studies have not been able to show a relationship between dust mite levels and allergic sensitization or disease activity, there is now general agreement that dust mite levels of greater than 2 μg of group 1 allergen per gram of dust should be considered a risk factor for sensitization[3,5-8] and that levels greater than 10 μg/g of dust are a risk factor for acute asthma.[9] Airborne sampling for dust mite allergen has proven difficult or impossible in the absence of substantial disturbance. This is a reflection of the fact that dust mite allergens are carried on relatively large particles, most ranging from 10 to 20 μ in mean aerodynamic diameter, which settle within minutes of disturbance.[10]

The prevalence of dust mite sensitivity in asthmatic patients varies considerably from one geographic area to another. For example, studies have demonstrated prevalence rates ranging from 5% in asthmatic children in Los Alamos, New Mexico, to 66% in Atlanta, Georgia, to 91% in Papua, New Guinea.[9,11,12] These differences are roughly proportional to differences in mite exposure in these areas of the world.

At least as significant as the relationship between mite exposure and mite sensitization is the evidence that mite exposure is capable of inducing not just sensitization but the asthmatic state itself. In a prospective trial, Sporik et al[8] demonstrated a significant increase in asthma, as well as mite sensitivity, in 11-year-old children who had experienced high mite exposure during infancy. Other studies have demonstrated a striking association between asthma development and mite sensitivity,[11,13-15] although these studies lacked a prospective evaluation of mite exposure. These studies are exciting in that they suggest that allergen avoidance early in life could prevent the development of asthma in some patients, an idea that has now been studied with encouraging results.[16]

Extensive evidence also exists to support a relationship between ongoing mite exposure and disease activity.[17-19] With regard to chronic symptoms, Vervloet et al[19] demonstrated a significant correlation between medication requirements and current mite exposure in a group of mite-sensitive adult asthma patients. Custovic et al[17] also demonstrated a relationship between mite exposure and asthma severity as evidenced by bronchial hyperreactivity (BHR), peak expiratory flow rate variability, and forced expiratory volume in 1 second (FEV_1). Several studies have also demonstrated mite exposure to be a risk factor for acute asthma and emergency room visits.[9,20] In a study by Call et al,[9] inner-city children in Atlanta were evaluated after presentation to the emergency room with acute asthma. Of these children, 72% were found to be allergic to either dust mite alone or both dust mite and cockroach allergen. The combination of mite exposure and mite sensitization was highly associated with the development of acute asthma (21 of 35 asthmatic patients versus 3 of 22 control subjects, $P < 0.001$).

The most compelling evidence for the role of dust mites in asthma comes from studies of allergen avoidance, either through environmental control in the home or the removal of mite-allergic patients from their homes. Two classic studies from the early 1980s provided dramatic evidence for the potential benefits of dust mite avoidance. Platts-Mills et al[21] investigated the effects of mite avoidance by placing nine young adults with mite-induced asthma in a hospital setting for a minimum of 2 months. All patients experienced reduced symptoms, seven patients had reduced medication requirements, and five patients showed at least an eightfold reduction in bronchial reactivity as measured by the concentration of histamine required to induce a 30% fall in FEV_1. In the second study Murray and Ferguson[22] studied 20 mite-allergic asthmatic children in a controlled trial of mite avoidance in the patients' homes. They found significant reductions in asthma symptoms, days on which wheezing was observed, days with low peak flow rates, and BHR in the group using active mite control measures.

The vast majority of subsequent trials of mite avoidance have yielded similar results.[23-27] Ehnert et al[25] studied 24 children with asthma and mite sensitivity in a 1-year trial of mite avoidance. The patients were divided into three groups. The first had their mattresses, pillows, and comforters covered with impermeable encasements; the second had their mattresses and carpets treated with an acaricide (benzyl benzoate); and the third had their mattresses and carpets treated with placebo. Significant reductions in dust mite allergen levels were found only in the group with mattress and pillow encasements. Similarly, a highly significant reduction in BHR was noted in that group compared with the other two.

One final study of mite avoidance deserves note. It has long been recognized that dust mite levels are significantly reduced at high altitude. Peroni et al[27] performed an extensive clinical study of mite avoidance by moving asthmatic children to a high-altitude environment. The study was divided into two groups, one with 22 children and the other with 23 children, who were admitted during successive years. They demonstrated significant reductions in total IgE levels, dust mite–specific IgE levels, methacholine reactivity, and response to dust mite bronchoprovocation. These differences were first detected after 3 months in the high-altitude setting and continued through the entire 9-month study. They were also able to study 14 of the 22 children from the first cohort 3 months after returning to their usual home environment. These children had experienced significant increases in their total IgE levels, methacholine reactivity, and response to exercise challenge. This important demonstration of reduced disease activity in the mite-free environment, followed by increased disease activity after returning to usual mite exposure, provides a remarkable demonstration of the power of both mite exposure and avoidance.

Dust Mite Control Measures

Although there should be no doubt as to the benefits of dust mite avoidance, there is still some controversy as to the specific measures that are necessary to sufficiently reduce mite exposure to control disease.[3] This controversy arises from three major factors. First, some environmental control measures have not been adequately studied to make any accurate conclusions. Second, for some measures studies of their efficacy have yielded conflicting results. Third, in many studies a combination of environmental control measures was used, making it difficult to determine which measures actually led to the benefit that was observed. Specific environmental control measures will therefore be reviewed individually and then summarized in Table 26-1.

TABLE 26-1 Environmental Control of House Dust Mites

First line (necessary and cost effective)
Replace mattress and pillow encasements
Wash bed linens every 1-2 weeks, preferably in hot water
Remove stuffed toys
Regularly vacuum carpeted surfaces
Regularly dust hard surfaces
Reduce indoor relative humidity (dehumidify and do not add humidity)

Second line (helpful but more expensive)
Remove carpets, especially in the bedroom
Remove upholstered furniture
Avoid living in basements

Third line (limited or unproven benefit)
Acaricides
Tannic acid
Air cleaners

It is very clear that allergen-proof encasements for mattresses and pillows significantly reduce dust mite exposure.[25,28,29] In the study by Ehnert et al,[25] polyurethane mattress encasements produced a 91% decrease in mite allergen by day 14 of treatment, which rose to 98% by month 12 of the study. In another study by Owen et al,[28] Der p 1 levels on encased mattresses were only 1% of those on control mattresses. These encasements should therefore be recommended for all patients with mite sensitivity. In addition, although encasements had been constructed of impermeable plastic or vinyl materials that were very uncomfortable, they are now also available in tightly woven fabrics that are considerably more comfortable to sleep on.

The effects of vacuum cleaning on mite levels have been extensively studied. Live mites are difficult to remove from carpeting, and it is clear that vacuum cleaning in the absence of other measures will provide only limited benefit. However, regular vacuum cleaning does remove significant amounts of dust from carpets, which will at least help to reduce the allergen reservoir. Patients should also be warned that vacuuming creates considerable disturbance, with transient increases in airborne mite levels. Vacuum cleaners equipped with special bags or filters to help prevent this problem are available and may be of some added benefit,[30] although it should be noted that because dust mite allergen is carried on large particles that settle quickly, it is not clear whether these specialized vacuums are of clinical importance. There is little evidence that wet vacuum cleaning or steam cleaning provides any additional benefit. One study found carpet shampooing to be no more effective than dry vacuum cleaning,[31] whereas another study showed that wet vacuum cleaning was shown to lead to a subsequent increase in mite numbers.[32] This was presumed to have occurred because of elevated humidity in the carpet after wet vacuuming.

A variety of carpet treatments have also been developed in an effort to control dust mite allergen exposure. These can be classified as either acaricides or denaturing agents. A variety of acaricides have been investigated and shown to kill house dust mites in laboratory conditions.[33,34] These range from caffeine[35] to potent and potentially toxic organophosphates.[36] Only one acaricide, benzyl benzoate, is available for use in the United States.

Although there is little doubt that benzyl benzoate is effective in killing dust mites, studies regarding the efficacy of this compound in home environments have provided varying results.[24,37-39] For example, while both Hayden et al[37] and Woodfolk et al[39] demonstrated significant reductions in dust mite allergen after treatment with benzyl benzoate, the changes were not always in a range that would be expected to produce clinical benefit and were relatively short-lived. In the Hayden study, mite levels were still reduced 2 months after treatment, but some increase was clearly evident compared to 1 month posttreatment, suggesting that repeat applications might be required every 2 to 3 months to maintain effect. In another study by Huss et al,[40] benzyl benzoate was compared to placebo in a group of 12 patients. The products were applied at baseline and after 6 months and allergen levels were measured at 0, 3, 6, 9, and 12 months. They detected no decrease in mite allergen in the benzyl benzoate group compared to the control group. Similarly, no effect on clinical asthma was detected. It should be noted that the application of benzyl benzoate every 6 months as performed in this study was based on the manufacturer's recommendations and that the lack of effect may have occurred simply because the product was not applied more often or because allergen levels were not measured sooner after application.

Tannic acid is a denaturing agent that has been extensively studied for the control of dust mite allergen. This product is designed to reduce allergen levels without affecting dust mite growth or allergen production. It has also been shown in the laboratory to be highly effective. Much like benzyl benzoate, however, its efficacy in home environments is less convincing. Woodfolk et al[41] evaluated the effects of tannic acid on 17 carpets. The carpets were treated on days 0 and 28 and dust samples were collected on days 0, 1, 7, 14, 28, and 42. The treated carpets exhibited reduced mite allergen levels compared to control carpets, although the effects were not dramatic and were not maintained for long periods.

The recommendation regarding the use of benzyl benzoate and tannic acid is therefore that these products may be useful adjuncts for the control of dust mite exposure in homes where carpets, particularly bedroom carpets, cannot be removed. Especially with benzyl benzoate, its use must be followed by intensive vacuum cleaning to remove residual allergen. It is likely that the combination of benzyl benzoate and tannic acid would produce the greatest effect, although even this could never be a substitute for carpet removal.[42]

Bed linens, stuffed animals, and other soft furnishings also provide excellent environments for dust mite growth. Objects such as stuffed animals should be removed whenever possible. The mite content of bedding materials and other objects that cannot be removed can typically be reduced by washing. Washing in hot water (greater than 55° C) is ideal in that it both removes allergen and kills dust mites.[43] These water temperatures, however, may not be available in many home environment because of safety concerns. It is important to note, therefore, that washing in cooler water does not kill mites but does remove mite allergens very effectively. Weekly washing of all bed linens in a hot cycle is therefore recommended for all mite-allergic patients. Dry cleaning also kills dust mites,[43,44] as does tumble drying at temperatures greater than 55° C for at least 20 minutes.[28]

Dust mites are susceptible to the effects of low as well as high temperatures. Freezing in a typical household freezer for 24 hours will kill most dust mites, although the mite allergen in the object will not necessarily be reduced.[45] Exposing carpets to direct sunlight for several hours will also kill dust mites because of the high temperature, the low humidity, or both.[46] It has also been shown that electric blankets will reduce mite growth.[47] None of these methods have been established in clinical trials.

Because of the reliance of dust mites on humidity for growth, it has been suggested that methods capable of reducing relative humidity would be useful in the control of mite exposure.[48,49] Korsgaard and Iversen[49] demonstrated that dust mite growth could be significantly reduced by keeping indoor humidity below 7 g/kg by ventilation, whereas Arlian[50] demonstrated that mite growth could be prevented by maintaining relative humidity below 35% for at least 22 hours a day. Air conditioning and dehumidification may also help to deter mite growth and should be used whenever possible.[51] It is clear, however, that such measures will be difficult or impossible in environments with very high relative humidity. A prime example of this fact is the difficulty in eliminating dust mites from carpets over cement slab floors in basements.

Finally, air filtration devices are frequently purchased by patients for the control of their dust mite allergies; however, there is little evidence to support their use.[52-55] In addition, one would not anticipate much effect because of the fact that dust mite allergens do not remain airborne for extended periods and would therefore not be available for filtration in most instances.

In summary, effective dust mite control can be accomplished in most homes with a combination of mattress and pillow covers, hot washing of bed linens, removal of stuffed animals and other soft furnishings, and carpet removal. In the absence of carpet removal, intense vacuum cleaning and the use of acaricides and denaturing agents may prove helpful in many homes. Because of the extraordinary benefits provided through dust mite avoidance in mite-sensitive asthmatic patients, these measures should be routinely recommended, and compliance with these recommendations should be reassessed at each subsequent visit.

ANIMAL ALLERGENS

Animal allergens are also potent causes of both acute and chronic asthma symptoms.[56] Cat and dog allergens are the most important, although significant exposure to a wide variety of other furred animals is not uncommon. Sensitivity to cat and dog allergens has been shown to occur in up to 67% of asthmatic children, and in some settings these are clearly the dominant indoor allergens.[12,57,58] This fact was best demonstrated in the study by Ingram et al[12] conducted in Los Alamos, New Mexico. In this environment, where cat and dog allergens are common but exposure to dust mite and cockroach allergens is rare, IgE antibody to cat and dog allergens was detected in 62% and 67% of asthmatic children, respectively. The presence of this IgE antibody was highly associated with asthma, whereas sensitivity to mite or cockroach allergen was not associated with asthma.

A number of studies have investigated the distribution of cat and dog allergens in the home and other environments.[12,58-61] Using settled dust analysis, it has been shown that levels of cat and dog allergens are clearly highest in homes housing these animals. However, it is also clear from a number of studies that the vast majority of homes contain cat and dog allergen even if a pet has never lived there. This widespread distribution of cat and dog allergens has also been documented in a variety of other settings, including office buildings and schools. Whereas most of the environments with no animals have relatively low allergen levels compared to those with a cat or dog, it is not uncommon to find rather high levels in some of these homes. This widespread distribution is presumed to occur primarily through passive transfer of allergen from one environment to another. The particles carrying animal allergens appear to be very sticky and, unlike dust mite allergens, can be found in high levels on walls and other surfaces within homes.[62]

The characteristics of airborne cat allergen have also been extensively studied. Cat allergen has been shown to be carried on particles that range from less than 1 μ to greater than 20 μ in mean aerodynamic diameter.[63,64] Although estimates have varied, studies agree that at least 15% of airborne cat allergen is carried on particles less than 5 μ. Less information is available for dog allergen, but evidence to date suggests that it is distributed very much like cat allergen, with about 20% of airborne dog allergen being carried on particles less than 5 μ in diameter.[65]

Cat allergen can also be detected in air samples from all homes with cats and from many homes without cats. Bollinger et al[66] detected airborne cat allergen in 10 out of 40 air samples from homes without cats. In addition, when a subset of those homes were reinvestigated on a weekly basis for 4 weeks, all of them had detectable airborne cat allergen on at least one occasion. In an attempt to determine the clinical significance of this unsuspected cat exposure, patients were challenged in an experimental cat exposure facility to varying levels of cat allergen. It was found that allergen levels of less than 100 ng/m^3 were capable of inducing upper and lower respiratory symptoms as well as significant pulmonary function changes. These levels are similar to those found in homes with cats as well as a subset of homes without cats, suggesting that even patients without known cat exposure may be exposed to clinically significant concentrations of airborne cat allergen on a regular basis.

Control of Animal Allergens

At the present time much less is known about the control of animal allergens than about the control of dust mite allergens.[56] In particular, there are still no convincing studies on the clinical benefit of environmental control measures for animal allergens. Although it is assumed that removing an animal from the home will lead to clinical improvement in patients who have disease related to their pets, this has not been proven. Even less data is available regarding the potential benefits of methods that might be used in lieu of animal removal. Cat allergen will be specifically discussed here because the most information is available regarding this important allergen. Most of the information should be applicable to other allergens, and the overall approach to the control of animal allergens is summarized in Table 26-2.

To begin, it should be stated that in any asthmatic patient who is known to be cat sensitive and whose asthma is believed to be related to a significant degree to a pet cat, the most

TABLE 26-2 Environmental Control of Animal Allergens

Remove source (e.g., find a new home for the pet).
  Allergen levels fall slowly—benefit would not be expected for weeks to months.
  Follow by aggressive cleaning to remove reservoirs of allergen.
  Possible role for tannic acid to augment allergen removal
If the pet is not removed:
  Install air cleaners, especially in the bedroom.
  Remove carpeting, especially in the bedroom.
  Replace mattress and pillow covers.
  Wash animals (not likely to help unless done at least twice a week).
  These may not reduce allergen levels enough to help highly allergic patients.

appropriate recommendation is to remove the cat from the home. This is clearly the correct advice from a medical standpoint, and it should be recommended strenuously. A number of potential alternative measures will also be discussed, however, because of the high proportion of patients who are either reluctant or completely unwilling to remove a household pet.

Once a cat has been removed from the home, it is important to recognize that the clinical benefit may not be seen for a period of at least several months because allergen levels fall quite slowly after cat removal.[61] In most homes levels in settled dust will have fallen to those seen in homes without cats within 4 to 6 months of cat removal. Levels may fall much more quickly if extensive environmental control measures are undertaken, such as removal of carpets, upholstered furniture, and other reservoirs from the home, whereas in other homes the process may be considerably slower. This information points to the fact that thorough and repeated cleaning will be required once the animal has been removed. It has also been shown that cat allergen may persist in mattresses for years after a cat has been removed from a home,[67] so new bedding or impermeable encasements must therefore also be recommended.

A number of studies have investigated other measures that might help to reduce cat allergen exposure without removing the animal from the home. De Blay et al[68] demonstrated significant reductions in airborne Fel d 1 with a combination of air filtration, cat washing, vacuum cleaning, and removal of furnishings, although these results were based on a small sample size and did not include any measure of clinical effect. When cat washing was evaluated separately in that study, dramatic reductions in airborne Fel d 1 were seen afterward. Subsequent studies, however, have presented conflicting results. Klucka et al[69] studied both cat washing and Allerpet/c (Allerpet, Inc., New York, New York) and found no benefit from either treatment. More recently, Avner et al[70] studied three different methods of cat washing and found transient reductions in airborne cat allergens after each. There was no sustained benefit, however, with levels returning to baseline within 1 week of washing.

Information is very limited as to the clinical benefits of these environmental control measures if one or more cats is allowed to remain in the home. Four studies have evaluated different combinations of control measures, and although all have shown reductions in allergen levels, clinical effect was less consistent.[71-74] Two studies showed a clear benefit, one showed benefit only in the group in which environmental control was done along with intranasal steroid treatment, and the fourth showed no clinical benefit whatsoever. It therefore still remains to be seen whether allergen exposure can be sufficiently reduced to produce a clinical effect in the absence of animal removal.

In families who insist on keeping their pets, the following should be recommended pending more definitive studies.[56] The animals should be restricted to one area of the home and certainly kept out of the patient's bedroom. HEPA or electrostatic air cleaners should be used, especially in the patient's bedroom. Carpets and other reservoirs for allergen collection should be removed whenever possible, again focusing on the patient's bedroom. Finally, mattress and pillow covers should be routinely used. Although tannic acid has been shown to reduce cat allergen levels, the effects are modest and short-lived when a cat is present, so this treatment should not be routinely recommended. Similarly, cat washing appears to be of such transient benefit that it is only likely to add significantly to the other avoidance measures if it is done at least twice a week.

COCKROACH ALLERGEN

The importance of cockroach allergen in asthma and allergy has been recognized only over the past 30 years. It is now clear that cockroach allergens represent a major cause of asthma, particularly in urban areas.[75] Significant cockroach exposure has been demonstrated in a number of cities, and the prevalence of cockroach sensitivity in urban patients with asthma has been shown to range from 23% to 60%.[9,76,77] In addition, the combination of cockroach exposure and cockroach sensitization has been shown to be a risk factor for acute asthma exacerbations.[9,20,61]

In the most comprehensive study to date on the problem of asthma in inner-city children, 1528 children with asthma from eight major inner-city areas were extensively investigated with regard to the factors, both allergic and otherwise, that contributed to their disease.[59] Although sensitivity to cockroaches, dust mites, and cats were all common (36.8%, 36.9%, and 22.7%, respectively), exposure to cockroach allergen was much more common than exposure to either dust mite or cat (50.2%, 9.7%, and 12.8%, respectively). The combination of cockroach sensitivity and high cockroach exposure was associated with significantly more hospitalizations, unscheduled medical visits for asthma, days of wheezing, missed days from school, and nights with sleep loss because of asthma. Such a correlation was not seen for dust mite or cat allergens. These data argue persuasively that cockroach allergen is a major factor, if not *the* major factor, in the high degree of morbidity seen in this patient population.

Although there are at least 50 cockroach species in the United States, only four or five are domiciliary.[75] Two species, the German cockroach (*Blatella germanica*), and the American cockroach (*Periplaneta americana*), are the most common causes of both household infestation and allergic sensitization. Several allergens from each species have been identified and characterized.[78,79] The most important among these are Bla g 1, Bla g 2, and Per a 1. There is significant cross reactivity between *B. germanica* and *P. americana*, although most patients in the United States appear to be primarily sensitized to *B. germanica*. The source of the major cockroach allergens is still not completely clear, although they do appear to be secreted or excreted, suggesting that they may also be digestive proteins.

The distribution of cockroach allergens has been studied in a number of settings. The highest levels tend to be found in kitchens, although the allergen is widely distributed through the home, including the bedroom.[59,77,79] In fact, in the inner-city asthma study noted above, the 50.2% exposure rate was found in bedroom dust samples.[59] It has been suggested that cockroach allergen levels of greater than 2 units per gram are associated with sensitization and levels greater than 8 units per gram are associated with disease activity. Cockroach allergen has also been detected at significant concentrations in schools in urban Baltimore.[80] Finally, limited study has suggested that cockroach allergen is very much like dust mite allergen with little or no measurable airborne cockroach allergen in the absence of significant disturbance.[75]

Cockroach Allergen Control

Extensive study has been performed on the chemical control of cockroach infestation, and a variety of pesticides and traps are readily available. These include chlorpyrifos (Dursban), diazanon, boric acid powder, and bait stations that contain hydranethylon. All of these agents, with the exception of boric acid, can reduce cockroach numbers by 90% or more, whereas boric acid reduces numbers by 40% to 50%. Very little is known, however, about the effects of extermination procedures on cockroach allergen levels. Several studies have shown that cockroach extermination is possible in most homes and that a combination of extermination and thorough cleaning can reduce cockroach allergen levels by 80% to 90%. There are still no studies, however, which prove that these methods are sufficient to reduce disease activity.[81-83]

Other measures that should help to reduce cockroach infestation include eliminating food sources and hiding and entry points (Table 26-3). All foods should be stored in sealed containers and the kitchen should be cleaned regularly. Finally, extensive cleaning should be performed after extermination to remove the cockroach debris as completely as possible. Even with the most aggressive measures, however, it is unlikely that cockroach exposure will be adequately reduced in some environments. This is particularly true of the older, multiple dwelling units that house a preponderance of inner-city asthma patients. It may be necessary to exterminate in the

---

TABLE 26-3 Environmental Control of Cockroach Allergen

Regular and thorough extermination
Thorough cleaning after extermination
Extermination of neighboring dwellings
Roach traps
Repair leaky faucets and pipes
Repair holes in walls and other entry points
Behavioral changes to reduce food sources
    Clean immediately after cooking
    Clean dirty dishes immediately
    Avoid open food containers
    Avoid uncovered trash cans

homes or apartments surrounding the patient's home to obtain maximum effect, and some patients may need to find new housing altogether. No studies have been reported to date on the clinical effects of extermination or other control measures.

MOLD ALLERGENS

A wide variety of mold species can be present in both indoor and outdoor environments. *Aspergillus* and *Penicillium* species are generally regarded as the most numerous indoor molds,[60,84-86] whereas *Alternaria* is important in both indoor and outdoor environments. Several mold allergens, including Alt n 1 and Asp f 1, have been identified and characterized.

Sensitivity to *Alternaria* has been shown to be associated with asthma in Tucson, Arizona,[87] and in an inland region in Australia.[6] In the Tucson study, sensitivity to *Alternaria* was demonstrated in 60.8% of 6-year-old children with persistent asthma, compared to only 11.8% for dust mite. In fact, *Alternaria* was the only allergen for which sensitivity was associated with an increased risk of asthma at both ages 6 and 11.

Molds tend to grow best in warm, moist environments and mold exposure is therefore roughly correlated with these conditions. Basements, window sills, shower stalls, and bathroom carpets are common sites of mold infestation. Air conditioners and humidifiers have also been shown to be sources of significant mold exposure.[88,89] To date, the assessment of mold exposure has been more difficult than for the other indoor allergens because of the lack of readily available immunoassays to measure major allergens. The currently available methods are very time consuming; these include culture and microscopic examination of air or dust samples. Airborne mold allergens have been shown to be carried on particles ranging in size from less than $2\ \mu$ to greater than $100\ \mu$.[85]

The control of mold allergens requires a concerted approach combining fungicides, measures to reduce humidity, and the removal of mold-infested items whenever possible[84] (Table 26-4). A variety of fungicides are commercially available that are highly effective as long as the sites of mold growth are carefully investigated. Any measures that can then be taken to reduce humidity should be recommended, including dehumidification, air-conditioning, increased ventilation, and a ban on the use of humidifiers and vaporizers. Moldy items, such as a basement carpet that has suffered water damage, should be removed altogether. Although no specific data are available, air filtration devices may also assist in reducing mold exposure; no clinical studies on the efficacy of mold avoidance measures have been undertaken.

TABLE 26-4 Environmental Control of Mold Allergens

Identify sites/sources of mold growth
Clean moldy areas with a fungicide
If cleaning is not possible, discard moldy items (e.g., carpets, furniture)
Dehumidify
Repair leaks and maximize drainage
Run vent in bathroom and kitchen
Clean refrigerator, dehumidifier, and humidifier with fungicide

---

INDOOR AIR POLLUTION

Although a detailed discussion of indoor air pollution is beyond the scope of this chapter, it should be emphasized that effective environmental control cannot be achieved without attention to a variety nonspecific irritants. The deleterious effects of passive cigarette smoke on pediatric asthma have been well documented in a number of studies.[90-92] No studies to date have assessed the clinical benefit of removal from a smoke-containing environment, but one would predict that this would have highly beneficial effects. In addition to passive cigarette smoke, a variety of other indoor pollutants, such as nitrous oxide and wood smoke, have been documented to exacerbate pediatric asthma. All patients must therefore be queried about these exposures and counseled about their control. Parents who are smokers and who have asthmatic children need to be reminded at each visit about the ongoing damage that they are causing.

OUTDOOR ALLERGENS

There is far less ability to control exposure to outdoor allergens than indoor allergens. Source control is rarely an option because the airborne pollens and molds travel so widely. Local mold control may be accomplished by ensuring good drainage, removing leaves and other debris as they accumulate, and limiting the use of mulch and other ground cover that might support mold growth. Otherwise, exposure may be reduced by staying indoors when pollen and mold counts are high, as long as windows and doors are kept closed. An air filter may help to reduce exposure, especially if windows are being left open; some activities, such as lawn mowing or plowing, may need to be avoided altogether. After being outside, it is important that allergic individuals wash their hands and faces immediately and that they wash their hair daily. When outside, masks and goggles can be very effective but there are very few children and adolescents willing to wear them.

CONCLUSIONS

Indoor allergens are of tremendous importance to pediatric allergic disease (Box 26-1). Exposure is a risk factor for the development of asthma as well as for more severe disease. Thankfully, there are measures that can help to reduce exposure to most allergens, which can significantly reduce symptoms and medication requirements. The guidelines for the management of asthma that were published in 1997[93] made a very clear statement regarding the importance of indoor allergens and environmental control, stating that for any patient with persistent asthma, the clinician should (1) identify allergen exposures; (2) use skin testing or *in vitro* testing to assess specific sensitivities to indoor allergens; and (3) implement environmental controls to reduce exposure to relevant allergens. They concluded by saying that "the first and most important step in controlling allergen-induced asthma is to reduce exposure to relevant indoor and outdoor allergens." With all the time, effort, and money put forth for the use of medications and immunotherapy for asthma and allergic rhinitis, it is very important that we do not lose sight of this logical and vitally important recommendation.

KEY CONCEPTS

Indoor Allergens Are Important Causes of Allergic Disease

- The major indoor allergens include dust mite, animal dander, cockroach, and mold.
- Indoor allergen exposure and sensitivity should be considered for all patients with chronic allergic symptoms, including asthma, allergic rhinitis, and atopic dermatitis.
- Allergen avoidance should be considered the first line of therapy for patients with indoor allergen sensitivities.
- Allergen avoidance should be approached with specific environmental control measures based on the patient's sensitivities and exposures.

HELPFUL WEBSITES

Allergy Web website (www.allergyweb.com)
The American Academy of Allergy, Asthma and Immunology website (www.aaaai.org/)
The American College of Allergy, Asthma and Immunology website (www.acaai.org/)
The Asthma and Allergy Foundation of America website (www.aafa.org/)

REFERENCES

1. Platts-Mills TAE, De Weck A: Dust mite allergens and asthma—a worldwide problem, *Bull WHO* 66:769-780, 1989.
2. Platts-Mills TAE, Thomas WR, Aalberse RC, et al: Dust mite allergens and asthma: report of a second international workshop, *J Allergy Clin Immunol* 89:1046-1060, 1992.
3. Arlian LG, Platts-Mills TAE: The biology of dust mites and the remediation of mite allergens in allergic disease, *J Allergy Clin Immunol* 107: S406-S413, 2001.
4. Arlian LG: Biology and ecology of house dust mites *Dermatophagoides* spp. and *Euroglyphus* spp, *Immunol Allergy Clin North Am* 9:339-356, 1989.
5. Kueher J, Frischer J, Meiner R, et al: Mite exposure is a risk factor for the incidence of specific sensitization, *J Allergy Clin Immunol* 94:44-52, 1994.
6. Lau S, Falkenhorst G, Weber A, et al: High mite-allergen exposure increases the risk of sensitization in atopic children and young adults, *J Allergy Clin Immunol* 84:718-725, 1989.
7. Peat JK, Tovey E, Mellis CM, et al: Importance of house dust mite and *Alternaria* allergens in childhood asthma: an epidemiological study in two climatic regions of Australia, *Clin Exp Allergy* 23:812-820, 1993.
8. Sporik R, Holgate ST, Platts-Mills TAE, et al: Exposure to house-dust mite allergen (Der p I) and the development of asthma in childhood: a prospective study, *N Engl J Med* 323:502-507, 1990.
9. Call RS, Smith TF, Morris E, et al: Risk factors for asthma in inner-city children, *J Pediatr* 121:862-866, 1992.
10. Platts-Mills TAE, Heymann PW, Longbottom JL, et al: Airborne allergens associated with asthma: particle sizes carrying dust mite and rat allergens measured with a cascade impactor, *J Allergy Clin Immunol* 77:850-857, 1986.
11. Dowse GK, Turner KJ, Stewart GA, et al: The association between *Dermatophagoides* mites and the increasing prevalence of asthma in village communities within the Papua New Guinea highlands, *J Allergy Clin Immunol* 75:75-83, 1985.
12. Ingram JM, Sporik R, Rose G, et al: Quantitative assessment of exposure to dog (Can f 1) and cat (Fel d 1) allergens: relationship to sensitization and asthma among children living in Los Alamos, New Mexico, *J Allergy Clin Immunol* 96:449-456, 1995.
13. Burrows B, Sears MR, Flannery EM, et al: Relations of bronchial responsiveness to allergy skin test reactivity, lung function, respiratory symptoms and diagnoses in thirteen-year-old New Zealand children, *J Allergy Clin Immunol* 95:548-556, 1995.
14. Peat JK, Tovey ER, Toelle BG, et al: House-dust mite allergens: a major risk factor for childhood asthma in Australia, *Am J Respir Crit Care Med* 153:141-146, 1996.
15. Sears MR, Herbison GP, Holdaway MD, et al: The relative risk of sensitivity to grass pollen, house dust mite, and cat dander in the development of childhood asthma, *Clin Exp Allergy* 19:419-424, 1989.
16. Hide DW, Matthews S, Tariq S, et al: Allergen avoidance in infancy and allergy at 4 years of age, *Allergy* 51:89-93, 1996.
17. Custovic A, Taggart SCO, Francis HC, et al: Exposure to house dust mite allergens and the clinical activity of asthma, *J Allergy Clin Immunol* 98: 64-72, 1996.
18. Kivity S, Solomon A, Soferman R, et al: Mite asthma in childhood: a study of the relationship between exposure to house dust mites and disease activity, *J Allergy Clin Immunol* 91:844-849, 1993.
19. Vervloet D, Charpin D, Haddi E, et al: Medication requirements and house dust mite exposure in mite-sensitive asthmatics, *Allergy* 46: 554-558, 1991.
20. Pollart SM, Chapman MD, Fiocco GP, et al: Epidemiology of acute asthma: IgE antibodies to common inhalant allergens as a risk factor for emergency room visits, *J Allergy Clin Immunol* 83:875-882, 1989.
21. Platts-Mills TAE, Tovey ER, Mitchell EB, et al: Reduction of bronchial hyperreactivity following prolonged allergen avoidance, *Lancet* ii:675-678, 1982.
22. Murray AB, Ferguson AC: Dust-free bedrooms in the treatment of asthmatic children with house dust or house dust mite allergy, *Pediatrics* 71:418-422, 1983.
23. Carswell F, Birmingham K, Weeks J, et al: The respiratory effects of reduction of mite allergen in bedrooms of asthmatic children: a double-blind controlled trial, *Clin Exp Allergy* 26:386-396, 1996.
24. Dietemann A, Bessot JC, Hoyet C, et al: A double-blind, placebo-controlled trial of solidified benzyl benzoate applied in dwellings of asthmatic patients sensitive to mites: clinical efficacy and effect on mite allergens, *J Allergy Clin Immunol* 1993:91:738-746.
25. Ehnert B, Lau-Schadendorf S, Weber A, et al: Reducing domestic exposure to dust mite allergen reduces bronchial hyperreactivity in sensitive children with asthma, *J Allergy Clin Immunol* 90:135-138, 1992.
26. Gillies DRN, Littlewood JM, Sarsfield JK: Controlled trial of house dust mite avoidance in children with mild to moderate asthma, *Clin Allergy* 105-111, 1987.
27. Peroni DG, Boner AL, Vallone G, et al: Effective allergen avoidance at high-altitude reduced allergen-induced bronchial hyerresponsiveness, *Am J Resp Crit Care Med* 149:1442-1446, 1994.
28. Owen S, Morganstern M, Hepworth J, et al: Control of house dust mite antigen in bedding, *Lancet* 335:396-397, 1990.
29. Tovey E, Marks G, Shearer M, et al: Allergens and occlusive bed covers, *Lancet* 342:126, 1993.
30. Kalra S, Owen SJ, Hepworth J, et al: Airborne house dust mite antigen after vacuum cleaning, *Lancet* 336:449, 1990.
31. de Bohr R: The control of house dust mite allergens in rugs, *J Allergy Clin Immunol* 86:808-814, 1990.
32. Wassenaar DP: Effectiveness of vacuum cleaning and wet cleaning in reducing house dust mites, fungi and mite allergen in a cotton carpet: a case study, *Exp Appl Acarol* 4:53-62, 1988.
33. Colloff MJ: House dust mites - part II. Chemical control, *Pestic Outlook* 1:3-8, 1990.
34. Colloff MJ, Ayres J, Carswell F, et al: The control of allergens of dust mites and domestic pets: a position paper, *Clin Exp Allergy* 22:1-28, 1992.
35. Russell DW, Fernandez-Caldas E, Swanson MC, et al: Caffeine, a naturally occurring acaricide, *J Allergy Clin Immunol* 87:107-110, 1992.
36. Mitchell EB, Wilkins S, Deighton J, et al: Reduction of house dust mite levels in the home: use of the acaricide, pirimiphos methyl, *Clin Allergy* 15:235-240, 1985.
37. Hayden ML, Rose G, Diduch KB, et al: Benzyl benzoate moist powder: investigation of acaricidal activity in cultures and reduction of dust mite allergens in carpets, *J Allergy Clin Immunol* 89:536-545, 1992.
38. Lau-Schadendorf S, Rusche AF, Weber AK, et al: Short-term effect of solidified benzyl benzoate on mite-allergen concentrations in house dust, *J Allergy Clin Immunol* 87:41-47, 1991.
39. Woodfolk JA, Hayden ML, Couture N, et al: Chemical treatment of carpets to remove allergen, *J Allergy Clin Immunol* 96:325-333, 1996.
40. Huss RW, Huss K, Squire EN, et al: Mite allergen control with acaricide fails, *J Allergy Clin Immunol* 94:27-32, 1994.
41. Woodfolk J, Hayden M, Miller J, et al: Chemical treatment of carpets to reduce allergen: a detailed study of the effects of tannic acid on indoor allergens, *J Allergy Clin Immunol* 94:19-26, 1994.

42. Tovey ER, Marks GB, Matthews M, et al: Changes in mite allergen *Der p 1* in house dust following spraying with a tannic acid/acaricide solution, *Clin Exp Allergy* 22:67-74, 1992.

43. McDonald LG, Tovey ER: The role of water temperature and laundry procedures in reducing house dust mite populations and allergen content of bedding, *J Allergy Clin Immunol* 90:599-608, 1992.

44. Vendenhove T, Soler M, Birnbaum J, et al: Effect of dry cleaning on the mite allergen levels in blankets, *Allergy* 48:264-266, 1993.

45. Dodin A, Rak H: Influence of low temperature on the different stages of the human allergy mite *Dermatophagoides pteronyssinus, J Med Entomol* 30:810-811, 1993.

46. Tovey E, Woolcock A: Direct exposure of carpets to sunlight can kill all mites, *J Allergy Clin Immunol* 93:1072-1074, 1993.

47. Mosbech H, Korsgaard J, Lind P: Control of house dust mites by electrical heating blankets, *J Allergy Clin Immunol* 81:706-710, 1988.

48. Colloff MJ: Dust mite control and mechanical ventilation: when the climate is right (editorial), *Clin Exp Allergy* 24:94-96, 1994.

49. Korsgaard J, Iversen M: Epidemiology of house dust mite allergy, *Allergy* 46:14-18, 1991.

50. Custovic A, Taggart S, Kennaugh J, et al: Portable dehumidifiers in the control of house dust mites and mite allergens, *Clin Exp Allergy* 25:312-316, 1995.

51. Arlian LG, Neal JS, Vyszenski-Moher HL: Reducing humidity to control the house dust mite *Dermatophagoides farinae, J Allergy Clin Immunol* 104:852-856, 1999.

52. Antonicelli L, Bilo MB, Pucci S, et al: Efficacy of an air-cleaning device equipped with a high-efficiency particulate air filter in house dust mite respiratory allergy, *Allergy* 46:594-600, 1991.

53. Nelson HS, Roger Hirsch S, Ohman JL Jr, et al: Recommendations for the use of residential air-cleaning devices in the treatment of respiratory diseases, *J Allergy Clin Immunol* 82:661-669, 1988.

54. Reisman R, Mauriello P, Davis G, et al: A double-blind study of the effectiveness of a high-efficiency particulate air (HEPA) filter in the treatment of patients with perennial allergic rhinitis and asthma, *J Allergy Clin Immunol* 85:1050-1059, 1990.

55. Warner JA, Marchant JL, Warner JO: Double-blind trial of ionisers in children with asthma sensitive to the house dust mite, *Thorax* 48:330-333, 1993.

56. Chapman MD, Wood RA: The role and remediation of animal allergens in allergic diseases, *J Allergy Clin Immunol* 107:S414-S421, 2001.

57. Sporik R, Ingram JM, Price W, et al: Association of asthma with serum IgE and skin-test reactivity to allergens among children living at high altitude: tickling the dragon's breath, *Am J Respir Crit Care Med* 151:1388-1392, 1995.

58. Munir AKM, Bjorksten B, Einarsson R, et al: Cat (Fel d I), dog (Can f 1) and cockroach allergens in homes of asthmatic children from three climatic zones in Sweden, *Allergy* 49:508-516, 1994.

59. Rosenstreich DL, Eggleston P, Kattan M, et al: The role of cockroach allergy and exposure to cockroach allergen in causing morbidity among inner-city children with asthma, *N Engl J Med* 336:1356-1363, 1997.

60. Wood RA, Eggleston PA, Ingemann L, et al: Antigenic analysis of household dust samples, *Am Rev Resp Dis* 137:358-363, 1988.

61. Wood RA, Chapman MD, Adkinson NF, et al: The effect of cat removal on allergen content in household dust samples, *J Allergy Clin Immunol* 83:730-734, 1989.

62. Wood RA, Mudd KE, Eggleston PA: The distribution of cat and dust mite allergens on wall surfaces, *J Allergy Clin Immunol* 89:126-130, 1992.

63. Wood RA, Laheri AN, Eggleston PA: The aerodynamic characteristics of cat allergen, *Clin Exp Allergy* 23:733-739, 1993.

64. Luczynska CM, Li Y, Chapman MD, et al: Airborne concentrations and particle size distribution of allergen derived from domestic cats (*Felis domesticus), Am Rev Respir Dis* 141:361-367, 1990.

65. Custovic A, Green R, Pickering CAC, et al: Major dog allergen Can f 1: distribution in homes, airborne levels, and particle sizing (abstract), *J Allergy Clin Immunol* 97:302, 1996.

66. Bollinger ME, Eggleston PA, Wood RA: Cat antigen in homes with and without cats may induce allergic symptoms, *J Allergy Clin Immunol* 97:907-914, 1996.

67. Van der Brempt X, Charpin D, Haddi E, et al: Cat removal and Fel d 1 levels in mattresses, *J Allergy Clin Immunol* 87:595-596, 1991.

68. De Blay F, Chapman MD, Platts-Mills TAE: Airborne cat allergen (Fel d 1): environmental control with the cat *in situ, Am Rev Respir Dis* 143:1334-1339, 1991.

69. Klucka CV, Ownby DR, Green J, et al: Cat shedding of Fel d 1 is not reduced by washings, Allerpet-C spray, or acepromazine, *J Allergy Clin Immunol* 95:1164-1171, 1995.

70. Avner DB, Perzanowski MS, Platts-Mills TAE, et al: Evaluation of different techniques for washing cats: quantitation of allergen removed from the cat and effect on airborne Fel d 1, *J Allergy Clin Immunol* 100:357-362, 1997.

71. Bjornsdottir US, Jakobinudottir S, Runarsdottir V, et al: Environmental control with cat *in situ* reduces cat allergen in house dust samples but does it alter clinical symptoms? *J Allergy Clin Immunol* 99:S389, 1997.

72. Soldatov D, De Blay F, Greiss P, et al: Effects of environmental control measures on patient status and airborne Fel d 1 levels with a cat *in situ, J Allergy Clin Immunol* 95:263, 1995.

73. Wood RA, Johnson EF, Van Natta ML, et al: A placebo-controlled trial of a HEPA air cleaner in the treatment of cat allergy, *Am J Resp Crit Care Med* 158:115-120, 1998.

74. Van der Heide S, van Aalderen WMC, Kaufmann HF, et al: Clinical effects of air cleaners in homes of allergic children sensitized to pet allergens, *J Allergy Clin Immunol* 104:447-451, 1999.

75. Eggleston PA, Arruda LK: Ecology and elimination of cockroaches and allergens in the home, *J Allergy Clin Immunol* 107:S422-S429, 2001.

76. Kang BC, Johnson J, Veres-Thorner C: Atopic profile of inner-city asthma with a comparative analysis on the cockroach-sensitive and ragweed-sensitive subgroups, *J Allergy Clin Immunol* 92:802-811, 1993.

77. Sarpong SB, Hamilton RG, Eggleston PA, et al: Socioeconomic status and race as risk factors for cockroach allergen exposure and sensitization in children with asthma, *J Allergy Clin Immunol* 97:1393-1401, 1996.

78. Arruda LK, Vailes LD, Mann BJ, et al: Molecular cloning of a major cockroach (*Blattella germanica*) allergen, Bla g 2, *J Biol Chem* 270:19563-19568, 1995.

79. Pollart S, Smith TF, Morris EC, et al: Environmental exposure to cockroach allergens: analysis with monoclonal antibody-based enzyme immunoassays, *J Allergy Clin Immunol* 87:505-510, 1995.

80. Sarpong S, Wood RA, Karrison T, et al: Cockroach allergen (Bla g 1) in school dust, *J Allergy Clin Immunol* 99:486-492, 1997.

81. Sarpong SB, Wood RA, Eggleston PA: Short-term effects of extermination and cleaning on cockroach allergen Bla g 2 in settled dust, *Ann Allergy Asthma Immunol* 76:257-260, 1996.

82. Eggleston PA, Wood Ra, Rand C, et al: Removal of cockroach allergen from inner-city homes, *J Allergy Clin Immunol* 104:842-846, 1999.

83. Wood RA, Eggleston PA, Rand C, et al: Cockroach allergen abatement with sodium hypochlorite in inner-city homes, *Annals Allergy* 87:60-64, 2001.

84. Bush RK, Portnoy JM: The role and abatement of fungal allergens in allergic diseases, *J Allergy Clin Immunol* 107:S430-S440, 2001.

85. Burge HA: Fungus allergens, *Clin Rev Allergy* 3:319-329, 1985.

86. Sporik RB, Arruda LK, Woodfolk J, et al: Environmental exposure to *Aspergillus fumigatus (Asp f I), Clin Exp Allergy* 23:326-331, 1993.

87. Halonen M, Stern D, Wright AL, et al: *Alternaria* as a major allergen for asthma in children raised in a desert environment, *Am J Respir Crit Care Med* 155:1356-1361, 1997.

88. Burge HA, Solomon W, Boise JR: Microbial prevalence in domestic humidifiers, *Appl Environ Microbiol* 39:840-844, 1980.

89. Kumar P, Lopez M, Fan W, et al: Mold contamination of automobile air conditioner systems, *Annals Allergy* 64:174-177, 1990.

90. Chilmonczyk BA, Salmun LM, Megathlin KN, et al: Association between exposure to environmental tobacco smoke and exacerbations of asthma in children, *N Engl J Med* 328:1665-1669, 1993.

91. Wright AL, Holberg C, Martinez FD, et al: Relationship of parental smoking to wheezing and nonwheezing lower respiratory tract illnesses in infancy, *J Pediatr* 118:207-214, 1991.

92. Cook DG, Strachan DP: Health effects of passive smoking, *Thorax* 54:357-366, 1999.

93. National Institutes of Health: Highlights of the Expert Panel Report 2: Guidelines for the diagnosis and management of asthma, 1997, Bethesda, Md, NIH Pub No. 97-4051A.

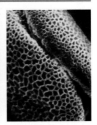

CHAPTER 27

Immunotherapy for Allergic Disease

ELIZABETH C. MATSUI ■ PEYTON A. EGGLESTON

In 1911, Noon[1] found that by administering increasing doses of grass pollen extract, he could induce a marked decrease in conjunctival sensitivity to grass pollen. It was this observation that eventually led to the widespread use of immunotherapy for the treatment of allergic disease.[1] *Immunotherapy* is the term used to describe a prolonged process of repeated injections of extracts of pollens or other allergens administered to patients with rhinitis or asthma who have a demonstrable allergic etiology for the purpose of reducing the symptoms of hay fever or asthma. It has also been called *desensitization* or *allergy injection therapy*. It is recommended in most discussions of the treatment of allergic airway disease, along with allergen avoidance and symptomatic drug therapy; a considerable proportion of the millions spent on the treatment of allergic disease each year goes to the manufacture and use of allergen extracts.

PRINCIPLES OF IMMUNOTHERAPY

In allergic rhinitis (AR), the effectiveness of immunotherapy has been demonstrated in many carefully conducted placebo-controlled trials. The results of a typical clinical trial are shown in Figure 27-1.[2] Three groups of patients matched on the basis of their allergic sensitivity to ragweed allergen were treated with injections of whole ragweed pollen extracts or placebo. Although everyone became symptomatic during the ragweed pollen season, it is obvious that those receiving placebo injections were more symptomatic than those receiving pollen extracts. It is important to recognize that in this clinical trial, the symptoms of hay fever from natural allergen exposure were effectively reduced. These trials have been reviewed in detail elsewhere and are addressed here only to review the principles learned for the safe and effective use of immunotherapy.

The first principle is that clinical effectiveness is dose dependent; that is, a certain minimal dose of allergen extract must be administered to produce effective symptomatic control.[3] These extracts are prepared by suspending source material (pollen, mold spores, dust mites, or animal pelts) in buffers to extract the water-soluble components into the buffer; they are now available commercially under license by the Food and Drug Administration. They are complex mixtures of dozens of proteins, of which only a few are allergenic. Clinical trials that compare treatment with purified allergens or with partially purified extracts containing high concentrations of allergens with treatment with currently available crude extracts have shown them to be equally effective. For instance, symptoms are reduced to a similar extent with immunotherapy with purified ragweed antigen E and with whole ragweed extract in the study illustrated in Figure 27-1. A corollary of this point is that only a limited number of materials are recommended for specific immunotherapy.

Another lesson from these studies is that therapeutic effectiveness increases with time. Significant improvement is generally not seen before 6 months or more of therapy.[4] It is not clear why such a long time is needed, but in part it reflects the time required to increase the injected dose from the very small dose that can be tolerated initially to the 10,000-fold higher dose that produces immunologic and clinical effects. Clinical benefit increases for several years after the maximal doses of antigens are achieved. Although the reason for the delayed effect of immunotherapy is not clear, it is important to discuss with patients so that their expectations will be realistic.

As shown in Figure 27-1, symptom scores in patients treated with active allergens are significantly lower than those treated with placebo. In other trials when symptom scores are compared with those in untreated patients, symptoms in those treated with placebo are reduced as well. This placebo effect is especially easy to see in the asthma trials in which most placebo-treated patients improve and 25% to 30% improve significantly.[4] For clinical investigators, this fact has made it absolutely essential to include a placebo group in any immunotherapy trial. For clinicians, it is important to recognize that there is a significant and powerful placebo effect associated with the repeated injections and frequent visits with sympathetic physicians and nurses. Only by administering concentrated antigen preparations to carefully selected patients are the benefits greater than those seen with sympathetic support.

For most patients, symptomatic improvement is partial and immunotherapy serves to decrease the severity of symptoms without totally eliminating them. In addition, a significant number of allergic patients, perhaps as many as 25%, do not benefit from therapy regardless of the potency of the antigen or the length of therapy. The reasons why certain patients are "nonresponders" are unclear, but the point is an important one to bear in mind when discussing immunotherapy with patients.

In clinical trials, a high incidence of systemic anaphylactic reactions is usually reported. These are usually mild and not life threatening but may require epinephrine therapy. Such reactions are not surprising because patients were selected who were clearly allergic on the basis of skin tests and radioallergosorbent

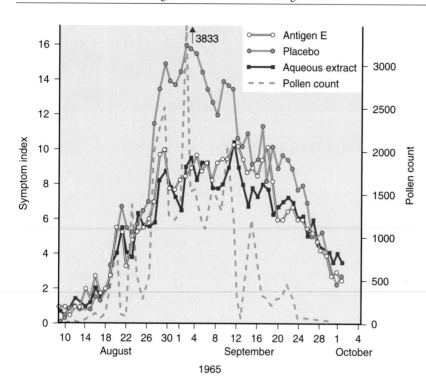

FIGURE 27-1 Typical result of an immunotherapy trial in patients allergic to ragweed pollen. (From Norman PS, Winkenwerder WL, Lichtenstein LM, et al: *J Allergy Clin Immunol* 42:93-108, 1968.)

tests (RASTs) and who had severe symptoms on allergen exposure and were administered repeated injections of the offending allergen. Although the patient population in clinical trials is more highly sensitive than that encountered in most clinical practices, even in a large clinical series 7% of patients experienced at least one systemic reaction, most of which were mild and responded to a single injection of epinephrine.[5] Therapy with newer, modified antigens is associated with much fewer systemic reactions, but they still occur. Thus the clinician should insist that the patient remain in the office for 20 to 30 minutes after an injection and should have the equipment and training to deal with an anaphylactic reaction.

The concept that efficacy of immunotherapy is dependent on dose and duration of dose has been known for decades. In fact, a movement to standardize allergen extracts is under way, in large part to ensure that patients receive adequate dosing during immunotherapy. There has also been much interest in accelerating the time to efficacy for immunotherapy, and many studies examining rush and ultrarush immunotherapy have been published. Investigators have also been studying adjuvants to improve efficacy of immunotherapy as well as modified allergens to reduce the risk of serious reactions to immunotherapy. Other routes of administering allergen extracts are also being studied, as well as the use of immunotherapy for other allergic diseases such as food allergy. Finally, therapies targeted at immune mediators are currently in clinical trials; these include agents such as anti-IgE and anticytokine therapies. All of these new directions are addressed in further detail in this chapter.

MECHANISMS OF ACTION

Many observations about patients' immunologic and cellular responses to immunotherapy have been made, but the precise mechanism of action of immunotherapy remains unknown.

Many studies have been published examining the effects of immunotherapy on allergen-specific antibody responses, inflammatory cells, and immune mediators and T cells. What is generally recognized is that skin test sensitivity decreases and allergen-specific IgG increases with immunotherapy.[6] It is not until after several years of immunotherapy that allergen-specific IgE decreases.[7] There has also been much speculation that immunotherapy acts on the T helper cell type 1 (Th1)/Th2 axis to shift the T cell phenotype away from the allergic Th2 phenotype.

Antibody Response and Immunotherapy

Studies have consistently demonstrated an increase in allergen-specific IgG and IgE within months of starting immunotherapy. One trial of ragweed immunotherapy in adults examined allergen-specific antibody responses. As can be seen in Figure 27-2, within months of starting immunotherapy, subjects demonstrated significant dose-dependent increases in ragweed-specific IgG long before symptom relief was seen. Ragweed-specific IgE initially increased and did not decrease until years into therapy.[7] Similar observations have been made by other investigators for both venom immunotherapy and inhalant allergen immunotherapy. It has been suggested that allergen-specific IgG acts as blocking antibody either by blocking antigen binding by IgE or by preventing aggregation of the high-affinity IgE receptor (FcERI) at the cell surface. To further confound the issue, the allergen-specific IgG response does not correlate with clinical efficacy, leaving many questions unanswered about the role, if any, of allergen-specific IgG in the clinical effectiveness of immunotherapy.[8] Another interesting observation is that in addition to the increase in allergen-specific IgE that accompanies immunotherapy, there is a blunting of the typical seasonal increase in allergen-specific IgE that is seen in untreated allergic patients.[9]

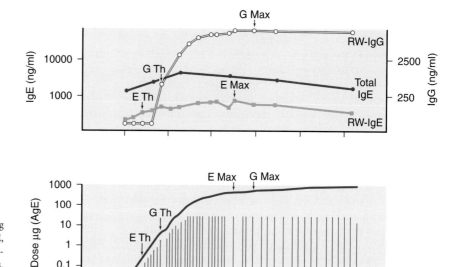

FIGURE 27-2 A profile of a typical patient receiving ragweed immunotherapy. **Top,** Ragweed-specific IgE, IgG, and total IgE responses during ragweed immunotherapy plotted against time expressed in days. **Bottom,** Cumulative dose *(curve)* and single doses *(lines)* plotted against time expressed in days. (From Creticos PS, Van Metre TE, Mardiney MR, et al: *J Allergy Clin Immunol* 73:94-104, 1984.)

Effects on T Cells

Because a Th2 phenotype has been associated with allergic disease and a Th1 phenotype with protection against allergic disease, it has been hypothesized that immunotherapy exerts its effects through modulation of the T helper phenotype. This modulation may result in either a shift from the Th2 to Th1 phenotype or through induction of CD8+ suppressor activity. Indeed, evidence has been published in support of both of these hypotheses. Rocklin et al[10] demonstrated the generation of allergen-specific suppressor cells during immunotherapy and provided evidence that the suppressor cells decrease IgE synthesis. Other studies have examined the cytokine profile of peripheral blood Th2 cells and demonstrated decreases in interleukin (IL)-4 production and, in some cases, concomitant increases in interferon (IFN)-γ production, suggesting a modulation of the T helper phenotype from Th2 to Th1. One study demonstrated an increase in IFN-γ production after allergen provocation in nasal mucosal biopsy specimens after 12 months of immunotherapy for seasonal AR, demonstrating a local phenotypic shift in T cells.[11]

Effects on Inflammatory Cells

There also is evidence that immunotherapy affects mast cells, basophils, and eosinophils. One study demonstrated a significant decrease in metachromatic cells (mast cells and basophils) in nasal scrapings after dust mite immunotherapy.[12] Ragweed immunotherapy has also been demonstrated to decrease peripheral blood basophil histamine release.[13] In addition, successful immunotherapy has been associated with a decrease in the numbers of eosinophils from nasal and bronchial specimens. Nasal eosinophils were significantly reduced before and 24 hours after nasal challenge in patients receiving ragweed immunotherapy.[14] Similar findings have been documented by other investigators in both nasal and pulmonary studies.[11,15]

SPECIFIC DISEASE INDICATIONS

Although immunotherapy has been demonstrated to be effective for stinging insect hypersensitivity, AR, and allergic asthma, appropriate patient selection is imperative. In the case of stinging insect hypersensitivity, children with a history of a life-threatening reaction combined with evidence of venom-specific IgE warrant treatment with immunotherapy. Immunotherapy should be considered for the treatment of AR in those patients with evidence of clinically relevant allergen-specific IgE, significant symptoms despite reasonable avoidance measures (e.g., dust mite allergen–proof mattress and pillow covers), and maximal medical therapy. Although similar criteria apply to patients with asthma, poorly controlled asthma is a contraindication for immunotherapy because of the risk of severe systemic reactions for these patients.

Allergic Rhinitis

Immunotherapy has been demonstrated to be quite effective in both seasonal and perennial AR. Several well-designed studies have examined the efficacy of immunotherapy for both ragweed- and grass-allergic patients with seasonal AR.[16,17] Both studies were randomized, controlled trials and demonstrated significant symptom relief for the treatment arms. Immunotherapy has also been shown to be effective for mite-induced perennial AR[18] and may also be effective in mold-induced rhinitis.[19] The duration of treatment is generally 3 to 5 years, and patients continue to have improvement in symptoms after discontinuing immunotherapy. Long-term efficacy was demonstrated for grass seasonal AR in a placebo-controlled, blinded study. Three years after discontinuing immunotherapy, the active treatment group continued to have decreased seasonal rhinitis symptoms and decreased medication use compared with the placebo arm.[20]

Asthma

Many studies in the past decade have examined the efficacy of immunotherapy for allergic asthma.[6,21-23] Certainly allergic sensitization and subsequent allergen exposure contribute significantly to asthma morbidity in children, making immunotherapy an appealing option for children with allergic asthma. However, IgE-mediated mechanisms are only part of the underlying pathophysiology of asthma, making the rationale for immunotherapy as a treatment option in allergic asthma less straightforward.

Results of clinical trials examining the efficacy of immunotherapy in allergic asthma have been conflicting. To complicate matters further, many studies have not included placebo arms, making it difficult to draw any conclusions about efficacy from those studies. Abramson et al[24] conducted a meta-analysis of randomized, controlled trials for immunotherapy in asthma. Twenty trials met inclusion criteria of being double blind, randomized, and placebo controlled. Nine trials examined dust mite immunotherapy; five, pollen; five, animal dander; and one, mold. After analysis of the combined results from these trials, immunotherapy was found to reduce bronchial hyperreactivity and medication use and to improve asthma symptoms. These results were statistically significant. The results were similar when the dust mite trials were analyzed separately. The effects of immunotherapy on pulmonary function were less pronounced.

A comprehensive review also concluded that immunotherapy is effective in the treatment of asthma but in carefully selected circumstances.[25] The authors concluded that immunotherapy is effective in grass pollen asthma but that results from studies for ragweed asthma were inconclusive. In addition, mite immunotherapy with standardized extracts was effective in reducing symptoms and increasing the threshold dose of mite extract needed to induce bronchial obstruction in bronchial challenges. The authors also make the point that children receiving mite immunotherapy benefited to a greater extent than adults.

Immunotherapy for animal-induced asthma has been more controversial. Some proponents of immunotherapy believe that there is a role for animal immunotherapy in the treatment of asthmatic patients who live with pets, but consensus statements from respected international organizations maintain that allergen avoidance is first-line therapy for these patients.[26] There have been carefully conducted, placebo-controlled trials demonstrating the efficacy of specific immunotherapy for cat asthma.[22] Studies have demonstrated a decrease in the quantitative airway responsiveness to cat allergen and decreased skin test reactivity in those treated with cat immunotherapy, but studies examining improvement in clinical symptoms have been inconclusive.

Clinical trials evaluating mold immunotherapy for asthma have been published for *Alternaria* and *Cladosporium*. One of the *Cladosporium* trials was conducted in children and demonstrated an increase in the *Cladosporium* provocative dose, causing a 20% drop in forced expiratory volume in 1 second (PD_{20} FEV_1) but did not provide good evidence of a decrease in symptoms or medication use.[19] Some studies evaluating *Alternaria* immunotherapy have demonstrated an improvement in asthma symptoms and a decrease in medication use. Although there is evidence to support the addition of certain mold extracts to an immunotherapy prescription, more

data are needed before any firm conclusions can be made about immunotherapy in mold asthma.

Many studies support a role for immunotherapy in the treatment of allergic asthma, but there have been some studies that have not demonstrated the efficacy of immunotherapy for asthma. One of these was a well-conducted, placebo-controlled trial of immunotherapy for children with allergic asthma, and the investigators found little evidence to support the efficacy of immunotherapy.[6] One hundred twenty-one children with moderate to severe asthma were randomly assigned to receive either polyvalent immunotherapy (i.e., a mixture of extracts of various allergens) or placebo. Both groups demonstrated statistically significant improvements in medication use and PD_{20} FEV_1. The improvement seen in the treatment group was not statistically significantly better than that seen in the placebo group. Despite the negative results of this well-conducted study, many other published studies have demonstrated the efficacy of immunotherapy for allergic asthma. One of the major differences in this trial is that multiple allergen extracts were included in the injections. Although this is the usual approach to immunotherapy for allergic asthma in the United States, European standards require therapy with a single allergen extract (e.g., dust mite, cat, *Alternaria*), and this trial is the only one dealing with polyvalent immunotherapy. It is possible that this approach differs in some important way from immunotherapy with single-allergen extracts. Perhaps the keys to efficacious immunotherapy include careful patient selection and the use of standardized extracts at therapeutic doses. Patients should have reversible obstructive lung disease and demonstrate allergic sensitization to allergens that is consistent with the clinical picture. Moreover, immunotherapy formulations should focus on those allergens for which evidence of efficacy exists. Duration of treatment has been addressed for immunotherapy for AR, but the appropriate duration for asthma immunotherapy remains unclear.

Stinging Insect

Immunotherapy for venom allergy is highly efficacious, affording protection for more than 95% of individuals undergoing treatment.[27] Although venom immunotherapy is indicated in adults with evidence of IgE to Hymenoptera venom and a history of a systemic reaction to Hymenoptera, the indications in children are somewhat different. Studies of the natural history of venom allergy in children indicate that the risk of a serious reaction from a subsequent sting for a child with a history of a cutaneous systemic reaction is small. There is an approximately 10% incidence of subsequent systemic reactions in this patient population and a 0.4% incidence of more severe reactions involving the respiratory and cardiovascular systems.[28] In light of these findings, venom immunotherapy has been reserved for those children who have had "life-threatening" reactions to Hymenoptera as well as evidence of IgE to Hymenoptera venom[29] (see also Chapter 59).

Food

Although immunotherapy is not a recommended treatment for food allergy, this treatment option is being actively investigated. One randomized trial of immunotherapy for peanut allergy demonstrated increased tolerance to peanut allergen, but the incidence of systemic reactions to the peanut immunotherapy was substantial.[30] The six patients receiving immunotherapy experienced a mean of 34.7 systemic reactions and required a mean of 9.8 epinephrine injections. The evidence of efficacy of immunotherapy for peanut allergy is encouraging, but the risk is substantial and remains the primary obstacle to immunotherapy becoming a viable treatment modality for food allergy.

PRACTICAL CONSIDERATIONS

Patient Selection

Allergic Rhinitis

Immunotherapy should be considered for patients with clear evidence of IgE-mediated symptoms who have not been adequately controlled with first-line medical therapy, including antihistamines, nasal corticosteroids, and ocular antihistamines or antiinflammatory medications. Other aspects of the patient's history should be taken into consideration. For example, successful immunotherapy requires that a patient be able to visit a physician's office weekly and spend a minimum of 30 minutes there. Certain medications, such as beta blockers, put a patient at higher risk for systemic reactions to immunotherapy.

Asthma

Although some of the same principles of patient selection apply, immunotherapy for asthma deserves separate commentary. Like AR, patients must have demonstrable IgE to allergens to which they are exposed and the clinical history should be consistent with exacerbation of asthma symptoms with exposure to the allergens. A patient's ability to visit a medical facility weekly, as well as his or her medications and age, should be taken into consideration. Immunotherapy may be appropriate for treating asthma that has been difficult to control, but it should not be prescribed for patients with unstable asthma and an FEV_1 less than 70% of that predicted, so it may be least appropriate for patients who continue to have clinical symptoms of asthma despite maximal medical therapy. It should be emphasized that every clinical situation is unique and guidelines cannot replace clinical judgment.

Allergen Extracts

Allergen Extracts for Immunotherapy

Allergen extracts are prepared by extracting bulk source materials (e.g., pollens, mite cultures, fungal cultures) in aqueous buffers; typically the potency of these extracts is expressed in a ratio of the weight of source material extracted

to the extraction volume, such as 1:10 wt/:v. Variations in the bulk sources and in the manufacturing process have led to vast differences in the quantity of active allergens in these extracts. A second approach to labeling is based on the total protein content of the extract and is expressed in protein nitrogen units (PNUs); this method has little relationship to allergenic potency but is still commonly used in the United States. Efforts to standardize extracts in Europe and the United States have produced fundamentally different approaches. One approach measures the content of the major allergen or allergens in the mixture using crossed immunoelectrophoresis, immunodiffusion, RAST inhibition, or enzyme-linked immunosorbent assay. Another approach compares the biologic activity of the material with the diameter of a control intradermal injection of histamine and expresses this as a BU (biologic unit). The U.S. Food and Drug Administration uses a slightly different approach to establish a BU, in which the wheal diameter of reference extract in a select group of allergic volunteers is compared with a reference extract and expresses the result in allergen units (AU) or bioequivalent allergen units (BAU). The results are somewhat confusing, and most commercially available extracts are labeled with more than one method to try to simplify administration of the materials. Studies that have established guidelines for effective maintenance doses for particular allergens report these doses in micrograms of major allergen, but translating wt/v, PNU, BU, AU, or BAU into microgram doses can be difficult. Fortunately, some products have also been standardized by the major allergen concentration expressed as micrograms per milliliter (μg/ml). There are also some data translating allergen content into micrograms of major allergen; this information may be helpful in guiding dosing decisions. Table 27-1 is adapted from a recent comparison of labeling methods.[31] Where they are available, standardized extracts should always be used for therapy.

Storage

Some loss of potency is usual over time; therefore, manufactured extracts are supplied with expiration dates. These expiration dates are based on the assumption that the extracts will be refrigerated because loss of activity is more rapid at temperatures above 5° C. Loss of potency is faster in more diluted solutions, but it can be decreased by the addition of 50% glycerol or 0.03% human serum albumin; because glycerol is irritating, most allergen solutions are diluted in albumin-containing buffers. Fungus, dust mite, and cockroach extracts have been found to have significant protease activity[32] and therefore may accelerate the deterioration of allergen solutions. Some experts recommend that when making up

TABLE 27-1 Major Allergen Content of Extracts

Source	Label	Allergen	N	Mean (μg)	Maximum (μg)	Minimum (μg)
Orchard grass	100,000 BAU/ml	Dac g 5	14	918	2414	294
Short ragweed	1:10 wt/v	Amb a 1	13	268	458	87
D. farinae	10,000 AU/ml	Der f 1	18	44	72	30
Cat hair	10,000 BAU/ml	Fel d 1	12	40	52	26
Dog hair	1:10 wt/v	Can f 1	4	5.4	7.2	2.7

Modified from Nelson HS: *J Allergy Clin Immunol* 106:41-45, 2000.

immunotherapy solutions, dust mite, cockroach, and fungal extracts should be placed in vials separate from other allergen extracts that do not contain protease activity.

Injection Regimens

A prescription for immunotherapy should reflect the patient's demonstrated specific IgE-mediated sensitization, as well as the clinical history of symptoms on exposure and other medical illnesses. The decision is a complex one and should be made by a trained allergist rather than a manufacturer or testing service. Typically, a prescription is written for a treatment set, with one vial containing a 1:10 dilution of concentrated material from a manufacturer and three or four other vials containing tenfold dilutions (i.e., 1:100, 1:1000, and so on). Each vial of the set should be clearly labeled with the patient's name, the allergens contained in the vial, the dilution, and an expiration date.

Administration and Dosing

Dosing instructions are shown in Table 27-2, modified from Nelson.[33] The principle is that a dose is administered that is in general tenfold smaller than the dose that will induce a positive skin test; then increasing doses are administered weekly until a dose 1000 to 10,000 times greater is tolerated. In the sample dosing regimen given in Table 27-2, a 0.1-ml dose of vial A (the 1:10,000 dilution of the concentrated extract supplied by the manufacturer) is the first dose, and each week the volume injected from vial A increases until the dose reaches 0.8 ml. The next week, the dose is 0.1 ml from vial B (the 1:1000 dilution of the concentrated extract). This progression continues until 0.5 ml of the 1:10 dilution is administered. This is the maximum dose according to this particular protocol, and the patient continues to receive this dose every other week for the first year. Generally, it takes 6 months of weekly doses to reach the maintenance dose. If a systemic reaction occurs, a lower dose may become the maximum tolerated dose. Immunologic and clinical changes are not generally seen until the highest doses are administered. Alternative dosing schedules have been proposed in which the buildup doses are administered every 20 to 30 minutes (rush immunotherapy) or 2 or 3 times a week (cluster immunotherapy). All of these regimens allow a patient to reach the maintenance dose in a shorter period of time, but each has a greater risk of allergic reactions to the injections.

Duration of Immunotherapy

Once maintenance doses have been reached, these are generally continued for 3 years or longer. Although experience in adults differs somewhat, if a child is able to tolerate two sequential pollen seasons with minimal symptoms or none at all, they are able to stop immunotherapy without a relapse the next season.

Reactions to Immunotherapy

The risks of immunotherapy are not trivial. Clinical surveys report 3% to 7% of patients experience systemic reactions and that one reaction occurs for every 250 to 1600 injections.[5] Reactions may be limited to urticaria, but 40% to 73% include respiratory reactions (stridor, rhinitis, wheezing) and almost 10% include hypotension; fatal reactions occur in 1 per 2 to 3 million injections.[34] From 70% to 90% of reactions begin within the first 30 minutes of an injection. The risk of reactions is greater during the buildup phase, but about half of the reactions occur during maintenance therapy. Reactions are more common in adolescents and young adults and during pollen or mold seasons. Risk factors for serious systemic reactions include severe asthma, age of less than 5 years, and use of a beta blocker.[35] For these reasons, injections should be given in a medical facility and by personnel who know how to recognize and treat a local and systemic reaction to allergenic extract and who are trained in basic cardiopulmonary resuscitation.[36] Resuscitation equipment should be available (minimal equipment is summarized in Table 27-3). Patients should remain in the facility for 30 minutes after an injection and should report immediately if a reaction begins. Injections should not be administered at home.

TABLE 27-2 Allergen Extract Prescription

Begin with vial A and progress to vial D, which is the most concentrated, or "maintenance," solution. Injections should be administered subcutaneously every week until the highest maintenance dose is administered, 0.5 ml of vial D. Then repeat this dose every other week for the next year. After the first year, maintenance doses can be given every 3 to 4 weeks.

- Call the center before resuming treatment if the treatment has lapsed by 4 weeks or more.
- During the buildup phase, repeat a dose if the last dose produced local swelling of more than 3 cm in diameter (the size of a silver dollar) or if treatment lapses for 1 to 2 weeks.
- Drop back twofold (i.e., from 0.4 to 0.2 ml) if the previous dose has produced local swelling of 5 cm or more in diameter, if a mild systemic reaction occurs, or if treatment lapses for more than 2 weeks.
- Drop back fourfold (i.e., from 0.4 to 0.1 ml) if a systemic reaction occurs.
- The patient should remain for observation for 30 minutes after each injection.

Vial A (1:10,000)	Vial B (1:1000)	Vial C (1:100)	Vial D (1:10)
0.1 ml	0.1 ml	0.1 ml	0.1 ml
0.2 ml	0.2 ml	0.2 ml	0.15 ml
0.4 ml	0.4 ml	0.4 ml	0.2 ml
0.8 ml	0.8 ml	0.8 ml	0.3 ml
			0.4 ml
			0.5 ml

Modified from Nelson HS: Immunotherapy for inhalant allergens. In Middleton EJ, Reed CE, Ellis EF, et al, eds: *Allergy: principles and practice*, ed 5, St Louis, 1998, Mosby.

TABLE 27-3 Minimum Resuscitation Equipment for Administering Immunotherapy

Stethoscope	Equipment for administering intravenous fluids
Sphygmomanometer	
Tourniquet	Aqueous epinephrine 1:1000
Syringes and needles (some 14 gauge)	Injectable and oral diphenhydramine
Equipment for administering oxygen by mask	Intravenous corticosteroids
Oral airway	Injectable vasopressor

FUTURE DIRECTIONS

Allergoids and Adjuvants

Allergoids are produced by chemically modifying or denaturing native allergens. The goal is to retain the ability of the allergen to elicit an immunologic response (specifically a T cell response) while decreasing the risk of anaphylaxis (the IgE-mediated response). Various chemical agents have been used, including urea, glutaraldehyde, and polyethylene glycol. Although some of these agents have appeared promising, the inability to standardize the process of chemical modification has made this approach impractical. Adjuvants are used with the allergen extract to boost immunologic response to immunotherapy in hopes of increasing its efficacy. Substances such as alum, tyrosine absorbate, and Freund's adjuvant have been used with the rationale that they have the ability to boost Th1-type immune responses.[37] It remains unclear whether adjuvants improve the efficacy of immunotherapy.

Peptides and Recombinant Allergens

In the modern era of cloning and sequencing, many allergens have been characterized at the molecular level. As a result, recombinant allergens and allergen peptides can be produced and may have a future role in immunotherapy. As more is discovered about T cell epitopes, peptides of major allergens can be produced and used as a means of decreasing the risk of IgE-mediated reactions while retaining immunologic potency. In fact, fragments of both the dust mite allergens Der p 1 and Der f 1 and the cat allergen Fel d 1 were found to contain epitopes that were capable of inducing tolerance in mice.[38] This led to clinical trials that showed that injections of mixtures of small synthetic peptides containing the Fel d 1 epitope modified T cell responsiveness in allergic patients and decreased symptoms on exposure to cats.[39] The effects were modest, and it is not clear whether this will be a clinically useful therapy.

Immunostimulatory DNA

Immunostimulatory sequences (ISSs) are short base-pair segments of DNA that are thought to enhance a Th1 immune response by inducing IL-12 production. Preclinical studies are under way and appear to be promising.[40] The activity of ragweed protein-linked ISSs was studied in peripheral blood mononuclear cultures from subjects with ragweed allergy. The ISS-tagged ragweed protein resulted in an IFN-γ–predominant cytokine profile, whereas Amb a 1 alone promoted a Th2 profile with increased IL-4 and IL-5 production. The addition of ISS may prove to be an effective strategy to enhance the efficacy and reduce the risk of immunotherapy.

Immune Modulators

Many immunomodulators are being actively investigated as therapeutic strategies for allergic disease; these include treatment strategies aimed at IgE as well as those aimed at cytokines. Two such therapies that have made it to human trials are an anti-IgE humanized monoclonal antibody and a humanized monoclonal antibody to IL-5. Anti-IgE has been evaluated as a treatment for allergic asthma and AR. Milgrom et al[41] conducted a randomized, placebo-controlled trial of anti-IgE in adolescent and adult patients with moderate to severe allergic asthma. Symptom scores in the active treatment groups were improved compared with the placebo arm, but perhaps the most striking result was the steroid-sparing effect of anti-IgE. Anti-IgE has also been shown to be effective in reducing the symptoms of seasonal AR in adolescents and adults with ragweed allergy.[42] One randomized, double-blinded study in children and adolescents examined its therapeutic value in seasonal AR when added to immunotherapy. Those subjects receiving anti-IgE in addition to specific immunotherapy had significant reduction in symptoms compared with those receiving immunotherapy alone.[43] Taken together, anti-IgE therapy appears to be effective for the treatment of allergic asthma and AR and will likely be used as an adjunctive treatment to first-line medications.

Monoclonal anti−IL-5 has been demonstrated in a placebo-controlled trial to significantly reduce peripheral and sputum eosinophilia without affecting the early- or late-phase responses with inhaled allergen challenges.[44] Despite serious methodologic concerns regarding this study,[45] it has tempered enthusiasm for anti−IL-5 therapy. It does, however, illustrate that anticytokine therapy is feasible and may in the future prove to be an effective treatment modality for allergic disease. Antagonists to IL-4 and IL-13 are also in development. Other cytokines, such as IL-12 and IL-10, are "antiallergic" in nature and may play a role in the treatment of allergic disease.[46]

Alternative Routes of Administration

Alternative routes for administering immunotherapy are also being actively investigated. Several clinical trials have examined the efficacy of sublingual swallow immunotherapy and demonstrated some efficacy in asthma and AR symptoms.[47] A double-blind, placebo-controlled trial of sublingual swallow immunotherapy with *Parietaria judaica* extract in children demonstrated a reduction in symptoms of AR with decreased risk of serious reactions.[48] The mechanisms of action of this route of immunotherapy remain unknown and may be different from those of conventional immunotherapy. Other routes under investigation include swallow, sublingual spit, and intranasal delivery.

Immunotherapy as Prevention

Immunotherapy has traditionally been used as a therapeutic intervention rather than a preventive one. However, some evidence suggests that specific immunotherapy may have a future role in the secondary prevention of allergic diseases. The Preventative Allergy Treatment Study is a European

> **BOX 27-1**
>
> **KEY CONCEPTS**
> *Principles of Immunotherapy*
>
> - Efficacy is dose dependent.
> - Clinical effectiveness occurs after maintenance doses are reached.
> - There is a significant placebo effect.
> - Approximately 75% of patients respond.
> - A major risk is systemic reaction.

multicenter, randomized trial of specific immunotherapy for seasonal AR. Among those children without asthma, those who had received 3 years of immunotherapy had significantly fewer asthma symptoms than those in the open control group.[49] In addition, a study evaluating dust mite immunotherapy in monosensitized children demonstrated a decreased risk of the development of additional sensitizations in the active treatment group compared with the control group.[50] The evidence is preliminary, but there is a suggestion that immunologic intervention at an early stage of immune development may alter the natural progression of the allergic phenotype.

CONCLUSIONS

Immunotherapy is an effective treatment option for pediatric patients with stinging insect hypersensitivity and AR (Box 27-1). It is also effective in selected patients with asthma. The adequate doses required to achieve efficacy may not be reached for 6 months. There is a small but definite risk of systemic allergic reactions; therefore facilities administering immunotherapy should be adequately prepared to handle such an event and patients should remain in the medical facility for 30 minutes after receiving the injection (Box 27-2).

Immunotherapy may act to suppress allergic symptoms through modification of antibody responses, lymphocyte responses, or target cell responses to allergen. Studies are under way to determine whether modifications of immunotherapy reagents or dosing route will improve its efficacy or reduce side effects. Immunotherapy is also being pursued as a

> **BOX 27-2**
>
> **THERAPEUTIC PRINCIPLES**
> **Clinical Principles of Allergen Immunotherapy**
>
> Immunotherapy is effective only in IgE-mediated diseases such as stinging insect anaphylaxis, allergic rhinitis, and asthma.
>
> Patients should be selected who have demonstrated specific IgE and in whom medical management has not adequately controlled disease.
>
> Successful therapy requires that maximal tolerated doses of allergen extracts be given and requires months to years to reach maximal benefit.
>
> Because of the risk of anaphylaxis during therapy, injections should be administered in a physician's office or other medical facility that can support cardiorespiratory resuscitation. Patients should be observed for 30 minutes after an injection is administered.

treatment option for food allergy, and there is some evidence to suggest that immunotherapy may alter the natural progression of sensitization. Immune modulators, such as anti-IgE and anti−IL-5, are also being actively pursued.

REFERENCES

1. Noon L: Prophylactic inoculation for hay fever, *Lancet* 1:1572, 1911.
2. Norman PS, Winkenwerder WL, Lichtenstein LM: Immunotherapy of hay fever with ragweed antigen E: comparisons with whole pollen extract and placebos, *J Allergy Clin Immunol* 42:93-108, 1968.
3. Johnstone DE: Study of the role of antigen dosage in the treatment of pollenosis and pollen asthma, *Am J Dis Child* 94:1, 1957.
4. Warner JO, Price JF, Southill JF, et al: Controlled trial of hyposensitization to *Dermatophagoides pteronyssinus* in children with asthma, *Lancet* 2:912, 1978.
5. Greenberg MA, Kaufman CR, Gonzalez GE, et al: Late and immediate systemic allergic reactions to inhalant allergen immunotherapy, *J Allergy Clin Immunol.* 77:865, 1986.
6. Adkinson NF, Eggleston PA, Eney D, et al: A controlled trial of immunotherapy for asthma in allergic children, *N Engl J Med* 336:324-331, 1997.
7. Creticos PS, Van Metre TE, Mardiney MR, et al: Dose response of IgE and IgG antibodies during ragweed immunotherapy, *J Allergy Clin Immunol* 73:94-104, 1984.
8. Durham SR, Till SJ: Immunologic changes associated with allergen immunotherapy, *J Allergy Clin Immunol* 102:157-164, 1998.
9. Gleich GJ, Jacob GL, Yuninger JW, et al: Measurement of the absolute levels of IgE antibodies in patients with ragweed hay fever: effect of immunotherapy on seasonal changes and relationship to IgG antibodies, *J Allergy Clin Immunol* 60:188-198, 1977.
10. Rocklin RE, Sheffer AL, Greineder DK, et al: Generation of antigen-specific suppressor cells during allergy sensitization, *N Engl J Med* 302:1213-1219, 1980.
11. Durham SR, Ying S, Varney VA, et al: Grass pollen immunotherapy inhibits allergen-induced infiltration of CD4+ T lymphocytes and eosinophils in the nasal mucosa and increase the number of cells expressing messenger RNA for interferon-γ, *J Allergy Clin Immunol* 97:1356-1365, 1996.
12. Otsuka H, Mezawa A, Ohnishi M, et al: Changes in nasal metachromatic cells during allergen immunotherapy, *Clin Exp Allergy* 21:115-119, 1991.
13. Creticos PS, Adkinson NF, Kagey-Sobotka A, et al: Nasal challenge with ragweed pollen in hay fever patients: effect of immunotherapy, *J Clin Invest* 76:2247-2253, 1985.
14. Furin MJ, Norman PS, Creticos PS, et al: Immunotherapy decreases antigen-induced eosinophil cell migration into the nasal cavity, *J Allergy Clin Immunol* 88:27-32, 1991.
15. Rak S, Lowhagen O, Venge P: The effect of immunotherapy on bronchial hyperresponsiveness and eosinophil cationic protein in pollen-allergic patients, *J Allergy Clin Immunol* 82:470-480, 1988.
16. Varney VA, Gaga M, Frew AJ, et al: Usefulness of immunotherapy in patients with severe summer hay fever uncontrolled by antiallergic drugs, *Br Med J* 302:265-269, 1991.
17. Lowell FC, Franklin W: A double-blind study of the effectiveness and specificity of injection therapy in ragweed hay fever, *N Engl J Med* 273:675-679, 1965.
18. Bousquet J, Hejjaoui A, Clauzel AM, et al: Specific immunotherapy with standardized *Dermatophagoides pteronyssinus* extract, *J Allergy Clin Immunol* 82:971-977, 1988.
19. Dreborg S, Agrell B, Foucard T, et al: A double-blind, multicenter immunotherapy trial in children using a purified and standardized *Cladosporium herbarum* preparation. I. Clinical results, *Allergy* 41:131-140, 1986.
20. Durham SR, Walker SM, Varga EM, et al: Long-term efficacy of grass pollen immunotherapy, *N Engl J Med* 341:468-475, 1999.
21. Ohman JL Jr: Allergen immunotherapy in asthma: evidence for efficacy, *J Allergy Clin Immunol* 84:133-140, 1989.
22. Van Metre TE, Marsh DG, Adkinson NF, et al: Immunotherapy for cat asthma, *J Allergy Clin Immunol* 82:1055-1068, 1988.
23. Bousquet J, Maasch A, Hejjaoui W, et al: Double blind placebo controlled immunotherapy with mixed grass pollen allergoids. III. Efficacy and safety of unfractionated and high molecular weight preparations in rhinoconjunctivitis and asthma, *J Allergy Clin Immunol* 84:546-556, 1989.
24. Abramson MJ, Puy RM, Weiner JM: Is allergen immunotherapy effective in asthma? *Am J Respir Crit Care Med* 151:969-974, 1995.

25. Bousquet J, Hejjaoui A, Michel FB: Specific immunotherapy in asthma, *J Allergy Clin Immunol* 86:292-305, 1990.

26. Thompson R, Bousquet J, Cohen S, et al: The current status of allergen immunotherapy (hyposensitization). Report of WHO/IUIS Working Group, *Lancet* 1:259-261, 1989.

27. Hunt KJ, Valentine MD, Sobotka AK, et al: A controlled trial of immunotherapy in insect sting hypersensitivity, *N Engl J Med* 299:157, 1978.

28. Valentine MD, Schuberth KC, Kagey-Sobotka A, et al: The value of immunotherapy with venom in children with allergy to insect stings, *N Engl J Med* 323:1601, 1990.

29. Golden DBK: Stinging insect vaccines: patient selection and administration of Hymenoptera venom immunotherapy, *Immunol Allergy Clin North Am* 20:553-570, 2000.

30. Nelson HS, Lahr J, Rule R, et al: Treatment of anaphylactic sensitivity to peanuts by immunotherapy with injections of aqueous peanut extract, *J Allergy Clin Immunol* 99:744-751, 1997.

31. Nelson HS: The use of standardized extracts in allergen immunotherapy, *J Allergy Clin Immunol* 106:41-45, 2000.

32. Stewart GA, Thompson PS, McWilliam AS: Biochemical properties of aeroallergens: contributory factors in allergic sensitization? *Pediatr Allergy Immunol* 4:163-172, 1993.

33. Nelson HS: Immunotherapy for inhalant allergens. In Middleton EJ, Reed CE, Ellis EF, et al, eds: *Allergy: principles and practice,* ed 5, St Louis, 1998, Mosby.

34. Tinkelman DG, Cole WQ III, Tunno J: Immunotherapy: a one-year prospective study to evaluate risk factors of systemic reactions, *J Allergy Clin Immunol* 95:8-14, 1995.

35. Reid MJ, Lockey RF, Turkeltaub PC, et al: Survey of fatalities from skin testing and immunotherapy 1985-1989, *J Allergy Clin Immunol* 92:6-13, 1993.

36. Executive Committee, American Academy of Allergy and Immunology: Personnel and equipment for allergenic extracts, *J Allergy Clin Immunol* 77:271-273, 1986.

37. Platts-Mills TAE, Mueller GA, Wheatley LM: Future directions for allergen immunotherapy, *J Allergy Clin Immunol* 102:335-343, 1998.

38. Briner TJM, Kuo M-C, Keating KM, et al: Peripheral T tolerance induced in naive and primed mice by subcutaneous injection of peptides from the major cat allergen Fel d 1, *Proc Natl Acad Sci U S A* 90:7608-7612, 1993.

39. Norman PS, Ohman JL Jr, Long AA, et al: Treatment of cat allergy with T-cell reactive peptides, *Am J Respir Crit Care Med* 154:1623-1628, 1996.

40. Marshall JD, Abtahi S, Eiden JJ, et al: Immunostimulatory sequence DNA linked to the Amb a 1 allergen promotes T(H)1 cytokine expression while downregulating T(H)2 cytokine expression in PBMCs from human patients with ragweed allergy, *J Allergy Clin Immunol* 108:191-197, 2001.

41. Milgrom H, Fick RB Jr, Su JQ: Treatment of allergic asthma with monoclonal anti-IgE antibody. rhuMAb-E25 Study Group, *N Engl J Med* 341:1966-1973, 1999.

42. Casale TB, Condemi J, LaForce C, et al: Effect of omalizumab on symptoms of seasonal allergic rhinitis: a randomized controlled trial, *JAMA* 286:2956-2967, 2001.

43. Kuehr J, Brauburger J, Zielen S, et al: Efficacy of combination treatment with anti-IgE plus specific immunotherapy in polysensitized children and adolescents with seasonal allergic rhinitis, *J Allergy Clin Immunol* 109:274-280, 2002.

44. Leckie MJ, ten Brinke A, Khan J, et al: Effect of an interleukin-5 blocking monoclonal antibody on eosinophils, airway hyper-responsiveness, and the late asthmatic response, *Lancet* 356:2144-2148, 2000.

45. O'Byrne PM, Inman MD, Parameswaran K: The trials and tribulations of IL-5, eosinophils, and allergic asthma (editorial), *J Allergy Clin Immunol* 108:503-508, 2001.

46. Barnes PJ: Cytokine-directed therapies for asthma, *J Allergy Clin Immunol* 108:S72-S76, 2001.

47. Frew AJ, Smith HE: Sublingual therapy, *J Allergy Clin Immunol* 107:441-444, 2001.

48. La Rosa M, Ranno C, Andre C, et al: Double-blind placebo-controlled evaluation of sublingual-swallow immunotherapy with standardized Parietaria judaica extract in children with allergic rhinoconjunctivitis, *J Allergy Clin Immunol* 104:425-432, 1999.

49. Moller C, Dreborg S, Ferdousi HA, et al: Pollen immunotherapy reduces the development of asthma in children with seasonal rhinoconjunctivitis (the PAT-study), *J Allergy Clin Immunol* 109:251-256, 2002.

50. Pajno GB, Barberio G, De Luca F, et al: Prevention of new sensitizations in asthmatic children monosensitized to house dust mite by specific immunotherapy. A six-year follow-up study, *Clin Exp Allergy* 31:1392-1397, 2001.

CHAPTER **28**

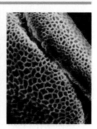

Allergic Rhinitis

DEBORAH A. GENTILE ■ GAIL G. SHAPIRO ■ DAVID P. SKONER

Rhinitis is defined as inflammation of the membranes lining the nose and is characterized by one or more of the following nasal symptoms: sneezing, itching, rhinorrhea, and nasal congestion. Rhinitis is frequently accompanied by symptoms that involve the eyes, ears, and throat.[1,2]

There are many different causes of rhinitis in children. Approximately 50% of all cases of rhinitis are caused by allergy. In allergic rhinitis, symptoms arise as a result of inflammation induced by an immunoglobulin E (IgE)–mediated immune response to specific allergens such as pollen, mold, animal dander, and dust mites. The immune response involves the release of inflammatory mediators and the activation and recruitment of cells to the nasal mucosa.[1,2]

A careful history and physical examination are the most effective diagnostic maneuvers for the identification of allergic rhinitis in children. Because allergic rhinitis and nonallergic rhinitis are frequently indistinguishable based on symptoms and because they require different management strategies and pharmacologic treatments, the value of an accurate differential diagnosis cannot be underestimated. Clinicians should pursue specific diagnostic testing when indicated. Management options for allergic rhinitis include treatment with pharmacologic agents and preventative measures such as environmental control and immunotherapy.

EPIDEMIOLOGY

Although allergic rhinitis reportedly occurs very frequently, data regarding the true underlying causes of rhinitis are difficult to interpret. Most population surveys rely on physician-diagnosed rhinitis for their data, possibly underestimating the actual frequency with which rhinitis occurs. Some population studies have been conducted by means of questionnaires administered to subjects, followed by telephone interviews to attempt to make a specific diagnosis of rhinitis. Results of such studies reflect a more accurate prevalence of rhinitis but are likely to continue to underreport this disease.[2-12]

Most epidemiologic studies have been directed toward the identification of seasonal allergic rhinitis because of the easy identification of the rapid and reproducible onset and offset of symptoms in association with pollen exposure. Perennial allergic rhinitis is more difficult to identify because its symptom complex often overlaps with chronic sinusitis, recurrent upper respiratory tract infections, and vasomotor rhinitis.

The reported prevalence of rhinitis in epidemiologic studies, conducted in various countries, ranges from 3% to 19%. Studies that have included the most information suggest that seasonal allergic rhinitis is found in approximately 10% of the general population and perennial rhinitis is found in 10% to 20% of the population.[2-12] Overall, allergic rhinitis affects 20 to 40 million people in the United States.[11,12]

The frequency of allergic rhinitis in the general population has risen in parallel with that of all IgE-mediated diseases during the past decade. Swedish army studies have shown that the prevalence of seasonal allergic rhinitis has increased from 4% to 8% in the 10-year period from 1971 to 1981.[13] In addition, atopic skin test reactivity increased from 39% to 50% in Tucson, Arizona, during an 8-year period of testing.[5,12]

The prevalence of allergic rhinitis in the pediatric population also appears to be rising. One study showed a prevalence of physician-diagnosed allergic rhinitis in 42% of 6-year-old children.[5] Another study conducted in Finland reported a near tripling of the prevalence from 1977 to 1991.[14] Currently, allergic rhinitis is the most common atopic disease and one of the leading chronic conditions in children younger than 18 years.[15] These figures relate to industrialized nations; there is generally less atopic disease in underdeveloped countries for reasons that are not entirely clear but involve genetic and environmental interactions.

Sex

In childhood, boys with allergic rhinitis outnumber girls, but, in general, equal numbers are affected during adulthood.

287

Age

Symptoms of allergic rhinitis develop before the age of 20 years in 80% of cases. Children in families with a bilateral family history of allergy generally have symptoms before puberty; those with a unilateral family history tend to have symptoms later in life or not at all.[5-7] Symptoms of allergic rhinitis develop in 1 of 5 children by 2 to 3 years of age and in approximately 40% by age 6 years. Approximately 30% develop symptoms during adolescence.

Risk Factors

Studies have shown that the frequency of allergic rhinitis increases with age and that positive allergy skin tests are significant risk factors for the development of new symptoms of allergic rhinitis. There appears to be a higher prevalence of rhinitis in higher socioeconomic classes, in nonwhites, in some polluted areas, in individuals with a family history of allergy, and in individuals born during the pollen season. Also, allergic rhinitis is more likely to occur in firstborn children. Studies in children in the first years of life have shown that the risk of rhinitis was higher in those with early introduction of foods or formula, heavy maternal cigarette smoking in the first year of life, exposure to indoor allergens such as animal dander and dust mites, higher serum IgE levels (> 100 IU/ml before age 6 years), the presence of positive allergen skin-prick tests, and parental allergic disorders.[5]

Socioeconomic Impact

Because of the high prevalence of allergic rhinitis, impaired quality of life, costs of treatment, and the presence of comorbidities such as asthma, sinusitis, and otitis media, allergic rhinitis has a tremendous impact on society.[16] The severity of allergic rhinitis ranges from mild to seriously debilitating. The cost of treating allergic rhinitis and indirect costs related to loss of workplace productivity resulting from the disease are significant and substantial. The estimated cost of allergic rhinitis, based on direct and indirect costs, was $2.7 billion for 1995, exclusive of costs for associated medical problems such as sinusitis and asthma.[17] In children with allergic rhinitis, the quality of life of both the parents and the child, including the ability to learn, may be affected.[17,18]

PATHOPHYSIOLOGY

Under normal conditions, the nasal mucosa quite efficiently humidifies and cleans inspired air. This is the result of orchestrated interactions of local and humoral mediators of defense.[19] In allergic rhinitis, these mechanisms do not function appropriately and contribute to signs and symptoms of the disorder.[20]

Components of the Allergic Response

The allergic sensitization that characterizes allergic rhinitis has a strong genetic component. The tendency to develop IgE, mast cell, and T helper cell type 2 (Th2) lymphocyte immune responses is inherited by atopic individuals. Exposure to threshold concentrations of dust mite fecal proteins; cockroach allergen; dog, cat, and other danders; pollen grains; or other allergens for prolonged periods of time leads to the presentation of the allergen by antigen-presenting cells to CD4+ T lymphocytes, which then release interleukin (IL)-3, -4, and -5 and other Th2 cytokines. These cytokines drive proinflammatory processes, such as IgE production, against these allergens through the mucosal infiltration and actions of plasma cells, mast cells, and eosinophils.

Once the patient has become sensitized to allergens, subsequent exposures trigger a cascade of events that result in the symptoms of allergic rhinitis. The response in allergic rhinitis can be divided into two phases: the immediate-, or early-, phase response and the late-phase response.

Early Phase

During periods of continuous allergen exposure, increasing numbers of IgE-coated mast cells traverse the epithelium, recognize the mucosally deposited allergen, and degranulate.[21] Products of this degranulation include preformed mediators such as histamine, tryptase (mast cell–specific marker), chymase (connective tissue mast cells only), kininogenase (generates bradykinin), heparin, and other enzymes. In addition, mast cells secrete several inflammatory mediators de novo (i.e., not preformed and stored in mast cell granules), including prostaglandin D_2 and sulfidopeptidyl leukotriene (LT) C_4, LTD_4, and LTE_4. These mediators cause blood vessels to leak and produce the mucosal edema and watery rhinorrhea that are characteristic of allergic rhinitis. Glands secrete mucoglycoconjugates and antimicrobial compounds and dilate blood vessels to cause sinusoidal filling and thus occlusion and congestion of nasal air passages. These mediators also stimulate sensory nerves, which convey the sensation of nasal itch and congestion, and recruit systemic reflexes such as sneezing. These responses develop within minutes of allergen exposure and thus constitute the early-phase, or "immediate," allergic response.[22] Sneezing, itching, and copious, clear rhinorrhea are characteristic symptoms during early-phase allergic responses, although some degree of nasal congestion can also occur.

Late Phase

The mast cell–derived mediators released during early phase responses are hypothesized to act on postcapillary endothelial cells to promote the expression of vascular adhesion molecule and E-selectin, which facilitate the adhesion of circulating leukocytes to the endothelial cells. Chemoattractant cytokines such as IL-5 promote the infiltration of the mucosa with eosinophils, neutrophils, and basophils; T lymphocytes; and macrophages.[23,24] During the 4- to 8-hour period after allergen exposure, these cells become activated and release inflammatory mediators, which in turn reactivate many of the proinflammatory reactions of the immediate response. This cellular-driven, late inflammatory reaction is termed the late-phase response. This reaction may be clinically indistinguishable from the immediate reaction, but congestion tends to predominate.[25] Eosinophil-derived mediators such as major basic protein, eosinophil cationic protein, and leukotrienes have been shown to damage the epithelium, leading ultimately to the clinical and histologic pictures of chronic allergic disease.

Subsets of the T helper lymphocytes are the likely orchestrators of the chronic inflammatory response to allergens. Th2 lymphocytes promote the allergic response by releasing IL-3,

IL-4, IL-5, and other cytokines that promote IgE production, eosinophil chemoattraction and survival in tissues, and mast cell recruitment.[26] Cytokines released from Th2 lymphocytes and other cells may circulate to the hypothalamus and result in fatigue, malaise, irritability, and neurocognitive deficits that are commonly noted in patients with allergic rhinitis. Cytokines produced during late phase allergic responses can be reduced by glucocorticoids.[27]

When subjects are challenged intranasally with allergen repeatedly, the amount of allergen required to produce an immediate response decreases.[28] This effect is termed "priming" and is hypothesized to be a result of the influx of inflammatory cells that occurs during late phase allergic responses. The response is clinically significant because exposure to an allergen may promote an exaggerated response to other allergens. Priming represents an increase in airway reactivity and highlights the importance of fully defining the spectrum of allergens for a given patient and the need to prevent this process by initiating preseasonal, prophylactic, antiinflammatory therapy.

Classification

On the basis of timing and duration of allergen exposure, and thus the allergen pathogenesis, allergic rhinitis is classified as seasonal or perennial. Overall, approximately 20% of all cases are strictly seasonal, 40% are perennial, and 40% are mixed (perennial with seasonal exacerbation).

Seasonal Allergic Rhinitis

Tree, grass, and weed pollens and outdoor mold spores are common seasonal allergens. The symptoms typically appear during a defined season in which aeroallergens are abundant in the outdoor air. The length of seasonal exposure to these allergens is dependent on geographic location. Therefore familiarity with the pollinating season of the major trees, grasses, and weeds of the locale makes the syndrome easier to diagnose.[29] Certain outdoor mold spores also display seasonal variation with the highest levels in the summer and fall months.[30]

Typical symptoms during pollen exposure include the explosive onset of profuse, watery rhinorrhea; itching; and sneezing, along with frequent allergic symptoms of the eye. Congestion also occurs but usually is not the most troubling symptom. The onset and offset of symptoms usually track the seasonal pollen counts. However, hyperresponsiveness to irritant triggers, which develops from the inflammatory reaction of the late phase and priming responses, often persists after cessation of the pollen season. Such triggers include tobacco smoke, noxious odors, changes in temperature, and exercise.

Perennial Allergic Rhinitis

Year-round exposure to dust mites, cockroaches, indoor molds, and cat, dog, and other danders leads to persistent tissue edema and infiltration with eosinophils, mast cells, Th2 lymphocytes, and macrophages.[31] Perennial allergic rhinitis can also be caused by pollen in areas where pollen is prevalent perennially.

A universally accepted definition of perennial rhinitis does not exist. Most often, it is defined as a disease that persists for longer than 9 months each year and produces two or more of the following symptoms: serous or seromucus hypersecretion, nasal blockage caused by a swollen nasal mucosa, and sneezing paroxysms. Nasal congestion and mucous production (postnasal drip) symptoms predominate in most patients, and sneezing, itching, and watery rhinorrhea may be minimal.[2] Because late phase reactivity is commonly ongoing, it becomes difficult to sort out early from late phase reactions; therefore the history of trigger factor exposure is often difficult to decipher.

Perennial Allergic Rhinitis with Seasonal Exacerbation

Symptoms of allergic rhinitis may also be perennial with seasonal exacerbation, depending on the spectrum of allergen sensitivities.

DIFFERENTIAL DIAGNOSIS

The causes of rhinitis are summarized in Table 28-1.[2] The most common form of nonallergic rhinitis in children is infectious rhinitis. Infectious rhinitis may be acute or chronic. Acute infectious rhinitis, such as the common cold, is usually caused by one of a large number of viruses, but secondary bacterial infection with sinus involvement may be a complication. Symptoms of chronic infectious rhinosinusitis include mucopurulent nasal discharge, facial pain and pressure, olfactory disturbance, and postnasal drainage with cough.

The symptoms of allergic rhinitis are frequently confused with those of infectious rhinitis when patients complain of a constant cold. Symptoms persisting longer than 2 weeks should prompt a search for a cause other than infection. If tests for atopy or airway disease (e.g., asthma) are negative, foreign body rhinitis should be considered in the differential diagnosis. In such cases, symptoms may be acute or chronic and unilateral or bilateral, and the nasal discharge may be bloodstained or foul smelling.

Exacerbation of rhinitis symptoms with predominant, clear rhinorrhea in patients with a known history of allergic rhinitis may be difficult to diagnose. The difference between active infection and allergy should be noted. When the history or physical examination is not diagnostic, a nasal smear should be obtained to aid in differentiation. The presence of more than 5% eosinophils suggests allergic disease, whereas a preponderance of neutrophils suggests infection.

Allergy, mucociliary disturbance, and immune deficiency may predispose certain individuals to the development of chronic infection.[32,33] Mucociliary abnormalities may be congenital, as in primary ciliary dyskinesia, Young syndrome, or cystic fibrosis, or they may be secondary to infection.[34,35] Similarly, immune deficiency may be congenital or acquired.

Tumors or nasal polyps (Figure 28-1) as well as other conditions (e.g., nasal septal deviation, adenoidal hypertrophy, hypertrophy of the nasal turbinates) can produce nasal airway obstruction.[36,37] Nasal polyps are common in children with cystic fibrosis but not in children with allergic rhinitis. Tumors as a cause of rhinitis are very uncommon in children; other anatomic anomalies are more common in children. Nasal septal deviation and nasal turbinate or adenoidal hypertrophy may block the flow of nasal secretions, leading to rhinorrhea or postnasal drip as well as causing nasal blockage. The most common acquired anatomic cause of nasal obstruction in infants and children is adenoidal hypertrophy.

Children with rhinitis should also be assessed for congenital and acquired anatomic causes of nasal obstruction.

TABLE 28-1 Causes of Rhinitis

Allergic rhinitis
   Seasonal
   Perennial
   Perennial with seasonal exacerbation
Nonallergic rhinitis
   Structural/mechanical factors
      Deviated septum/septal wall anomalies
      Hypertrophic turbinates
      Adenoidal hypertrophy
      Foreign bodies
      Nasal tumors
         Benign
         Malignant
      Choanal atresia
   Infectious
      Acute
      Chronic
   Inflammatory/immunologic
      Wegener granulomatosis
      Sarcoidosis
      Midline granuloma
      Systemic lupus erythematosus
      Sjögren's syndrome
      Nasal polyposis
   Physiologic
      Ciliary dyskinesia syndrome
      Atrophic rhinitis
      Hormonally induced
         Hypothyroidism
         Pregnancy
         Oral contraceptives
         Menstrual cycle
         Exercise
         Atrophic
   Drug induced
      Rhinitis medicamentosa
      Oral contraceptives
      Antihypertensive therapy
      Aspirin
      Nonsteroidal antiinflammatory drugs
   Reflex induced
      Gustatory rhinitis
      Chemical or irritant induced
      Posture reflexes
      Nasal cycle
   Environmental factors
      Odors
      Temperature
      Weather/barometric pressure
      Occupational
Nonallergic rhinitis with eosinophilia syndrome
Perennial nonallergic rhinitis (vasomotor rhinitis)
Emotional factors

From Skoner DP: *J Allergy Clin Immunol* 108:S2-S8, 2001.

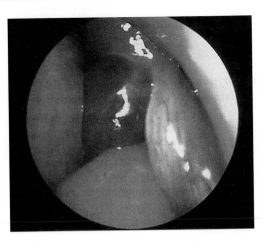

FIGURE 28-1 Appearance of nasal polyps on rhinoscopy. (Courtesy of Dr. Sylvan Stool, Department of Otolaryngology, Children's Hospital, Denver, Colo.)

referred to an otolaryngologist for a complete examination of the upper respiratory tract.

EVALUATION AND MANAGEMENT

History and Physical Examination

A careful history and physical examination are the most effective diagnostic maneuvers for the identification of allergic rhinitis in children.[2] The key to accurate and timely diagnosis in children is a heightened awareness of the condition and its potential comorbidities. Allergic rhinitis in children is often undiagnosed or misdiagnosed as other disorders such as recurrent colds. When cough is predominant, especially at night, allergic rhinitis may be misdiagnosed as "cough-variant asthma." To make a correct diagnosis with appropriate accuracy and timeliness, the clinician must be knowledgeable of and attentive to the symptoms and signs of rhinitis, ask specific questions directed at the presence and cause of rhinitis symptoms at each well-child visit, and understand the differential diagnosis of allergic rhinitis in children[2,38] (see Table 28-1). One must be aware of the comorbidities of allergic rhinitis (asthma, sinusitis, otitis media), pursue specific diagnostic tests when indicated, and often administer therapeutic trials of antiinflammatory medications.[39,40]

Parents must also be aware of signs and symptoms and report them to physicians because the more subtle case presentations may otherwise go undiagnosed. Such underdiagnosis may be responsible for substantial morbidity in children, who often do not report their symptoms. Unfortunately, children who live with allergic symptoms on a daily basis for prolonged periods of time may mistakenly assume that their altered state is normal.

The signs and symptoms of allergic rhinitis are summarized in Table 28-2. Typical symptoms of allergic rhinitis include sneezing, itching, clear rhinorrhea, and congestion. Congestion may be bilateral or unilateral and may alternate from side to side. It is generally more pronounced at night. With nasal obstruction, the patient is likely to be a mouth breather, and snoring can be a nocturnal symptom. As such, sleep disturbances may indicate the presence of an allergic disorder. With chronic disease, abnormalities of facial

Reduced airflow through the nasal passages in infants may be caused by congenital choanal atresia.

Refractory, clear rhinorrhea may be caused by cerebrospinal fluid leak, even in the absence of trauma or recent surgery. Any case of suspected tumor should be promptly

TABLE 28-2 Signs and Symptoms of Allergic Rhinitis

Itching of the nose, ears, palate, or throat
Sneezing episodes
Thin, clear rhinorrhea
Nasal congestion
Sinus headache
Eustachian tube dysfunction
Mouth breathing or snoring
Chronic postnasal drip
Chronic, nonproductive cough
Frequent throat clearing
Sleep disturbance
Daytime fatigue

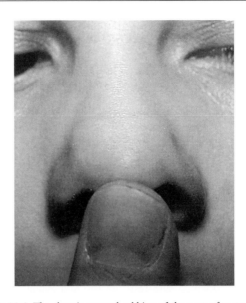

FIGURE 28-2 The chronic upward rubbing of the nose often results in a nasal crease in patients with allergic rhinitis. (From Zitelli BJ, Davis HW: *Atlas of pediatric physical diagnosis*, St Louis, 1987, Mosby.)

development, dental malocclusion, and the allergic facies may ensue, with an open mouth and gaping habitus.

Older children blow their noses frequently, whereas younger children do not. Instead, they sniff, snort, and repetitively clear their throats. Their voices may be abnormally hyponasal. Nasal pruritis may stimulate grimacing and twitching and picking of the nose. The latter may result in epistaxis. Children often have the allergic salute, an upward rubbing of the nose with the palm of the hand. This often produces an allergic nasal crease, which is an accentuated, horizontal skin fold over the lower third of the nose (Figure 28-2). Children with allergic rhinitis may also have recurrent sinusitis or otitis media, eczema, or asthma.

Patients may also complain of red, itchy eyes, along with itchy throat and ears. They may also lose their senses of smell and taste. Increased symptoms are frequently noted with increased exposure to the responsible allergen, such as after grass is cut.

With development of the allergic reaction, clear nasal secretions will be evident, and the nasal mucous membranes will become edematous without much erythema. The mucosa appears boggy and blue-gray. With continued exposure to the allergen, the turbinates will appear swollen and can obstruct the nasal airway. Conjunctival edema, itching, tearing, and hyperemia are frequent findings in patients with associated allergic conjunctivitis. Allergic rhinitis patients, particularly children with significant nasal obstruction and venous congestion, may also demonstrate edema and darkening of the tissues beneath the eyes. These "shiners" are not pathognomonic for allergic rhinitis because they can also be seen in patients with chronic rhinitis and/or sinusitis.

In severe cases, especially during the peak pollen season, mucous membranes of the eyes, eustachian tube, middle ear, and paranasal sinuses may be involved. This produces conjunctival irritation (itchy, watery eyes), redness and tearing, ear fullness and popping, itchy throat, and pressure over the cheeks and forehead. Malaise, weakness, and fatigue may also be present. The coincidence of other allergic syndromes, such as atopic eczema or asthma, and a positive family history of atopy point toward an allergic pathology. Approximately 20% of cases are accompanied by symptoms of asthma.[4]

When a clear relation between onset of pollination and the typical rhinitis symptoms is present, the diagnosis of allergic rhinitis is relatively simple. However, when all of the typical

rhinitis symptoms are not expressed, the diagnosis is more difficult. Chronic nasal obstruction alone may be the major symptom of perennial allergic rhinitis as a result of ongoing inflammation and late phase allergic reactions.[25]

Distinct temporal patterns of symptom production may aid in the diagnosis. Symptoms of rhinitis, which occur each time the patient is exposed to a furry pet, suggest IgE-mediated sensitivity to that pet. Furthermore, patients who are sensitive to animal proteins may develop symptoms of rhinitis and asthma when entering a house, even though the animal was removed several hours earlier. Exposure to airborne allergens in the school or work environment may produce symptoms only during the week, with a symptom-free period during weekends. Likewise, vacations may be notably symptom free.

Several processes and anomalies in presentation may complicate the diagnosis of allergic rhinitis. For example, the symptoms on any particular day of pollen exposure will be influenced by exposure on that day but also on previous days because of the *priming phenomenon*. As a consequence, at the end of the pollen season, the decline of symptoms usually takes place more slowly than the decline of pollen counts.[41] In cases of perennial rhinitis, the symptoms are chronic and persistent, and patients may have secondary complaints of mouth-breathing, snoring sinusitis, otitis media, or a "permanent cold."[42]

Diagnostic Tests

Laboratory confirmation of the presence of IgE antibodies to specific allergens such as dust mites, pollens, and animal dander is helpful in establishing a specific allergic diagnosis, especially if the history of specific allergen exposure is not clear cut. In many patients, it is necessary to test for specific allergens to convince the family and patient of an allergic diagnosis and to reinforce the importance of environmental control measures.

Although skin testing can be performed on any child of any age, children younger than 1 year may not display a positive reaction. Often the child with seasonal respiratory allergy will not have a positive test until after two seasons of exposure. Clinicians should be selective in the use of allergens for skin testing and should use only common allergens of potential clinical importance. The most useful allergens for testing in the child with perennial inhalant allergy are dust mite, animal dander, and fungi. Allergens important in the diagnosis of seasonal allergic rhinitis are weed, grass, and tree pollen. Because there is a significant geographic specificity with regard to pollens, the importance of these seasonal allergens varies not only by season of the year but also by geographic distribution. Therefore allergens used for skin testing must be individualized and should be selected on the basis of prevalence in the patient's geographic area of the country and the home and school environment in which they live and play.

There are two methods for specific IgE antibody testing: *in vivo* skin testing and *in vitro* serum testing. Each has advantages and disadvantages[43] (Table 28-3). At the present time, properly performed skin tests are the best available method for detecting the presence of allergen-specific IgE. The skin prick, which is also called the *puncture* or *epicutaneous skin test,* is the preferred method of IgE antibody testing. Scratch testing has been abandoned as too traumatic. If skin prick test results are negative and allergy is highly suspected, then intradermal testing, which is more sensitive but less specific, may be used if indicated.

In vitro tests are acceptable substitutes for skin tests in the following circumstances: (1) the patient has abnormal skin conditions such as dermatographism or extensive dermatitis, (2) the patient cannot or did not discontinue antihistamines or other interfering medications, (3) the patient is very allergic by history and anaphylaxis is a possible risk, and (4) the patient is noncompliant for skin testing.

To avoid false-negative tests, most antihistamine medications should be withheld for 72 hours because antihistamines suppress the skin results. Longer-acting antihistamines, such as astemizole, should be withheld for 4 to 6 weeks before skin tests are performed.

Physicians must remember that positive tests for allergen-specific IgE themselves are not sufficient for a diagnosis of allergic disease. These tests only indicate the presence of IgE molecules with a particular immunologic specificity. A decision of whether the specific IgE antibodies are responsible for clinically apparent disease must be based on the physician's assessment of the entire clinical picture. The ultimate standard

for the diagnosis of allergic disease remains the combination of (1) positive history, (2) the presence of specific IgE antibodies, and (3) demonstration that the symptoms are the result of IgE-mediated inflammation.

Blood eosinophilia and total serum IgE levels have been proposed as screening tests for allergies, but they have relatively low sensitivity and should not be used routinely for the diagnosis of allergic rhinitis. The nasal secretions or sputum of patients with respiratory allergy contains increased numbers of eosinophils, which form the basis of a useful nonspecific test (nasal smear for eosinophils) but one that will not identify any specific allergen etiology. Nasal smears for eosinophil/neutrophil counts can be useful in the differential diagnosis when the diagnosis is unclear.

Guidelines for Diagnosis and Management

Recently, evolving evaluation and management trends were delineated in an algorithm proposed by the Joint Task Force on Practice Parameters in Allergy, Asthma and Immunology[1] (Figure 28-3). It suggests that the initial evaluation of a patient with rhinitis symptoms (e.g., rhinorrhea, nasal congestion, sneezing, nasal pruritus, postnasal drainage, and conjunctivitis) be performed by a primary care physician, who should pay particular attention to the nature and history of the symptoms, the presence of complications and comorbid conditions, the identification and timing of factors that trigger symptoms, the effect on rhinitis symptoms of medications taken for rhinitis and for other conditions, and the effects of rhinitis symptoms on the patient's ability to function and have a good quality of life. Based on findings at the initial evaluation, the patient may be treated empirically in the primary care setting or referred to an allergist/immunologist for consultation. The indications for referral are summarized in Table 28-4.

In the proposed algorithm, the management of patients with mild or moderate rhinitis who do require referral includes the avoidance of suspected triggers and treatment with a single agent or combination therapy. Routine assessment of response to therapy includes evaluation of improvements in nasal symptoms, functional ability, quality of life, and comorbid conditions. Follow-up of patients is important when treatment is successful to ensure continued control of symptoms, absence of side effects, and maintenance of improved quality of life. Patients who do not respond well to treatment or who are unable to maintain improvements should be referred to an allergist/immunologist for further evaluation and treatment. Consultation should also be considered when patients can benefit from immunotherapy, when identification of allergic triggers could facilitate implementation of avoidance measures that require patient education, or when complications or comorbidities persist or worsen.

One of the primary purposes of a consultation with an allergist/immunologist is the differential diagnosis of allergic rhinitis based on the combined results of a detailed medical history, physical examination of the airway, and ancillary tests, particularly skin tests. Effective management of allergic rhinitis may require a combination of aggressive avoidance measures, patient education regarding allergen avoidance and the administration of pharmacologic therapy, allergen immunotherapy, management of coexisting conditions, and

TABLE 28-3 Comparison of *In Vivo* Skin Tests and *In Vitro* Serum IgE Antibody Immunoassay in Allergic Diagnosis

Skin Test	Serum Immunoassay
Less expensive	No patient risk
Greater sensitivity	Patient-doctor convenience
Wide allergen selection	Not suppressed by antihistamines
Results available immediately	Results are quantitative
	Preferable to skin testing in:
	Dermatographism
	Widespread dermatitis
	Uncooperative children

From Skoner DP: *J Allergy Clin Immunol* 108:S2-S8, 2001.

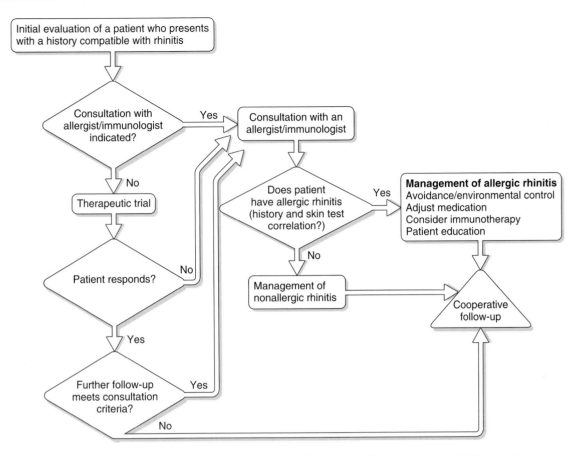

FIGURE 28-3 Algorithm for diagnosis and management of rhinitis. (Modified from Dykewicz MS, Fineman S, Skoner DP, et al: *Ann Allergy Asthma Immunol* 81:478-518, 1998.)

adjustments in pharmacologic therapy. Cooperative follow-up is an essential part of the successful management of allergic rhinitis and ideally includes the patient, the family, and all health care providers (e.g., primary care provider, allergist/immunologist, and otolaryngologist). With the common goal of reducing symptoms and improving functional ability, all involved would cooperatively manage exacerbations and complications through the optimal use of environmental avoidance measures, medications, and immunotherapy in appropriately selected patients. Periodic assessments and continued patient education should also be included in the follow-up protocol.

TABLE 28-4 Indications for Referral to an Allergist/Immunologist

Prolonged history of rhinitis

Presence of complications or comorbid conditions including asthma, otitis media, and sinusitis

Prior corticosteroid use or prolonged treatment with multiple medications

Treatment that is either ineffective or produces adverse events

Symptoms that significantly interfere with the patient's functional ability or reduce the quality of life

Need to further define allergic/environmental triggers of rhinitis

Management

Specific treatment options include environmental control for allergen avoidance, pharmacotherapy, and immunotherapy. In all cases, the primary goal of treatment is to control the symptoms and to improve the quality of life without altering the patient's ability to function. A second but equally important goal is to prevent the development of sequelae of allergic rhinitis, including sinusitis and otitis media.[1,40]

Environmental Control for Allergen Avoidance

Educating families about avoiding exposure to allergens is an essential part of the treatment of allergic rhinitis (Table 28-5). Unfortunately, the specific measures are often highly impractical; moreover, they may have negative psychosocial ramifications for children that should not be ignored. Avoiding outdoor sports in the springtime and banishing furred pets from the home, for example, may have adverse effects on children that range beyond allergen control. Nevertheless, families should be taught about the importance of environmental control measures and advised to adhere to them to the extent possible.[1]

Oral Antihistamines

The Joint Task Force on Practice Parameters in Allergy, Asthma and Immunology recently published guidelines on the diagnosis and management of allergic rhinitis.[1] These guidelines review the considerations in selecting an antihistamine for the

TABLE 28-5 Environmental Control of Allergen Exposure

Allergens	Control Measures
Dust mites	Encase bedding in airtight covers
	Wash bedding in water at temperatures > 130° F
	Remove wall-to-wall carpeting
	Remove upholstered furniture
Animal dander	Avoid furred pets
	Keep animals out of patient's bedroom
Cockroaches	Control available food supply
	Keep kitchen/bathroom surfaces dry and free of standing water
	Professionally exterminate
Mold	Destroy moisture-prone areas
	Avoid high humidity in patient's bedroom
	Repair water leaks
	Check basements, attics, and crawl spaces for standing water and mold
Pollen	Keep automobile and house windows closed
	Control timing of outdoor exposure
	Restrict camping, hiking, and raking leaves
	Drive in air-conditioned automobile
	Air-condition the home
	Install portable, high-efficiency particulate air filters

treatment of allergic rhinitis. As with any medication, the choice of an antihistamine should be considered in the context of an individual patient's needs and response to a given agent regarding the benefit obtained versus the risk of adverse effects. Adherence issues are also important because treatment is usually administered chronically.

Three generations of antihistamines are available: the first-generation (sedating) antihistamines, which are available without prescription; the second-generation (hyposedating or nonsedating) agents, most of which require a prescription; and the third-generation (nonsedating metabolites of second-generation agents), all of which require a prescription in the United States at this time (Table 28-6). Antihistamines act primarily by blocking the H_1-histamine receptor, but several of the newer agents have also been shown to have mild antiinflammatory properties. The problems of sedation and frequent dosing that limited treatment with the first-generation antihistamines have been in large part eliminated by the second- and third-generation agents. The second- and third-generation agents have several advantages over the first-generation agents, including preferential binding to peripheral H_1-receptors, which results in minimal penetration of the central nervous system; minimal antiserotinergic, anticholinergic, and α-adrenergic blocking activities; and minimal sedative and performance-impairing effects.[44-46]

As a general rule, antihistamines reduce symptoms of sneezing, pruritis, and rhinorrhea but have little or no effect on nasal congestion. Consequently, a topical or oral decongestant may have to be added. Many antihistamine/decongestant formulations are available. The major advantage of these combinations is their convenience. Disadvantages are intolerance of the fixed dose of decongestant in certain patients and an inability to titrate each agent independently.[45]

Patients should be educated about the appropriate use of antihistamines. For optimal results, antihistamines should be administered prophylactically (2 to 5 hours before allergen exposure) or on a regular basis if needed chronically. Although antihistamines are effective on an as-needed basis, these agents work best when they are administered in a maintenance fashion.[45]

Decongestants

Decongestants produce vasoconstriction within the nasal mucosa through α-adrenergic receptor activation and therefore are effective in relieving the symptoms of nasal obstruction. However, these agents have no effect on other symptoms such as rhinorrhea, pruritis, or sneezing and may be most effective when used in combination with other agents, such as antihistamines.[45]

A number of decongestants are available for oral use, but the most commonly used decongestant is pseudoephedrine. The most common side effects of oral decongestants are central nervous system (nervousness, insomnia, irritability, headache) and cardiovascular (palpitations, tachycardia) effects. In addition, these drugs may elevate blood pressure, raise intraocular pressure, and aggravate urinary obstruction.[45]

Topical intranasal decongestants are sometimes used by patients with allergic rhinitis. However, when these agents are

TABLE 28-6 Second- and Third-Generation Antihistamines

Medication	Onset of Action (hrs)	Formulations	Recommended Dosage
Azelastine	3	Nasal spray	≥ 12 yr: 2 sprays per nostril bid
			5-11 yr: 1 spray per nostril bid
Cetirizine	1-2	Tablets 10 mg	≥ 12 yr: 10 mg qd
		Syrup 5 mg/5 ml	6-11 yr: 5-10 mg qd
			2-5 yr: 5 mg qd
Fexofenadine	1-2	Capsules 60 mg	≥ 12 yr: 60 mg bid or 180 mg qd
		Tablets 30 mg	6-11 yr: 30 mg bid
		Tablets 60 mg	
		Tablets 180 mg	
Loratadine	1-2	Tablets 10 mg	≥ 12 yr: 10 mg qd
		Syrup 5 mg/5 ml	6-11 yr: 5-10 mg qd
			2-5 yr: 5 mg qd
Desloratadine	1-2	Tablets 5 mg	≥ 12 yr: 5 mg qd

used for longer than 3 to 5 days, many patients experience rebound congestion after withdrawal of the drug. If patients continue to use these medications over several months, a form of rhinitis, rhinitis medicamentosa, will develop, which can be difficult to treat effectively.[45]

Intranasal Corticosteroids

Topical intranasal corticosteroids represent the most efficacious agents for the treatment of allergic rhinitis and are useful in relieving symptoms of nasal pruritis, rhinorrhea, sneezing, and congestion. These drugs exert their effects through multiple mechanisms, including vasoconstriction and reduction of edema, suppression of cytokine production, and inhibition of inflammatory cell influx. Physiologically, prophylactic treatment before nasal allergen challenge reduces both the early and late phase allergic responses.[46]

These agents work best when taken regularly on a daily basis or prophylactically in anticipation of an imminent pollen season. However, because of their rapid onset of action (within 12 to 24 hours for many agents), there is increasing evidence that they may also be effective when used intermittently. A number of glucocorticoid compounds are available for intranasal use in both aerosol and aqueous formulations (Table 28-7). Although the topical potency of these agents varies widely, clinical trials have been unable to demonstrate significant differences in efficacy.[47,48]

The most important pharmacologic characteristic differentiating these agents is systemic bioavailability. After intranasal administration, the majority of the dose is swallowed. Most of the available compounds, including beclomethasone dipropionate, budesonide, flunisolide, and triamcinolone acetonide, are absorbed readily from the gastrointestinal tract into the systemic circulation and subsequently undergo significant first-pass hepatic metabolism. The resulting bioavailabilities can be as high as 50%. However, neither fluticasone propionate nor mometasone furoate is well absorbed through the gastrointestinal tract, and the small amount of drug that reaches the portal circulation is rapidly and thoroughly metabolized. The low systemic availabilities of these two newer agents may be most important in growing children and in patients who are already using inhaled corticosteroids for asthma. Nevertheless, there are no studies to document the comparative effects of nasal corticosteroids on growth and development at this time.[47-51]

Patients who use intranasal corticosteroids experience dryness and irritation of the nasal mucous membranes in 5% to 10% of mild cases and mild epistaxis in approximately 5%. For mild symptoms, the dose of intranasal corticosteroid may be reduced if tolerated, and/or saline nasal spray should be instilled before the drug is sprayed.

Mast Cell Stabilizers

Mast cell stabilizers, such as cromolyn sodium, can be useful in relieving nasal pruritis, rhinorrhea, and sneezing; however, they have minimal effects on congestion. Cromolyn sodium is generally well tolerated and is most efficacious when taken prophylactically, well in advance of allergen exposure. In addition, because of its short duration of action, it should be taken 4 times a day; as a result, compliance is difficult for many patients.[1]

Ipratropium Bromide

Topical intranasal ipratropium bromide 0.03% and 0.06% solution reduces the volume of watery secretions but has little or no effect on other symptoms. Therefore this agent is most helpful in allergic rhinitis, when rhinorrhea is refractory to topical intranasal corticosteroids and/or antihistamines. The most common side effects include nasal irritation, crusting, and mild epistaxis. This drug can be helpful for blocking reflex-mediated rhinitis, which occurs in people with profuse rhinorrhea after the ingestion of spicy foods or in those with cold-air exposure.[1]

Allergen Immunotherapy

Specific-allergen immunotherapy continues to be a useful and important treatment for many patients with severe allergic rhinitis.[52,53] Research performed during the past decade has demonstrated that allergen immunotherapy induces a state of allergen-specific T-lymphocyte tolerance with a subsequent reduction in mediator release and tissue inflammation. When administered to appropriately selected patients, immunotherapy is effective in most cases. In addition to short-term benefits, recently published data suggest that the improvement in rhinitis symptoms persists for several years after the treatment is discontinued. Immunotherapy should be considered in patients who (1) do not respond to a combination of environmental control measures and medications, (2) experience substantial side effects with medications, (3) have symptoms

TABLE 28-7 Intranasal Corticosteroid Sprays

Corticosteroid	Dose per Actuation (μg)	Recommended Dosage
Beclomethasone dipropionate	42	$\geq$ 6 yr: 168-336 μg/day qd or bid
	84	
Budesonide	32	$\geq$ 12 yr: 64-256 μg/day qd
		6-11 yr: 64-128 μg/day qd
Flunisolide	25	$\geq$ 14 yr: 200-400 μg/day bid
		6-14 yr: 15-200 μg/day bid
Fluticasone propionate	50	$\geq$ 4 yr: 100-200 μg/day qd or bid
Mometasone furoate	50	$\geq$ 12 yr: 200 μg/day qd
		3-11 yr: 100 μg/day qd
Triamcinolone acetonide	55	$\geq$ 12 yr: 220-440 μg/day qd or bid
		6-11 yr: 220 μg/day qd

for a significant portion of the year that require daily therapy, or (4) prefer long-term modulation of their allergic symptoms. In making the decision to prescribe this therapy, the clinician should consider the positive and potentially negative effects of regular office visits for the administration of injections. If the decision is made to prescribe immunotherapy, it must be administered by a physician who is experienced in its use and whose office is set up to deal with the management of adverse allergic reactions, including anaphylaxis should this rare, untoward event occur.

CONCLUSIONS

Despite the high prevalence of allergic rhinitis in the pediatric population, this disease is often overlooked or undertreated. Untreated allergic rhinitis impairs the quality of life of the child and his or her parents. Accurate and timely diagnosis of allergic rhinitis in children relies on awareness of the symptoms and signs of the disease and its comorbidities, including asthma, sinusitis, and otitis media. Clinicians should understand the differential diagnosis of allergic rhinitis in children and pursue specific diagnostic testing when indicated. Treatment options include environmental controls and the use of intranasal corticosteroids, nonsedating antihistamines, and immunotherapy. The key concepts of allergic rhinitis in children are summarized in Box 28-1.

HELPFUL WEBSITES

The American Academy of Allergy, Asthma, and Immunology website (www.aaaai.org)

The American College of Allergy, Asthma and Immunology website (www.allergy.mcg.edu)

The Journal of Allergy and Clinical Immunology website (www.jaci@aaaai.org)

The Annals of Allergy, Asthma and Immunology website (www.annallergy.org)

BOX 28-1	**KEY CONCEPTS** *Allergic Rhinitis*

- Allergic rhinitis is one of the most common chronic disorders of childhood.
- Allergic rhinitis in children is an inflammatory airway disease.
- The distinction between allergic and nonallergic forms of rhinitis is important in children.
- Treatment should be individualized, aggressive, and targeted toward decreasing inflammation.
- Attention should be given to decreasing environmental exposures (e.g., allergens, tobacco smoke) and the use of intranasal corticosteroids and nonsedating antihistamines.
- Intranasal steroids constitute very effective therapy for allergic rhinitis and are safe despite a potential small drug-specific effect on growth rates.
- Allergic rhinitis in children may predispose to the development of otitis media, sinusitis, and asthma.

REFERENCES

1. Dykewicz MS, Fineman S, Skoner DP, et al: Diagnosis and management of rhinitis: complete guidelines of the Joint Task Force on Practice Parameters in Allergy, Asthma and Immunology. American Academy of Allergy, Asthma and Immunology, *Ann Allergy Asthma Immunol* 81: 478-518, 1998.
2. Skoner DP: Allergic rhinitis: definition, epidemiology, pathophysiology, detection and diagnosis, *J Allergy Clin Immunol* 108:S2-S8, 2001.
3. Linna O, Kokkonen J, Lukin M: A 10-year prognosis for childhood allergic rhinitis, *Acta Paediatr* 81:100-102, 1992.
4. Evans R: Epidemiology and natural history of asthma, allergic rhinitis, and atopic dermatitis (eczema). In Middleton E, Reed C, Ellis E, eds: *Allergy: principles and practice*, ed 4, St Louis, 1993, Mosby.
5. Wright AL, Holberg CJ, Martinez FD, et al: Epidemiology of physician-diagnosed allergic rhinitis in childhood, *Pediatrics* 94:895-901, 1994.
6. Aberg N, Engstrom I: Natural history of allergic diseases in children, *Acta Paediatr Scand* 79:206-211, 1990.
7. Tang RB, Tsai LC, Hwang HM, et al: The prevalence of allergic disease and IgE antibodies to house dust mite in schoolchildren in Taiwan, *Clin Exp Allergy* 20:33-38, 1990.
8. Schachter J, Higgins MW: Median age at onset of asthma and allergic rhinitis in Tecumseh, Michigan, *J Allergy Clin Immunol* 57:342-351, 1976.
9. Aberg N: Familial occurrence of atopic disease: genetic vs environmental factors, *Clin Exp Allergy* 23:829-843, 1993.
10. Gerrard JW, Vickers P, Gerrard CD: The familial incidence of allergic disease, *Ann Allergy* 36:10-15, 1976.
11. Fireman P: Allergic rhinitis. In Fireman P, Slavin R, eds: *Atlas of allergies*, Philadelphia, 1991, JB Lippincott.
12. Meltzer EO: The prevalence and medical and economic impact of allergic rhinitis in the United States, *J Allergy Clin Immunol* 99:S805-S828, 1997.
13. Aberg N: Asthma and allergic rhinitis in Swedish conscripts, *Clin Exp Allergy* 19:59-63, 1989.
14. Rimpela AH, Savonius B, Rimpela MK, et al: Asthma and allergic rhinitis among Finnish adolescents in 1977-1991, *Scand J Soc Med* 23:60-65, 1995.
15. Newacheck PW, Stoddard JJ: Prevalence and impact of multiple childhood chronic illnesses, *J Pediatr* 124:40-48, 1994.
16. Fineman SM: The burden of allergic rhinitis: beyond dollars and cents, *Ann Allergy Asthma Immunol* 88:2-7, 2002.
17. McMenamin P: Costs of hay fever in the United States in 1990, *Ann Allergy* 73:35-39, 1994.
18. Vuurman EF, van Vaggel LM, Uiterwijk MM, et al: Seasonal allergic rhinitis and antihistamine effects on children's learning, *Ann Allergy* 71: 121-126, 1993.
19. Raphael GD, Baraniuk JN, Kaliner MA: How and why the nose runs, *J Allergy Clin Immunol* 87:457-467, 1991.
20. Baraniuk J, Kaliner M: Functional activity of upper airway nerves. In Busse W, Holgate S, eds: *Mechanisms in asthma and rhinitis: implications for diagnosis and treatment*, London, 1995, Blackwell Scientific.
21. Naclerio RM: Allergic rhinitis, *N Engl J Med* 325:860-869, 1991.
22. Mygind N, Naclerio R: *Allergic and nonallergic rhinitis*, Philadelphia, 1993, WB Saunders.
23. Naclerio RM, Proud D, Togias AG, et al: Inflammatory mediators in late antigen-induced rhinitis, *N Engl J Med* 313:65-70, 1985.
24. Bascom R, Pipkorn U, Lichtenstein LM, et al: The influx of inflammatory cells into nasal washings during the late response to antigen challenge: effect of systemic steroid pretreatment, *Am Rev Respir Dis* 138:406-412, 1988.
25. Skoner D, Doyle W. Boehm S, et al: Late phase eustachian tube and nasal allergic responses associated with inflammatory mediator elaboration, *Am J Rhinol* 2:155-161, 1988.
26. Durham SR, Ying S, Varney VA, et al: Cytokine messenger RNA expression for IL-3, IL-4, IL-5, and granulocyte/macrophage-colony-stimulating factor in the nasal mucosa after local allergen provocation: relationship to tissue eosinophilia, *J Immunol* 148:2390-2394, 1992.
27. Sim TC, Reece LM, Hilsmeier KA, et al: Secretion of chemokines and other cytokines in allergen-induced nasal responses: inhibition by topical steroid treatment, *Am J Respir Crit Care Med* 152:927-933, 1995.
28. Connell JT: Quantitative intranasal pollen challenges, III: the priming effect in allergic rhinitis, *J Allergy* 43:33-44, 1969.
29. Jelks M: *Allergy plants that cause sneezing and wheezing*, London, 1986, Worldwide Publications.
30. Platts-Mills TA, Hayden ML, Chapman MD, et al: Seasonal variation in dust mite and grass-pollen allergens in dust from the houses of patients with asthma, *J Allergy Clin Immunol* 79:781-791, 1987.

31. Bradding P, Feather IH, Wilson S, et al: Immunolocalization of cytokines in the nasal mucosa of normal and perennial rhinitic subjects: the mast cell as a source of IL-4, IL-5, and IL-6 in human allergic mucosal inflammation, *J Immunol* 151:3853-3865, 1993.

32. MacKay I, Cole P: Rhinitis, sinusitis, and associated chest disease. In MacKay I, Null T, eds: *Scott-Brown's otolaryngology,* London, 1987, Butterworths.

33. Lund VJ, Scadding GK: Immunologic aspects of chronic sinusitis, *J Otolaryngol* 20:379-381, 1991.

34. Afzelius BA: A human syndrome caused by immotile cilia, *Science* 193:317-319, 1976.

35. Young D: Surgical treatment of male infertility, *J Reprod Fertil* 23:541-542, 1970.

36. Skoner D, Casselbrant M: Diseases of the ear. In Bierman C et al, eds: *Allergy, asthma, and immunology from infancy to adulthood,* ed 3, Philadelphia, 1996, WB Saunders.

37. Gentile DA, Michaels MG, Skoner DP: Pediatric allergy and immunology. In Davis H, Zitelli B, eds: *Atlas of pediatric physical diagnosis,* ed 4, St Louis, 2002, Mosby.

38. Settipane RA, Lieberman P: Update on nonallergic rhinitis, *Ann Allergy Asthma Immunol* 86:494-508, 2001.

39. Gideon Lack: Pediatric allergic rhinitis and comorbid conditions, *J Allergy Clin Immunol* 108:9-15, 2001.

40. Skoner DP: Complications of allergic rhinitis, *J Allergy Clin Immunol* 105:S605-S609, 2000.

41. Brostrom G, Moller C: A new method to relate symptom scores with pollen counts: a dynamic model for comparison of treatments of allergy, *Grana* 28:123-128, 1990.

42. Lucente FE: Rhinitis and nasal obstruction, *Otolaryngol Clin North Am* 22:307-318, 1989.

43. Bernstein IL, Storms WW: Practice parameters for allergy diagnostic testing: Joint Task Force on Practice Parameters for the Diagnosis and Treatment of Asthma. The American Academy of Allergy, Asthma and Immunology and the American College of Allergy, Asthma and Immunology, *Ann Allergy Asthma Immunol* 75:543-625, 1995.

44. Berger WE: Treatment update: allergic rhinitis, *Allergy Asthma Proc* 22:191-198, 2001.

45. Gentile DA, Friday GA, Skoner DP: Management of allergic rhinitis: antihistamines and decongestants, *Immunol Allergy Clin North Am* 20:355-368, 2000.

46. Mygind N, Nielsen LP, Hoffman HJ, et al: Mode of action of intranasal corticosteroids, *J Allergy Clin Immunol* 108:S16-S25, 2001.

47. Szefler SJ: Pharmacokinetics of intranasal corticosteroids, *J Allergy Clin Immunol* 108:S26-S31, 2001.

48. Scadding GK: Corticosteroids in the treatment of pediatric allergic rhinitis, *J Allergy Clin Immunol* 108:S26-S31, 2001.

49. Schenkel EJ, Skoner DP, Bronsky EA, et al: Absence of growth retardation in children with perennial allergic rhinitis following 1 year of treatment with mometasone furoate aqueous nasal spray, *Pediatrics* 105:E22, 2000.

50. Skoner DP, Rachelefsky GS, Meltzer EO, et al: Detection of growth suppression in children during treatment with intranasal beclomethasone dipropionate, *Pediatrics* 105:E23, 2000.

51. Pederson S: Assessing the effect of intranasal steroids on growth, *J Allergy Clin Immunol* 108:S26-S31, 2001.

52. DuBuske L: Appropriate and inappropriate use of immunotherapy, *Ann Allergy Asthma Immunol* 87:56-67, 2001.

53. Bousquet J, Demoly P, Michel FB: Specific immunotherapy in rhinitis and asthma, *Ann Allergy Asthma Immunol* 87:38-42, 2001.

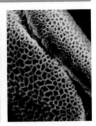

CHAPTER 29

Otitis Media

PHILIP FIREMAN

Otitis media (OM), with the potential resultant otitis media with effusion (OME), is the most common disease, except for viral upper respiratory infections, that requires care by pediatricians in the first decade of life. The costs of primary and specialty care, as well as the indirect costs incurred by the family in providing care for these patients, are enormous. The primary care costs of treating OM are in excess of $1 billion per year, surgical and specialty care costs are approximately $1 billion per year, and indirect costs of care are approximately $500 million per year, with total annual costs of more than $2.5 billion.[1] Even though there have been significant advances in the past 20 years in understanding the pathogenesis, pathophysiology, and immunopathology of OM, there has not been a decrease in the expression of this illness. In fact, there is a clinical impression that OM is occurring more frequently than previously. In addition, there are major questions and even disagreements among clinicians as to various medical and surgical management regimens used in the care of these patients.

The possibility that allergy contributes to OM is not a new concept, and its role has been debated for years.[2] Therefore this illness is of considerable interest to the allergist. If a causal relationship between allergy and middle ear (ME) disease were to be established, then one might anticipate that antiallergic therapy would reduce the morbidity and health care costs associated with OM. This chapter provides a review of the epidemiology, pathogenesis, eustachian tube (ET) physiology, and immunology of OM and the medical and surgical therapies to treat it.

DEFINITIONS

OM is characterized by an acute or chronic inflammation of the ME.[3] Although it can occur at any age, OM occurs most commonly in infants and children younger than 4 years. The clinical presentation and course of OM can vary, and a clinical classification of OM is presented in Table 29-1. Acute OM is typically preceded by or associated with a viral upper respiratory tract infection (URI), and a suppurative process in the ME is usually manifest. In about 50% of cases, when recognized and appropriately treated with antibiotics, the acute process resolves in less than 3 to 4 weeks.[4] Some children may experience repeated episodes of acute symptomatology and are classified as recurrent acute OM. When the acute process occurs more than six times, the child is considered "otitis prone."

The inflammation of acute OM manifests or evolves into an effusion, referred to as OME. Although frequently recognized as sequelae of acute OM, OME may also be recognized as an occult condition associated with a subclinical or protracted inflammation of the ME. OME may persist for weeks, but, when the duration exceeds 12 weeks without resolution, the process is termed *chronic OME*. Many synonyms have been used during the past 50 years to designate OM and OME, including serous OM, secretory OM, mucoid otitis, "glue ear," and suppurative and nonsuppurative OM. These descriptive terms have created much confusion. It is difficult to determine through visual inspection of the tympanic membrane the nature and characteristics of the ME effusion. Without a diagnostic tympanocentesis, the clinician cannot define the physical or microbial nature of the effusion. Because tympanocentesis is not currently recommended for most patients at the time of initial diagnosis, the generic OM or OME terminology is preferred, as listed in Table 29-1. The use of other terminology is to be discouraged because it may mislead the clinician and is not helpful in understanding the pathogenesis and potential etiology of OM.

EPIDEMIOLOGY

OM appears to be multifactorial in terms of those factors that increase the risk of disease expression, and a list of those epidemiologic factors is presented in Table 29-2. Males are affected more than females in all studies from many different countries and cultures. North American Indian, Inuit, and certain Polynesian children have a much higher incidence than white children.[5] There is a difference of opinion as to whether there is more otitis in white children than in African American children. Compared with bottle-feeding, breast-feeding is associated with a decreased risk of acute otitis or recurrent otitis during the first year of life.[6] Cigarette smoking by the parents, especially the mother, poses a significant risk factor for acute otitis during the first year of life.[7] Children whose parents or siblings have had a history of chronic otitis have a higher incidence than those with no family history of disease.[8] Studies by Rockley in the British Commonwealth suggest a genetic predisposition to OME, as well as an effect related to socioeconomic status, family size, and cigarette smoking in the family.[9] A prospective study of 175 sets of twins and triplets from birth has documented a genetic component to susceptibility to OM.[10] The estimate of discordance

TABLE 29-1 Classification of Otitis Media

Acute otitis media
Recurrent acute otitis media
Otitis media with effusion
Chronic otitis media with effusion

of acute OM in monozygotic twins was 0.04 compared with 0.49 in dizygotic twins ($P = 0.005$).

Allergy has also been incriminated as an epidemiologic risk factor, especially in studies of children with OME or chronic OME necessitating surgical intervention.[11] Several large Scandinavian and U.S. studies show that during the first 3 years of life, the association with allergic disease does not predispose to increased acute episodes of OM and suggest that allergy is not a risk factor in this age group.[12] Because the seasonal expression of acute otitis is greatest in the winter months, many authors suggest that this winter seasonality refutes an association with pollen-provoked seasonal allergic rhinitis. However, this would not refute an association of otitis with dust mite—provoked perennial allergic rhinitis. Studies of children with chronic OM who were referred to otolaryngologists and were also evaluated for allergy before surgical placement of a ventilation tube indicate that 40% to 50% of children were diagnosed with allergic rhinitis as confirmed by positive allergy skin tests or increased serum immunoglobulin E (IgE) antibodies to specific allergens.[13] Many of these children were older than 3 years. If the expression of allergic rhinitis in the 3- to 6-year-old pediatric population is estimated to be approximately 10% to 20%, then there is a twofold to fourfold greater expression of allergic rhinitis in children with chronic OME than in the general pediatric population. Japanese investigators reported that allergic rhinitis was found in 50% of 259 patients (mean age, 6 years) being treated for OME and that OME was found in 21% of 605 patients being treated for allergic rhinitis. However, in a comparison group of 108 school-aged children in whom neither condition had been diagnosed, the incidences of allergic rhinitis, OME, and both conditions were 17%, 6%, and 2%, respectively.[14] An association of OM with food allergy, based on clinical improvement after the avoidance of certain foods, especially milk, has been proposed in several anecdotal and inadequately designed surveys[15]; therefore, a definitive association of OM with food allergy requires better-designed studies before food allergy can be accepted as a risk factor for otitis.

TABLE 29-2 Risk Factors for Otitis Media

Viral upper respiratory tract infection (winter months)
Allergic rhinitis
Genetic predisposition
Eustachian tube dysfunction
Cigarette smoke (passive)
Not breast-fed
Male gender
Immunologic deficiency
Cilia dysfunction
Cleft palate disease

The best-defined risk factor in the development of acute OM is a preceding viral URI. A prospective telephone epidemiologic survey by Wald et al[16] reported that 25% to 40% of URIs in children from birth to 3 years of age were accompanied by an episode of OM. This survey also showed that otitis was more frequently associated with a URI in children 1 year of age or less than in 2- or 3-year-old children. These studies reported that URI, as well as acute otitis, was much more frequent in children who were in day care programs with other children than in those cared for in small groups or alone by a caretaker in the home. This study may be criticized because not all of these episodes of OM were confirmed by an examination of the patients and no viral cultures or laboratory studies were performed. Several other specific diseases have been associated with an increased expression of URI and OM. These illnesses include Down's syndrome, ciliary dysfunction syndromes, and immune deficiency syndromes, including isolated IgA deficiency and agammaglobulinemia.[17]

Based on a number of epidemiologic studies, by 1 year of age almost 50% of children surveyed have had a least one episode of acute otitis.[18] By 3 years of age, two thirds of children have had at least one otitis event. Three or more episodes of OM occur in 10% of children by 1 year of age and in 33% by 3 years of age. Tos et al[19] reported a prevalence of OME in 13% during the first 2 years of life. In the 4- to 6-year-old children, prevalence decreased to 7% and in the 8- to 10-year-old children to 2% to 4%.[19] Surveys of otherwise healthy children for the presence of ME ear fluid, with the use of tympanometry, have been conducted in several day care and school settings.[20] These surveys indicate that ME effusion (supposedly asymptomatic) is relatively frequent, especially in the winter months compared with the summer months. Repeated evaluations indicate that many of these effusions resolve spontaneously without therapy, and the effusions may shift from one ear to another and may persist for up to 6 months without overt symptoms. Yet children with persistent ME effusion or recurrent acute OM may manifest a conductive hearing loss with potential defects in speech and language development.[21]

PATHOPHYSIOLOGY

Structure and Function

OM should be considered a disease of the upper respiratory tract. Ventilation of the ME is accomplished via the ET from the posterior nasopharynx. As discussed later, OM and OME appear to be related by abnormal functioning of the ET.

Understanding and diagnosing this disease require familiarity with the anatomy and physiology of the upper airway, which is made up of the nasal cavity, nasopharynx, ET, ME, and mastoid air cells. The ET provides an anatomic communication between the nasopharynx and the ME and is in a unique position to effect changes in the ME secondary to reactions in the nose. In relation to the ME and the nasopharynx, the ET may be considered to be analogous in part to the bronchial tree in relation to the lung and nasopharynx. Like mucosa elsewhere in the respiratory tract, the mucosa lining the ET contains mucus-producing cells, ciliated cells, plasma cells, and mast cells.[22] Unlike the bronchial tree, the ET is usually collapsed and thus closed to the nasopharynx and its contents. Active opening of the ET is accomplished through contraction of the tensor veli palatine (TVP) muscle during swallowing, yawning, crying, or sneezing. In this regard the

ET, like the bronchial airway, serves several physiologic functions—protection, drainage, and ventilation: protection from nasopharyngeal secretions, drainage into the nasopharynx of secretions produced within the ME, and ventilation of the ME to equilibrate air pressure with atmospheric pressure and to replenish oxygen that has been absorbed.

In normal tubal function, intermittent opening of the ET maintains near-ambient pressure in the ME cavity. It is suspected that in cases in which active swallowing is inadequate to overcome tubal resistance, the tube remains persistently collapsed, resulting in progressively negative ME pressure. This type of ventilation appears to be common in children because moderate to high negative ME pressures have been identified with tympanometry in many children who are apparently normal. However, periodic or persistently high negative pressure may be pathologic and has been associated with abnormal function of the ET. Persistently high negative ME pressure with severe retraction of the tympanic membrane has been termed *atelectasis of the tympanic membrane* and results in acute OM. If effective ventilation does not occur because of persistent ET obstruction, transudation of sterile ME effusion in the tympanum can result as a consequence of the constant absorption of oxygen by the ME epithelium. Because tubal opening is possible in an ME with an effusion, aspiration of nasopharyngeal secretions might occur, thus creating the clinical condition in which persistent effusion and recurrent acute OM occur together. Thus abnormal ET function may predispose the ME to atelectasis, infection, or effusion.[23]

Eustachian Tube Obstruction

Two types of ET obstruction, mechanical and functional, could result in acute or chronic OME. Table 29-3 lists the common conditions associated with ET obstruction. Intrinsic mechanical obstruction may result from the inflammation of infection or allergy, whereas extrinsic obstruction may result from enlarged adenoids or, in rare instances, nasopharyngeal tumors. Experimentally, allergic rhinitis provoked in patients with a history of allergy has been associated with the development of ET obstruction.[24] This obstruction, related to edema and inflammation of the posterior nasopharynx, could be both extrinsic and intrinsic. A persistent collapse of the ET during swallowing may result in functional obstruction, which appears to be related to increased tubal compliance; an inefficient, active opening mechanism by the TVP muscle; or both. Functional ET obstruction is common in infants and younger children because the amount and stiffness of the cartilage support of the ET are less than in older children and adults. Also, there appear to be marked age differences in the angulation of the craniofacial base, which renders the TVP muscle less efficient before puberty. The incidence of OME, which is very frequent in infants and children with cleft palate, is related to a functional obstruction of the ET.[25]

PATHOGENESIS

The development of rational treatment and prevention strategies for OM is dependent on a fundamental understanding of disease pathogenesis. In this regard, the etiology of OM has been shown to be multifactorial, with ET dysfunction, bacterial or viral infection of the ME, and nasal inflammation resulting from allergic rhinitis or viral URI acknowledged as being contributing factors. However, investigations of pathogenic mechanisms based on individual factors in isolation are not consistent with the results of epidemiologic studies, suggesting that the pathogenesis of OM involves significant interactions between these factors.[26]

The suggested role of allergic rhinitis in the pathogenesis of OM was supported by experiments conducted in sensitized monkeys, which showed that the ME mucosa is capable of sustaining an allergic reaction; however, the extent and duration of inflammation were limited and OME was not observed.[27] Alternatively, it was hypothesized that nasal inflammation resulting from allergic rhinitis could cause ET dysfunction and OM by hydrops ex vacuo. Intranasal relevant allergen challenge in adult allergic rhinitis subjects and in sensitized primates caused classic signs and symptoms of allergic rhinitis as well as ET dysfunction, and challenge of allergic rhinitis patients with irrelevant allergens or of nonallergic rhinitis subjects with allergens did not provoke these responses.[24,28] These signs and symptoms could be reproduced using intranasal challenges with chemicals released or synthesized during an allergic reaction.[29] Two response domains were documented, with significant relationships established between sneezing and secretion production and between nasal congestion and ET dysfunction.[30] However, none of these studies resulted in the prerequisite events for OM by hydrops ex vacuo (i.e., sustained ME underpressures). Additional studies have documented ET dysfunction and ME underpressures in allergic rhinitis patients during natural allergen exposure, but the development of OM was a rare event.[31]

In contrast to an allergic etiology, convincing data exist with respect to a viral etiology of OM. Viral URIs are the most common infections that affect humans; they occur between 2 and 4 times per year in adults and significantly more frequently in children.[32] The primary etiologic agents identified during viral URI include rhinovirus, adenovirus, influenzavirus, parainfluenza virus, coxsackievirus, and respiratory syncytial virus (RSV), among others.[33] For OM, approximately 50% of new episodes are diagnosed immediately after or concurrent with a viral URI.[34] A causal relationship between the two disease entities is supported by the results of experimental studies that reported OM resulting from adenovirus and influenzavirus infections in the chinchilla.[35] Using adult volunteers, OM was reported to be a complication of experimental infections in human volunteers with rhinovirus 39 and influenza A (INF-A) virus in approximately 3% and 20% of the subjects, respectively.[36,37] In addition, a significantly lower incidence of acute OM was reported for infants and children immunized with an

TABLE 29-3 Types of Eustachian Tube Obstruction

Mechanical obstruction
  Intrinsic
    Infectious inflammation
    Allergic inflammation
  Extrinsic (peritubular)
    Adenoidal hypertrophy
    Nasopharyngeal tumor
Functional obstruction
  Poor tensor veli palatini muscle function
  Increased tubal compliance

influenzavirus vaccine than nonimmunized controls during a seasonal influenza epidemic.[38]

Both viral URI and nasal allergic reactions provoke nasal inflammation, ET dysfunction, and enhanced nasal protein transudation and secretion in association with the release of a variety of bioactive substances.[39,40] The provoked nasal and tubal effects are probably initiated, sustained, and modulated by inflammatory mediators, cytokines, and proteins. Indeed, these effects have been reproduced by provocative challenges with histamine, and some of the responses were augmented in allergic rhinitis subjects.[29] Others reported that allergic rhinitis patients with rhinovirus URI had significantly enhanced lower airway responsiveness and basophil histamine release to ragweed challenge.[41] These data suggest that allergic rhinitis patients may be physiologically hyperresponsive to various mediators of inflammation elaborated during a viral URI and that this could be potentiated by the priming of a preceding allergen exposure or URI. To test this hypothesis, allergic and nonallergic rhinitis subjects were experimentally infected with rhinovirus 39 and were monitored for the development of nasal and otologic symptoms, signs, and pathophysiologies.[42] The results failed to support a physiologic hyperresponsiveness in allergic rhinitis subjects, but *in vitro* studies documented augmented IgE synthesis and increased basophil histamine release in allergic rhinitis subjects only.[43] After experimental infection with INF-A virus, allergic rhinitis subjects manifested enhanced release of histamine from their peripheral blood basophils.[44] In other studies, the hypothesis that viral URIs could prime the nasal response to specific and nonspecific stimuli was tested. In one study, paired histamine and cold air challenges were performed before infection with rhinovirus 39 and after acute symptoms subsided. The results showed greater provoked sneezing and secretion responses for both allergic rhinitis and nonallergic rhinitis subjects to these stimuli for the sessions conducted after virus infection.[45] Similar results were documented for histamine challenges conducted before and after infection with INF-A virus.[46] These observations show that preexisting viral infection primes certain responses of the nose in both allergic rhinitis and nonallergic rhinitis subjects to challenges with a mediator of inflammation (histamine) and a stimulus (cold air) that causes the release of mediators of inflammation.[47] These data support the hypothesized interaction between virus infection and nasal allergy in enhancing certain responses. Such an interaction could explain the mechanism by which allergic rhinitis is expressed as a risk factor for OM, thereby defining a target population for therapeutic interventions focused on risk reduction.

An *in situ* infection of the ME mucosa by viruses has been suggested, and experiments using the chinchilla showed that the ME mucosa can be infected with influenzavirus and adenovirus after direct challenge.[35] Although cultures of ME effusions from children with persistent and acute OM have recovered viruses in relatively few cases,[48] indirect assays of effusions for viral proteins or nuclei and sequences have documented these chemicals in relatively high frequencies.[49] However, a significant role for an acute virus infection of the ME mucosa is difficult to reconcile, with ME effusion bacterial recovery rates of 70% for acute OM and 30% to 50% for persistent OM.[50] As with viruses, these rates are significantly increased when diagnostic polymerase chain reaction (PCR) is used.[51] These and other observations have led investigators to suggest that viral URIs interact with bacterial pathogens in promoting OM. Viral effects that could promote bacterial infections include altered bacterial adherence modulation of the host immune/inflammatory response and impaired ET function.

Viruses causing URI have been shown to alter respiratory epithelial receptors, thereby differentially affecting bacterial adherence and thus the bacterial flora of the nasopharynx. These changes may promote the development of a secondary bacterial infection of the ME. Rhinovirus infections have been shown to alter the immune response of the host.[41] Others showed that influenzavirus infection suppresses polymorphonuclear chemotactic activity and perhaps phagocytic activity.[52] Giebink et al[53] reported impaired polymorphonuclear chemotactic bactericidal and chemiluminescent activity in 15% to 23% of children with persistent OM. These effects could compromise host defenses and increase susceptibility to a secondary bacterial infection.

A role for ET dysfunction in the pathogenesis of OM during a viral URI is supported by the results of a variety of clinical and experimental studies. Studies reported tubal dysfunction in children and adults with natural viral URI,[54] in adults experimentally infected with respiratory viruses,[55] and in animals infected with influenzavirus.[56] URIs have been shown to result in the local release of inflammatory mediators, which provoke tubal dysfunction when applied to the nasal mucosa.[29] Sustained tubal dysfunction results in ME underpressures and OM that is sterile for pathogens,[57] and intermittent tubal opening during ME underpressures can promote bacterial or viral infection of the ME through aspiration of nasopharyngeal secretions containing pathogens.[58]

A model of disease pathogenesis that synthesizes these observations with respect to the mechanism by which viral URI could cause an otologic disease was supported by research involving experimental virus infection of adult volunteers. Initial studies concentrated on rhinovirus infection because this virus is the most common cause of colds. These studies showed that rhinovirus infection results in significant increases in nasal inflammation, impaired tubal function in a majority of subjects, abnormal ME pressures in more than 40% of subjects, and asymptomatic OM in approximately 2% of subjects.[55] These events occurred sequentially and in descending frequency, supporting a causal pathway. Using a smaller number of subjects, this pattern was generalizable in infection with rhinovirus 39, influenza A virus, and coxsackievirus A.[59] Later studies showed that infection of adult volunteers with influenzavirus caused significant nasal, throat, and general symptoms; ET dysfunction; and ME underpressures in the majority of subjects and OM in approximately 20%.[37] In the majority of cases, the OM episode was asymptomatic and the recovered effusion for one symptomatic episode was negative by culture for viruses and bacteria but positive for genomic sequences of INF-A and *Streptococcus pneumoniae* by diagnostic PCR.[51] Assay of the peripheral blood from adult subjects infected with either rhinovirus or influenzavirus documents infection-related changes in lymphocyte subpopulations and response to mitogens.[60] Also, during the acute INF-A virus infection, depressed neutrophil chemotaxis and enhanced superoxide production in the resting state and when exposed to an opsonized stimuli were observed. Serial throat cultures of the subjects during experimental influenza documented an increase in the frequency of recovery of S. *pneumoniae* in the other suspected pathogens or in the commensal bacterial flora.[61] These results indicate that the various components of OM pathogenesis are indeed realized during a viral URI, which may also potentiate the allergic inflammatory response.

ETIOLOGY

Infection and Otitis Media Effusion

Bacteria have been cultured from approximately 70% of ME effusions obtained via tympanocentesis in children with acute OM, and the microbiology has been shown to be similar to that found in the sinus aspirates of children with acute sinusitis.[50] As illustrated in Table 29-4, S. *pneumoniae* has been cultured from approximately 35% of ME effusion and is clearly the most common infectious agent in all age groups. Penicillin-resistant S. *pneumoniae* has been recognized as a significant clinical problem and has increased from approximately 1% to 8% to 34% of organisms cultured from acute OM.[62] Interestingly, isolates from the ME are more likely to be resistant to penicillin than those from other sites, such as the blood, central nervous system, and lungs. *Haemophilus influenzae*, nontypable, has been found in approximately 23% of the ear effusions. About 30% of the H. *influenzae* organisms were β-lactamase producing, and the percentage of this amoxicillin-resistant organism has gradually increased during the past several years. In the past, the incidence of *Moraxella catarrhalis* has been about 15%, but it is now 20% or higher in certain localities. About 75% of M. *catarrhalis* strains are β-lactamase producing and amoxicillin resistant. These increases in amoxicillin resistance have had an important impact on the choice of antibiotics for therapy. The frequency of group A β-hemolytic *Streptococcus* was 3%, and *Staphylococcus aureus* was present in fewer than 2%.

Based on epidemiologic surveys, episodes of acute otitis are preceded by or associated with a clinical illness typical of a viral URI. However, as discussed in the "Pathogenesis" section, viruses have been difficult to culture from ME aspirates of children who have acute OM, but viral antigens have been identified using immunoassay in 10% to 20% of ME effusions. Why viruses have been difficult to culture or identify from ME effusions is not known. This is especially important, because many episodes of acute otitis are preceded by a viral URI, which sets the stage for the secondary bacterial infection (see section on pathogenesis).

Previously it had been assumed, incorrectly, that chronic EF effusions were sterile, especially after apparently adequate antimicrobial therapy. In several studies, about 50% of the chronic, persistent ME effusions had positive cultures for bacteria, whose microbiology was similar to that found in acute otitis. An inadequate host defense can contribute to recurrent respiratory infections as well as OME. The most common of these unusual problems is IgA deficiency, but other Ig or cellular immune deficiencies, as well as the immotile cilia syndrome, cannot be overlooked.

ALLERGY AND OTITIS MEDIA EFFUSION

That IgE-mediated allergic reactions participate in the pathogenesis of chronic OME has been suggested by clinical observations reporting a higher prevalence of chronic OME in allergic patients, but these studies were retrospective and lacked appropriate controls and experimental design. The role of allergy in OME may involve one or more of the following mechanisms: (1) ME mucosa functioning as a target organ, (2) inflammatory swelling of the ET with resultant obstruction, (3) inflammatory obstruction of the nose and nasopharynx, and (4) reflux, insufflation, or aspiration of bacteria-laden allergic nasopharyngeal secretions into the ME cavity. The latter three mechanisms would be associated with abnormal function of the ET. Although histamine and other mediators of inflammation are present in ME effusions, there is minimal evidence that the ME mucosa functions as the allergic "shock organ" via IgE antibody and allergen reaction.[11,13]

Nasal obstruction through infection, allergy, or both may also be involved in the pathogenesis of OME. Swallowing when the nose is obstructed (inflammation or obstructive adenoids) creates a closed nasopharyngeal chamber. During swallowing, an initial positive nasopharyngeal air pressure is followed by a negative pressure phase within the closed system. There are two possible effects of these pressures on a pliant tube: (1) with positive nasopharyngeal pressure, secretions might be insufflated in the ME, especially when the ME has a high negative pressure, or (2) with negative nasopharyngeal pressures, such a tube could be prevented from opening and become further functionally obstructed. This has been termed the *Toynbee phenomenon*.

The following sequence of events is postulated to occur in patients who have respiratory allergy and OM. Most probably, a basic ET dysfunction is present in certain infants and children whose tubal function becomes compromised in the presence of upper respiratory tract allergy, similar to or in association with ET obstruction caused by a URI. Upper respiratory tract allergy may cause some intrinsic as well as extrinsic mechanical obstruction in patients who have normal ET function, but their normal active opening mechanisms, that is, TVP muscle pull, is able to overcome the obstruction. Therefore patients who have functional obstruction because of poor muscular opening would be at the highest risk for development of sufficient mechanical obstruction to give rise to ME disease. Many children, as part of normal development, have difficulty in actively opening their ET; they are the population most at risk for manifesting OME, especially in association with respiratory allergy, URI, or both.

DIAGNOSIS OF OTITIS MEDIA

Signs and Symptoms

The earliest signs of OM are most frequently ear pain and discomfort, which may be difficult to discern in a child who is too young to speak. The child may be irritable and pull on the

TABLE 29-4	Bacteria Cultured from Middle Ear Effusion Tympanocentesis of Acute Otitis Media

Bacteria	Percentage
Streptococcus pneumoniae	30
Haemophilus influenzae	20
Moraxella catarrhalis	15
Streptococci (group A)	3
Staphylococcus aureus	2
No growth	30

affected ear. There may be an associated conductive hearing deficit, which, if not recognized or if neglected for a prolonged period of time, may predispose the child to subsequent speech pathology.

Most children with OM will have an associated rhinitis, and it is important to decide whether the rhinitis is infectious or allergic. The differentiation between infection and perennial allergic rhinitis can be difficult. Symptoms of a URI, such as fever and malaise with profuse active rhinorrhea, would suggest an infection. The presence of a similar acute illness in immediate family members or contacts would also indicate an infection. Of course, a purulent rhinorrhea or pharyngitis would suggest an infection. A prolonged perennial or recurrent seasonal rhinitis with itching and sneezing would suggest an allergic basis, as would bilateral red, itchy, swollen, nonpurulent inflammation of the eyes, all of which are manifestations of allergic rhinoconjunctivitis.

Even if ET obstruction is minimal, patients with allergic rhinitis may have mild symptoms of ET dysfunction, such as "popping" and "snapping" sounds in the ear. These symptoms may be aggravated during airplane travel. Many of these patients will experience these symptoms and go on to have more problems, such as hearing loss, ear discomfort, tinnitus, and, rarely, vertigo during the worst periods of their allergic rhinitis. These symptoms may not be manifest in the nonverbal child. A family history of allergy along with a seasonal runny nose or constant "cold" should raise suspicions of an allergic diathesis. Other allergic conditions associated with allergic rhinitis include atopic dermatitis and allergic asthma. Seasonal allergic rhinitis occurs episodically, most typically in temperate climate during the tree, grass, and weed pollen seasons, whereas perennial allergic rhinitis evokes symptoms all year. These perennial allergens can be caused by pollens or fungi in a tropical climate or nonseasonal allergens present in the home, especially the bedroom, or in the workplace. These indoor perennial allergens include house dust, dust mites, cockroach, storage mold spores, pet animal products, or occupational allergens.

Diagnostic Techniques

Pneumatic Otoscopy

Recognition of OME during the physical examination requires the use of pneumatic otoscopy. The physician must choose the correct size of speculum to fit each patient's ear canal. It is necessary to obtain a good pneumatic seal during an otoscopic examination to ascertain the motility of the tympanic membrane by the gentle application of air pressure via the hand-held bulb. The loss of normal movement of the eardrum during this procedure indicates a loss of compliance of the eardrum as a result of either ME effusion behind the drum or increased stiffness from scarring or thickening of an inflamed eardrum.

Otoscopic inspection requires visualization of the tympanic membrane, and frequently cerumen may have to be removed from the external ear canal to permit an adequate examination. The normal tympanic membrane is thin, translucent, neutrally positioned, and mobile. The bony ossicles, particularly the malleus, are generally visible through the tympanic membrane. Adequate assessment requires that the physician take note of the major characteristics of the tympanic membrane—its thickness, degree of translucence, position, and mobility to applied pressure.

A bulging eardrum indicates the presence of excessive ME fluid and documents effusion. The presence of marked erythema and hyperemia points to a clinical diagnosis of acute OM. Sometimes the presence of air bubbles and fluid levels documents OME. The presence of a retracted eardrum suggests negative pressure and possibly atelectasis within the ME. Acute OM may, by virtue of increased ME pressure, result in acute perforation of the tympanic membrane. On presentation, the canal may be filled with pus. Careful removal of the pus with a cotton wick will usually reveal an inflamed drum, with perforation. The outcome of neglected otitis with recurrent inflammation may be the development of a cholesteatoma.

The persistence of OME despite adequate therapy for more than 4 to 6 months and the presence of a hearing deficit are indications for a myringotomy and the insertion of ventilation tubes. These will facilitate hearing and reduce the frequency of recurrent otitis.

Tympanometry

The use of the tympanometer in the assessment of potential ear disease has been recognized as a valuable adjunct in the management of OME. When otoscopic findings are unclear or otoscopy is difficult to perform, tympanometry can be very useful in evaluating children older than 6 months. This instrument, which measures the compliance of the eardrum as well as ME pressure, is also helpful in clinical practice in confirming the diagnosis of OME. Thus besides otolaryngologists, many pediatricians and allergists have incorporated tympanometry into their consulting practices. An audiogram is also necessary for the management of recurrent and chronic OME. The evaluation of a potential conductive hearing deficit as a complication of this disease is an important aspect of patient management that must not be ignored.

DIFFERENTIAL DIAGNOSIS

Allergy

If allergy, specifically allergic rhinitis, is suspected on the basis of the history and confirmed by physical examination as a risk factor for the development of OME, then an allergic evaluation is suggested to confirm this suspicion. Skin prick testing is preferred to serologic anti-IgE antibody tests for the detection of IgE antibodies to specific allergens because of the increased sensitivity and lower cost of these tests. Total serum IgE levels are usually not especially helpful for the evaluation of allergic rhinitis because only a third of these allergic individuals have elevated total serum IgE. In addition, total serum IgE does not assist in defining specific allergen sensitivity.

Immunodeficiency Syndrome

The possibility of an immune deficiency syndrome should be included in the differential diagnosis if the physician decides that the child has undue susceptibility to infection. When a child with chronic recurrent or persistent OME has also had recurrent sinusitis, pneumonia, or other infections in addition to the recurrent URI, then immunologic assessment is indicated to evaluate potential immune deficiency syndromes. The initial laboratory tests performed should include quantification of serum IgG, IgA, and IgM, as well as a complete blood count, including a total leukocyte count and leukocyte differential count to ascertain the absolute lymphocyte count.

A delayed skin test to *Candida*, mumps, or tetanus can be applied to assess cell-mediated immunity. Whether additional immunologic laboratory tests should be performed to assess specific functional serum antibodies, serum Ig subclasses, and T and B lymphocytes, as well as complement function, will depend on the other signs and symptoms of recurrent infection.

TREATMENT

The therapy for acute OM is outlined in Figure 29-1. If there are no potential or documented complications, the initial management consists of choosing appropriate antibiotics. If there has been no acute OM in the previous month, the antibiotic of choice is amoxicillin. Because of the increased penicillin resistance, an increased dose of 80 to 90 mg/kg/day of amoxicillin is recommended. If symptoms persist for longer than 3 days, this is considered a clinically defined treatment failure and an alternative second-line antibiotic should be selected, considering the likelihood of infection with resistant organisms; these include an amoxicillin-clavulanate mixture or cephalosporins such as oral cefuroxime.[62] If the patient has had acute OM in the previous month, then the second-line antibiotic should be prescribed. If the symptoms improve, the patient should be examined in 4 to 6 weeks to determine whether the acute OM has resolved or if an ME effusion (OME) has persisted. If an ME effusion is present, then additional management is indicated and the clinician should follow therapy as outlined in Figure 29-2. If the acute OM is complicated, it may be appropriate to perform tympanocentesis to obtain ME fluid for culture and identification of antibiotic sensitivities because of the high incidence of antibiotic resistance. Of course, antibiotic therapy should be instituted and modified when culture results are available. If the patient has a history of recurrent acute OM, which is defined as three episodes of acute OM in 6 months or four episodes of acute OM in 12 months, these patients deserve additional evaluation and follow-up as indicated in Algorithm A. Environmental risk factors and immune deficiency should be considered. Pneumococcal and influenza vaccines have been shown to reduce frequency of acute OM. Antimicrobial prophylaxis for recurrent acute OM has demonstrated efficacy, but because of the problem of increased bacterial resistance, this should be limited to selected cases. Surgical management of recurrent acute OM with myringotomy and tube placement may be helpful, but adenoidectomy or tonsillectomy is not recommended as first-line surgical therapy for recurrent acute OM. Analgesics are appropriate. Decongestants are widely used, but their efficacy has not been documented in controlled studies.

The management of OME is outlined in Figure 29-2. As indicated earlier, OME may be an unresolved complication of an acute OM or it may be detected as an occult condition without previous signs or symptoms of an infection, perhaps a subclinical infection. OME is frequently asymptomatic but may cause a hearing loss or balance disturbance. As indicated previously, the cause is multifactorial. If the patient is identified as not at high risk, the OME is present for less than 3 months, and the patient is asymptomatic, then antibiotic therapy is optional but environmental risk factors should be considered. However, these patients need to be examined at 4 to 6 weeks to determine whether the effusion has resolved. If the effusion has persisted for longer than 3 months, then hearing evaluation with audiometry should be considered. If normal hearing is present in at least one ear, then antibiotic therapy should be considered and the patient should be rechecked periodically. If there is bilateral hearing loss and no recent antibiotic therapy, then oral antibiotic therapy should be initiated as described earlier. If the child with hearing loss has persistent effusion despite appropriate antibiotic therapy, then surgery consultation should be obtained. An additional indication for a surgical consultation is the presence of OME for longer than 6 months. The presence of a high risk as outlined in Figure 29-2 deserves more aggressive antibiotic therapy and more frequent examination by the clinician. The presence of persistent effusion deserves a more prompt surgical consultation.

In all patients with OME in whom nasal obstruction, persistent rhinitis, or recurrent rhinitis is documented, allergy should be considered and the patient evaluated as discussed earlier. If allergic rhinitis is documented in association with OME, then allergy management should include antihistamine therapy and the avoidance of offending allergens. If these are not effective, then intranasal topical steroids should be initiated. Allergen immunotherapy may also be considered. Even though allergen immunotherapy has shown efficacy for allergic rhinitis, there are no placebo-controlled trials that document efficacy in reduction of frequency or resolution of OME. The roles of oral steroids in the management of chronic OME and recurrent OM have been suggested and appear promising but require better definition and additional study.

The surgical management of OME includes the insertion of tympanostomy (ventilation) tubes to promote drainage of persistent unresolved effusions and improve hearing. With the recognition of the sequelae of chronic OME, this surgical procedure has become the most frequently performed operation in the United States. Many physicians have questioned the increasing popularity of this surgery and have cautioned against its potential abuse. Indications for consultation with an otolaryngologist to consider insertion of tympanostomy tubes include the following: (1) appropriate medical management has not been successful in alleviating the OME; (2) the OME was documented as recurrent, with three or more episodes in the preceding 6 months; (3) OME has persisted for more than 4 to 6 months; and (4) persistent conductive hearing deficiency was documented. Adenoidectomy has also been recommended to relieve extrinsic ET obstruction caused by peritubular lymphoid tissue. Both of these surgical procedures appear to be beneficial in certain patients, but better documentation of their efficacy needs to be established and confirmed in controlled, double-blind studies.

CONCLUSIONS

OM is a multifactorial illness that affects many children as either an acute or a chronic and recurrent disease. The roles of infection, ET obstruction, allergy, and host defense defects have been delineated and discussed. Infection and ET obstruction are the principal contributing factors in acute OM; however, the role of allergy in the child with chronic or recurrent OM should not be ignored. It is anticipated that better definition of the pathogenesis of OME will provide the basis for more appropriate medical management, which will reduce the need for and frequency of insertion of myringotomy tubes and other surgical procedures. This will also reduce the health care costs, as well as increase the well-being of these children (Box 29-1).

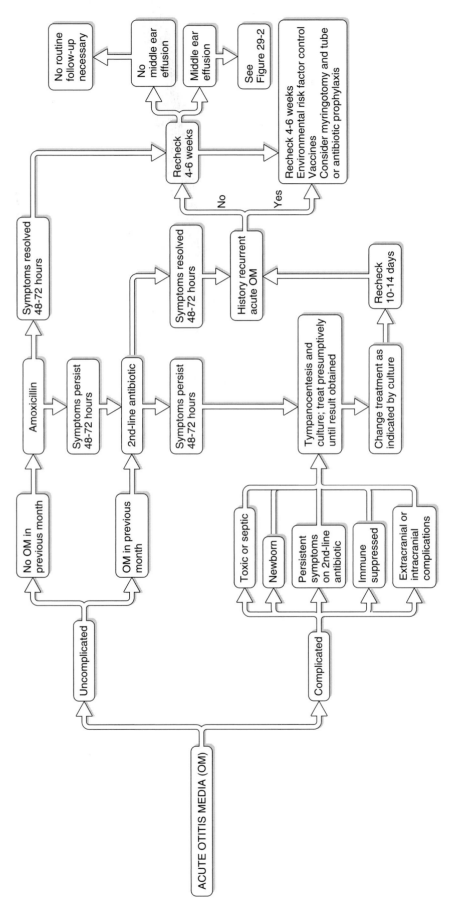

FIGURE 29-1 Algorithm for management of acute otitis media. (Modified from Mandel EM, Casselbrant ML: *Acute otitis media in decision making*. In Alper CM, Myers EN, Eibling DE, eds: *Ear, nose, and throat disorders*, Philadelphia, 2001, WB Saunders.)

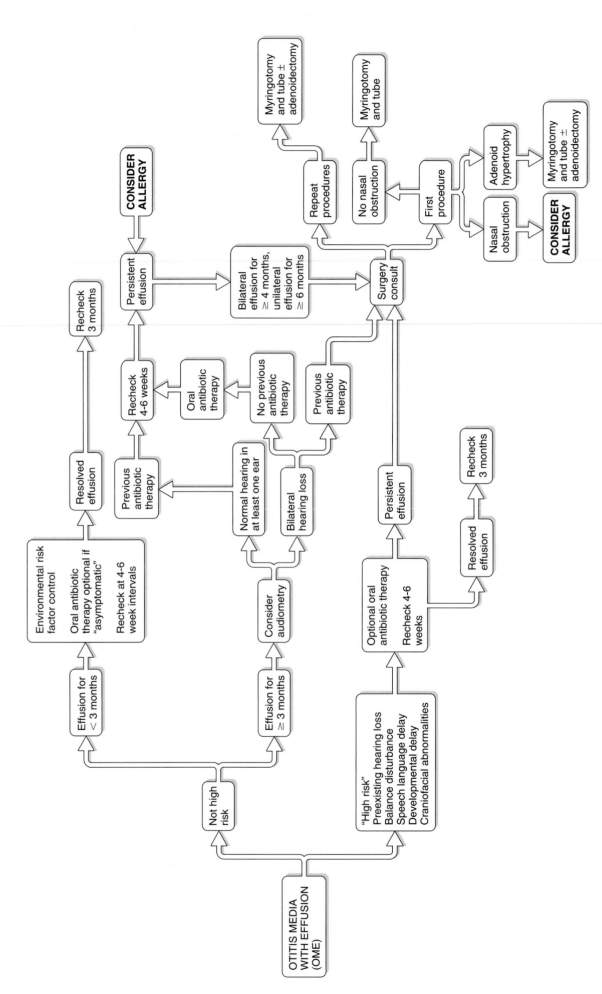

FIGURE 29-2 Algorithm for management of otitis media with effusion. (Modified from Mandel EM, Casselbrant ML: Acute otitis media in decision making. In Alper CM, Myers EN, Eibling DE, eds: *Ear, nose, and throat disorders,* Philadelphia, 2001, WB Saunders.)

- Acute otitis media, a frequent multifactorial illness of early childhood, can evolve into a chronic otitis media with effusion associated with obstruction of the eustachian tube.

- Viral upper respiratory infection often precedes acute otitis media with bacteria cultured in 70% of patients with acute otitis media and 50% of patient with otitis media with effusion.

- Chronic otitis media with effusion of more than 3 months' duration promotes a conduction hearing deficit with potential speech pathology.

- Increased frequency of bacterial resistance to antibiotics requires judicious selection of antibiotics without excessive use.

- Epidemiologic and experimental studies suggest a role for allergic rhinitis in the patient with chronic otitis media with effusion and nasal obstruction but not in acute otitis media.

REFERENCES

1. Stool SE, Field MJ: The impact of otitis media, *Pediatr Infect Dis* 8: S11-S14, 1990.
2. Fireman P: Eustachian tube obstruction and allergy: a role in otitis media with effusion, *J Allergy Clin Immunol* 76:137-139, 1985.
3. Bernstein JM: Recent advances of immunologic reactivity in otitis media with effusion, *J Allergy Clin Immunol* 81:1004, 1982.
4. Teele DW, Klein JO, Rosner BA: Middle ear disease during the first five years of life, *JAMA* 249:1026-1029, 1983.
5. Bluestone CD, Klein JO: Otitis media, atelectasis and eustachian tube dysfunction. In Bluestone CD, Stool SE, Alper CM, et al, eds: *Pediatric otolaryngology,* ed 2, Philadelphia, 1990, WB Saunders.
6. Teele DW, Klein JO, Greater Boston Collaborative Group: Beneficial effects of breast feeding on the duration of middle ear effusion after first episode of acute otitis media, *Pediatr Res* 14:94-101, 1980.
7. Kraemer MJ, Richardson MA, Weiss NS: Risk factors for persistent middle-ear effusion, *JAMA* 249:1022-1025, 1983.
8. Teele DW, Klein JO, Rosner BA: Epidemiology of otitis media in children, *Ann Otol Rhinol Laryngol* 89:5, 1980.
9. Rockley TJ: Family studies in serous otitis media. In Lim D, Bluestone C, Klein J, et al, eds: *Recent advances in otitis media,* Toronto, 1988, BC Decker.
10. Casselbrant ML, Mandel EM, Fall PA, et al: The hereditability of otitis media: a twin and triplet study, *JAMA* 282:2125-2130, 1999.
11. Bernstein JM, Lee J, Conboy K, et al: The role of IgE-mediated hypersensitivity in recurrent otitis media with effusion, *Am J Otol* 10:566, 1983.
12. Pukander JS, Karma PH: Persistence of middle ear effusion and its risk factors after an acute attack of otitis media with effusion. In Lim D, Bluestone C, Klein J, et al, eds: *Recent advances in otitis media,* Toronto, 1988, BC Decker.
13. Bernstein JM, Lee L, Conboy K, et al: Further observations on the role of IgE-mediated hypersensitivity in recurrent otitis media with effusion, *Otolaryngol Head Neck Surg* 93:611, 1985.
14. Tomonaga K, Kurono Y, Mogi G: The role of nasal allergy in otitis media with effusion: a clinical study, *Acta Otolaryngol (Stockh) Suppl* 458: 41-47, 1998.
15. Buccafogli A, Vicentini L, Camerani A, et al: Adverse food reactions in patients with grass pollen allergic respiratory disease, *Ann Allergy* 73: 301-308, 1994.
16. Wald ER, Guerra N, Byers C. Upper respiratory tract infections in young children: duration of and frequency of complications, *Pediatrics* 98: 129-137, 1991.
17. Stiehm ER: Immunodeficiency disorders: general considerations. In Stiehm ER, ed: *Immunologic disorders in infants and children,* Philadelphia, 1992, WB Saunders.
18. Teele DW, Klein JO, Rosner BA: Epidemiology of otitis media during the first seven years of life in children in Greater Boston: a perspective cohort study, *J Infect Dis* 160:83, 1989.
19. Tos M, Stangerup SE, Hvid G, et al: Epidemiology of natural history of secretory otitis. In Sade J, ed: *Acute and secretory otitis media,* Amsterdam, 1986, Kugler Publications.
20. Casselbrant ML, Brostoff LM, Cantekin EI, et al: Otitis media in preschool children in United States. In Lim DJ, Bluestone CD, Klein JO, et al, eds: *Otitis media with effusion,* Toronto, 1986, BC Decker.
21. Lehmann KD, Charron K, Kummer L, et al: The effects of chronic middle ear effusion on speech and language development: a descriptive study, *Int J Pediatr Otorhinolaryngol* 1:137, 1979.
22. Ishi T, Toriyama M, Suzuki J: Histopathological study of otitis media with effusion, *Ann Otol Rhinol Laryngol* 89:83, 1985.
23. Bluestone CD: Role of eustachian tube function: physiology and role in otitis media, *Ann Otol Rhinol Laryngol Suppl* 120:1-60, 1985.
24. Friedman RA, Doyle WJ, Casselbrant M, et al: Immunologic mediated eustachian tube obstruction: a double blind crossover study, *J Allergy Clin Immunol* 71:442-447, 1983.
25. Paradise JL, Bluestone CD, Felder H: The university of otitis media in 50 infants with cleft plate, *Pediatrics* 44:35, 1969.
26. Bernstein L, Doyle WJ: The role of IgE-mediated hypersensitivity in otitis media with effusion: pathophysiological considerations, *Ann Otol Rhinol Laryngol* 103:15-19, 1994.
27. Doyle WJ, Takahara T, Fireman P: Eustachian tube obstruction in passively sensitized rhesus monkey following provocative nasal antigen challenge, *Arch Otolaryngol* 110:508-511, 1984.
28. Skoner DP, Doyle WJ, Chamovitz AH, et al: Eustachian tube obstruction after intranasal challenge with house dust mite, *Arch Otolaryngol* 112:840-842, 1986.
29. Doyle WJ, Boehm S, Skoner DP: Physiologic responses to intranasal dose-response challenges with histamine, methacholine, bradykinin and prostaglandin in adult volunteers with and without nasal allergy, *J Allergy Clin Immunol* 86:924-935, 1990.
30. Skoner DP, Doyle WJ, Boehm S, et al: Effect of terfenadine on nasal, eustachian tube and pulmonary function after provocative intranasal histamine challenge, *Ann Allergy* 67:619-624, 1991.
31. Skoner DP, Lee L, Doyle WJ, et al: Nasal physiology and inflammatory mediators during natural pollen exposure, *Ann Allergy* 65:206-210, 1990.
32. Gwaltney JM, Jordan WS: Rhinovirus and respiratory illness in university students, *Am Rev Respir Dis* 93:362-371, 1966.
33. Henderson FW, Collier AM, Sanya MA, et al: A longitudinal study of respiratory viruses and bacteria in the etiology of acute otitis media with effusion, *N Engl J Med* 306:1377-1383, 1982.
34. Clements DA, Henderson FW, Neebe EC: The relationship of viral isolation to otitis media with a research day care center 1978-88. In Proceedings of the 5th International Symposium on Recent Advances in Otitis Media, Toronto, 1993, BC Decker.
35. Bakaletz LO, Daniels RJ, Lim DJ: Modeling adenovirus type 1-induced otitis media in the chinchilla: effect on ciliary activity and fluid transport function of eustachian tube mucosal epithelium, *J Infect Dis* 168:865-872, 1993.
36. Buchman CA, Doyle WJ, Skoner D, et al: Otologic manifestations of experimental rhinovirus infection, *Laryngoscope* 104:1295-1299, 1994.
37. Doyle WJ, Skoner DP, Jeroky JR, et al: Nasal and otologic effects of experimental influenza A virus infection, *Ann Otol Rhinol Laryngol* 103: 59-69, 1994.
38. Heikkinen T, Ruuskanen O, Waris M, et al: Influenza vaccination in the prevention of acute otitis media, *Am J Dis Child* 145:445-448, 1991.
39. Proud D, Naclerio RM, Gwaltney JM, et al: Kinins are generated in nasal secretions during rhinovirus colds, *J Infect Dis* 164:120-123, 1990.
40. Naclerio RM, Meier HL, Kagy-Sabotka A, et al: Mediator release after nasal airway challenge with allergen, *Am Rev Respir Dis* 112:597-602, 1993.
41. Busse W: Respiratory infections and bronchial hyperactivity, *J Allergy Clin Immunol* 81:770-775, 1988.
42. Doyle WJ, Skoner DP, Fireman P, et al: Rhinovirus 39 infection in allergic and non-allergic subjects, *J Allergy Clin Immunol* 89:968-978, 1992.
43. Skoner DP, Doyle WJ, Tanner EP, et al: Reproducibility of the effects of intranasal ragweed challenges in allergic subjects, *Ann Allergy Asthma Immunol* 74:171-176, 1995.
44. Fireman P, Skoner D, Tanner E, et al: Effect of influenza A virus (FLU) and rhinovirus 39 (RV-39) infections on leukocyte histamine in allergic rhinitis and non-allergic rhinitis subjects, *J Allergy Clin Immunol* 93:194, 1994.

45. Doyle WJ, Skoner DP, Hayden F, et al: Effect of experimental rhinovirus 39 infection on the nasal response to histamine and cold air challenges in allergic and non-allergic subjects, *J Allergy Clin Immunol* 92:534-542, 1994.

46. Doyle WJ, Skoner DP, Seroky J, et al: Effect of experimental influenza infection in nasal response to histamine challenge in allergic and non-allergic subjects, *Am J Rhinol* 7:227-235, 1993.

47. Togias AG, Naclerio RM, Proud D, et al: Nasal challenges with cold dry air results in release of inflammatory mediators: mast cell involvement, *J Clin Invest* 76:1375-1381, 1985.

48. Arola M, Ruuskanen O, Ziegler T, et al: Clinical role of respiratory virus infection in acute otitis media, *Pediatrics* 86:848-855, 1990.

49. Okamoto Y, Kudo K, Ishikawa K, et al: Presence of respiratory syncytial virus genomic sequences in middle ear fluid and its relationships to expression of cytokines and cell adhesion molecules, *J Infect Dis* 168:177-184, 1993.

50. Giebink GS: The microbiology of otitis media, *Pediatr Infect Dis J* 8:518-520, 1989.

51. Post JC, Preston RA, Aul JJ, et al: Molecular analysis of bacterial pathogens in otitis media with effusion, *JAMA* 273:1598-6041, 1995.

52. Warshauer D, Goldstein E, Akers T, et al: Effect of influenza viral infection in the ingestion and killing of bacteria by alveolar macrophages, *Am Rev Respir Dis* 115:269-277, 1977.

53. Giebink GS, Mills EL, Cates KL, et al: Polymorphonuclear leukocyte dysfunction in children with recurrent otitis media, *J Pediatr* 94:13-18, 1979.

54. Bylander A: Upper respiratory tract infection and eustachian tube in children, *Acta Otolaryngol* 97:342-349, 1984.

55. McBride TP, Doyle WJ, Hayden FG, et al: Alteration of eustachian tube function, middle ear pressure and nasal patency in response to an experimental rhinovirus challenge, *Arch Otol* 115:1054-1059, 1989.

56. Giebink GS, Ripley ML, Wright PF: Eustachian tube histopathology during experimental influenza A virus infection in the chinchilla, *Ann Otol Rhinol Laryngol* 96:199-206, 1987.

57. Casselbrant ML, Cantekin EI, Dirkmaat DC, et al: Experimental paralysis of tensor veli palatini muscle, *Acta Otolaryngol (Stockh)* 106:178-185, 1988.

58. Giebink GS, Berzins IK, Marker SG, et al: Experimental otitis media after nasal inoculation of Streptococcus pneumoniae and influenza A virus in chinchillas, *Infect Immunol* 30:445-450, 1980.

59. Reuman PD, Swarts JD, Maddern BD, et al: In Proceedings of the 5th International Symposium on Recent Advances in Otitis Media, The effects of influenza A H3N2, rhinovirus 39 and coxsackie A 21 infection on nasal and middle ear function in adult subjects, Toronto, 1993, BC Decker.

60. Skoner DP, Whiteside TL, Wilson JW, et al: Effect of rhinovirus 39 (RV-39) infection on cellular immune parameters in allergic and non-allergic subjects, *J Allergy Clin Immunol* 92:732-743, 1993.

61. Wadowsky RM, Mietzner SM, Skoner DP, et al: Effect of experimental influenza A virus infection on the isolation of Streptococcus pneumoniae and other aerobic bacteria from the oropharynx of allergic and non-allergic adult subjects, *Infect Immunol* 63:1153-1157, 1995.

62. Dowel SF, Butler JC, Giebink GS: Acute otitis media: management and surveillance in an era of pneumococcal resistance, *Pediatr Infect Dis* 18:1-9, 1999.

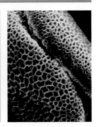

CHAPTER 30

Sinusitis

KENNY H. CHAN ■ MARK J. ABZUG ■ SAMER FAKHRI ■ QUTAYBA A. HAMID ■ ANDREW H. LIU

This chapter on sinusitis in children will provide a current overview of the pathogenesis and management of acute and chronic sinus disease. The goals of sinusitis treatment are to relieve sinusitis symptoms and signs and to prevent complications. Although acute sinusitis has been substantially investigated, relatively little is known about chronic sinusitis in children.

SINUS DEVELOPMENT IN CHILDHOOD

There are four pairs of paranasal sinuses in humans: maxillary, ethmoid, frontal, and sphenoid. The maxillary and ethmoid sinuses are present at birth and invaginate to become radiographically visible in the first 1 to 2 years of life (Figure 30-1). In comparison, frontal and sphenoid sinuses begin to develop in the first few years of life and gradually become pneumatized and radiographically visible between 7 to 15 years of age. The maxillary, anterior ethmoid, and frontal sinus ostia enter the nasal cavity through the middle meatus, under the middle turbinate (i.e., osteomeatal complex; see Figure 30-1). The sphenoid and posterior ethmoid ostia join the nasal cavity through the superior meatus, above the middle turbinate.

CLINICAL DEFINITIONS OF SINUSITIS

Several descriptive modifiers for sinusitis are commonly used, although the pathogenic and therapeutic relevance of the differences between subgroups has not been well clarified. In terms of sinusitis duration, (1) *acute* sinusitis refers to sinus symptoms of 10 to 30 days, with complete resolution of symptoms,[1] (2) *subacute* sinusitis refers to symptoms that last 30 to 90 to 120 days, and (3) *chronic* sinusitis is used for symptoms that last more than 90 to 120 days. *Recurrent* sinusitis occurs in patients who improve with sinus therapy but experience multiple episodes. *Refractory* sinusitis refers to patients who do not respond to conventional therapy for sinusitis.

The uses of the term *sinusitis* and *rhinosinusitis* have been debated; *sinusitis* implies that the disease is the manifestation of an infectious process of the sinuses.[2] In comparison, the term *rhinosinusitis* implies that the nasal and sinus mucosae are involved in similar and concurrent pathogenic (e.g., inflammatory) processes.[1] In this chapter the two terms will be used interchangeably, although the bias of the authors is that sinusitis is both pathogenically and clinically linked to rhinitis.

EPIDEMIOLOGY

Sinusitis is a common problem in childhood, but only a few epidemiologic studies have assessed its prevalence and natural history in childhood. In a study of 1- to 5-year-old children seen in pediatric practices, 9.3% met the clinical criteria of sinusitis (i.e., ≥ 10 days of symptoms).[3] In a large birth cohort study primarily intended to study the natural history of childhood asthma (Children's Respiratory Study, Tucson, Arizona), 13% of 8-year-old children reported physician-diagnosed sinusitis within the past year.[4] Of children with sinusitis, 50%, 18%, and 11% had sinusitis diagnosed for the first time at ages 6 years, 3 years, and 2 years, respectively. The main risk factors for sinusitis were current allergic rhinitis and grass pollen hypersensitivity.

The National Center for Health Statistics in the United States reported that from 1980 to 1992, sinusitis was the fifth leading diagnosis for which antibiotics were prescribed.[5] The annual outpatient visit rates for sinusitis increased about threefold over this period and the use of amoxicillin and cephalosporin antibiotics for sinusitis also increased significantly. Antibiotic resistance of bacterial pathogens from the sinuses of children with acute sinusitis[6] and chronic sinusitis[7] is currently common. Severe alterations in quality of life can result from chronic recurrent sinusitis in children. Using a standardized child health questionnaire, children with chronic sinusitis and their parents reported more bodily pain and greater limitation in their physical activity than those typically reported by children with asthma or juvenile rheumatoid arthritis.[8] Complications of sinusitis, such as intracranial or intraorbital extension of bacterial infection from the sinuses, are medical emergencies that are life-threatening and carry a high risk of morbidity and mortality.

ETIOLOGY

A combination of anatomic, mucosal, microbial, and immune pathogenic processes is believed to underlie sinusitis in children. Children with congenital mucosal diseases (e.g., cystic fibrosis, ciliary dyskinesias) and lymphocyte immune deficiencies (congenital and acquired) typically have chronic recurrent sinus disease. Also, allergic airway diseases in children have both epidemiologic and pathogenic links to sinusitis.

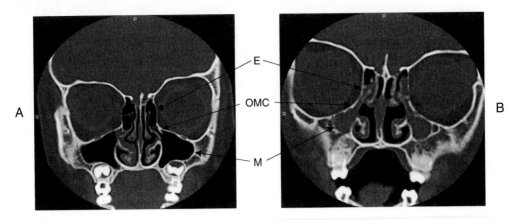

FIGURE 30-1 Computed tomography scans of the paranasal sinuses. Coronal views of a 4-year-old child with (**A**) normal maxillary and ethmoid sinuses and patent osteomeatal complex and (**B**) opacified maxillary and ethmoid sinuses consistent with sinusitis. *E*, Ethmoid sinus; *M*, maxillary sinus; *OMC*, osteomeatal complex.

Anatomic Pathogenesis

Anatomic obstructions of the sinus ostia in the nasopharynx have long been suspected causes of sinusitis. The pathophysiology of osteomeatal obstruction leading to sinusitis is believed to be similar to that of otitis media.[9] For the middle ear space, animal model studies reveal that a lack of ventilation (i.e., oxygenation) of the middle ear results in negative pressure in the closed space, leading to mucosal vascular leakage, edema, inflammation, and middle ear fluid accumulation.[10,11] Both anatomic obstructive lesions and mucosal disorders such as mucosal injury from viral upper respiratory tract infections (URTIs), inhalant allergies, cystic fibrosis, and ciliary dyskinesias may begin this cascade of pathogenic events. Anatomic variations associated with sinusitis in children in uncontrolled studies include concha bullosa (10%), paradoxical turbinates (4% to 8%), lateralized uncinate process with hypoplastic maxillary sinus (7% to 17%); Haller cell (5% to 10%), and septal deviation (10%).[12,13] However, because these anatomic variations are commonly found in asymptomatic infants and children, surgical intervention is not recommended on the basis of these anatomic variations alone.

Microbial Pathogenesis

Both viral and bacterial infections have integral roles in the pathogenesis of sinusitis. Viral URTIs commonly cause sinus mucosal injury and swelling, resulting in osteomeatal obstruction, loss of ciliary activity, and mucous hypersecretion. Indeed, radiologic sinus imaging studies of adults with common colds revealed that sinus mucosal abnormalities are the norm, and even air-fluid levels in the maxillary sinuses and opacification of the maxillary sinuses are common.[14,15] Specifically, coronal sinus computed tomography (CT) scans of adults with URTIs revealed that 87% had abnormalities of one or both maxillary sinuses, 77% had obstruction of the ethmoid infundibulum, 65% had abnormal ethmoid sinuses, 32% had abnormal frontal sinuses, and 39% had abnormal sphenoid sinuses.[15]

Sneezing and nose blowing are thought to introduce nasal flora into the sinuses. Bacterial growth conditions are favorable in obstructed sinuses, reflected by bacterial concentrations of up to 10^7 bacterial colony-forming units (cfu)/ml in sinus aspirates. White blood cell counts in excess of 10,000 cells/ml in sinus aspirates are evidence of a robust inflammatory response to infection. The combination of infection and this inflammatory reaction can be directly destructive, resulting in intense epithelial damage and transmucosal injury.[16,17]

Microbiology of Acute and Subacute Sinusitis

The gold standard for microbiologic diagnosis of bacterial sinusitis has been the recovery of $\geq 10^4$ cfu/ml of pathogenic bacteria from a sinus aspirate.[1,18] Studies employing sinus aspirates indicate that the pathogens responsible for acute and subacute sinusitis are similar to each other and mirror those responsible for acute otitis media[18-23] (Table 30-1). *Streptococcus pneumoniae* is recovered in approximately 30% of cases, nontypable *Haemophilus influenzae* in approximately 20%, and *Moraxella catarrhalis* in approximately 20%. A significant proportion of *S. pneumoniae* isolates have intermediate or high-level resistance to penicillin, and *H. influenzae* and *M. catarrhalis* isolates are frequently β-lactamase positive. Actual resistance rates vary with time period, geographic region, and the prevalence of risk factors for resistance (e.g., age < 2 years, day care attendance, recent antibiotic exposure). *Streptococcus pyogenes* and other streptococcal species are recovered in a small number of cases. *Staphylococcus aureus* and anaerobes are uncommon causes of acute and subacute pediatric sinusitis; however, they are more frequently identified in severe, complicated disease, or, in the case of anaerobes, associated with dental disease.[24] Less commonly recovered bacteria include gram-negative organisms such as *Eikenella corrodens* and other *Moraxella* and *Neisseria* species. Fungi are uncommonly recovered in acute sinusitis except in immunocompromised patients.[19] The protozoan *Acanthamoeba* has also been identified as a rare cause of sinusitis in severely immunosuppressed hosts.[25,26] Sinus aspirates are sterile in approximately 30% to 35% of children with clinically and/or radiographically diagnosed sinusitis.[1,18,22,27] Respiratory viruses are recovered from approximately 10% of sinus aspirates; whether they play a direct pathogenic role in the sinus is poorly understood.

Microbiology of Chronic Sinusitis

Infection is a key component in most cases of pediatric chronic sinusitis. In numerous studies, 65% to 100% of children with chronic sinusitis have positive cultures of sinus aspirates.[7,28-32] Rates of recovery of specific organisms vary among studies; this variability is likely explained by differences in patient populations, sinuses evaluated, specimen collection methods, and microbiologic culture techniques. Despite these differences, certain general observations can be made. *S. pneumoniae, H. influenzae,* and *M. catarrhalis* are frequently isolated from children with chronic sinusitis and mirror common pathogens in acute and subacute sinusitis[7,29,33] (see Table 30-1). With increasing chronicity, other organisms may also be recovered, including *S. aureus, S. pyogenes,* alpha streptococci, group D streptococci, diphtheroids, coagulase-negative staphylococci, neisseria species, gram-negative aerobic rods, and anaerobes.[28,30-32] *S. aureus* and anaerobes tend to be disproportionately associated with protracted, severe, or complicated disease.[34-37] Recovery of anaerobes (e.g., peptococcus, peptostreptococcus, *Propionibacterium acnes,* prevotella, veillonella, fusobacterium, bacteroides, and actinomyces) has varied widely from less than 5% to more than 90%, depending on the populations and sinuses evaluated and microbiologic methods employed.[28-32,38,39] Many anaerobic isolates are β-lactamase producing.[35] Fungi, including Aspergillus, Alternaria, and other dematiaceous species, and zygomycetes are occasionally isolated, although invasive disease is uncommon except in immunocompromised children.[31] In young adults, fungi may be a trigger for allergic fungal sinusitis.[40] Respiratory viruses are occasionally identified in sinus mucosal or lavage specimens.[41,42] Interestingly, bilateral cultures of the sinuses are often discordant.[7,32]

Antibiotic resistance has emerged as an important factor in the microbiology of chronic sinusitis. For example, in a 4-year retrospective review of maxillary sinus aspirates from children with sinusitis for more than 8 weeks, rates of nonsusceptibility of *S. pneumoniae* (recovered in 19% of cultures) were 64% for penicillin, 40% for cefotaxime, and 18% for clindamycin.[7] Of *H. influenzae* isolates (recovered in 24%), 44% were nonsusceptible to ampicillin, and all *M. catarrhalis* isolates (recovered in 17%) were β-lactamase positive.

Immune Pathogenesis

There are very few studies in the literature on the immunopathology of sinusitis in children. Most of our knowledge is derived from studies conducted on adults with chronic hyperplastic sinusitis and nasal polyposis (CHS/NP). Chronic sinusitis is characterized by mucosal thickening, goblet cell hyperplasia, subepithelial fibrosis, and persistent inflammation[43] (Figure 30-2). Although not fully understood, the fibrotic changes are thought to be driven by activated eosinophils and their products, including the profibrotic transforming growth factor-β,[44] GM-CSF,[45,46] and interleukin (IL)-11.[47] Tissue fibroblasts are stimulated to increase the synthesis and deposition of collagen and matrix products, resulting in thickening of the sub-basement membrane layer. Subepithelial collagen deposition has also been reported in children with chronic sinusitis, but to a lesser degree than that seen in adults.[48]

Current views implicate sensitivity to aeroallergens as a primary pathologic mechanism in the development of chronic sinusitis in both adults[49,50] and children.[51] Many studies have shown that the composition of the inflammatory substrate in chronic sinusitis is similar to that seen in allergic rhinitis and the late-phase response to antigen challenge.[49,52]

Th2-Mediated Eosinophilic Inflammation

Although many immune cell types are involved in the pathogenesis of chronic sinusitis, a specific subclass of T lymphocytes (i.e., T helper cell type 2 [Th2] lymphocytes) and eosinophils appear to have a central role. Th2 cells differentiate in response to IL-4 and are primarily associated with allergy.[53] The orchestration of cellular recruitment and activation of the

TABLE 30-1 Microbiology of Acute, Subacute, and Chronic Sinusitis

Microorganism	Frequency		
	Common	Occasional	Uncommon
Streptococcus pneumoniae	A*, C†		
Haemophilus influenzae, nontypable	A, C		
Moraxella catarrhalis	A, C		
Streptococcus pyogenes		A, C	
Other streptococcal species		A, C	
Staphylococcus aureus	C		A
Diphtheroids	C		
Coagulase-negative staphylococci	C		
Other gram-negatives, moraxella, neisseria	C		A
Anaerobes	C		A
Respiratory viruses		A, C	
Fungi (aspergillus, alternaria, other dematiaceous fungi, zygomycetes)‡	C		A
Acanthamoeba§			A

*Acute and subacute sinusitis.
†Chronic sinusitis.
‡Primarily in immunocompromised hosts or associated with allergic fungal sinusitis.
§Primarily in immunocompromised hosts.

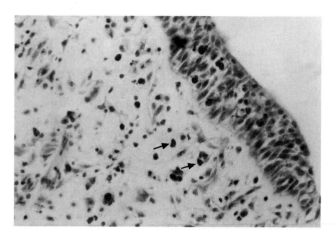

FIGURE 30-2 Chronic sinusitis: sinus mucosal biopsy. Colocalization of major basic protein immunoreactivity to eosinophils (*arrows*). Also note hyperplasia and squamous metaplasia of the epithelium (hematoxylin counterstain, original magnification ×400).

inflammatory infiltrate in CHS/NP have been largely attributed to the Th2 cells and their cytokines (i.e., IL-3, IL-4, IL-5, IL-9, IL-13, GM-CSF). Among immune cell types, eosinophils are the most characteristic and are found in 80% to 90% of nasal polyps.[54] Two histopathologic studies have investigated the inflammatory cells in pediatric chronic sinusitis and reported similar findings: the numbers of eosinophils, and to a much lesser extent mast cells and T lymphocytes, are significantly increased in children with chronic sinusitis compared to control subjects[48,55] (see Figure 30-2). In these studies, the degree of tissue eosinophilia was not affected by the allergic status of patients. This is in agreement with published studies on chronic sinusitis in the adult population where the level of eosinophilic infiltration was found to be similar between allergic and nonallergic patients with either chronic sinusitis without nasal polyps[56,57] or CHS/NP.[58,59] Levels of neutrophils are also increased in the sinus lavage fluid of adults with chronic sinusitis, particularly in nonallergic patients.[60] In contrast, the level of neutrophilia in pediatric chronic sinusitis is not increased when compared to controls.[48]

This implies that IgE-dependent interactions are not the only Th2 mechanism in recruiting eosinophils to sites of inflammation in chronic sinusitis. In fact, Th2 cells produce IL-3, IL-5, and GM-CSF, which are important cytokines in the recruitment, differentiation, activation, and survival of eosinophils.[58] The upregulation of IL-4, IL-5, and GM-CSF in chronic sinusitis is paralleled by an increase in the expression of their receptors on inflammatory cells. Wright et al[57] demonstrated that IL-4 receptor mRNA expression was increased in the epithelium and lamina propria of patients with allergic chronic sinusitis. Similarly, IL-5 receptor mRNA expression was up-regulated in the lamina propria of patients with chronic sinusitis compared to controls, with the highest expression in allergic compared to nonallergic patients. Conversely, expression of GM-CSF receptors was predominantly increased in nonallergic chronic sinusitis.

The process of recruiting and facilitating the transendothelial migration of inflammatory cells into the nasal mucosa following allergen challenge requires the activation of adhesion molecules including VCAM and selectins, as well as the expression of chemokines. The adhesion molecule VCAM-1, specific for eosinophils, lymphocytes, and basophils, is up-regulated in CHS/NP.[61] A number of chemokines are up-regulated in the nasal mucosa of both allergic patients after allergen challenge and patients with CHS/NP. Hamilos et al[61] found an increased expression of RANTES and eotaxin in the epithelial and submucosal cells of patients with CHS/NP compared with controls. Wright et al[62] demonstrated an increase in the expression of monocyte chemotactic proteins (MCP-3 and MCP-4) in the sinus mucosae of patients with chronic sinusitis compared with controls. The elaboration of chemokines MCP-3, MCP-4, RANTES, and eotaxin, as well as the adhesion molecule VCAM-1, is up-regulated by cytokines, particularly IL-4, IL-13, and tumor necrosis factor (TNF)-α.[61,63]

It seems therefore that the immunopathologic mechanisms underlying the development of some forms of chronic sinusitis, especially CHS/NP, are largely related to the effects of Th2 cytokines and their receptors, such that the final pathologic profile of intense eosinophilic infiltration is a common finding of chronic sinusitis in both atopic and nonatopic patients.

Asthma and Allergy Risk Factors

Along with histologic evidence that the immune pathologic processes of chronic sinusitis and asthma are similar, radiographic and clinical studies also link sinusitis with asthma. Using plain radiography of the sinuses, the prevalence of radiographic sinus abnormalities was significantly higher in asthmatic children (31%) than nonasthmatic controls (0%).[64] In asthmatic children who were hospitalized for an acute exacerbation, significant radiographic abnormalities of the sinuses were revealed in 87% of the patients.[65] A study of patients undergoing surgery for chronic sinusitis found that sinus CT evidence of extensive disease was associated with asthma, allergen sensitization, and peripheral blood eosinophilia.[66] Of those with eosinophilia, 87% had extensive sinus disease.

Allergic rhinitis and inhalant allergen sensitization have also been associated with sinusitis in children. In a large birth cohort study (Children's Respiratory Study, Tucson, Arizona), both allergic rhinitis and grass pollen sensitization were significant and independent risk factors for sinusitis in childhood (i.e., age 8 years).[4] Experimentally, in allergic rhinitis subjects, nasal provocation with allergen induced sinus radiographic changes (i.e., mucosal thickening, sinus opacification) and symptoms of headache and pressure in the maxillary sinuses.[67]

Genetic Risk Factors

Association studies between chronic sinusitis and genetic markers in a few candidate genes have been reported. Chronic sinusitis and nasal polyposis are hallmark features of cystic fibrosis (CF). In some chronic sinusitis patients without CF, mutations in the cystic fibrosis transmembrane regulator (CFTR) gene have been recently observed. In a cohort of 147 white adults with chronic sinusitis, the proportion of chronic sinusitis patients who were found to have a CFTR mutation (7%) was significantly higher than in nonsinusitis controls (2%).[68] Furthermore, 9 of the 10 CF carriers also had the CFTR polymorphism M470V. M470V homozygotes were also overrepresented in the remaining sinusitis patients. A similar study in children with chronic sinusitis found that 12% were carrying CFTR mutations compared with the expected 3% to 4% in the nonsinusitis control group.[69] However, if a CFTR mutation carrier is susceptible to chronic sinusitis, then one would expect the siblings of CF patients to have a higher incidence of chronic sinusitis. A questionnaire survey failed to detect a difference in the prevalence of rhinosinusitis between 261 obligate CF heterozygotes and 201 control subjects.[70]

Two other susceptibility gene investigations for chronic sinusitis have been reported. In a study of 82 Japanese adults with chronic sinusitis, the major histocompatibility B54 haplotype was increased (29%) when compared with nonsinusitis controls (11%).[71] The same investigators reported a significant increase of a polymorphism in the TNF-β gene in 38 Japanese adults with chronic sinusitis (74%) when compared with nonsinusitis controls (56%).[72]

Other Risk Factors

Medical conditions that render children susceptible to acute and chronic sinus disease include immune deficiencies (especially T- and B-lymphocyte defects and acquired immune deficiencies, such as AIDS, and patients receiving immunosuppressive medications) and primary ciliary dyskinesias. The association of gastroesophageal reflux disease (GERD) with chronic sinusitis has also received attention. GERD, diagnosed by pH-monitored nasopharyngeal acid reflux[73] or esophageal biopsy,[74] was associated with rhinosinusitis in children. Phipps et al[75] also reported significantly increased nasopharyngeal reflux in children with chronic sinusitis when compared with a historical control group. Antireflux treatment of their GERD-positive cohort resulted in a 79% improvement in chronic sinusitis symptoms. However, a randomized, controlled trial demonstrating posttreatment improvement in sinus disease by radiographic imaging and resolution of GERD by pH studies is currently lacking.

SINUSITIS MANAGEMENT

Overview

Medical histories and physical examinations can help to distinguish sinusitis in children from URTIs and other masqueraders and to identify complications from sinusitis and underlying risk factors for chronic recurrent disease. Radiographic imaging studies are particularly helpful in evaluating children with chronic, recurrent, or complicated sinusitis. Sinus washings for bacterial culture and targeted antimicrobial therapy, while ideal, are surgical procedures (e.g., antral irrigation) that require general anesthesia in children. Therefore, their use is generally reserved for (1) children with chronic sinusitis that does not adequately improve with multiple courses of antibiotics, (2) sinusitis with complications, and (3) sinusitis in immunocompromised hosts. Differential diagnostic considerations are provided in Table 30-2.

Consensus-based guidelines on the management of sinusitis in children have been recently published,[1,76] including a report from a subcommittee of the American Academy of Pediatrics in conjunction with the American Academy of Allergy, Asthma and Immunology, the American Academy of Otolaryngology—Head and Neck Surgery, and the American College of Emergency Physicians. Their comprehensive literature review and expert panels acknowledged that consistent evidence (i.e., randomized, controlled trials) to support management guidelines is generally lacking and at times controversial, especially for chronic disease. This consensus report provided recommendations (but not a protocol) for the management of acute bacterial sinusitis that have been considered in the following discussion.

History and Physical Examination

Acute Sinusitis

Nasal discharge (77%) and cough (80%) lasting longer than 10 to 14 days are the common symptoms of sinusitis in children.[18] Nasal discharge can be of any quality, and cough can be daytime, nighttime, or both. Fever may accompany the illness. Although headaches and sinus tenderness are generally believed to be the hallmarks of sinusitis, a study of 200 sinusitis patients did not find a significant correlation of facial pain or headache with abnormal findings on sinus CT.[77] Additionally, the reported regions of facial pain did not correlate with radiographically identified sinus abnormalities. The nasal cavity is usually filled with discharge and the nasal muscosa and turbinates are generally edematous. Following decongestion of the nasal cavity, purulent drainage coming from the middle meatus can sometimes be observed in older children. Tenderness over the frontal sinus in older children may indicate frontal sinus disease, but tenderness in general is rare in children with acute disease. Transillumination, considered by some to be a useful tool in adults, is unreliable in children.

TABLE 30-2 Differential Diagnosis and Risk Factors for Acute and Chronic Sinusitis in Children

Acute sinusitis
Prolonged viral upper respiratory tract infection
Foreign body in the nose
Acute exacerbation of inhalant allergies
Acute adenoiditis or adenotonsillitis

Chronic sinusitis
Rhinitis, allergic and nonallergic
Anatomic causes of nasopharyngeal obstruction
  Turbinate hypertrophy
  Adenoid hypertrophy
  Nasal polyps
  Severe septal deviation
  Choanal atresia
Asthma
Neoplasms of the nose and nasopharynx
  Juvenile angiofibroma
  Rhabdomyosarcoma
  Lymphoma
  Dermoid cyst
Cystic fibrosis
Lymphocyte immune deficiencies:
  B lymphocytes—antibody deficiencies
  T lymphocyte deficiencies—congenital and acquired
Primary ciliary dyskinesias
Wegener's granulomatosis
Churg-Strauss vasculitis
Dental caries/abscess
Gastroesophageal reflux disease with nasopharyngeal reflux

Chronic Sinusitis

The most common symptoms associated with chronic sinusitis in children are nasal discharge (59%), facial pain/discomfort (33%), nasal congestion (30%), cough (19%), and wheezing (19%).[76] Nasal discharge can be of any quality, but purulent discharge is the most common. Daytime mouth-breathing and snoring are common complaints. Examination of the nasal cavity may or may not reveal nasal discharge. The nasal turbinates are generally enlarged and can be edematous or erythematous. Although facial pain or discomfort may be a common complaint, tenderness over the sinuses is an uncommon finding in children.

Radiographic Imaging

A recent consensus report provided by the American College of Radiology[78] provided appropriateness criteria of various radiographic imaging modalities in assessing pediatric sinus disease. Currently, coronal CT is the recommended examination for imaging persistent or chronic sinusitis in patients of any age. Plain sinus radiographs (Waters and Caldwell projections), although widely available, can both underdiagnose and overdiagnose sinus soft tissue changes. Magnetic resonance imaging provides superlative soft tissue delineation; however, it is expensive, has limited availability, and does not provide bony details of the osteomeatal complex. Conventional tomography, nuclear medicine studies, and ultrasound have significant limitations for imaging the sinuses.

It is tempting to consider sinus mucosal abnormalities and associated anatomic variations seen in imaging studies in symptomatic patients as clear indications for sinusitis therapy (e.g., sinus surgery). However, the clinical importance of such findings is challenged by studies that have revealed a high prevalence of such soft tissue findings in people without sinusitis symptoms or with URTIs.[14,15] In these studies, URTI symptoms and associated radiographic sinus abnormalities have improved without specific sinusitis therapy (i.e., no antibiotics or surgery for sinusitis).

The American College of Radiology consensus report has the following recommendations: (1) the diagnoses of acute and chronic sinusitis should be made clinically and not on the basis of imaging findings alone; (2) no imaging studies are indicated for acute sinusitis except for cases where complications are suspected or cases that are not responding to therapy; and (3) if imaging information in patients with chronic sinusitis is desired, coronal sinus CT is recommended. The use of plain radiographs of the sinuses (i.e., Waters and Caldwell views) is generally discouraged in this report, except in children younger than 4 years of age. The use of Waters view radiographs in children is supported by a study in which the sensitivity and specificity of a Waters view radiograph to diagnose chronic sinusitis in children were 76% and 81%, respectively.[79] In the same study, limited coronal CT scans were better than sinus x-rays and nearly as good as full sinus CT evaluations.

Sinusitis Complications

Complications of sinusitis (Table 30-3) are generally believed to be acute events that result from a combination of outflow obstruction and pathogenic bacteria in the sinuses. Intracranial extension of infection is by direct erosion, thrombophlebitis, or extension through preformed pathways (e.g., fracture lines). The incidence of intracranial complications in children hospitalized for sinusitis was 3%.[80]

Orbital complications from sinusitis are primarily the result of acute ethmoid disease but could occasionally be extensions of frontal disease.[81] A classic description of the progression of sinusitis to orbital complications is as follows: inflammatory edema, orbital cellulitis, subperiosteal abscess, orbital abscess, and cavernous sinus thrombosis.[82] The most common presentations of orbital complications include eyelid edema, orbital pain, diplopia, proptosis, and chemosis, as well as fever, nasal discharge, and headache.[83] In a cohort of children with orbital complications from sinusitis, 72% of hospitalized children had a history of a URTI, and 24% had received oral antibiotic therapy prior to their presentation with orbital complications.[83] It can be difficult to differentiate between preseptal cellulitis and orbital cellulitis on clinical parameters alone (i.e., based on lid edema and pain without an imaging study). In orbital cellulitis, proptosis progresses and leads to chemosis and ophthalmoplegia. Fortunately, orbital abscesses and cavernous sinus thrombosis caused by sinusitis are rarely seen today.

Intracranial complications from sinusitis are primarily the result of frontal sinus disease.[80] There are many similarities

TABLE 30-3 Sinusitis Complications (by Sinus Involvement)

Complication	Maxillary Sinus	Ethmoid Sinus	Frontal Sinus	Sphenoid Sinus
Osteomyelitis	+		++	
Mucocele	++	++	++	+
Preseptal cellulitis		+++		
Orbital cellulitis		+++	+	
Subperiosteal abscess		+++		
Orbital abscess		+		
Meningitis			++	
Epidural abscess			++	
Subdural abscess			+	
Brain abscess			+	
Cavernous sinus thrombosis		+		+
Toxic shock syndrome	+	+	+	+

+++, Frequent; ++, less frequent; +, least frequent.

between the pathogenesis of intracranial extension of frontal sinusitis and that of otitis media. The classic presentations of the progression from meningitis to the various intracranial abscesses will not be discussed here. Intracranial complications in the preantibiotic era were devastating, with mortality rates of up to 75%. Current mortality rates for these complications are between 10% to 20%. Cavernous sinus thrombosis is a unique intracranial complication of ethmoid and sphenoid sinusitis by direct extension. This complication is characterized by a toxic-appearing patient with infectious/inflammatory involvement of the third, fourth, and sixth cranial nerves, resulting in ophthalmoplegia. Progressive disease within the cavernous sinus can lead to carotid artery thrombosis and mycotic aneurysm formation, resulting in neurologic sequelae and death.

Complications of maxillary sinusitis are rare. Mucoceles in the maxillary sinus are occasionally encountered in children with cystic fibrosis, but they are unusual in the general pediatric population. Osteomyelitis of the maxillary sinus was more prevalent in the preantibiotic era and in adults with dental disease. This appears to be a rare complication today—there have been no reported cases in the literature since the 1950s.

SINUSITIS TREATMENT

Antimicrobial Therapy

Acute and Subacute Sinusitis

The goals of therapy for acute and subacute sinusitis are to hasten clinical improvement, prevent intracranial and orbital complications, and prevent mucosal damage that may predispose to chronic sinus disease[19,20] (Box 30-1). The actual benefit of antibiotics in achieving these goals has not been conclusively proven. A pivotal randomized trial showed that antibiotic therapy (amoxicillin or amoxicillin-clavulanic acid) for acute sinusitis, defined by clinical and plain radiograph criteria, was associated with symptom resolution in 66% of children at 10 days, significantly greater than the 43% rate of resolution among placebo-treated subjects.[84] A subsequent meta-analysis of five randomized, controlled trials similarly suggested benefit of antibiotics in reducing persistence of symptoms; benefit was modest, however, with approximately six children requiring therapy to achieve one additional cure.[85] A more recent randomized trial comparing amoxicillin, amoxicillin-clavulanate, and placebo in children with clinically diagnosed acute sinusitis found no differences among groups in symptom improvement at 14 days (79% to 81% in each) nor in relapse and recurrence rates.[86] Differences in inclusion criteria among studies may account for their differing results.[1] This discrepancy mirrors the published experience in adults, in which some placebo-controlled studies have demonstrated faster recovery with antibiotic treatment,[87,88] whereas others have shown no antibiotic benefit.[89,90] As in children, meta-analyses of studies in adults with acute sinusitis favor antibiotic therapy, but note that benefits are modest.[91,92] Because studies suggest that about two thirds of adults with acute sinusitis improve without antibiotic treatment,[91] recent practice guidelines for acute sinusitis in adults question the need for antibiotic treatment except in moderate to severe disease.[93-95]

Despite lack of definitive proof of efficacy, antibiotic treatment is recommended for most children with acute and subacute sinusitis because bacterial pathogens are recoverable from the majority of affected sinuses,[1,19] and preventing sinusitis complications is a major concern. There is a paucity of trial data to indicate which antibiotics may be superior. Antibiotic selection is commonly directed by typical susceptibility profiles of frequently isolated bacteria and pharmacokinetic properties of candidate antibiotics[19,20] (Table 30-4). Because their microbiology is similar, the approach to antibiotic selection for acute and subacute sinusitis is similar. Amoxicillin is commonly recommended for previously untreated, mild, and uncomplicated acute sinusitis based on its excellent tolerability, low cost, narrow spectrum, and track record for both sinusitis and otitis media.[1,94,96] This parallels recommendations for adults, in whom meta-analyses of randomized trials support the efficacy of amoxicillin (and penicillin) for acute sinusitis.[91,92,97] However, a 5% to 20% failure rate can be expected with amoxicillin because of resistant *S. pneumoniae, H. influenzae,* and *M. catarrhalis.*[1,23] High-dose amoxicillin (80 to 90 mg/kg/day) can be used to improve eradication of potentially resistant *S. pneumoniae* in children with risk factors for antibiotic resistance (e.g., antibiotic therapy within the preceding 30 to 90 days, day care attendance, and/or age < 2 years).[1,19] Initial therapy with a broader antibiotic targeting β-lactamase–producing organisms and resistant *S. pneumoniae* should be considered in the following circumstances: a history of poor response to amoxicillin; moderate-severe, complicated, or potentially complicated disease (including frontal or sphenoidal involvement); protracted or recurrent disease; and high risk for antibiotic resistance.[23,96] Options include amoxicillin-clavulanic acid (80 to 90 mg/kg/day of amoxicillin component if risk factors for resistance are present), cefuroxime, and oral third-generation cephalosporins (especially cefpodoxime and cefdinir). Macrolides such as clarithromycin, azithromycin, and

---

BOX 30-1

KEY CONCEPTS

Use of Antimicrobials in Sinusitis

- For acute and subacute sinusitis, target therapy toward the same pathogens responsible for acute otitis media: *Streptococcus pneumoniae, Haemophilus influenzae,* and *Moraxella catarrhalis.*
- Broad-spectrum antibiotics targeting β-lactamase–producing organisms and resistant *S. pneumoniae* should be used when there is:
  - Poor response to first-line antibiotics
  - Moderate-severe, chronic, or recurrent disease
  - Complicated or potentially complicated disease (including frontal or sphenoidal involvement)
  - High risk for first-line antibiotic-resistant organisms: Antibiotic therapy within the preceding 30-90 days
  - Day care attendance.
- Treat until asymptomatic plus an additional 7 days (at least 10 days).
- Consider sinus aspiration for microbiologic identification and targeted antimicrobial therapy if disease is:
  - Severe
  - Associated with orbital or intracranial complications
  - Unresponsive to multiple antibiotic courses
  - In immunocompromised patients.

TABLE 30-4 Selected Antibiotics for Acute, Subacute, and Chronic Sinusitis

Antibiotic	Comments
Penicillins	
Amoxicillin	Untreated, mild, uncomplicated disease; high dose targets resistant *Streptococcus pneumoniae*
Amoxicillin-clavulanate	Poor response to amoxicillin or moderate-severe, complicated, or protracted disease; high dose of amoxicillin component targets resistant *S. pneumoniae*
Cephalosporins	Poor response to amoxicillin or moderate-severe, complicated, or protracted disease; intravenous agents
Cefuroxime	for severe or complicated disease or disease unresponsive to oral antibiotics
Cefpodoxime	
Cefdinir	
Cefotaxime	
Ceftriaxone	
Macrolides	Option if significant β-lactam allergy; increasing resistance of *S. pneumoniae* and marginal activity
Clarithromycin	against *Haemophilus influenzae*
Azithromycin	
Erythromycin-sulfisoxazole	
Trimethoprim-sulfamethoxazole	Option if significant beta-lactam allergy; increasing resistance of *S. pneumoniae* and marginal activity against *H. influenzae*
Clindamycin	Activity against gram-positive aerobes (including *S. pneumoniae, Staphylococcus aureus, and streptococci*) and anaerobes
Vancomycin	Intravenous; severe or complicated disease or disease unresponsive to oral antibiotics

erythromycin-sulfisoxazole are less useful because of increasing resistance of *S. pneumoniae* and marginal *in vivo* activity versus *H. influenzae* unless other options are limited by the patient being allergic to β-lactam.[1,19,96] The role of trimethoprim-sulfamethoxazole has been reduced by increasing resistance of both *S. pneumoniae* and *H. influenzae;* it remains an option in patients with beta-lactam allergy.[1,19,20,96] Clindamycin can be useful if there is a known or suspected gram-positive (e.g., *S. pneumoniae* or *S. aureus*) and/or anaerobic pathogen but offers no activity against *H. influenzae* or *M. catarrhalis.* Newer quinolones (e.g., levofloxacin, moxifloxacin, gatifloxacin) are active against the most frequent pathogens and have excellent sinus penetration and demonstrated efficacy in adults; however, evaluation of their safety and efficacy in children is needed.[19,98,99] In some cases, combinations of antimicrobial agents targeting gram-positive and gram-negative organisms may be appropriate.[20]

If amoxicillin is chosen for initial therapy, lack of clinical response within 48 to 72 hours should prompt a change to a broader agent if sinusitis is still considered the correct diagnosis.[20,23] If the disease becomes severe, protracted, associated with orbital or intracranial complications, or unresponsive to multiple antibiotic trials, sinus aspiration for microbiologic diagnosis and/or intravenous antibiotics (e.g., cefotaxime, ceftriaxone, vancomycin, clindamycin) should be considered.[1,19,96] In immunocompromised hosts, closer follow-up and sinus aspiration should be considered because of their increased risk for atypical and resistant organisms and their impaired immune response to them.[23,96]

There has been no systematic evaluation of the optimal duration of antibiotic therapy for acute sinusitis in children. Data obtained in adults suggest that treatment for 10 days affords microbiologic cure rates in excess of 90%, whereas 7-day courses are associated with microbiologic failure in 20%. However, treatment courses as short as 3 to 5 days in adults and children have had encouraging clinical results in a limited number of trials.[100,101] In general, a 10- to 14-day treatment course is recommended for the majority of children, tailored to a patient's response (e.g., treat until asymptomatic plus an additional 7 days).[1,23,96,102] Longer courses (e.g., 3 to 4 weeks) should be considered if resolution is unusually slow.[19,96,102]

Chronic Sinusitis

As for acute and subacute disease, the roles of antibiotics in hastening clinical improvement from and preventing complications of chronic sinusitis are unproven. In a study of atopic children with chronic sinusitis, antibiotics such as amoxicillin and trimethoprim-sulfamethoxazole were associated with higher response rates than either erythromycin or an oral antihistamine/decongestant without antibiotic.[103] However, in other studies of subacute or chronic sinusitis, response rates with antibiotic therapy plus decongestant were not greater than those with decongestant plus nasal saline[104] or with placebo or drainage procedures.[33]

Despite lack of firm evidence of efficacy, antibiotics are generally prescribed for chronic sinusitis because pathogenic bacteria in the sinuses have been well documented. Broad-spectrum antibiotics are chosen for empirical therapy, with the choice dependent on previous treatments (see Table 30-4). Favorable options include amoxicillin-clavulanic acid, cefuroxime, and third-generation cephalosporins such as cefpodoxime and cefdinir. If these agents are unsuccessful, a trial of clindamycin to target β-lactam–resistant *S. pneumoniae, S. aureus,* and anaerobes is reasonable.[19,105,106] The roles of oxazolidinones (e.g., linezolid) and newer quinolones for pediatric chronic sinusitis are yet to be determined. After multiple failed antibiotic courses, concern for resistant organisms increases, and sinus aspiration for culture and susceptibilities should be considered to facilitate targeted antibiotic treatment.[7,23,29,96,107] Nasal swabs have insufficient positive predictive value to accurately guide antibiotic therapy.[27,32,41,108] Middle meatus swabs may have better, although still imperfect, correlation with sinus cultures.[32,41,109] Patients with very resistant isolates and/or extremely refractory disease may benefit from intravenous therapy with agents such as cefotaxime, ceftriaxone, cefuroxime, ampicillin-sulbactam, ticarcillin-clavulanate, vancomycin, or clindamycin.[29,96,107] For invasive fungal sinusitis, surgical debridement and systemic antifungal therapy are indicated.[110]

The optimal duration of therapy is unknown. A minimum of 14 days is generally recommended if there is a prompt response. Longer courses (e.g., 3 to 6 weeks) can be considered for slower responses.[96,102] Antibiotic prophylaxis with agents such as amoxicillin or sulfonamides has been used for children with recurrent sinusitis by analogy with recurrent otitis media.[23,76] However, increasing rates of antibiotic resistance have prompted warnings to reduce antibiotic exposure, suggesting that prolonged prophylaxis should be restricted.[1,111] An alternative approach is short-term, preemptive prophylaxis with the onset of a URTI in children who have frequently recurrent sinusitis triggered by URTIs, a strategy that has been beneficial for recurrent otitis media.[112]

Sinus Surgery

Acute Sinusitis

The indications to perform sinus surgery on a child with acute and uncomplicated sinusitis are limited. Acute sinusitis symptoms are generally relieved by medical therapy consisting of antibiotics and adjunctive medical therapy. However, acute frontal or sphenoidal sinusitis in an adolescent may benefit from emergent surgical drainage for pain relief. In immunocompromised hosts, sinus irrigations to obtain specimens for microbial staining and culturing may be needed to identify potentially unusual, opportunistic pathogens.

Chronic Sinusitis

Endoscopic sinus surgery (ESS) was popularized after sinus surgery using endoscopes was imported from Europe by American surgeons in the 1980s. The safety and efficacy of this procedure in pediatric sinusitis cases have been reported, based primarily on satisfaction questionnaires.[113-115] A meta-analysis using data from eight published studies and personal data on the outcomes of pediatric ESS concluded that ESS is a safe and effective treatment of chronic sinusitis in children.[116] However, it is important to note that all the studies included in this analysis lack an untreated control group, and all except one of the nine data sources used were retrospective chart reviews.

Others have reported symptomatic and clinical improvements following ESS in special populations such as children with severe asthma[117] and cystic fibrosis.[118] Opposing this trend have been sporadic commentaries challenging the impression that pediatric sinusitis is a surgical disease.[111,119] Indeed, in a cohort of children who have undergone ESS at an early age, a markedly higher rate of revision surgeries (50%) was required (e.g., for postsurgical osteomeatal scarring), in comparison with a control group of young, chronic sinusitis patients who had not had prior sinus surgery (9%).[120]

Despite its unproven clinical efficacy and uncertain indications, ESS has safety attributes that surpass those of its predecessors. ESS with pediatric instrumentation can provide sinus drainage and sinus ablation. Specifically, the ostium of the maxillary sinuses can be widened by endoscopic antrostomy. By performing endoscopic ethmoidectomy, the ethmoid cells and polypoid tissue can be removed, frontal duct drainage can be enhanced, and the sphenoid sinus can be entered and drained.

Surgery for Sinusitis Complications

The type of sinusitis complication dictates whether an otolaryngologist will need the additional expertise of an ophthalmologist or a neurosurgeon. Generally, the participation of a pediatrician or an infectious disease consultant in the care of a child with sinusitis complications is beneficial.

Subperiosteal and orbital abscesses can be drained through either an external or endoscopic approach. Small epidural abscesses may be treated medically. Other intracranial abscesses are usually drained by a neurosurgeon. Complicated frontal sinusitis (e.g., mucocele, osteomyelitis of the frontal bone) is treated through an external approach, with the intent to achieve drainage and debridement. Severe cases in which long-term antimicrobial therapy has failed may need sinus obliteration, cranialization, and/or other reconstructive procedures. Mucoceles of the ethmoid and sphenoid sinuses can be drained endoscopically. Children with toxic shock syndrome from sinusitis should undergo sinus irrigation for culture and drainage.

Adjunctive Surgical Procedures

Adenoid hypertrophy as a cause of chronic sinusitis and the benefits of adenoidectomy for chronic sinusitis have been suggested by uncontrolled studies.[121,122] Chronic sinusitis patients with severe nasal obstruction from adenoid hypertrophy are likely to have some symptomatic benefit from an adenoidectomy.

Inferior turbinate hypertrophy causing nasal obstruction is also found in some children with chronic sinusitis. There are no published reports on the efficacy of inferior turbinate cauterization or reduction in the treatment of chronic sinusitis. In subjects in whom intranasal corticosteroid therapy for nasal obstructive symptoms associated with inferior turbinate hypertrophy has failed, a turbinate reduction procedure for symptomatic relief may be considered.

Adjunctive Medical Therapy

Empirically, clinicians have used an assortment of agents in conjunction with oral antibiotics for the treatment of both acute and chronic sinusitis in children. These agents include nasal saline (isotonic and hypertonic) washes, topical and oral decongestants, topical and oral antihistamines, topical anticholinergic agents, leukotriene receptor antagonists, and corticosteroids (intranasal and oral). The use of these agents is currently based on their theoretical benefits of improving associated rhinitis and rhinorrhea by decreasing mucosal inflammation and edema, which increases mucociliary transport, thereby improving nasal patency and presumably ostial drainage, with little support from randomized clinical trials. Similarly, managing comorbid medical conditions (i.e., allergic rhinitis, asthma, GERD) has theoretical benefits and may help to improve symptoms shared with sinusitis. Recently, a randomized, controlled trial compared cefuroxime with intranasal fluticasone propionate with cefuroxime alone for the treatment of acute sinusitis in 95 adults.[123] Patients receiving fluticasone achieved a significantly higher degree and a more rapid rate of symptomatic improvement. However, although all these subjects had a history of chronic sinusitis, the efficacy of this regimen on chronic outcomes or on radiographic abnormalities was not addressed.

Allergic Fungal Sinusitis

Allergic fungal sinusitis is characterized by an intense and chronic allergic reaction to fungi growing in allergic mucin within the sinus cavities and is believed to be pathogenically similar to allergic bronchopulmonary mycoses (ABPMs).[124,125] Mostly dematiaceous fungi (e.g., *Aspergillus, Alternaria, Curvularia, Bipolaris*) have been cultured from affected sinuses. In a large adult cohort of 67 allergic fungal sinusitis patients in Phoenix, Arizona, *Bipolaris spicifera* was cultured from 67% of the patients' sinus cultures.[125] Although this disease is believed to be more prevalent in adults, two series of pediatric subjects have been reported. One cohort of 6 patients (ages 8 to 16 years) all had nasal polyposis, facial deformity, and fungal hyphae in allergic mucin filling the sinuses; 4 of 6 patients had bony erosion of the sinuses.[126] In another series, 10 pediatric subjects with allergic fungal sinusitis were reported (mean age, 14 years).[127] The management of this condition with oral corticosteroids after surgical debridement has been adapted from treatment regimens for ABPM.[124] Antifungal therapy (e.g., itraconazole) has been used in a small number of reported cases.[40]

CONCLUSIONS

Sinusitis in children is a common problem of widely varying duration. Unfortunately, symptoms, physical examination, and radiographic findings of sinusitis are blurred with those of common URTIs, without clearly distinguishing features. Sinusitis rarely leads to severe, life-threatening complications, which are usually the result of direct extension of bacterial infection from the sinuses.

Management of uncomplicated sinusitis consists of antimicrobial and medical adjunctive treatment aiming for symptom relief and prevention of complications and recurrence. Radiographic imaging studies may be helpful in chronic and/or recurrent sinusitis. In uncomplicated cases, limited coronal sinus CT scans are generally preferred. In complicated cases, complete coronal sinus CT series are recommended. Antral irrigation can provide sinus specimens for bacterial culture and targeted antimicrobial therapy in patients with chronic, refractory, and complicated disease. Sinus surgery in uncomplicated sinusitis, especially in young children, should generally be avoided. Great reductions in mortality caused by sinusitis complications coincide with improvements in antimicrobial and surgical therapy.

Dr. Liu's work was supported by NIH No. K23-HL-04272 and the American Academy of Allergy, Asthma and Immunology (Education & Research Trust).

REFERENCES

1. American Academy of Pediatrics: Clinical practice guideline: management of sinusitis, *Pediatrics* 108:798-808, 2001.
2. Clement PA, Gordts F: Epidemiology and prevalence of aspecific chronic sinusitis, *Int J Pediatr Otorhinolaryngol* 49:S101-S103, 1999.
3. Aitken M, Taylor JA: Prevalence of clinical sinusitis in young children followed up by primary care pediatricians, *Arch Pediatr Adolesc Med* 152:244-248, 1998.
4. Lombardi E, Stein RT, Wright AL, et al: The relation between physician-diagnosed sinusitis, asthma, and skin test reactivity to allergens in 8-year-old children, *Pediatr Pulmonol* 22:141-146, 1996.
5. McCaig LF, Hughes JM: Trends in antimicrobial drug prescribing among office-based physicians in the United States, *JAMA* 273:214-219, 1995.
6. Doern GV, Brueggemann AB, Huynh H, et al: Antimicrobial resistance with *Streptococcus pneumoniae* in the United States, 1997-1998, *Emerg Infect Dis* 5:757-765, 1999.
7. Slack CL, Dahn KA, Abzug MJ, et al: Antibiotic-resistant bacteria in pediatric chronic sinusitis, *Pediatr Infect Dis J* 20:247-250, 2001.
8. Cunningham JM, Chiu EJ, Landgraf JM, et al: The health impact of chronic recurrent rhinosinusitis in children, *Arch Otolaryngol Head Neck Surg* 126:1363-1368, 2000.
9. Parsons DS, Wald ER: Otitis media and sinusitis: similar diseases, *Otolaryngol Clin North Am* 29:11-25, 1996.
10. Swarts JD, Alper CM, Seroky JT, et al: *In vivo* observation with magnetic resonance imaging of middle ear effusion in response to experimental underpressures, *Ann Otol Rhinol Laryngol* 104:522-528, 1995.
11. Piltcher OB, Swarts JD, Magnuson K, et al: A rat model of otitis media with effusion caused by eustachian tube obstruction with and without *Streptococcus pneumoniae* infection: methods and disease course, *Otolaryngol Head Neck Surg* 126:490-498, 2002.
12. Milczuk HA, Dalley HA, Wessbacher RW, et al: Nasal and paranasal sinus anomalies in children with chronic sinusitis, *Laryngoscope* 103:247-252, 1993.
13. Lusk RP, McAlister B, el Fouley A: Anatomic variation in pediatric chronic sinusitis: a CT study, *Otolaryngol Clin North Am* 29:75-91, 1996.
14. Puhakka T, Makela MJ, Alanen A, et al: Sinusitis in the common cold, *J Allergy Clin Immunol* 102:403-408, 1998.
15. Gwaltney JMJ, Phillips CD, Miller RD, et al: Computed tomographic study of the common cold, *N Engl J Med* 330:25-30, 1994.
16. Bolger WE, Leonard D, Dick JEJ, et al: Gram negative sinusitis: a bacteriologic and histologic study in rabbits, *Am J Rhinol* 11:15-25, 1997.
17. Gwaltney JM: *Principles and practice of infectious diseases*, Philadelphia, 2000, Churchill Livingstone.
18. Wald ER, Milmoe GJ, Bowen A, et al: Acute maxillary sinusitis in children, *N Engl J Med* 304:749-754, 1981.
19. Brook I, Gooch WM, Jenkins S, et al: Medical management of acute bacterial rhinosinusitis, *Ann Otol Rhinol Laryngol* 109:S2-S20, 2000.
20. Sinus and Allergy Health Partnership: Antimicrobial treatment guidelines for acute bacterial rhinosinusitis, *Otolaryngol-Head Neck Surg* 123:S1-S32, 2000.
21. Tinkleman DG, Silk HJ: Clinical and bacteriologic features of chronic sinusitis in children, *Am J Dis Child* 143:938-941, 1989.
22. Wald ER, Byers C, Guerra N, et al: Subacute sinusitis in children, *J Pediatr* 115:28-32, 1989.
23. Wald ER: Sinusitis, *Pediatr Ann* 27:811-818, 1998.
24. Brook I, Frazier EH, Gher ME: Microbiology of periapical accesses and associated maxillary sinusitis, *J Periodontol* 67:608-610, 1996.
25. Kim SY, Syms MJ, Holtel MR, et al: Acanthamoeba sinusitis with subsequent dissemination in an AIDS patient, *Ear Nose Throat J* 79:168-174, 2000.
26. Teknos TN, Poulin MD, Laruentano AM, et al: Acanthamoeba rhinosinusitis: characterization, diagnosis, and treatment, *Am J Rhinol* 14:387-391, 2000.
27. Arruda LK, Mimica IM, Sole D, et al: Abnormal maxillary sinus radiographs in children: do they represent bacterial infection? *Pediatrics* 85:553-558, 1990.
28. Brook I: Bacteriologic features of chronic sinusitis in children, *JAMA* 246:967-969, 1981.
29. Don DM, Yellon RF, Casselbrant ML, et al: Efficacy of a stepwise protocol that includes intravenous antibiotic therapy for the management of chronic sinusitis in children and adolescents, *Arch Otolaryngol Head Neck Surg* 127:1093-1098, 2001.
30. Erkan M, Ozcan M, Arslan S, et al: Bacteriology of antrum in children with chronic maxillary sinusitis, *Scand J Infect Dis* 28:283-285, 1996.
31. Muntz HR, Lusk RP: Bacteriology of the ethmoid bullae in children with chronic sinusitis, *Arch Otolaryngol Head Neck Surg* 117:179-181, 1991.
32. Orobellow PW, Park RI, Belcher LJ, et al: Microbiology of chronic sinusitis in children, *Arch Otolaryngol Head Neck Surg* 117:980-983, 1991.
33. Otten FWA, Grote JJ: Treatment of chronic maxillary sinusitis in children, *Int J Pediatr Otorhinolaryngol* 15:269-278, 1988.

34. Brook I, Frazier EH, Foote PA: Microbiology of the transition from acute to chronic maxillary sinusitis, *J Med Microbiol* 45:372-375, 1996.

35. Brook I, Yocum P, Frazier EH: Bacteriology and beta-lactamase activity in acute and chronic maxillary sinusitis, *Arch Otolaryngol Head Neck Surg* 122:418-423, 1996.

36. Brook I, Frazier EH: Microbiology of subperiosteal orbital abscess and associated maxillary sinusitis, *Laryngoscope* 106:1010-1013, 1996.

37. Frederick J, Braude A: Anaerobic infection of the paranasal sinuses, *N Engl J Med* 290:135-137, 1974.

38. Brook I: Bacteriology of chronic maxillary sinusitis in adults, *Ann Otol Rhinol Laryngol* 98:426-428, 1989.

39. Erkan M, Aslan T, Ozcan M, et al: Bacteriology of antrum in adults with chronic maxillary sinusitis, *Laryngoscope* 104:321-324, 1994.

40. Andes D, Proctor R, Bush RK, et al: Report of successful prolonged antifungal therapy for refractory allergic fungal sinusitis, *Clin Infect Dis* 31:202-204, 2000.

41. Chan KH, Liu A, Abzug MJ, et al: Unpublished data.

42. Ramadan HH, Farr RW, Wetmore SJ: Adenovirus and respiratory syncytial virus in chronic sinusitis using polymerase chain reaction, *Laryngoscope* 107:923-925, 1977.

43. Van Nostrand AWP, Goodman WS: Pathologic aspects of mucosal lesions of the maxillary sinus, *Otolaryngol Clin North Am* 9:21-27, 1976.

44. Rochester CL, Ackerman SJ, Zheng T, et al: Eosinophil-fibroblast interactions: granule major basic protein interacts with IL-1 and transforming growth factor-beta in the stimulation of lung fibroblast IL-6-type cytokine production, *J Immunol* 156:4449-4456, 1996.

45. Broide DH, Paine MM, Firestein GS: Eosinophils express interleukin 5 and granulocyte macrophage-colony-stimulating factor mRNA at sites of allergic inflammation in asthmatics, *J Clin Invest* 90:1414-1424, 1992.

46. Kita H, Ohnishi T, Okubo Y, et al: Granulocyte/macrophage colony-stimulating factor and interleukin 3 release from human peripheral blood eosinophils and neutrophils, *J Exp Med* 174:745-748, 1991.

47. Minshall E, Chakir J, Laviolette M, et al: IL-11 expression is increased in severe asthma: association with epithelial cells and eosinophils, *J Allergy Clin Immunol* 105:232-238, 2000.

48. Sobol SE, Fukakusa M, Christodoulopoulos P, et al: Inflammation and remodeling of the sinus mucosa in children and adults with chronic sinusitis, *Laryngoscope* (in press).

49. Durham SR, Ying S, Varney VA, et al: Cytokine messenger RNA expression for IL-3, IL-4, IL-5 and granulocyte/macrophage-colony-stimulating factor in the nasal mucosa after local allergen provocation: relationship to tissue eosinophilia, *J Immunol* 148:2390-2394, 1992.

50. Hamilos DL, Leung DYM, Wood R, et al: Evidence for distinct cytokine expression in allergic versus nonallergic chronic sinusitis, *J Allergy Clin Immunol* 96:537-544, 1995.

51. Rachelefsky GS: Chronic sinusitis: a disease of all ages, *Am J Dis Child* 143:886-888, 1989.

52. Varney VA, Jacobson MR, Sudderick RM, et al: Immunohistology of the nasal mucosa following allergen-induced rhinitis: identification of activated T lymphocytes, eosinophils and neutrophils, *Am Rev Respir Dis* 146:170-176, 1992.

53. Romagnani S: Biology of human TH1 and TH2 cells, *J Clin Immunol* 15:121-129, 1995.

54. Settipane GA: Epidemiology of nasal polyps, *Allergy Asthma Proc* 17:231-236, 1996.

55. Baroody FM, Hughes T, McDowell PR, et al: Eosinophilia in chronic childhood sinusitis, *Arch Otolaryngol Head Neck Surg* 121:1396-1402, 1995.

56. Demoly P, Crampette L, Mondain M, et al: Assessment of inflammation in noninfectious chronic maxillary sinusitis, *J Allergy Clin Immunol* 94:95-108, 1994.

57. Wright ED, Frenkiel S, Al-Ghamdi K, et al: Interleukin-4, interleukin-5, and granulocyte-macrophage colony-stimulating factor receptor expression in chronic sinusitis and response to topical steroids, *Otolaryngol Head Neck Surg* 118:490-495, 1998.

58. Hamilos DL, Leung DYM, Wood R, et al: Chronic hyperplastic sinusitis: association of tissue eosinophilia with mRNA expression of granulocyte-macrophage colony-stimulating factor and interleukin-3, *J Allergy Clin Immunol* 92:39-48, 1993.

59. Hamilos DL: Chronic sinusitis, *J Allergy Clin Immunol* 106:213-227, 2000.

60. Demoly P, Crampette L, Mondain M, et al: Myeloperoxidase and interleukin-8 levels in chronic sinusitis, *Clin Exp Allergy* 27:672-675, 1997.

61. Hamilos DL, Leung DYM, Wood R, et al: Eosinophil infiltration in non-allergic chronic hyperplastic sinusitis with nasal polyposis (CHS/NP) is

62. Wright ED, Hamid Q, Frenkiel S: *Cilia, mucus, and mucociliary interactions,* New York, 1998, Marcel Dekker.

63. Christodoulopoulos P, Cameron L, Durham S, et al: Molecular pathology of allergic disease II: upper airway disease, *J Allergy Clin Immunol* 105:211-223, 2000.

64. Zimmerman B, Stinger D, Feanny S, et al: Prevalence of abnormalities found by sinus x-rays in childhood asthma: lack of relation to severity of asthma, *J Allergy Clin Immunol* 80:268-273, 1987.

65. Rossi OVJ, Pirila T, Laitinen J, et al: Sinus aspirates and radiographic abnormalities in severe attacks of asthma, *Int Arch Allergy Immunol* 103:209-213, 1994.

66. Newman LJ, Platts-Mills TAE, Phillips CD, et al: Chronic sinusitis: relationship of computed tomographic findings to allergy, asthma, and eosinophilia, *JAMA* 271:363-367, 1994.

67. Pelikan Z, Pelikan-Filipek M: Role of nasal allergy in chronic maxillary sinusitis-diagnostic value of nasal challenge with allergen, *J Allergy Clin Immunol* 86:484-491, 1990.

68. Wang X, Moylan B, Leopold DA, et al: Mutation in the gene responsible for cystic fibrosis and predisposition to chronic rhinosinusitis in the general population, *JAMA* 284:1814-1819, 2000.

69. Raman V, Clary R, Siegrist KL, et al: Increased prevalence of mutations in the cystic fibrosis transmembrane conductance regulator in children with chronic rhinosinusitis, *Pediatrics* 109:E13, 2002.

70. Castellani C, Quinzii C, Altieri S, et al: A pilot survey of cystic fibrosis clinical manifestations in CFTR mutation heterozygotes, *Genet Test* 5:249-254, 2001.

71. Takeuchi K, Majima Y, Shimizu T, et al: Analysis of HLA antigens in Japanese patients with chronic sinusitis, *Laryngoscope* 109:275-278, 1999.

72. Takeuchi K, Majima Y, Shimizu T: Tumor necrosis factor gene polymorphism in chronic sinusitis, *Laryngoscope* 110:1711-1714, 2000.

73. Contencin P, Narcy P: Nasopharyngeal pH monitoring in infants and children with chronic rhinopharyngitis, *Int J Pediatr Otorhinolaryngol* 22:249-256, 1991.

74. Yellon RF, Coticchia J, Dixit S: Esophageal biopsy for the diagnosis of gastroesophageal reflux-associated otolaryngologic problems in children, *Am J Med* 108:131S-138S, 2000.

75. Phipps CD, Wood WE, Gibson WS, et al: Gastroesophageal reflux contributing to chronic sinus disease in children: a prospective analysis, *Arch Otolaryngol Head Neck Surg* 126:831-836, 2000.

76. Chan KH, Winslow CP, Levin MJ, et al: Clinical practice guidelines for the management of chronic sinusitis in children, *Otolaryngol Head Neck Surg* 120:328-334, 1999.

77. Mudgil SP, Wise SW, Hopper KD, et al: Correlation between presumed sinusitis-induced pain and paranasal sinus computed tomographic findings, *Ann Allergy Asthma Immunol* 88:223-226, 2002.

78. McAlister WH, Parker BR, Kushner DC, et al: Sinusitis in the pediatric population: American College of Radiology. ACR appropriateness criteria, *Radiology* 215(suppl):811-818, 2000.

79. Garcia DP, Corbett ML, Eberly SM, et al: Radiographic imaging studies in pediatric chronic sinusitis, *J Allergy Clin Immunol* 94:523-530, 1994.

80. Lerner DN, Zalzal GH, Choi SS, et al: Intracranial complications of sinusitis in childhood, *Ann Otol Rhinol Laryngol* 104:288-293, 1995.

81. Garcia CE, Cunningham MJ, Clary RA, et al: The etiologic role of frontal sinusitis in pediatric orbital abscesses, *Am J Otolaryngol* 14:449-452, 1993.

82. Chandler JR, Lanenbrunner DJ, Steven ER: The pathogenesis of orbital complications in acute sinusitis, *Laryngoscope* 141:1414-1428, 1970.

83. Samad I, Riding K: Orbital complications of ethmoiditis: B.C. Children's Hospital experience, *J Otolaryngol* 20:400-403, 1991.

84. Wald ER, Chiponis D, Ledesma-Medina J: Comparative effectiveness of amoxicillin and amoxicillin-clavulanate potassium in acute paranasal sinus infections in children: a double-blind, placebo-controlled trial, *Pediatrics* 77:795-800, 1986.

85. Morris P: Antibiotics for persistent nasal discharge (rhinosinusitis) in children, *Cochrane Database Syst Rev* 3:CD001094, 2000.

86. Garbutt JM, Goldstein M, Gellman E, et al: A randomized, placebo-controlled trial of antimicrobial treatment for children with clinically diagnosed acute sinusitis, *Pediatrics* 107:619-625, 2001.

87. Hansen JG, Schmidt H, Grinsted P: Randomized, double-blind, placebo-controlled trial of penicillin V in the treatment of acute maxillary sinusitis in adults in general practice, *Scand J Prim Health Care* 18:44-47, 2000.

associated with endothelial VCAM-1 upregulation and expression of TNF-alpha, *Am J Respir Cell Mol Biol* 15:443-450, 1996.

88. Lindbaek M, Hjortdahl P, Johnsen UL: Randomized, double-blind, placebo-controlled trial of penicillin V and amoxicillin in treatment of acute sinusitis infections in adults, *Br Med J* 313:325-329, 1996.

89. Stalman W, van Essen GA, van der Graaf Y, et al: The end of antibiotic treatment in adults with acute sinusitis-like complaints in general practice? A placebo-controlled double-blind randomized doxycycline trial, *Br J Gen Pract* 47:794-799, 1997.

90. Van Buchem FL, Knottnerus JA, Schrijnemaekers VJ, et al: Primary-care-based randomized placebo-controlled trial of antibiotic treatment in acute maxillary sinusitis, *Lancet* 349:683-687, 1997.

91. Benninger MS, Sedory Holzer SE, Lau J: Diagnosis and treatment of uncomplicated acute bacterial rhinosinusitis: summary of the Agency for Health Care Policy and Research evidence-based report, *Otolaryngol Head and Neck Surg* 122:1-7, 2000.

92. Williams JWJ, Aguilar C, Makela M, et al: Antibiotics for acute maxillary sinusitis, *Cochrane Database Syst Rev* 2:CD000243, 2000.

93. Hickner JM, Bartlett JG, Besser RE, et al: Principles of appropriate antibiotic use for acute rhinosinusitis in adults: background, *Ann Intern Med* 134:498-505, 2001.

94. Piccirillo JF, Mager DE, Frisse ME, et al: Impact of first-line vs. second-line antibiotics for the treatment of acute uncomplicated sinusitis, *JAMA* 286:1849-1856, 2001.

95. Snow V, Mottur-Pilson C, Hickner JM: Principles of appropriate antibiotic use for acute sinusitis in adults, *Ann Intern Med* 134:495-497, 2001.

96. Clement PAR, Bluestone CD, Gordts F, et al: Management of rhinosinusitis in children, *Arch Otolaryngol Head Neck Surg* 124:31-34, 1998.

97. Williams JW Jr, Aguilar C, Makela M: Which antibiotics lead to higher clinical cure rates in adults with acute maxillary sinusitis? *West J Med* 173:42, 2000.

98. Rakkar S, Roberts K, Towe BF, et al: Moxifloxacin versus amoxicillin clavulanate in the treatment of acute maxillary sinusitis: a primary care experience, *Int J Clin Pract* 55:309-315, 2001.

99. Siegert R, Gehanno P, Nikolaidis P, et al: A comparison of the safety and efficacy of moxifloxacin (BAY 12-8039) and cefuroxime axetil in the treatment of acute bacterial sinusitis in adults: the sinusitis study group, *Respir Med* 94:337-344, 2000.

100. Ng DK, Chow PY, Leung I, et al: A randomized controlled trial of azithromycin and amoxicillin/clavulanate in the management of subacute rhinosinusitis, *J Paediatr Child Health* 36:378-381, 2000.

101. Pichichero M: Short course antibiotic therapy for respiratory infections: a review of the evidence, *Pediatr Infect Dis J* 19:929-937, 2000.

102. Zacharisen MC, Kelly KJ: Allergic and infectious pediatric sinusitis, *Pediatr Ann* 27:759-766, 1998.

103. Rachelefsky GS: Chronic sinusitis in children with respiratory allergy: the role of antimicrobials, *J Allergy Clin Immunol* 69:382-387, 1982.

104. Dohlman AW, Hemstreet MP, Odrezin GT, et al: Subacute sinusitis: are antimicrobials necessary? *J Allergy Clin Immunol* 91:1015-1023, 1993.

105. Brook I, Yocum P: Antimicrobial management of chronic sinusitis in children, *J Laryngol Otol* 109:1159-1162, 1995.

106. Bussey MF: Acute sinusitis, *Pediatr Rev* 20:142, 1999.

107. Buchman CA, Yellon RF, Bluestone CD: Alternative to endoscopic sinus surgery in the management of pediatric chronic rhinosinusitis refractory to oral antimicrobial therapy, *Otolaryngol-Head Neck Surg* 120:219-224, 1999.

108. Sener B, Hascelik G, Onerci M, et al: Evaluation of the microbiology of chronic sinusitis, *J Laryngol Otol* 110:547-550, 1996.

109. Vogan JC, Bolger WE, Keyes AS: Endoscopically guided sinonasal cultures: a direct comparison with maxillary sinus aspirate cultures, *Otolaryngol Head Neck Surg* 122:370-373, 2000.

110. Rizk SS, Kraus DH, Gerresheim G, et al: Aggressive combination treatment for invasive fungal sinusitis in immunocompromised patients, *Ear Nose Throat J* 79:278-280, 282, 284-285, 2000.

111. Baroody FM: Pediatric sinusitis, *Arch Otolaryngol Head Neck Surg* 127:1099-1101, 2001.

112. Prellner K, Fogle-Hansson M, Jorgensen F: Prevention of recurrent acute otitis media in otitis-prone children by intermittent prophylaxis with penicillin, *Acta Otolaryngol* 114:182-187, 1994.

113. Parsons DS, Phillips SE: Functional endoscopic surgery in children: a retrospective analysis of results, *Laryngoscope* 103:899-903, 1993.

114. Lazar RH, Younis RT, Long TE: Functional endonasal sinus surgery in adults and children, *Laryngoscope* 103:1-5, 1993.

115. Gross CW, Gurucharri MJ, Lazar RH, et al: Functional endonasal sinus surgery (FESS) in the pediatric age group, *Laryngoscope* 99:272-275, 1989.

116. Hebert RL, Bent JP III: Meta-analysis of outcomes of pediatric functional endoscopic sinus surgery, *Laryngoscope* 108:796-799, 1998.

117. Manning SC, Wasserman RL, Silver R, et al: Results of endoscopic sinus surgery in pediatric patients with chronic sinusitis and asthma, *Arch Otolaryngol Head Neck Surg* 120:1142-1145, 1994.

118. Rosbe KW, Jones DT, Rahbar R, et al: Endoscopic sinus surgery in cystic fibrosis: do patients benefit from surgery? *Int J Pediatr Otorhinolaryngol* 61:113-119, 2001.

119. Poole MD: Pediatric sinusitis is not a surgical disease, *Ear Nose Throat J* 71:622-623, 1992.

120. Chan KH, Winslow CP, Abzug MJ: Persistent rhinosinusitis in children following endoscopic sinus surgery, *Otolaryngol Head Neck Surg* 121:577-580, 1999.

121. Vandenberg SJ, Heatley DG: Efficacy of adenoidectomy in relieving symptoms of chronic sinusitis in children, *Arch Otolaryngol Head Neck Surg* 123:675-678, 1997.

122. Rosenfeld RM: Pilot study of outcomes in pediatric rhinosinusitis, *Arch Otolaryngol Head Neck Surg* 121:729-736, 1995.

123. Dolor RJ, Witsell DL, Hellkamp AS, et al: Comparison of cefuroxime with or without intranasal fluticasone for the treatment of rhinosinusitis. The CAF trial: a randomized controlled trial, *JAMA* 286:3097-3105, 2001.

124. Schubert MS, Goetz DW: Evaluation and treatment of allergic fungal sinusitis. II. Treatment and follow-up, *J Allergy Clin Immunol* 102:395-402, 1998.

125. Schubert MS, Goetz DW: Evaluation and treatment of allergic fungal sinusitis. I. Demographics and diagnosis, *J Allergy Clin Immunol* 102:387-394, 1998.

126. Manning SC, Vuitch F, Weinberg AG, et al: Allergic aspergillosis: a newly recognized form of sinusitis in the pediatric population, *Laryngoscope* 99:681-685, 1989.

127. Kupferberg SB, Bent JP: Allergic fungal sinusitis in the pediatric population, *Arch Otolaryngol Head Neck Surg* 122:1381-1384, 1996.

CHAPTER 31

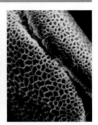

Chronic Cough

HENRY MILGROM

Cough, a decidedly familiar yet distinctive phenomenon, is the most conspicuous and often most distressing manifestation of respiratory disease.[1] Twenty-four million annual physician visits for cough took place in the United States from 1995 through 1996, the largest number documented for a single symptom.[2] Of these patients, 47.7% were younger than 15 years old. In this young cohort cough accounted for 8.5% of all medical appointments, exceeded only by well-baby visits.[2] In Great Britain, cough without colds has a prevalence of 28.5% in boys and 30.3% in girls[3]; other surveys around the world also have reported high occurrence rates.[2,4] Two studies have used electronic recorders to determine how often normal children cough.[5,6] Average frequency over 24 hours was 11.3, with a range of 1 to 34 coughs in children who were free from respiratory infection for at least 1 month and had normal physical and spirometric findings, and only 2 of 41 children coughed at night.[5] Chang et al[6] found that median cough frequency was 65 per day in children with chronic cough and 10 per day in normal controls. Unfortunately, most studies rely on parents to report their children's cough, a method that has been shown to provide inaccurate information.[7,8] When data from questionnaires administered to parents were compared with overnight cough recordings performed in 145 homes, the agreement was low, with kappa statistics ranging from 0.02 to 0.10,[9] a discrepancy that causes misgivings about clinical strategies based on studies that use parents' recall or paper diaries.

Respiratory symptoms are often caused by self-limiting illnesses, but in some children, persistent cough indicates the presence of congenital malformations or chronic disorders. Pediatric texts generally describe chronic cough as a condition that persists for longer than 3 weeks. This definition leads to the observation that chronic cough is likely to improve in time without treatment.[10] A better-founded classification by Irwin and Madison[11] divides cough into three categories: acute, lasting less than 3 weeks; subacute, lasting 3 to 8 weeks; and chronic, lasting longer than 8 weeks. Irwin and Madison's definitions exclude a greater proportion of self-limiting cases, and chronic cough by their criteria tends to last longer and to require medical intervention. Viral infections of the upper respiratory tract are the most common cause of acute cough. In adults the prevalence of cough due to the common cold ranges from 83% in the first 48 hours to 26% on day 14.[12] Acute bronchitis, usually a brief and self-limiting illness, follows the symptoms of an upper respiratory tract infection such as rhinitis or pharyngitis. Typically the symptoms resolve after 10 to 14 days. Patients with subacute cough most often present with a history of recent upper respiratory tract infection or seasonal allergic rhinitis. Other common conditions to consider are postinfectious cough, bacterial sinusitis, and asthma.

Patients with chronic or recurrent episodes of cough that is nonproductive and lasts for weeks or months are frequently seen in pediatric practice.[2,13] This type of cough, the subject of this chapter, calls for a careful evaluation (Figure 31-1). It is often a manifestation of an underlying disorder, and it invariably is an exhausting process that contributes to the child's morbidity and affects both the patient and the family. Many children with chronic cough have experienced repeated treatment failure, and the families have come to regard the condition as permanent and irremediable. Fortunately, in most cases this perception is incorrect. However, a systematic approach to the diagnosis is necessary, and effective therapy should be directed at all identified cough mechanisms at the same time.

DIFFERENTIAL DIAGNOSIS
(Table 31-1)

The differential diagnosis of cough in childhood varies with the age of the patient; the duration, character, and time of occurrence of the cough; associated signs and symptoms; and the patient's exposure and family history. In the neonatal period, congenital abnormalities, above all pulmonary or cardiac, must be considered. Prematurity, especially in a patient who had required mechanical ventilation, may lead to bronchopulmonary dysplasia or the development of tracheal or bronchial stenosis. Vomiting and regurgitation may be the presenting signs and symptoms of esophageal reflux or a tracheoesophageal fistula. Recurrent choking or cough associated with difficulty in sucking or swallowing suggests aspiration. Cough may occur during or after resolution of a respiratory infection. Attendance in day care increases the risk of upper respiratory symptoms and infections in young children. In the toddler the list of causes grows longer to include foreign body aspiration and cystic fibrosis. A history of fever and/or presentation in winter suggests a viral etiology; seasonal occurrence may indicate asthma or seasonal allergic rhinitis; and year-round symptoms point to perennial allergic rhinitis and exposure to house dust mites, pets, molds, or cigarette smoke. Maternal smoking in particular appears to influence the development of respiratory symptoms in young children.[14] In the older child, immune deficiency, tuberculosis

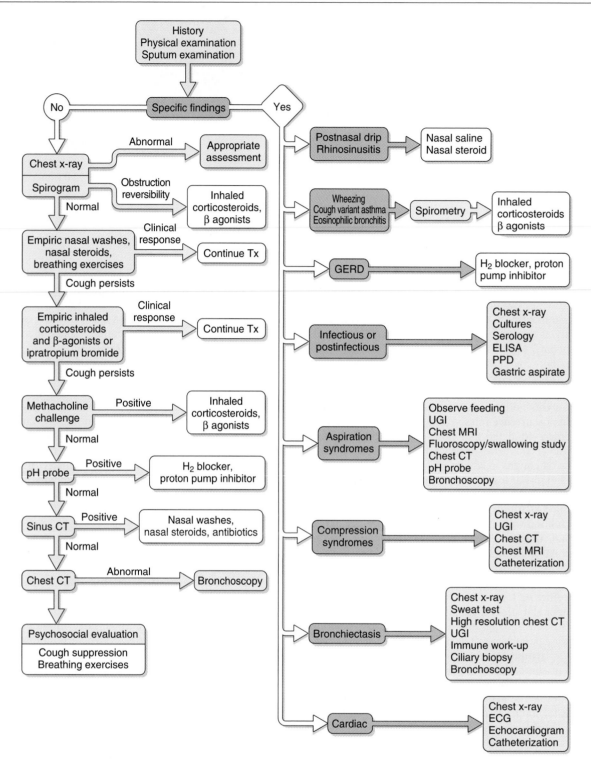

FIGURE 31-1 Algorithm for the evaluation and treatment of chronic cough in childhood. *CT,* Computed tomography; *Tx,* therapy; *GERD,* gastroesophageal reflux disease; *ELISA,* enzyme-linked immunosorbent assay; *PPD,* purified protein derivative; *UGI,* upper gastrointestinal series; *MRI,* magnetic resonance imaging; *ECG,* electrocardiogram.

TABLE 31-1 Differential Diagnosis of Chronic Cough

Congenital anomalies
  Connection of the airway to the esophagus
    Laryngeal cleft
    Tracheoesophageal fistula
  Laryngotracheomalacia
    Primary laryngotracheomalacia
    Laryngotracheomalacia secondary to vascular or other
      compression
  Bronchopulmonary foregut malformation
  Congenital mediastinal tumors
  Congenital heart disease with pulmonary congestion
Infectious or postinfectious cough
  Recurrent viral infection (infants and toddlers)
  Chlamydial infection (infants)
  Whooping cough–like syndrome
    Bordetella pertussis infection
    Chlamydial infection
    Mycoplasma infection
    Cystic fibrosis (infants and toddlers)
  Granulomatous infection
    Mycobacterial infection
    Fungal infection
  Suppurative lung disease (bronchiectasis and lung abscess)
    Cystic fibrosis
    Foreign body aspiration with secondary suppuration
    Ciliary dysfunction
    Immunodeficiency
      Primary immunodeficiency
      Secondary immunodeficiency (acquired immune deficiency
        syndrome)
  Paranasal sinus infection
Asthma related
  Asthma
  Cough-variant asthma
  Eosinophilic bronchitis
Rhinitis related
  Allergic rhinitis
  Rhinosinusitis
  Vasomotor rhinitis
  Postnasal drip
Gastroesophageal reflux without aspiration
Vocal cord dysfunction
Aspiration (fluid material)
  Dyskinetic swallowing with aspiration
    General neurodevelopmental problems
    Möbius' syndrome
  Bottle-propping and bottle in bed (infant and toddlers)
  Gastroesophageal reflux
Foreign body aspiration (solid material)
  Upper airway aspiration (tonsillar, pharyngeal, laryngeal)
  Tracheobronchial aspiration
  Esophageal foreign body with an obstruction or aspiration result-
    ing from dysphagia
Physical and chemical irritation
  Smoke from tobacco products (active and passive)
  Wood smoke from stoves and fireplaces
  Dry, dusty environment (hobbies and employment)
  Volatile chemicals (hobbies and employment)
  Dampness
  Mold
Psychogenic cough
Habit cough

Modified from Brown MA, Morgan WJ: Clinical assessment and diagnostic approach to common problems. In Taussig LM, Landau LI, eds: *Pediatric respiratory medicine*, St Louis, 1999, Mosby.

(TB), and psychogenic cough enter into the differential diagnosis. The most common causes of chronic cough in the adolescent are asthma, postnasal drip, and gastroesophageal reflux (GER), but cigarette smoking and psychogenic causes require consideration.[1,15]

PATHOPHYSIOLOGY

Henry Hyde Salter[16] wrote on the subject of cough in 1882:

> It is the constituted mechanism of expulsion of any particles of foreign matter which may at any time be introduced with the respired air, and against whose ingress the stricture function of the glottis so imperfectly provides. . . . Cough is, no doubt, often a phenomenon of disease, but it becomes pathological from the material on which it is exercised and not from the essential action of the act.

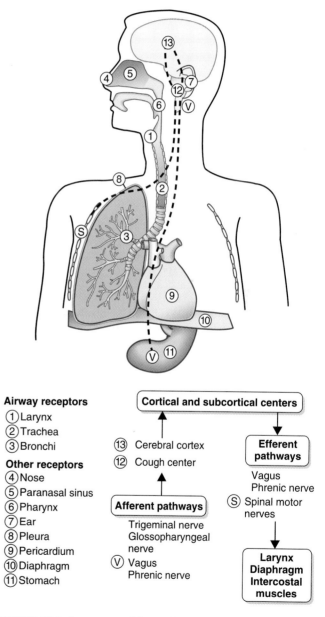

FIGURE 31-2 Components of the cough reflex. (Modified from Karlsson J-A, Sant'Ambroggio G, Widdicombe J: *J Appl Physiol* 65:1007-1023, 1988; Korpas J: Cough. In Korpas J, Tomori Z, eds: *Cough and other respiratory reflexes*, Basel, Switzerland, 1979, S. Karger.)

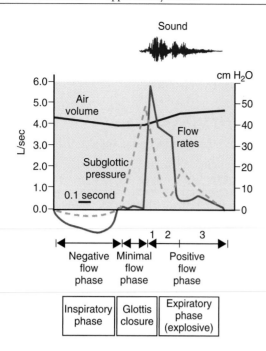

FIGURE 31-3 Changes in flow rate, air volume, subglottic pressure, and sound level generated during the act of coughing. (From Bianco S, Robuschi M: Mechanics of cough. In Braga PC, Allegra L, eds: *Cough,* New York, 1989, Raven.)

Cough serves as a protective mechanism that clears the respiratory tract and defends against the aspiration of noxious materials.[17] Two associated processes, bronchoconstriction and mucus secretion, add to its effectiveness. Although mechanical barriers limit the exposure of the respiratory tract to inhaled pathogens, the mucociliary apparatus and cough act to expel any organisms that may have bypassed the primary defenses.[18] Recurrent partial collapse or incomplete inflation of the lungs and pneumonia in conditions characterized by ineffective cough give weight to its importance.[19] Cough is executed as a complex reflex, an autonomic response to a stimulus, completed by the afferent and efferent pathways and a putative cough center in the brain but at least in part under voluntary control intensified or restrained at will (Figures 31-2 and 31-3). The main afferent pathways of cough originate in nerve receptors immediately beneath the respiratory epithelium in the larynx and the tracheobronchial tree and at extrapulmonary sites: the nose, paranasal sinuses, pharynx, ear canals and eardrums, pleura, stomach, pericardium, and diaphragm. Nerve impulses from the tracheobronchial tree are carried by the vagus nerve, the principal afferent pathway,[18,20,21] and cough may result from direct stimulation of the vagus nerve.[22] The trigeminal, glossopharyngeal, and phrenic nerves conduct impulses from extrapulmonary sites.[21] Axon reflexes traveling through branches of sensory end organs may cause the release of neuropeptides and subsequent smooth muscle contraction, mucus secretion, and epithelial injury. Thus sensory signals taking part in cough may trigger or enhance bronchospasm. Reflexes regulate the parasympathetic nervous system, and chronic cough lowers the threshold for sensory signals. Efferent impulses of the cough reflex are transmitted to the respiratory musculature through the phrenic and other spinal motor nerves and to the larynx through the recurrent laryngeal branches of the vagus nerve.[21] The vagus nerve also provides efferent innervation to the tracheobronchial tree where its branches mediate bronchoconstriction.

COUGH AND BRONCHOSPASM

Cough and bronchospasm are two closely related reflexes that enhance one another, but neither depends on the other for its action.[23] Cough clears the airways effectively only at high lung volumes; sufficient air velocity to shear mucus from bronchial walls can be achieved only down to the sixth or seventh generation of airway branching.[17] Coexisting bronchoconstriction adds to the effectiveness of cough by extending peripherally the region of rapid and turbulent airflow. Challenge with either methacholine or histamine provokes both cough and bronchoconstriction.[24] However, the receptors for both reflexes are functionally distinct, and either response can arise independently. Challenge with hyperosmolar solutions causes both cough and bronchoconstriction, but hypo-osmolar solutions tend to bring about cough alone.[25] Pretreatment sets apart induced cough and bronchoconstriction.[26,27] When aerosolized water serves as a provoking agent, inhaled lidocaine blocks cough but not bronchoconstriction, whereas the opposite is true for cromolyn.[26] When inhaled capsaicin is used, opiates administered systemically suppress cough, whereas the same agents administered by inhalation suppress bronchoconstriction.[27] Bronchoconstriction, but not the urge to cough, can be blocked by pretreatment with intravenous atropine,[28] consistent with the role of cholinergic pathways in the efferent limb of reflex bronchoconstriction. The mechanisms that trigger cough and bronchospasm after exercise or exposure to cold air appear to be different. Cough results mainly from excessive water loss, whereas bronchoconstriction follows airway rewarming.[29] Cold air–induced bronchoconstriction can be blocked by β-adrenergic agents, but cough cannot.[30] Cough most often results from excitation of receptors concentrated in the larynx and proximal airways, whereas bronchoconstriction can be triggered from the lower airways as well.[31] And finally, inflammatory changes in the airways may result in cough without simultaneously giving rise to bronchospasm.[32]

COUGH-VARIANT ASTHMA AND EOSINOPHILIC BRONCHITIS

Childhood asthma is a syndrome of inflammation in medium and small airways that gives rise to hyperresponsiveness and constriction of the bronchial smooth muscle, edema and disruption of the mucosa, and obstruction of the airway lumen.[33,34] Inflammation may lead to airway remodeling with proliferation of smooth muscle and deposition of matrix proteins. Cough-variant asthma is associated with the same disordered physiologic processes and clinical signs, but overt wheezing is absent, and cough is the most evident clinical manifestation. However, substantial evidence shows that the awareness of symptoms by children with asthma is poor,[35] and pulmonary function abnormalities have been documented in asymptomatic individuals.[18] Perceptual accuracy varies markedly with correlations between subjective and objective indices ranging from 0.86 to 0.16.[36] The most frequent presenting signs of asthma in children are cough (92%), wheeze (90%), shortness of breath (83%), and recurrent "pneumonia" (35%).[37] Cough stands out as the most common presenting symptom of asthma,[37] the most obvious and perhaps the least subjective. For this reason some patients or their parents may recognize and report cough more readily than other symptoms of airway obstruction. It is important to note that the three studies that in the 1970s established the clinical entity now known as cough-variant asthma all reported observations made in patients who in addition to cough also had documented episodes of bronchospasm and whose symptoms were controlled by treatment with prednisone or inhaled beta agonists.[38-40] In most cases the patients' cough was triggered by exercise, and either exercise or cough precipitated exacerbations of asthma.[38-40]

In 1979 Corrao et al[41] described a group of adult patients who had chronic cough but no dyspnea or wheezing. Their baseline spirometry was normal; however they demonstrated airway hyperresponsiveness after methacholine challenge. All patients improved after therapy with theophylline or terbutaline and relapsed when the therapy was withdrawn. Two patients later developed overt wheezing. Experience among pediatric patients has been similar.[18] Cloutier and Loughlin[42] evaluated 15 children with chronic cough. Ten had normal pulmonary function studies, and minor abnormalities were found in 5, but exercise challenge revealed evidence of exercise-induced bronchospasm (EIB) in all 15. All improved with theophylline therapy. When theophylline was discontinued, cough recurred in 11 patients. Nine were studied again and were found to have recurrence of EIB. Reinstitution of theophylline eliminated the symptoms yet again. More recently, Koh et al[43] performed annual methacholine challenges for 4 years in 36 children between 7 and 15 years old with cough-variant asthma. Sixteen of 29 patients available for follow-up had developed clinical wheezing and a decrease in methacholine PD_{20}. McKenzie et al[44] measured airway resistance by the interrupter technique (Rint) before and after albuterol treatment in 82 children with recurrent wheeze, 58 with isolated cough, and 48 control subjects. Median baseline Rint was higher in children who wheezed than in either those who coughed or control subjects. Median ratios of baseline to postalbuterol measurements in the groups differed significantly, with the cough patients occupying an intermediate position. The investigators concluded that those patients with cough who had high bronchodilator responses may have had cough-variant asthma.[44] As a result of such clinical observations, cough has come to be regarded as the first or the only clinical manifestation of asthma in some patients.

Still, a debate persists on whether cough-variant asthma is a real clinical entity, one that constitutes an indication for therapy with controller medications. Much disagreement arises from the indiscriminate diagnosis of asthma on the basis of cough alone, which accounts not only for exaggerated occurrence rates of this disease but also for an unsustainable identification of cough-variant asthma.[45] In 1991, 10% of children with cough as the only symptom were diagnosed as having asthma; 2 years later, the figure jumped to 22.6%.[45] Whereas in the past cough may have been underrecognized as a sign of asthma, at present the opposite appears to be true.[19,46]

This is borne out by the report that inhaled albuterol and beclomethasone in children with cough but without wheezing were no more effective than placebo in reducing cough frequency.[47] A study of nocturnal cough showed that in the absence of wheeze, shortness of breath, or tightness of the chest, cough did not connote hidden or atypical asthma in most children.[48] A prospective study of infants followed up to the age of 11 years showed that recurrent cough present early in life resolved in the majority of children. Children with recurrent cough but without wheeze did not have airway hyperresponsiveness or atopy and significantly differed from those with classic asthma with or without cough.[49] Brooke et al[50] reassessed a cohort of children during the early school years identified as having recurrent cough in the preschool period. Seventy of 125 (56.0% [95% confidence interval (CI), 47.3% to 64.5%]) were symptom free at follow-up, 46 (36.8% [95% CI, 28.7% to 45.5%]) continued to have recurrent cough in the absence of colds, and only 9 (7.2% [95% CI, 3.6% to 12.8%]) reported recent wheezing. The authors concluded that there are children with long-term recurrent cough consistent with the diagnosis of cough-variant asthma but that few progress to develop asthma characterized by wheeze.

Isolated cough is rarely caused by asthma and often fails to respond to asthma medications.[19,45,46] On the other hand, patients with a prolonged history of cough who respond to treatment with asthma medications or show evidence of bronchospasm or hyperresponsiveness without concurrent wheezing should be considered to have cough-variant asthma. Patients may be free of bronchoconstriction at the time of their evaluation. Their history of respiratory disease may be difficult to assess, and physical findings and routine pulmonary function tests may disclose no evidence of airway obstruction. In such cases, evaluation of airway function by bronchial provocation with methacholine, histamine, or exercise is recommended. In children too young to perform pulmonary function testing, the diagnosis of cough-variant asthma may be confirmed by the patient's development of unequivocal evidence of reversible airway obstruction later in the clinical course and by his or her response to asthma therapy.

Gibson et al[51] reported on patients who may have no clinical evidence of asthma or increased airway responsiveness but whose sputum contains eosinophils and metachromatic cells in proportions similar to those of patients with asthma. They proposed the term *eosinophilic bronchitis* (EB) for this condition and reported that although wheeze is a good discriminator of EB, persistent cough and recurrent chest colds without wheeze occur in a significant minority of cases. The causes, mechanisms, and treatment of EB appear to be similar to those of asthma. The prognosis of EB is not known, but authors suggest that it may be a precursor of asthma and that its recognition may permit effective treatment and reduction in the rising prevalence of this latter disease. They recommend that analysis of induced sputum for eosinophils to aid in the diagnosis of EB should become part of clinical evaluation of airway diseases.[51] A recent comparison of biopsy specimens from patients with asthma and others with EB revealed a striking increase in the numbers of mast cells in smooth muscle bundles from the patients with asthma that correlated with airway hyperresponsiveness.[52] Tissue from patients with EB contained increased numbers of eosinophils, but EB was not associated with airway hyperresponsiveness.

COUGH DURING AND AFTER RESPIRATORY INFECTION

Children have an average of six to eight respiratory infections per year, and the number may be higher in those with siblings or in day care. Repeated infections common in winter months may result in a chronic cough.[53] Cough associated with infection with respiratory syncytial virus (RSV), other respiratory viruses, and cytomegalovirus; *Mycoplasma pneumoniae, Chlamydia trachomatis, Ureoplasma urealyticum,* and *Pneumocystis carinii; Corynebacterium diphtheriae;* and *Bordetella pertussis* often lasts beyond the acute stage. Measles causes cough with coryza, conjunctivitis, and fever. In the immunized patient, atypical measles is more likely to cause cough or pneumonia than the characteristic rash.[53]

The pathogenesis of persistent postinfectious cough is not known. Patients do not have airway eosinophilia typical of untreated asthma, but some manifest increased reactivity of the airways. These observations suggest that postinfectious cough has different pathophysiologic features than asthma.[54] The infection in most cases remains unidentified. The diagnosis is clinical and one of exclusion. It should be considered in patients with normal chest radiographs who cough only after respiratory tract infections. Postinfectious cough generally regresses over time, but it often recurs. Its resolution may be accelerated by the administration of corticosteroids or ipratropium bromide.[53]

Acute Viral Bronchiolitis

Bronchiolitis occurs in epidemics during the winter months in temperate regions and during the hottest months and the rainy season in tropical climates. Cough set off by microorganisms contributes to their spread and survival. RSV is the leading cause of epidemic bronchiolitis, accounting for more than 40% of cases. Influenza, parainfluenza type 3, and adenovirus are responsible for most of the remaining cases.[55] The risk of RSV illness in the first year is greater than 60%, and it infects nearly all children by the age of 2 years.[56] RSV lower respiratory tract infections lead to 125,000 hospital admissions per year in the United States. Eighty percent occur in infants, with a peak incidence at 2 to 8 months.[55] RSV accounts for 25% of all acute hospitalizations in children younger than 5 with chronic lung disease.[57] Between 0.5% and 3.2% of children with RSV infection require hospitalization, and there are approximately 4500 deaths per year.

The typical clinical picture is that of an infant who presents with 1 to 3 days of rhinorrhea, an irritating cough, respiratory distress, and difficulty nursing. On physical examination there is hyperinflation of the lungs, and fine crackles are heard throughout both lung fields, often with a high-pitched wheeze. Hyperinflation, bilateral perihilar and patchy parenchymal infiltrates, peribronchial cuffing, and atelectasis are seen on chest radiography. The diagnosis of RSV infection can be established promptly with commercially available enzyme immunoassay kits or immunofluorescent staining and detection of RSV antigen.

It has been proposed that RSV may affect substance P, a neuropeptide known to mediate neurogenic inflammation in asthma.[58] There is a general consensus that after even mild RSV bronchiolitis, children are at increased risk of repeated bouts of respiratory symptoms during the first 3 years of life; there is evidence of increased bronchial reactivity; and there has been speculation about a role of early RSV infection in the subsequent development of asthma.[59] Ehlenfield et al[60] reported that only those infants with RSV bronchiolitis who had associated eosinophilia had a higher risk of asthma later in childhood. Pifferi et al[61] evaluated 48 previously healthy children who had acute bronchiolitis with documented RSV infection before 18 months of age to determine whether serum eosinophil cationic protein (s-ECP) concentrations predict later development of persistent respiratory symptoms. Initial values of s-ECP in children with bronchiolitis were higher (16.1 ± 18.7 g/L) than in a control group of healthy infants (3.9 ± 1.5 g/L) and showed a correlation with peripheral eosinophil counts but not with total IgE levels. At 5-year follow up, the s-ECP values were 19.2 ± 11.8 versus 8.4 ± 4.2 g/L for the study and control groups, respectively. High s-ECP values during the acute attack significantly correlated with later persistent respiratory symptoms but not with allergic sensitization. Of the children in the study, 52% had asthma symptoms during the follow-up period.[61] Stein et al,[62] who followed the patients for the longest time, reported a relationship to recurrent respiratory symptoms up to 6 years of age but not to asthma after the age of 13.

Ribavirin does not appear to be effective in the treatment of moderately severe acute bronchiolitis.[63] Some infants, who cannot be identified before treatment, show significant response to bronchodilator therapy.[64] There is little evidence to support the use of inhaled corticosteroids in conventional doses in the treatment of bronchiolitis or for the prevention of subsequent long-term respiratory symptoms.[55] However, the use of systemic corticosteroids shortens the duration of illness, and outpatients with moderate to severe acute bronchiolitis have been shown to derive significant benefit from oral dexamethasone treatment at the relatively high dose of 1 mg/kg in the initial 4 hours of therapy.[65]

Two products have been approved for prevention of RSV disease in children younger than 24 months—RSV immune globulin and palivizumab (Synagis; MedImmune, Gaithersburg, MD)—the latter a monoclonal antibody, but neither has been approved for the treatment of established infection. RSV immune globulin is given intravenously once a month just before and monthly throughout the RSV season at a dose of 15 ml/kg (or 750 mg/kg). Palivizumab is administered intramuscularly once a month during the season at a dose of 15 mg/kg.[66] Several candidate vaccines against RSV are under investigation. Most inauspiciously, vaccination with formalin-treated RSV has been linked to a severe pulmonary eosinophilic response.[67] To be effective, a vaccine against RSV must be safely administered shortly after birth and must provide better immunity than natural disease.[68] Another approach may be to immunize the mother during pregnancy to achieve transfer of the protective antibody during gestation.

For most patients, treatment for RSV bronchiolitis, other than supportive therapy such as hydration, supplemental oxygen, and, when required, mechanical ventilation, remains limited and controversial.[66,68] However, it appears prudent to administer both inhaled bronchodilators and oral dexamethasone to infants with severe bronchiolitis and to patients with bronchiolitis superimposed over cardiopulmonary disorders, malignancy, immunodeficiency, or underlying pulmonary diseases in whom infection with RSV may be life threatening.

Mycoplasma pneumoniae

Most infections with *M. pneumoniae* in infants and young children are asymptomatic or are associated only with upper respiratory symptoms.[69] However, it is the most frequent cause of pneumonia in children between 5 and 15 years of age[70] and a cause of bronchiolitis in all age groups. Pneumonia caused by this agent presents with a gradual onset of malaise, fever, and headache. Cough begins several days after the onset of illness and often persists for weeks. It may be productive of white or blood-tinged sputum. Physical findings include crackles, rhonchi, and bronchial breath sounds. The incidence of wheezing with the acute infection has been reported to be 40%. Radiographic findings, although not diagnostic, frequently show unilateral lower lobe involvement. Initially the pattern is reticular and interstitial; later, patchy segmental consolidation is seen. Hilar adenopathy and pleural effusions may be present. In 10% of the children, an exanthem develops, and 36% have elevated hepatic transaminases. The diagnosis can be made by measuring specific IgM antibody. A rise in IgG antibody takes between 1 and 2 weeks. Cold agglutinins are positive in 40% to 60% of patients, but the results are not specific. There is little evidence that treatment with antibiotics is helpful during the acute illness; however, macrolide antibiotics may shorten the duration of fever and respiratory symptoms.[15]

Clinical evidence suggests a role for mycoplasma in airway hyperresponsiveness. In subjects with no prior history of asthma, a significant response to bronchodilators has been observed 1 month after infection. Moreover, abnormal forced expiratory volume in 1 second and forced expiratory flow after 50% of the expired vital capacity have been noted as long as 3 years after initial infection.[15,71]

Bordetella pertussis

Whooping cough caused serious morbidity and mortality among infants and children before the introduction of whole cell pertussis vaccine.[72] It continues to be the main cause of postinfectious bronchiectasis in underdeveloped countries. The widespread use of the vaccine in combination with diphtheria and tetanus toxoids starting in the United States in the late 1940s led to a historic low point of 1010 cases of pertussis in 1976. However, since the early 1980s, cases of pertussis have increased with cyclical peaks every 3 to 4 years. In 1996, the U.S. Centers for Disease Control and Prevention reported 7796 cases, almost half among individuals aged 10 years or older. In the same year acellular pertussis vaccines were licensed and recommended for the routine immunization of infants.[72] The effectiveness of the complete vaccination series is 80% (95% CI, 66% to 88%). Having received fewer than three doses constitutes a significant risk factor (relative risk, 5.1; 95% CI, 3 to 8.6).[73] As many as 90% of nonimmune household contacts acquire the disease. Infection in immunized children and older persons is often mild.[74] The burden of disease, assessed by rates of complications and death, remains greatest in the youngest patients, but there has been a recent resurgence of pertussis in adolescents and adults. These groups represent a major source of disease transmission to younger children. Increased exposure to pertussis in the community, delay in identification and treatment, and high contact rates among children attending school or day care contribute to the spread of the disease.

In the nonimmunized child infection with *B. pertussis* leads to a catarrhal phase with rhinitis, conjunctivitis, low-grade fever, and cough. *B. pertussis* infection causes infiltration of airway mucosa by lymphocytes and polymorphonuclear leukocytes, necrosis of the midzonal layers of the mucosa, and injury to the ciliated epithelium of the respiratory tract.[72] A stage of tracheobronchitis ensues, with episodes of paroxysmal cough that increase in number and severity. Repetitive, forceful coughs during a single expiration are followed by an abrupt inspiration that produces the characteristic whoop. Many children experience posttussive emesis. Fever is absent or minimal. The duration of classic pertussis is 6 to 10 weeks. Pertussis is more severe in the first year of life. A clinical case is defined as an acute cough illness lasting a minimum of 14 days in a person with at least one pertussis-associated symptom (i.e., paroxysmal cough, posttussive vomiting, or inspiratory whoop) or 14 days of cough during an established outbreak. A confirmed case is a cough illness of any duration in a person from whom *B. pertussis* has been isolated or a case that meets the clinical definition and is confirmed by polymerase chain reaction or by an epidemiologic connection to a laboratory-confirmed case.[72] A whooping cough syndrome also may be caused by *B. pertussis, B, bronchiseptica, M. pneumoniae, C. trachomatis, Chlamydia pneumoniae,* and certain adenoviruses.[74]

There is growing evidence that *B. pertussis* is an important cause of persistent cough in adolescents and adults. Pertussis has been implicated in 16% of cases of chronic cough of adults in Denmark. Susceptibility to infection with *B. pertussis* recurs several years after vaccination. Moreover, cases of laboratory-proven reinfection have been reported.[75] *B. pertussis* should be considered in patients with symptoms of typical or atypical whooping cough, regardless of their vaccination status or past history of the disease.[75] By demonstrating *B. pertussis* in an adult, one can reassure the patient that the symptoms will subside without the need for extensive evaluation and treatment and can recommend measures to protect others, especially unvaccinated infants.[76] Droplet precautions are recommended for 5 days after initiation of effective therapy or until 3 weeks after the onset of paroxysms if appropriate antimicrobial therapy has not been given. Erythromycin or clarithromycin eliminates pertussis from the nasopharynx in 3 to 4 days, decreasing the spread of the disease.[77] Given within 14 days of onset, these antibiotics may abort pertussis. Once paroxysms of cough develop, antibiotics have little effect on the course of illness. An association between erythromycin and idiopathic hypertrophic pyloric stenosis has been reported in infants younger than 6 weeks.[78] There are no such reports for clarithromycin, but its use in infants has been limited.

In addition to maintaining high vaccination rates among preschool children, effort must be directed at identification and treatment of pertussis cases to prevent further spread. Erythromycin (40 to 50 mg/kg/day orally in four divided doses, maximum 2 g/day) for 14 days is recommended for all close contacts regardless of age or immunization status. Exposure of infants to children and adults with cough illnesses should be minimized.[72] A major public health challenge at present is to address the illness in adolescents and adults. A rational strategy might call for a universal booster vaccination of adolescents and a program targeted at those adults most likely to come in contact with infants.[79]

Mycobacterium tuberculosis

Pediatric pulmonary TB remains a major cause of morbidity and mortality worldwide.[80] From 1985 to 1992, the number of cases of childhood TB increased; however, between 1992 and 1998, the figures declined substantially in all age groups.[81] The incidence of TB among children is lower than that among adults. Most of the pediatric morbidity and mortality occurs in children younger than 5 years. In the United States the groups with the highest rates include immigrants from Asia, Africa, and Latin America; the homeless; and residents of correctional facilities.[82] Children from Asia and Africa, where TB is endemic, may have a cough that mimics TB, often with hemoptysis and without fever, as a result of an infestation with a fluke of the genus *Paragonimus* acquired by eating undercooked freshwater crab or crayfish.

Children contract TB from adults and adolescents; disease transmission among youngsters is uncommon. Most infections with *M. tuberculosis* in children are asymptomatic when the tuberculin skin test converts to positive. The radiographs at that time are usually negative, and the primary infection progresses slowly. Early manifestations become evident 1 to 6 months after initial infection; they include fever, weight loss, cough, night sweats, and chills. Chest radiographs may show lymphadenopathy of the hilar and mediastinal nodes, involvement of a lung segment or lobe with atelectasis or infiltrate, cavitary lesions, and military disease. Tuberculous meningitis may be an early finding. Later extrapulmonary manifestations may involve the middle ear, the mastoid, bones, joints, skin, and kidneys.[82] The recommended treatment regimen for TB disease consists of an initial 2-month phase of four drugs—isoniazid, rifampin, pyrazinamide, and ethambutol—followed by a 4-month continuation phase of isoniazid and rifampin. Ethambutol is generally not used for young children whose visual acuity cannot be monitored. Streptomycin may be substituted for ethambutol but must be given by injection. Ethambutol (or streptomycin) can be discontinued when drug susceptibility results show the infecting organism to be fully drug susceptible.[81]

ALLERGIC RHINITIS, CHRONIC SINUSITIS, AND POSTNASAL DRIP

Allergic rhinitis and sinusitis, both described elsewhere in the text, are associated with cough that results from postnasal drip and irritation of the larynx.[83] Sinusitis may be an early manifestation of immunodeficiency or ciliary dysfunction. Irwin and Madison[11] identified postnasal drip as the most common cause of chronic cough among their patients. The diagnosis can be established by history. Mucoperiosteal changes on radiographs or sinus computed tomography (CT) scans of an atopic child in the absence of opacification or air-fluid levels and acute symptoms do not constitute an indication for treatment with antibiotics or sinus surgery. A most effective treatment is once- or twice-daily nasal irrigation with normal saline buffered by bicarbonate followed by the instillation of a nasal corticosteroid spray.

COMPRESSION SYNDROMES

Tracheomalacia or Bronchomalacia

Tracheomalacia or bronchomalacia is characterized by flaccidity or congenital absence of the cartilaginous rings supporting the trachea and/or the bronchi. Although most infants are asymptomatic, some present with cough, paroxysmal dyspnea, wheezing, and stridor. Recurrent "pneumonia" on chest radiographs results from the collapse of segments of the airway during expiration. The caliber of the airways on chest radiographs varies from normal to markedly reduced depending on the phase of respiration. Consolidation most often reflects atelectasis, but secondary infection of the collapsed lung may occur. A prolonged expiratory phase and retractions are common. The diagnosis is established by observation of the collapse of tracheal or bronchial walls on fluoroscopy or bronchoscopy. Intrinsic airway stenosis or extrinsic compression exaggerates the manifestation of tracheomalacia or bronchomalacia (Figure 31-4). If associated bronchospasm is present, it must be treated aggressively. Although the symptoms usually subside by 12 to 18 months of age, some infants require a trial of continuous positive airway pressure or mechanical ventilation.[15,84]

Vascular Rings

The trachea can become partially obstructed by a vascular abnormality involving a right aortic arch with left ligamentum arteriosum or persistent ductus arteriosus, double aortic arch, anomalous innominate artery, or left carotid artery (see Figure 31-4). These abnormalities are generally referred to as *vascular rings*. Typical symptoms include inspiratory stridor, expiratory wheezing, and a barking cough. Respiratory distress may be present especially during feeding or when infection intervenes. Feeding difficulties may be present in the first few weeks of life. There may be recurrent pneumonia and atelectasis.

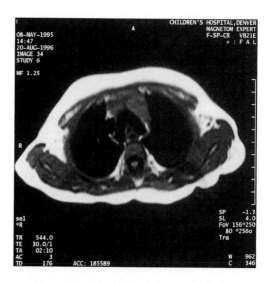

FIGURE 31-4 A 15-month-old infant had a history of cough, hoarseness, and wheezing. Magnetic resonance imaging performed after an abnormal esophagram shows both limbs of the double aortic arch compressing the trachea. Diminished caliber of the trachea points to tracheomalacia. (From Milgrom H, Wood R, Ingram D: *Immunol Allergy Clin North Am* 18:113-132, 1998.)

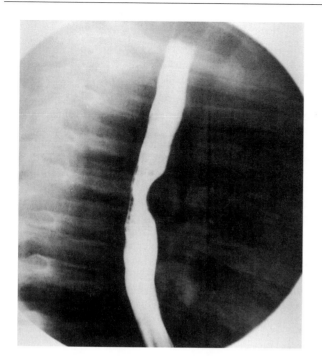

FIGURE 31-5 A 6-month-old infant has persistent croupy cough and wheezing. The esophagram shows an anterior indentation of the esophagus and a posterior indentation of the trachea typical of pulmonary sling in which the left pulmonary artery arises from the right pulmonary artery. (From Milgrom H, Wood R, Ingram D: *Immunol Allergy Clin North Am* 18:113-132, 1998.)

The presence of vascular rings must be considered in any infant with stridor. The chest radiograph may show a right or an indeterminate aortic arch. Tracheal compression by an anomalous innominate artery causes a curvilinear indentation of the anterior trachea. Although barium esophagrams may show characteristic indentations from various anomalies of the aortic arch (Figure 31-5), magnetic resonance imaging (MRI) with its multiplanar images has become the procedure of choice at many institutions. Laryngotracheobronchoscopy is useful in excluding upper airway obstruction. Tracheal compression viewed endoscopically may be recognizable as a pulsatile, extrinsic mass. Vascular rings may be life threatening, but with prompt recognition and surgical treatment, they are usually completely correctable.[15,85]

Mediastinal Masses

Mediastinal masses may be manifested at birth. Children younger than 2 years are likely to present with respiratory symptoms, including dyspnea, cough, stridor, and chest pain. Additional signs and symptoms may include cyanosis, atelectasis, superior vena cava syndrome, Horner's syndrome, dysphagia, spinal cord compression, intercostal nerve neuralgia, and cervical lymphadenopathy. These masses may be categorized as congenital or neoplastic. Most neoplastic tumors are malignant, and prompt diagnosis and treatment are required. In a large number of older children, the masses are asymptomatic and are recognized coincidentally on chest radiographs. The asymptomatic masses are often benign. Chest radiographs provide information about the presence, location, and size of calcifications (Figure 31-6). A barium swallow may be helpful in defining the anatomy. CT and MRI provide the

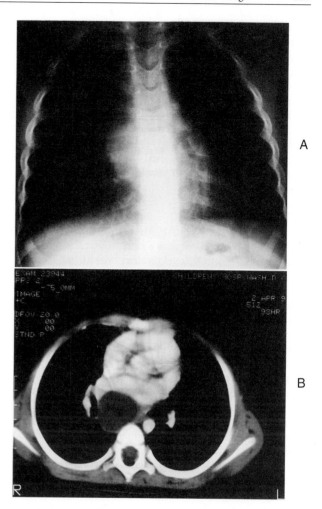

FIGURE 31-6 A, Chest radiograph of a 2-year-old child shows a subcarinal mass uplifting and compressing the right main stem bronchus. **B,** Contrast-enhanced computed tomography scan shows a round fluid-filled mass in the subcarinal region. A bronchogenic cyst was removed at surgery. (From Milgrom H, Wood R, Ingram D: *Immunol Allergy Clin North Am* 18:113-132, 1998.)

most useful information for further diagnosis and treatment; other valuable tests include percutaneous biopsy, bone marrow aspiration, urinary catecholamines, and a skeletal survey. Monoclonal antibodies have been used for the diagnosis, assessment of response to therapy, and monitoring for relapse.[85]

Bronchial Stenosis

Bronchial stenosis is a fixed narrowing of the bronchus that is not usually associated with other congenital malformations, although coexisting segmental bronchomalacia, most commonly of the left main bronchus, has been reported. In the past, TB was a common cause of bronchial stenosis. It can occur at any level along the bronchial tree, although it most commonly involves a main bronchus, just distal to the carina. The degree of stenosis varies. Wheezing, both inspiratory and expiratory, is a typical presenting symptom. It may be associated with cough, dyspnea, and stridor. Chest radiographs reveal recurrent atelectasis that may become secondarily infected. Hyperinflation is usually noted on the radiographs of patients with stenosis of the main bronchus. In patients with segmental bronchomalacia, the involved lung is usually hyperlucent. If the orifices of the upper lobes or right middle lobe are involved, there may be an associated collapse. Recurrent consolidation or persistent collapse is a common radiologic finding of stenosis of a lobar bronchus. Diagnosis is accomplished by endoscopy. Treatment varies with the severity of obstruction. In some cases, the administration of bronchodilators and chest physical therapy are sufficient; more severe cases may require positive-pressure ventilation or surgery to remove the stenotic segment. Lobar resection may be necessary to control persistent infection.[15,86]

Tracheal Stenosis

Signs and symptoms of congenital tracheal stenosis include persistent cough and respiratory distress in the newborn period. Patients may have expiratory stridor and wheezing. History of feeding difficulties is common. Chest radiographs and fluoroscopy may disclose a missing segment of the trachea. Highly penetrated films of the neck may show tracheal narrowing. In congenital tracheal stenosis, there is intrinsic narrowing of the tracheal lumen caused by complete cartilaginous rings. The size of the lumen can be assessed by CT or MRI; the definitive diagnosis is made by endoscopy. The differential diagnosis includes extrinsic compression of the trachea by vascular rings or mediastinal masses. Tracheotomy may be necessary to maintain a patent airway. Endoscopic procedures may be used to treat thin tracheal webs and unilateral lesions. Conservative management of patients with mild symptoms should be attempted. Dilation of tracheal stenosis may provide a temporary solution until definitive surgical repair can be accomplished. Surgical treatment is associated with significant morbidity and mortality.[15,85]

ASPIRATION SYNDROMES

Aspiration pneumonia is a common disorder frequently mistaken for nonspecific respiratory infection, whereas aspiration bronchitis is mistaken for asthma. In infants, these conditions are most commonly associated with the inhalation of milk as a result of one of three conditions: impairment of sucking or swallowing, GER, or tracheoesophageal fistula.

The initial step in diagnosis is to observe the nursing child for difficulty with sucking or swallowing or for associated cough or choking. Gross structural abnormalities of the mouth, jaw, or palate can be noted. Placing a finger in the baby's mouth can assess the act of sucking. Radiographs of children with aspiration bronchitis typically show perihilar thickening and increased bronchovascular markings, whereas those of children with aspiration pneumonia show patchy areas of uniform opacity that may have a segmental or lobar distribution. In infants, the posterior parts of the upper and lower lobes are most commonly involved, with the right side predominant. Fluoroscopy is used to evaluate the anatomy of the upper airway and esophagus and the swallowing function. Esophageal pH probe monitoring establishes the presence of reflux. Bronchoscopy and the examination of the aspirate for lipid-laden macrophages substantiate the diagnosis of aspiration.

Tracheoesophageal fistulas require prompt surgical repair. The management of a child with a swallowing disorder requires the assistance of those at a clinic who specialize in this problem.

GASTROESOPHAGEAL REFLUX

GER (discussed in Chapters 38 and 41) is one of most common causes of chronic cough in individuals of all ages and of apnea in infants even without coexisting aspiration. Its most likely mode of action is through vagal stimulation, although aspiration must be considered. GER has been documented in about half of the adults with chronic cough, and it commonly occurs in children.[87] The respiratory manifestations of GER—cough, wheezing, sore throat, hoarseness, throat clearing, choking, and throat irritation—often persist in the absence of more familiar symptoms such as heartburn and regurgitation. Proton pump inhibitors or H_2 blockers effectively reduce the respiratory complications of GER. However, higher-than-standard doses may be necessary, and therapy may need to be continued for several months before a therapeutic effect is achieved. Laparoscopic fundoplication has been performed safely even in high-risk children.[88]

FOREIGN BODY

A foreign body may lodge in the hypopharynx, larynx, trachea, bronchus, or esophagus. Aspiration of a foreign body into the airway typically causes stridor. It is a pediatric emergency requiring immediate management by a specialist, even though unsuspected bronchial foreign bodies may be present for a long time and lead to chronic bronchitis and bronchiectasis. Unrecognized esophageal foreign bodies resulting in tracheal compression have caused recurrent wheezing or cough without dysphagia for as long as 1 year. Cough, wheezing, or dyspnea may date from the time of aspiration or may begin later, after edema and inflammation have set in and reflex bronchospasm has resulted. The majority of aspirated foreign bodies are foods such as peanuts or sunflower seeds, but a remarkable variety of objects have been removed at bronchoscopy. It is of note that peanuts release oils that are irritating to the bronchial mucosa, causing inflammation and edema. Other organic solids such as beans, peas, corn, and seeds can absorb water and increase considerably in size.

In one third of children with foreign body aspiration, the actual event goes unobserved by caretakers.[89] The diagnosis may be suspected on the basis of history and physical findings. Classic signs are wheezing, coughing, and decreased breath sounds. Use of a differential stethoscope may be helpful in detecting localized airway obstruction. The diagnosis is established by radiographic findings and ultimately by bronchoscopy. Chest radiographs show atelectasis in cases of complete obstruction of a bronchus. In cases of partial obstruction, the foreign body may act as a valve that allows air entry but impedes exhalation from a portion of the lung. Observation of inspiratory and expiratory films shows a hyperinflated obstructed portion in comparison with the unaffected lung after expiration. On decubitus films and fluoroscopy, the dependent lung should show less inflation unless obstructive hyperinflation from the valve-like mechanism is present. Bronchoscopy provides decisive evidence for diagnosis and treatment. Rigid bronchoscopy is preferred because it can be used to remove the foreign body at the time of diagnosis. Alternative treatment with bronchodilators, postural drainage, and chest physical therapy is no longer recommended.

CYSTIC FIBROSIS

Cystic fibrosis is diagnosed with increasing frequency during neonatal screening. The presenting symptoms of this disease are cough, poor weight gain, and abnormal stools. The earliest symptom is usually a loose cough. Most patients experience recurrent lower respiratory infection before 12 months, but the age of onset is variable. Purulent bronchitis may be associated with wheezing and cough, and the diagnosis of asthma is often made in error.

ALLERGIC BRONCHOPULMONARY ASPERGILLOSIS

Allergic bronchopulmonary aspergillosis (ABPA) is described in Chapter 41. Timely diagnosis is important because untreated ABPA results in progressive, irreversible lung damage. ABPA is a disease differentiated by recurrent infiltrates on chest radiography, bronchiectasis on the chest CT, markedly elevated serum IgE concentrations, eosinophilia, and underlying asthma. Clinically, it is characterized by afebrile episodes of cough, sputum production, dyspnea, and wheezing.

HYPERSENSITIVITY LUNG DISEASE

Hypersensitivity pneumonitis, or extrinsic allergic alveolitis, is a syndrome that results from sensitization to inhaled organic dusts; in children, these are most often avian antigens. Bird fancier's disease has been reported to occur in families. During acute attacks, patients have both respiratory and systemic symptoms, including cough, dyspnea, temperature as high as 40° C, chills, and myalgia.

VOCAL CORD DYSFUNCTION

Vocal cord dysfunction (VCD) (discussed in Chapters 38 and 41) is a condition characterized by a paradoxical adduction of the vocal cords on inspiration that causes shortness of breath, cough, and stridor.[90] VCD in children commonly occurs during exertion and must be differentiated from EIB. VCD has been documented in adolescents, usually female athletes.[91] Among these patients, perfectionism, depression, and anxiety are common.

The chest radiographs in uncomplicated VCD are normal. Spirometry shows blunting or truncation of the inspiratory portion of the flow-volume curve. However, the flow rate patterns vary, and during asymptomatic periods, normal flow-volume curves are likely to be found. It is possible to replicate symptoms and spirometric findings of VCD by exercise or inhalation challenge, but negative results do not rule out the diagnosis. Observation of the vocal cords of a patient experiencing either spontaneous or induced symptoms by flexible fiberoptic rhinolaryngoscopy documents the presence of VCD.[90] The examination can be videotaped or photographed for the medical record. Complications are rare and discomfort is minimal. In VCD, the vocal cords adduct anteriorly from the vocal process, and the posterior glottic chink remains open. The adduction occurs during inspiration or in both the inspiratory and expiratory phases. The adduction of vocal cords with an open glottic chink in a symptomatic patient unequivocally establishes the diagnosis of VCD.

In the author's experience, the most successful treatment of VCD is derived from breathing exercises used for hyperfunctional voice disorders to decrease the laryngeal muscle tone.[92] In some extreme cases, hypnosis, biofeedback, and psychotherapy have been used successfully. An approach reserved for acute attacks is the administration of a mixture of helium and oxygen. More aggressive therapies under study for patients with intractable, recurrent symptoms include the injection of botulinum toxin directly into one vocal cord or sectioning of the laryngeal nerve. In our experience, the injection of botulinum toxin has not been effective.[90]

PSYCHOGENIC COUGH

In some cases, complete evaluation of chronic cough may require an assessment of the psychosocial factors that influence its origin, progression, persistence, or exacerbation. Some children derive secondary gain from chronic cough in the form of greater attention or emotional support from their parents. Cough is typically very disruptive and may negatively affect a broad spectrum of social and interpersonal experiences. This may range from distress at school to exclusion from play, social functions, or participation in sports. A psychologic evaluation may focus on such specific detrimental effects of the cough. As in other chronic medical conditions, emotional responses to the symptom may need to be addressed. Depression and frustration are the most common adjustment reactions, but negative responses may range over the entire affective spectrum.

Occasionally, it is difficult to reconcile the parents' or child's accounts with clinical findings. Although wholly psychogenic cough is rare, children and/or parents may exaggerate some or all aspects of the cough. The parents may demand inappropriate treatment and may instill in the child the belief that he or she is physically disabled. When clinical findings differ from the history, confirmation of the cough by the use of a recording device or admission to the hospital for observation may be invaluable. The circumstances call for sympathy and understanding; the physician's responsibility to the child must take precedence over the physician-parent relationship.

EVALUATION (see Figure 31-1)

Information about the history of onset, character of the cough (e.g., harsh, dry, productive, paroxysmal), triggers, time of occurrence, and accompanying symptoms or sensations offers clues about its etiology. A detailed health history must be obtained with attention to the neonatal period; feeding problems; congenital malformations affecting the heart, great vessels, nasopharynx, upper respiratory tract, and gastrointestinal tract; respiratory infections; signs and symptoms of chronic illness; respiratory symptoms including those related to the upper airway tract such as postnasal drip or irritation and lower respiratory tract such as wheezing, dyspnea, and reduced exercise tolerance; heartburn; nocturnal symptoms; and environmental exposures, including cigarette smoke at home, at school, at day care, and at the homes of close playmates, exposure to aeroallergens by older children, and dietary experience of infants and toddlers. Social history provides information about family or school problems that may contribute to psychogenic cough. The physical examination focuses on the head and neck and the respiratory and cardiovascular systems. We look for signs of allergic rhinitis, stridor, tachypnea, hyperinflation, wheezing, crackles, rhonchi (with special attention paid to unilateral or asymmetric findings), heart murmurs, gallops, and congestive heart failure. Eosinophils on the nasal smear suggest allergic rhinitis, neutrophils, and infectious sinusitis. Eosinophils in the sputum are an indication of EB. Pulmonary function testing should be used in any child capable of performing the necessary maneuvers. Other useful data include a complete blood count with differential, serum IgE, allergy skin tests, an examination of the vocal cords, chest and sinus radiographs or CT, bronchial challenge, and esophageal pH monitoring. Additional laboratory tests are based on clinical findings related to conditions discussed in the earlier sections. They include sputum culture, immunoglobulins, purified protein derivative, sweat test, and ciliary biopsy. Bronchoscopy is indicated in cases of compression, aspiration, or hemoptysis. For dynamic evaluation of compression syndromes, flexible bronchoscopy provides the best detail, but if a foreign body aspiration is likely, rigid bronchoscopy should be used. Cough with hemoptysis is an indication for a chest radiograph, chest CT scan, and bronchoscopy.

ENVIRONMENT

It is important to obtain an environmental history of children with chronic cough because it may be possible to make improvements in their surroundings. A survey of respiratory symptoms in children aged 12 to 14 years was conducted throughout Great Britain as part of the International Study of Asthma and Allergies in Childhood (ISAAC). The response rate was 79.3%, and 25,393 children in 93 schools participated[3] (see Table 31-1). Interestingly, the presence of pets and the choice of fuel used for cooking did not predispose to cough in these relatively mature children. Cough and phlegm were strongly associated with active and passive smoking. The prevalence of both tended to be higher in the metropolitan areas; the opposite trend applied to asthma. Exposure to any passive smoking raises the odds ratio (OR) for night cough (OR, 1.8), snoring (OR, 1.4), and respiratory infections (OR, 1.3) during the first 2 years of life. Other reports provide evidence of a further increase in cough and related symptoms in children whose mothers or both parents smoke.[14] All respiratory symptoms are more prevalent in homes with reported mold or dampness.[93] Adjusted odds ratios ranged from 1.32 (95% CI, 1.06 to 1.39) for bronchitis to 1.89 (95% CI, 1.58 to 2.26) for cough.[93] There is an association between coal fires and nocturnal cough.[94] There are opposing views regarding the association of respiratory symptoms with indoor exposure to nitrogen dioxide.

TREATMENT

Clinical studies in patients, especially children, with chronic cough have been performed on a rather small scale. In acute cough, a systematic review of six trials involving 438 children found that antitussives, antihistamine-decongestant combinations, other fixed drug combinations, and antihistamines were no more effective than placebo.[95] Antitussive medications, sold for the most part over the counter, are generally inadequate for chronic cough, and neither codeine nor dextromethorphan is superior to placebo in treating night cough in children.[96] Health information on the Internet related to treatment of cough is generally unreliable. Of the 19 website pages identified, 10 received a negative score because they contained more incorrect than correct information; only 1 received a high score.[97] The fear of excessive respiratory secretions caused by antitussive medications is appropriate only in those patients with preexisting chronic lung disease whose cough is associated with copious sputum production (i.e., bronchiectasis and cystic fibrosis).[98] The main limitation to treatment is the lack of effective medications. The best antitussive drugs presently available are potent opioids such as hydrocodone acting at the putative cough center in the central nervous system and inhaled local anesthetics suppressing afferent neural activity. The side effects of opioids reduce their usefulness to a small number of patients with severe symptoms. Lidocaine, a local anesthetic, can be administered by nebulization to older children and teenagers to offer them some relief from severe cough. We generally use 2 ml of 4% solution. It should not be administered for 2 hours before meals.

Antiasthma drugs are not reliably effective in patients with chronic dry cough; however, a 2-week course of a potent inhaled corticosteroid should be administered to children with prolonged cough without wheeze who have not already received such therapy, especially if they have obstructive pulmonary function tests or positive bronchial challenge results. Inhaled corticosteroids should be discontinued in children who have taken high-dose therapy for several weeks and are continuing to cough and whose pulmonary function tests are normal. Failure to improve after 4 weeks of inhaled corticosteroids and/or normal pulmonary function tests call for consideration of alternative diagnoses and for proceeding with the clinical evaluation described earlier. New treatment should be directed at all conditions identified that may be responsible for the patient's cough and should include breathing exercises.[92]

Patient education plays an important role in the management of chronic cough. The patient and family who understand how individual mechanisms may contribute to the cough and where each form of treatment fits carry out their regimen with greater adherence and reduced anxiety. They cope more effectively with the symptoms, especially during periods of exacerbation. On rare occasions, it may be necessary to enlist the help of a psychotherapist to help the patient and the family accept the diagnosis and to comply with therapy.

CONCLUSIONS

Two decades ago, thoughtful pediatricians writing on chronic cough in childhood observed that clear definitions of the etiology, natural history, therapy, and prognosis had not been described for this condition.[99] They questioned whether it was a single disease and recommended a therapeutic approach that would rule out more specific diagnoses and would seek to prevent further airway disease by limiting exogenous causes of airway damage and treating those endogenous factors that could be identified. The same judgment and recommendations hold true today. Although major new pharmacologic approaches

KEY CONCEPTS

Evaluation of Chronic Cough

- Cough is a common manifestation of disease in childhood.
- Cough is an important defense mechanism.
- Cough functions as a complex neurologic reflex.
- Cough may be classified as acute (lasting < 3 weeks), subacute (lasting 3 to 8 weeks), or chronic (lasting ≥ 8 weeks).
- The cause of chronic cough can be determined in most patients; specific therapy based on a systematic evaluation is usually successful.
- A chest radiograph should be obtained in children with chronic cough to rule out lower respiratory tract and cardiac pathology.
- Postnasal drip, acting alone or with other conditions, is the most common cause of chronic cough.
- Asthma is very often associated with chronic cough, but few children with chronic cough develop asthma.
- Cough-variant asthma is suggested by (1) airway obstruction and reversibility, (2) airway hyperresponsiveness, and/or (3) clinical improvement after treatment with asthma medications.
- Eosinophilic bronchitis may be clinically expressed as chronic cough without airway hyperresponsiveness. Histologically, it is characterized by increased numbers of eosinophils in the airways without increased mast cells in the smooth muscle bundles.
- Gastroesophageal reflux may cause or intensify chronic cough through a vagal reflex or as a result of aspiration of stomach contents.
- Postinfectious cough resolves over time; the use of oral or inhaled corticosteroids or ipratropium bromide may shorten its duration.
- Congenital anomalies and aspiration are relatively uncommon causes of chronic cough in children.
- Bronchiectasis is a rare cause of chronic cough in children.
- Psychogenic cough and habit cough are diagnoses of exclusion.

and expert consensus guidelines have emerged for the treatment of asthma and chronic obstructive pulmonary disease, no such unanimity exists regarding the management of chronic cough in childhood. We need to conduct a thorough review of available information, gain knowledge of the condition and the underlying pathologic processes, and perform rigorous clinical trials using precise criteria for the inclusion of subjects and objective, quantifiable study outcomes. As the ability to perform pulmonary function testing in infants and toddlers expands and surrogate markers of disease become identified, serial studies in very young children will become feasible, and it will become possible to assess both immediate and long-term consequences of cough and its treatment. The ultimate goal must be to find effective remedies for this common condition causing so much distress to children (Box 31-1).

REFERENCES

1. Hart M, Kercsmar C: Chronic cough in children: a systematic approach, *J Respir Dis Pediatr* 3:155-163, 2001.
2. Vital and Health Statistics: *National Ambulatory Medical Care Survey: 1995-96 summary. Series 13: data from the National Health Care Survey No. 142*, Hyattsville, Md, 1999, U.S. Department of Health and Human Services, Centers for Disease Control and Prevention, National Center for Health Statistics.
3. Burr ML, Anderson HR, Austin JB, et al: Respiratory symptoms and home environment in children: a national survey, *Thorax* 54:27-32, 1999.
4. Singh D, Arora V, Sobti PC: Chronic/recurrent cough in rural children in Ludhiana, Punjab, *Indian Pediatr* 39:23-29, 2002.
5. Munyard P, Bush A: How much coughing is normal? *Arch Dis Child* 74:531-534, 1996.
6. Chang AB, Phelan PD, Robertson CF, et al: Frequency and perception of cough severity, *J Paediatr Child Health* 37:142-145, 2001.
7. Shann F: How often do children cough? *Lancet* 348:699-700, 1996.
8. Falconer A, Oldman C, Helms P: Poor agreement between reported and recorded nocturnal cough in asthma, *Pediatr Pulmonol* 15:209-211, 1993.
9. Dales RE, White J, Bhumgara C, et al: Parental reporting of children's coughing is biased, *Eur J Epidemiol* 13:541-545, 1997.
10. Powell CV, Primhak RA: Stability of respiratory symptoms in unlabelled wheezy illness and nocturnal cough, *Arch Dis Child* 75:385-391, 1996.
11. Irwin RS, Madison JM: The diagnosis and treatment of cough, *N Engl J Med* 343:1715-1721, 2000.
12. Curley FJ, Irwin RS, Pratter MR, et al: Cough and the common cold, *Am Rev Respir Dis* 138:305-311, 1988.
13. Chang AB, Asher MI: A review of cough in children, *J Asthma* 38:299-309, 2001.
14. Lister SM, Jorm LR: Parental smoking and respiratory illnesses in Australian children aged 0-4 years: ABS 1989-90 National Health Survey results, *Aust N Z J Public Health* 22:781-786, 1998.
15. Milgrom H, Wood RI, Ingram D: Respiratory conditions that mimic asthma, *Immunol Allergy Clin North Am* 18:113-132, 1998.
16. Salter HH: *On asthma: its pathology and treatment*, New York, 1882, William Wood.
17. Leith DE, Butler JP, Sneddon SL, et al: Cough. In Mead J, Macklem PT, eds: *Handbook of physiology: section 3: the respiratory system. volume III. mechanics of breathing, part 1*, Bethesda, Md, 1986, American Physiological Society.
18. Milgrom H: Cough variant asthma. In Weiss E, Stein M, eds: *Bronchial asthma: mechanisms and therapeutics*, Boston, 1993, Little, Brown.
19. Chang AB: Cough, cough receptors, and asthma in children, *Pediatr Pulmonol* 28:59-70, 1999.
20. Widdicombe J: Sensory mechanisms, *Pulm Pharmacol* 9:383-387, 1996.
21. Irwin RS, Rosen MJ, Braman SS: Cough: a comprehensive review, *Arch Intern Med* 137:1186-1191, 1977.
22. Helmers SL, Wheless JW, Frost M, et al: Vagus nerve stimulation therapy in pediatric patients with refractory epilepsy: retrospective study, *J Child Neurol* 16:843-848, 2001.
23. Anonymous: Cough and wheeze in asthma: are they interdependent? *Lancet* 1:447-448, 1988.
24. Chausow AM, Banner AS: Comparison of the tussive effects of histamine and methacholine in humans, *J Appl Physiol* 55:541-546, 1983.
25. Eschenbacher WL, Boushey HA, Sheppard D: Alteration in osmolarity of inhaled aerosols cause bronchoconstriction and cough, but absence of a permeant anion causes cough alone, *Am Rev Respir Dis* 129:211-215, 1984.
26. Sheppard D, Rizk NW, Boushey HA, et al: Mechanism of cough and bronchoconstriction induced by distilled water aerosol, *Am Rev Respir Dis* 127:691-694, 1983.
27. Fuller RW, Karlsson JA, Choudry NB, et al: Effect of inhaled and systemic opiates on responses to inhaled capsaicin in humans, *J Appl Physiol* 65:1125-1130, 1988.
28. Simonsson BG, Jacobs FM, Nadel JA: Role of autonomic nervous system and the cough reflex in the increased responsiveness of airways in patients with obstructive airway disease, *J Clin Invest* 46:1812-1818, 1967.
29. McFadden ER Jr, Nelson JA, Skowronski ME, et al: Thermally induced asthma and airway drying, *Am J Respir Crit Care Med* 160:221-226, 1999.
30. Banner AS, Chausow A, Green J: The tussive effect of hyperpnea with cold air, *Am Rev Respir Dis* 131:362-367, 1985.

31. Karlsson JA, Sant'Ambrogio G, Widdicombe J: Afferent neural pathways in cough and reflex bronchoconstriction, *J Appl Physiol* 65:1007-1023, 1988.

32. Chang AB, Harrhy VA, Simpson J, et al: Cough, airway inflammation, and mild asthma exacerbation, *Arch Dis Child* 86:270-275, 2002.

33. American Academy of Allergy, Asthma and Immunology: *Pediatric asthma: promoting best practice,* 1999, http://www.aaaai.org/members/resources/initiatives/pediatricasthma.stm.

34. Lemanske RF Jr: Inflammation in childhood asthma and other wheezing disorders, *Pediatrics* 109:368-372, 2002.

35. Baker RR, Mishoe SC, Zaitoun FH, et al: Poor perception of airway obstruction in children with asthma, *J Asthma* 37:613-624, 2000.

36. Fritz GK, Klein RB, Overholser JC: Accuracy of symptom perception in childhood asthma, *J Dev Behav Pediatr* 11:69-72, 1990.

37. Parks DP, Ahrens RC, Humphries CT, et al: Chronic cough in childhood: approach to diagnosis and treatment, *J Pediatr* 115:856-862, 1989.

38. Stanescu DC, Teculescu DB: Exercise- and cough-induced asthma, *Respiration* 27:377-383, 1970.

39. Glauser FL: Variant asthma, *Ann Allergy* 30:457-459, 1972.

40. McFadden ER Jr: Exertional dyspnea and cough as preludes to acute attacks of bronchial asthma, *N Engl J Med* 292:555-559, 1975.

41. Corrao WM, Braman SS, Irwin RS: Chronic cough as the sole presenting manifestation of bronchial asthma, *N Engl J Med* 300:633-637, 1979.

42. Cloutier MM, Loughlin GM: Chronic cough in children: a manifestation of airway hyperreactivity, *Pediatrics* 67:6-12, 1981.

43. Koh YY, Jeong JH, Park Y, et al: Development of wheezing in patients with cough variant asthma during an increase in airway responsiveness, *Eur Respir J* 14:302-308, 1999.

44. McKenzie SA, Bridge PD, Healy MJ: Airway resistance and atopy in preschool children with wheeze and cough, *Eur Respir J* 15:833-838, 2000.

45. Kelly YJ, Brabin BJ, Milligan PJ, et al: Clinical significance of cough and wheeze in the diagnosis of asthma, *Arch Dis Child* 75:489-493, 1996.

46. McKenzie S: Cough—but is it asthma? *Arch Dis Child* 70:1-2, 1994.

47. Chang AB, Phelan PD, Carlin JB, et al: A randomised, placebo controlled trial of inhaled salbutamol and beclomethasone for recurrent cough, *Arch Dis Child* 79:6-11, 1998.

48. Ninan TK, Macdonald L, Russell G: Persistent nocturnal cough in childhood: a population based study, *Arch Dis Child* 73:403-407, 1995.

49. Wright AL, Holberg CJ, Morgan WJ, et al: Recurrent cough in childhood and its relation to asthma, *Am J Respir Crit Care Med* 153:1259-1265, 1996.

50. Brooke AM, Lambert PC, Burton PR, et al: Recurrent cough: natural history and significance in infancy and early childhood, *Pediatr Pulmonol* 26:256-261, 1998.

51. Gibson PG, Fujimura M, Niimi A: Eosinophilic bronchitis: clinical manifestations and implications for treatment, *Thorax* 57:178-182, 2002.

52. Brightling CE, Bradding P, Symon FA, et al: Mast-cell infiltration of airway smooth muscle in asthma, *N Engl J Med* 346:1699-1705, 2002.

53. Irwin RS, Boulet LP, Cloutier MM, et al: Managing cough as a defense mechanism and as a symptom. A consensus panel report of the American College of Chest Physicians, *Chest* 114:133S-181S, 1998.

54. Zimmerman B, Silverman FS, Tarlo SM, et al: Induced sputum: comparison of postinfectious cough with allergic asthma in children, *J Allergy Clin Immunol* 105:495-499, 2000.

55. Schlesinger C, Koss MN: Bronchiolitis: update 2001, *Curr Opin Pulm Med* 8:112-116, 2002.

56. Simoes EA, Groothuis JR: Respiratory syncytial virus prophylaxis—the story so far, *Respir Med* 96 (Suppl B):S15-S24, 2002.

57. Griffin MR, Coffey CS, Neuzil KM, et al: Winter viruses: influenza- and respiratory syncytial virus-related morbidity in chronic lung disease, *Arch Intern Med* 162:1229-1236, 2002.

58. Tripp RA, Moore D, Winter J, et al: Respiratory syncytial virus infection and G and/or SH protein expression contribute to substance P, which mediates inflammation and enhanced pulmonary disease in BALB/c mice, *J Virol* 74:1614-1622, 2000.

59. McBride JT, McConnochie KM: RSV, recurrent wheezing, and ribavirin, *Pediatr Pulmonol* 25:145-146, 1998.

60. Ehlenfield DR, Cameron K, Welliver RC: Eosinophilia at the time of respiratory syncytial virus bronchiolitis predicts childhood reactive airway disease, *Pediatrics* 105:79-83, 2000.

61. Pifferi M, Ragazzo V, Caramella D, et al: Eosinophil cationic protein in infants with respiratory syncytial virus bronchiolitis: predictive value for subsequent development of persistent wheezing, *Pediatr Pulmonol* 31:419-424, 2001.

62. Stein RT, Sherrill D, Morgan WJ, et al: Respiratory syncytial virus in early life and risk of wheeze and allergy by age 13 years, *Lancet* 354:541-545, 1999.

63. Everard ML, Swarbrick A, Rigby AS, et al: The effect of ribavirin to treat previously healthy infants admitted with acute bronchiolitis on acute and chronic respiratory morbidity, *Respir Med* 95:275-280, 2001.

64. Shay DK, Holman RC, Roosevelt GE, et al: Bronchiolitis-associated mortality and estimates of respiratory syncytial virus-associated deaths among US children, 1979-1997, *J Infect Dis* 183:16-22, 2001.

65. Schuh S, Coates AL, Binnie R, et al: Efficacy of oral dexamethasone in outpatients with acute bronchiolitis, *J Pediatr* 140:27-32, 2002.

66. American Academy of Pediatrics: Respiratory syncytial virus. In Pickering L, ed: *2000 Red Book: report of the Committee on Infectious Diseases,* Elk Grove Village, Ill, 2000, The Academy.

67. Openshaw PJ, Culley FJ, Olszewska W: Immunopathogenesis of vaccine-enhanced RSV disease, *Vaccine* 20:S27-S31, 2001.

68. Hall CB: Respiratory syncytial virus: a continuing culprit and conundrum, *J Pediatr* 135:2-7, 1999.

69. Fernald GW, Collier AM, Clyde WA Jr: Respiratory infections due to *Mycoplasma pneumoniae* in infants and children, *Pediatrics* 55:327-335, 1975.

70. Murphy TF, Henderson FW, Clyde WA Jr, et al: Pneumonia: an eleven-year study in a pediatric practice, *Am J Epidemiol* 113:12-21, 1981.

71. Sabato AR, Martin AJ, Marmion BP, et al: *Mycoplasma pneumoniae:* acute illness, antibiotics, and subsequent pulmonary function, *Arch Dis Child* 59:1034-1037, 1984.

72. Centers for Disease Control and Prevention. Pertussis—United States, 1997-2000, *JAMA* 287:977-979, 2002.

73. Khetsuriani N, Bisgard K, Prevots DR, et al: Pertussis outbreak in an elementary school with high vaccination coverage, *Pediatr Infect Dis J* 20:1108-1112, 2001.

74. American Academy of Pediatrics: Pertussis. In Pickering L, ed: *2000 Red Book: report of the Committee on Infectious Diseases,* Elk Grove Village, Ill, 2000, The Academy.

75. Versteegh FG, Schellekens JF, Nagelkerke AF, et al: Laboratory-confirmed reinfections with *Bordetella pertussis, Acta Paediatr* 91:95-97, 2002.

76. Birkebaek NH: *Bordetella pertussis* in the aetiology of chronic cough in adults: diagnostic methods and clinic, *Dan Med Bull* 48:77-80, 2001.

77. Lebel MH, Mehra S: Efficacy and safety of clarithromycin versus erythromycin for the treatment of pertussis: a prospective, randomized, single blind trial, *Pediatr Infect Dis J* 20:1149-1154, 2001.

78. Centers for Disease Control and Prevention. Hypertrophic pyloric stenosis in infants following pertussis prophylaxis with erythromycin—Knoxville, Tennessee, 1999, *JAMA* 283:471-472, 2000.

79. Campins-Marti M, Cheng HK, Forsyth K, et al: Recommendations are needed for adolescent and adult pertussis immunisation: rationale and strategies for consideration, *Vaccine* 20:641-646, 2001.

80. Eamranond P, Jaramillo E: Tuberculosis in children: reassessing the need for improved diagnosis in global control strategies, *Int J Tuberc Lung Dis* 5:594-603, 2001.

81. Centers for Disease Control and Prevention, National Center for HIV, STD and TB Prevention, Division of Tuberculosis Elimination. *Reported tuberculosis in the United States, 2000,* http://www.cdc.gov/nchstp/tb/surv/surv.htm.

82. American Academy of Pediatrics: Tuberculosis. In Pickering L, ed: *2000 Red Book: report of the Committee on Infectious Diseases,* Elk Grove Village, Ill, 2000, The Academy.

83. Lack G: Pediatric allergic rhinitis and comorbid disorders, *J Allergy Clin Immunol* 108:S9-S15, 2001.

84. Filler RM, de Fraga JC: Tracheomalacia, *Semin Thorac Cardiovasc Surg* 6:211-215, 1994.

85. Andrews T, Myer C, Bailey W: Intrathoracic lesions involving the tracheobronchial tree. In Myer C, Cotton R, Shott S, eds: *The pediatric airway: an interdisciplinary approach,* Philadelphia, 1995, JB Lippincott.

86. Oermann CM, Moore RH: Foolers: things that look like pneumonia in children, *Semin Respir Infect* 11:204-213, 1996.

87. McGeady S: GERD and airways disease in children and adolescents. In Stein M, ed: *Gastroesophageal reflux disease and airway disease,* New York, 1999, Marcel Dekker.

88. Rothenberg SS, Bratton D, Larsen G, et al: Laparoscopic fundoplication to enhance pulmonary function in children with severe reactive airway disease and gastroesophageal reflux disease, *Surg Endosc* 11:1088-1090, 1997.

89. Cohen SR, Herbert WI, Lewis GB Jr, et al: Foreign bodies in the airway. Five-year retrospective study with special reference to management, *Ann Otol Rhinol Laryngol* 89:437-442, 1980.

90. Wood RP II, Milgrom H: Vocal cord dysfunction, *J Allergy Clin Immunol* 98:481-485, 1996.

91. Landwehr LP, Wood RP II, Blager FB, et al: Vocal cord dysfunction mimicking exercise-induced bronchospasm in adolescents, *Pediatrics* 98:971-974, 1996.

92. Blager F, Gay M, Wood RI: Voice therapy techniques adapted to treatment of habit cough: a pilot study, *J Commun Disord* 21:393-400, 1988.

93. Dales RE, Zwanenburg H, Burnett R, et al: Respiratory health effects of home dampness and molds among Canadian children, *Am J Epidemiol* 134:196-203, 1991.

94. Strachan DP, Elton RA: Relationship between respiratory morbidity in children and the home environment, *Fam Pract* 3:137-142, 1986.

95. Schroeder K, Fahey T: Should we advise parents to administer over the counter cough medicines for acute cough? Systematic review of randomised controlled trials, *Arch Dis Child* 86:170-175, 2002.

96. Taylor JA, Novack AH, Almquist JR, et al: Efficacy of cough suppressants in children, *J Pediatr* 122:799-802, 1993.

97. Pandolfini C, Impicciatore P, Bonati M: Parents on the web: risks for quality management of cough in children, *Pediatrics* 105:e1, 2000.

98. Morice AH, Kastelik JA, Thompson R: Cough challenge in the assessment of cough reflex, *Br J Clin Pharmacol* 52:365-375, 2001.

99. Morgan WJ, Taussig LM: The chronic bronchitis complex in children, *Pediatr Clin North Am* 31:851-864, 1984.

ASTHMA

STANLEY J. SZEFLER

CHAPTER **32**

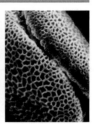

Immunology of the Asthmatic Response

CLAUDIA MACAUBAS ▪ ROSEMARIE H. DeKRUYFF ▪ DALE T. UMETSU

Asthma is an immunologic disease in which adaptive immunity plays a major role. Asthma, as a complex trait, develops after environmental exposures, such as to innocuous allergens, infectious agents, and air pollutants, in genetically susceptible individuals.[1] These events induce an immune response associated with a specific type of inflammation in the lungs that causes asthma and is characterized by the presence of T helper cell type 2 (Th2) lymphocytes, eosinophils, and basophils. This Th2-biased immune response results in increased mucus production, mucosal edema as well as reversible airway obstruction, bronchial hyperresponsiveness (BHR) and remodeling, and the symptoms of asthma. In addition, the inflammatory response in asthma is associated with sensitization to indoor and outdoor allergens[2-4] and with elevated serum IgE levels,[5,6] which have been shown to be major risk factors for the development of asthma and persistent wheezing.

COMPONENTS OF THE ALLERGIC INFLAMMATORY RESPONSE

The Th2-biased inflammatory response that results in asthma is complex and involves a number of cell types producing a large number of cytokines and chemokines (Figure 32-1). Together, these cell types and mediators are responsible for the *immediate-phase response* (IPR), as well as the *late-phase response* (LPR). The IPR occurs within minutes after allergen challenge due to binding of allergen to IgE on the surface of mast cells, resulting in mast cell degranulation and causing increased vascular permeability and extravasation of fluid into the tissues. The LPR occurs 4 to 12 hours later as a result of the accumulation of eosinophils, basophils, and activated T cells that typify the allergic inflammatory response. The LPR and its accompanying inflammation are associated with BHR, a cardinal feature of asthma.

Th2 Lymphocytes

CD4+ T lymphocytes producing Th2 cytokines play a prominent role in asthma and are present in lung biopsy specimens and bronchoalveolar lavage (BAL) fluid from patients with asthma.[7] Several studies showed a correlation between the presence of CD4+ Th2 cells and Th2 cytokine levels with the severity of asthma.[8] Although several cell types produce Th2 cytokines, including mast cells, basophils, and natural killer (NK) T cells, Th2 lymphocytes are considered fundamental in asthma because, in animal models, CD4+ T cell depletion prevents the development of asthma. In fact, B cell–, IgE-, and mast cell–deficient mice can still develop asthma, whereas CD4−, STAT-6−, and interleukin (IL)-13–deficient mice cannot. The signature Th2 cytokine IL-4 plays an important initiator role. IL-4 is essential for the differentiation of Th2 lymphocytes, and in the absence of IL-4, Th2 cell differentiation is severely impaired. IL-4 is critical for the induction of IgE synthesis and for the up-regulation of IgE receptor expression on B cells (low affinity, CD23), mast cells, and basophils (high affinity, FcεRI). Inhalation of recombinant IL-4 leads to BHR and eosinophil recruitment in asthmatic people.[9] IL-4 also increases the production of cysteinyl leukotrienes from IgE-primed mast cells[10] and induces expression of adhesion molecules like vascular cell adhesion molecule-1 (VCAM-1) on pulmonary endothelium, which is involved in the migration of eosinophils, basophils, and lymphocytes. IL-4 induces expression of eotaxin by lung cells, although IL-13, another Th2 cytokine, is more potent in this regard. In addition, IL-4 increases mucus production and may have direct effects on smooth muscle cells, but the exact role of IL-4 in causing BHR and mucus production is complex and overlaps with that of IL-13 (see later).

IL-5 is another central Th2 cytokine that is coordinately produced with IL-4. IL-5, together with IL-3 and granulocyte-macrophage colony-stimulating factor (GM-CSF), promotes

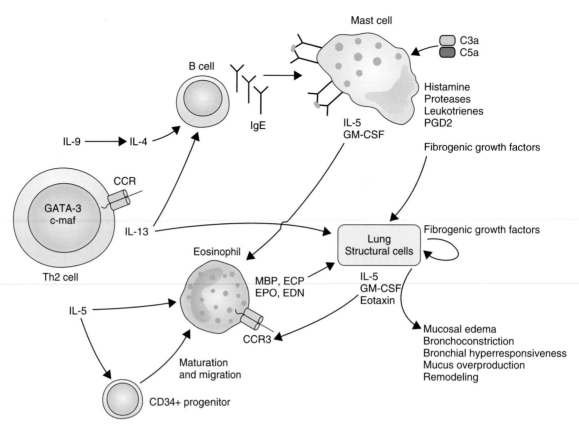

FIGURE 32-1 Schematic representation of the effector phase in asthma. Cytokines derived from CD4+ Th2 T cells orchestrate the asthmatic response through effects on other cells such as B cells, mast cells, and eosinophils and by direct interactions with lung structural cells.

the differentiation and maturation of eosinophil progenitors (CD34+ cells) in the bone marrow and induces the release of mature eosinophils from the bone marrow into the circulation. Although IL-3 and GM-CSF also promote the differentiation of multiple cell lineages, IL-5 promotes only the terminal differentiation of eosinophils. IL-5 has also been shown to be important for the survival of eosinophils once in the tissues and for priming eosinophils for response to several stimuli. Clinically, the presence of eosinophils in the airways (and in the circulation) is closely associated with the presence of asthma, suggesting that eosinophil-induced damage to the pulmonary epithelium causes BHR and asthma. However, recent studies showed that BHR in both mice and humans was not reduced after the depletion of eosinophils through neutralization of IL-5 with anti–IL-5 monoclonal antibody,[11,12] suggesting that eosinophils play only a minor role in asthma pathogenesis. Eosinophils may enhance the production of IL-13,[13] which appears to be primarily responsible for BHR. Although migration of the eosinophils into the lungs may be dependent on chemokines such as eotaxin as well as IL-5, these studies suggest that while eosinophils and IL-5 may exacerbate BHR, eosinophils may not be an essential component of the allergic inflammatory response required for the development of asthma.

Another Th2 cytokine, IL-13, has been shown to play a critical role in asthma. IL-13 has 30% homology with IL-4, and the receptors for both cytokines share one receptor chain, the IL-4Rα, involved in signal transduction. Accordingly, IL-4 and IL-13 share several functions, including the promotion of IgE switch, and use the same transduction pathways (STAT-6). However, IL-13 is not able to induce Th2 differentiation because of the absence of the IL-13 receptor on the surface of T lymphocytes. Nevertheless, IL-13 directly increases mucus production by epithelial cells in the lung and directly causes BHR by binding to IL-13 receptors on airway smooth muscle cells.[14,15] High IL-13 levels are observed in bronchial biopsy samples from patients with asthma and in BAL fluid and serum of atopic asthmatic subjects. IL-13–deficient mice fail to develop BHR, even though they develop pulmonary eosinophilia.[16] Selective overexpression of IL-13 in the lungs results in pulmonary inflammation, airway epithelial and goblet cell hyperplasia with increased mucus production, increased collagen deposition, an increase in eotaxin, and an increase in BHR in response to methacholine. These findings indicate that IL-13 is the most critical cytokine required for the development of asthma.

IL-9, another cytokine produced by Th2 cells, also contributes to the development of asthma. IL-9 has a role in hematopoiesis, participates in mast cell maturation, and potentiates IgE production elicited by IL-4.[17] The expression of IL-9 and IL-9 receptor is increased in bronchial tissue of atopic asthmatic subjects,[18] and constitutive overexpression of IL-9 is associated with several manifestations of experimental asthma, such as BHR, inflammation, mucus production, and increased number of tissue mast cells.[19] IL-9–deficient mice have significantly decreased goblet cell hyperplasia and mast cell proliferation in a pulmonary granuloma model, although they have minimal reductions in a model of allergen sensitization.[20,21] The effects of IL-9 are mediated through IL-4 and IL-5 because the effects of IL-9 are inhibited by the neutralization of IL-4 and IL-5 and IL-13 in a model of experimental asthma where IL-9 was inducibly overexpressed.[22] IL-9 and IL-13 may mediate goblet cell hypertrophy via induction of Gob-5 expression (human equivalent, hCLCA1).[23]

IL-25, a newly identified cytokine, which is produced by Th2 cells, is a member of the IL-17 cytokine family, and has structural similarity to IL-17E (see later), has functions similar to those of IL-4. IL-25 therefore may play an important role in asthma by promoting an increase in IgE synthesis, an increase in Th2 cytokine production, and an increase in blood eosinophils, epithelial hypertrophy, and mucus production. Like IL-9, IL-25 mediates its effects through the induction of Th2 cytokine production (IL-4, IL-5, and IL-13). IL-25 also induces Th2 cytokine production by a subset of antigen-presenting cells (APCs), which express high levels of major histocompatibility complex (MHC) class II, and are CD11c[dull] and lineage[−],[24] indicating that IL-25 amplifies allergic-type inflammatory responses by effects on several cell types.

Members of the IL-17 family also show important proinflammatory properties, especially IL-17E, which induces a Th2-type cytokine production, as well as eosinophilia, increased IgE and IgG1 production, and higher levels of Th2-type cytokines.[25] The precise cell types that produce IL-17E are not clear, but it is detected at very low levels in several tissues, including brain, kidney, lung, prostate, testis, spinal cord, adrenal gland, and trachea by reverse transcription–polymerase chain reaction. IL-17 is expressed in high amounts in sputum and BAL of asthmatic subjects,[26] and the administration of human IL-17 in rat tracheas induces airway epithelial cells to produce MIP-2/CXCL2 (a C-X-C chemokine), resulting in the attraction of neutrophils to the airways.[27]

Human epithelial cells in the lung and skin produce another cytokine, thymic stromal lymphopoietin (TSLP), which triggers dendritic cells (DCs) to induce T cell production of IL-4, IL-5, and IL-13 while down-regulating IL-10 and interferon (IFN)-γ.[28] Bronchial epithelial cells are known to also produce several mediators, including cytokines (IL-5 and GM-CSF), chemokines (RANTES/CCL5, eotaxin/CCL11, and MCP-1/CCL2), growth factors (platelet-derived growth factor, β-fibroblast growth factor, and endothelins), and other mediators such as nitric oxide that increase airway inflammation.[29] TSLP appears to be unique in that it activates DCs to induce Th2 cytokine production and to produce the Th2-attracting chemokines TARC and MDC. These functions of TSLP may help localize allergic inflammatory responses to the respiratory mucosa and skin of atopic individuals.

INTRACELLULAR EVENTS IN Th1 AND Th2 CELL DIFFERENTIATION

The binding of cytokines such as IL-4 or IL-12 to cell surface receptors induces a cascade of transcription factors and translocation events that leads to the development of polarized T cells.[30] The most important transcription factors in Th2 and Th1 cells include GATA-3 and T-bet.

The differentiation of Th2 cells requires the presence of IL-4, which binds to IL-4R, composed of the IL-4Rα and the common

γ chain (also part of the receptors for IL-2, IL-7, IL-9, and IL-15). Binding of IL-4 to its surface receptor activates STAT-6. Mice deficient in STAT-6 have reduced BHR, eosinophilic infiltration, and IgE production,[31] and BHR can be partially restored in these mice by adoptive transfer of T cells expressing STAT-6.[32] The binding of IL-13 to its receptors, which consist of IL-13Rα1 and IL-13Rα2 and the IL-4Rα chain, also results in phosphorylation of STAT-6. Increased expression of STAT-6 in bronchial mucosa of asthmatic patients has been observed.[33] STAT-6 may directly translocate to the nucleus and bind to STAT-6 transcriptional elements or interact with additional Th2-associated transcription factors such as GATA-3. In contrast to STAT-6, GATA-3 is selectively expressed in Th2 cells and is critical for Th2 cytokine expression. GATA-3 functions as a chromatin remodeling factor, making the *IL-4/IL-13/IL-5* locus accessible to other transcription factors. Overexpression of GATA-3 induces IL-4 and inhibits IFN-γ production, even in Th1 cells,[34] although IL-4 production is enhanced by the transcription factor c-Maf. GATA-3–deficient mice have decreased production of Th2 cytokines and reduced eosinophilic infiltrates. GATA-3 is expressed in higher levels in the bronchial mucosa of asthmatic people,[35] and a dominant negative mutant of GATA-3 severely attenuates all key features of asthma.[36]

The development of Th1 cells requires IL-12, which binds to the IL-12R, formed by the two chains IL-12Rβ1 and IL-12Rβ2. IL-12 production has been reported to be decreased in patients with asthma and allergy[37]; in addition, IL-12Rβ2 expression may be decreased in atopic asthma.[38] Signaling through the IL-12 receptor activates STAT-4, but STAT-4 alone cannot directly activate the IFN-γ production. In contrast, the transcription factor T-bet greatly increases IFN-γ production and directs Th1 cell commitment.[39] Mice deficient in T-bet exhibits spontaneously some characteristic of asthmatic phenotype, such as BHR and inflammation, and increased production of IL-4, IL-13, and transforming growth factor (TGF)-β1.[40] In addition, T-bet expression is decreased in the airways of patients with asthma.

A series of factors are also involved in the negative regulation of cytokine signaling. Because many activating steps involve phosphorylation, the expression of phosphatases such as SHP-1 is an important negative mechanism. Cytokine production is also negatively regulated by two other protein families, the protein inhibitors of STATs (PIAS) and the cytokine-inducible suppressor of cytokine signaling (SOCS), which has been shown to inhibit the Jak/STAT pathway.[41]

OTHER CELL TYPES THAT AFFECT THE IMMUNE RESPONSE IN ASTHMA

The IPR is IgE dependent and mediated by mast cells, which migrate from the bone marrow as precursors to the tissues where they mature locally in response to stem cell factor. The number of mast cells infiltrating smooth muscle cells in the airways in asthmatic compared with nonasthmatic individuals is increased, suggesting that mast cells contribute to the development of BHR via direct effects on smooth muscle cells.[42]

The LPR is characterized by an inflammatory infiltrate that includes mainly eosinophils but also basophils, neutrophils, and activated T cells. Recent work has suggested that neutrophilic infiltration is an important feature of severe asthma,[43] and basophils are an important source of IL-4 and

IL-13.[44] The LPR is dependent on the IPR and is thought to be responsible for the development of BHR and the chronic symptoms of asthma.

CD8+ T Cells

CD8+ T cells producing IL-4 and IL-5 (type 2 CD8+ cells) in the lungs and blood of asthmatic individuals may contribute to asthma pathogenesis.[45] CD8+ cells producing IFN-γ (type 1 CD8+ cells) may also contribute to asthma symptoms and to asthma exacerbation,[46] although they may protect against asthma, by eliminating allergen-specific Th2 cells. The precise role of CD8+ cells in asthma is not clear and may depend on the relative number of type 1 versus type 2 CD8 T+ cells present. Allergen-specific CD8+ cells respond to exogenous allergens cross-presented through class I pathways. In addition, virus-specific CD8+ cells producing type 2 cytokines may develop during certain viral infections, suggesting a mechanism for virus-induced asthma exacerbation.[47,48]

γδ T Cells

T cells expressing γδ T cell receptors (γδ T cells) have been shown to promote allergic sensitization in models of systemic sensitization.[49,50] These cells, which are found in high numbers in mucosal tissue, are thought to be involved in the initiation of immune response to bacterial antigens in mucosal epithelium. It is thought that subsets of γδ T cells producing Th2-type cytokines develop after allergen challenge.[51] Increased γδ T cell numbers have been reported in BAL fluid from patients with asthma,[52] suggesting that these cells exacerbate asthma symptoms. However, the precise role of γδ T cells in asthma is controversial, and other studies show that atopic asthmatics have decreased numbers of peripheral blood γδ cells.[53] γδ T cells may promote tolerance to inhaled antigen[54] and inhibit BHR independent of induction of eosinophilia.[55]

Natural Killer and Natural Killer T Cells

NK cells, which are lymphocytes that do not express CD3, CD4, or CD8, are important in controlling certain microbial infections and killing virus-infected cells and tumors. NK cells rapidly produce IFN-γ and may produce other cytokines, including tumor necrosis factor (TNF)-α, TGF-β1, IL-5, and IL-10. Depletion of NK cells in a murine model resulted in a reduction in pulmonary eosinophilia, suggesting that NK cells normally exacerbate airway inflammation and increase Th2 cytokine production.[56] However, the activation of NK cells, such as that with CpG oligonucleotides, greatly increases NK cell production of IFN-γ, which may protect against the development of asthma.[57]

NK T cells are a subset of NK cells that express both NK markers and αβ T cell receptors. NK T cells are part of the innate immune system and rapidly (within hours of stimulation) produce cytokines and therefore have been thought to direct the adaptive immune system. It has been proposed that CD4+ NK1.1 T cells provide the initial source of IL-4 for Th2 differentiation, but animals deficient in this subset still develop normal Th2 responses.[58] However, subsets of NK T cells exist, some producing IFN-γ but not IL-4, whereas others produce IL-4, IL-13, and IFN-γ. The activated NK T cells that inhibit Th2 differentiation[59] may be the former subset, whereas the latter NK T cell subset may exacerbate asthma.

Complement and Asthma

Complement appears to be important in the development of asthma, although its precise role is controversial. Activated C5a and C3a fragments are called *anaphylatoxins* because they participate in anaphylaxis reaction. They induce smooth muscle contraction, increase the permeability of blood vessels, and cause the release of histamine from mast cells and basophils. The C5a fragment, in addition, is a chemoattractant for neutrophils and monocytes. A pathogenic role for complement has been demonstrated using C3a receptor–deficient mice, which have reduced BHR, although they develop airway inflammation and increased IgE levels and produce Th2-type cytokines.[60] Similar results were observed in a naturally occurring guinea pig strain with a defective C3a receptor, in which the animals have reduced BHR but no reductions in eosinophil infiltration.[61] Furthermore, mice deficient in C3 have partially reduced BHR and partially reduced eosinophil infiltrate, concomitant with an increase in neutrophils and macrophages. In addition, production of IL-4 in the lungs was partially reduced, as were IgE and IgG1 levels (both isotypes controlled by IL-4).[62] Consistent with the possibility that complement exacerbates airways disease, increased levels of complement factors C3a and C5a after allergen challenge are found in BAL from asthmatic people,[63] and receptors for C3a and C5a are expressed in murine and human lungs.[64] However, complement may protect against asthma, because C5 deficiency in mice is associated with susceptibility toward BHR.[65]

EPITHELIAL-MESENCHYMAL TROPHIC UNIT AND AIRWAY REMODELING

Although the development of asthma depends to a great extent on immunologic components such as allergic sensitization and Th2-biased inflammation, not all individuals with allergic sensitization develop asthma, suggesting that mechanisms that are intrinsic to the lung also contribute to asthma pathogenesis.

A factor intrinsic to the lung that may contribute to the development of asthma involves epithelial and mesenchymal cell interactions and the epithelial cell response to injury. Under normal circumstances, the pulmonary epithelium and underlying mesenchymal cells communicate with each other through cytokines and growth factors (TGF-β and epithelial growth factor [EGF]) and coordinate growth and the response to damage after injury from the environment in this epithelial-mesenchymal unit.[66] In asthma, the mesenchymal cells differentiate into myofibroblasts that deposit interstitial collagens, resulting in thickening of the subepithelial basement membrane (lamina reticularis). These structural remodeling changes are only partially reversible and account for a portion of the deterioration in lung function associated with persistent disease.[66,67] The alterations observed in the airways include thickening of the bronchial wall, subepithelial fibrosis, mucus hypersecretion, hyperplasia and hypertrophy of the smooth muscle layer, and neovascularization.[67]

The extent of these remodeling changes and their effects on the development of asthma may be dependent on the degree

KEY CONCEPTS

Allergic Inflammatory Response

- Inflammation is mediated by Th2 lymphocytes, IgE and mast cells, eosinophils, basophils, neutrophils, and structural cells.
- The inflammatory response is associated with an increase in mucus production, mucosal edema, reversible obstruction, hyperresponsiveness, and remodeling of the airways.
- Bronchial hyperresponsiveness can be induced independent of eosinophilic inflammation through the Th2 cytokine interleukin (IL)-13.
- CD8 T cells, natural killer (NK) and NK T cells, γδ T cells, and the complement components C3a and C5a may also contribute to asthma pathology.

Clinical Relevance
- Neutralization of some components of the inflammatory response is being investigated as asthma treatments (e.g., anti-IgE monoclonal antibody, anti–IL-5 monoclonal antibody).
- Antagonism of IL-13 may be a powerful therapy in asthma.

of the Th2 inflammatory response and on abnormalities in the epithelial repair mechanisms. Genetic polymorphisms in asthma susceptibility genes may affect both of these pathways and result in the development of asthma. Recently, the *ADAM33* gene was identified through positional cloning as a major asthma susceptibility gene.[68] This gene codes for a metalloprotease, which may regulate the response of the respiratory epithelium to damage and stress, and asthma-inducing alleles of *ADAM33* may amplify repair mechanisms, leading to greater inflammation, airway remodeling, and the development of asthma (Box 32-1).

INITIATION OF ALLERGEN-SPECIFIC IMMUNE RESPONSE IN THE LUNGS

Antigen Presenting Cells

Environmental allergens are taken up by specialized APCs, processed, and presented to cells in the adaptive immune system. DCs, B cells, and macrophages are all able to present antigen to T cells, but DCs, which line the mucous membranes of the airways,[69] are the most potent stimulators of naive T cells. In contrast, alveolar macrophages, which are abundant in the lung, phagocytize antigen but appear normally to actively tolerize CD4+ T cells.[70] Alveolar macrophages fail to up-regulate expression of CD80 (B7.1) and CD86 (B7.2) co-stimulatory antigens and consequently are not competent in inducing T cell–mediated immune responses in the pulmonary compartment. On the other hand, DCs, which are derived from bone marrow progenitors, populate most peripheral tissues, including the lung in small numbers, but are extremely effective in activating T cells. DCs in the periphery and in the lung survey the environment by constantly sampling and capturing antigens. These tissue DCs are considered "immature" because they lack expression of co-stimulatory molecules and cannot stimulate T cells well. However, these immature DCs migrate

to regional lymph nodes, and in the process they mature and express chemotactic receptors as well as co-stimulatory molecules, such as MHC class II, CD80, and CD86. The maturation and migration of DCs are greatly enhanced by the presence in the lungs or tissue of necrotic cells or pathogens. After reaching the regional lymph nodes, the mature DCs encounter T and B cells, which they efficiently activate (Figure 32-2).

Based on the expression of distinct cell surface markers, cell culture requirements, and functional differences, DCs have been classified into distinct subsets.[71] In humans, one subset, called DC1, derives from blood monocytes, whereas another subset, called DC2, appears as plasmacytoid cells and expresses high levels of CD123 (IL-3 receptor α chain). DC1 cells induce naive CD4+ T cells to produce large quantities of IFN-γ but few Th2 cytokines, such as IL-4 and IL-5, whereas DC2 induce CD4+ T cells to produce large amounts of Th2 cytokines but not IFN-γ. It is not clear whether DC1 and DC2 cells are of different lineages or represent different maturation/differentiation steps of a single lineage. Plasmacytoid preDC2s express Toll-like receptors (TLRs) 7 and 9 and respond to microbial TLR9 ligand CpG-oligodeoxynucleotides (ODNs containing unmethylated CpG motifs) by producing IFN-α. In contrast, pre-DC1 express TLR1, 2, 4, 5, and 8 and respond to microbial ligands for TLR2 (peptidoglycan, lipoteichoic acid) and TLR4 (lipopolysaccharide [LPS]) by producing TNF-α and IL-6. The expression of distinct sets of TLRs and the difference in reactivity to microbial molecules support the concept that DC1s and DC2s developed through distinct evolutionary pathways to recognize different microbial antigens.[72] In the respiratory tract, DCs are recruited to the airway epithelium after the administration of infectious agents or challenge with soluble protein allergens. DC2 are thought to be preferentially recruited to the respiratory mucosa during allergic-type responses.[73]

CO-STIMULATORY REQUIREMENTS FOR THE DEVELOPMENT OF SENSITIZATION

DCs present the processed allergen to naive T cells in a process that requires co-stimulation (Figure 32-3). The best characterized co-stimulatory molecule expressed on T cells is CD28, which binds to CD80 (B7-1) and CD86 (B7-2) expressed on APCs.[74] CD28 is essential for the development of experimental asthma, and inhibition of CD28-B7 interactions using CTLA-4-Ig fusion proteins inhibited BHR, inflammatory infiltration, and IL-4 production.[75,76] Human studies with isolated peripheral blood mononuclear cells also indicate that blockage of CD28-B7 interactions with CTLA-4-Ig inhibits allergen-induced proliferation and production of IL-5 and IL-13.[77] However, spontaneous or constitutive production of these cytokines by effector T cells within airway tissues could not be inhibited with CTLA-4-Ig,[78] indicating that CD28-B7 interactions are important primarily for the development but not for the function of effector cells.

Another more recently described member of the CD28 family, called inducible T cell co-stimulator (ICOS), is expressed by activated T cells and germinal center T cells[74] and appears to be important for both the development and effector function of Th2 cells. ICOS binds to the B7-related protein ICOS ligand (ICOSL) or B7RP-1, expressed on DCs, monocytes, B cells, and endothelial cells. In the absence of ICOS-ICOSL signaling, such as that in ICOS-deficient mice, the

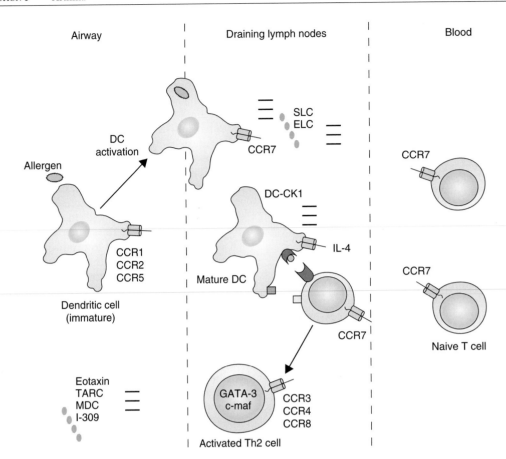

FIGURE 32-2 Cell trafficking and the initiation of allergic response. Immature dendritic cells *(DCs)* survey the airways and capture allergen. Allergen-loaded DCs migrate to draining regional lymph nodes on influence of chemoattractants such as secondary lymphoid tissue chemokine *(SLC)* and EBL-1−ligand chemokine *(ELC)*. These chemokines are also involved in attracting naive T cells from the circulation into lymph nodes. Other chemoattractants such as DC-CK1 are also important in bringing close together DCs and T cells. Activated Th2 cells express distinct chemokine receptors that bind to Th2-associated chemokines such as eotaxin, TARC, MDC, and I-309, expressed in sites of allergic inflammation.

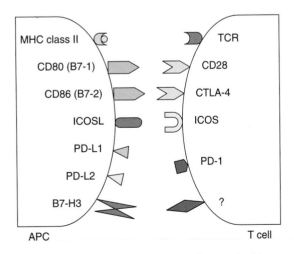

FIGURE 32-3 Antigen presentation and co-stimulation. Major histocompatibility complex class II molecules on the surfaces of antigen-presenting cells present processed allergen to the T cell receptor. Co-stimulatory signals are also necessary to modulate the T cell response. Known members of the best characterized co-stimulatory family, the B7/CD28, are represented in the figure.

production of IL-4 and IgE is greatly reduced.[79] ICOS is expressed by naive T cells on activation but is preferentially expressed on Th2 but not Th1 cells. Inhibition of ICOS signaling decreases Th2 effector activity but not Th1 responses and blocks both the development and expression of experimental asthma.[80] These results suggest that interruption of the ICOS-ICOSL pathway could be a potential target in asthma therapy by blocking pathways in both acute and chronic asthma.

Other co-stimulatory pathways for T cells include CTLA-4-B7, which induces T cell inhibitory signals. Consistent with this, treatment with a neutralizing anti–CTLA-4 monoclonal antibody increased IgE production, eosinophilic inflammation and BHR, and Th2 cytokine production but decreased TGF-β production in mice.[81] Another member of the CD28 family is the PD-1 (programmed death) receptor, which interacts with the B7 family members PD-L1 and PD-L2.[82] PD-1 expression is up-regulated in T, B, and myeloid cells on activation. Binding of PD-1 to both PD-L1 and PD-L2 has been associated mainly with inhibition of T cell function in both CD4+ and CD8+ T cells, although some studies reported T cell stimulation, especially production of IL-10. Nevertheless, studies with PD-1–deficient mice exhibited the characteristic of autoimmunity, suggesting its involvement in the regulation of T and B cell tolerance. Involvement of PD-1 in allergic responses remains to be investigated. Finally, the latest identified member of the B7 family is B7-H3.[74] B7-H3 expression is induced on DCs and monocytes by proinflammatory cytokines. The receptor for B7-H3 is still unknown and is distinct from CD28, CTLA-4, ICOS, and PD-1. B7-H3 co-stimulation induces proliferation in both CD4+ and CD8+ T cells, induces cytotoxic activity, and selectively increases expression of IFN-γ[83] (Box 32-2).

THE ROLE OF CELL TRAFFICKING IN PULMONARY INFLAMMATION

The development of asthma and lung inflammation depends not only on the mounting of Th2-biased immune responses but also on the homing of the inflammatory cells to the lung (see Figure 32-2). This cell trafficking process involves several families of proteins, including cytokines, chemokines, adhesion molecules, and matrix metalloproteinases (MMPs), in processes that are complex and redundant.

The first cells to be recruited to the lungs during allergic inflammation are basophils (expressing the chemokine receptors CCR2, 3, and 4) by chemokines MCP-1/CCL2, MCP-2/CCL8, and eotaxin/CCL11, which are produced by several cells in the lung. Eosinophils (expressing CCR3, CXCR4, and α4β1/VLA-4 and α4β7/LPAM-1 integrins) are also recruited

BOX 32-2	**KEY CONCEPTS**
	Initiation of Allergic Sensitization

- Initiation of immune response to allergens requires presentation by specialized antigen-presenting cells (APCs); APC/T cell interactions may determine the development of an allergic or a tolerant response.
- Dendritic cells (DCs) are the main APCs lining the airways.
- Two subtypes of DCs have been identified: DC1 and DC2; asthmatic subjects may have a higher proportion of DC2 in the blood than nonasthmatic subjects.
- Beyond major histocompatibility complex/T cell receptor interactions, co-stimulatory signals are necessary for efficient T cell priming and activation; co-stimulatory signals are also involved in cellular inhibition.
- Interleukin (IL)-4 and IL-13 cytokine receptors are heterodimers; both IL-4 and IL-13 receptors use the IL-4Rα subunit.
- Distinct transcription factors have been associated with T helper subsets: GATA-3 and c-*maf* with Th2 cells and T-bet with Th1 cells.

Clinical Relevance
- DCs could be manipulated to induce allergen tolerance.
- Inhibition or activation of co-stimulatory signals could be used for asthma therapy, such as inhibition of inducible T cell co-stimulator ligand/inducible T cell co-stimulator interaction.
- Soluble receptors may be used as cytokine antagonists, and soluble IL-4R is under investigation for asthma treatment. Another interesting possibility is the use of soluble IL-13R to neutralize IL-13.

into the lung by chemokines MCP-3/CCL7, MCP-4/CCL13, and VCAM-1 and MadCAM-1.[84] Expression of CCR3 and eotaxin/CCL11 is increased in atopic asthma, demonstrating the importance of these chemokines.[85] Th2 cells express CCR4 and CCR8 and are recruited into the lungs by MDC/CCL22, TARC/CL17, and I-309/CCL1 and by specific antigen. Expression of the CCR4 ligands MDC and TARC is up-regulated in epithelial cells after allergen challenge but not of the CCR8 ligand I-309/CCL1. Th1 cells express CXCR3 and CCR5 and migrate to the lungs in response to MiG/CXCL9, IP-10/CXCL10, and ITAC/CXCL11, all of which are induced by IFN-γ and interact with CXCR3. CCR5 interacts with MIP-1α/CCL3, MIP-1β/CCL4, and RANTES/CCL5, and CCR5 expression is associated, although not exclusively, with Th1 responses.

After recruitment to the lungs, migration of cells into the tissues requires integrin-mediated, firm adhesion. Chemokine-mediated activation of lymphocytes, which increases expression of and activates integrins, assists in this process. Chemokines and cytokines are also involved in lymphocyte extravasation/diapedesis by regulating the expression of proteinases such as MMPs, matrix-degrading enzymes that allow the leukocytes to penetrate through the basement membrane and into the tissue stroma. Recent studies showed that MMPs, especially MMP2 and possibly MMP9, are important in airway inflammation. MMP2 and MMP9 are increased in BAL fluid after allergen challenge in experimental asthma.[86] If MMP2 inhibitor TIMP-2 was administered, egression of eosinophils out of the lungs into airway lumen would be blocked, causing greater airway inflammation. These results were extended in an MMP2-deficient mouse model, in which allergen challenge resulted in severe airway inflammation and death of mice by asphyxia.[87]

INCREASED PREVALENCE IN ASTHMA AND ENVIRONMENTAL FACTORS

During the past several decades in industrialized countries, atopic diseases, including asthma, have increased dramatically in both prevalence and severity. Because the environment in westernized cultures has also changed significantly, particularly in terms of the prevalence of infectious diseases, it is thought that infections may affect the immune system in ways that protect against the development of asthma (hygiene hypothesis). However, the specific infectious pathogens that can protect against asthma have not been identified, and thus the link between asthma pathogenesis and infections remains nebulous. Nevertheless, identification of how the environment affects the immune system and asthma will greatly improve understanding of the immunology of asthma.

Infections with several pathogens, such as *Mycobacteria tuberculosis* or respiratory viruses, may enhance Th1 responses and limit Th2-driven responses and therefore may be important in asthma. Thus skin test reactivity to tuberculosis in children in Japan correlated inversely with the likelihood of having asthma, suggesting that exposure and response to *M. tuberculosis* inhibit the development of asthma.[88] However, this observation could be explained more directly by the fact that individuals in whom asthma and atopy develop genetically may have less robust cell-mediated immune responses to most antigens, including *M. tuberculosis*, but have increased humoral (IgE-mediated) responses to allergens and helminths.[89] A link between infection with specific respiratory viruses and asthma has been recognized for decades, in which respiratory viruses precipitate acute airway obstruction and wheezing in patients with asthma. However, although reduced asthma prevalence in children who enter day care early or in those who have older siblings suggests otherwise, frequent respiratory viral infections appear to exacerbate rather than prevent the development of asthma.

In contrast to respiratory viral infection, gastrointestinal exposure to bacteria and bacterial products may have a significant effect on the maturation of the immune system and indeed protect against the development of asthma. Recent studies have shown that increased incidence of allergy is associated with reduced prevalence of colonization of the gastrointestinal tract in children with *Bifidobacteria* and *Lactobacillus* strains, two gram-positive commensal bacteria.[90] Furthermore, exposure of infants to *Lactobacillus* in the neonatal period appears to protect against the development of atopy.[91] The effect of gastrointestinal bacteria on the developing immune system may be mediated through TLRs, which may inhibit the development of Th2-biased immune responses. "Improved" hygiene may eliminate exposure and the protective effects of these commensal gastrointestinal bacteria. The specific TLRs that may protect against asthma are not clear, although several investigators suggest that based on epidemiologic studies of farm environments as discussed earlier, TLR4 and exposure to bacterial LPS may be protective against asthma.[92] However, examination of the specific effects of LPS and TLR4 on T cell differentiation and cytokine production indicates that LPS may in fact exacerbate rather than limit Th2 cell development.

HEPATITIS A VIRUS AND THE *Tim1* GENE

In addition to gastrointestinal bacteria, several other gastrointestinal pathogens appear to have potent effects in the protection against the development of asthma. For example, evidence of infection with hepatitis A virus (HAV) is strongly associated with protection against the development of asthma.[93] Infection with other gastrointestinal pathogens such as *Helicobacter pylori* and *Toxoplasma gondii* may protect against the development of asthma, although to a lesser extent.[94] However, because HAV, *H. pylori,* and *T. gondii* are not respiratory pathogens and because HAV is transmitted via fecal-oral routes, clinical investigators have assumed that infections with these agents are merely markers of poor hygiene and that other infectious pathogens, possibly involving the respiratory tract, are more directly involved in protecting against asthma.

The mechanisms by which HAV infection prevents the development of asthma may be more direct than previously suspected. The positional cloning of a novel asthma susceptibility gene, *Tim1,* provides evidence for a direct role of HAV in the prevention of atopic disease.[95] In humans and other primates, the *Tim1* gene, which lies at human chromosome 5q33.2, a region that has been repeatedly linked to asthma, codes for the cellular receptor for HAV. By interacting with HAV, human TIM-1 may directly alter the helper T cell balance of the infected individual. Because *Tim1* is associated with the development of Th2-biased immune responses and may be selectively expressed on Th2 cells, infection with HAV may selectively eliminate allergen-specific Th2 cells by clonal deletion and thus specifically protect against the development of atopy. Alternatively, HAV may alter T cell development and enhance the development of immune responses that protect against asthma.

DO Th1 RESPONSES PROTECT AGAINST ASTHMA?

Until recently, specific pathogens that were suspected of limiting the development of asthma were those that could induce Th1 responses because the primary mechanism thought to protect against asthma involved Th1 cells, as predicted by the Th1-Th2 paradigm. Th1 responses were thought to protect against allergic disease by dampening the activity of Th2 responses, as has been shown in models of parasite infection. In accordance with this idea, infection in infants has been proposed to stimulate the immune system nonspecifically to mature and convert the predominantly Th2 bias of infants toward a Th1 bias by increasing the production of IFN-γ.

In reality, however, Th1 cells may exacerbate asthma and allergy because human asthma is associated with the production of IFN-γ, which appears to contribute to disease pathogenesis.[96] Allergen-specific Th1 cells, when adoptively transferred into naive recipients, migrate to the lungs but fail to counterbalance Th2 cell–induced BHR. Instead, allergen-specific Th1 cells cause severe airway inflammation.[97] Thus, although Th2 cells play a critical role in the pathogenesis of asthma, the binary Th1-Th2 paradigm in which Th1 cells balance Th2 cells cannot explain all of the immunologic processes that occur in asthma. These processes in asthma may be much more complex than those predicted by the Th1-Th2 paradigm, and "unhygienic" environments may protect against asthma by inducing additional non–Th1-Th2 immunologic regulatory mechanisms. This is consistent with the fact that Th1-mediated autoimmune diseases such as type 1 diabetes and inflammatory bowel disease have also increased in prevalence in westernized cultures during the past two decades. If improved hygiene in westernized cultures has reduced Th1 responses, then the prevalence of autoimmune diseases should decrease rather than increase, suggesting that mechanisms other than pure Th1 responses must be involved in protection against asthma.

T CELL TOLERANCE AND ASTHMA

One immune mechanism that may protect against and regulate the development of asthma, which could be significantly affected by changes in the environment in westernized cultures, is immune tolerance induced by mucosal (respiratory and gastrointestinal) exposure to antigen. In support of this possibility, investigators showed that peripheral CD4+ T cell tolerance, induced by respiratory exposure to allergen, prevents the development of Th2-biased responses and allergen-induced BHR.[98,99] In humans, the degree of allergen exposure appears to affect the induction of tolerance, with high exposure inducing greater tolerance.[100] The mechanisms by which respiratory antigens induce T cell tolerance include T cell clonal deletion, anergy, or active suppression mediated by regulatory cells secreting IL-10 or TGF-β, as is thought to occur in oral tolerance.[101,102]

The development of respiratory tolerance is initiated by the uptake of antigen in the lungs by immature DCs, followed by maturation and migration of the DCs to the bronchial lymph nodes. These DCs produce IL-10 transiently and express high levels of the co-stimulatory molecules CD80 and CD86 and stimulate the development of CD4+ regulatory T (T_R) cells that also produce high amounts of IL-10.[103] Antigen-specific B cells also play a role in this process because in the absence of B cells, respiratory tolerance cannot be induced.[104] Allergen-specific CD4 T_R cells may mediate T cell tolerance that inhibits airway inflammation and BHR.[105] In addition the development of the tolerance process and the function of the T_R effector cells depend on ICOS-ICOSL pathways, on CD28-B7-2 pathways, and on IL-10 because block of the ICOS interactions or neutralization of IL-10 inhibits their function.[105] TGF-β producing T cells may also be involved in inhibiting the development of BHR,[106,107] and mice overexpressing Smad7, which inhibits TGF-β signaling pathways, showed enhanced BHR and airway inflammation, suggesting that TGF-β is important for modulation of the allergic response.[108] However, TGF-β producing Th3 cells may be more important in the gastrointestinal tract rather than in pulmonary diseases.[109]

The role of IL-10 in limiting BHR and inflammation has been controversial, and IL-10 has been found to be increased or decreased in patients with asthma.[110,111] IL-10 has been considered to be an essential Th2 cytokine, particularly because IL-10 inhibits Th1 cytokine production by inhibiting IL-12 synthesis, and IL-10$^{-/-}$ mice develop poor Th2 responses and resist the development of BHR.[112] However, IL-10 may have several roles in asthma, not only by playing a critical function in initiating the development of Th2-polarized responses but also by playing an important regulatory role late during immune responses, by down-modulating Th2-driven inflammation.[113-115] The administration of IL-10 inhibits BHR, and T_R cells producing IL-10 prevent the development of BHR even in allergen-sensitized mice, suggesting that T_R cells normally develop during respiratory exposure to allergen and protect against allergic asthma.[105]

The idea that ICOS-ICOSL interactions co-stimulate the development of both Th2-driven inflammation and T_R cell–mediated tolerance suggests that these distinct processes are related. Both Th2 and T_R cells are associated with respiratory mucosal responses, require co-stimulation through CD28 and ICOS for induction, and produce both IL-4 and IL-10, although in relatively different quantities. Th2 cells produce primarily IL-4, IL-13, and IL-10, whereas T_R cells produce primarily IL-10 and low levels of IL-4[116] but not IL-13.[105] Moreover, the functions of T_R and Th2 cells in asthma are clearly distinct, because T_R cells, but not Th2 cells, block the development of BHR. Pulmonary DCs from mice exposed to intranasal OVA induce T cell production of both IL-4 and IL-10 initially, but with subsequent stimulation, IL-4 production wanes, whereas production of IL-10 is maintained. The specific signals that preferentially induce the development of T_R cells rather than Th2 cells are not entirely clear but may involve IL-10 production by DCs. In the presence of IL-10–producing DCs (or in the presence of exogenously derived IL-10), T_R cells develop, whereas in the absence of IL-10, T_R cells fail to develop. The development of Th2 cells and allergic diseases may represent an aberration of T_R cell development, possibly due to inadequate production of IL-10.[117] Thus Th2 cells in allergic asthma may develop as a consequence of limited IL-10 and enhanced IL-4 and IL-13 production and from the failure to develop allergen-specific

T_R cells, or "modified Th2 cells," rather than from a failure to develop Th1 cells.

LOSS OF TOLERANCE AND THE HYGIENIC HYPOTHESIS

It thus appears that the natural environment in the past (before widespread industrialization) maintained the respiratory and gastrointestinal mucosal systems in a state that favored the development of T cell tolerance to nonreplicating antigens encountered on mucosal surfaces, such as in food and in inhaled material. The establishment of these tolerance mechanisms at mucosal surfaces may require the presence of commensal bacteria in the gastrointestinal and upper respiratory tracts because immune tolerance induced by mucosal exposure to antigen does not occur in germ-free animals.[118,119] Commensal bacteria may enhance the production of IL-10 through mechanisms involving the innate immune system and receptors such as nucleotide-binding oligomerization domain 2 (NOD2). NOD2 is a member of the NOD family of proteins involved in the regulation of programmed cell death and host defense against pathogens[120] and is associated with the development of Crohn's disease.[121] NOD2 expression is highly restricted to monocytes, and when activated by LPS from some bacteria, it induces nuclear translocation of nuclear factor kappa B (NFκB) in a manner that appears to down-modulate inflammation. The antiinflammatory effects induced in the gastrointestinal tract by NOD2 may be related to the enteric "immunosuppressive" effects observed with nonvirulent *Salmonella* strains, which block NFκB activation by inhibiting IκB degradation.[122] Infection with high levels of helminths may also favor the development of tolerance to nonreplicating environmental antigens by enhancing IL-10 production.[123,124] Therefore some microorganisms may diminish inflammation at mucosal surfaces, and changes in the environment in westernized societies limit exposure to these types of organisms and thereby diminish the normal tolerance-inducing state of mucosal surfaces, resulting in enhanced mucosal inflammation. These changes prevent the development of allergen-specific T_R cells in some individuals, resulting in an aberrant form of T_R cells developing in atopic individuals (i.e., Th2 cells) that induces the development of allergy. The responsible environmental changes may include frequent use of antibiotics or changes in diet,[125] which alter the normal gastrointestinal flora, resulting in reduced IL-10 and TGF-β production by epithelial cells, DCs, and B cells in the mucosa, causing increased development of Th2 cells and allergy.

HOW CAN ASTHMA BE TREATED TO INDUCE PROTECTIVE IMMUNITY?

Most available treatments for asthma are effective at controlling symptoms, but none so far are curative. If the increase in asthma could be ascribed to alterations in tolerance, then procedures to induce tolerance to environmental allergens could be used to better treat asthma. Several strategies are possible. Conventional immunotherapy, although efficient in controlling symptoms and even reversing established disease,[126] is burdensome to administer. Strategies to increase the efficiency of conventional immunotherapy are being developed. For example, DNA vaccination with plasmids encoding specific allergens has been shown to prevent, although not reverse, the development of experimental asthma.[127] Reversal of previously established experimental asthma is achieved by the use of a fusion of cytokine and allergen genes, specifically IL-18.[128] This approach is antigen specific, can change the course of the disease, and can provide long-lasting remission. The success of the antigen-specific strategy in reversing asthmatic features further supports the importance of allergen sensitization in the development of asthma. Another possibility is the use of modifiers of conventional immunotherapy by conjugating allergen with CpG oligonucleotide motifs. CpG motifs bind to TLR9; induce the production of IL-12, IFN-γ, and IL-10; and have been shown to inhibit development of several asthmatic features, including BHR and eosinophil infiltration in a model of asthma. Importantly, CpG-allergen conjugates prevent inflammation and BHR in animals already sensitized. Another possible strategy is the induction of T_R cells, either by DC manipulation or by administration of other agents, such as mycobacteria.[129] Oral immunotherapy through the oral administration of allergens could be used to stimulate the mucosal mechanisms of tolerance. Oral tolerance has been shown to be able to prevent development of experimental asthma. Finally, because intestinal flora has been shown to be essential for the establishment of tolerance in animal models,[119] the administration of probiotics such as *Lactobacillus* may also be helpful in altering the immune system and inducing protective immunity[91] (Box 32-3).

CONCLUSIONS

Our understanding of the immunology of asthma has progressed rapidly during the past decade and is radically changing the focus of therapy for this disease. Although past therapies were based on relieving airway obstruction in asthma, current therapy focuses on reducing airway inflammation and neutralizing the effects of mast cell mediators. As even more is learned about the underlying immunologic mechanisms that enhance and prolong airway inflammation and the immunologic processes that prevent and reverse airways disease, therapies will become more specific and effective. Thus knowledge of critical mediators involved in the Th2-biased asthmatic immune response (e.g., IL-4, IL-13, chemokines, and integrins) and in airway remodeling (e.g., metalloproteases [ADAM33] and EGF) has spurred the development of strategies to limit the activity of these mediators as therapies for asthma. Furthermore, as our understanding of innate immunity and other specific mechanisms involved in regulating and reversing Th2-driven response becomes more complete (e.g., of microbial exposure, HAV infection, and the *Tim1* gene), additional preventive, and potentially curative, immunotherapies are likely to develop in the near future, bringing about a new era in asthma management.

BOX 32-3	**KEY CONCEPTS**
	Increase in Asthma, Tolerance, and Immunotherapy

- Changes in microbial load may underlie the increase in asthma prevalence, but the mechanisms involved are largely unknown.
- Identification of an asthma susceptibility gene (*Tim1*) in mice, of which the human homologue is the hepatitis A receptor, may explain the inverse relationship between hepatitis A infection and susceptibility to atopy.
- Although some microbes are good inducers of T helper cell type 1 (Th1) function and interferon-gamma may inhibit certain aspects of the asthmatic response, several lines of evidence suggest that polarization toward Th1 may not be the main mechanism involved in protection against allergic diseases.
- Respiratory tolerance is initiated by interleukin-10–producing dendritic cells, which induce the development of T-regulatory cells.

Clinical Relevance

- Understanding of the relationship among *Tim1*. Polymorphisms and asthma susceptibility may open new ways to treat asthma.
- Induction of tolerance by manipulating dendritic cells and/or by inducing T-regulatory cells could be used to reverse asthma.
- Modified forms of allergen immunotherapy, such as those in combination with CpG motifs, may be more effective than conventional immunotherapy.

REFERENCES

1. Holt PG, Macaubas C, Stumbles PA, et al: The role of allergy in the development of asthma, *Nature* 402:B12-B17, 1999.
2. Sporik R, Holgate ST, Platts-Mills TA, et al: Exposure to house-dust mite allergen (Der p I) and the development of asthma in childhood. A prospective study, *N Engl J Med* 323:502-507, 1990.
3. O'Hollaren MT, Yunginger JW, Offord KP, et al: Exposure to an aeroallergen as a possible precipitating factor in respiratory arrest in young patients with asthma, *N Engl J Med* 324:359-363, 1991.
4. Martinez FD, Wright AL, Taussig LM, et al: Asthma and wheezing in the first six years of life. The Group Health Medical Associates, *N Engl J Med* 332:133-138, 1995.
5. Burrows B, Martinez FD, Halonen M, et al: Association of asthma with serum IgE levels and skin-test reactivity to allergens, *N Engl J Med* 320:271-277, 1989.
6. Sears MR, Burrows B, Flannery EM, et al: Relation between airway responsiveness and serum IgE in children with asthma and in apparently normal children, *N Engl J Med* 325:1067-1071, 1991.
7. Robinson DS, Hamid Q, Ying S, et al: Predominant Th2-like bronchoalveolar T-lymphocyte population in atopic asthma, *N Engl J Med* 326:298-304, 1992.
8. Robinson DS, Ying S, Bentley AM, et al: Relationships among numbers of bronchoalveolar lavage cells expressing messenger ribonucleic acid for cytokines, asthma symptoms, and airway methacholine responsiveness in atopic asthma, *J Allergy Clin Immunol* 92:397-403, 1993.
9. Shi HZ, Deng JM, Xu H, et al: Effect of inhaled interleukin-4 on airway hyperreactivity in asthmatics, *Am J Respir Crit Care Med* 157:1818-1821, 1998.
10. Hsieh FH, Lam BK, Penrose JF, et al: T helper cell type 2 cytokines coordinately regulate immunoglobulin E-dependent cysteinyl leukotriene production by human cord blood-derived mast cells: profound induction of leukotriene C(4) synthase expression by interleukin 4, *J Exp Med* 193:123-133, 2001.
11. Corry DB, Folkesson HG, Warnock ML, et al: Interleukin 4, but not interleukin 5 or eosinophils, is required in a murine model of acute airway hyperreactivity, *J Exp Med* 183:109-117, 1996.
12. Leckie MJ, ten Brinke A, Khan J, et al: Effects of an interleukin-5 blocking monoclonal antibody on eosinophils, airway hyper-responsiveness, and the late asthmatic response, *Lancet* 356:2144-2148, 2000.
13. Mattes J, Yang M, Mahalingam S, et al: Intrinsic defect in T cell production of interleukin (IL)-13 in the absence of both IL-5 and eotaxin precludes the development of eosinophilia and airways hyperreactivity in experimental asthma, *J Exp Med* 195:1433-1444, 2002.

14. Wills-Karp M, Luyimbazi J, Xu X, et al: Interleukin-13: central mediator of allergic asthma, *Science* 282:2258-2261, 1998.

15. Grunig G, Warnock M, Wakil AE, et al: Requirement for IL-13 independently of IL-4 in experimental asthma, *Science* 282:2261-2263, 1998.

16. Walter DM, McIntire JJ, Berry G, et al: Critical role for IL-13 in the development of allergen-induced airway hyperreactivity, *J Immunol* 167:4668-4675, 2001.

17. Demoulin JB, Renauld JC: Interleukin 9 and its receptor: an overview of structure and function, *Int Rev Immunol* 16:345-364, 1998.

18. Shimbara A, Christodoulopoulos P, Soussi-Gounni A, et al: IL-9 and its receptor in allergic and nonallergic lung disease: increased expression in asthma, *J Allergy Clin Immunol* 105:108-115, 2000.

19. Temann UA, Geba GP, Rankin JA, et al: Expression of interleukin 9 in the lungs of transgenic mice causes airway inflammation, mast cell hyperplasia, and bronchial hyperresponsiveness, *J Exp Med* 188:1307-1320, 1998.

20. Townsend JM, Fallon GP, Matthews JD, et al: IL-9-deficient mice establish fundamental roles for IL-9 in pulmonary mastocytosis and goblet cell hyperplasia but not T cell development, *Immunity* 13:573-583, 2000.

21. McMillan SJ, Bishop B, Townsend MJ, et al: The absence of interleukin 9 does not affect the development of allergen-induced pulmonary inflammation nor airway hyperreactivity, *J Exp Med* 195:51-57, 2002.

22. Temann UA, Ray P, Flavell RA: Pulmonary overexpression of IL-9 induces Th2 cytokine expression, leading to immune pathology, *J Clin Invest* 109:29-39, 2002.

23. Nakanishi A, Morita S, Iwashita H, et al: Role of gob-5 in mucus overproduction and airway hyperresponsiveness in asthma, *Proc Natl Acad Sci U S A* 98:5175-5180, 2001.

24. Fort MM, Cheung J, Yen D, et al: IL-25 induces IL-4, IL-5, and IL-13 and Th2-associated pathologies *in vivo, Immunity* 15:985-995, 2001.

25. Pan G, French D, Mao W, et al: Forced expression of murine IL-17E induces growth retardation, jaundice, a Th2-biased response, and multiorgan inflammation in mice, *J Immunol* 167:6559-6567, 2001.

26. Molet S, Hamid Q, Davoine F, et al: IL-17 is increased in asthmatic airways and induces human bronchial fibroblasts to produce cytokines, *J Allergy Clin Immunol* 108:430-438, 2001.

27. Laan M, Cui ZH, Hoshino H, et al: Neutrophil recruitment by human IL-17 via C-X-C chemokine release in the airways, *J Immunol* 162:2347-2352, 1999.

28. Soumelis V, Reche PA, Kanzler H, et al: Human epithelial cells trigger dendritic cell mediated allergic inflammation by producing TSLP, *Nat Immunol* 3:673-680, 2002.

29. Holgate ST, Lackie P, Wilson S, et al: Bronchial epithelium as a key regulator of airway allergen sensitization and remodeling in asthma, *Am J Respir Crit Care Med* 162:S113-S117, 2000.

30. Murphy KM, Ouyang W, Farrar JD, et al: Signaling and transcription in T helper development, *Annu Rev Immunol* 18:451-494, 2000.

31. Akimoto T, Numata F, Tamura M, et al: Abrogation of bronchial eosinophilic inflammation and airway hyperreactivity in signal transducers and activators of transcription (STAT)6-deficient mice, *J Exp Med* 187:1537-1542, 1998.

32. Tomkinson A, Duez C, Lahn M, et al: Adoptive transfer of T cells induces airway hyperresponsiveness independently of airway eosinophilia but in a signal transducer and activator of transcription 6-dependent manner, *J Allergy Clin Immunol* 109:810-816, 2002.

33. Mullings RE, Wilson SJ, Puddicombe SM, et al: Signal transducer and activator of transcription 6 (STAT-6) expression and function in asthmatic bronchial epithelium, *J Allergy Clin Immunol* 108:832-828, 2001.

34. Zheng W,Flavell RA: The transcription factor GATA-3 is necessary and sufficient for Th2 cytokine gene expression in CD4 T cells, *Cell* 89:587-596, 1997.

35. Nakamura Y, Ghaffar O, Olivenstein R, et al: Gene expression of the GATA-3 transcription factor is increased in atopic asthma, *J Allergy Clin Immunol* 103:215-222, 1999.

36. Zhang DH, Yang L, Cohn L, et al: Inhibition of allergic inflammation in a murine model of asthma by expression of a dominant-negative mutant of GATA-3, *Immunity* 11:473-482, 1999.

37. Tang L, Benjaponpitak S, DeKruyff RH, et al: Reduced prevalence of allergic disease in patients with multiple sclerosis is associated with enhanced IL-12 production, *J Allergy Clin Immunol* 102:428-435, 1998.

38. Rogge L, Papi A, Presky DH, et al: Antibodies to the IL-12 receptor beta 2 chain mark human Th1 but not Th2 cells *in vitro* and *in vivo, J Immunol* 162:3926-3932, 1999.

39. Szabo SJ, Kim ST, Costa GL, et al: A novel transcription factor, T-bet, directs Th1 lineage commitment, *Cell* 100:655-669, 2000.

40. Finotto S, Neurath MF, Glickman JN, et al: Development of spontaneous airway changes consistent with human asthma in mice lacking T-bet, *Science* 295:336-338, 2002.

41. Greenhalgh CJ,Hilton DJ: Negative regulation of cytokine signaling, *J Leukoc Biol* 70:348-356, 2001.

42. Brightling CE, Bradding P, Symon FA, et al: Mast-cell infiltration of airway smooth muscle in asthma, *N Engl J Med* 346:1699-1705, 2002.

43. Ordonez CL, Shaughnessy TE, Matthay MA, et al: Increased neutrophil numbers and IL-8 levels in airway secretions in acute severe asthma: clinical and biologic significance, *Am J Respir Crit Care Med* 161:1185-1190, 2000.

44. Schroeder JT, Lichtenstein LM, Roche EM, et al: IL-4 production by human basophils found in the lung following segmental allergen challenge, *J Allergy Clin Immunol* 107:265-271, 2001.

45. Stanciu LA, Shute J, Promwong C, et al: Increased levels of IL-4 in CD8+ T cells in atopic asthma, *J Allergy Clin Immunol* 100:373-378, 1997.

46. Magnan AO, Mely LG, Camilla CA, et al: Assessment of the Th1/Th2 paradigm in whole blood in atopy and asthma. Increased IFN-gamma-producing CD8(+) T cells in asthma, *Am J Respir Crit Care Med* 161:1790-1796, 2000.

47. Coyle AJ, Erard F, Bertrand C, et al: Virus-specific CD8+ cells can switch to interleukin 5 production and induce airway eosinophilia, *J Exp Med* 181:1229-1233, 1995.

48. O'Sullivan S, Cormican L, Faul JL, et al: Activated, cytotoxic CD8(+) T lymphocytes contribute to the pathology of asthma death, *Am J Respir Crit Care Med* 164:560-564, 2001.

49. Zuany-Amorim C, Ruffie C, Haile S, et al: Requirement for gammadelta T cells in allergic airway inflammation, *Science* 280:1265-1267, 1998.

50. Schramm CM, Puddington L, Yiamouyiannis CA, et al: Proinflammatory roles of T-cell receptor (TCR) gammadelta and TCRalphabeta lymphocytes in a murine model of asthma, *Am J Respir Cell Mol Biol* 22:218-225, 2000.

51. Krug N, Erpenbeck VJ, Balke K, et al: Cytokine profile of bronchoalveolar lavage-derived CD4(+), CD8(+), and gammadelta T cells in people with asthma after segmental allergen challenge, *Am J Respir Cell Mol Biol* 25:125-131, 2001.

52. Spinozzi F, Agea E, Bistoni O, et al: Increased allergen-specific, steroid-sensitive gamma delta T cells in bronchoalveolar lavage fluid from patients with asthma, *Ann Intern Med* 124:223-227, 1996.

53. Chen KS, Miller KH, Hengehold D: Diminution of T cells with gamma delta receptor in the peripheral blood of allergic asthmatic individuals, *Clin Exp Allergy* 26:295-302, 1996.

54. McMenamin C, Pimm C, McKersey M, et al: Regulation of IgE responses to inhaled antigen in mice by antigen-specific gamma delta T cells, *Science* 265:1869-1871, 1994.

55. Lahn M, Kanehiro A, Takeda K, et al: Negative regulation of airway responsiveness that is dependent on gammadelta T cells and independent of alphabeta T cells, *Nat Med* 5:1150-1156, 1999.

56. Korsgren M, Persson CG, Sundler F, et al: Natural killer cells determine development of allergen-induced eosinophilic airway inflammation in mice, *J Exp Med* 189:553-562, 1999.

57. Broide D, Schwarze J, Tighe H, et al: Immunostimulatory DNA sequences inhibit IL-5, eosinophilic inflammation, and airway hyperresponsiveness in mice, *J Immunol* 161:7054-7062, 1998.

58. Smiley ST, Kaplan MH, Grusby MJ: Immunoglobulin E production in the absence of interleukin-4-secreting CD1-dependent cells, *Science* 275:977-979, 1997.

59. Cui J, Watanabe N, Kawano T, et al: Inhibition of T helper cell type 2 cell differentiation and immunoglobulin E response by ligand-activated Valpha14 natural killer T cells, *J Exp Med* 190:783-792, 1999.

60. Humbles AA, Lu B, Nilsson CA, et al: A role for the C3a anaphylatoxin receptor in the effector phase of asthma, *Nature* 406:998-1001, 2000.

61. Bautsch W, Hoymann HG, Zhang Q, et al: Cutting edge: guinea pigs with a natural C3a-receptor defect exhibit decreased bronchoconstriction in allergic airway disease: evidence for an involvement of the C3a anaphylatoxin in the pathogenesis of asthma, *J Immunol* 165:5401-5405, 2000.

62. Drouin SM, Corry DB, Kildsgaard J, et al: Cutting edge: the absence of C3 demonstrates a role for complement in Th2 effector functions in a murine model of pulmonary allergy, *J Immunol* 167:4141-4145, 2001.

63. Krug N, Tschernig T, Erpenbeck VJ, et al: Complement factors C3a and C5a are increased in bronchoalveolar lavage fluid after segmental allergen provocation in subjects with asthma, *Am J Respir Crit Care Med* 164:1841-1843, 2001.

64. Drouin SM, Kildsgaard J, Haviland J, et al: Expression of the complement anaphylatoxin C3a and C5a receptors on bronchial epithelial and smooth muscle cells in models of sepsis and asthma, *J Immunol* 166:2025-2032, 2001.

65. Karp CL, Grupe A, Schadt E, et al: Identification of complement factor 5 as a susceptibility locus for experimental allergic asthma, *Nat Immunol* 1:221-226, 2000.

66. Holgate ST, Davies DE, Lackie PM, et al: Epithelial-mesenchymal interactions in the pathogenesis of asthma, *J Allergy Clin Immunol* 105:193-204, 2000.

67. Elias JA, Zhu Z, Chupp G, et al: Airway remodeling in asthma, *J Clin Invest* 104:1001-1006, 1999.

68. van Eerdewegh P, Little RD, Dupuis J, et al: Association of the ADAM33 gene with asthma and bronchial hyperresponsiveness, *Nature* 418:426-430, 2002.

69. McWilliam AS, Holt PG: Immunobiology of dendritic cells in the respiratory tract: steady-state and inflammatory sentinels? *Toxicol Lett* 102-103:323-329, 1998.

70. Blumenthal R, Campbell D, Hwang P, et al: Human alveolar macrophages induce functional inactivation of antigen-specific CD4+ T cells, *J Allergy Clin Immunol* 107:258-264, 2001.

71. Shortman K, Liu YJ: Mouse and human dendritic cell subtypes, *Nat Rev Immunol* 2:151-161, 2002.

72. Kadowaki N, Ho S, Antonenko S, et al: Subsets of human dendritic cell precursors express different Toll-like receptors and respond to different microbial antigens, *J Exp Med* 194:863-869, 2001.

73. Jahnsen FL, Lund-Johansen F, Dunne JF, et al: Experimentally induced recruitment of plasmacytoid (CD123high) dendritic cells in human nasal allergy, *J Immunol* 165:4062-4068, 2000.

74. Sharpe AH, Freeman GJ: The B7-CD28 superfamily, *Nat Rev Immunol* 2:116-126, 2002.

75. Krinzman SJ, De Sanctis GT, Cernadas M, et al: Inhibition of T cell costimulation abrogates airway hyperresponsiveness in a murine model, *J Clin Invest* 98:2693-2699, 1996.

76. Keane-Myers A, Gause WC, Linsley PS, et al: B7-CD28/CTLA-4 costimulatory pathways are required for the development of T helper cell 2-mediated allergic airway responses to inhaled antigens, *J Immunol* 158:2042-2049, 1997.

77. Larche M, Till SJ, Haselden BM, et al: Costimulation through CD86 is involved in airway antigen-presenting cell and T cell responses to allergen in atopic asthmatics, *J Immunol* 161:6375-6382, 1998.

78. Lordan JL, Davies DE, Wilson SJ, et al: The role of CD28-B7 costimulation in allergen-induced cytokine release by bronchial mucosa from patients with moderately severe asthma, *J Allergy Clin Immunol* 108:976-981, 2001.

79. McAdam AJ, Greenwald RJ, Levin MA, et al: ICOS is critical for CD40-mediated antibody class switching, *Nature* 409:102-105, 2001.

80. Gonzalo JA, Tian J, Delaney T, et al: ICOS is critical for T helper cell-mediated lung mucosal inflammatory responses, *Nat Immunol* 2:597-604, 2001.

81. Hellings PW, Vandenberghe P, Kasran A, et al: Blockade of CTLA-4 enhances allergic sensitization and eosinophilic airway inflammation in genetically predisposed mice, *Eur J Immunol* 32:585-594, 2002.

82. Freeman GJ, Long AJ, Iwai Y, et al: Engagement of the PD-1 immunoinhibitory receptor by a novel B7 family member leads to negative regulation of lymphocyte activation, *J Exp Med* 192:1027-1034, 2000.

83. Chapoval AI, Ni J, Lau JS, et al: B7-H3: a costimulatory molecule for T cell activation and IFN-gamma production, *Nat Immunol* 2:269-274, 2001.

84. Kunkel EJ, Butcher EC: Chemokines and the tissue-specific migration of lymphocytes, *Immunity* 16:1-4, 2002.

85. Lamkhioued B, Renzi PM, Abi-Younes S, et al: Increased expression of eotaxin in bronchoalveolar lavage and airways of asthmatics contributes to the chemotaxis of eosinophils to the site of inflammation, *J Immunol* 159:4593-4601, 1997.

86. Kumagai K, Ohno I, Okada S, et al: Inhibition of matrix metalloproteinases prevents allergen-induced airway inflammation in a murine model of asthma, *J Immunol* 162:4212-4219, 1999.

87. Corry DB, Rishi K, Kanellis J, et al: Decreased allergic lung inflammatory cell egression and increased susceptibility to asphyxiation in MMP2-deficiency, *Nat Immunol* 3:347-353, 2002.

88. Shirakawa T, Enomoto T, Shimazu S, et al: The inverse association between tuberculin responses and atopic disorder, *Science* 275:77-79, 1997.

89. Lynch NR, Hagel IA, Palenque ME, et al: Relationship between helminthic infection and IgE response in atopic and nonatopic children in a tropical environment, *J Allergy Clin Immunol* 101:217-221, 1998.

90. Bjorksten B, Naaber P, Sepp E, et al: The intestinal microflora in allergic Estonian and Swedish 2-year-old children, *Clin Exp Allergy* 29:342-346, 1999.

91. Kalliomaki M, Salminen S, Arvilommi H, et al: Probiotics in primary prevention of atopic disease: a randomised placebo-controlled trial, *Lancet* 357:1076-1079, 2001.

92. Gehring U, Bolte G, Borte M, et al: Exposure to endotoxin decreases the risk of atopic eczema in infancy: a cohort study, *J Allergy Clin Immunol* 108:847-854, 2001.

93. Matricardi PM, Rosmini F, Ferrigno L, et al: Cross sectional retrospective study of prevalence of atopy among Italian military students with antibodies against hepatitis A virus, *Br Med J* 314:999-1003, 1997.

94. Matricardi PM, Rosmini F, Riondino S, et al: Exposure to foodborne and orofecal microbes versus airborne viruses in relation to atopy and allergic asthma: epidemiological study, *Br Med J* 320:412-417, 2000.

95. McIntire JJ, Umetsu SE, Akbari O, et al: Identification of Tapr (an airway hyperreactivity regulatory locus) and the linked Tim gene family, *Nat Immunol* 2:1109-1116, 2001.

96. Cembrzynska-Nowak M, Szklarz E, Inglot AD, et al: Elevated release of tumor necrosis factor-alpha and interferon-gamma by bronchoalveolar leukocytes from patients with bronchial asthma, *Am Rev Respir Dis* 147:291-295, 1993.

97. Hansen G, Berry G, DeKruyff RH, et al: Allergen-specific Th1 cells fail to counterbalance Th2 cell-induced airway hyperreactivity but cause severe airway inflammation, *J Clin Invest* 103:175-183, 1999.

98. Seymour BW, Gershwin LJ, Coffman RL: Aerosol-induced immunoglobulin (Ig)-E unresponsiveness to ovalbumin does not require CD8+ or T cell receptor (TCR)-gamma/delta+ T cells or interferon (IFN)-gamma in a murine model of allergen sensitization, *J Exp Med* 187:721-731, 1998.

99. Tsitoura DC, Blumenthal RL, Berry G, et al: Mechanisms preventing allergen-induced airways hyperreactivity: role of immune deviation and tolerance, *J Allergy Clin Immunol* 106:239-246, 2000.

100. Platts-Mills T, Vaughan J, Squillace S, et al: Sensitisation, asthma, and a modified Th2 response in children exposed to cat allergen: a population-based cross-sectional study, *Lancet* 357:752-756, 2001.

101. Chen Y, Kuchroo VK, Inobe J, et al: Regulatory T cell clones induced by oral tolerance: suppression of autoimmune encephalomyelitis, *Science* 265:1237-1240, 1994.

102. Chen Y, Inobe J, Marks R, et al: Peripheral deletion of antigen-reactive T cells in oral tolerance, *Nature* 376:177-180, 1995.

103. Akbari O, DeKruyff RH, Umetsu DT: Pulmonary dendritic cells producing IL-10 mediate tolerance induced by respiratory exposure to antigen, *Nat Immunol* 2:725-731, 2001.

104. Tsitoura DC, Yeung VP, DeKruyff RH, et al: Critical role of B cells in the development of T cell tolerance to aeroallergens, *Int Immunol* 14:659-667, 2002.

105. Akbari O, Freeman GJ, Meyer EH, et al: Antigen-specific regulatory T cells develop via the ICOS-ICOS-ligand pathway and inhibit allergen-induced airway hyperreactivity, *Nat Immunol* 8:1024-1032, 2002.

106. Hansen G, McIntire JJ, Yeung VP, et al: CD4(+) T helper cells engineered to produce latent TGF-beta1 reverse allergen-induced airway hyperreactivity and inflammation, *J Clin Invest* 105:61-70, 2000.

107. Haneda K, Sano K, Tamura G, et al: TGF-beta induced by oral tolerance ameliorates experimental tracheal eosinophilia, *J Immunol* 159:4484-4490, 1997.

108. Nakao A, Miike S, Hatano M, et al: Blockade of transforming growth factor beta/Smad signaling in T cells by overexpression of Smad7 enhances antigen-induced airway inflammation and airway reactivity, *J Exp Med* 192:151-158, 2000.

109. Weiner HL: The mucosal milieu creates tolerogenic dendritic cells and Tr1 and Th3 regulatory cells, *Nat Immunol* 2:671-672, 2001.

110. Borish L, Aarons A, Rumbyrt J, et al: Interleukin-10 regulation in normal subjects and patients with asthma, *J Allergy Clin Immunol* 97:1288-1296, 1996.

111. Robinson DS, Tsicopoulos A, Meng Q, et al: Increased interleukin-10 messenger RNA expression in atopic allergy and asthma, *Am J Respir Cell Mol Biol* 14:113-117, 1996.

112. Makela MJ, Kanehiro A, Borish L, et al: IL-10 is necessary for the expression of airway hyperresponsiveness but not pulmonary inflammation after allergic sensitization, *Proc Natl Acad Sci U S A* 97:6007-6012, 2000.

113. Akdis CA, Blesken T, Akdis M, et al: Role of interleukin 10 in specific immunotherapy, *J Clin Invest* 102:98-106, 1998.

114. Oh JW, Seroogy CM, Meyer EH, et al: CD4 T helper cells engineered to produce IL-10 prevent allergen-induced airway hyperreactivity and inflammation, *J Allergy Clin Immunol* 110:460-468, 2002.

115. Jeannin P, Lecoanet S, Delneste Y, et al: IgE versus IgG4 production can be differentially regulated by IL-10, *J Immunol* 160:3555-3561, 1998.

116. Groux H, O'Garra A, Bigler M, et al: A CD4+ T-cell subset inhibits antigen-specific T-cell responses and prevents colitis, *Nature* 389:737-742, 1997.

117. Umetsu DT, McIntire JJ, Akbari O, et al: Asthma: an epidemic of dysregulated immunity, *Nat Immunol* 3:715-720, 2002.

118. Wannemuehler MJ, Kiyono H, Babb JL, et al: Lipopolysaccharide (LPS) regulation of the immune response: LPS converts germfree mice to sensitivity to oral tolerance induction, *J Immunol* 129:959-965, 1982.

119. Sudo N, Sawamura S, Tanaka K, et al: The requirement of intestinal bacterial flora for the development of an IgE production system fully susceptible to oral tolerance induction, *J Immunol* 159:1739-1745, 1997.

120. Ogura Y, Inohara N, Benito A, et al: NOD2, a Nod1/Apaf-1 family member that is restricted to monocytes and activates NF-kappaB, *J Biol Chem* 276:4812-4818, 2001.

121. Hugot JP, Chamaillard M, Zouali H, et al: Association of NOD2 leucine-rich repeat variants with susceptibility to Crohn's disease, *Nature* 411:599-603, 2001.

122. Neish AS, Gewirtz AT, Zeng H, et al: Prokaryotic regulation of epithelial responses by inhibition of IkappaB-alpha ubiquitination, *Science* 289:1560-1563, 2000.

123. Mahanty S, Mollis SN, Ravichandran M, et al: High levels of spontaneous and parasite antigen-driven interleukin-10 production are associated with antigen-specific hyporesponsiveness in human lymphatic filariasis, *J Infect Dis* 173:769-773, 1996.

124. Yazdanbakhsh M, Kremsner PG, van Ree R: Allergy, parasites, and the hygiene hypothesis, *Science* 296:490-494, 2002.

125. Diez-Gonzalez F, Callaway TR, Kizoulis MG, et al: Grain feeding and the dissemination of acid-resistant Escherichia coli from cattle, *Science* 281:1666-1668, 1998.

126. Moller C, Dreborg S, Ferdousi HA, et al: Pollen immunotherapy reduces the development of asthma in children with seasonal rhinoconjunctivitis (the PAT-study), *J Allergy Clin Immunol* 109:251-256, 2002.

127. Hsu CH, Chua KY, Tao MH, et al: Immunoprophylaxis of allergen-induced immunoglobulin E synthesis and airway hyperresponsiveness *in vivo* by genetic immunization, *Nat Med* 2:540-544, 1996.

128. Maecker HT, Hansen G, Walter DM, et al: Vaccination with allergen-IL-18 fusion DNA protects against, and reverses established, airway hyperreactivity in a murine asthma model, *J Immunol* 166:959-965, 2001.

129. Zuany-Amorim C, Sawicka E, Manlius C, et al: Suppression of airway eosinophilia by killed Mycobacterium vaccae-induced allergen-specific regulatory T-cells, *Nat Med* 8:625-629, 2002.

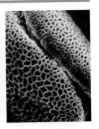

CHAPTER 33

Guidelines for Treatment of Asthma

JOHN O. WARNER

Clinical guidelines have been described as "systematically developed statements to assist practitioner and patient decisions about appropriate health care for specific clinical circumstances."[1] The justification for generating guidelines must be based on a number of key criteria, which include the degree of importance of the condition by both its prevalence and seriousness, its relevance to child health practice, the availability of evidence-based clinical information and supporting data, and the potential for health gain from the intervention. Finally, there should be a wide variation in clinical practice dealing with the disorder.[2] It is apparent that asthma fulfills virtually all of these criteria. This condition is common, with a progressively increasing prevalence during the past three to four decades. It is sometimes underdiagnosed and undertreated. Conversely, in some parts of the developed world, mild episodic disease is overtreated. Occasionally the condition is life threatening even in childhood, and there is good evidence that effective intervention improves quality of life and long-term health. However, evidence that interventions modify long-term outcomes is rather less secure.[3]

Asthma has a wide spectrum of manifestations and severity, and therefore management must be tailored to the individual's requirements. To some extent, the ideal combination of therapies is achieved through a process of trial and error, using a rational sequence of therapeutic approaches. Most guidelines have been based on this principle, involving progressive step-up sequences in treatment until disease control is attained. Some have advocated a more aggressive approach, commencing with high doses of inhaled corticosteroids (ICSs) with or without oral steroids until perfect lung function is achieved, with slow step-down of treatment thereafter. However, with experience it is often possible to assess severity and to identify the therapeutic strategy immediately without resorting to a series of therapeutic trials. A prerequisite for effective application of guidelines is accurate diagnosis in the first place. Indeed, it has been asserted that most of the problems of undertreatment of the condition are a consequence of failed diagnosis. An additional requirement in applying guidelines is objective monitoring of appropriate outcome indicators. The goal of treatment must be to return the child to a normal existence with participation in all normal childhood activities. This is possible in all but a minority of cases.

Therapy must be based on a clear understanding of the natural history of the disease and its various manifestations, a full understanding of the pharmacokinetics of drugs being administered, which will vary by age; and a complete knowledge of the pathophysiology of the disease. The pediatrician must also understand the complexities of the child within his or her environment and should be equipped to provide appropriate support to families and all other agencies involved on a day-to-day basis with the child.

It is incumbent on the developers of guidelines to construct them in such a way that they allow deviation and do not suffocate initiative that might bring further improvements in care. Updates should be frequent when changes in prevailing opinions occur as a consequence of newly published data.

It is, however, clear that clinical guidelines are very important tools to be used by clinicians when professional judgment dictates, but they should not be considered a compulsory recipe. They should merely provide a template in which clinicians can exercise their own judgment as the clinical situation dictates.[4]

EVIDENCE-BASED MEDICINE

Many of the original guidelines generated for the management of any disease, and this includes asthma, were based on a procedure that has been amusingly described as "good old boys sat around the table" (GOBSAT). It has become clear that it is necessary to use a much more systematic approach, as emphasized earlier, in the definition of *clinical practice guidelines*. Many now consider this to be synonymous with referral to at least one meta-analysis of randomized clinical trials. However, even the original and oft-quoted definition of *evidence-based medicine* takes a far broader perspective. "The practice of evidence-based medicine means integrating individual clinical expertise with the best available external clinical evidence from systematic research. By individual clinical expertise, we mean the proficiency and judgement that individual clinicians acquire through clinical experience and clinical practice."[5] This concept takes into account clinical judgment, experience, qualitative factors, and attitudes of the physician. To this must be added the attitudes of the patients and their caregivers, which become ever more important in this era of consumer health informatics in which clinicians must accept the patients and their caregivers as partners in the generation of an individualized management strategy.[6] One suspects that the latter is the most important in achieving an effective outcome. Successive studies scrutinizing the application of the guidelines has shown that they have failed, probably because of a failure to account for the views of patients and caregivers.[7]

AIMS OF MANAGEMENT

The strategy for managing asthma in all guidelines is based on the paradigm that the fundamental pathology of the disease is airway inflammation, particularly involving eosinophils and mast cells. Indeed, the current dogma suggests that eosinophilic inflammation progressively damages the airway epithelium, thereby initiating an exuberant repair process. This eventually leads to a phenomenon known as "remodeling," with increased collagen deposition below the basement membrane and in the lamina propria and hypertrophy of smooth muscle. It therefore follows that early and aggressive use of therapy that suppresses inflammation should prevent the chronic "remodeling" process that is associated with some degree of irreversibility of airflow limitation. However, there is little or no evidence that any therapy alters the natural history of asthma. Until there is clear evidence that the early introduction of high-dose antiinflammatory therapy is both safe and effective in changing long-term outcomes, it is more appropriate to use a more circumspect approach that addresses the patient's symptoms and signs.

It should be possible to return the overwhelming majority of children with asthma to a normal life comparable to that of nonasthmatic subjects. Clearly this must be achieved without producing undue side effects as a result of the interventions, which must include the maintenance of normal growth and development. Once these aims cannot be achieved, it is important to reconsider the initial diagnosis, establish whether there has been adequate adherence to the recommended regimen, identify whether there are any persisting avoidable triggers, and consider whether any comorbidities such as allergic rhinitis might be impairing the ability to control the lower airway disease. Psychosocial issues may figure very prominently as factors that impair the ability to control the disease. The single most common reason for failed treatment is the prescription of inappropriate medications and in particular inappropriate inhalation devices for children of different ages and with different abilities.

ASTHMA GUIDELINES

The first pediatric asthma guidelines were published in 1989 and were followed by updates in 1992 and 1998.[8] All of these were generated by the GOBSAT system. The same has, to a certain extent, been true of the Global Initiative for Asthma[9] and national guidelines from many countries. However, recently updated asthma guidelines from the United States and the United Kingdom can now claim to be truly systematic. The National Asthma Education and Prevention Programme 2002 update used an evidence-based approach to address six major questions related to therapeutic recommendations. For details, see the website (www.nhlbi.nih.gov). The 2002 U.K. guidelines are a collaboration between the British Thoracic Society and other representative bodies with the Scottish Intercollegiate Guidelines Network (SIGN).

Evidence review groups are established to generate the list of key words required for a comprehensive literature search. All papers are then scrutinized by the review group, having been trained in SIGN methodology and critical appraisal. This is based on an 8-level grading (1++ to 4) as seen in Table 33-1. Once the evidence tables have been constructed, considered judgment proformas are then completed for each key

question from which graded recommendations are produced on a 4-point scale (A to D) (see Table 33-1). Clearly, however, there are situations in which either it is impossible to conduct randomized trials or such studies have yet to be performed. Under such circumstances, it should not be considered that the recommendations from the guidelines are necessarily of less value but just that at present they are based on the best recommended practice from clinical experience. Thus once the draft guidelines have been produced, they are released for comment to as large a constituency as possible. Throughout this chapter, the levels of evidence and grades of recommendation will therefore be annotated as indicated in Table 33-1. If the recommendation is based on a so-called *good practice point* (i.e., clinical experience rather than controlled trials), this will be annotated in the text as GPP.

Most guidelines consider pharmacotherapeutic interventions in two groups: "preventers" and "relievers." The former are taken regularly and on a long-term basis to sustain consistent control of disease. In general, these are considered to be synonymous with medications that have been demonstrated to have some form of antiinflammatory effect, and many would

---

TABLE 31-1 Levels of Evidence and Grades of Recommendation

Levels of Evidence

1++   High-quality meta-analyses, systematic reviews, or randomized clinical trials (RCTs) with a very low risk of bias

1+   Well-conducted meta-analyses, systematic reviews, or RCTs with a low risk of bias

1−   Meta-analyses, systematic reviews, or RCTs with a high risk of bias

2++   High-quality systematic reviews of case-control or cohort studies or high-quality case-control or cohort studies with a very low risk of confounding or bias and a high probability that the relationship is causal

2+   Well-conducted case-control or cohort studies with a low risk of confounding or bias and a moderate probability that the relationship is causal

2−   Case-control or cohort studies with a high risk of confounding or bias and a significant risk that the relationship is not causal

3   Nonanalytical studies such as case reports or case series

4   Expert opinion

Grades of Recommendation

A   At least one meta-analysis, systematic review, or RCT rated as 1++ and directly applicable to the target population or a body of evidence consisting principally of studies rated as 1+, directly applicable to the target population, and demonstrating overall consistency of results

B   A body of evidence including studies rated as 2++, directly applicable to the target population, and demonstrating overall consistency of results or extrapolated evidence from studies rated as 1++ or 1+

C   A body of evidence including studies rated as 2+, directly applicable to the target population, and demonstrating overall consistency of results or extrapolated evidence from studies rated as 2++

D   Evidence level 3 or 4 or extrapolated evidence from studies rated as 2+

view this as being a primary focus on ICSs. The second category of drugs, namely relievers, predominantly alleviate bronchospasm associated with acute wheezing and may sometimes have some impact on other symptoms such as cough and chest tightness. In general, this focuses on short-acting beta agonists. However, lately a number of medications have been introduced that do not quite fit into either of the two groups. Indeed, theophyllines as a member of the reliever medications have been shown to have some degree of antiinflammatory as well as bronchodilating effects. The leukotriene receptor antagonist drugs clearly achieve bronchodilation and also have some degree of antiinflammatory effect. Although long-acting beta agonists have no clear-cut antiinflammatory effects, they certainly improve long-term control in patients with more difficult asthma.[3] These latter medications are termed "controllers" or "add-on therapies" (Table 33-2). Given the potential for ICSs to have systemic effects in high doses, the controller medications are sometimes used as steroid-sparing agents. This dictates their current position in the algorithm as add-on therapy if low-dose ICSs are ineffective.

All guidelines present the pharmacologic treatment strategy in the form of an algorithm (Figure 33-1). In the Third International Pediatric Consensus Statement,[8] asthma is divided into severity categories: infrequent episodic disease, frequent episodic disease, and persistent asthma, the latter of which can be further subdivided into mild, moderate, and severe.

In infrequent episodic disease, where there is normal spirometry between episodes, such problems may be treated with intermittent short-acting beta-agonist inhalants alone. There is no evidence that this strategy will have any long-term adverse effects.[10]

Level of Evidence for Beta Agonists Alone in Intermittent Asthma: 1++.

Grade of Recommendation: A.

With more frequent episodic disease, in which wheezing and coughing occur more often than once every 4 weeks, it is appropriate to consider the introduction of prophylaxis, even if spirometry is relatively normal between episodes. The first prophylactic compound recommended is either a cromolyn sodium or nedocromil sodium or low-dose ICS ($\leq$ 400 µg/day of beclomethasone dipropionate [BDP] or equivalent).[11]

Level of Evidence for Use of ICSs in Frequent Intermittent Asthma: 1++.

Grade of Recommendation: A.

There is no evidence that starting with very high doses of ICSs and stepping down confers additional benefits: 1+.

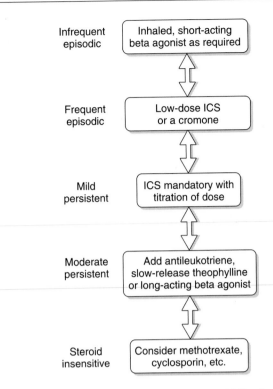

FIGURE 33-1 Therapeutic algorithm for asthma in childhood.

As soon as a patient is identified with any degree of abnormal spirometry between episodes, the classification of persistent asthma is used, and ICSs are mandatory.[3,8]

Level of Evidence: 1++.

Grade of Recommendation: A.

Once it is not possible to control the problem with BDP at a dose of at least 400 µg/day or the equivalent, which might be indicated by the need for inhaled, short-acting beta agonists more frequently than three times a week, then either the dose of ICSs is increased or an additional therapeutic intervention is required with leukotriene receptor antagonists, long-acting beta agonists, or slow-release theophylline. The choice will depend on availability, suitability, compliance issues, patient preferences, cost, and individual clinicians' experience.

Level of Evidence: 2+.

Grade of Recommendation: D.

As the disease becomes progressively more severe with poor response to ICSs, the patients are often classified as having

TABLE 33-2 The Three Groups of Commonly Used Asthma Medication in Childhood

Group	Specific Drugs	Administration	Comments
Relievers	Short-acting beta agonists	Inhaled preferred	Best used as needed
	Muscarinic receptor antagonists	Inhaled only	Less effective than beta agonists
Preventers	Cromolyn sodium and nedocromil sodium	Inhaled only	Very safe but only weakly antiinflammatory
	Inhaled corticosteroids	Inhaled	Systemic effects in high doses
Controllers	Leukotriene antagonists	Oral	Good safety profile
	Slow-release theophyllines	Oral	Narrow therapeutic window
	Long-acting beta agonists	Inhaled (salmeterol and formoterol)	Not antiinflammatory but can be
		Oral (bambuterol)	steroid sparing

steroid-insensitive or -resistant asthma. Alternative strategies include a range of treatments such as immunosuppression with methotrexate or cyclosporin, continuous subcutaneous infusion of beta agonists, and intravenous immunoglobulin.

Level of Evidence: 4.
Grade of Recommendation: GPP—use of highly speculative additional therapy for steroid-insensitive asthma should be in a center with experience in use of these drugs.

ROUTE OF ADMINISTRATION OF MEDICATIONS

It has become a truism that there are considerable advantages to using the inhaled route of medication administration because this delivers the drug directly to the source of the problem in the airways, in high concentrations (Table 33-3). There is often a much more rapid onset of action, which is clearly the case for the use of short-acting beta agonists. Systemic side effects are therefore minimized or at times even avoided. Furthermore, some medications are actually effective only via inhalation because of inadequate absorption via the oral route. However, it is evident from a number of adherence studies that the oral route is preferred by patients.[12]

In general, it is important to use one variety of device in any individual patient to avoid confusion; thus the preventers and relievers should be administered in the same type of device.

Level of Evidence: 4.
Grade of Recommendation: GPP—to avoid confusion, use only one inhaler type for both reliever and preventer medications, at least in young children.
The National Institute for Clinical Excellence in the United Kingdom has recently issued guidelines for inhaler devices in the management of chronic asthma in childhood.[13] The guidance is based on a systematic review of evidence. The recommendation is that in addition to the therapeutic need of a particular drug at a particular dose, there are a number of factors to be taken into account when choosing an inhaler device for an individual child. These factors are as follows.

- The ability of the child to develop and maintain an effective technique with the specific device
- The suitability of a device for individual children and their caregivers
- The child's preference for and willingness to use the device
- When more than one device suffices, cost can then become a consideration

The general recommendation is that a press-and-breathe, pressurized, metered-dose inhaler (pMDI) with a suitable spacer device is the first line of choice for ICSs because this maximizes benefits and minimizes side effects. However, for beta agonists a wide range of devices may be considered to take into account frequency of use, portability, cost, and personal preference.

Once the selection of an inhaler device has been made, there is an additional essential step, as follows:

- Practical training and demonstration that it can be used efficiently.[14] Indeed, many studies have shown that mistakes in inhaler technique are common and that training can improve techniques.

Level of Evidence: 1+.
Grade of Recommendation: B.

- Regular monitoring of technique and adherence to therapy
- Annual review of inhaler needs, which will change over time

Level of Evidence (for above two steps): 3.
Grade of Recommendation: D (GPP).
For the administration of beta agonists, the use of a pMDI and spacer is at least as good as a nebulizer to administer bronchodilators in children aged 5 years and older.[15] There are no controlled trials of the use of spacers in children younger than 2 for either acute or chronic asthma. However, low-volume (250-ml) spacers have been shown to have at least some beneficial effects.[16]

Level of Evidence: 1++ for the administration of bronchodilators for acute asthma in children. A large-volume (750-ml) spacer is as good as a nebulizer.
Grade of Recommendation: A—children with exacerbation of asthma should be treated with pMDI and a large-volume spacer.
Level of Evidence: 2+ in infants with acute asthma; low-volume (250-ml) spacers with pMDI for bronchodilators achieve some clinical benefit.
Grade of Recommendation: D (GPP)—low-volume spacers with pMDI may be used to administer bronchodilators in infants.
For the delivery of antiinflammatory drugs, several studies have examined different devices in childhood and on balance suggest that the use of a pMDI and spacer is as effective as any dry powder inhaler (DPI) and better than pMDI alone.

TABLE 33-3 First and Second Choices of Recommended Inhaler Devices for Asthmatic Children of Different Ages

Age	Device	Medication
0 to 5 yr	Pressurized metered-dose inhaler and low-volume spacer with mask (< 3 yr)	Beta agonist Cromolyn sodium and nedocromil sodium Inhaled corticosteroids
	Nebulizer	Beta agonist Cromolyn sodium and nedocromil sodium Budesonide
5 to 15 yr	Pressurized metered-dose inhaler and 750-ml spacer	All medications
	Dry powder inhaler	All medications

Level of Evidence: 2+ for the delivery of inhaled steroids for stable asthma in children, a pMDI plus large-volume spacer is effective.
Grade of Recommendation: C (GPP)—there is some suggestion that a pMDI and spacer for the administration of ICSs reduces oropharyngeal deposition and therefore oral candidiasis and increases the proportion of medication reaching the airways; thus this should be a preferred delivery option.[14,17] *Optimal use of spacers has been extensively investigated; being inexpensive and easy to use, they overcome many of the problems of poor technique and coordination with actuation and inspiration associated with the use of pMDIs alone.*[18,19]

For the administration of ICSs in infants, the majority of studies have investigated nebulized therapy using budesonide, which has at least demonstrated efficacy but high doses are required.[20] If extrapolations from observations of the effects of beta-2 agonists by a pMDI and low volume spacer are to be accepted, then it may be appropriate to administer ICSs through the same device, thus avoiding the need for the very high doses required by a nebulizer.

In general, DPIs cannot be reliably used in young children. However, DPIs can achieve higher airway deposition in older children, provided that the child generates an adequate inspiratory flow, than even a pMDI with spacer, although there is little evidence to suggest an advantage of DPI in this situation.[8,21] Breath-actuated pMDIs are sometimes preferred by older children. Although the automatic actuation removes some of the difficulties of coordination, the sound from the device and the sensation of the actuation may hamper inspiration in some children and increase oropharyngeal deposition.[14] Thus in general, they would not be the system of first choice but must be available for those children who prefer them.

The advent of nonchlorofluorocarbon (CFC) propellants for pMDIs has created some confusion. The dose equivalence for CFC and non-CFC inhalers with beta agonists is a 1:1 ratio,[22] but this is not the case for ICSs. In CFC inhalers, the corticosteroid was in a suspension and airway delivery depended on particle size. However, in the non-CFC propellants, the steroid is soluble, and therefore in solution the particle size is dependent on the device itself. This means that for some devices the proportion of steroid in small particles is higher and airway delivery is increased, increasing both efficacy and systemic activity. It is therefore essential that, in converting from CFC to non-CFC inhalers, there be a titration of the dose against the clinical effect.[23,24]

There also is confusion about which ICS is most appropriate to use because dose equivalence cannot be assumed. Indeed, fluticasone is twice as potent as BDP and budesonide but also twice as likely to produce systemic effects.[25] Comparisons of BDP with budesonide are complicated by the use of different devices. Thus, although the two ICSs are equipotent in terms of antiinflammatory effects, there is some evidence that budesonide administered via Turbuhaler is more effective than BDP administered via pMDI or Rotahaler.[26]

NONPHARMACOLOGIC MANAGEMENT

It is important to consider that there are a host of nonpharmacologic approaches to the management of asthma that should have equal importance in the overall management strategy.

Allergen Avoidance

Increased allergen exposure in sensitized individuals is associated with an increase in asthma symptoms, bronchial hyperresponsiveness, and a reduction in lung function. Increases in treatment requirements, hospital attendance, and acute admissions are associated with exposure to high concentrations, particularly of indoor allergens. Indeed, for a number of allergens, a threshold concentration has been found beyond which sensitive individuals have a significantly higher risk of acute exacerbation.[27] Despite these compelling data, evidence that reducing allergen exposure can reduce morbidity is tenuous. Uncontrolled studies of children and adults being transferred to very low allergen environments demonstrate very considerable improvement.[28] However, the benefits in such circumstances cannot necessarily be attributed to allergen avoidance alone.

House Dust Mite Avoidance Measures

There have been two Cochrane reviews on house mite control measures for the management of asthma. The first suggested that all methods were ineffective and that such approaches could not be recommended as part of the long-term management strategy for house mite–sensitive asthmatic subjects.[29] This has undergone an amendment, which concluded that physical methods may reduce asthma symptoms.[30] Thus there is some justification for recommending complete barrier bed covering systems, removal of carpets, removal of soft toys from the bed, high temperature washing of bed linen, application of acaracides to soft furnishings, and the use of dehumidifiers.

Level of Evidence: 2—for physical methods of house mite reduction.
Grade of Recommendation: C (GPP)—use of bed barrier systems, carpet removal, and dehumidification.

Other Allergens

Cat and dog allergies have been identified as common associations with asthma. Indeed, there is ubiquitous exposure to these allergens even among children who do not have a pet in their homes. It has been shown that children exposed in school via the clothing of other children who have pets can have increased bronchial hyperresponsiveness, abnormalities in lung function, and symptoms.[31] Observational studies have found that removing a pet from a home fails to improve asthma control, in part because of ubiquitous exposure and because reduction in allergen after removal of a pet is very slow. Furthermore, there is even a possibility that the maintenance of a high exposure to such allergens in the domestic environment might actually induce some degree of tolerance.[32] A randomized, controlled trial of high-efficiency vacuuming in homes that did not contain a cat or dog showed both a reduction in cat allergen levels and an improvement in bronchial hyperresponsiveness in cat-sensitive asthmatic subjects.[33] Thus on balance it seems sensible to recommend removal of pets from homes and the use of high-efficiency vacuuming where individuals with asthma are identified as having an allergy to pets.

Level of Evidence: 2—cat or dog removal from home of sensitized asthmatic subjects.
Grade of Recommendation: C (GPP).
Similar issues relate to cockroach allergy. One controlled avoidance study did not achieve a reduction in cockroach allergen despite an improvement in asthma. It may be that in this study it was the reduction in mite allergen levels that achieved the small benefit.[34] There are no controlled trials of any other form of allergen avoidance, and therefore other than recommendations on house mite avoidance and cat and dog allergen avoidance, no other recommendations can be made.

Other Environmental Triggers

There is an association between exposure to environmental tobacco smoke and increased respiratory symptoms. This mostly relates to wheezing associated with viral infections in infants and young children. The degree to which this affects asthma is not so clear. However, the U.S. Institute of Medicine identified a causal relationship between environmental tobacco smoke exposure and exacerbation of asthma in preschool children, with a 30% increased risk of symptoms in exposed children.[35] One small study suggested that by stopping smoking, parents can decrease the severity of asthma in their children.[36] Furthermore, starting smoking as a teenager increases the risk of persisting asthma.

Level of Evidence: 2++—exposure to environmental tobacco smoke in the home increases the frequency of respiratory illnesses in children.
Grade of Recommendation: B (GPP)—parents who smoke should not do so because of danger to themselves and their children.
No studies have investigated in detail whether a reduction in other domestic pollutants, such as nitrogen oxides and volatile organic compounds, can make any difference to asthma control. There is limited evidence that exposure to these factors might actually potentiate asthma, but further research is required before recommendations can be made.

Immunotherapy

Allergen-specific immunotherapy by subcutaneous injection of slowly increasing doses of allergen extract has undergone several systematic reviews, the last of which was Cochrane based.[37] A consistent beneficial effect of treatment compared with placebo was demonstrated in well-conducted, double-blind, controlled trials specifically in relation to house dust mite, grass pollen, and cat and dog allergies. No controlled trials have yet made direct comparisons between conventional pharmacotherapy and allergen immunotherapy.

Thus immunotherapy undoubtedly has beneficial effects in allergic asthmatic subjects, but its place in the therapeutic algorithm is impossible to define. When other reasons exist for providing this therapy, such as associated seasonal rhinoconjunctivitis, it can be recommended and will have additional benefits for asthma.

Level of Evidence: 1+—house mite, pollen, cat, or dog allergy immunotherapy in asthma.
Grade of Recommendation: A—to use immunotherapy primarily for allergic rhinitis, with additional benefits for asthma.

Other Nonpharmacologic Treatments

A host of other treatments have at various times been recommended for the management of asthma, including herbal and traditional Chinese medicine, acupuncture, homeopathy, hypnosis, various forms of manual therapy, physical exercise, and breathing exercises—none have generated sufficient evidence from trials to justify recommendation.[38-43] For air ionizers, there is some evidence of an adverse effect and therefore their use should be discouraged.[44]

Level of Evidence: 21—to avoid the use of alternative therapies.
Grade of Recommendation: C.
Various forms of psychotherapy have also been investigated, and there is a Cochrane review of family therapy.[45] However, this identified only two trials with 55 children that could be assessed, and these trials suggested that family therapy might be a useful adjunct to medication.

Level of Evidence: 2—in childhood asthma there may be a role for family psychotherapy.
Grade of Recommendation: GPP—psychotherapy may be an adjunct to pharmacotherapy.

Treatment of Gastroesophageal Reflux

A Cochrane review of 12 double-blind, controlled trials revealed that the treatment of gastroesophageal reflux had no benefit on asthma symptoms or lung function when the two conditions coexisted, although there was some reduction in cough, probably not originally the result of asthma.[46] Thus gastroesophageal reflux should be treated if present, but this will have no impact on asthma control.

Level of Evidence: 1+—treatment of gastroesophageal reflux does not improve asthma.
Grade of Recommendation: A—treat when present but continue all other asthma therapy.

CONCLUSIONS

Asthma is the most common chronic disease of childhood for which there is wide variation in diagnostic ascertainment and management. Thus the development of guidelines for the diagnosis and management of childhood asthma is clearly justified. Published guidelines vary in the degree to which evidence is assessed in an unbiased and systematic way. However, the most recent from the United States and the United Kingdom used evidence-based approaches. The small differences between them are a consequence of the need to take account of the patients' and caregivers' wishes and expectations, which will vary from country to country. Indeed, failure to accept the patient and caregiver as partners in the planning of management could be the primary reason why guidelines often do not achieve as much as what might be expected. It is furthermore incumbent on guideline developers to produce frequent updates whenever new information appears.

The main focus of asthma management tends to be on pharmacotherapy, which is usually presented in the form of an algorithm, with increasing intensity of treatment when the disease is more severe. The emphasis is on a steady stepwise increase in treatment as the disease severity dictates. Stepping down of therapy when the clinical situation improves is equally important but should be monitored with great care.

Nonpharmacologic approaches should not be forgotten. The avoidance of precipitants seems to be a sensible and logical approach, but the evidence of efficacy is rather weak. Conversely, there is a strong evidence base for the use of allergen immunotherapy in asthma, but its place in the therapeutic algorithm has still not been clearly defined because of concerns about the risk/benefit ratio. Head-to-head control trials that compare standard pharmacotherapy with immunotherapy are required. Finally, while so-called complementary medicine has become very fashionable, there is no evidence base to support its use.

REFERENCES

1. Field MJ, Lohr KN, eds: *Guidelines for clinical practice: from development to use.* Washington, DC, 1992, National Academy Press.
2. Warner JO: Sanity and management guidelines, *Pediatr Allergy Immunol* 12:177-178, 2001.
3. Spahn JD, Szefler SJ: Childhood asthma: New insights into management, *J Allergy Clin Immunol* 109:3-13, 2002.
4. Tingle JH: Do guidelines have legal implications? *Arch Dis Child* 86:387-388, 2002.
5. Sackett DL, Rosenberg WMC, Muir Gray JH, et al: Evidence based medicine: what it is and what it isn't, *Br Med J* 312:71-72, 1996.
6. Edwards A, Elwyn G, eds: *Evidence based patient choice (inevitable or impossible?),* Oxford, UK, 2001, Oxford University Press.
7. Doerschug KC, Peterson MW, Dayton CS, et al: Asthma guidelines. An assessment of physician understanding and practice, *Am J Respir Crit Care Med* 159:1735-1741, 1999.
8. Warner JO, Naspitz CK: Third International Pediatric Consensus Statement on the management of childhood asthma, *Pediatr Pulmonol* 25:1-17, 1998.
9. National Heart, Lung, and Blood Institute/World Health Organization Workshop Report: *Global strategy for asthma management and prevention,* NIH Pub No. 02-3659, Bethesda, Md, 2002.
10. Oswald H, Phelan PD, Lanigan A, et al: Childhood asthma and lung function in mid-adult life, *Pediatr Pulmonol* 23:14-20, 1997.
11. The Childhood Asthma Management Programme Research Group: Long term effects of budesonide or nedocromil in children with asthma, *N Engl J Med* 343:1054-1063, 2000.
12. Kelloway JS, Wyatt RA, Adlis SA: Comparison of patients' compliance with prescribed oral and inhaled asthma medications, *Arch Intern Med* 154:1349-1352, 1994.
13. National Institute for Clinical Excellence: *Inhaler devices for routine treatment of chronic asthma in older children (aged 5-15 years),* London, March 2002, The Institute, Technology Appraisal Guidance No. 38.
14. Pedersen S, Mortensen S: Use of different inhalation devices in children, *Lung* 168(suppl):653-657, 1990.
15. Dewar AL, Stewart A, Cogswell JJ, et al: A randomised controlled trial to assess the relative benefits of large volume spacers and nebulisers to treat acute asthma in hospital, *Arch Dis Child* 80:421-423, 1999.
16. Wildahaber JH, Devadason SG, Hayden MJ, et al: Aerosol delivery to wheezy infants: a comparison between a nebuliser and 2 small volume spacers, *Pediatr Pulmonol* 23:212-216, 1997.
17. Dolovich MB, Everard ML: Delivery of aerosols to children: devices and inhalation techniques. In Naspitz CK, Szefler SJ, Tinkelman DG, eds: *Textbook of pediatric asthma: an international perspective,* London, UK, 2001, Martin Dunitz.
18. Wildahaber JH, Devadason SG, Eber E, et al: Effect of electrostatic charge, flow, delay and multiple actuations on the *in vitro* delivery from different small volume spacers for infants, *Thorax* 51:985-988, 1996.
19. Barry PW, Robertson C, O'Callaghan C: Optimal use of spacer devices, *Arch Dis Child* 69:693-694, 1993.
20. Ilangovan P, Godfrey S, Noviski N, et al: Nebulised budesonide suspension in severe steroid dependent pre-school asthma, *Arch Dis Child* 68:356-359, 1993.
21. Pedersen S, Hansen OR, Fuglsang G: Influence of inspiratory flow rate upon the effect of a turbohaler, *Arch Dis Child* 65:308-310, 1990.
22. Ram FSF, Brocklebank DM, White J, et al: Pressurized metered dose inhalers vs. all other hand held inhaler devices to deliver beta-2 agonist bronchodilators for non-acute asthma (Cochrane Review). In *The Cochrane Library,* Oxford, UK, 2002, Update Software
23. Szefler S, Warner J, Staab D, et al: Switching from conventional to extrafine aerosol beclomethasone dipropionate formulations: an open-label, randomised comparison of extrafine and conventional aerosols in children with asthma, *J Allergy Clin Immunol* 110:445-450, 2002.
24. June D: Achieving the change: challenges and successes in the formulation of CFC-free MDIs, *Eur Respir Rev* 7:32-34, 1997.
25. Adams N, Bestall JM, Jones PW: Fluticasone vs. beclomethasone or budesonide for chronic asthma (Cochrane Review). In *The Cochrane Library,* Oxford, UK, 2002, Update Software.
26. Adams N, Bestall JM, Jones PW: Inhaled beclomethasone vs. budesonide for chronic asthma (Cochrane Review). In *The Cochrane Library,* Oxford, UK, 2002, Update Software.
27. Gelber LE, Seltzer LH, Bouzoukis JK: Sensitization and exposure to indoor allergens as risk factors for asthma among patients presenting to hospital, *Am Rev Respir Dis* 147:57-58, 1993.
28. Peroni DG, Boner AL, Vallone G, et al: Effective allergen avoidance at high altitude reduces allergen induced bronchial hyperresponsiveness, *Am J Respir Crit Care Med* 149:1442-1446, 1994.
29. Gotzsche PC, Hammarquist C, Burr M: House dust mite control measures in the management of asthma: meta-analysis, *Br Med J* 317:1105-1110, 1998.
30. Gotzsche PC, Johansen HK, Hammarquist C, et al: House dust mite control measures for asthma (Cochrane Review). In *The Cochrane Library,* Oxford, UK, 2001, Update Software.
31. Warner JA: Controlling indoor allergens, *Pediatr Allergy Immunol* 11:208-219, 2000.
32. Platts-Mills T, Vaughan J, Squillace S, et al: Sensitization, asthma and a modified Th-2 response in children exposed to cat allergens: a population based cross-sectional study, *Lancet* 357:752-756, 2001.
33. Popplewell EJ, Innes VA, Lloyd-Hughes S, et al: The effect of high efficiency and standard vacuum cleaners on mite cat and dog allergen levels and clinical progress, *Pediatr Allergy Immunol* 11:142-148, 2000.
34. Gergen PJ, Mortimer KM, Eggleston PA, et al: Results of the National Cooperative Intercity Asthma Study (NCICAS). Environmental intervention to reduce cockroach allergen exposure in inner city homes, *J Allergy Clin Immunol* 103:501-506, 1999.
35. Committee on the Assessment of Asthma & Indoor Air: Exposure to indoor tobacco smoke. In *Clearing the air: asthma & indoor exposures,* Washington, DC, 2000, National Academy Press.
36. Murray AB, Morrison BJ: The decrease in severity of asthma in children of parents who smoke since the parents have been exposing themselves to less cigarette smoke, *J Allergy Clin Immunol* 91:102-110, 1993.
37. Abramson M, Puy R, Weiner J: Immunotherapy and asthma: an updated systematic review, *Allergy* 54:1022-1041, 1999.
38. Huntley A, Ernst E: Herbal medicines for asthma: a systematic review, *Thorax* 55:925-929, 2000.
39. Linde K, Jobst K, Panton J: Acupuncture for chronic asthma (Cochrane Review). In *The Cochrane Library,* Oxford, UK, 2000, Update Software.
40. Linde K, Jobst KA: Homeopathy for chronic asthma (Cochrane Review). In *The Cochrane Library,* Oxford, UK, 2000, Update Software.
41. Hondras MA, Linde K, Jones AP: Manual therapy for asthma (Cochrane Review). In *The Cochrane Library,* Oxford, UK, 2000, Update Software.
42. Ram FSF, Robinson SM, Black PN: Physical training for asthma (Cochrane Review). In *The Cochrane Library,* Oxford, UK, 2001, Update Software.
43. Holloway E, Ram FSF: Breathing exercises for asthma (Cochrane Review). In *The Cochrane Library,* Oxford, UK, 2001, Update Software.
44. Warner JA, Marchant JL, Warner JO: A double blind trial of ionisers in house dust mite sensitive asthmatic children, *Thorax* 48:330-333, 1993.
45. Panton J, Barley EA: Family therapy for asthma in children (Cochrane Review). In *The Cochrane Library,* Oxford, UK, 2001, Oxford Update Software.
46. Cockland JL, Gibson PG, Henry RL: Medical treatment for reflux oesophagitis does not consistently improve asthma control: a systematic review, *Thorax* 56:198-204, 2001.

CHAPTER 34

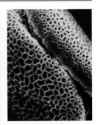

Functional Assessment of Asthma

GARY L. LARSEN ■ GWENDOLYN S. KERBY ■ THERESA W. GUILBERT ■ WAYNE J. MORGAN

Asthma is characterized in part by intermittent airway obstruction. Signs and symptoms commonly seen as obstruction increases include shortness of breath, cough, wheezing, and chest tightness. However, even moderate degrees of obstruction may not be clinically apparent. In asthmatic subjects, airflow limitation may vary from mild and self-limited to life threatening in degree. Between these extremes are gradations of obstruction that should be quantified if the patient is to be optimally assessed and managed. This chapter deals with functional assessments of asthma in the pediatric patient, with an emphasis on tests that reflect airway and lung function. Although the primary focus is on studies that can be easily performed in an office or a clinic setting, tests that require more sophisticated equipment than usually found in these locations are also noted. Furthermore, because the onset of this disease is often in preschool children, tests of lung function that may be performed in the youngest patients are also mentioned. Many of the latter studies are not usually available within the scope of general clinical practice, but they may be performed in centers with expertise in pediatric pulmonary medicine. In addition, knowledge of airway function close to the onset of disease is an important subject of ongoing investigations into the pathogenesis of the disorder.

Because structural changes within airways may relate to the functional assessments, this chapter initially addresses the pathology of asthma. This is relevant for several reasons. For example, an understanding of the pathologic findings in severe asthma identifies components contributing to obstruction that are poorly responsive to acute treatment and take time to resolve. This will be reflected in tests of airway function. At the other end of the clinical spectrum of disease activity, tests that define airway responsiveness may also correlate with lung pathology in subjects in whom the disease is clinically quiescent. Thus this chapter first focuses on a brief review of asthma pathology and then on physiologic correlates before a discussion of functional assessments of the disease. The use of tests of lung function to identify diseases that may mimic asthma is then presented. The ways in which pulmonary function tests may be helpful in guiding therapy in both acute and chronic settings are also considered. Studies involving infants, children, and adolescents are cited whenever possible because of the focus of this text and chapter on childhood asthma. Investigations into structural and functional assessments of the disease in adults are cited when they provide additional insight into the process and when no comparable studies exist within the pediatric population.

THE PATHOLOGY OF ASTHMA

Fatal asthma is associated with marked airway inflammation with mucus and cellular debris, epithelial desquamation, subepithelial collagen deposition, and airway wall thickening resulting in luminal obstruction.[1-3] Airway wall thickening occurs as a result of a combination of factors, including smooth muscle hypertrophy, edema, goblet cell hyperplasia, and infiltration of inflammatory cells into airway walls. These features have been noted in autopsy material not only from adults but also from pediatric patients of varying ages.[4] We also know that severe asthma can be characterized by similar pathologic findings. For example, Cutz et al[5] found that biopsy samples obtained from children with severe but clinically stable asthma had features that were also found when the disease led to death. This observation is especially important to keep in mind when considering the length of time it may take for the functional assessment of airway mechanics to return to an acceptable level after an acute episode of the disease.

With the more recent use of bronchoalveolar lavage (BAL) and endobronchial biopsies to address asthma pathogenesis, it is apparent that even clinically mild asthma is also characterized by airway inflammation.[6,7] The most frequent features of this inflammation include infiltration of airways by eosinophils, activation of T cells within airways, an increase in mast cell numbers, and desquamation of airway epithelium.[8] These invasive studies have been performed primarily in adults, with a loose correlation found between indices of inflammation and the level of airway responsiveness to agents such as histamine and methacholine (see later). Although information on pediatric patients is more limited, work using BAL in older children and adolescents suggests that findings within their lungs are similar to some of the abnormalities described in adults.[9,10] For example, Ferguson et al[10] reported an association between the level of airway responsiveness to histamine and both eosinophil numbers and mast cell tryptase within BAL fluid of 6- to 16-year-old children. The characteristics of the inflammation present in lungs of preschool children with wheezing are not as clearly defined. However, this is an area being addressed through research involving analysis of lavage fluid.[11,12] Wheezing phenotypes have been characterized physiologically in infants and small children,[13] but the association between pulmonary inflammation and objective measures of airway function in this group of subjects has not been addressed.

THE PHYSIOLOGY OF ASTHMA

Asthma is defined by physiologic abnormalities. As noted earlier, these abnormalities include increased responsiveness of airways, variable airflow limitation, and reversible airway obstruction. Given these features, asthma is a disease that is best characterized in a quantitative manner by tests of lung function. Several measures of lung mechanics have been used to describe asthma during both symptomatic and asymptomatic phases of the disease.[14] These measures include lung volumes, the pressure-volume characteristics of the lung, resistance to airflow, and flow rates. A discussion of each of these measures in severe childhood asthma is presented.[15] This discussion focuses on measures most likely to be used by practicing physicians to assess asthma of varying severity in children; therefore the emphasis is primarily on flow rates and lung volumes. These considerations follow a general discussion of airway hyperresponsiveness, a fundamental feature of this disease.[16,17] This chapter also includes a review of the changes that occur in arterial blood gases as the severity of obstruction increases.

Heightened Airway Responsiveness

Airway responsiveness is commonly defined as the ease with which airways narrow in response to various nonallergic and nonsensitizing stimuli, including inhaled pharmacologic agents (e.g., histamine, methacholine) as well as natural physical stimuli (e.g., exercise, exposure to cold air). Heightened airway responsiveness to several stimuli is a hallmark of asthma.[16,17] At a time when conventional assessments of lung function are normal in children with chronic stable asthma, the airways commonly exhibit this heightened responsiveness. The most common method of quantifying airway responsiveness is to assess lung function (usually forced expiratory volume in 1 second [FEV_1]) before and after inhaling increasing concentrations of methacholine. The test is concluded when a defined decrease in lung function has been achieved; for the FEV_1, this is usually a 20% decrease from baseline values. The more responsive the airways, the less methacholine is needed to decrease lung function.

The level of airway responsiveness to pharmacologic agents has been noted to roughly correlate with the severity of disease in both adults[16] and children.[18,19] Thus asthmatic subjects who are the most responsive are generally the most symptomatic (wheeze, cough, chest tightness) and require the most medications to control their disease. Although there can be great variability in responsiveness within groups of patients classified by disease severity,[20] the concept that the level of responsiveness correlates with disease severity is important when considering factors that lead to loss of control of the disease. In this respect, the level of airway responsiveness is not static in either normal individuals or asthmatic subjects but may increase or decrease in response to various stimuli. When responsiveness increases, control of the disease is often lost in that this is when asthmatic subjects develop signs and symptoms of their disease. In general, stimuli that increase responsiveness are found in our environment and induce or exacerbate airway inflammation. For children, these stimuli commonly include various viral respiratory infections, air pollutants (including cigarette smoke), and allergens.[21]

A viral respiratory infection is a common antecedent to acute episodes of asthma in children.[22] This has been documented for several respiratory viruses, including respiratory syncytial virus[23] and rhinovirus.[24] In terms of air pollutants, both nitrogen dioxide[25] and ozone[26] have been shown to enhance airway responsiveness. Cigarette smoke is arguably the most serious environmental air pollutant in terms of the respiratory health of children and has been implicated in the onset as well as the perpetuation of the disease.[27-29] In addition, exposure of atopic individuals to relevant allergens can lead to significant increases in airway responsiveness that persist for days to months.[30,31] These classes of precipitants are usually considered separately, but they likely interact in an asthmatic subject's airways in ways that lead to instability of the disease.[24]

Just as airway responsiveness will increase in response to certain stimuli that lead to airway inflammation, the level of responsiveness will also decrease if measures are taken to decrease inflammation within airways.[21] These measures include use of medications with antiinflammatory properties (e.g., inhaled corticosteroids) and the avoidance of relevant allergens (atopic asthmatic subjects) and cigarette smoke.[17]

Flow Rates

The usual method of measuring the degree of airflow limitation is to assess lung function during a maximal forced exhalation.[32] The subject exhales forcibly from total lung capacity (TLC) to residual volume (RV) into either a spirometer or through a flow meter by which flow is integrated to give volume. The results are usually expressed as either a time-based recording of expired volume (spirogram) or a plot of instantaneous airflow against lung volume (maximal expiratory flow-volume [MEFV] curve). The tests of lung function derived from a spirogram are the forced vital capacity (FVC), the FEV_1, and the forced expiratory flow from 25% to 75% of the FVC (FEF_{25-75}). From the flow-volume curve, the maximal expiratory flow rate (MEFR) achieved approximates the peak expiratory flow rate (PEFR) obtained from a flow meter. Flow at 50% of the vital capacity (VC) and flows at lower lung volumes are also obtained as part of this maneuver. Because airflow is related to lung volume, plethysmography combined with the MEFV maneuver plotted as a flow-volume curve or loop allows assessment of the relationship between airflow and absolute lung volumes (Figure 34-1). Measurement of flow rates in this manner may be informative when an isovolumetric shift occurs (discussed later).

In subjects with asthma, the expected pattern of altered flow rates during an exacerbation has been described. On spirometry, both the FEV_1 and FEF_{25-75} are diminished, although the former is more preserved as a percent of predicted than the latter. On the MEFV curve, the overall shape of the flow-volume loop usually changes and there is a "scooping out" of the distal portion of the loop as one of the first abnormalities (see Figure 34-1) due to a greater decrease in flows at low lung volumes. These flows are the first to decrease and the last to return to normal. The MEFR, like its counterpart, the

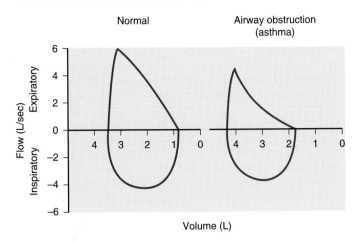

FIGURE 34-1 Maximal inspiratory and expiratory curves that together constitute a flow-volume loop are shown in a patient with asthma when the disease is under control *(left loop)* and when control is lost *(right loop)*. Flow is shown on the y-axis, whereas absolute lung volume is displayed on the x-axis. The point of maximal inspiration (TLC) is the point of zero flow on the left side of the loops while the point of maximal expiration (RV) is at the point of zero flow at the right side of the loops. When asthma control is lost, hyperinflation is noted, with an increase in RV. In addition, expiratory flow rates decrease, as demonstrated in the maximal expiratory portion of the curve, which becomes concave. With milder instability, as shown in this example, the inspiratory portion of the loop is fairly well preserved. With more severe obstruction, inspiratory flows will be more compromised. (From Wenzel SE, Larsen GL: Assessment of lung function: pulmonary function testing. In Bierman CW, Pearlman DS, Shapiro GS, et al, eds: *Allergy, asthma, and immunology from infancy to adulthood,* ed 3, Philadelphia, 1996, WB Saunders.)

FEV_1, is more preserved during the acute attacks and likewise is quicker to normalize.

In a minority of episodes of asthma, the spirogram or MEFV curve alone will not reflect significant airway obstruction. However, if subjects are studied with both an MEFV maneuver and plethysmography to assess lung volumes, they will have a displacement of the flow-volume curve to a higher lung volume without a change in the configuration of the curve itself.[33] Thus if flow is measured as a percent of the VC, no change in flow is appreciated. However, when the same curve is plotted as a function of the absolute lung volumes present before and after onset of symptoms, substantial changes in flow become apparent at the same lung volume, that is, at an isovolume. This represents an isovolumetric shift to a higher lung volume. The factors responsible for isovolumetric shifts are poorly defined but may include closure of some airways with loss of the contribution of these more-obstructed units to the flow-volume pattern.

In acute asthma, loss of symptoms and signs of asthma do not mean that lung function has returned to normal. Classic studies by McFadden et al[34] demonstrated that when patients with severe, acute asthma became asymptomatic, the overall mechanical function of their lungs in terms of the FEV_1 was still only 40% to 50% of predicted normal values. Thus loss of clinical signs of airway obstruction does not mean there has been physiologic recovery.

The use of peak flow meters within the home is an inexpensive method of monitoring a flow rate to assess asthma stability.[35] Although there are limitations in that the PEFR may be normal while other spirometric indices are abnor-

mal,[36] home monitoring with this lung function can still contribute to the care of selected patients. In this respect, significant changes in PEFR may be manifest before symptoms are evident. These devices may be especially helpful in defining the presence and severity of nocturnal asthma in individual patients.[37] Given that excessive diurnal variations in lung function during recovery from status asthmaticus have been associated with an increased risk of sudden death,[38] this vulnerable period of time may be monitored very closely within both the hospital and home environment. In the more severe patients, monitoring the PEFR as part of their daily routine may allow for earlier recognition of loss of control with more timely intervention. The diurnal variation of PEFR (i.e., the difference between morning and evening measurements) is normally less than 10%. A PEFR variability of greater than 15% to 20% has been used as one defining feature of nocturnal asthma, a common clinical manifestation of more severe asthma in both children and adults. Patients with nocturnal asthma should be regarded as having more severe disease as well as loss of asthma control.

Lung Volumes

During the exacerbation of asthma, all of the various capacities and volumes of gas contained in the lung may be altered to some extent. The RV, functional residual capacity (FRC), and TLC are usually increased (RV >> FRC >TLC), whereas the VC and its subdivisions are decreased (see Figure 34-1). These alterations have been described during natural exacerbation of asthma in adults[39] and children.[40] Although laboratory-induced changes in lung volumes (exercise, histamine challenge) may be immediately normalized with inhalation of a bronchodilator, it may take weeks after an episode of severe, acute asthma for the RV to return to a normal range.[14] The mechanisms responsible for the increases in RV, FRC (hyperinflation), and TLC (overdistension) are not completely understood. However, several factors have been identified that may contribute, including a generalized decrease in the elastic properties of the lung, a ball-valve phenomenon caused by swollen and mucus-plugged airways, and tonic activity in the intercostal muscles and diaphragm during episodes of obstruction.[14]

Arterial Blood Gases

The primary function of the lung is to provide for gas exchange such that oxygen is taken up and delivered to the body while carbon dioxide is eliminated. This function may be altered when control of asthma is lost. Several studies of acute asthma have correlated arterial blood gases with the level of airway obstruction. One of the classic descriptions is the work of McFadden and Lyons.[41] These authors studied a large population (101 subjects) who, because of age (14 to 45 years old) and medical history, were unlikely to have their asthma complicated by bronchitis and emphysema. This study and others (cited later) provide an important description of the expected abnormalities in gas exchange as a function of the degree of airway obstruction.

Oxygen Tension

McFadden and Lyons[41] found that the characteristic blood gas pattern in patients who were experiencing acute asthma was hypoxemia associated with respiratory alkalosis. The hypoxemia was the most consistent abnormality found in subjects in the study. An approximately linear correlation was found between values of FEV$_1$ and arterial oxygen tension (Figure 34-2, *top*). Patients with an FEV$_1$ of 50% to 85% of their predicted normal values were arbitrarily classified as having mild airway obstruction; those with values of 26% to 50%, moderate obstruction; and those with values of less than 25%, severe obstruction. The mean values of arterial oxygen tension (in mm Hg as measured at sea level) ranked by disease severity were 82.8, 71.3, and 63.1, respectively. Thus there was almost a 20-mm Hg difference in arterial oxygen tensions between the mild and severe groups. Just as important, it was also noted that some degree of hypoxemia was encountered at all levels of airway obstruction. In terms of studies in children, Weng et al[42] noted similar findings in asthmatic subjects who were 14 months to 14 years old. The study found that all symptomatic asthma patients were hypoxemic, with the level of hypoxemia correlating with the degree of airflow obstruction.

Several mechanisms likely contribute to the hypoxemia just described. The primary mechanism is thought to be an alteration in ventilation-perfusion ratios.[41,42] In severely obstructed subjects in whom atelectatic alveoli are still being perfused, transitory anatomic shunts may also contribute to the hypoxemia. In the most severely obstructed subjects, alveolar hypoventilation is also likely to be important.

The normal response of the body to a decrease in arterial oxygen is to increase ventilation. A reduced chemosensitivity to hypoxia coupled with a blunted perception of dyspnea may predispose patients to fatal asthma attacks. Kikuchi et al[43] found that adult patients with a history of near-fatal asthma had respiratory responses to hypoxia that were significantly lower than responses in normal subjects and in asthmatic subjects without near-fatal attacks. The lower hypoxic response was seen in conjunction with a blunted perception of dyspnea. These abnormalities could occur because of preexisting genetic factors as well as adaptation of the body to recurrent hypoxia. The relative importance of these and other factors is undefined. Children with poor perception of airway obstruction may be at risk for fatal or near-fatal asthma.[44]

Carbon Dioxide Tension

McFadden and Lyons[41] demonstrated that the characteristic blood gas pattern found in asthmatic subjects experiencing acute attacks was hypoxemia associated with respiratory alkalosis. In terms of carbon dioxide tensions, their study suggested that most attacks were associated with alveolar hyperventilation and that hypercapnia was not likely to occur until extreme degrees of obstruction were reached. Plotting airways obstruction (percent predicted FEV$_1$) against the carbon dioxide tension indicated that hypercapnia was not seen until the FEV$_1$ fell to less than 20% of its predicted value (see Figure 34-2, *bottom*). Thus a "normal" or elevated PaCO$_2$ in a patient with acute asthma is cause for concern.

Arterial Values of pH

Values of arterial pH in acute asthma have generally reflected the respiratory alkalosis noted earlier. In the study of McFadden and Lyons,[41] 73 of the 101 subjects had a respiratory alkalosis (mean pH 7.46); 21, normal pH; and 7, respiratory acidosis (mean pH 7.32). Weng et al[42] reported similar results in children. A metabolic acidosis may also be seen in acute asthma. Although this is not commonly seen in adults, it has been noted in combination with a respiratory acidosis in children with severe asthma.[42,45] When this disturbance in acid-base balance is present, it is usually associated with very severe airway obstruction.[46] Although the mechanisms responsible for the metabolic acidosis remain to be clarified, subjects with this pattern on arterial blood gas are in imminent danger of respiratory failure.[42]

FUNCTIONAL ASSESSMENTS OF ASTHMA IN INFANTS AND SMALL CHILDREN

Assessment of lung function in a quantitative manner in infants and small children is very challenging. Noninvasively assessing arterial oxygenation and gas exchange may be relatively straightforward (see later), but measuring pulmonary mechanics, including airflow and lung volumes, is more problematic. Foremost among the problems encountered in working with young subjects is that many are unable to cooperate in the performance of respiratory maneuvers needed to measure conventional respiratory mechanics. There has been progress in addressing spirometric lung function in healthy preschool children,[47] but limits remain related to the age and developmental level of the child. Thus many assessments must

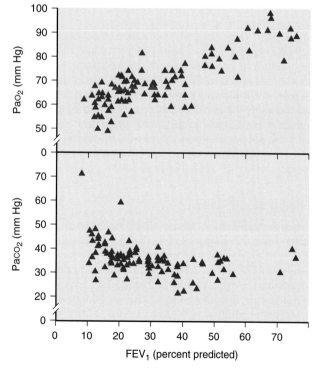

FIGURE 34-2 The relationship between arterial oxygen (mm Hg) and degree of airway obstruction (FEV$_1$ as a percent of predicted) **(top)** and the relationship between arterial carbon dioxide (mm Hg) and FEV$_1$ **(bottom)**. Although the level of hypoxemia correlates with the level of airway obstruction, an elevation in carbon dioxide levels is seen only when the FEV$_1$ is markedly compromised. (Data from McFadden ER Jr, Lyons HA: *N Engl J Med* 278:1027-1032, 1968.)

be done while the youngest subjects are sedated and asleep. In this respect, methods exist for assessing lung function in infants using spirometric techniques in which the patient is passive and forced exhaled flows are generated from near TLC to RV through rapid compression of the chest.[48] When this is accomplished, tests similar to those that can be performed in older children and adults may also be measured in young subjects. Although it is beyond the scope of this chapter to discuss in detail the methods that are used for these studies, it is important to point out that insight into normal maturation of airway function has been gained by this and similar approaches. For example, the highest flow rates corrected for lung size are found in newborns and healthy premature infants, with size-corrected flows decreasing to values found in older children and adults by the end of the first year of life.[49] In addition, studies have demonstrated that normal infants bronchoconstrict when exposed to low concentrations of bronchoreactive agents such as methacholine[50] and histamine[51] as well as to the physical stimulus of cold, dry air.[52] Goldstein et al[53] also found that the response in infants to the inhaled bronchodilator albuterol as assessed by forced expiratory flows was greatest in the youngest subjects. These observations have led to speculation that the level of responsiveness is normally quite high and decreases with postnatal maturation. Although there is an age-dependent variability in the levels of airway responsiveness in normal individuals,[54] higher levels of responsiveness in infants may also reflect technical factors inherent in the administration of a bronchoconstricting stimulus to a small airway. Nevertheless, there is information suggesting that an insult to an airway at a young age may interfere with this normal age-related decrease in responsiveness.[55,56] In this respect, the cross-sectional and longitudinal data of Montgomery and Tepper[57] demonstrate that normal infants and young children have a decrease in airway responsiveness to methacholine as they become older.

The onset of asthma is commonly during the early years of life. This has been noted in several studies, including work from Europe[58] as well as the United States.[59,60] Investigations of asthma are beginning to focus on disease pathogenesis closer to the time of onset. One practical consequence of this is that younger subjects must be assessed, given that the onset of disease is often in preschool children. In terms of quantitative assessments that help categorize disease severity as well as the effects of any intervention, measurements of lung function become essential. However, conventional methods of assessing lung function are neither technically feasible nor practical when considering multicenter studies involving large numbers of infants and preschool children. In addition, conventional lung functions are impractical in the day-to-day care of young asthmatic subjects within many clinical settings, yet other techniques offer promise when the assessment must be done in a time-effective manner in subjects with limited ability to cooperate.

Forced oscillation is one of several newer techniques that have been used to obtain lung function measures in young subjects.[49,61] This method involves the application of sine waves to the airway opening via a mouthpiece while the child breathes normally (tidal breathing). Several variables can be assessed, including resistance and reactance of the respiratory system. Although use of this technique has not been applied to large populations of children, results from a published study demonstrate a reasonable agreement with more traditional measures of lung function.[62] There are reports of the use of this technique in young children with acute asthma.[63] This technique has also been used to quantify the response to bronchoconstrictor agents, including methacholine,[62,63] in young asthmatic subjects when clinically stable. In addition, the bronchodilator response in healthy and stable asthmatic children has been addressed.[64] The results of these studies suggest that this approach may be feasible for assessing lung function to evaluate responses to therapy. This technique may also prove useful in following the course of the disease.

USES OF ASSESSMENTS OF LUNG FUNCTION

The preceding paragraphs have provided an overview of the tests of lung function that are commonly used to provide a functional assessment of asthma. Reference has been made to pathologic and physiologic correlates in the disease. This section is provided to address practical ways in which these functional assessments are commonly used. In this respect, we concentrate on lung function in diseases that may masquerade as asthma and therefore must be considered in the differential diagnosis of children with wheezing and other nonspecific pulmonary symptoms. We also address how these tests may be used to assess and follow asthma once that diagnosis has been established. In terms of the latter, the value of functional assessments during both acute and chronic phases of the disease is considered.

Functional Assessments of Diseases that Masquerade as Asthma

Shortness of breath, cough, wheezing, and chest tightness are not specific for asthma. Thus children who present in this manner may have medical problems other than asthma. The differential diagnosis of wheezing and dyspnea in pediatric subjects is influenced by the age of the patient. The younger the child, the more one has to consider congenital problems involving the airways. This is especially true for infants and toddlers. In terms of older children and adolescents, the confounding conditions will be more analogous to the problems seen in adults. We next discuss disorders that mimic asthma in which an assessment of lung function will help arrive at the correct diagnosis.

Children with bronchiolitis obliterans have experienced insults to their lungs (e.g., adenovirus infection, Stevens-Johnson syndrome with pulmonary involvement) that have led to scarring within small airways and severe airway obstruction.[65] They may present with dyspnea and/or wheezing, leading to the impression that they have asthma. On assessment of lung function, they demonstrate an obstructive pattern with evidence of hyperinflation with a decrease in flow rates. The same pattern is seen in other obstructive processes, including asthma and cystic fibrosis. The correct diagnosis may be suggested by the lack of significant reversal of the airway obstruction with therapy that includes corticosteroids. A chest radiograph and computed tomography examination of the chest may also suggest the correct diagnosis.

Pediatric patients with interstitial lung disease (ILD) may also present with dyspnea by history and poor air exchange on physical examination.[66,67] These patients have an FEV_1 that is diminished, but the FEV_1/FVC ratio is normal. In addition, lung volumes are decreased in classic presentations of ILD. This pattern is restrictive in nature compared with the obstructive pattern seen in asthma. The disease processes that lead to ILD are diverse.[66,67] Because the causes and treatments, as well as the prognosis, are much different than those of asthma, it is critical to be able to recognize this pattern on assessment of lung function and to address the potential causes that lead to interstitial disease.

Vocal cord dysfunction (VCD), a functional disorder of vocal cords that mimics attacks of asthma and/or upper airway obstruction, has received widespread attention.[68,69] Paroxysms of wheezing and dyspnea seen with VCD are refractory to standard therapy for asthma. During symptomatic episodes, the maximal expiratory and inspiratory flow-volume loop resembles a variable extrathoracic obstruction (Figure 34-3). The diagnosis is confirmed by laryngoscopy results, which demonstrate that the wheezing and/or stridor is associated with paradoxic adduction of the vocal cords during inspiration and sometimes during the entire respiratory cycle. Both the flow-volume loops and the laryngoscopic findings are completely normal when the subjects are asymptomatic. In the vast majority of patients, VCD is subconscious and may be associated with stress. In pediatric patients as young as 4 years, underlying factors such as stress related to athletic or academic performance may be found.[70-72] It must be noted that VCD and asthma frequently coexist in children.[71] Truncation of the inspiratory portion of the flow-volume loop together with a concave shape of the expiratory curve may then be found. Treatment of VCD is primarily accomplished through speech therapy together with psychotherapy in selected patients.[69] Although rarely needed, breathing a mixture of 70% helium/30% oxygen can relieve dyspnea and abort acute attacks.

Just as flow-volume loops may be helpful in making a diagnosis of VCD, they can also aid in the diagnosis of other types of obstructive lesions in the proximal airways (larynx and trachea) that may present with wheezing. For example, with a lesion that is circumferential, preventing either compression or dilation of the airway with respiratory efforts, a "fixed" pattern is seen (see Figure 34-3) with truncation of both the inspiratory and expiratory curves. Subglottic stenosis and vascular rings that surround an airway might present with such a pattern. If a lesion permits compression or dilation with respiration, the pattern will depend on the location of the lesion (intrathoracic or extrathoracic). With an extrathoracic problem, a picture like that noted previously regarding VCD is seen. With an intrathoracic lesion, more of an effect on expiratory flow rates will be found.[32] One example of such an intrathoracic lesion is tracheomalacia.

Functional Assessment of Acute Asthma

The severity of acute asthma may be gauged by findings on physical examination as well as through tests of lung function and the adequacy of oxygenation and ventilation (oximetry, arterial blood gases). In terms of the examination, use of the accessory muscles of respiration, particularly the sternocleidomastoid muscle, is an indication of significant airflow obstruction.[73] The presence of a pulsus paradoxus of greater than 20 mm Hg is also a useful indicator of severe airflow limitation in children with acute asthma.[74,75] The finding of a "quiet chest" in an anxious patient struggling to breathe is an ominous finding.

Although it is critical to recognize and appreciate the importance of these physical findings, quantitative assessments are also of great value in the patient with acute asthma. In asthmatic subjects who are extremely breathless, tests of lung mechanics, although highly desirable, may be difficult or impossible to obtain. Repeated spirometry alone may lead to greater airway obstruction in some children with moderate to severe acute asthma, precluding this manner of assessing the subject. When tests can be performed, assessments commonly include PEFR and FEV_1. Flow rates on presentation are important to record, but a lack of improvement in lung function

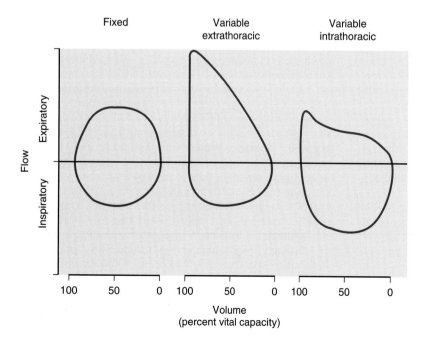

FIGURE 34-3 Flow-volume loops are displayed for various types of obstructive lesions in the proximal airways (larynx and trachea) that may present with wheezing. For comparison, the normal contour of a flow-volume loop is shown (see left side of Figure 34-1). With a lesion that is circumferential, preventing either compression or dilation of the airway with respiratory efforts, a "fixed" pattern is seen with truncation of both the inspiratory and expiratory curves. Subglottic stenosis and vascular rings that surround an airway might present with such a pattern. If a lesion permits compression or dilation with respiration, the pattern will depend on whether the lesion is intrathoracic or extrathoracic. With extrathoracic lesions (vocal cord dysfunction) *(middle)*, the inspiratory curve is more affected. An intrathoracic lesion (mass that compresses only part of the airway, tracheomalacia) *(right)* will have more of an effect on expiratory flow rates. (From Wenzel SE, Larsen GL: Assessment of lung function: pulmonary function testing. In Bierman CW, Pearlman DS, Shapiro GS, et al, eds: *Allergy, asthma, and immunology from infancy to adulthood,* ed 3, Philadelphia, 1996, WB Saunders.)

after initial treatment may be a better predictor of the need for hospitalization than the pretreatment value.[76]

In critically ill children, arterial blood gases may need to be performed at presentation and then serially as dictated by abnormalities in gas exchange and clinical status. The expected abnormalities in terms of arterial oxygen and carbon dioxide levels as a function of the level of obstruction (FEV_1) were discussed earlier and are displayed in Figure 34-2. In most clinical settings, advances made in noninvasive monitoring allow for relatively quick assessments in patients with acute asthma regardless of age or degree of obstruction; these methods include pulse oximetry and transcutaneous measurements of oxygen and/or carbon dioxide. The latter has been applied primarily to infants and children, but it has also been used in older pediatric patients.[77] Oximetry has become the most widely applied and clinically useful tool for assessing oxygenation in emergent situations. Oximeters offer a rapid and reliable noninvasive method of assessing the most vital physiologic consequence of obstructed breathing. Physical signs of hypoxemia, such as irritability, pallor, and cyanosis, are variable and may not be present at mild to moderate levels of oxygen desaturation. In children, oximetry provides a gauge of the acuity of their asthma and may be helpful in decision-making regarding the need for hospitalization. In a study from Australia, Geelhoed et al[78] found that the initial arterial oxygen saturation was highly predictive of outcome in pediatric asthma patients in an emergency department. A saturation of 91% was found to discriminate between favorable and unfavorable outcomes as defined in part by the need for subsequent care after the initial visit. In addition, continuous measurements of oxygen saturation during therapy help to minimize fluctuations in oxygenation that may be the consequence of both the disease and the therapy provided to the patient. In terms of the latter, lung mechanics may improve after inhalation of a bronchodilator while oxygenation deteriorates.[79] This phenomenon has been attributed in part to the vasodilatory effect of the drugs on the pulmonary vessels, counteracting local vasoconstrictive factors in the lung. Both oximetry and electrodes that assess transcutaneous oxygen provide a noninvasive approach that allows quick responses to fluctuating oxygen needs.

In instances when the episode is mild and the therapy is initiated early within the home environment, administration of one respiratory treatment via metered-dose inhaler (two actuations) or by nebulization (0.5 ml of a 5 mg/ml solution in 3 ml of normal saline) may lead to substantial and prolonged bronchodilation. A good response is commonly defined as a return of the PEFR to greater than 80% of that predicted or personal best, with the response sustained for 4 hours.[35] Children who improve with home bronchodilator therapy may then safely repeat this treatment as frequently as every 4 hours. Serial measurements of peak flow before and after therapy are useful not only to assess the severity of acute asthma but also to monitor the response to treatment. A lack of response or an incomplete response to inhalation of a β_2-adrenergic agonist in a patient with asthma should always be a concern and is reason for evaluation and treatment by a physician.

Functional Assessment of Chronic Asthma

As noted earlier, airway obstruction may be present in children with asthma who are asymptomatic. In a subset of subjects who deny symptoms, the degree of obstruction can be quite remarkable. When this is encountered on a child's initial evaluation, the significance of the findings is difficult to assess. Therefore serial tests of lung function in subjects with chronic asthma will be helpful in several respects. First, when several determinations are made over time, the child's personal best lung functions are defined and serve as a point of reference for that child. Second, serial tests of lung function will help support the diagnosis of asthma if fluctuations in PEFR or FEV_1 are noted spontaneously or as a result of therapy. When this lability is not seen, other diagnoses may need to be considered. Third, the functional response to therapy (or lack thereof) provides important information on the degree of reversibility in the individual child. When little or no reversibility of lung function is found in the face of significant obstruction, a disease such as bronchiolitis obliterans may be present. Fourth, simple tests of lung function may help identify subjects with increased risk of future asthma attacks[80] or subjects at the most risk for the persistence of respiratory symptoms.[81]

CONCLUSIONS

Asthma is characterized by increased responsiveness of airways to various stimuli, variable airflow limitation, and reversible airway obstruction (Box 34-1). Given these features, asthma is a disease that is best characterized in a quantitative manner by tests of lung function. During acute episodes of asthma, marked decreases in flow rates together with hyperinflation of the lungs are seen in tests of lung mechanics. In addition, hypoxemia is a common finding in subjects with wheezing, whereas hypercapnia develops as a late consequence of severe airflow obstruction. Clinical signs and symptoms of obstruction resolve long before tests of lung function, which may not normalize for some time. In a subgroup of asthmatic patients, lung function will never completely normalize. In the chronic phase of the disease, serial tests of lung function help define a child's personal best lung functions, help support the diagnosis of asthma, give clues to alternate diagnoses and complicating problems, and help identify subjects with increased risk of future asthma attacks. A fundamental knowledge of the pathophysiology of acute and chronic asthma is necessary to provide effective treatment for

---

BOX 34-1	KEY CONCEPTS
	Functional Assessment of Asthma in Pediatric Patients

- Asthma is defined by physiologic abnormalities.
- Asthma pathology has physiologic correlates.
- Inflammatory stimuli may increase airway responsiveness.
- Decreases in airflow plus hyperinflation are seen in acute asthma.
- Normalization of lung function lags behind clinical recovery in acute asthma.
- Hypoxemia correlates with the level of airway obstruction in acute asthma.
- Carbon dioxide in arterial blood increases when airway obstruction is severe.
- Serial tests of lung function are valuable in following the course of asthma.

patients with this common yet potentially life-threatening condition.

Acknowledgments

This work was supported in part by National Institutes of Health grants HL-36577 and HL-67818.

REFERENCES

1. Dunnill MS: The pathology of asthma, with special reference to changes in the bronchial mucosa, *J Clin Pathol* 13:27-33, 1960.
2. Dunnill MS, Massarella GR, Anderson JA: A comparison of the quantitative anatomy of the bronchi in normal subjects, in status asthmaticus, in chronic bronchitis, and in emphysema, *Thorax* 24:176-179, 1969.
3. Persson CGA: Centennial notions of asthma as an eosinophilic, desquamative, exudative, and steroid-sensitive disease, *Lancet* 350:1021-1024, 1997.
4. Richards W, Patrick JR: Death from asthma in children, *Am J Dis Child* 110:4-23, 1965.
5. Cutz E, Levison H, Cooper DM: Ultrastructure of airways in children with asthma, *Histopathology* 2:407-421, 1978.
6. Beasley R, Roche WR, Roberts JA, et al: Cellular events in the bronchi in mild asthma and after bronchial provocation, *Am Rev Respir Dis* 139:806-817, 1989.
7. Vignola AM, Chanez P, Campbell AM, et al: Airway inflammation in mild intermittent and in persistent asthma, *Am J Respir Crit Care Med* 157:403-409, 1998.
8. Djukanović R, Roche WR, Wilson JW, et al: Mucosal inflammation in asthma, *Am Rev Respir Dis* 142:434-457, 1990.
9. Ferguson AC, Wong FW: Bronchial hyper-responsiveness in asthmatic children. Correlation with macrophages and eosinophils in bronchoïlavage fluid, *Chest* 96:988-991, 1989.
10. Ferguson AC, Whitelaw M, Brown H: Correlation of bronchial eosinophil and mast cell activation with bronchial hyperresponsiveness in children with asthma, *J Allergy Clin Immunol* 90:609-613, 1992.
11. Marguet C, Jouen-Boedes F, Dean TP, et al: Bronchoalveolar cell profiles in children with asthma, infantile wheeze, chronic cough, or cystic fibrosis, *Am J Respir Crit Care Med* 159:1533-1540, 1999.
12. Krawiec ME, Westcott JY, Chu HW, et al: Persistent wheezing in very young children is associated with lower respiratory inflammation, *Am J Respir Crit Care Med* 163:1338-1343, 2001.
13. Stein RT, Holberg CJ, Morgan WJ, et al: Peak flow variability, methacholine responsiveness and atopy as markers for detecting different wheezing phenotypes in childhood, *Thorax* 52:936-937, 1997.
14. McFadden ER Jr: Development, structure, and physiology in the normal lung and in asthma. In Middleton E Jr, Reed CE, Ellis EF, et al, eds: *Allergy: principles and practice*, ed 5, St Louis, 1998, Mosby.
15. Larsen GL, Brugman SM: Severe asthma in children. In Barnes PJ, Grunstein MM, Leff A, eds: *Asthma*, Philadelphia, 1997, Lippincott-Raven.
16. Hargreave FE, Dolovich J, O'Byrne PM, et al: The origin of airway hyper-responsiveness, *J Allergy Clin Immunol* 78:825-832, 1986.
17. Colasurdo GN, Larsen GL: Airway hyperresponsiveness. In Busse WW, Holgate ST, eds: *Asthma and rhinitis*, ed 2, London, 2000, Blackwell Science.
18. Murray AB, Ferguson AC, Morrison B, et al: Airway responsiveness to histamine as a test for overall severity of asthma in children, *J Allergy Clin Immunol* 68:119-124, 1981.
19. Avital A, Noviski N, Bar-Yishay E, et al: Nonspecific bronchial reactivity in asthmatic children depends on severity but not on age, *Am Rev Respir Dis* 144:36-38, 1991.
20. Amaro-Galvez R, McLaughlin FJ, Levison H, et al: Grading severity and treatment requirements to control symptoms in asthmatic children and their relationship with airway hyperreactivity to methacholine, *Ann Allergy* 59:298-302, 1987.
21. Larsen GL: Asthma in children, *N Engl J Med* 326:1540-1545, 1992.
22. Rakes GP, Arruda E, Ingram JM, et al: Rhinovirus and respiratory syncytial virus in wheezing children requiring emergency care, *Am J Respir Crit Care Med* 159:785-790, 1999.
23. Hall WJ, Hall CB, Speers DM: Respiratory syncytial virus infection in adults. Clinical, virologic, and serial pulmonary function studies, *Ann Intern Med* 88:203-205, 1978.
24. Lemanske RF Jr, Dick EC, Swenson CA, et al: Rhinovirus upper respiratory infection increases airway hyperreactivity and late asthmatic reactions, *J Clin Invest* 83:1-10, 1989.
25. Bauer MA, Utell MJ, Morrow PE, et al: Inhalation of 0.3 ppm nitrogen dioxide potentiates exercise-induced bronchospasm in asthmatics, *Am Rev Respir Dis* 134:1203-1208, 1986.
26. Zwick H, Popp W, Wagner C, et al: Effects of ozone on the respiratory health, allergic sensitization, and cellular immune system in children, *Am Rev Respir Dis* 144:1075-1079, 1991.
27. Martinez FD, Antognoni G, Macri F, et al: Parental smoking enhances bronchial responsiveness in nine-year-old children, *Am Rev Respir Dis* 138:518-523, 1988.
28. Fielder HMP, Lyons RA, Heaven M, et al: Effect of environmental tobacco smoke on peak flow variability, *Arch Dis Child* 80:253-256, 1999.
29. Burr ML, Anderson HR, Austin JB, et al: Respiratory symptoms and home environment in children: a national survey, *Thorax* 54:27-32, 1999.
30. Boulet LP, Cartier A, Thomson NC, et al: Asthma and increases in nonallergic bronchial responsiveness from seasonal pollen exposure, *J Allergy Clin Immunol* 71:399-406, 1983.
31. Mussaffi H, Springer C, Godfrey S: Increased bronchial responsiveness to exercise and histamine after allergen challenge in children with asthma, *J Allergy Clin Immunol* 77:48-52, 1986.
32. Wenzel SE, Larsen GL: Assessment of lung function: pulmonary function testing. In Bierman CW, Pearlman DS, Shapiro GS, et al, eds: *Allergy, asthma, and immunology from infancy to adulthood*, ed 3, Philadelphia, 1996, WB Saunders.
33. Olive JT Jr, Hyatt RE: Maximal expiratory flow and total respiratory resistance during induced bronchoconstriction in asthmatic subjects, *Am Rev Respir Dis* 106:366-376, 1972.
34. McFadden ER Jr, Kiser R, deGroot WJ: Acute bronchial asthma. Relations between clinical and physiologic manifestations, *N Engl J Med* 288:221-225, 1973.
35. National Asthma Education and Prevention Program, Expert Panel Report II: *Guidelines for the diagnosis and management of asthma*, Bethesda, Md, April 1997, National Heart, Lung, and Blood Institute, NIH publication No. 97-4051.
36. Bye MR, Kerstein D, Barsh E: The importance of spirometry in the assessment of childhood asthma, *Am J Dis Child* 146:977-978, 1992.
37. Martin RJ: Nocturnal asthma, *Clin Chest Med* 13:533-550, 1992.
38. Hetzel MR, Clark TJH, Branthwaite MA: Asthma: analysis of sudden deaths and ventilatory arrests in hospitals, *Br Med J* 1:808-811, 1977.
39. Woolcock AJ, Read J: Lung volumes in exacerbations of asthma, *Am J Med* 41:259-273, 1966.
40. Weng TR, Levison H: Pulmonary function in children with asthma at acute attack and symptom-free status, *Am Rev Respir Dis* 99:719-728, 1969.
41. McFadden ER Jr, Lyons HA: Arterial-blood gas tension in asthma, *N Engl J Med* 278:1027-1032, 1968.
42. Weng TR, Langer HM, Featherby EA, et al: Arterial blood gas tensions and acid-base balance in symptomatic and asymptomatic asthma in childhood, *Am Rev Respir Dis* 101:274-282, 1970.
43. Kikuchi Y, Okabe S, Tamura G, et al: Chemosensitivity and perception of dyspnea in patients with a history of near-fatal asthma, *N Engl J Med* 330:1329-1334, 1994.
44. Baker RR, Mishoe SC, Zaitourn FH, et al: Poor perception of airway obstruction in children with asthma, *J Asthma* 37:613-624, 2000.
45. Downes JJ, Wood DW, Striker TW, et al: Arterial blood gas and acid-base disorders in infants and children with status asthmaticus, *Pediatrics* 42:238-249, 1968.
46. Appel D, Rubenstein R, Schrager K, et al: Lactic acidosis in severe asthma, *Am J Med* 75:580-584, 1983.
47. Eigen H, Bieler H, Grant D, et al: Spirometric pulmonary function in healthy preschool children, *Am J Respir Crit Care Med* 163:619-623, 2001.
48. Jones MH, Castile RG, Davis SD, et al: Forced expiratory flows and volumes in infants: normative data and lung growth, *Am J Respir Crit Care Med* 161:353-359, 2000.
49. Martinez FD, Morgan WJ, Holberg CJ, et al: Initial airway function is a risk factor for recurrent wheezing respiratory illnesses during the first three years of life, *Am J Respir Crit Care Med* 143:312-316, 1991.
50. Tepper RS: Airway reactivity in infants: a positive response to methacholine and metaproterenol, *J Appl Physiol* 62:1155-1159, 1987.
51. Lesouëf PN, Geelhoed GC, Turner DJ, et al: Response of normal infants to inhaled histamine, *Am Rev Respir Dis* 139:62-66, 1989.
52. Geller DE, Morgan WJ, Cota KA, et al: Airway responsiveness to cold, dry air in normal infants, *Pediatr Pulmonol* 4:90-97, 1988.
53. Goldstein AB, Castile RG, Davis SD, et al: Bronchodilator responsiveness in normal infants and young children, *Am J Respir Crit Care Med* 164:447-454, 2001.

54. Hopp RJ, Bewtra A, Nair NM, et al: The effect of age on methacholine response, *J Allergy Clin Immunol* 76:609-613, 1985.

55. Young S, LeSouëf PN, Geelhoed GC, et al: The influence of a family history of asthma and parental smoking on airway responsiveness in early infancy, *N Engl J Med* 324:1168-1173, 1991.

56. Tepper RS, Rosenberg D, Eigen H: Airway responsiveness in infants following bronchiolitis, *Pediatr Pulmonol* 13:6-10, 1992.

57. Montgomery GL, Tepper RS: Changes in airway reactivity with age in normal infants and young children, *Am Rev Respir Dis* 142:1372-1376, 1990.

58. Croner S, Kjellman N-IM: Natural history of bronchial asthma in childhood. A prospective study from birth up to 12-14 years of age, *Allergy* 47:150-157, 1992.

59. Yunginger JW, Reed CE, O'Connell EJ, et al: A community-based study of the epidemiology of asthma. Incidence rates, 1964-1983, *Am Rev Respir Dis* 146:888-894, 1992.

60. Halonen M, Stern DA, Lohman C, et al: Two subphenotypes of childhood asthma that differ in maternal and paternal influences on asthma risk, *Am J Respir Crit Care Med* 160:564-570, 1999.

61. Desager KN, Marchal F, van de Woestijne KP: Forced oscillation technique. In Stocks J, Sly PD, Tepper RS, et al, eds: *Infant respiratory function testing*, New York, 1996, Wiley-Liss.

62. Duiverman EJ, Neijens HJ, Van der Snee-van Smaalen M, et al: Comparison of forced oscillometry and forced expirations for measuring dose-related responses to inhaled methacholine in asthmatic children, *Bull Eur Physiopathol Respir* 22:433-436, 1986.

63. Klug B, Bisgaard H: Measurement of lung function in awake 2-4-year-old asthmatic children during methacholine challenge and acute asthma: a comparison of the impulse oscillation technique, the interrupter technique, and transcutaneous measurement of oxygen versus whole-body plethysmography, *Pediatr Pulmonol* 21:290-300, 1996.

64. Hellinckx J, De Boeck K, Bande-Knops J, et al: Bronchodilator response in 3-6.5 years old healthy and stable asthmatic children, *Eur Respir J* 12:438-443, 1998.

65. Hardy KA, Schidlow DV, Zaeri N: Obliterative bronchiolitis in children, *Chest* 93:460-466, 1988.

66. Fan LL, Mullen ALW, Brugman SM, et al: Clinical spectrum of chronic interstitial lung disease in children, *J Pediatr* 121:867-872, 1992.

67. Fan LL, Langston C: Chronic interstitial lung disease in children, *Pediatr Pulmonol* 16:184-196, 1993.

68. Christopher KL, Wood RP, Eckert C, et al: Vocal-cord dysfunction presenting as asthma, *N Engl J Med* 308:566-570, 1983.

69. Martin RJ, Blager FB, Gay ML, et al: Paradoxic vocal cord motion in presumed asthmatics, *Semin Respir Med* 8:332-337, 1987.

70. O'Connell MA, Sklarew PR, Goodman DL: Spectrum of presentation of paradoxical vocal cord motion in ambulatory patients, *Ann Allergy Asthma Immunol* 74:341-344, 1995.

71. Gavin LA, Wamboldt M, Brugman S, et al: Psychological and family characteristics of adolescents with vocal cord dysfunction, *J Asthma* 35:409-417, 1998.

72. Powell DM, Karanfilov BI, Beechler KB, et al: Paradoxical vocal cord dysfunction in juveniles, *Arch Otolaryngol Head Neck Surg* 126:29-34, 2000.

73. Commey JOO, Levison H: Physical signs in childhood asthma, *Pediatrics* 58:537-541, 1976.

74. Galant SP, Groncy CE, Shaw KC: The value of pulsus paradoxus in assessing the child with status asthmaticus, *Pediatrics* 61:46-51, 1978.

75. Martell JAO, Lopez JGH, Harker JEG: Pulsus paradoxus in acute asthma in children, *J Asthma* 29:349-352, 1992.

76. Schuh S, Johnson D, Stephens D, et al: Hospitalization patterns in severe acute asthma in children, *Pediatr Pulmonol* 23:184-192, 1997.

77. Holmgren D, Sixt R: Transcutaneous and arterial blood gas monitoring during acute asthmatic symptoms in older children, *Pediatr Pulmonol* 14:80-84, 1992.

78. Geelhoed GC, Landau LI, LeSouëf PN: Predictive value of oxygen saturation in emergency evaluation of asthmatic children, *Br Med J* 297:395-396, 1988.

79. Holmgren D, Sixt R: Effects of salbutamol inhalations on transcutaneous blood gases in children during the acute asthmatic attack: from acute deterioration to recovery, *Acta Paediatr* 83:515-519, 1994.

80. Fuhlbrigge AL, Kitch BT, Paltiel AD, et al: FEV_1 is associated with risk of asthma attacks in a pediatric population, *J Allergy Clin Immunol* 107:61-67, 2001.

81. Bahçeciler NN, Barlan IB, Nuhoglu Y, et al: Risk factors for the persistence of respiratory symptoms in childhood asthma, *Ann Allergy Asthma Immunol* 86:449-455, 2001.

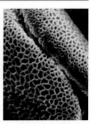

CHAPTER 35

Infections and Asthma

JAMES E. GERN ■ LEONARD B. BACHARIER ■ ROBERT F. LEMANSKE, JR.

Respiratory tract infections caused by viruses,[1,2] chlamydia,[3-7] or mycoplasma[8] have been implicated in the pathogenesis of asthma. Of these respiratory pathogens, viruses have been demonstrated to be epidemiologically associated with asthma in at least three ways (Figure 35-1). First, during infancy, certain viruses have been implicated as potentially being responsible for the inception of the asthmatic phenotype. Second, in patients with established asthma, particularly children, viral upper respiratory tract infections (URIs) play a significant role in producing acute exacerbations of airway obstruction that may result in frequent outpatient visits or in hospitalizations.[1,6,9,10] The increased propensity for viral infections to produce lower airway symptoms in asthmatic individuals may be related, at least in part, to interactions among allergic sensitization, allergen exposure, and viral infections acting as cofactors in the induction of acute episodes of airflow obstruction.[11,12] Third, and paradoxically, certain infections have been considered to have the potential of actually preventing the development of allergic respiratory tract diseases, including asthma.[13,14] For infections with other microbial agents, recent attention has focused on chlamydia[15,16] and mycoplasma[8] as potential contributors to both exacerbations and the severity of chronic asthma in terms of loss of lung function or medication requirements. Finally, infections involving the upper airways have been considered to contribute to asthma control instability, evoking the concept of a unified airway[17] in relation to inflammatory responses and alterations in airway physiology. We review these various associations as they pertain to both the pathogenesis and treatment of childhood asthma.

EPIDEMIOLOGY

Relationship of Virus-Induced Wheezing in Infancy to Childhood Asthma

In infants, infection with respiratory syncytial virus (RSV) has received much attention because of its predilection to produce a pattern of symptoms termed "bronchiolitis," which parallels many of the features of childhood and adult asthma. From 1980 to 1996, the rates of hospitalization of infants with bronchiolitis increased substantially, as did the proportion of total hospitalizations and those for lower respiratory tract infection (LRI) associated with bronchiolitis[18]; RSV causes about 70% of these episodes. However, RSV bronchiolitis represents only the most severe fraction of cases in that by age 1, 50% to 65%

of children will have been infected with this virus and by age 2 nearly 100%.[19] Children aged 3 to 6 months are most prone to the development of lower respiratory tract symptoms, suggesting that a developmental component (e.g., lung and/or immunologic maturation) may be involved as well.[19] Although controversy exists regarding the relevance of antecedent RSV infections and the development of recurrent wheezing,[20] a recent long-term prospective study of large numbers of children has demonstrated that RSV bronchiolitis is a significant independent risk factor for subsequent frequent wheezing, at least within the first decade of life.[21] It remains to be established, however, how RSV infections produce these outcomes because of the fact that virtually all children have been infected with this virus before their second birthday. Some of the factors that have been evaluated include the immune response (both innate and adaptive) to the virus and host-related differences (gender, lung size, passive smoke exposure[22]) that may predispose an infant or child to lower airway physiologic alterations as a consequence of the infection.

Recently, additional insight into these areas was provided by the results of an 11-year prospective study involving 880 children who were enrolled at birth, followed for the development of LRIs in the first 3 years of life, and then evaluated for the presence or absence of physician-diagnosed asthma and/or a history of current wheezing at the ages of 6 and 11 years.[23] Most important, lung function was evaluated in the first few months of life in a subset of these children before the development of a documented LRI. During the first 3 years of life, 7.4% had pneumonia documented radiographically and 44.7% had a significant LRI without pneumonia. RSV and parainfluenza virus were identified in 36.4% and 7.3%, respectively, of the subjects with pneumonia and in 35.6% and 15.2%, respectively, of the subjects with LRI. At age 6, physician-diagnosed asthma was present in 13.6% (odds ratio [OR] = 3.3), 10.2% (OR = 2.4), and 4.6% of the subjects with pneumonia, LRI, and no LRI, respectively. By age 11, these values increased to 25.9% (OR = 2.8), 16.1% (OR = 1.6), and 11%, respectively. Mean values of maximal volume at functional residual capacity before any LRI were lower in children with pneumonia and with LRIs than in children without LRIs. These latter results favor the hypothesis that inherent abnormalities in pulmonary function predispose infants to more severe lower respiratory tract symptoms (i.e., association vs. causation[24]). When pulmonary function measurements were evaluated at ages 6 and 11, similar group

FIGURE 35-1 Infections and asthma. Infections can influence the pathophysiology of asthma in a number of ways. First, they may be involved in the inception of the asthmatic phenotype within the first decade of life. Second, once asthma is clinically recognized, viral infections may cause disease exacerbations in patients with both intermittent and persistent phenotypes. Third, if asthma goes into remission, it is possible that certain infections may contribute to disease relapse. Fourth, infections may contribute to disease chronicity and/or severity over time. Fifth, infections (based on their type, frequency, target organ involvement, and/or timing) may actually prevent the development of allergic sensitization and perhaps asthma as well. Finally, allergic sensitization and allergen exposures may act as important cofactors in the clinical expression of the asthmatic response to various infections.

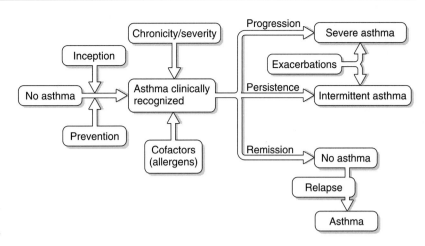

relationships persisted. Interestingly, despite the persistence of lowered baseline lung function in both the pneumonia and LRI groups, many of these deficits were markedly (but not completely) reduced after the administration of albuterol.

In a second report, further follow-up of this large cohort of children demonstrated that the risk for both frequent (> 3 episodes per year) and infrequent (≤ 3 episodes per year) wheezing in relation to RSV LRIs decreased markedly with age and became nonsignificant by age 13.[21] A decrease in the frequency of wheezing with increasing age after documented RSV infections has been observed by other investigators as well.[25,26] These data suggest that although RSV infections contribute substantially to the expression of the asthmatic phenotype, other cofactors (e.g., genetic, environmental, developmental) also appear to contribute in terms of either its initial expression or modification of the phenotype over time.

From a number of epidemiologic observations, it appears that other viral infections during infancy and early childhood that have a predisposition for lower airway involvement (e.g., parainfluenza and influenza A viruses) can also be associated with chronic lower respiratory tract symptoms, including asthma.[23,27-29] As previously stated, premorbid measurements of lung function indicate that children with reduced levels of lung function in infancy appear to be at an increased risk of the development of chronic lower respiratory tract sequelae after viral infections.[23] Whether this defect is alone responsible for these developments is presently unknown. Further, the ability of one virus (i.e., RSV) to be more likely responsible for these outcomes (because of either virus- or host-specific factors) has not been well defined.[26] Indeed, recent data indicate that rhinovirus (RV)-induced bronchiolitis, although less frequent than that induced by RSV, may cause more severe patterns of disease during infancy.[30]

Can Infections Cause Acute Exacerbations of Asthma?

The relationship between viral infections and wheezing illnesses in older children and adults has been clarified by the advent of sensitive diagnostic tests, based on the polymerase chain reaction (PCR), for picornaviruses such as RV. With the advent of these more sensitive diagnostic tools, information linking common cold infections with exacerbations of asthma has come from a number of sources. Prospective studies of subjects with asthma have demonstrated that up to 85% of

exacerbations of asthma in children and close to half of such episodes in adults are caused by viral infections.[10] Although many respiratory viruses can provoke acute asthma symptoms, RVs are most often detected, especially during the spring and fall RV seasons. In fact, the spring and fall peaks in hospitalizations because of asthma closely coincide with patterns of RV isolation within the community.[6] Influenza and RSV are somewhat more likely to trigger acute asthma symptoms in the wintertime but appear to account for a smaller fraction of asthma flares. RV infections are also frequently detected in children older than 2 years who present to emergency departments with acute wheezing,[12,31] and in adults, RV infections account for approximately half of asthma-related acute care visits.[32] Together, these studies provide evidence of a strong relationship between viral infections, particularly those because of RV, and acute exacerbations of asthma.

It is interesting that individuals with asthma do not necessarily have more colds, and neither the severity nor the duration of virus-induced *upper* respiratory symptoms is enhanced by respiratory allergies or asthma.[33,34] In contrast to findings in the upper airway, a prospective study of colds in couples consisting of one asthmatic and one normal individual demonstrated that colds cause greater duration and severity of *lower* respiratory symptoms in subjects with asthma.[34] These findings suggest that there are fundamental differences in the lower airway effects of respiratory viral infections related to asthma.

Although viral infections alone can promote lower airway symptoms, there is evidence that viral infections may exert synergistic effects together with other known triggers for asthma. For example, there is evidence that the effects of colds on asthma may be amplified by exposure to allergens[11] and possibly by exposure to greater levels of air pollutants.[35] In addition to provoking asthma, RV infections can increase lower airway obstruction in individuals with other chronic airway diseases (e.g., chronic obstructive pulmonary disease and cystic fibrosis). Thus common cold viruses that produce relatively mild illnesses in most people can cause severe pulmonary problems in selected individuals.

Can Infections Reduce the Subsequent Risk of Allergies and Asthma?

It has been suggested that some viral or bacterial infections might actually *protect* against the subsequent development of allergies and asthma. This controversial theory, termed the "hygiene hypothesis," was first suggested by David Strachan, who noted that the risk of the development of allergies and asthma is inversely related to the number of children in the family,[36] an observation that has been duplicated in a number of subsequent studies.[37,38] This finding has led to speculation that infectious diseases, which are more likely to be transmitted in large families, could modulate the development of the immune system in a manner to reduce the chances of developing allergies. This hypothesis implies that the immune system is skewed toward a T helper cell type 2 (Th2)–like response pattern at birth; in support of this concept, there is experimental evidence to show that Th1-like interferon responses are depressed at birth.[39] According to this hypothesis, each viral infection would provide a stimulus for the development and/or activation of Th1-like immune responses. The result of this repetitive stimulation would be to change the polarization of the Th system away from a Th2 overexpression and thus reduce the risk for developing allergies (Figure 35-2).

Since the 1990s, a number of epidemiologic variables have been evaluated in terms of their contribution to the hygiene hypothesis. Presently, the evidence most strongly supports a reduction in the incidence of allergic sensitization in individuals from large families, particularly the youngest in the family (birth order effect), and those living in a less-affluent environment.[14] Interestingly, these relationships are much stronger for allergic sensitization than for asthma.[40,41] Other epidemiologic and biologic factors that have been considered to influence the development of allergic sensitization and/or asthma are reviewed in detail in Chapters 1 and 2.

Can Infections Cause Chronic Asthma?

In contrast to viral illnesses, the imprecision of current diagnostic laboratory tests in temporally correlating certain microbial infections with the onset of *acute* asthma symptom exacerbations has made the verification of any etiologic relationship challenging. However, because bacterial infections are known to impair mucociliary clearance and increase

mucous production in the lung,[8] it has been proposed that certain bacterial infections may contribute to the *chronic* lower airway inflammation in asthma. Organisms primarily implicated in this process include *Chlamydia pneumoniae*[15] and *Mycoplasma pneumoniae*.[8,16] As will be discussed, if these agents contribute to asthma pathogenesis, evidence thus far most closely links them with disease *chronicity*, severity, and/or instability.

Data to support a potential role for these agents in asthma are most convincing for *C. pneumoniae*. Historically, the first potential association between asthma and *C. pneumoniae* was reported in 1991 in 19 wheezing adult asthmatic patients, of whom 9 were found to have serologic evidence of current or recent infection with this organism.[3] These initial findings were later extended by the demonstration that adults with recently diagnosed asthma had serologic evidence of chronic respiratory infection with *C. pneumoniae*.[42] It was additionally found that acute wheezing illnesses because of *C. pneumoniae* infection could herald the development of chronic asthma in previously asymptomatic individuals.[43]

In school-age children with wheezing, an unexpectedly high prevalence of low-grade *C. pneumoniae* infection has also been reported.[5] In this study, one hundred eight children (ages 9 to 11 years) with asthma symptoms longitudinally maintained (13 months) a daily diary of respiratory symptoms and peak flow rates. Nasal aspirates were obtained when respiratory symptoms were reported. The presence of *C. pneumoniae* infection was determined by PCR and serology (secretory IgA). The detection of *C. pneumoniae* infection was similar during symptomatic and asymptomatic episodes (23% vs. 28%, respectively). Children who reported multiple episodes also tended to remain PCR positive for *C. pneumoniae*, suggesting chronic infection. Further, *C. pneumoniae*-specific secretory IgA antibodies were more than 7 times greater in subjects who reported four or more exacerbations in the study compared with those who reported just one. Although there was no evidence linking acute infection with *C. pneumoniae* and acute exacerbations of asthma, these findings suggest that chronic infection with *C. pneumoniae* was more common in children with higher rates of exacerbation. It is interesting to speculate that chronic chlamydial infection promotes ongoing airway inflammation that increases susceptibility to other exacerbating stimuli such as viruses, allergens, or both.

Thus far the most comprehensive evaluation of the role of both chlamydial and mycoplasmal infections in chronic asthma was recently reported by Martin et al.[16] This group of investigators evaluated 55 adult patients with chronic asthma (percent predicted forced expiratory volume in 1 second [FEV_1] = 69.3 [2.1%]) and 11 controls for infection with *Mycoplasma*, *C. pneumoniae*, and viruses. Bronchoalveolar lavage cell count and differential, as well as tissue morphometry, were also evaluated. Of the asthmatic patients, 56% had a positive PCR for *M. pneumoniae* ($N = 25$) or *C. pneumoniae* ($N = 7$), which was mainly found in lavage fluid or biopsy samples. Only 1 of 11 control subjects had a positive PCR for *Mycoplasma*. A distinguishing feature between patients with positive and negative PCR results was the significantly greater number of tissue mast cells in the group of patients who were positive on PCR. Cultures for both organisms were negative in all patients, and serologic confirmation correlated poorly with PCR results. Although these intriguing findings suggest that these organisms may play a role in the pathophysiology of

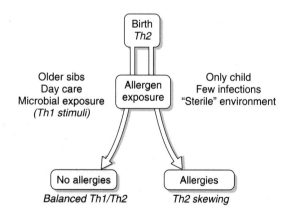

FIGURE 35-2 The hygiene hypothesis. According to this hypothesis, children are born with an immature immune system that is skewed toward T helper cell type 2 (Th2) responses. Exposure to infections or microbial products soon after birth provides Th1-like stimuli that help the immune system to develop balanced T cell responses. In the absence of these stimuli, the Th2 skewing persists, and with exposure to allergens in the environment, allergy and atopic disorders are likely to develop. (Modified from Gern JE, Busse WW: *J Allergy Clin Immunol* 106:201-212, 2000.)

asthma in some patients, the specificity of these findings to asthma and the phenotypic and genotypic characteristics of the at-risk patient need further delineation.

To further substantiate the contribution of *C. pneumoniae* to asthma, the results of pharmacologic intervention trials are noteworthy. Recently, roxithromycin was administered for 6 weeks to a group of adult asthmatic patients who had serologic evidence of concurrent infection with *C. pneumoniae*.[44] After treatment, a small but significant improvement was observed in both morning and evening peak expiratory flow rates. Although these short-term effects were statistically significant, the clinical relevance of the changes is questionable (15 L/min in the treated group vs. 3 L/min in the control group). In addition, these improvements were not sustained when evaluated 3 and 6 months after the discontinuation of therapy. Finally, because a *C. pneumoniae*−negative population of asthmatic patients was not evaluated in parallel, it is difficult to ascertain if the observed positive effects were related to an antimicrobial effect, an antiinflammatory effect, or both.[45]

If *C. pneumoniae* infection does indeed contribute to asthma chronicity, disease severity, and instability, what mechanisms may contribute to these effects? In this regard, some investigators have proposed that the development of *C. pneumoniae*−specific IgE antibody causes the release of mediators that lead to bronchospasm, airway inflammation, and airway reactivity.[46] Unless the organism were eradicated with antibiotic therapy, antigenic stimulation leading to specific IgE production would persist, thereby explaining the protracted course of asthma in some patients that is unresponsive to the aggressive use of bronchodilators and steroids.[46] In addition, as indicated previously, a major *C. pneumoniae* antigen is heat shock protein 60 (cHSP60). This protein has been implicated in the induction of deleterious immune responses in human chlamydial infections and has been found to co-localize with infiltrating macrophages in atheromatous lesions. Recently, cHSP60 was found to be a potent inducer of macrophage inflammatory responses mediated through the innate immune receptor complex TLR4-MD2 (Toll-like receptor 4).[47] These latter findings suggest that chronic asymptomatic chlamydial infections may perpetuate ongoing airway inflammatory responses through both innate and adaptive immune responses.

As briefly introduced previously, *M. pneumoniae* also has been associated with both acute and chronic asthma. Various investigators have not been able to uniformly establish the potential for mycoplasmal infections to induce acute exacerbations of asthma. Although some have reported infection in up to 25% of children with wheezing,[48] others have not been able to substantiate these observations.[5] Indeed, when the same population of children was evaluated for the relative contributions of mycoplasmal (and chlamydial) infections to acute exacerbations, viral etiologies were by far the most frequently implicated.[5] It is possible that these data may be altered in the future as more sensitive and specific serologic diagnostic tests become available and/or culture techniques improve.

In contrast to the effects of pathogenic *Mycoplasma* species on acute asthma exacerbations, associations of this microbe with chronic asthma have been more securely established. Using PCR techniques on bronchial biopsy specimens, *Mycoplasma* species have been detected in 25 of 55 adult asthmatic subjects and only 1 of 11 controls.[8] Case reports of chronic asthma beginning with *M. pneumoniae* infection suggest that this infection is potentially a causative agent in some

patients.[49] In this regard, possible causal mechanisms of *Mycoplasma*-induced airway inflammation have been investigated, including increased Th2 responses and inflammatory neuropeptides. Children with acute *M. pneumonia* have an elevated interleukin (IL)-4/interferon (IFN)-γ ratio compared with children with pneumococcal pneumonia or controls,[50] and mice experimentally infected with *M. pneumoniae* develop airway hyperresponsiveness (AHR), which is associated with decreased production of mRNA for IFN-γ.[51] In addition, asthmatic patients with *M. pneumoniae* infection detected by PCR have elevated levels of neurokinin 1, which responds to treatment with a macrolide antibiotic.[52]

One additional mechanism implicated in the pathogenesis of chronic asthmatic symptoms is latent adenovirus infection. A latent infection occurs when a virus incorporates itself into the host cell DNA and continues to periodically express viral genes. Respiratory disease caused by adenoviruses can be followed by latent infection that persists for many years.[53] A Slovenic study demonstrated that 94% of children with steroid-resistant asthma had detectable adenovirus antigens compared with 0% of controls.[54] In adults both with and without asthma, evidence of adenoviral infection has been reported to be as high as 50% of the individuals tested.[16] Although these preliminary results are intriguing, additional studies are needed to establish causality and the specificity of these observations to asthma pathogenesis and to define immunoinflammatory mechanisms contributing to these associations in both adult and pediatric patients.

WHAT IS THE RELATIONSHIP BETWEEN SINUS INFECTIONS AND ASTHMA?

The nature of the association between asthma and sinusitis in children (and adults) has been the subject of debate for many years. Recently, the concept of "one airway, one disease" has been emphasized in the diagnosis and treatment of allergic respiratory tract diseases.[17] As reviewed in Chapter 26, untreated sinus disease may contribute to unstable asthma control in some patients. Because bacterial infections are clearly involved in acute and chronic sinus disease, the mechanisms by which these microbes may promote AHR in the lower airway have been of great interest. These relationships are covered in depth elsewhere in this text and therefore are note further reviewed in this chapter.

THE IMMUNE RESPONSE TO RESPIRATORY VIRAL INFECTIONS
Immune Responses to Viral Infections

Role of Epithelial Cells
The epithelial cell is a focal point in the pathogenesis of viral respiratory infections because it serves as the host cell for viral replication and initiates innate immune responses (Figure 35-3). It has been hypothesized that other cells may become infected during viral infections. For example, airway smooth muscle cells can be infected by virus in tissue culture, suggesting a potential mechanism for viral infections to cause bronchospasm and AHR,[55,56] although this has not been verified *in vivo* (Box 35-1).

Damage to the epithelial cells can disturb airway physiology via a number of different pathways. For example, epithelial edema and shedding together with mucus production can

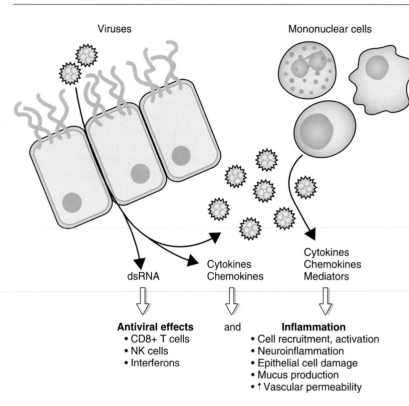

Viruses

Mononuclear cells

dsRNA

Cytokines
Chemokines

Cytokines
Chemokines
Mediators

Antiviral effects
- CD8+ T cells
- NK cells
- Interferons

and

Inflammation
- Cell recruitment, activation
- Neuroinflammation
- Epithelial cell damage
- Mucus production
- ↑ Vascular permeability

FIGURE 35-3 Virus-induced inflammation. Airway epithelial cells are the principal host cells for viral replication and, through the release of cytokines and chemokines, help to initiate the immune response to viral infection. In turn, these factors recruit mononuclear cells into the airway, and after the initial round of viral replication, these cells are activated by virus. Virus-induced cytokines, together with unique viral products such as double-stranded RNA (dsRNA), are potent inducers of antiviral responses. In addition, many of these factors promote airway inflammation and dysfunction through a number of mechanisms, as shown in the figure.

cause airway obstruction and wheezing. The immune response to the virus can also contribute to the pathogenesis of respiratory symptoms. For viruses such as RV, which infect relatively few cells in the airway, this may be the primary mechanism for airway symptoms and lower airway dysfunction.[57] Virus-induced epithelial damage can also increase the permeability of the mucosal layer,[58,59] perhaps facilitating allergen contact with immune cells and exposing neural elements to promote neurogenic inflammation.

The processes associated with viral replication trigger both innate and adaptive immune responses within the epithelial cell. Virus attachment to cell surface receptors may initiate some immune responses. For example, RSV infection activates signaling pathways in airway epithelial cells through the surface molecule TLR4.[60] There also is evidence of receptor-independent pathways for virus activation of epithelial cells, such as the generation of oxidative stress.[61]

Replication of viral RNA can also stimulate antiviral responses in epithelial cells. Double-stranded RNA (dsRNA) that is synthesized in virus-infected cells can bind to cell surface receptors and directly activate intracellular enzymes, such as the dsRNA-dependent protein kinase (PKR) and 2,5-oligoadenylate synthase, which are important components of the innate antiviral immune response.[62] Via this mechanism, viral replication induces innate antiviral activity through the generation of nitric oxide, activation of RNase L, and inhibition of protein synthesis within infected cells. In addition, dsRNA generated during viral infections promotes the activation of chemokine genes such as IL-8 and RANTES (regulated on activation, normal T cells expressed and secreted), which recruit inflammatory cells into the airway.[63] Thus host cell recognition of dsRNA is an important pathway for the initiation of multiple and antiviral and proinflammatory pathways within the cell.

Proinflammatory and Antiviral Leukocyte Responses

During natural infection, the initial inoculum that transmits the illness is presumed to be quite small; however, during sampling, viral titers in respiratory secretions can attain 10^6 infectious units/ml, even after dilution by nasal lavage.[64] At this point it is likely that mononuclear cells are activated by these high titers of virus. Monocytes, macrophages, and presumably dendritic cells can be activated by viruses to secrete proinflammatory cytokines such as IL-1, IL-8, IL-10, tumor necrosis factor (TNF)-α, and IFN-γ.[65-67] These cytokines activate other cells in the environment and are potent inducers of adhesion molecules. Together with chemokines generated by epithelial cells, this response provides a potent stimulus for inflammatory cell recruitment.

Acute respiratory viral infections are often accompanied by neutrophilia of upper and lower respiratory secretions, and it is likely that products of neutrophil activation are involved in obstructing the airways and causing lower airway symptoms.[68,69] Of particular interest is evidence that activated neutrophils, through the release of the potent secretagogue elastase, can up-regulate goblet cell secretion of mucus.[70] In addition, changes in IL-8 levels in nasal secretions have been related to respiratory symptoms and virus-induced increases in AHR.[71,72] These findings suggest that neutrophils and neutrophil activation products contribute to airway obstruction and symptoms during viral infections and exacerbations of asthma.

Relationship of Mononuclear Cell Responses to Outcome of Viral Infections

Lymphocytes are recruited into the upper and lower airways during the early stages of a viral respiratory infection, and it is presumed that innate and adaptive immune responses serve to limit the extent of infection and to clear virus-infected epithelial cells. This is consistent with reports of severe viral LRIs in immunocompromised patients.[73]

For RSV, the G (attachment) and F (fusion) proteins are the major surface glycoproteins against which neutralizing antibody is directed. Interestingly, in both murine[74] and human[75] *in vitro* experiments, it has been noted that the G protein elicits a predominant Th2 immune response, whereas the F protein and infectious RSV produce a predominant Th1 response. This property of the G protein has led to speculation that this may be a mechanism by which RSV promotes allergen sensitization.

In murine models, RSV infections are associated with the development of AHR and an augmented allergic airway response.[77] Some[78] but not all[79] investigators have demonstrated that these alterations are related to increased production of the Th2-like cytokine IL-13 in the airway.

These and other animal models of respiratory viral infection suggest that cellular immune responses and patterns of cytokine production may be related to the outcome of respiratory infections. This same concept has been tested in a limited number of studies involving humans. For example, reduced peripheral blood mononuclear cell (PBMC) production of IFN-γ both during and months after RSV has been observed in only those children who developed subsequent asthma.[80] In contrast, concentrations of IFN-γ in upper airway secretions are increased during episodes of virus-induced wheezing compared with URIs.[81]

Additional information has been obtained by evaluating immune responses in volunteers inoculated with a strain of RV. PBMC responses to RV-16 *in vitro* were assessed in a group of volunteers who were then inoculated with the same virus. Individuals who had strong IFN-γ responses to virus in peripheral blood cells shed less virus during the peak of the cold.[82] In addition, cytokine patterns in sputum have been compared with the outcome of experimentally induced RV infection. A stronger Th1-like response in sputum cells (higher IFN-γ/IL-5 mRNA ratio) during the acute cold was associated with milder cold symptoms and more rapid clearance of the virus.[64] Together, these experimental findings suggest that the cellular immune response to respiratory viruses, IFN-γ production in particular, can influence the clinical and virologic outcomes of infection.

Finally, PBMC secretion of the antiinflammatory cytokine IL-10 has also been evaluated in relation to RSV-induced

bronchiolitis resulting in hospitalization.[83] During the convalescent phase (3 to 4 weeks after illness onset), IL-10 responses were significantly increased in patients compared with those in healthy control subjects. At follow-up, 58% of the children had recurrent episodes of wheezing. IL-10 levels, measured during the convalescent phase, were significantly higher in patients who developed recurrent wheezing during the year after RSV bronchiolitis than in patients without recurrent episodes of wheezing. Moreover, IL-10 responses during the convalescent phase correlated significantly with the number of wheezing episodes. Interestingly, no association was found between IFN-γ responses, IL-4 responses, or IFN-γ/IL-4 ratios and recurrent wheezing. Unfortunately, in all of the studies reported thus far, the pattern of cytokine response these infants had *before* infection was not evaluated, begging the question as to which of the observed results may be the cause and which may be the effect.

MECHANISMS OF VIRUS-INDUCED WHEEZING AND ASTHMA

Interactions between Viral Infections and Allergy

In addition to premorbid lung function, the influence of atopy on the development of the asthmatic phenotype in relation to viral infections has been evaluated. Interactions between these two factors appear to be bidirectional and dynamic in that the atopic state can influence the lower airway response to viral infections,[22,84] viral infections can influence the development of allergen sensitization,[85,86] and interactions can occur when individuals are exposed simultaneously to both allergens and viruses[87,88] (Box 35-2).

Atopy can be defined as the genetic predisposition to the preferential development of an IgE antibody response to a variety of environmental allergens. As stated previously, atopy has been considered to be a risk factor for the development of childhood asthma, and its influence on the pattern of responses after viral infections has been of interest to many investigative groups. It has also been suggested that atopy could be a significant predisposing factor for the development of

BOX 35-2	**KEY CONCEPTS**
	Mechanisms of Virus-Induced Asthma and Wheezing

- Upper respiratory tract infections (common "colds") frequently cause exacerbations of asthma in children.
- Interactions between respiratory viral infections and allergic sensitization followed by relevant allergen exposure can be bidirectional and dynamic in their ability to influence asthma symptom development and control.
- Respiratory viral infections may enhance underlying airway inflammation in asthma in at least two ways.
  Directly through viral infection of lower airway epithelial cells
  Indirectly after infection of the upper airway through the generation of systemic immune responses
- A characteristic feature of respiratory viral infections is their ability to enhance airway responsiveness in both normal and asthmatic individuals.

acute bronchiolitis during RSV epidemics.[89] Although some have found that those children most likely to have persistent wheezing were children born to atopic parents,[89-91] others have not found this.[92,93] Although some have found that personal atopy is not more prevalent in symptomatic children *after* bronchiolitis,[21,93] others have found that documented RSV bronchiolitis significantly increases a child's chances (32% vs. 9% in controls) of subsequent development of IgE antibody[85] or lymphocyte proliferative responses[94] to both food and aeroallergens.

RSV infections may interact with immunoinflammatory mechanisms involved in immediate hypersensitivity responses in a number of ways.[95] First, it has been suggested that viruses capable of infecting lower airway epithelium may lead to enhanced absorption of aeroallergens across the airway wall, predisposing to subsequent sensitization.[96,97] Second, RSV-specific IgE antibody formation may lead to mast cell mediator release within the airway, resulting in the development of bronchospasm and the ingress of eosinophils.[98-100] Third, airway resident and inflammatory cell generation of various cytokines (TNF-α, IL-10, IL-12, IL-6),[101-104] chemokines (MIP-1α, RANTES, MCP-1, IL-8),[105,106] leukotrienes,[81] and adhesion molecules (intracellular adhesion molecule [ICAM]-1)[101] may further up-regulate the ongoing inflammatory response. Finally, similar to various allergenic proteins,[107] the processing of RSV antigens and their subsequent presentation to lymphocyte subpopulations may provide a unique mechanism of interaction to promote a Th2-like response in a predisposed host.

Studies have been performed using the techniques of bronchoscopy and experimental viral inoculation to understand RV-induced inflammation in the lower airway and interactions with allergen-induced inflammation. These studies have demonstrated that RV infections can enhance lower airway histamine responses and eosinophil recruitment in response to allergen challenge.[88,108] In addition, during an RV infection, study subjects had enhanced immediate responses to allergen and were more likely to have a late asthmatic response after allergen challenge.[87] These findings suggest that RV can enhance both the immediate- and the late-phase responses to allergen.

Other interactions between allergy and RV infections have been observed in clinical studies involving natural infections. In these studies, risk factors for developing acute wheezing episodes were ascertained in children who presented to an emergency department.[12] Individual risk factors for developing wheezing included detection of a respiratory virus, most commonly RV; positive allergen-specific IgE as detected by radioallergosorbent testing (RAST); and either eosinophilia or evidence of eosinophil degranulation in nasal secretions. Notably, there also was evidence of a synergistic effect between viral infections and allergic inflammation (eosinophilia or positive RASTs) in determining the risk of wheezing.[12] Furthermore, other studies have shown that experimental inoculation with RV is more likely to increase airway responsiveness in allergic individuals than in nonallergic individuals.[109] Finally, the risk of hospitalization among virus-infected individuals is increased in patients who are both sensitized and exposed to respiratory allergens.[11] When considered together, these findings provide strong evidence that individuals with either respiratory allergies or eosinophilic airway inflammation have an increased risk for wheezing with viral infections.

Mechanisms of Virus-Induced Exacerbations of Asthma

Extension of Common Cold Infections into the Lower Airway

By damaging the epithelium and inducing inflammatory responses, viral infections have the potential to induce airway inflammation and respiratory symptoms in anyone, yet individuals with asthma and other chronic lung diseases are at a greater risk for virus-induced lower airway compromise.[34] Efforts to account for this heightened sensitivity to lower airway effects of common cold infections led to the hypothesis that common cold infections, which were initially thought to be restricted to upper airway tissues, extend to involve the lower airways.

RV has traditionally been considered to be an upper airway pathogen because of its association with common cold symptoms and the observation that RV replicates best at 33° to 35° C, which approximates temperatures in the upper airway. There is evidence to indicate, however, that temperature may not be a barrier to RV replicating in lower airway tissues. In fact, lower airway temperatures have been directly mapped using a bronchoscope equipped with a thermister.[110] During quiet breathing at room temperature, airway temperatures are conducive to RV replication down to second-generation bronchi and exceed 35° C only in the periphery of the lung. Moreover, RV appears to replicate equally well in cultured epithelial cells derived from either upper or lower airway epithelium.[63] Finally, although RV has been difficult to culture from the lower airway, it has been detected in lower airway cells and secretions by both reverse transcription–PCR and *in situ* hybridization of mucosal biopsies after experimental inoculation.[111,112] These findings establish that RV can replicate in the lower airway epithelium at temperatures found in large airways of the lung. This concept is further supported by evidence that RV infections can produce lower airway inflammation, including increased neutrophils in bronchial lavage fluid,[113] influx of T cells and eosinophils into lower airway epithelium,[114] and enhanced epithelial expression of ICAM-1.[115]

Remaining challenges include determining how much virus is present in the lower airway and establishing whether viral replication in the lower airway is a sufficient stimulus to provoke exacerbations of asthma. If the degree of RV infection in the lower airway is trivial and therefore insufficient to trigger small airway obstruction, this implies that there are alternate mechanisms for the deterioration of asthma during viral URI. Mechanisms that have been proposed include systemic immune activation, the existence of reflex bronchospasm triggered by upper airway inflammation, and the aspiration of inflammatory cells and mediators that are generated in the upper airway.[116]

Effects of Viral Infections on Airway Hyperresponsiveness

Information derived from animal models, as well as clinical studies of natural or experimentally induced viral infections, indicates that viruses can enhance AHR, which is one of the key features of asthma. The clinical studies have generally shown that viral infections cause mild increases in airway responsiveness during the time of peak cold symptoms and that these changes can sometimes last for several weeks. A heightened sensitivity to inhaled irritants and greater maximum bronchoconstriction in response to these stimuli have been observed. The mechanism of virus-induced airway responsiveness is likely to be multifactorial, and contributing factors are likely to include impairment in the inactivation of tachykinins, viral effects on nitric oxide production, and virus-induced changes in neural control of the airways.[117]

Tachykinins, which are synthesized by sensory nerves, are potent bronchoconstrictors and vasodilators and, through these effects, have the potential to cause severe airway obstruction. Because airway epithelial cells help to regulate tachykinin levels through the production of the enzyme neutral endopeptidase, loss of this enzyme activity in epithelium that has been damaged by viral infection could lead to airway obstruction.[118] Nitric oxide can regulate both vascular and bronchial tone and can interfere with the replication of some viruses.[119] Nitric oxide synthesis is enhanced by viral infections,[120] but because of the many potential effects of nitric oxide on the lower airways, it is uncertain as to whether this is beneficial to lower airway function in asthma.

Viruses can also affect airway tone and responsiveness by enhancing vagally mediated reflex bronchoconstriction, and this has been demonstrated in humans and in animal models. One potential mechanism for this effect is virus interference in the function of the M2 muscarinic receptor.[121] The M2 receptors are part of an important negative feedback loop that limits the release of acetylcholine from vagal nerve endings. When the M2 receptor is damaged by viral infection or virus-induced interferon,[122,123] bronchoconstriction is enhanced, leading to increased airway obstruction. Further delineation of this pathway may lead to novel treatments for virus-induced asthma symptoms that are refractory to standard therapy.

TREATMENT

Virus-Induced Wheezing in Infancy

Standard therapy for virus-induced wheezing in young children generally includes a stepwise addition of medications, typically commencing with a bronchodilator. If lower respiratory tract symptoms become increasingly severe or respiratory distress develops, oral corticosteroids are often added. Recent clinical trials in the management of these wheezing episodes also have included the use of high-dose inhaled corticosteroids (ICSs) (both prophylactically and as an acute intervention) and leukotriene receptor antagonists (Box 35-3).

The efficacy of various therapeutic interventions for the acute symptoms of wheezing, tachypnea, retractions, and hypoxemia that occur as a result of bronchiolitis has been controversial because of variations in study design, the inability to rapidly and conveniently measure pulmonary physiologic variables, the confounding of results by the inclusion of children with a history of multiple wheezing episodes (i.e., asthmatic phenotypes), and the choice of outcome measures that have been evaluated. In a recent Cochrane meta-analysis of this subject,[124] bronchodilators were found to produce modest short-term improvements in clinical features of mild or moderately severe bronchiolitis; no differences in the rate or duration of hospitalization were noted. However, given the high costs and uncertain benefit of this therapy, the authors concluded that bronchodilators could not be recommended for routine management of first-time wheezers. They further recommended that before conducting future treatment trials, an

---

BOX 35-3

KEY CONCEPTS

Treatment of Virus-Induced Asthma: Prevention and Intervention

- Inhaled corticosteroid (ICS) treatment after respiratory syncytial virus bronchiolitis does not significantly decrease the development of chronic lower airway symptomatology.
- Chronic treatment with ICS does not reduce the frequency or severity of intermittent virus-induced wheezing episodes.
- Treatment of virus-induced asthma exacerbations with oral corticosteroids significantly improves a number of outcome measures.
    The overall and comparative efficacy of the treatment of similar episodes with either high-dose ICS or leukotriene modifiers warrants further study.

---

outcome measure that reflects pulmonary status independent of the level of alertness needs to be validated.

The efficacy of therapy with either oral or parenteral corticosteroids was recently reviewed in a meta-analysis of studies that sought to evaluate this form of intervention.[125] Of 12 relevant publications, 6 met the selection criteria and had relevant data available. Corticosteroid therapy (prednisone, prednisolone, methylprednisone, hydrocortisone, or dexamethasone, with routes of administration being oral, intramuscular, or intravenous; dose ranges, 0.6 to 6.3 mg/kg/day of prednisone equivalents) was associated with a statistically significant reduction in clinical symptom scores and length of hospital stay. The effects of corticosteroids on improving clinical symptom scores were apparent within 24 hours of treatment initiation. The authors also indicated that their analyses suggested that corticosteroid treatment might have its greatest effects in more severe cases.

Effect of Corticosteroids for the Prophylactic Treatment of Chronic Respiratory Tract Symptoms Associated with Respiratory Syncytial Virus—Induced Bronchiolitis

Several placebo-controlled trials that address the question of whether corticosteroid treatment can influence the degree of respiratory sequelae after RSV bronchiolitis were recently reviewed.[26] The majority (7 of 10) of these trials did not show any long-term effects (follow-up time, 6 months to 5 years) on postbronchiolitic wheezing, the development of various wheezing phenotypes (transient, persistent, or late onset), or a subsequent diagnosis of asthma. In the trials that did show some benefit, the positive effects observed were mainly over shorter time intervals after infection. One study[126] concluded that the greatest benefit was more likely to be seen in atopic children.

Role of Oral Corticosteroids in Acute Exacerbations of Asthma in Young Children

Numerous studies have been undertaken to assess the role of corticosteroid therapy in acute episodes of asthma in children and adults. A meta-analysis of these studies supports the early use of systemic corticosteroids in acute exacerbations based on a reduction in the admission rate for asthma and prevention of relapse in the outpatient treatment of exacerbations.[127] As a reflection of such information, the most recent National Heart, Lung, and Blood Institute Guidelines for the Diagnosis and Management of Asthma recommends the addition of corticosteroids for asthma exacerbations unresponsive to bronchodilators. These guidelines suggest either doubling the dose of maintenance ICSs for mild episodes unresponsive to bronchodilators or adding oral corticosteroids for the management of moderate and severe exacerbations.[128] Unfortunately, the applicability of these recommendations to young children and infants whose acute wheezing episodes are primarily related to viral respiratory tract infections has not been as thoroughly evaluated.

However, results from a few clinical trials are noteworthy. Brunette et al[129] explored the role of early intervention with oral corticosteroid therapy in 32 children under the age of 6 years (mean age, 38.4 months) with asthma typically provoked by viral URI. During the first year of this 2-year study, acute exacerbations were treated with oral bronchodilators initially, with the addition of prednisone for more severe attacks. In the second year, oral prednisone was administered at the first sign of a URI to a group of patients whose parents and caretakers were unblinded to the treatment intervention. The group receiving prednisone during the second year experienced fewer attacks, a 65% reduction in the number of wheezing days, a 61% decrease in emergency department visits, and a 90% decrease in hospitalizations. The administration of prednisone at the first sign of URI was not associated with greater overall prednisone use. Although this study suggests that early intervention with oral corticosteroids has the potential to significantly affect the morbidity associated with acute virus-induced asthma episodes, the unblinded study design makes these results less convincing.

Tal et al[130] conducted an emergency department–based, double-blind, placebo-controlled trial of administration of a single dose of methylprednisolone intramuscularly and demonstrated a statistically significant decrease in hospitalization rate (20% in the methylprednisolone group vs. 43% in the control group, $P < 0.05$); this effect was most pronounced in the group less than 24 months old (18% in methylprednisolone group vs. 50% in control group, $P < 0.050$). Taken together, the results of these two studies suggest that early corticosteroid therapy, ideally started at home, should have an impact on the progression of asthma episodes and decrease the rate of hospitalization for asthma.

Role of Inhaled Corticosteroids in the Treatment of Acute Asthma Exacerbations

Young children who experience frequent exacerbations of asthma may receive several short courses of systemic corticosteroids during each viral season. Individual courses of oral corticosteroids may be associated with behavioral side effects. In addition, Dolan et al[131] reported that 20% of children who received four or more short courses of oral corticosteroids in the past year had impaired responses to insulin-induced hypoglycemia. The potential toxicity of repeated courses of oral corticosteroids is a significant clinical concern and likely influences the behaviors of pediatricians faced with young children who wheeze after having URI symptoms. The use of top-

ical ICSs in the treatment of acute exacerbations is likely to be accompanied by a greater safety profile and parental acceptance.

The efficacy of ICS intervention has been evaluated by at least six different research groups. First, Wilson and Silverman[132] examined the use of beclomethasone dipropionate (750 μg 3 times daily for 5 days administered via metered-dose inhaler [MDI]) at the first sign of an asthma episode in children 1 to 5 years of age. Although failing to alter the need for additional therapy, ICS therapy was associated with improvement in asthma symptoms during the first week of the episode. Second, Daugbjerg et al[133] conducted a double-blind, placebo-controlled trial comparing the effects of inhaled bronchodilator alone or in combination with either high-dose ICS (budesonide nebulization 0.5 mg every 4 hours until discharge) or systemic corticosteroid (prednisolone) in children younger than 18 months who were admitted to a hospital with acute wheezing. Their results demonstrated earlier discharge from the hospital in both the inhalation and systemic corticosteroid–treated groups, as well as a significantly accelerated rate of clinical improvement in the budesonide-treated group compared with the oral corticosteroid– and noncorticosteroid-treated groups. Third, Connett and Lenney[134] compared the efficacy of two doses of budesonide (800 or 1600 μg twice daily) via MDI and a spacer device initiated at the onset of upper respiratory tract symptoms in preschool-aged children with recurrent wheezing with URIs. Therapy was continued for up to 7 days or until patients were asymptomatic for 24 hours. Budesonide therapy was associated with decreased symptom scores during the first week of infection. Fourth, a double-blind, placebo-controlled crossover study by Svedmyr et al[135] involved the administration of budesonide (200 μg 4 times daily for 3 days, 3 times daily for 3 days, and then twice daily for 3 days) via MDI and spacer or placebo to children 3 to 10 years of age with a history of URI-associated deterioration of asthma. Although budesonide therapy had no significant impact on symptom scores, it was associated with significantly higher peak expiratory flow rates. Fifth, in a recent emergency department–based study, Volovitz et al[136] compared the effects of inhaled budesonide and oral prednisolone in children aged 6 to 16 years with acute asthma exacerbations. Patients received either budesonide 1600 μg by Turbuhaler or 2 mg/kg of oral prednisolone in the emergency department followed by a tapering dose of medication over the next 6 days. Both treatment groups had similar rates of improvement in the emergency department in terms of symptom scores and peak expiratory flow. However, over the next week, the budesonide-treated group had a more rapid improvement in asthma symptoms. Serum cortisol levels and response to corticotropin were significantly decreased in the prednisolone-treated group at the end of the week of therapy compared with the budesonide-treated group but returned to the normal range 2 weeks later. This study suggests that high-dose therapy with a potent ICS may be as effective as oral prednisolone and avoids hypothalamic-pituitary-adrenal axis suppression. Sixth, a recent study comparing the effects of high-dose ICSs and oral corticosteroids in children seen in an emergency department for severe, acute asthma (mean FEV_1, < 40% predicted on presentation) found oral corticosteroids to be superior in terms of improvement in lung function and hospitalization rate.[137] However, these patients were clearly in the middle of severe exacerbations, and ICSs were not used early in the course of the illness.

In summary, ICSs appear to improve asthma symptoms when administered for acute exacerbations of asthma. Although all of these studies provide useful information, they are limited by small numbers of patients and do not delineate features predictive of patients who would be expected to respond to a given therapy. In addition, the ideal drug, dosage, delivery system, and duration of therapy remain unclear. Improved delivery of a potent drug to the lower airways may be associated with a more favorable clinical response.

Role of Leukotrienes in Virus-Induced Wheezing

The cysteinyl leukotrienes have been identified as important mediators in the complex pathophysiology of asthma. Leukotrienes are detectable in the blood, urine, nasal secretions, sputum, and bronchoalveolar lavage fluid of patients with chronic asthma. In addition, leukotrienes are released during acute asthma episodes. Volovitz et al[99] demonstrated elevated levels of leukotriene C_4 (LTC_4) in nasopharyngeal secretions from infants with acute bronchiolitis because of RSV compared with children with upper respiratory illnesses alone. A recent study by van Schaik et al[81] also examined leukotriene levels in nasopharyngeal samples from infants and young children with URIs without wheezing, bronchiolitis (first-time wheezers), or acute episodes of wheezing in children with prior wheezing episodes. These investigators found elevated levels of leukotrienes in nasopharyngeal samples from both first-time and recurrent viral wheezers compared with children with nonwheezing URIs. Finally, bronchoalveolar lavage samples obtained from recurrently wheezing young children (median age, 14.9 months) have been found to contain not only an increase in the numbers of epithelial and inflammatory cells but also increased levels of cyclooxygenase and lipoxygenase pathway mediators.[138] Interestingly, the levels of these cells and mediators were unaffected by concurrent treatment with ICSs. These studies, when combined with *in vitro* data demonstrating increased 5-lipoxygenase activity with RSV infection of bronchial epithelial cell lines[139] or reductions in RSV-induced airway edema in rats after treatment with a leukotriene receptor antagonist,[140] suggest a potential role of leukotrienes in acute, episodic, viral-induced wheezing.

CONCLUSIONS

As reviewed, respiratory tract infections have the potential to influence the pathophysiology of asthma in a number of ways, including inception, exacerbation, and disease chronicity and severity over time (see Figure 35-1). As such, current research initiatives have focused on therapeutic interventions that may attenuate or abrogate these relationships. Given the close relationship between viral infections and wheezing illnesses in children, it would be attractive to apply antiviral strategies to the prevention and treatment of asthma, and both RV and RSV are obvious targets. Unfortunately, attempts at developing an RSV vaccine have so far been unsuccessful, and vaccination to prevent RV infection does not seem to be feasible because of the large number of serotypes. As an alternative, several types of antiviral agents are in development, and several compounds with activity against RV have been tested in clinical trials. These include molecules such as soluble ICAM

and capsid-binding agents, which either hinder RV binding to cellular receptors or inhibit uncoating of the virus to release RNA inside the cell,[141-144] and inhibitors of RV 3C protease. One problem with the use of antiviral medications is that once the clinical signs and symptoms appear, viral replication is well under way. As a result, reductions in respiratory symptoms or the duration of illness are modest.[144] Studies of neuraminidase inhibitors for the treatment of influenza have yielded similar results.[145] In fact, these medications are most effective when given prophylactically because they prevent 85% of clinically apparent cases of influenza.[146] For influenza, this approach has no advantage over the less costly alternative of immunization, but preventive use of an antiviral medication may be a viable strategy for viruses for which vaccines are not available.

The other potential therapeutic approach for respiratory viral infections would be to inhibit proinflammatory immune responses induced by the virus. This approach has proved to be effective because the systemic administration of glucocorticoids can reduce acute airway obstruction and the risk of hospitalization for virus-induced exacerbations of asthma. It should be noted that oral corticosteroids are ineffective at relieving upper airway symptoms of RV infections, indicating that there are differences in the pathogenesis of these two clinical syndromes.[147] It remains to be demonstrated whether more focused inhibition of specific components of virus-induced inflammation, such as proinflammatory cytokines (e.g., IL-8) or mediators (leukotrienes, bradykinin), will be successful in reducing the severity of viral respiratory infections or exacerbations of asthma.

Acknowledgments

This work was supported by National Institutes of Health grants AI-34891, HL-56396, 1RO1-HL-61879, and P01-HL-070831.

HELPFUL WEBSITES

The National Heart, Lung and Blood Institute website (www.nhlbi.nih.gov)
The American Academy of Allergy Asthma and Immunology website (www.aaaai.org)
The Childhood Asthma Research and Education Network website (www.asthma-carenet.org)
The Asthma Clinical Research Network website (www.acrn.org)

REFERENCES

1. Folkerts G, Busse WW, Nijkamp FP, et al: Virus-induced airway hyperresponsiveness and asthma, *Am J Respir Crit Care Med* 157:1708-1720, 1998.
2. Lemanske RF Jr, Lemen RJ, Gern JE: Infections in childhood. In Barnes PJ, Grunstein MM, Leff AR, et al, eds: *Asthma*, Philadelphia, 1997, Lippincott-Raven.
3. Hahn DL, Dodge RW, Golubjatnikov R: Association of *Chlamydia pneumoniae* (strain TWAR) infection with wheezing, asthmatic bronchitis, and adult-onset asthma, *JAMA* 266:225-230, 1991.
4. Cook PJ, Davies P, Tunnicliffe W, et al: *Chlamydia pneumoniae* and asthma, *Thorax* 53:254-259, 1998.
5. Cunningham AF, Johnston SL, Julious SA, et al: Chronic *Chlamydia pneumoniae* infection and asthma exacerbations in children, *Eur Respir J* 11:345-349, 1998.
6. Johnston SL, Pattemore PK, Sanderson G, et al: The relationship between upper respiratory infections and hospital admissions for asthma: a time-trend analysis, *Am J Respir Crit Care Med* 154:654-660, 1996.

7. Von Hertzen L, Töyrylä M, Gimishanov A, et al: Asthma, atopy and *Chlamydia pneumoniae* antibodies in adults, *Clin Exp Allergy* 29: 522-528, 1999.

8. Kraft M, Cassell GH, Henson JE, et al: Detection of *Mycoplasma pneumoniae* in the airways of adults with chronic asthma, *Am J Respir Crit Care Med* 158:998-1001, 1998.

9. Johnston SL, Pattemore PK, Sanderson G, et al: Role of virus infections in children with recurrent wheeze or cough, *Thorax* 48:1055-1060, 1993.

10. Johnston SL, Pattemore PK, Sanderson G, et al: Community study of role of viral infections in exacerbations of asthma in 9-11 year old children, *Br Med J* 310:1225-1229, 1995.

11. Green RM, Custovic A, Sanderson G, et al: Synergism between allergens and viruses and risk of hospital admission with asthma: case-control study, *Br Med J* 324:763, 2002.

12. Rakes GP, Arruda E, Ingram JM, et al: Rhinovirus and respiratory syncytial virus in wheezing children requiring emergency care. IgE and eosinophil analyses, *Am J Respir Crit Care Med* 159:785-790, 1999.

13. Gern JE, Lemanske RF Jr, Busse WW: Early life origins of asthma, *J Clin Invest* 104:837-843, 1999.

14. Strachan DP: Family size, infection and atopy: the first decade of the "hygiene hypothesis," *Thorax* 55(suppl 1):S2-S10, 2000.

15. Von Hertzen LC: Role of persistent infection in the control and severity of asthma: focus on *Chlamydia pneumoniae, Eur Respir J* 19:546-556, 2002.

16. Martin RJ, Kraft M, Chu HW, et al: A link between chronic asthma and chronic infection, *J Allergy Clin Immunol* 107:595-601, 2001.

17. Simons FER: Allergic rhinobronchitis: the asthma-allergic rhinitis link, *J Allergy Clin Immunol* 104:534-540, 1999.

18. Shay DK, Holman RC, Newman RD, et al: Bronchiolitis-associated hospitalizations among US children, 1980-1996, *JAMA* 282:1440-1446, 1999.

19. Openshaw PJM: Immunological mechanisms in respiratory syncytial virus disease, *Springer Semin Immunopathol* 17:187-201, 1995.

20. Reijonen TM, Kotaniemi-Syrjänen A, Korhonen K, et al: Predictors of asthma three years after hospital admission for wheezing in infancy, *Pediatrics* 106:1406-1412, 2000.

21. Stein RT, Sherrill D, Morgan WJ, et al: Respiratory syncytial virus in early life and risk of wheeze and allergy by age 13 years, *Lancet* 354: 541-545, 1999.

22. Martinez FD, Wright AL, Taussig LM, et al: Asthma and wheezing in the first six years of life, *N Engl J Med* 332:133-138, 1995.

23. Castro-Rodríguez JA, Holberg CJ, Wright AL, et al: Association of radiologically ascertained pneumonia before age 3 yr with asthmalike symptoms and pulmonary function during childhood: a prospective study, *Am J Respir Crit Care Med* 159:1891-1897, 1999.

24. McBride JT: Pulmonary function changes in children after respiratory syncytial virus infection in infancy, *J Pediatr* 135:28-32, 1999.

25. Kneyber MCJ, Steyerberg EW, De Groot R, et al: Long-term effects of respiratory syncytial virus (RSV) bronchiolitis in infants and young children: a quantitative review, *Acta Paediatr* 89:654-660, 2000.

26. Wennergren G, Kristjansson S: Relationship between respiratory syncytial virus bronchiolitis and future obstructive airway diseases, *Eur Respir J* 18:1044-1058, 2001.

27. Eriksson M, Bennet R, Nilsson A: Wheezing following lower respiratory tract infections with respiratory syncytial virus and influenza A in infancy, *Pediatr Allergy Immunol* 11:193-197, 2000.

28. Korppi M, Reijonen T, Poysa L, et al: A 2- to 3-year outcome after bronchiolitis, *Am J Dis Child* 147:628-631, 1993.

29. Wennergren G, Amark M, Amark K, et al: Wheezing bronchitis reinvestigated at the age of 10 years, *Acta Paediatr* 86:351-355, 1997.

30. Papadopoulos NG, Moustaki M, Tsolia M, et al: Association of rhinovirus infection with increased disease severity in acute bronchiolitis, *Am J Respir Crit Care Med* 165:1285-1289, 2002.

31. Ingram JM, Rakes GP, Hoover GE, et al: Eosinophil cationic protein in serum and nasal washes from wheezing infants and children, *J Pediatr* 127:558-564, 1995.

32. Atmar RL, Guy E, Guntupalli KK, et al: Respiratory tract viral infections in inner city asthmatic adults, *Arch Intern Med* 158:2459, 1998.

33. Skoner DP, Doyle WJ, Seroky J, et al: Lower airway responses to rhinovirus 39 in healthy allergic and nonallergic subjects, *Eur Respir J* 9:1402-1406, 1996.

34. Corne JM, Marshall C, Smith S, et al: Frequency, severity, and duration of rhinovirus infections in asthmatic and non-asthmatic individuals: a longitudinal cohort study, *Lancet* 359:831-834, 2002.

35. Tarlo SM, Broder I, Corey P, et al: The role of symptomatic colds in asthma exacerbations: influence of outdoor allergens and air pollutants, *J Allergy Clin Immunol* 108:52-58, 2001.

36. Strachan DP: Hay fever, hygiene, and household size, *Br Med J* 299: 1259-1260, 1989.

37. von Mutius E, Martinez FD, Fritzsch C, et al: Skin test reactivity and number of siblings, *Br Med J* 308:692-695, 1994.

38. von Mutius E: The influence of birth order on the expression of atopy in families: a gene-environment interaction? *Clin Exp Allergy* 28: 1454-1456, 1998.

39. Prescott SL, Macaubas C, Smallacombe T, et al: Development of allergen-specific T-cell memory in atopic and normal children, *Lancet* 353:196-200, 1999.

40. Lewis S, Butland B, Strachan D, et al: Study of the etiology of wheezing illness at age 16 in two national British birth cohorts, *Thorax* 51: 670-676, 1996.

41. Butland BK, Strachan DP, Lewis S, et al: Investigation into the increase in hay fever and eczema at age 16 observed between the 1958 and 1970 British birth cohorts, *Br Med J* 315:717-721, 1997.

42. Hahn DL, Anttila T, Saikku P: Association of *Chlamydia pneumoniae* IgA antibodies with recently symptomatic asthma, *Epidemiol Infect* 117:513-517, 1996.

43. Hahn DL, McDonald R: Can acute *Chlamydia pneumoniae* respiratory tract infection initiate chronic asthma? *Ann Allergy Asthma Immunol* 81:339-344, 1998.

44. Black PN, Blasi F, Jenkins CR, et al: Trial of roxithromycin in subjects with asthma and serological evidence of infection with *Chlamydia pneumoniae, Am J Respir Crit Care Med* 164:536-541, 2001.

45. Avila PC, Boushey HA: Macrolides, asthma, inflammation, and infection, *Ann Allergy Asthma Immunol* 84:565-568, 2000.

46. Emre U, Sokolovskaya N, Roblin PM, et al: Detection of anti-*Chlamydia pneumoniae* IgE in children with reactive airway disease, *J Infect Dis* 172:265-267, 1995.

47. Bulut Y, Faure E, Thomas L, et al: Chlamydial heat shock protein 60 activates macrophages and endothelial cells through Toll-like receptor 4 and MD2 in a MyD88-dependent pathway, *J Immunol* 168:1435-1440, 2002.

48. Henderson FW, Clyde WA Jr, Collier AM, et al: The etiologic and epidemiologic spectrum of bronchiolitis in pediatric practice, *J Pediatr* 95:183-190, 1979.

49. Yano T, Ichikawa Y, Komatu S, et al: Association of *Mycoplasma pneumoniae* antigen with initial onset of bronchial asthma, *Am J Respir Crit Care Med* 149:1348-1353, 1994.

50. Koh YY, Park Y, Lee HJ, et al: Levels of interleukin-2, interferon-gamma, and interleukin-4 in bronchoalveolar lavage fluid from patients with *Mycoplasma pneumonia:* implication of tendency toward increased immunoglobulin E production, *Pediatrics* 107:E39, 2001.

51. Martin RJ, Chu HW, Honour JM, et al: Airway inflammation and bronchial hyperresponsiveness after *Mycoplasma pneumoniae* infection in a murine model, *Am J Respir Cell Mol Biol* 24:577-582, 2001.

52. Chu HW, Kraft M, Krause JE, et al: Substance P and its receptor neurokinin 1 expression in asthmatic airways, *J Allergy Clin Immunol* 106:713-722, 2000.

53. Matsuse T, Hayashi S, Kuwano K, et al: Latent adenoviral infection in the pathogenesis of chronic obstructive pulmonary disease, *Am Rev Respir Dis* 146:177-184, 1992.

54. Macek V, Sorli J, Kopriva S, et al: Persistent adenoviral infection and chronic airway obstruction in children, *Am J Respir Crit Care Med* 150:7-10, 1994.

55. Hakonarson H, Carter C, Maskeri N, et al: Rhinovirus-mediated changes in airway smooth muscle responsiveness: induced autocrine role of interleukin-1β, *Am J Physiol Lung Cell Mol Physiol* 277:L13-L21, 1999.

56. Grunstein MM, Hakonarson H, Whelan R, et al: Rhinovirus elicits proasthmatic changes in airway responsiveness independently of viral infection, *J Allergy Clin Immunol* 108:997-1004, 2001.

57. Hendley JO: The host response, not the virus, causes the symptoms of the common cold, *Clin Infect Dis* 26:847-848, 1998.

58. Hedlin G, Svedmyr J, Ryden A-C: Systemic effects of a short course of betamethasone compared with high-dose inhaled budesonide in early childhood asthma, *Acta Paediatr* 88:48-51, 1999.

59. Ohrui T, Yamaya M, Sekizawa K, et al: Effects of rhinovirus infection on hydrogen peroxide-induced alterations of barrier function in the cultured human tracheal epithelium, *Am J Respir Crit Care Med* 158: 241-248, 1998.

60. Kurt-Jones EA, Popova L, Kwinn L, et al: Pattern recognition receptors TLR4 and CD14 mediate response to respiratory syncytial virus, *Nat Immunol* 1:398-401, 2000.

61. Kaul P, Biagioli MC, Singh I, et al: Rhinovirus-induced oxidative stress and interleukin-8 elaboration involves p47-*phox* but is independent of attachment to intercellular adhesion molecule-1 and viral replication, *J Infect Dis* 181:1885-1890, 2000.

62. Williams BRG: PKR: a sentinel kinase for cellular stress, *Oncogene* 18:6112-6120, 1999.

63. Konno S, Grindle KA, Lee WM, et al: Interferon-gamma enhances rhinovirus-induced RANTES secretion by airway epithelial cells, *Am J Respir Cell Mol Biol* 26:594-601, 2002.

64. Gern JE, Vrtis R, Grindle KA, et al: Relationship of upper and lower airway cytokines to outcome of experimental rhinovirus infection, *Am J Respir Crit Care Med* 162:2226-2231, 2000.

65. Gern JE, Vrtis R, Kelly EAB, et al: Rhinovirus produces nonspecific activation of lymphocytes through a monocyte-dependent mechanism, *J Immunol* 157:1605-1612, 1996.

66. Panuska JR, Merolla R, Rebert NA, et al: Respiratory syncytial virus induces interleukin-10 by human alveolar macrophages: suppression of early cytokine production and implications for incomplete immunity, *J Clin Invest* 96:2445-2453, 1995.

67. Johnston SL, Papi A, Monick MM, et al: Rhinoviruses induce interleukin-8 mRNA and protein production in human monocytes, *J Infect Dis* 175:323-329, 1997.

68. Gern JE, Busse WW: Relationship of viral infections to wheezing illnesses and asthma, *Nat Rev Immunol* 2:132-138, 2002.

69. McNamara PS, Smyth RL: The pathogenesis of respiratory syncytial virus disease in childhood, *Br Med Bull* 61:13-28, 2002.

70. Cardell LO, Agusti C, Takeyama K, et al: LTB(4)-induced nasal gland serous cell secretion mediated by neutrophil elastase, *Am J Respir Crit Care Med* 160:411-414, 1999.

71. Grünberg K, Timmers MC, Smits HH, et al: Effect of experimental rhinovirus 16 colds on airway hyperresponsiveness to histamine and interleukin-8 in nasal lavage in asthmatic subjects *in vivo*, *Clin Exp Allergy* 27:36-45, 1997.

72. Gern JE, Martin MS, Anklam KA et al: Relationships among specific viral pathogens, virus-induced interleukin-8, and respiratory symptoms in infancy, *Pediatr Allergy Immunol* 13:386-393, 2002.

73. Malcolm E, Arruda E, Hayden FG, et al: Clinical features of patients with acute respiratory illness and rhinovirus in their bronchoalveolar lavages, *J Clin Virol* 21:9-16, 2001.

74. Alwan WH, Record FM, Openshaw PJM: Phenotypic and functional characterization of T cell lines specific for individual respiratory syncytial virus proteins, *J Immunol* 150:5211-5218, 1993.

75. Jackson M, Scott R: Different patterns of cytokine induction in cultures of respiratory syncytial (RS) virus-specific human T$_H$ cell lines following stimulation with RS virus and RS virus proteins, *J Med Virol* 49:161-169, 1996.

76. Peebles RS Jr, Sheller JR, Johnson JE, et al: Respiratory syncytial virus infection prolongs methacholine-induced airway hyperresponsiveness in ovalbumin-sensitized mice, *J Med Virol* 57:186-192, 1999.

77. Lukacs NW, Tekkanat KK, Berlin A, et al: Respiratory syncytial virus predisposes mice to augmented allergic airway responses via IL-13-mediated mechanisms, *J Immunol* 167:1060-1065, 2001.

78. Tekkanat KK, Maassab HF, Cho DS, et al: IL-13-induced airway hyperreactivity during respiratory syncytial virus infection is STAT6 dependent, *J Immunol* 166:3542-3548, 2001.

79. Peebles RS Jr, Sheller JR, Collins RD, et al: Respiratory syncytial virus infection does not increase allergen-induced type 2 cytokine production, yet increases airway hyperresponsiveness in mice, *J Med Virol* 63:178-188, 2001.

80. Renzi PM, Turgeon JP, Marcotte JE, et al: Reduced interferon-γ production in infants with bronchiolitis and asthma, *Am J Respir Crit Care Med* 159:1417-1422, 1999.

81. van Schaik SM, Tristram DA, Nagpal IS, et al: Increased production of IFN-γ and cysteinyl leukotrienes in virus-induced wheezing, *J Allergy Clin Immunol* 103:630-636, 1999.

82. Parry DE, Busse WW, Sukow KA, et al: Rhinovirus-induced PBMC responses and outcome of experimental infection in allergic subjects, *J Allergy Clin Immunol* 105:692-698, 2000.

83. Bont L, Heijnen CJ, Kavelaars A, et al: Monocyte IL-10 production during respiratory syncytial virus bronchiolitis is associated with recurrent wheezing in a one-year follow-up study, *Am J Respir Crit Care Med* 161:1518-1523, 2000.

84. Bardin PG, Fraenkel DJ, Sanderson G, et al: Amplified rhinovirus colds in atopic subjects, *Clin Exp Allergy* 24:457-464, 1994.

85. Sigurs N, Bjarnason R, Sigurbergsson F, et al: Asthma and immunoglobulin E antibodies after respiratory syncytial virus bronchiolitis: a prospective cohort study with matched controls, *Pediatrics* 95:500-505, 1995.

86. Frick OL: Effect of respiratory and other virus infections on IgE immunoregulation, *J Allergy Clin Immunol* 78:1013-1018, 1986.

87. Lemanske RF Jr, Dick EC, Swenson CA, et al: Rhinovirus upper respiratory infection increases airway hyperreactivity and late asthmatic reactions, *J Clin Invest* 83:1-10, 1989.

88. Calhoun WJ, Dick EC, Schwartz LB, et al: A common cold virus, rhinovirus 16, potentiates airway inflammation after segmental antigen bronchoprovocation in allergic subjects, *J Clin Invest* 94:2200-2208, 1994.

89. Laing I, Riedel F, Yap PL, et al: Atopy predisposing to acute bronchiolitis during an epidemic of respiratory syncytial virus, *Br Med J* 284:1070-1072, 1982.

90. Rooney JC, Williams HE: The relationship between proved viral bronchiolitis and subsequent wheezing, *J Pediatr* 79:744-747, 1971.

91. Zweiman B, Schoenwetter WF, Pappano JE, et al: Patterns of allergic respiratory disease in children with a past history of bronchiolitis, *J Allergy Clin Immunol* 48:283-289, 1971.

92. Pullan CR, Hey EN: Wheezing, asthma, and pulmonary dysfunction 10 years after infection with respiratory syncytial virus in infancy, *Br Med J* 284:1665-1669, 1982.

93. Murray M, Webb MS, O'Callaghan C, et al: Respiratory status and allergy after bronchiolitis, *Arch Dis Child* 67:482-487, 1992.

94. Noma T, Yoshizawa I: Induction of allergen-specific IL-2 responsiveness of lymphocytes after respiratory syncytial virus infection and prediction of onset of recurrent wheezing and bronchial asthma, *J Allergy Clin Immunol* 98:816-826, 1997.

95. Welliver RC: Immunologic mechanisms of virus-induced wheezing and asthma, *J Pediatr* 135:S14-S20, 1999.

96. Sakamoto M, Ida S, Takishima T: Effect of influenza virus infection on allergic sensitization to aerosolized ovalbumin in mice, *J Immunol* 132:2614-2617, 1984.

97. Freihorst J, Piedra PA, Okamoto Y, et al: Effect of respiratory syncytial virus infection on the uptake of and immune response to other inhaled antigens, *Proc Soc Exp Biol Med* 188:191-197, 1988.

98. Garofalo R, Kimpen JLL, Welliver RC, et al: Eosinophil degranulation in the respiratory tract during naturally acquired respiratory syncytial virus infection, *J Pediatr* 120:28-32, 1992.

99. Volovitz B, Welliver RC, De Castro G, et al: The release of leukotrienes in the respiratory tract during infection with respiratory syncytial virus: role in obstructive airway disease, *Pediatr Res* 24:504-507, 1988.

100. Rabatic S, Gagro A, Lokar-Kolbas R, et al: Increase in CD23+ cells in infants with bronchiolitis is accompanied by appearance of IgE and IgG4 antibodies specific for respiratory syncytial virus, *J Infect Dis* 175:32-37, 1997.

101. Patel JA, Kunimoto M, Sim TC, et al: Interleukin-1α mediates the enhanced expression of intercellular adhesion molecule-1 in pulmonary epithelial cells infected with respiratory syncytial virus, *Am J Respir Cell Mol Biol* 13:602-609, 1995.

102. Arnold R, König B, Galatti H, et al: Cytokine (IL-8, IL-6, TNF-α) and soluble TNF receptor-I release from human peripheral blood mononuclear cells after respiratory syncytial virus infection, *Immunology* 85:364-372, 1995.

103. Tsutsumi H, Matsuda K, Sone S, et al: Respiratory syncytial virus-induced cytokine production by neonatal macrophages, *Clin Exp Immunol* 106:442-446, 1996.

104. Takeuchi R, Tsutsumi H, Osaki M, et al: Respiratory syncytial virus infection of neonatal monocytes stimulates synthesis of interferon regulatory factor 1 and interleukin-1β (IL-1β)-converting enzyme and secretion of IL-1β, *J Virol* 72:837-840, 1998.

105. Olszewska-Pazdrak B, Casola A, Saito T, et al: Cell-specific expression of RANTES, MCP-1, and MIP-1α by lower airway epithelial cells and eosinophils infected with respiratory syncytial virus, *J Virol* 72:4756-4764, 1998.

106. Harrison AM, Bonville CA, Rosenberg HF, et al: Respiratory syncytial virus-induced chemokine expression in the lower airways: eosinophil recruitment and degranulation, *Am J Respir Crit Care Med* 159:1918-1924, 1999.

107. Comoy EE, Pestel J, Duez C, et al: The house dust mite allergen, *Dermatophagoides pteronyssinus*, promotes type 2 responses by modulating the balance between IL-4 and IFN-γ, *J Immunol* 160:2456-2462, 1998.

108. Calhoun WJ, Swenson CA, Dick EC, et al: Experimental rhinovirus 16 infection potentiates histamine release after antigen bronchoprovocation in allergic subjects, *Am Rev Respir Dis* 144:1267-1273, 1991.

109. Gern JE, Calhoun W, Swenson C, et al: Rhinovirus infection preferentially increases lower airway responsiveness in allergic subjects, *Am J Respir Crit Care Med* 155:1872-1876, 1997.

110. McFadden ER Jr: Improper patient techniques with metered dose inhalers: clinical consequences and solutions to misuse, *J Allergy Clin Immunol* 96:278-283, 1995.

111. Gern JE, Galagan DM, Jarjour NN, et al: Detection of rhinovirus RNA in lower airway cells during experimentally induced infection, *Am J Respir Crit Care Med* 155:1159-1161, 1997.

112. Papadopoulos NG, Bates PJ, Bardin PG, et al: Rhinoviruses infect the lower airways, *J Infect Dis* 181:1875-1884, 2000.

113. Jarjour NN, Gern JE, Kelly EAB, et al: The effect of an experimental rhinovirus 16 infection on bronchial lavage neutrophils, *J Allergy Clin Immunol* 105:1169-1177, 2000.

114. Fraenkel DJ, Bardin PG, Sanderson G, et al: Lower airways inflammation during rhinovirus colds in normal and asthmatic subjects, *Am J Respir Crit Care Med* 151:879-886, 1995.

115. Grünberg K, Sharon RF, Hiltermann TJN, et al: Experimental rhinovirus 16 infection increases intercellular adhesion molecule-1 expression in bronchial epithelium of asthmatics regardless of inhaled steroid treatment, *Clin Exp Allergy* 30:1015-1023, 2000.

116. Bardin PG, Johnston SL, Pattemore PK: Viruses as precipitants of asthma symptoms. II. Physiology and mechanisms, *Clin Exp Allergy* 22:809-822, 1992.

117. Jacoby DB: Virus-induced asthma attacks, *JAMA* 287:755-761, 2002.

118. Jacoby DB, Tamaoki J, Borson DB, et al: Influenza infection causes airway hyperresponsiveness by decreasing enkephalinase, *J Appl Physiol* 64:2653-2658, 1988.

119. Sanders SP: Asthma, viruses, and nitric oxide, *Proc Soc Exp Biol Med* 220:123-132, 1999.

120. Sanders SP, Siekierski ES, Richards SM, et al: Rhinovirus infection induces expression of type 2 nitric oxide synthase in human respiratory epithelial cells *in vitro* and *in vivo*, *J Allergy Clin Immunol* 107:235-243, 2001.

121. Fryer AD, Jacoby DB: Parainfluenza virus infection damages inhibitory M2 muscarinic receptors on pulmonary parasympathetic nerves in the guinea pig, *Br J Pharmacol* 102:267-271, 1991.

122. Bowerfind WML, Fryer AD, Jacoby DB: Double-stranded RNA causes airway hyperreactivity and neuronal M_2 muscarinic receptor dysfunction, *J Appl Physiol* 92:1417-1422, 2002.

123. Fryer AD, Costello RW, Jacoby DB: Muscarinic receptor dysfunction in asthma, *Allergy Clin Immunol Int* 12:63-67, 2000.

124. Kellner JD, Ohlsson A, Gadomski AM, et al: Bronchodilators for bronchiolitis, *Cochrane Database Syst Rev* CD001266, 2000.

125. Garrison MM, Christakis DA, Harvey E, et al: Systemic corticosteroids in infant bronchiolitis: a meta-analysis, *Pediatrics* 105:E44, 2000.

126. Reijonen T, Korppi M, Kuikka L, et al: Anti-inflammatory therapy reduces wheezing after bronchiolitis, *Arch Pediatr Adolesc Med* 150:512-517, 1996.

127. Rowe BH, Keller JL, Oxman AD: Effectiveness of steroid therapy in acute exacerbations of asthma: a meta-analysis, *Am J Emerg Med* 10:301-310, 1992.

128. Murphy S, Bleecker ER, Boushey H, et al: *Guidelines for the diagnosis and management of asthma: National Asthma Education and Prevention Program,* ed 2, Bethesda, Md, 1997, National Institutes of Health.

129. Brunette MG, Lands L, Thibodeau L-P: Childhood asthma: prevention of attacks with short-term corticosteroid treatment of upper respiratory tract infection, *Pediatrics* 81:624-628, 1988.

130. Tal A, Levy N, Bearman JE: Methylprednisolone therapy for acute asthma in infants and toddlers: a controlled clinical trial, *Pediatrics* 86:350-356, 1990.

131. Dolan L, Kesarwala HH, Holroyde J, et al: Short-term, high-dose, systemic steroids in children with asthma: the effect on the hypothalamic-pituitary-adrenal axis, *J Allergy Clin Immunol* 80:81-87, 1987.

132. Wilson NM, Silverman M: Treatment of acute, episodic asthma in preschool children using intermittent high dose inhaled steroids at home, *Arch Dis Child* 65:407-410, 1990.

133. Daugbjerg P, Brenoe E, Forchhammer H, et al: A comparison between nebulized terbutaline, nebulized corticosteroid and systemic corticosteroid for acute wheezing in children up to 18 months of age, *Acta Paediatr* 82:547-551, 1993.

134. Connett G, Lenney W: Prevention of viral induced asthma attacks using inhaled budesonide, *Arch Dis Child* 68:85-87, 1993.

135. Svedmyr J, Nyberg E, Asbrink-Nilsson E, et al: Intermittent treatment with inhaled steroids for deterioration of asthma because of upper respiratory tract infections, *Acta Paediatr* 84:884-888, 1995.

136. Volovitz B, Bentur L, Finkelstein Y, et al: Effectiveness and safety of inhaled corticosteroids in controlling acute asthma attacks in children who were treated in the emergency department: a controlled comparative study with oral prednisolone, *J Allergy Clin Immunol* 102:605-609, 1998.

137. Schuh S, Reisman J, Alshehri M, et al: A comparison of inhaled fluticasone and oral prednisone for children with severe acute asthma, *N Engl J Med* 343:689-694, 2000.

138. Krawiec ME, Westcott JY, Chu HW, et al: Persistent wheezing in very young children is associated with lower respiratory inflammation, *Am J Respir Crit Care Med* 163:1338-1343, 2001.

139. Behera AK, Kumar M, Matsuse H, et al: Respiratory syncytial virus induces the expression of 5-lipoxygenase and endothelin-1 in bronchial epithelial cells, *Biochem Biophys Res Commun* 251:704-709, 1998.

140. Wedde-Beer K, Hu C, Rodriguez MM, et al: Leukotrienes mediate neurogenic inflammation in lungs of young rats infected with respiratory syncytial virus, *Am J Physiol Lung Cell Mol Physiol* 282:L1143-L1150, 2002.

141. Rotbart HA: Pleconaril treatment of enterovirus and rhinovirus infections, *Infect Med* 17:488-494, 2000.

142. Rotbart HA: Treatment of picornavirus infections, *Antiviral Res* 53:83-98, 2002.

143. Turner RB, Dutko FJ, Goldstein NH, et al: Efficacy of oral WIN 54954 for prophylaxis of experimental rhinovirus infection, *Antimicrob Agents Chemother* 37:297-300, 1993.

144. Turner RB, Wecker MT, Pohl G, et al: Efficacy of tremacamra, a soluble intercellular adhesion molecule 1, for experimental rhinovirus infection: a randomized clinical trial, *JAMA* 281:1797-1804, 1999.

145. Treanor JJ, Hayden FG, Vrooman PS, et al: Efficacy and safety of the oral neuraminidase inhibitor oseltamivir in treating acute influenza: a randomized controlled trial: US Oral Neuraminidase Study Group, *JAMA* 283:1016-1024, 2000.

146. Hayden FG, Gubareva LV, Monto AS, et al: Inhaled zanamivir for the prevention of influenza in families: Zanamivir Family Study Group, *N Engl J Med* 343:1282-1289, 2000.

147. Farr BM, Gwaltney JMJ, Hendley JO, et al: A randomized controlled trial of glucocorticoid prophylaxis against experimental rhinovirus infection, *J Infect Dis* 162:1173-1177, 1990.

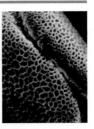

Special Considerations for Infants and Young Children

RONINA A. COVAR ■ JOSEPH D. SPAHN ■ STANLEY J. SZEFLER

Recent advances in the etiology, mechanisms, and management of asthma have led to a better understanding of this disease and may in part be responsible for the stabilization of the steady increase in asthma morbidity and mortality noted since the 1980s.[1] The need to better understand the natural history of early-onset wheezing is urgent, especially given the fact that the majority of asthma patients have onset of their disease in the first 4 years of life. In addition, epidemiologic studies suggest that the cumulative prevalence of asthma is as high as 22% by the age of 4 years.[2,3] It is worrisome that some studies have hinted that pulmonary development in infancy can be adversely affected by asthma, resulting in a decrease in lung function of approximately 20% by adulthood.[4] An equally important reason why asthma in infants and younger children

deserves a closer look comes from the fact that infants and young children are at particular risk for asthma morbidity. Admission rates for asthmatic children under the age of 4 years are greater than those of all other age groups, and they account for some of the high annual rate of asthma mortality.[1] In addition, younger children with asthma are also more likely to be readmitted to the hospital for acute exacerbations.[5] In this observational study of 1034 children admitted to a large hospital in Australia for acute asthma, the investigators found that over half of the children were readmitted over a 2-year period. Lastly, in a retrospective analysis of 49 asthmatic children whose mean age was 5.2 years (range 2 months to 16 years) admitted to a community-based pediatric intensive care unit over a 10-year period, as many as 75% were 6 years or younger.[6]

Asthma in young children places a significant burden on health care utilization, especially when one considers the significant number of missed work days parents incur in order to care for an acutely ill child. Several clinical practice guidelines developed in recent years have attempted to address special issues in the management of asthma peculiar to this age group.[7,8] Many issues are unique to this age group that deserve special consideration such as the presence of confounding factors or disease masqueraders, who and when to treat with controller therapy, what medications to use, how best to deliver the medications, and how to monitor the response to treatment (Box 36-1).

CONFOUNDING FACTORS

The first practical consideration in approaching the wheezing child is to ensure that an alternative diagnosis is not being overlooked. Inherent in this age group are several factors that mimic asthma, thereby contributing to poor asthma control. In addition, infants and small children have a greater degree of bronchial hyperresponsiveness, which may predispose them to wheeze.[9]

The differential diagnosis of wheezing in infants and young children includes conditions such as foreign body aspiration, congenital airway anomalies, abnormalities of the great vessels, congenital heart disease, cystic fibrosis, recurrent aspiration, immunodeficiency, infections, ciliary dyskinesia, and mediastinal masses. Other systemic features, such as a neonatal onset of symptoms, associated failure to thrive, diarrhea or vomiting, and even focal lung or cardiovascular findings, suggest an alternative diagnosis and require

---

BOX 36-1

KEY CONCEPTS

Challenging Issues Pertinent to the Management of Recurrent Wheezing

- There is an urgent need to focus research efforts on the care of infants and small children with suspected asthma because of the potential to modulate the disease process early on and the significant morbidity associated with uncontrolled asthma in this age group.
- The clinical presentation of asthma in this age group is often similar to those of other conditions seen in early childhood.
- After confounders and masqueraders of asthma have been excluded in the evaluation of children with suspected asthma, recurrent wheezing in infants and young children still comprises a heterogeneous group of conditions with different risk factors and prognoses.
- The diagnosis of asthma in infants and small children is often based on clinical grounds and fraught with lack of clinically available tools that meet the criteria for the definition of asthma used in older children and adults such as airway inflammation, bronchial hyperresponsiveness, and airflow limitation.
- The difficulties in the management of asthma include limited effective and convenient delivery devices, complete dependence on the caregivers to carry out the treatment regimen, and inadequate selection of medications completely devoid of adverse effects.

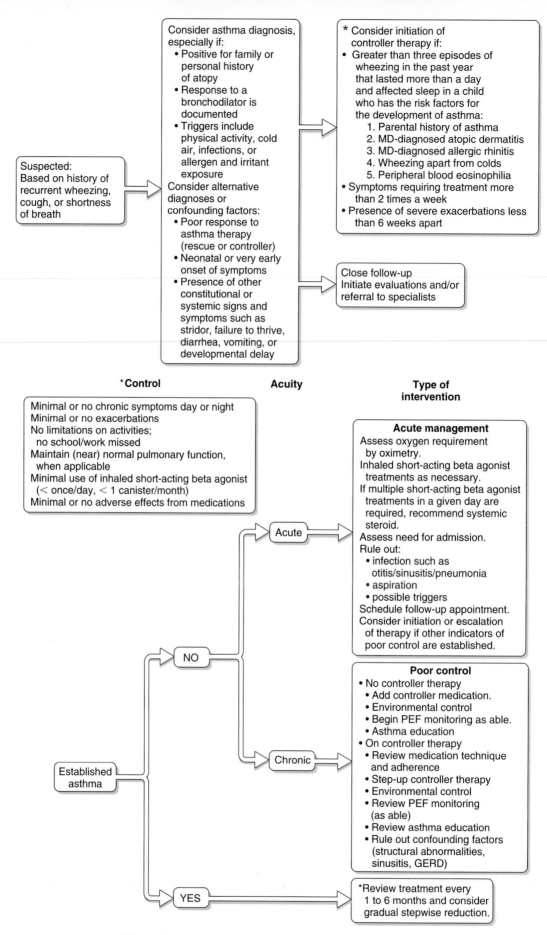

Suspected: Based on history of recurrent wheezing, cough, or shortness of breath

Consider asthma diagnosis, especially if:
- Positive for family or personal history of atopy
- Response to a bronchodilator is documented
- Triggers include physical activity, cold air, infections, or allergen and irritant exposure

Consider alternative diagnoses or confounding factors:
- Poor response to asthma therapy (rescue or controller)
- Neonatal or very early onset of symptoms
- Presence of other constitutional or systemic signs and symptoms such as stridor, failure to thrive, diarrhea, vomiting, or developmental delay

* **Consider initiation of controller therapy if:**
- Greater than three episodes of wheezing in the past year that lasted more than a day and affected sleep in a child who has the risk factors for the development of asthma:
  1. Parental history of asthma
  2. MD-diagnosed atopic dermatitis
  3. MD-diagnosed allergic rhinitis
  4. Wheezing apart from colds
  5. Peripheral blood eosinophilia
- Symptoms requiring treatment more than 2 times a week
- Presence of severe exacerbations less than 6 weeks apart

Close follow-up Initiate evaluations and/or referral to specialists

***Control**

- Minimal or no chronic symptoms day or night
- Minimal or no exacerbations
- No limitations on activities; no school/work missed
- Maintain (near) normal pulmonary function, when applicable
- Minimal use of inhaled short-acting beta agonist ($<$ once/day, $<$ 1 canister/month)
- Minimal or no adverse effects from medications

Acuity

Type of intervention

Established asthma

NO → **Acute**

Chronic

YES

Acute management
Assess oxygen requirement by oximetry.
Inhaled short-acting beta agonist treatments as necessary.
If multiple short-acting beta agonist treatments in a given day are required, recommend systemic steroid.
Assess need for admission.
Rule out:
- infection such as otitis/sinusitis/pneumonia
- aspiration
- possible triggers
Schedule follow-up appointment.
Consider initiation or escalation of therapy if other indicators of poor control are established.

Poor control
- No controller therapy
  - Add controller medication.
  - Environmental control
  - Begin PEF monitoring as able.
  - Asthma education
- On controller therapy
  - Review medication technique and adherence
  - Step-up controller therapy
  - Environmental control
  - Review PEF monitoring (as able)
  - Review asthma education
  - Rule out confounding factors (structural abnormalities, sinusitis, GERD)

*Review treatment every 1 to 6 months and consider gradual stepwise reduction.

*Adapted from the NHLBI-NAEPP 2002 Quick Reference

FIGURE 36-1 Algorithm for suggested management of infants and young children with suspected or established asthma. *PEF,* Peak expiratory flow; *GERD,* gastroesophageal reflux disease. (Modified from National Asthma Education Prevention Program Expert Panel: *Guidelines for the diagnosis and management of asthma—update on selected topics 2002,* Bethesda, Md, 2002, U.S. Department of Health and Human Services National Heart, Lung, and Blood Institute.)

extensive investigations. Clinical features in addition to age at onset of symptoms that should be taken into consideration include triggers for the respiratory symptoms and aggravating factors associated with respiratory distress such as nighttime occurrences, environmental exposure, physical exertion, feeding, and infections. Clearly, making the correct diagnosis is essential because the treatment for these conditions can vary substantially. For example, in children with significant gastroesophageal reflux, improvement in asthma symptoms with concomitant reduction in asthma medication use occurred after a prokinetic agent was instituted.[10] A practical approach that can be considered for a young child in whom asthma is strongly suspected is an empiric trial of asthma controller therapy while other evaluations are still being pursued (Figure 36-1).

DIAGNOSTIC AND MONITORING TOOLS TO EVALUATE ASTHMA IN YOUNG CHILDREN

Given the complexity of asthma and the many conditions that can masquerade as asthma, the diagnosis can be difficult to make, especially in young children.[7] Werk et al[11] sought to determine the factors primary care pediatricians believe are important in establishing an initial diagnosis of asthma. Questionnaires on asthma diagnosis consisting of 20 factors obtained from the National Heart, Lung, and Blood Institute (NHLBI) National Asthma Education Prevention Program (NAEPP) guidelines[7] and an expert local panel of subspecialists were sent to 862 active members of the Massachusetts American Academy of Pediatrics.[11] Over 80% of the respondents rated 5 factors as necessary or important in establishing the diagnosis of asthma. These factors included recurrent wheezing, symptomatic improvement following bronchodilator use, presence of recurrent cough, exclusion of other diagnoses, and suggestive peak expiratory flow rate findings. It is noteworthy that 27% of the respondents indicated that a child had to be older than 2 years; 18% indicated that fever must be absent during an exacerbation.

The diagnosis of asthma in young children is based largely on clinical judgment and an assessment of symptoms and physical findings. Because lung function measurements in infants and small children are difficult to perform, a trial of treatment is often a practical way to make a diagnosis of asthma in young children.

Monitoring Response and Disease Activity

Monitoring response to therapy can be difficult to objectively assess. Thus subjective measures including asthma symptom scoring systems,[12] the need for rescue bronchodilator or oral glucocorticoid therapy, and emergent care visits/hospitalizations are used to judge efficacy of therapy. At present there are no easily performed lung function measures[13] that serve as the gold standard in adults and older children or noninvasive markers of airway inflammation that can be used to help make the diagnosis of asthma or to help guide response to therapy. The following section will highlight "cutting-edge" techniques that hold the potential to revolutionize how lung function and airway inflammation are monitored in the young child with asthma.

Forced Oscillometry

Forced oscillometry is a newly developed pulmonary function technique that measures respiratory system resistance (Rrs) and reactance (Xrs) at several frequencies.[14] Some investigators believe that Xrs at low frequencies is a potential measure of peripheral airways function.

Using three different lung function measures, Nielsen and Bisgaard[15] evaluated the bronchodilator response of 92 children 2 to 5 years old, 55 of whom had asthma. Children with asthma had diminished lung function compared to nonasthmatic children in all measures evaluated, including specific airway resistance (sRaw) utilizing whole body plethysmography, respiratory resistance utilizing an interrupter technique (Rint), and respiratory resistance utilizing the impulse oscillation technique at 5 Hz (Rrs5). All children, including nonasthmatics, responded to terbutaline, although children with asthma improved to a significantly greater extent than the nonasthmatic children. The investigators found sRaw utilizing body plethysmography to be the best pulmonary function measure for distinguishing the asthmatics from nonasthmatics based on bronchodilator response. They concluded that assessment of bronchodilator responsiveness using sRaw as a measure of lung function may help define asthma in young children.

Noninvasive Measures of Inflammation

Exhaled nitric oxide (eNO) levels are elevated in patients with asthma.[16,17] In addition, they rise during acute exacerbations and fall following oral or inhaled glucocorticoid therapy.[18,19] Lastly, eNO levels correlate positively with sputum eosinophilia.[20,21] As a result, eNO measurement has been described as an easily performed, noninvasive marker of airway inflammation. Buchvald and Bisgaard[22] recently published findings suggesting that eNO levels can be reliably obtained in children as young as 2 years of age.

Another study by Baraldi et al[23] in infants and young children found significantly higher mean ($\pm$SEM) eNO levels (14.1 $\pm$ 1.8 ppb) in 13 infants and young children aged 7 to 33 months presenting with an acute wheeze and a history of at least three prior wheezing episodes compared to six first-time viral wheezers aged 9 to 14 months of age (8.3 $\pm$ 1.3 ppb, $P < 0.05$) and nine healthy matched controls (5.6 $\pm$ 0.5 ppb, $P < 0.001$). No differences in eNO measurements were seen between the two latter groups. In addition, eNO levels were reduced by 52% after steroid therapy to a level comparable to those of the healthy controls and first-time wheezers.[23]

Unlike sophisticated measures of lung function and bronchial hyperresponsiveness, which are time-consuming and limited to research institutions, eNO can be easily and quickly measured. At present, its biggest disadvantage comes from the initial cost associated with buying the equipment.

In one of the few studies designed to specifically address the role of eosinophil cationic protein (ECP) in recurrently wheezing children less than 2 years old, Carlsen et al[24] found a strong correlation between serum ECP and response to albuterol/salbutamol using the tidal flow volume loop technique in children 0 to 2 years of age. These investigators suggested that ECP may be measuring airway inflammation and that it may have some prognostic value in diagnosing asthma in infants and toddlers with recurrent wheezing. The major drawback for ECP comes from its lack of sensitivity and difficulties preparing the sample following collection.

PREDICTING WHO IS LIKELY TO DEVELOP PERSISTENT ASTHMA

After confounders and masqueraders have been excluded, recurrent wheezing in infants and young children still comprises a heterogeneous group of conditions with different risk factors and prognoses. Atopy appears to be the single most important risk factor in the development of persistent wheezing and subsequent asthma. Other factors or exposures early in life such as fetal nutrition, duration of pregnancy, viral lower respiratory tract infections in the first years of life, cigarette smoke exposure, air pollution, postnatal nutrition, breast-feeding, family size, maternal age, socioeconomic status, and allergen exposure have been implicated to varying degrees. Most of what is known about the natural history of asthma comes from large population-based studies. This is summarized in Chapter 2.

From these available studies it has become clear that there are several subtypes of "recurrent wheezers."[25-29] The investigators from the Tucson Children's Respiratory Group enrolled over 1000 newborns served by a large health maintenance organization to evaluate factors involved in early-onset wheezing in relationship to persistent wheezing at 6 years of life.[8] Nearly one third of the cohort had had at least one episode of wheezing by 3 years of age. However, only 40% of these early wheezers persisted to wheeze by 6 years of age. Of the children, 15% did not wheeze during the first 3 years of life but had wheezing at 6 years. These late-onset wheezers had a percentage of atopic children similar to that of persistent wheezers and were likely to have mothers with asthma. Hence, there seems to be a similar genetic predisposition for the asthma phenotype characterizing both persistent and late-onset wheezers. Of the total group, 20 had at least one episode of wheezing associated with a respiratory tract infection during the first 3 years of life but had no wheezing at 6 years. These children who had early-onset (transient) wheezing were more likely to have diminished airway function and a history of maternal smoking and were less likely to be atopic. Although these data suggest the coexistence of different "phenotypes," it remains to be determined whether the late-onset wheezers are a group distinct from the persistent wheezers.

Only a few studies have attempted to quantitate the likelihood of children developing persistent asthma and to offer a tool to select accurately the patients who are likely to need treatment or to benefit from early-intervention studies. One such study came from Southampton General Hospital, where 107 infants (mean age 10.9 months) with a history of wheeze within 12 weeks and at least one parent having a history of asthma or eczema and current allergen prick skin test reactivity were evaluated over a 12-month period to determine which factors or combination of factors would predict persistent asthma.[30] Infants with their first episodes of wheeze secondary to a presumed or established respiratory syncytial virus (RSV) bronchiolitis were excluded. The diagnosis of persistent asthma was based on the need for prophylactic asthma medication upon completion of the 12-month follow-up period; 50% of the children required a controller asthma medication. Using univariate logistic regression analysis, atopy, older age, and a history of atopy in both parents were risk factors for need

for controller treatment. Using multivariate logistic regression and modeling techniques, the only risk factors were an increased age at presentation and elevated serum-soluble interleukin-2R levels, accounting for a positive predictive value of 76% and a negative predictive value of 92%. This study has many limitations, including a short duration of follow-up, a small sample size, and inadequate diagnostic criteria for persistent asthma (i.e., need for controller medication).

A more clinically useful study comes from the Tucson Children's Respiratory Group, who sought to define an asthma predictive index using a combination of clinical and easily obtainable laboratory data to help identify preschool-age children who are at risk of developing persistent asthma. Information on parental asthma diagnosis and prenatal maternal smoking status was obtained at enrollment, while the child's history of asthma and wheezing and physician-diagnosed allergic rhinitis or eczema, along with measurements of blood eosinophil count, were obtained at the follow-up visits. Two indices were used to classify the children. The stringent index required recurrent wheezing in the first 3 years plus one major (parental history of asthma or physician-diagnosed eczema) or two of three minor (eosinophilia, wheezing without colds, allergic rhinitis) risk factors, whereas the loose index required any episode of wheezing in the first 3 years plus one major or two of three minor risk factors. The authors concluded that the subsequent development of asthma could be predicted with a reasonable degree of accuracy by using a simple, clinically based index.[31] The asthma predictive index may serve as a useful tool in assessing the role of early intervention in disease modification. Children with a positive loose index were 2.6 to 5.5 times more likely to have active asthma sometime during the school years. In contrast, risk of asthma increased to 4.3 to 9.8 times when the stringent criteria were used. In addition, at least 90% of young children with a negative "loose" or "stringent" index will not develop "active asthma" in the school age years.

PATIENT SELECTION AND TIMING OF TREATMENT

There has been a recent trend toward intervening early in the course of the disease with the hope that by inhibiting or suppressing the inflammatory reaction before it becomes established, the natural history of asthma can be altered. To have any chance for success, early intervention will require identifying high-risk infants and establishing effectiveness of the intervention strategy in young children while minimizing the potential for adverse effects.

Two studies have evaluated the effects of ketotifen and cetirizine, respectively, in preventing the onset of asthma in genetically prone children.[32,33] In a double-blind, placebo-controlled, parallel study, Bustos et al[32] randomized children up to 2 years of age with a family history of asthma or allergic rhinitis and presence of elevated serum IgE but without a prior history of wheezing to receive either ketotifen (0.5 to 1 mg twice daily) ($N = 45$, mean age 11.5 months) or placebo ($N = 40$, mean age 10.8 months) for 3 years. The percentage of patients developing at least three episodes of wheezing during the study period was significantly lower in the active treatment group than the placebo group (9% vs. 35%, $P = 0.003$).[32] The other study, called the Early Treatment of the Atopic Child, was a randomized, double-blind, parallel group trial that compared cetirizine (0.25 mg/kg twice daily) and placebo.[33] The medications were administered for 18 months to infants between 1 and 2 years of age with atopic dermatitis and outcome in the next 18 months after discontinuation of treatment was evaluated. All the infants had a family history of atopy. There was no significant difference in the percentage of patients in either the cetirizine (52%) or placebo (50%, $P = 0.7$) groups who developed asthma (defined as three episodes of wheezing during the 36 months of followup). The primary outcome, which was the time to the onset of asthma, was also not different between the two groups (median time was 26.5 and 27.1 months for cetirizine and placebo, respectively). However, in the cetirizine group, infants with evidence of dust mite or grass pollen sensitivity were less likely to have asthma over the 18 months of treatment with a sustained effect for grass-sensitized infants over the 36 months of follow-up compared with those treated with placebo. Furthermore, in the placebo group there was an increased risk of developing asthma in those with baseline sensitivity to egg, house dust mite, grass pollen, or cat allergen. These two studies support the role of easily administered secondary preventive measures in delaying or even preventing the development of asthma in genetically predisposed children.

Reijonen et al[34] sought to determine if early antiinflammatory therapy would protect against subsequent development of asthma and to identify the effects of allergic sensitization and RSV infection on the development of asthma. Eighty-nine children 2 years old or younger who were hospitalized for infection associated with wheezing were enrolled to receive 4 months of budesonide, cromolyn, or no treatment and followed for 3 years. The investigators found that a 4-month course of antiinflammatory therapy did not change the occurrence of asthma 3 years later with 48% of the children on cromolyn, 48% of the children on budesonide, and 55% of the control children with current asthma. Significant risk factors for asthma were age older than 12 months at the initial wheezing episode (risk ratio [RR] 4.1), a history of prior wheezing (RR 6.8), atopic dermatitis on study entry (RR 3.4), and positive allergen skin test reactivity at 16 months (RR 9.5). Hence, all 18 subjects who were sensitized to a furred pet went on to develop asthma. Of note, allergic sensitization became the most important risk factor for subsequent asthma, whereas RSV infection appeared to actually "protect" against subsequent asthma. This finding is quite unexpected, especially when compared to the findings of Sigurs et al,[35] who showed in a case-controlled study that RSV infection is a major risk factor for subsequent asthma and a risk factor for atopy as well.

A large multicenter trial, the NHLBI Childhood Asthma Research and Education Network Prevention of Early Asthma in Kids study, is currently under way and will attempt to determine whether long-term antiinflammatory therapy can indeed alter the natural history of wheezing in toddlers predisposed to the development of asthma.

Adult and pediatric studies have demonstrated the beneficial effects of introduction of inhaled glucocorticoids closer to the time of asthma diagnosis or onset of symptoms, suggesting an amelioration of the disease process.[36,37] At present, multiple issues around the cost of controller medications, optimal delivery of medications, and safety of long-term inhaled glucocorticoid treatment remain unresolved.

MANAGEMENT

Issues Related to the Delivery of Medications to Infants and Small Children

There are unique challenges relating to the delivery of medications (both oral and inhaled) to infants and young children with asthma. Obviously, liquid preparations are better tolerated than tablets/pills, especially for infants. Montelukast is available as a chewable tablet and there are several liquid prednisone/prednisolone preparations available for use in infants and small children. With regard to inhaled medications, certain anatomic and physiologic properties inherent in children younger than 6 years are worth considering. First, because infants display preferential nasal breathing and have small airways, low tidal volume, and high respiratory frequency, delivery of the drug to the lower airways is often inadequate.[38] Second, it is difficult if not impossible for young children to perform the maneuvers specified for optimal delivery of aerosol therapy such as slow inhalation through the mouth with a period of breath-holding for pressurized metered-dose inhalers (pMDIs) or rapid and forceful inhalation required in the case of dry-powder inhalers (DPIs). Third, delivery devices appropriate for the young child are limited to those that require a minimum of skills and cooperation from the child and must allow ease of administration for the caregivers. Although at present there are at least three basic inhaled aerosol delivery systems available for older children and adults, only two are used in this age group: the nebulizer and the pMDI with spacer/holding chamber and facemask. Within these two general types of delivery systems there are numerous products available that vary widely in performance. The pMDI with spacer or holding chamber is portable and inexpensive, takes less time to administer, and is likely to be better tolerated than delivery with a nebulizer.

The NHLBI NAEPP guidelines in 1997 mention the use of inhaled short-acting β agonist either by MDI or nebulizer treatment as an initial asthma exacerbation home intervention.[7] The recent Global Initiative for Asthma (GINA) guidelines[8] recommend the use of short-acting inhaled β agonist by MDI (ideally with a spacer) for home management of mild, moderate, and severe exacerbations. The GINA guidelines also recommend nebulized treatments for severe exacerbations at home and for hospital-based management of acute asthma.

Data in young children clearly support the use of β agonists administered via a pMDI with spacer for acute asthma.[39,40] In a study of 60 children between 1 and 5 years of age hospitalized for an asthma exacerbation, Parkin et al[39] found salbutamol (400 to 600 μg, 4 to 6 puffs, based on weight) and ipratropium bromide (40 μg, 2 puffs), both delivered via pMDI with an Aerochamber and mask, to be as effective as nebulized salbutamol (0.15 mg/kg) and ipratropium bromide (125 μg) suspended in 3 ml of normal saline administered over 15 minutes by facemask. However, nearly one third of the subjects randomized to MDI eventually required a nebulized β agonist.

Two studies have evaluated lower respiratory tract deposition of a radiolabeled salbutamol/albuterol mixture administered to young children. Tal et al[41] showed that on average, less than 2% of the nominal dose of the albuterol given by a pMDI with a spacer and mask to children less than 5 years old was deposited in the lower respiratory tract with most of the drug remaining in the spacer.

Wildhaber et al[42] compared the lung deposition of radiolabeled salbutamol from a nebulizer and a pMDI and spacer in 17 asthmatic children aged 2 to 9 years. Both delivery devices were delivering roughly 5% of the nominal dose to the lower airways. Because of the larger doses of salbutamol administered via the nebulizer (2000 μg vs. 400 μg) than the pMDI, a larger amount of drug was deposited in the airways using the nebulizer (108 μg vs. 22 μg, respectively). In addition, both devices were approximately 50% less efficient in children less than 4 years old than the older children.

In general, β agonist administration by nebulization is still the delivery system of choice in the treatment of infants and young children with severe, acute asthma because it requires the simple technique of relaxed tidal breathing. In addition, oxygen can be used to power the nebulizer providing β agonist and supplemental oxygen simultaneously, and it does offer the capability to administer a controller agent and rescue β agonist at the same time. Although evidence exists that demonstrates comparable efficacy of short-acting β agonists delivered either by nebulizer or pMDI with a holding chamber for the treatment of acute asthma in infants and young children that supports the recommendations of the GINA guidelines,[8] no similar data exist comparing inhaled glucocorticoids administered via nebulizer and pMDI with spacer and mask.

Adherence

The issue of adherence in infants and small children is complicated because the child is entirely dependent on the caregiver to administer the medication. In an observational study of preschool children, Gibson et al[43] sought to evaluate adherence with inhaled prophylactic medications delivered through a large volume spacer using an electronic timer device. Adherence was only 50% with a range of 0% to 94%. In addition, only 42% of the subjects received the prescribed medication on each study day, and reporting of symptoms in the diary cards did not correlate with good compliance with the prophylactic medication, nor was a correlation found between frequency of administration and adherence. In another study, parental reporting of symptom scores correlated with measured bronchodilator use in only 63% of preschool children.[44]

A few studies have attempted to determine why caregivers are unable to administer medications as prescribed. Lim et al[45] asked parents why they were reluctant to administer prophylactic medications (such as inhaled glucocorticoids) to their young children with asthma. Reasons cited included hesitancy to use medications for fear of dependence, side effects, and overdosage. Fortunately, patient education programs developed for parents of small children with asthma improve asthma morbidity and self-management outcome.[46,47]

Controller Therapy for Small Children with Persistent Asthma

The NHLBI NAEPP released an update on selected topics included in the clinical guidelines for the diagnosis and management of asthma.[48] The NAEPP report considers initiation of a controller therapy "in infants and young children who have had more than three episodes of wheezing in the past year that lasted more than 1 day and affected sleep and who

TABLE 36-1 Stepwise Approach for Managing Infants and Young Children (5 Years of Age or Younger) with Acute or Chronic Asthma

Classify Severity of Clinical Features Before Treatment or Adequate Control of Symptoms/ Day (Symptoms/Night)	Medications Required to Maintain Long-term Control
Step 4: Severe persistent continual (frequent)	*Preferred treatment:* High-dose inhaled corticosteroids and long-acting inhaled β₂ agonists And, if needed, corticosteroid tablets or syrup long-term (2 mg/kg/day; generally do not exceed 60 mg/day); make repeated attempts to reduce systemic corticosteroids and make control with high-dose inhaled corticosteroids
Step 3: Moderate persistent daily (> 1 night/wk)	*Preferred treatment:* Low-dose inhaled corticosteroids and long-acting inhaled β₂ agonists or medium-dose inhaled corticosteroids *Alternative treatment:* Low-dose inhaled corticosteroids and either leukotriene receptor antagonist or theophylline If needed (particularly in patients with recurring severe exacerbations): *Preferred treatment:* Medium-dose inhaled corticosteroids and long-acting inhaled β₂ agonists *Alternative treatment:* Medium-dose inhaled corticosteroids and either leukotriene receptor antagonist or theophylline
Step 2: Mild persistent > 2/wk but < 1/day (> 2 nights/mo)	*Preferred treatment:* Low-dose inhaled corticosteroid (with nebulizer or metered-dose inhaler [MDI] with holding chamber with or without facemask or dry-powder inhaler) *Alternative treatment (listed alphabetically):* Cromolyn (nebulizer is preferred or MDI with holding chamber) or leukotriene receptor antagonist
Step 1: Mild intermittent ≤ 2 days/wk (≤ 2 nights/mo)	No daily medication needed

have risk factors for the development of asthma (parental history of asthma or physician-diagnosed atopic dermatitis or two of the following: physician-diagnosed allergic rhinitis, wheezing apart from colds, and peripheral blood eosinophilia)." These criteria are based largely on the asthma predictive index using the stringent criteria cited earlier from the Tucson Respiratory Study Group.[26] Apart from these, other recommended indications for initiating long-term controller therapy include use of symptomatic treatment more than twice a week or presence of severe exacerbations less than 6 weeks apart.

The stepwise approach to asthma management in small children is still based largely on the frequency of daily and nighttime symptoms, similar to that used for older children and adults except for the exclusion of lung function tests (Table 36-1). This new version recommends the use of inhaled corticosteroids (administered either by the nebulizer or by MDI with holding chamber with or without a facemask or DPI) as the preferred therapy for all levels of persistent asthma severity. The leukotriene receptor antagonists (LTRAs) are now clearly placed as alternative medications, along with cromolyn and nedocromil for infants and young children with mild persistent asthma. Combination therapy of a low-medium–dose inhaled corticosteroid with a long-acting β_2 agonist (preferred) or a leukotriene modifier or theophylline (considered alternative add-on medications to the inhaled corticosteroid) is now a mainstay therapy for moderate persistent asthma in children and adults. Nedocromil is no longer placed as an adjunct therapy for moderate persistent asthma in younger children. In addition, for infants and younger children, the use of medium-dose inhaled corticosteroids by itself is also considered a preferred treatment for moderate persistent asthma, whereas this is just an alternative therapy for older children and adults with moderate persistent severity. Recommended medications for severe persistent asthma are limited to high-dose inhaled corticosteroids and long-acting β_2 agonists and systemic corticosteroids, if warranted.

The GINA guidelines[8] has also been recently updated. There is no specific section devoted to the management of infants and young children with asthma, although a paragraph on this group of children is included that states: "Although there are no well-conducted clinical trials to provide scientific evidence for the proper treatment of asthma at each step of severity in these age groups, a treatment algorithm similar to that used in schoolchildren is recommended for preschool children and infants." There are a few differences between the GINA[8] and the NHLBI NAEPP guidelines.[48] The GINA guidelines do not strongly recommend LTRAs to be used as monotherapy in patients with mild persistent asthma in that there is insufficient data on this class of medications in children with mild persistent asthma to justify their use. The GINA guidelines acknowledge that the LTRAs are moderately effective in children and adults with moderate and severe asthma and, by extrapolation, likely to be effective in mild asthma. Second, although escalation of the dose of the inhaled glucocorticoid therapy is recommended with increasing disease severity, the new GINA guidelines encourage the addition of other controller agents such as theophylline, long-acting β agonists, or LTRAs over increasing the dose of inhaled corticosteroid for moderate persistent asthma. Lastly, these add-on controller medications are recommended not only for moderate but also for severe persistent asthma.

Inhaled Glucocorticoids

Inhaled glucocorticoids have been shown to reduce asthma symptoms, improve baseline pulmonary function, and reduce bronchial hyperresponsiveness in adults and older children with asthma.[49,50] In addition, they reduce the need for prednisone and decrease the number of urgent-care visits and hospitalizations for acute asthma.[51] Most recently, they have been shown to reduce the risk of death from asthma.[52] Much of the following discussion will focus on nebulized budesonide, the most extensively studied inhaled glucocorticoid in young children.

Efficacy and Safety of Nebulized Budesonide.

The initial studies with nebulized budesonide in young children with moderate to severe persistent asthma found nebulized budesonide to be superior to placebo in improving symptoms, reducing prednisone use, or improving overall asthma control.[53,54] DeBlic et al,[53] in a double-blind, placebo-controlled parallel study, evaluated the efficacy of high-dose nebulized budesonide (1 mg twice daily) or placebo for 12 weeks in 40 toddlers with severe asthma (mean age 17 months). Budesonide therapy resulted in approximately 50% fewer exacerbations, less need for prednisone, less daytime and nighttime wheezing, and greater asthma control than placebo. Ilangovan et al[54] evaluated the effect of 1 mg of budesonide or placebo twice daily for 8 weeks in 36 toddlers (mean age 27 months) who required chronically administered oral glucocorticoids. There was an 80% reduction in the mean oral glucocorticoid requirement in the budesonide-treated group compared to a 41% reduction in the placebo-treated group ($P < 0.05$). Over 60% of the children on budesonide were completely tapered off oral glucocorticoid versus only 12.5% randomized to placebo. Budesonide also significantly improved symptom scores and overall health status compared with placebo.

Recent studies evaluated the efficacy and safety of nebulized budesonide in children with mild to moderate persistent asthma. In general, these studies included older children and evaluated multiple budesonide dosages administered once or twice daily given over a 3-month period. Shapiro et al[55] studied three doses of budesonide (0.25 mg, 0.5 mg, and 1 mg) administered twice daily over a 12-week period in a randomized, placebo-controlled, double-blind, parallel group study of 178 children, 4 to 8 years old, on chronic inhaled glucocorticoid therapy. Budesonide was superior to placebo in reducing both daytime and nighttime symptoms and in significantly improving morning peak expiratory flow rates. Budesonide was associated with significantly fewer withdrawals from the study secondary to poorly controlled asthma (9% vs. 36% for budesonide and placebo, respectively). Budesonide therapy did not result in any linear growth suppression, nor was it associated with basal or adrenocorticotropic hormone (ACTH)–stimulated cortisol suppression. Of note, all doses of budesonide were found to be equally effective based on the parameters studied.

Kemp et al[56] sought to evaluate the efficacy of nebulized budesonide administered once daily (0.25, 0.5, or 1 mg) in a 12-week randomized, double-blind, placebo-controlled study of 359 children 6 months to 8 years old (mean age 4.7 years) with mild persistent asthma not on inhaled glucocorticoid therapy. All dosing regimens were more effective than placebo in improving symptoms scores, reducing rescue medication use, and improving morning peak expiratory flow rates in patients who could adequately perform the procedure.

In a study of 480 children ages 6 months to 8 years (mean age 4.6 years) over a 12-week period, Baker et al[57] again found several budesonide doses administered once or twice daily (0.25 mg or 1 mg once daily, 0.25 mg or 0.5 mg twice daily) to be superior to placebo. Of note, improvement in symptom scores occurred as early as 2 weeks after starting budesonide. Twice-daily dosing of 0.5 mg appeared to be somewhat more effective than 1 mg administered once daily. The investigators suggested that a dose of 0.25 mg/day may be sufficient for mild asthma, whereas subjects with moderate asthma should be treated with 0.5 to 1 mg/day and those with severe asthma dependent on oral steroids should be treated with 1 to 2 mg/day. No significant differences in basal cortisol levels or ACTH-stimulated cortisol levels were found between any of the active treatment groups and placebo.

Pharmacokinetics of Nebulized Budesonide in Small Children. Little is known regarding the amount of drug delivered, by any inhaled device and with any drug, to infants and young children with asthma. Inhaled glucocorticoids have the potential for adverse effects, so it is of critical importance to deliver the smallest amount of drug required for response. To address this issue, Agertoft et al[58] evaluated the systemic availability and pharmacokinetics of nebulized budesonide in a group of preschool children (mean age 4.7 years) with chronic asthma. Ten children underwent pharmacokinetic studies of both intravenously administered (125 μg) and inhaled budesonide (1 mg delivered by nebulization). The amount of nebulized budesonide delivered to the patient was calculated by subtracting the amount of drug remaining in the nebulizer, the amount emitted into the ambient air, and the amount found in the mouth after rinsing from the initial amount of budesonide in the nebulizer (the nominal dose). The mean dose to the subject was found to be 23% of the nominal dose (231 μg), while the systemic availability was only 6.1% of the nominal dose, or 61 μg. The clearance of budesonide was calculated to be 0.54 L/min with a $t_{1/2}$ of 2.3 hours, and V_{dss} of 55 L. It is noteworthy that the systemic availability in these small children was approximately half that seen in adults. In addition, the clearance of budesonide in these children was twice that of adults.

Efficacy of Inhaled Glucocorticoids Administered via MDI with Holding Chamber and Mask. The GINA guidelines prefer the administration of inhaled glucocorticoids via MDI with a spacer and facemask in small children with asthma, yet there is a paucity of studies that document the effectiveness of chronically administered inhaled glucocorticoids delivered by this method in this age group. Bisgaard et al[59] sought to determine whether fluticasone delivered via a pMDI with holding chamber and facemask was superior to placebo in improving asthma symptoms in young children with frequent asthma symptoms. Of the children, 32% had previously been hospitalized for an acute exacerbation and 24% were receiving cromolyn before the study. Children (N = 237) with a mean age of 28 months were enrolled to receive fluticasone (100 μg/day or 200 μg/day) or placebo for 12 weeks following a 4-week run-in phase. Fluticasone resulted in a dose-related improvement in asthma symptoms with fluticasone 200 μg/day more effective than placebo in 8 out of 10 diary card parameters (including wheezing, cough, and breathlessness), whereas fluticasone 100 μg/day resulted in significant improvements in five parameters. In addition,

fewer children on fluticasone required a prednisolone burst and fewer experienced asthma exacerbations. Fluticasone delivered via a holding chamber and mask may be effective in this population of small children as a result of its high potency and its long retention time within the lung. These properties, which are present to lesser degrees with the other inhaled glucocorticoids, may explain why there are so few studies published demonstrating efficacy with the other inhaled glucocorticoids in this age group. It may not be advisable to extrapolate the results obtained using the Nebuhaler or the Babyhaler to the currently available devices in the United States such as the Aerochamber with facemask because aerosol delivery is significantly different for the various devices.[60] The authors state that a brief trial of fluticasone can be attempted, and if a response is not seen, therapy should be discontinued. Further, in those that do respond, the dose should be titrated to the lowest effective dose.

Whether or not children with recurrent wheezing will respond to long-term controller therapy is an important question that has yet to be answered. A recent study by Roorda et al[61] using data from two large placebo-controlled studies evaluated the clinical features of preschool children likely to respond to fluticasone administered via a pMDI with holding chamber and facemask. The investigators identified two clinical features that predicted a positive response to inhaled glucocorticoid therapy—those being frequent symptoms (≥ 3 days/wk) and a family history of asthma. In contrast, children with fewer symptoms, no family history of asthma, or both did not appear to respond to fluticasone. The presence of rhinitis or eczema in the child and the number of previous exacerbations were not associated with response to fluticasone.

Children with frequent symptoms and/or a positive family history of asthma are good candidates for inhaled glucocorticoid therapy. It is surprising that the presence of eczema and the number of previous acute exacerbations were not associated with response to fluticasone. The presence of eczema predisposes a child with recurrent wheezing to subsequent asthma,[31] but it does not appear to predict response to inhaled glucocorticoid therapy. It should be noted that a lack of response over a short course of treatment (12 weeks) does not necessarily mean that a response would not be seen over a much longer period of time (months to years).

Inhaled Glucocorticoids and Growth in Small Children. Recent studies evaluating the safety of long-term inhaled glucocorticoid therapy in school-age children with asthma have not shown inhaled glucocorticoid therapy to be associated with significant growth suppression.[51,62] Few published studies evaluate the effects of inhaled glucocorticoids on the linear growth of preschool children. Reid et al,[63] in an open-label study, measured linear growth velocity in 40 children (mean age 1.4 years) before and during treatment with nebulized budesonide. All of the children had "troublesome" asthma despite treatment with an inhaled glucocorticoid administered with a pMDI with spacer and facemask or nebulized cromolyn before entry into the study. They were then administered 1 to 4 mg/day of nebulized budesonide depending on their level of asthma severity. The median intervals of time for linear growth determinations during the run-in period and nebulized budesonide treatments were 6 months and 1 year, respectively. The height standard deviation scores (SDSs) for the group during the run-in period were −0.21, at baseline −0.46, and after at least 6 months of nebulized budesonide

−0.17. Note that an SDS of less than 0 denotes impaired growth velocity. Thus the subjects were growing at less than an impaired rate before nebulized budesonide therapy, and the institution of nebulized budesonide did not result in further growth suppression. In fact, there was a trend toward improved growth velocity while on nebulized budesonide.

Skoner et al[64] recently evaluated the growth of children enrolled in 52-week open-label extension studies of the three efficacy studies of budesonide by Drs. Shapiro, Kemp, and Baker previously discussed. The dose of budesonide was either 0.5 mg once or twice daily with a taper to the lowest tolerated dose, and conventional asthma therapy consisted of any available therapy including inhaled glucocorticoids in two of the studies; in total, 670 children participated. The investigators found a modest impairment in growth in only one of the three extension studies. The extension study where a decline in growth was noted consisted primarily of young children with milder asthma who had not been on inhaled glucocorticoids before entry into the initial study. In contrast, the two extension studies that did not find growth impairment consisted of children with more severe disease and had allowed for inhaled glucocorticoid use as part of the conventional asthma therapy algorithm. The Skoner study suggests that modest growth suppression can occur in young children receiving nebulized budesonide who have not required inhaled glucocorticoid therapy in the past and that children with milder asthma may be at greater risk for growth suppression secondary to increased intrapulmonary deposition. Alternatively, the findings may be attributable to the fact that over twice as many children randomized to the conventional asthma therapy arm withdrew from the study because of poor asthma control.

Poor asthma control can negatively impact growth. The growth of 58 children (mean age 3.5 years for males, 4.4 years for females) with asthma was followed over a 5-year period.[65] Each child's asthma was classified as being in good, moderate, or poor control according to asthma symptoms during a 2-year observational period before the institution of inhaled glucocorticoid therapy. The group as a whole had diminished growth velocity to start the study, with a mean height velocity standard deviation (HVSD) score of −0.51. Children whose asthma was in good control had the least evidence for growth suppression before inhaled glucocorticoid therapy was instituted and continued to grow at the same rate as when on therapy (HVSD score −0.01 pre- vs. −0.07 during treatment). In contrast, the subjects whose asthma was poorly controlled grew poorly before and after institution of inhaled glucocorticoid therapy (HVSD score −1.50 pre- vs. −1.55 during treatment). Of interest, those with moderately controlled asthma demonstrated improved growth velocity while on inhaled glucocorticoid therapy, with their HVSD score increasing from −0.83 to −0.49. The investigators concluded that poor asthma control adversely impacts linear growth to a greater extent than inhaled glucocorticoid therapy.

Alternative and/or Adjunct Medications

The NHLBI NAEPP recently updated version,[47] the newly revised GINA guidelines,[8] the British guidelines,[66] and the International Pediatric Consensus Statement[67] all recommend use of adjunct controller medications for children with moderate to severe persistent asthma in an attempt to limit the dose of inhaled corticosteroid in moderate asthma and oral corticosteroids in severe asthma.

Cromolyn and Nedocromil. Cromolyn (Intal) and nedocromil (Tilade) are related compounds having similar effects on inhibiting mediator release from mast cells. They inhibit both the early- and late-phase pulmonary components of the allergic response following inhalation of an allergen in sensitized subjects.[68] Cromolyn (5 mg four times daily by pMDI) has also been shown in a 6-week double-blind, placebo-controlled crossover trial of 16 ex-premature infants (given at 15 months postnatally) with recurrent episodes of wheezing to reduce symptom scores and β-agonist rescue use and to increase lung function measurement by functional residual capacity (FRC).[69]

Cromolyn and nedocromil are now considered alternative monotherapy for children with mild persistent asthma.[8,48] A few studies have shown no added benefit with the use of cromolyn over placebo in young children with more severe disease.[70-72] Several efficacy studies that have found cromolyn to have beneficial effects were short-term trials and employed small numbers of young children.[73,74]

In a 12-month double-blind, placebo-controlled crossover study, Cogswell and Simpkiss[75] found nebulized cromolyn (20 mg) administered four times daily in a group of young children (mean age 33 months) to be superior to placebo in terms of reducing nighttime cough score, improving daily activity score, increasing the percentage of symptom-free days (60% vs. 50%), and improving asthma overall severity score. Of note, cromolyn did not prevent nor did it modify severe, acute asthma attacks requiring hospitalization. The authors concluded that nebulized cromolyn "is a tedious prophylactic treatment for the young asthmatic, but it is useful when other treatments fail."[75]

Unfortunately, many recent larger studies have failed to find nedocromil[51] or cromolyn[70] to be more effective than placebo for most parameters studied. A recent meta-analysis of 22 control studies evaluating cromolyn in childhood asthma found it no better than placebo.[76] One of the largest studies evaluating the efficacy of cromolyn in young children was by Tasche et al,[70] who enrolled 218 children 1 to 4 years old to receive cromolyn (10 mg) or placebo three times a day administered via pMDI with a holding chamber for 5 months following a 1-month baseline period. Cromolyn and placebo were equally effective in improving symptoms during treatment compared with the baseline period with no differences between the groups in terms of symptom-free days or any other outcome measure. The authors concluded that in the majority of small children, long-term prophylactic cromolyn therapy is no more effective than placebo. A possible shortcoming of this study was the fact that cromolyn was administered via a pMDI and not by nebulization. It is possible that lung deposition of cromolyn may have been enhanced had it been delivered by nebulization. There is one study that attempted to compare the delivery of cromolyn via the nebulizer and the pMDI with holding chamber. In a small study of males aged 9 to 36 months, the amount of cromolyn deposited into the lungs given either via a jet nebulizer compared to a pMDI with a valved spacer was accessed by measuring the urinary sodium cromoglycate.[77] Greater cumulative urinary excretion of sodium cromoglycate was observed when the children were treated with a nebulizer than with a pMDI and spacer. They calculated twice the nominal dose of sodium cromoglycate absorbed via the nebulizer (0.76%) compared with that obtained by the pMDI and spacer (0.30%). This difference may be clinically insignificant because the dose delivered by either method was poor. Hence some of the problems of treatment in young children are the result of inadequate medication reaching the lungs and the differences in the manner by which the medication is delivered.

A multicenter, randomized, parallel-group, 52-week, open-label study in preschool children found nebulized cromolyn (20 mg four times daily) (N = 335) to be inferior to nebulized budesonide suspension (0.5 mg daily) (N = 168) using several outcome parameters. The primary outcome was the rate of asthma exacerbation during the study period. A full dose of the study drug was given for at least 8 weeks and a taper or elevation of the dose was allowed thereafter at physician discretion.[78] Inhaled budesonide suspension was found to significantly reduce the rate of asthma exacerbations per year compared to nebulized cromolyn (median 0.99 vs. 1.85, respectively; $P < 0.001$). In addition, inhaled budesonide was superior to inhaled cromolyn on the other outcome measures evaluated, including longer times to first asthma exacerbation (median 248 vs. 94 days) and first use of additional long-term controller therapy (364.0 vs. 297.5 days); nearly doubled improvements in nighttime and daytime symptom scores by the second week of treatment; and significantly reduced use of rescue medications by the second week of treatment sustained through the rest of the study period. Although there were no significant differences in the rates of hospitalization and emergency room visits between the two groups, significantly lower urgent-care or unscheduled physician visits and oral corticosteroid use were found in children who received the inhaled corticosteroid. There were no clinically significant differences in the adverse events reported. However, mean height increases from baseline in children randomized to inhaled budesonide and inhaled cromolyn were 6.69 and 7.55 cm, respectively. This difference of 0.86 cm is similar to the difference in height measurements seen in other studies with inhaled corticosteroid therapy after 1 year of treatment in older children.[51,79,80]

Leukotriene Modifying Agents.

Leukotrienes are potent proinflammatory mediators that induce bronchospasm, mucus secretion, and airway edema. In addition, they may be involved in eosinophil recruitment into the asthmatic airway.[81] Two classes of leukotriene modifiers have been developed—those that inhibit the production of leukotrienes (synthesis inhibitors) and those that block the binding of leukotrienes to their receptors (receptor antagonists). Leukotriene modifiers have beneficial effects in terms of reducing asthma symptoms and supplemental β agonist use while improving baseline pulmonary function.[82-84] The receptor antagonists prevent the binding of LTD_4 to its receptor. These agents can also block both the early- and late-phase allergic response following allergen challenge. Zafirlukast (Accolate) and montelukast (Singulair) are the only members of this class of drugs currently approved for use in the United States. Zafirlukast is administered twice daily and is approved for children 7 years and older; montelukast is approved for children 2 years of age or older. The recent NHLBI NAEPP update[48] and the GINA guidelines[8] have positioned the LTRAs as an alternative monotherapy for children with mild persistent asthma and as an alternative add-on therapy to low- and medium-dose inhaled corticosteroids for patients with moderate persistent asthma. GINA guidelines recommend LTRAs as a supplemental therapy to high-dose inhaled corticosteroids for severe persistent asthma.

In general, few studies have evaluated the efficacy of the LRTAs in children with any level of asthma severity. Knorr et al[85] evaluated the safety and effectiveness of 8 weeks of montelukast (5 mg once daily) or matching placebo in a large cohort of children (6 to 14 years old) with moderate asthma. Upon entry into the study, the children had a mean forced expiratory volume in 1 second (FEV_1) of 72% of that predicted, and approximately one third of the children remained on an inhaled glucocorticoid during the study. The mean AM FEV_1 for the children randomized to montelukast increased by 8.23% compared with an increase of 3.6% in the placebo group, for a difference of roughly 5% between the two groups. In addition, montelukast therapy was associated with significant decreases in β agonist use and circulating eosinophils. There were no differences in patient-reported daytime or nighttime peak expiratory flows, nocturnal awakening, discontinuations because of worsening asthma, or rescue prednisone use.

Safety and efficacy studies with the 4-mg chewable montelukast tablet in children aged 2 to 5 years with asthma have just been published.[86] Almost 700 children 2 to 5 years of age were enrolled to receive montelukast or placebo for 12 weeks in a double-blind, multicenter, multinational study at 93 centers worldwide. Montelukast was well tolerated and was not associated with any significant adverse effects. Montelukast was superior to placebo in reducing daytime symptoms including improvements in cough, wheeze, difficulty breathing, and activity level, and it effectively reduced nighttime cough. In addition, montelukast therapy was associated with a reduction in rescue β agonist use and reduced need for prednisone for acute severe exacerbations.

Long-acting Inhaled β Agonists.

The current NHLBI NAEPP update summary[48] has placed long-acting inhaled $β_2$ agonists such as salmeterol (Serevent) and formoterol (Foradil) as the preferred add-on therapy for children and adults with moderate and severe persistent asthma. However, no studies in younger children have evaluated their efficacy as a supplemental therapy. Salmeterol delivered using the Diskus device is FDA approved for use in children as young as 4 years of age (50 μg blister every 12 hours), whereas formoterol delivered using the Aerolizer is approved for use in children 6 years of age and older (12 μg capsule every 12 hours). The long-acting $β_2$ agonists are not viewed as "rescue" medications for acute episodes of bronchospasm, nor are they meant to replace inhaled antiinflammatory agents. Salmeterol has a prolonged onset of action with maximal bronchodilation approximately 1 hour following administration; formoterol has an onset of effect within minutes. Both medications have a prolonged duration of action of at least 12 hours. As such, they are especially well suited for patients with nocturnal asthma[87] and for individuals who require frequent use of short-acting β agonist inhalations during the day to prevent exercise-induced asthma.[88]

Preschool children may deserve an extended bronchodilatory coverage for exercise because they are constantly active. There is one study that has evaluated single-dose bronchoprotective effects of salmeterol given through a Babyhaler spacer device using a methacholine provocation challenge in infants less than 4 years old with recurrent episodes of wheezing. Originally 42 preschool children (age range 8 to 45 months) received one of the 25-, 50-, or 100-μg dose of salmeterol and a placebo dose 2 to 7 days apart in a double-blind, randomized fashion, but only 33 completed the study. All the subjects had reactivity to methacholine at or below 8 mg/ml on both visits. The investigators found a dose-dependent bronchoprotective effect of salmeterol measured by treatment/placebo methacholine dose ratios. Significant improvements from placebo were found only for the 50 (2.5 fold) and 100 (fourfold) μg doses.[89]

Few studies that have been performed in older children have found salmeterol to be effective in blocking exercise-induced asthma[88] and in improving lung function.[90] Of note, adding either salmeterol or increasing the dose of beclomethasone in a study of older children failed to result in any further benefit in FEV_1, PD_{20} methacholine, symptom scores, and exacerbation rates after 1 year.[91] This is in marked contrast to several studies in adults.[92-94]

Theophylline. The NHLBI NAEPP 2002 guidelines[48] only mention theophylline as an alternative add-on treatment to low- and medium-dose inhaled glucocorticoid for small children with moderate asthma, whereas the GINA guidelines[8] also extend its use as an add-on medication to severe persistent asthma and as an alternative monotherapy to mild persistent asthma in children. Theophylline is an effective medication in children with asthma.[95,96] Recently published studies in adults with asthma have suggested that the modest antiinflammatory effects from bronchial biopsy specimens of low doses of theophylline were associated with clinical response.[97,98] The NHLBI EPR-2 guidelines state that "theophylline may have particular risks of adverse side effects in infants, and theophylline should only be considered if serum concentration levels are carefully monitored."[7] Theophylline has a narrow therapeutic window and consequently, levels need to be routinely monitored, especially if the child has a viral illness associated with a fever or is placed on a medication known to delay theophylline clearance, such as macrolide antibiotics (erythromycin, clarithromycin), cimetidine, antifungal agents, and ciprofloxacin.[99] Further complicating the use of theophylline in small children is the variability in theophylline metabolism from infancy through childhood requiring frequent dose monitoring and dose adjustments; lastly, sustained-release theophylline can be erratically absorbed.[100]

Nonpharmacologic Intervention

The nonpharmacologic measures may be as important not only for young children with established respiratory symptoms, allergies, and passive smoke exposure but also in the primary and secondary prevention of asthma.[101,102] The first and likely the most important step toward controlling asthma in sensitized children is to avoid or reduce the patient's exposure to the offending allergen. The environmental interventions that seem to hold the most promise are those that target reducing exposure to indoor allergens and tobacco smoke. Specific environmental control measures are covered in Chapter 23.

Lastly, yearly influenza immunization is also strongly recommended for children 6 months of age and older with chronic pulmonary diseases, including asthma. Kramarz et al[103] recently evaluated the effectiveness of influenza vaccination in preventing influenza-related asthma exacerbations in children 1 to 6 years of age using a retrospective cohort study with the Vaccine Safety Datalink, which contains data on more than 1 million children enrolled in four large health maintenance organizations. Of note, less than 10% of children with asthma were vaccinated against influenza in any of the years studied. Although the incidence rates of asthma exacerbation in those who were vaccinated were found to be higher in the vaccinated group than in those who were not vaccinated, the difference was thought to be largely confounded by asthma severity in the vaccinated group. Using a "self-control" analysis to correct for this confounder, the risks of asthma exacerbation during each of the influenza seasons were reduced by 22% to 41% with influenza vaccination.

CONCLUSIONS

There exists a tremendous gap in our knowledge regarding the pathogenesis and management of asthma in older children and adults compared to the information available on this disease in infants and younger children. The findings of large population-based studies that included preschool children with recurrent wheezing demonstrate that they constitute a heterogeneous group. It remains to be determined who should be treated and with what controller medication. The diagnosis and management of infants and small children with asthma remain problematic, and numerous areas need to be explored. Currently no clinically available objective measure of lung function, bronchial hyperresponsiveness, or airway inflammation exists that is applicable to this age group. There is an urgent need to evaluate objectively the efficiency of the various delivery devices available for administration of inhaled therapies to infants and young children. Again, this may be partly the result of the difficulty in evaluating lung deposition because it may require radiolabeled material or invasive techniques for pharmacokinetic analysis. Only a few medications have been approved for use in this population, and none of them have been investigated in long-term studies to evaluate safety and efficacy in controlling the underlying inflammatory reaction and reducing significant exacerbations. In addition, there is a need to conduct large prospective studies to evaluate the impact of early pharmacologic intervention on the natural history of infantile asthma. The NHLBI-sponsored Childhood Asthma Research and Education Network is conducting an early intervention study to specifically look at the role of inhaled glucocorticoids in preventing the development of asthma. The National Institute of Child Health and Human Development's Pediatric Pharmacology Research Unit (PPRU) is a consortium of centers participating with the FDA and the pharmaceutical industry in an attempt to gain labeling of all asthma medications used in small children. A concerted effort by government and industry should drive the impetus in carrying out studies that will fill the gaps in the understanding and treatment of this challenging group of patients.

HELPFUL WEBSITES

The National Heart, Lung, and Blood Institute website (www.nhlbi.nih.gov)

REFERENCES

1. Mannino DM, Homa DM, Akinbami LJ, et al: *Surveillance for asthma—United States, 1980-1999*, Atlanta, 2002, Epidemiology Program Office.
2. Croner S, Kjellman N-I: Natural history of bronchial asthma in childhood, *Allergy* 47:150-157, 1992.

3. Tariq SM, Matthews SM, Hakim EA, et al: The prevalence of and risk factors for atopy in early childhood: a whole population birth cohort study, *J Allergy Clin Immunol* 101:587-593, 1998.

4. Martin AJ, Landau LI, Phelan PD: Lung function in young adults who had asthma in childhood, *Am Rev Respir Dis* 122:609-616, 1980.

5. Mitchell EA, Bland JM, Thompson JMD: Risk factors for readmission to hospital for asthma in childhood, *Thorax* 49:33-36, 1994.

6. Paret G, Kornecki A, Szeinberg A, et al: Severe acute asthma in a community hospital pediatric intensive care unit: a ten years' experience, *Ann Allergy Asthma Immunol* 80:339-344, 1998.

7. Expert Panel Report II: *Guidelines for the diagnosis and management of asthma*, Bethesda, Md, 1997, National Heart, Lung, and Blood Institute/National Institutes of Health.

8. National Heart, Lung and Blood Institute/World Health Organization Workshop: *Global strategy for asthma management and prevention*, Bethesda, Md, 2002, National Institutes of Health.

9. Young S, Le Souef PN, Geelhoed GC, et al: The influence of a family history of asthma and parental smoking on airway responsiveness in early infancy, *N Engl J Med* 324:1168-1173, 1991.

10. Ibero M, Ridao M, Artigas R, et al: Cisapride treatment changes the evolution of infant asthma with gastroesophageal reflux, *Invest Allergol Clin Immunol* 8:176-179, 1998.

11. Werk LN, Steinbach S, Adams WG, et al: Beliefs about diagnosing asthma in young children, *Pediatrics* 105:585-590, 2000.

12. Wilson N, van Bever H: Overall symptom measurement: which approach? *Eur Respir J* S9:8s-11s, 1996.

13. Stocks J, Sly PD, Tepper RS, et al: *Infant respiratory function testing*, New York, 1996, Wiley-Liss & Sons.

14. Hellinckx J, Boeck K, Bande-Knops J, et al: Bronchodilator response in 3-6.5 years old healthy and stable asthmatic children, *Eur Respir J* 12:438-443, 1998.

15. Nielsen KG, Bisgaard H: Discriminitive capacity of bronchodilator response measured with three different lung function techniques in asthmatic and healthy children aged 2 to 5 years, *Am J Respir Crit Care Med* 164:554-559, 2001.

16. Artlich A, Busch T, Lewandowski K, et al: Childhood asthma: exhaled nitric oxide in relation to clinical symptoms, *Eur Respir J* 13:1396-1401, 1999.

17. Dotsch J, Demirakca S, Terbrack HG, et al: Airway nitric oxide in asthmatic children and patients with cystic fibrosis, *Eur Respir J* 9:2537-2540, 1996.

18. Baraldi E, Azzolin NM, Zanconato S, et al: Corticosteroids decrease exhaled nitric oxide in children with acute asthma, *J Pediatr* 131:381-385, 1997.

19. Carra S, Gagliardi L, Zanconato S, et al: Budesonide but not nedocromil sodium reduces exhaled nitric oxide levels in asthmatic children, *Respir Med* 95:734-739, 2001.

20. Mattes J, Storm van's Gravesande K, Reining U, et al: NO in exhaled air is correlated with markers of eosinophilic airway inflammation in corticosteroid-dependent childhood asthma, *Eur Respir J* 13:1391-1395, 1999.

21. Piacentini GL, Bodini A, Costella S, et al: Exhaled nitric oxide and sputum eosinophil markers of inflammation in asthmatic children, *Eur Respir J* 13:1386-1390, 1999.

22. Buchvald F, Bisgaard H: FeNO measured at fixed exhalation flow rate during controlled tidal breathing in children from the age of 2 yr, *Am J Respir Crit Care Med* 163:699-704, 2001.

23. Baraldi E, Dario C, Ongaro R, et al: Exhaled nitric oxide concentrations during treatment of wheezing exacerbation in infants and young children, *Am J Respir Crit Care Med* 159:1284-1288, 1999.

24. Carlsen KCL, Halvorsen R, Ahlstedt S, et al: Eosinophil cationic protein and tidal flow volume loops in children 0-2 years of age, *Eur Respir J* 8:1148-1154, 1995.

25. Brooke AM, Lambert PC, Burton PR, et al: The natural history of respiratory symptoms in preschool children, *Am J Respir Crit Care Med* 152:1872-1878, 1995.

26. Martinez FD, Wright AL, Taussig LM, et al: Asthma and wheezing in the first six years of life, *N Engl J Med* 332:133-138, 1995.

27. Sporik R, Holgate ST, Cogswell JJ: Natural history of asthma in childhood—a birth cohort study, *Arch Dis Child* 66:1050-1053, 1991.

28. Rhodes HL, Thomas P, Sporik R, et al: A birth cohort study of subjects at risk of atopy. Twenty-two-year follow-up of wheeze and atopic status, *Am J Respir Crit Care Med* 165:176-180, 2002.

29. Delacourt C, Benoist M-R, Waernessycle S, et al.: Relationship between bronchial responsiveness and clinical evolution in infants who wheeze, *Am J Respir Crit Care Med* 164:1382-1386, 2001.

30. Clough JB, Keeping KA, Edwards LC, et al: Can we predict which wheezy infants will continue to wheeze? *Am J Respir Crit Care Med* 160:1473-1480, 1999.

31. Castro-Rodriguez JA, Holberg CJ, Wright AL, et al: A clinical index to define risk of asthma in young children with recurrent wheezing, *Am J Respir Crit Care Med* 162:1403-1406, 2000.

32. Bustos GJ, Bustos D, Bustos GJ, et al: Prevention of asthma with ketotifen in preasthmatic children: a three-year follow-up study, *Clin Exp Allergy* 25:568-573, 1995.

33. Warner JO, Early Treatment of the Atopic Child Group: A double-blinded, randomized, placebo-controlled trial of cetirizine in preventing the onset of asthma in children with atopic dermatitis: 18 months' treatment and 18 months' posttreatment follow up, *J Allergy Clin Immunol* 108:929-937, 2001.

34. Reijonen TM, Kotaniemi-Syrajanen A, Korhonen K, et al: Predictors of asthma three years after hospital admission for wheezing in infancy, *Pediatrics* 106:1406-1412, 2000.

35. Sigurs N, Bjarnason R, Sigurbergsson F, et al: Respiratory syncytial virus bronchiolitis in infants is an important risk factor for asthma and allergy at age 7, *Am J Respir Crit Care Med* 161:1501-1507, 2000.

36. Agertoft L, Pedersen S: Effects of long-term treatment with an inhaled corticosteroid on growth and pulmonary function in asthmatic children, *Respir Med* 88:373-381, 1994.

37. Haahtela T, Jarvinen M, Kava T, et al: Effects of reducing or discontinuing inhaled budesonide in patients with mild asthma, *N Engl J Med* 331:700-705, 1994.

38. Newhouse MT: Pulmonary drug targeting with aerosols: principles and clinical applications in adults and children, *Am J Asthma Allergy Pediatr* 7:23-35, 1993.

39. Parkin PC, Saunders NR, Diamond SA, et al: Randomized trial spacer vs nebulizer for acute asthma, *Arch Dis Child* 72:239-240, 1995.

40. Closa RM, Ceballos JM, Gomez-Papi A, et al.: Efficacy of bronchodilators administered by nebulizers versus spacer devices in infants with acute wheezing, *Pediatr Pulmonol* 26:344-348, 1998.

41. Tal A, Golan H, Grauer N, et al: Deposition pattern of radiolabeled salbutamol inhaled from a metered-dose inhaler by means of a spacer with mask in young children with airway obstruction, *J Pediatr* 128:479-484, 1996.

42. Wildhaber JH, Dore ND, Wilson JM, et al: Inhalation therapy in asthma: nebulizer or pressurized metered-dose inhaler with holding chamber? *In vivo* comparison of lung deposition in children, *J Pediatr* 135:28-33, 1999.

43. Gibson NA, Ferguson AE, Aitchison TC, et al: Compliance with inhaled asthma medication in preschool children, *Thorax* 50:1274-1279, 1995.

44. Ferguson AE, Gibson NA, Aitchison TC, et al: Measured bronchodilator use in preschool children with asthma, *Br Med J* 310:1161-1164, 1995.

45. Lim SH, Goh DYT, Tan AYS, et al: Parents' perceptions towards their child's use of inhaled medications for asthma therapy, *J Paediatr Child Health* 32:306-309, 1996.

46. Mesters I, Meertens R, Kok G, et al: Effectiveness of a multidisciplinary education protocol in children with asthma (0-4 years) in primary health care, *J Asthma* 31:347-359, 1994.

47. Wilson SR, Latini D, Starr NJ, et al: Education of parents of infants and very young children with asthma: a developmental evaluation of the Wee Wheezers program, *J Asthma* 33:239-254, 1996.

48. National Asthma Education Prevention Program Expert Panel: *Guidelines for the diagnosis and management of asthma—update on selected topics 2002*, Bethesda, Md, 2002, US Department of Health and Human Services National Heart, Lung, and Blood Institute www.nhlbi.nih.gov.

49. Haahtela T, Jarvinen M, Kava T, et al: Comparison of a β_2-agonist, terbutaline, with an inhaled corticosteroid, budesonide, in newly detected asthma, *N Engl J Med* 325:388-392, 1991.

50. van Essen-Zandvliet EE, Hughes MD, Waalkens HJ, et al: Effects of 22 months of treatment with inhaled corticosteroids and/or beta-agonists on lung function, airway responsiveness, and symptoms in children with asthma, *Am Rev Respir Dis* 146:547-554, 1992.

51. The Childhood Asthma Management Program Research Group: Long-term effects of budesonide or nedocromil in children with asthma, *N Engl J Med* 343:1054-1063, 2000.

52. Suissa S, Ernst P, Benayoun S, et al: Low-dose inhaled corticosteroids and the prevention of death from asthma, *N Engl J Med* 343:332-336, 2000.

53. DeBlic J, Delacourt C, LeBourgeois M, et al: Efficacy of nebulized budesonide in treatment of severe infantile asthma: a double blind study, *J Allergy Clin Immunol* 98:14-20, 1996.

54. Ilangovan P, Pedersen S, Godfrey S, et al: Treatment of severe steroid-dependent preschool asthma with nebulized budesonide suspension, *Arch Dis Child* 68:356-359, 1993.

55. Shapiro G, Mendelson L, Kraemer MJ, et al: Efficacy and safety of budesonide inhalation suspension (Pulmicort Respules) in young children with inhaled steroid-dependent, persistent asthma, *J Allergy Clin Immunol* 102:789-796, 1998.

56. Kemp JP, Skoner DP, Szefler SJ, et al: Once-daily budesonide inhalation suspension for the treatment of persistent asthma in infants and young children, *Ann Allergy Asthma Immunol* 83:231-239, 1999.

57. Baker JW, Mellon M, Wald J, et al: A multiple-dosing, placebo-controlled study of budesonide inhalation suspension given once or twice daily for treatment of persistent asthma in young children and infants, *Pediatrics* 103:414-421, 1999.

58. Agertoft L, Andersen A, Weibull E, et al: Systemic availability and pharmacokinetics of nebulized budesonide in preschool children, *Arch Dis Child* 80:241-247, 1999.

59. Bisgaard H, Gillies J, Groenewald M, et al: The effect of inhaled fluticasone propionate in the treatment of young asthmatic children: a dose comparison study, *Am J Respir Crit Care Med* 160:126-131, 1999.

60. Agertoft L Pedersen S: Influence of spacer device on drug delivery to young children with asthma, *Arch Dis Child* 71:217-220, 1994.

61. Roorda RJ, Mezei G, Bisgaard H, et al: Response of preschool children with asthma symptoms to fluticasone propionate, *J Allergy Clin Immunol* 108:540-546, 2001.

62. Agertoft L, Pedersen S: Effect of long-term treatment with inhaled budesonide on adult height in children with asthma, *N Engl J Med* 343:1064-1069, 2000.

63. Reid A, Murphy C, Steen HJ, et al: Linear growth of very young asthmatic children treated with high-dose nebulized budesonide, *Acta Paediatr* 85:421-424, 1996.

64. Skoner DP, Szefler SJ, Welch M, et al: Longitudinal growth in infants and young children treated with budesonide inhalation suspension for persistent asthma, *J Allergy Clin Immunol* 105:259-268, 2000.

65. Ninan TK, Russell G: Asthma, inhaled corticosteroid treatment, and growth, *Arch Dis Child* 67:703-705, 1992.

66. British Thoracic Society, British Paediatric Association, Royal College of Physicians of London, The King's Fund Centre, National Asthma Campaign: Asthma in children under five years of age, *Thorax* 52:S9-S21, 1997.

67. Warner JO, Naspitz CK, Cropp GJA: Third international pediatric consensus statement on the management of childhood asthma, *Pediatr Pulmonol* 25:1-17, 1998.

68. Dahl R, Pedersen S: Influence of nedocromil sodium on the dual asthmatic reaction after antigen challenge: a double blind, placebo-controlled study, *Eur Respir J* 69 (suppl 147):263-267, 1986.

69. Yuskel B, Greenough A: Inhaled sodium cromoglycate for pre-term children with respiratory symptoms at follow up, *Respir Med* 86:131-134, 1992.

70. Tasche MJ, Van Der Wouden JC, Uijen JH, et al: Randomized placebo-controlled trial of inhaled sodium cromoglycate in 1-4 year old children with moderate asthma, *Lancet* 350:1060-1064, 1997.

71. Bertelsen A, Andersen JB, Busch P, et al: Nebulized sodium cromoglycate in the treatment of wheezy bronchitis, *Allergy* 41:266-270, 1986.

72. Furfaro S, Spier S, Drblik SP, et al: Efficacy of cromoglycate in persistently wheezing infants, *Arch Dis Child* 71:331-334, 1994.

73. Hiller EJ, Milner AD, Lenney W: Nebulized sodium cromoglycate in young asthmatic children: double-blind trial, *Arch Dis Child* 52:875-876, 1977.

74. Glass J, Archer LNJ, Adams W, et al: Nebulized cromoglycate, theophylline, and placebo in preschool asthmatic children, *Arch Dis Child* 56:648-651, 1981.

75. Cogswell JJ, Simpkiss MJ: Nebulized sodium cromoglycate in recurrently wheezy preschool children, *Arch Dis Child* 60:736-738, 1985.

76. Tasche MJ, Uijen JH, Bernsen RM, et al: Inhaled disodium cromoglycate (DSCG) as maintenance therapy in children with asthma: a systematic review, *Thorax* 55:913-920, 2000.

77. Salmon B, Wilson NM, Silverman M: How much aerosol reaches the lungs of wheezy infants and toddlers? *Arch Dis Child* 65:401-403, 1990.

78. Leflein JG, Szefler SJ, Murphy KR, et al: Nebulized budesonide inhalation suspension compared with cromolyn sodium nebulizer solution for asthma in young children: results of a randomized outcomes trial, *Pediatrics* 109:866-872, 2002.

79. Simons FE: A comparison of beclomethasone, salmeterol, and placebo in children with asthma. Canadian Beclamethasone Dipropionate-Salmeterol Xinafoate Study Group, *N Engl J Med* 337:1659-1665, 1997.

80. Verberne AA, Frost C, Roorda RJ, et al: One year treatment with salmeterol compared with beclomethasone in children with asthma. The Dutch Paediatric Asthma Study Group, *Am J Respir Crit Care Med* 156:688-695, 1997.

81. Chung KF: Leukotriene receptor antagonists and biosynthesis inhibitors: potential breakthrough in asthma therapy, *Eur Respir J* 8:1203-1213, 1995.

82. Israel E, Rubin P, Kemp JP, et al: The effect of inhibition of 5-lipoxygenase by zileuton in mild-to-moderate asthma, *Ann Int Med* 119:1059-1066, 1993.

83. Liu MC, Dube LM, Lancaster J: Acute and chronic effects of a 5-lipoxygenase inhibitor in asthma: a 6-month randomized multicenter trial. Zileuton Study Group, *J Allergy Clin Immunol* 98:859-871, 1996.

84. Spector SL, Smith LJ, Glass M: Effects of 6 weeks of therapy with oral doses of ICI 204,219, a leukotriene D4 receptor antagonist, in subjects with bronchial asthma. ACCOLATE Asthma Trialists Group, *Am J Respir Crit Care Med* 150:618-623, 1994.

85. Knorr B, Matz J, Bernstein JA, et al: Montelukast for chronic asthma in 6- to 14-year-old children, *JAMA* 279:1181-1186, 1998.

86. Knorr B, Franchi LM, Bisgaard H, et al: Montelukast, a leukotriene receptor antagonist, for the treatment of persistent asthma in children aged 2 to 5 years, *Pediatrics* 108:E48, 2001.

87. Fitzpatrick MF, Mackay T, Driver H, et al: Salmeterol in nocturnal asthma: a double-blind, placebo controlled trial of a long-acting inhaled beta 2 agonist, *Br Med J* 301:1365-1368, 1990.

88. Green CP, Price JF: Prevention of exercise-induced asthma by inhaled salmeterol xinafoate, *Arch Dis Child* 67:1014-1017, 1992.

89. Primhak RA, Smith CM, Yong SC, et al: The bronchoprotective effect of inhaled salmeterol in preschool children: a dose-ranging study, *Eur Respir J* 13:78-81, 1999.

90. Von Berg A, De Blic J, La Rosa M, et al: A comparison of regular salmeterol vs. 'as required' salbutamol in asthmatic children, *Respir Med* 92:292-299, 1998.

91. Verberne AA, Frost C, Duiverman EJ, et al: Addition of salmeterol versus doubling the dose of beclomethasone in children with asthma: the Dutch Asthma Study Group, *Am J Respir Crit Care Med* 158:213-219, 1998.

92. Greening AP, Ind PW, Northfield M, et al: Added salmeterol versus higher-dose corticosteroid in asthma patients with symptoms on existing inhaled corticosteroid, *Lancet* 344:219-224, 1994.

93. O'Byrne PM, Barnes PJ, Rodriguez-Roisin R, et al: Low-dose inhaled budesonide and formoterol in mild persistent asthma, *Am J Respir Crit Care Med* 164:1392-1397, 2001.

94. Woolcock A, Lundback B, Ringdal N, et al: Comparison of addition of salmeterol to inhaled steroids with doubling the dose of inhaled steroids, *Am J Respir Crit Care Med* 153:1481-1488, 1996.

95. Neijens HJ, Duiverman EJ, Graatsma BH, et al: Clinical and bronchodilating efficacy of controlled-release theophylline as a function of its serum concentrations in preschool children, *J Pediatr* 107:811-815, 1985.

96. Stratton D, Carswell F, Hughes AO, et al: Double-blind comparisons of slow-release theophylline, ketotifen, and placebo for prophylaxis of asthma in young children, *Br J Dis Chest* 78:163-167, 1984.

97. Kidney J, Dominguez M, Taylor PM, et al: Immunomodulation by theophylline in asthma, *Am J Respir Crit Care Med* 151:1907-1914, 1995.

98. Sullivan P, Bekir S, Jaffar Z, et al: Anti-inflammatory effects of low-dose oral theophylline in atopic asthma, *Lancet* 343:1006-1008, 1994.

99. Hendeles L, Weinberger M, Szefler SJ, et al: Safety and efficacy of theophylline in children with asthma, *J Pediatrics* 120:177-183, 1992.

100. Haltom JR, Szefler SJ: Theophylline absorption in young asthmatic children receiving sustained-release formulation, *J Pediatr* 107:805-810, 1985.

101. Boner AL, Bodini A, Piacentini GL: Environmental allergens and childhood asthma, *Clin Exp Allergy* 28(suppl 5):76-81, 1998.

102. Peat J, Bjorksten B: Primary and secondary prevention of allergic asthma, *Eur Respir J* 27:28s-34s, 1998.

103. Kramarz P, Destefano F, Gargiullo PM, et al: Does influenza vaccination prevent asthma exacerbations in children? *J Pediatr* 138:306-310, 2001.

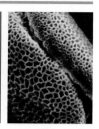

CHAPTER 37

Inner City Asthma

CRAIG A. JONES ■ LORAN T. CLEMENT

During the past 20 years, inner city asthma has emerged as a story about the influence of modern society on health and disease. Although asthma prevalence and morbidity have increased in many countries worldwide, a disproportionate increase has occurred in westernized urban settings. Extensive multidisciplinary research efforts have been directed toward understanding the causes of this epidemic. In the United States a desire to mitigate health care–related financial pressures has certainly provided one important motivation. In 1995 the direct costs of asthma care in the United States were estimated to be $6.2 billion, with 65% related to emergency department (ED)–or hospital-based care. Considerable effort has been focused on understanding and correcting a pattern of resource utilization that is considered expensive and episodic.

However, investigation of the urban asthma epidemic that has taken place goes beyond the motivations stemming from escalating health care costs. To some degree, the study of inner city asthma offers a fundamental look at the way in which modern living and an urban environment influence the functions of the immune system. It is also a look at the way in which environmental, social, and economic factors can converge to influence health status and the course of a chronic disease. In addition, research studies of urban asthma have provided a novel view of the ways that modern societies prioritize, structure, and fund health care delivery, as well as the way in which social and economic factors influence health care utilization.

PREVALENCE, MORBIDITY, AND MORTALITY OF ASTHMA IN INNER CITIES

Asthma Prevalence

The International Study of Asthma and Allergies in Childhood Steering Committee has reported that the 12-month prevalence of symptoms of asthma among children 13 to 14 years of age in countries around the world varies from 1.6% to 36.8%, with the highest prevalence rates generally found in economically developed, "westernized" societies.[1] In the United States the principal source of national asthma prevalence data has been the National Health Interview Survey conducted by the National Center for Health Statistics. In 1995 the overall age-adjusted prevalence rate for asthma in the United States was estimated to be 5.38%.[2] Among children,

prevalence rates are considerably higher. Of U.S. children, 11% have been diagnosed with asthma at some time in their lives,[3] and the highest age-specific prevalence rate for any age group (7.4%) is found for children 5 to 14 years of age.[2]

From 1980 through 1995, the overall age-adjusted asthma prevalence rate in the United States increased by 75%.[2] Similar, albeit smaller, increases have been noted in a number of other countries.[4] Demographic analyses have consistently shown that the increased prevalence and morbidity of asthma have been disproportionate among various segments of the population.[2,5-7] The populations in the United States that have been most affected include the following:

- Children: Although increases in prevalence and morbidity across time have occurred in all age groups, the greatest proportionate rise has occurred in children.[2,6] From 1980 through 1995, asthma prevalence increased by 160% in children younger than 5 years and by 74% in children 5 to 14 years old. Significant increases in ED visits and hospitalizations due to asthma have also occurred, and the number of children dying from asthma increased almost threefold from 1979 to 1996.
- Urban populations: The prevalence of asthma for people living in an urban setting in the United States (7.1%) is higher than that found for those living in rural areas (5.7%).
- Ethnic minorities: Racial differences in asthma prevalence, morbidity, and mortality have consistently been found. The greatest increases in asthma prevalence have been seen among African Americans and people of Puerto Rican heritage. In 2000 the prevalence of asthma among African Americans (8.5%) exceeded that reported for whites (7.1%) or persons of other race/ethnicity (5.6%).
- Low socioeconomic status (SES) populations: The prevalence of asthma is inversely correlated with family income; asthma prevalence varied from 9.8% among persons with family incomes of less than $15,000 to 5.9% in those with family incomes of greater than $75,000.[6]

Numerous efforts have been made to determine asthma prevalence rates for children living in various U.S. cities.[8-12] The disparate, and often staggering, prevalence rates reported for several U.S. inner city populations are shown in Table 37-1. It is important to note that accurate measurements of asthma prevalence in inner city populations are problematic.

392

Woolcock[13] has described five areas of difficulty: (1) the lack of a uniform definition of asthma, (2) the absence of a standardized questionnaire, (3) the nonspecific nature of bronchial provocation tests, (4) the variable nature of the disease at different ages, and (5) the seasonal nature of the illness. Because there also is no uniform definition of the term *inner city*, further variation in the environmental or demographic characteristics of different urban areas can be expected. As a result, it remains difficult to ascertain, interpret, or compare asthma prevalence rates reported for different inner city populations, and establishing coordinated and systematic local, state and national systems for asthma surveillance is one of the 5-year priorities of the Action Against Asthma initiative in the United States.[14] Although precise prevalence figures may be lacking, the evidence that asthma has disproportionately affected inner city children is compelling.

Asthma Morbidity

The increased prevalence of asthma has been accompanied by a significant rise in the number of ED visits and hospitalizations due to asthma. In 1998 there were an estimated 2 million ED visits for asthma in the United States.[15] The ED visit rate for children was substantially higher than that for adults, and the rate for African Americans was more than three times higher than rates for non-Hispanic whites.[15] Factors associated with recurrent or increased use of the ED for asthma care included lower education, single-parent families, African American race, and residence in an urban setting.[16,17]

Comparable increases in the estimated number of asthma-related hospitalizations have been reported.[2] Although recent data suggest that hospitalization rates may have stabilized or even been reduced, there were still 423,000 asthma hospitalizations in the United States in 1998.[15] Rates have consistently been higher for children and African Americans than for other age or ethnic groups.[15] The most striking increases have occurred in inner city neighborhoods inhabited by ethnic minorities and/or persons of low SES.[18,19]

Asthma Mortality

From 1960 to 1978, the overall mortality rate for asthma in the United States declined by 7.8% per annum. Declining rates were observed for all age, gender, and ethnic groups.[2,20] Since 1979, however, U.S. asthma mortality rates have been steadily increas-ing, and the overall age-adjusted mortality rate in 1998 was 55.6% higher than the rate reported in 1978.[21] Neither more frequent diagnosis nor aging of the population could account for this change.[20] Fortunately, the number of children who die from asthma remains low; in 1998 only 246 children in the United States were reported to have died because of asthma.[21]

Although asthma mortality has increased for all major demographic groups since 1978, certain populations are at strikingly increased risk. In the United States, deaths from asthma occur predominantly in large cities. Among urban dwellers, those who are at particularly high risk include persons of low SES and ethnic minorities.[2,22-24] Asthma mortality rates for African Americans are particularly disturbing: age-adjusted mortality rates are more than three times greater for urban African Americans (particularly young African American males) than for whites.[23] Among children, the disparity appears to be even greater: from 1993 through 1995, African American children were more than four times as likely to die from asthma as were white children.[25] In one U.S. city, asthma mortality remained stable among non-Hispanic whites from 1968 to 1991 but increased by 337% for African Americans.[24]

CAUSATIVE OR CONTRIBUTORY FACTORS

Urbanization

From the earliest analyses, it has been apparent that the pace and magnitude of the increases in asthma prevalence and morbidity (in the United States and elsewhere) have been greatest among urban populations.[26,27] The hypothesis that the "urbanization" of a discrete population results in an increase in the prevalence and morbidity of asthma has stimulated considerable interest in identifying transcultural facets of urban life that may alter the prevalence and/or morbidity of this disease. Perhaps the most striking revelation from the hundreds of elegant, yet frequently inconclusive, analyses that have been conducted is the complexity of this issue. Potential sources of variability and/or contradiction include the following:

- There are inconsistent definitions of asthma and variations in methodology.
- "Inner cities" are not uniform, either in the United States or globally. The largest U.S. cities differ considerably in climate, ethnic composition, air pollution, cultural practices, and a broad range of other attributes that have been implicated as possible risk factors.
- Most of the putative risk factors for inner city populations are prevalent in other settings. For example, the poverty rate in rural areas of the United States exceeds that found in metropolitan areas and closely approaches the rate found for inner city populations.[28] Rural children with asthma (from every ethnic group) face many of the same barriers that have been proposed to adversely affect the health of their urban counterparts; indeed, the prevalence and/or magnitude of these barriers is often greater for rural children, who are less likely to have health insurance, face greater geographic barriers to health care, and are less likely to see an asthma specialist or be treated with long-term controllers.[29-31]

Some of the factors that have been most frequently found to be associated with the increased prevalence, morbidity, and mortality from asthma among inner city dwellers are

Urban Area	Prevalence of Diagnosed Asthma	Prevalence of Undiagnosed (Probable) Asthma	Reference
Bronx County, New York	14.3%	4.2%	9
San Diego, California	14.7%	12.5%	10
Detroit, Michigan	17.4%	11.7%	11
Chicago, Illinois	10.8%	ND	12
Chicago, Illinois	16.0%	ND	13

TABLE 37-1 Asthma Prevalence Rates for Children Living in U.S. Inner Cities

ND, Not determined.

discussed later. Although certain attributes, either individually or in combination, identify populations at risk, there continues to be uncertainty or even controversy concerning the role of these factors in the inner city asthma epidemic. Taken together, it appears quite likely that a variable array of different risk factors and barriers, which are probably unique to each child or family, combine to increase the risk of morbidity from this treatable disease.

Putative Factors in the Physical Environment

Since genetic change seems highly unlikely in the short time span attending the inner city asthma explosion, exposures to environmental factors, including allergens and indoor and outdoor pollutants, have been postulated to have contributory roles.

Increased Allergen Exposure and Sensitization

Although little indication exists that the mechanisms involved in allergen sensitization are qualitatively different for those living in the inner city, a number of studies have suggested that sensitization and subsequent reexposure to high levels of certain allergens more commonly found in the inner city may play an important role in the inner city asthma epidemic. Three allergens (cockroach, dust mite, and cat) have been most extensively studied.

Cockroach Allergens. One allergen of particular interest is cockroach allergen.[32] High levels of this allergen have been demonstrated in many inner city homes in the United States, and cockroach allergy is common among poor inner city dwellers.[32-35] The risk of sensitization appears to be related to the concentration of allergen in bedrooms.[36] Although cockroach infestation, allergen exposure, and sensitization is certainly not unique to urban dwellings,[37] the number of homes with elevated allergen concentrations appears to be greater in urban settings; thus children living in the inner city may be more likely to be exposed and sensitized.[36]

Important information about the possible role of inner city allergens has come from studies conducted by the National Cooperative Inner-City Asthma Study (NCICAS) group. Children with asthma symptoms who lived in urban neighborhoods where more than 30% of the households had incomes below the poverty level were enrolled. In a study investigating allergen sensitization and exposure, cockroach allergy was found to be a particularly significant factor in the morbidity of inner city asthma.[35] The asthma hospitalization rate for children who were cockroach sensitive and exposed to high levels of this allergen was more than threefold higher than seen for other children in this cohort. These children also had 78% more unscheduled visits to health care facilities and significantly more days and nights with asthma symptoms. Both allergen sensitivity and exposure to high levels of cockroach allergen were required to produce increased asthma morbidity. Although comparable numbers of children were allergic to other common inner city allergens, such as dust mite and cat, no significant associations between any measure of asthma morbidity and high exposure to these allergens was noted.

House Dust Mite Allergens. Exposure and sensitization to dust mite allergen are frequently high in inner city areas, where human crowding, high indoor humidity, and older carpeting or bedding provide ideal conditions for mite proliferation.[34,38] Exposure to high levels of dust mite allergen has been shown to be associated with asthma,[39] and in a recent analysis of 27 environmental agents that have been reported to play a role in the development of asthma, the Institute of Medicine concluded that exposure to dust mites was one of only two exposures (along with tobacco smoke) for which there was sufficient evidence to establish an etiologic role.[40] In both case-control and prospective cohort studies conducted in a variety of geographic settings, reducing dust mite allergen exposure has been found to mitigate asthma morbidity in sensitized subjects.[41-43] Although dust mite sensitization and exposure were not shown to affect asthma symptom frequency or the rate of hospitalization in one inner city cohort,[35] it nonetheless seems likely that dust mite allergy plays an important role in inner city asthma, particularly in locales that promote dust mite proliferation.

Cat Allergens. Cat allergens are commonly detected in urban settings; indeed, significant concentrations are found in 25% of inner city residences without pets and in about 25% of urban airborne samples.[44] Although it is clear that exposure to cat allergen can trigger asthma symptomatology in sensitized individuals, several studies have failed to detect a strong correlation between cat allergen exposure and increased asthma morbidity in inner city populations.[35,36,45]

Although the hypothesis that allergen sensitization and exposure are responsible for the increased morbidity of asthma in the inner city remains popular, some have questioned whether the epidemiologic evidence in support of this premise is sufficient.[46,47] They argue that the data from population studies are equivocal and provide little consistent evidence that allergen exposure is associated with the asthma prevalence at the population level. They also point out that there have been no longitudinal studies in which allergen exposure during infancy in a random population sample has been related to asthma risk after the age of six years. Indeed, two longitudinal studies that were conducted in selected populations chosen on the basis of a family history of asthma or allergy failed to show an association between allergen exposure and current asthma.[46,47] Others have suggested that factors unrelated to atopy are of primary importance because preschool wheezing disorders distinct from atopic asthma, such as virus-induced wheezing, have also increased in recent years.[48] Finally, there is little evidence that allergen concentrations, sensitization rates, or the magnitude of allergen exposure has increased during the 25 years in which the prevalence and morbidity of asthma in U.S. cities has so dramatically increased. Cockroaches and dust mites have been present (and shown to be allergenic) in inner city environments for many decades.[49] It remains to be established whether changes in allergen sensitization and/or exposure *per se* have contributed to the increases in asthma prevalence and morbidity that have been observed.

Air Pollution

The possible role that air pollution may play in the inner city asthma epidemic has been the subject of a number of recent reviews.[50-53] The outdoor air pollutants that have been most widely studied include ozone, sulfur dioxide, nitrogen dioxide, volatile organic compound emissions, diesel exhaust particles, and particulate matter, a complex mixture of particles containing many components, including endotoxin. Laboratory and epidemiologic studies have linked high concentrations of many of these air pollutants with signs of increased asthma morbidity (bronchial hyperreactivity, pulmonary function decrements, and increases in medication use, ED visits, and asthma-related hospitalizations). Indoor air pollution has received less attention, and environmental tobacco smoke (ETS; discussed later) is the only indoor air pollutant that has consistently been linked to disease activity.

Studies seeking to define the role of air pollutants in the increasing morbidity of inner city asthma have focused on two questions. What initiates (or induces) the appearance of asthma in an unaffected individual? What triggers (or provokes) asthma attacks among persons who already have the disease? A number of different investigators have concluded that, with the possible exception of tobacco smoke, it appears unlikely that either outdoor or indoor air pollution has contributed substantially to the initiation of asthma in healthy subjects or to the increases in asthma prevalence or morbidity that have been observed in recent decades, in the inner cities or elsewhere.[50-53] Exposure to pollutant levels that evoke acute respiratory responses is uncommon in community air pollution. Furthermore, temporal correlations between the concentrations of most air pollutants and signs of increasing asthma morbidity have generally been poor. The striking increase in inner city asthma has occurred during a time when the concentrations of all major outdoor air pollutants have declined substantially, a trend apparent since the mid-1960s. Taken together, these data suggest that air pollution has not been a major factor in the increasing morbidity of asthma in inner city populations during the past 25 years.

Environmental Tobacco Smoke Exposure

Numerous studies have shown that children exposed to ETS have a considerably higher-than-average risk of developing asthma.[54] As noted previously, the Institute of Medicine has concluded that exposure to tobacco smoke was one of only two exposures (along with dust mite exposure) for which there was sufficient evidence to establish an etiologic role.[40] Exposure to ETS has also been shown to increase airway reactivity, the frequency of ED visits, and the risk of hospitalization for children with asthma.[54-56] Although the level of cigarette smoking has declined in the United States during the past two decades, smoking rates remain relatively high in many inner city populations.[56,57] The role that ETS exposure may play in the increased morbidity of asthma in the inner cities has not been precisely defined, but it is likely that exposure to ETS contributes to this problem.

Socioeconomic, Cultural, and Ethnic Factors

Low Socioeconomic Status

Almost all analyses of the risk factors associated with increased asthma morbidity in the United States have shown that inner city residents of low SES are disproportionately affected, in terms of both increased disease prevalence and increased rates of adverse clinical sequelae (ED use, hospitalization, and mortality). This relationship has been the subject of numerous reviews or commentaries.[26,58-60] The measures used to define low SES have varied somewhat; low family income has been the primary variable in almost all U.S. studies, whereas occupational social class has been used more

frequently in Great Britain.[60] Other parameters that have been used as indicators of low SES include low parental or personal education levels, health insurance status, or enrollment in Medicaid programs.

Although increased asthma morbidity has consistently been associated with low SES in most studies of urban populations in the United States, a review of 22 questionnaire-based studies of asthma in children from other countries revealed little consistency in the relationship between SES and asthma morbidity, although children with severe asthma generally had lower SES.[61] In addition, atopy, which continues to be the single most significant risk factor for the development of asthma, has frequently been found to be more prevalent among those of higher SES groups, and asthma severity and morbidity do not appear to be increased in individuals of lower SES (of any ethnicity) who live in rural environments of the United States. Thus it appears that the association of increased asthma morbidity with lower SES may be largely restricted to the inner cities of the United States.

Many of the problems faced by poor families are directly related to their economic privation. However, a number of other factors that have been linked to asthma (smoking, obesity, large family size, low birth weight, and minority ethnic background) are also more prevalent in populations of lower SES in the United States. In Table 37-2, some of the environmental, socioeconomic, cultural, and psychosocial factors that have been reported to contribute to the morbidity of asthma in inner city children from families of lower SES are listed.

Asthma in Ethnic Minorities

During the latter half of the twentieth century, the percentage of inner city residents belonging to ethnic minorities increased significantly in the United States. According to the 2000 U.S. Census, the non-Hispanic white share of population in the largest 100 cities declined to 44%, the lowest level on record. Almost half of these cities no longer have majority white populations. Because these demographic changes correlated temporally with the increased asthma morbidity and mortality noted for inner city residents, numerous studies have been done to assess the basis for the disproportionate burdens borne by various ethnic minorities living in the inner cities.

The difficulties experienced by African Americans have been particularly well documented. As noted previously, the prevalence of asthma in African American children and adults is higher than that found for other ethnic populations.[2,5,7] Disproportionately increased rates of ED use and hospital admissions for asthma have also been repeatedly observed for inner city African American populations, and disturbing differences in asthma mortality rates (particularly for young African American males) have been well documented.[19,21-24,62,63] Whether these substantial differences are the result of independent ethnic factors or reflect the coexisting burdens resulting from lower SES or inner city environmental factors has been the subject of some debate. A number of epidemiologic studies have reported that the increased prevalence or morbidity of asthma is still significantly associated with race (African-American versus white) after adjusting for socioeconomic factors, environmental exposures, and other confounding factors.[23,63-65] In contrast, others have found that the increased risks in African-American children lost significance when other risk factors were included in multivariate linear

TABLE 37-2 Factors Reported to Contribute to Asthma Morbidity in Children of Lower Socioeconomic Status

Suboptimal access to medical care
No health insurance
Limited access to primary care physicians
Limited access to asthma specialists
Lack of transportation to outpatient health care facilities
Poor access to asthma support groups
Unable to afford medications

Inadequate medical care
Improper diagnosis or underdiagnosis
Lack of recognition of asthma severity by physician
Underprescription of controller medications

Increased frequency of other contributory or comorbid medical conditions
Obesity
Low birth weight, preterm delivery
More frequent upper respiratory infections

Inadequate asthma education
Lack of understanding of the role of bronchial inflammation
Lack of understanding of the importance of early intervention
Overuse or inappropriate use of asthma medications
Poor adherence to therapeutic regimens

Low level of education or illiteracy

Psychosocial dysfunction of patient and family
Depression
Mood and anxiety disorders
Hopelessness and despair
Stress from exposure to violence and crime
Illicit drug use

Lack of social support
Young maternal age
Single-parent families
Social isolation of caregivers
Lack of child care resources

Increased exposure to indoor or outdoor environmental agents
Dust mites
Cockroaches
Air pollutants
Maternal cigarette smoking and/or exposure to tobacco smoke

Deprived living conditions
Overcrowded living conditions
Decrepit housing and physical decay

regression models.[7,12,18] At the present time, an unequivocal explanation for the increased problems faced by African Americans remains elusive.

Increased asthma prevalence and morbidity rates have also been reported for inner city Hispanic populations.[9,59,65-68] The Hispanic population (a grouping defined solely by cultural heritage) is racially and culturally diverse, and the prevalence and impact of asthma appear to vary among subgroups. In the United States, asthma prevalence, hospitalization, and mortality rates are highest for Hispanics of Puerto Rican ancestry.[9,66,67] Rates for Mexican Americans appear to be considerably lower, approaching those reported for non-Hispanic whites in some studies[67,68] but not others.[9] This variability may at least in part reflect the fact that asthma is often underdiagnosed in this population.[9,68] The basis for the increased morbidity of asthma in inner city Hispanics appears to be multifactorial. Many of the factors that have been reported (low SES and lower educational attainment[60]) parallel those identified for other ethnic minorities. In addition, Hispanics are particularly likely to have poor access to medical care. In many areas of the United States, medical insurance coverage is considerably lower for Hispanic children than for African American or non-Hispanic white children.[9,69] Language barriers and/or social or culturally based beliefs about health and illness appear to be of greater significance than low SES or environmental exposures.[66,70]

Little is currently known about the prevalence or morbidity of asthma in inner city Asian populations. However, recent survey data suggest that the prevalence and morbidity of asthma among Asian Americans is lower than that seen in other ethnic minorities and approximates that seen in non-Hispanic white populations.[65,68]

When analyzing data from studies examining the disproportionate morbidity of asthma among ethnic minorities, it is important to note that epidemiologic studies cannot adequately quantify a variety of highly subjective factors that may nonetheless be extremely important. These include numerous cultural factors, habits, traditions, or beliefs that may differ significantly among populations grouped by ethnicity. In addition, ethnicity may be a surrogate measure of discrimination that affects the nature or quality of health care, even within systems where access is not a variable.[63,71] Finally, as discussed later, asthma-related medical care for ethnic minorities and the poor living in the inner cities of the United States may be inaccessible, inappropriate, or substandard in quality.

Inadequacies of the Health Care Delivery System

Although many of the risk factors associated with inner city asthma extend beyond the traditional purview of U.S. health care systems, deficiencies in the availability or quality of the medical care received by inner city residents play a major and perhaps primary role in the increased morbidity of asthma experienced by this population. Although almost every attribute, process, and component of asthma care for inner city populations has been studied and described in detail, the current status of asthma care in the inner city can best be understood when it is first viewed in a broader context. The functions of urban health care delivery systems and the manner in which they are used are influenced by a number of complex issues that converge to define life in the urban United States. These include the logistics of daily living for people of lower SES, interactions among people of diverse ethnic and cultural backgrounds, and the financial incentives that influence health care providers and health service models.

From almost any perspective, the picture of asthma care that emerges from this mix of social, cultural, and economic influences is unsettling. In the United States it is largely a picture of African American and Hispanic children living in an environment that is defined and dominated by their lower socioeconomic standing. They often have only episodic contact with health care professionals, and this typically occurs when they are acutely ill in a setting, such as an ED, that is neither structured nor inclined to provide disease-specific education, prescribe long-term antiinflammatory medications, or engage in other preventative care practices. When inner city children do have contact with health care providers in a more appropriate setting, their asthma severity may be underestimated, and they are often undertreated. Even if antiinflammatory medications are prescribed, adherence and outcomes are poor for those patients who do not have routine follow-up with a single, knowledgeable provider. Poor compliance is accentuated by the fact that many of these children are from single-parent households, and they are frequently responsible for their own daily care.

Appropriate, effective care for children with chronic diseases is typically a complex process that requires coordinated interactions among different components of the health care delivery system. For inner city children with asthma, almost every link in the health care delivery chain has been shown to be broken or deficient.

Inadequate Access to Health Care

Lack of Health Insurance. A significant fraction (as high as 25%) of children in some urban areas do not have health insurance.[69,72] In comparison with children with insurance, uninsured children are more likely to lack a regular source of care, to rely on EDs for their care, and to go without needed care for chronic health conditions, including asthma.[72,73] The Institute of Medicine has cited lack of adequate health insurance as the single most important barrier to health care services for children in the United States.[74]

Poor Access to Asthma Specialists. Patients receiving their asthma care from specialists have higher health-related quality of life measures and are considerably more likely to report using asthma controller therapy.[75-77] Access to care from asthma specialists is reduced for those who are poor (and, independently, for those who belong to an ethnic minority).[71]

Inappropriate Utilization of Health Care Resources

Numerous studies have shown that EDs are frequently the main source of health care for inner city asthmatics.[78,79] In part, this can be directly attributed to the increased prevalence and/or severity of asthma among inner city residents. In addition, asthma patients without insurance or a primary caregiver may use the ED as a last resort, when asthma symptoms or exacerbations can no longer be ignored and emergency care is essential.

The need for repetitive emergency care has a number of untoward consequences. First, this may become habitual: the ED can become a familiar surrogate for a primary care provider. In one study, poor asthmatic subjects were four times more likely to attend an ED than other asthmatics with similar severity.[80] This pattern of inappropriate utilization, which is independent of health insurance status, may continue, even when more appropriate sources of outpatient care are available.[16,81,82] In addition, a wide variety of other socioeconomic barriers (e.g., transportation difficulties or

problems in paying copayments) have been shown to discourage the use of nonurgent health care resources and to increase the number of ED visits for asthma care.[81] Certain "cultural" attributes of the medical care delivery system also contribute to this phenomenon. Patterns of reimbursement by insurance companies or other payers, which often reimburse care provided in an ED more readily or fully than regular outpatient care, is likely to perpetuate this process. This "crisis management" approach to care contributes to the higher admission rates for inner city asthmatics that are seen in urban EDs.[81,83]

Reliance on an ED for asthma care has numerous other shortcomings. Children who receive care in an ED seldom receive any significant education about long-term asthma control. They rarely receive written action plans and are unlikely to be started on controller medications, and provisions for follow-up care in regular facilities are sporadic and are associated with poor adherence. What happens after a child leaves the ED, and why is the transition to regular outpatient preventive care so unusual? Detailed insight emerges from an NCICAS study examining follow-up care for inner city children who were seen in an ED for an acute exacerbation of asthma.[84] Only 29% of the patients were provided a follow-up appointment at the time of the ED visit; 69% of these appointments were kept. An additional 39.9% were told to make an appointment. More than 78% of the caretakers tried to make an appointment, and 63% were able to do so: 95% of these appointments were kept. In contrast, for the 31% who were neither given an appointment nor told to make one, only 28% made a follow-up appointment. Caretaker-reported barriers to making an appointment included (1) their child was well, (2) lack of a suitable appointment time, (3) not knowing an appointment was needed, (4) busy telephone, (5) busy parent, and (6) cost. It is important to focus on the lessons learned from "real world" studies such as this because children will not have improved health status unless they become engaged in routine preventive health care practices.

Inadequate Medical Care

Studies like NCICAS demonstrate that it is essential to develop strategies that transition families from episodic care to routine outpatient care. However, at the present time, it is not clear that this would improve the health status of inner city children with asthma because it has been repeatedly documented that the quality of care delivered to poor inner city children who do gain access to primary medical care is typically suboptimal.[79,85-87] Frequently, the diagnosis of asthma is not made, even when children are experiencing daily respiratory symptoms.[10] Inner city children with asthma are rarely treated in accordance with nationally accepted standards of asthma care. Primary care physicians frequently report that they are unable to devote the time needed to provide disease-specific education, and written treatment plans outlining the steps that should be taken when an asthma exacerbation commences are seldom provided or explained.

The failure to prescribe antiinflammatory medications for children with persistent asthma is particularly common and consequential. It is widely accepted that the daily use of controller medications, such as inhaled corticosteroids, can reduce the number of asthma exacerbations and ED visits.[88] A large number of studies have shown that patients with persistent asthma (in all areas of the country, including the inner cities) are frequently not using the controller medications indicated for controlling disease activity. This may result because these medications are not prescribed, because prescriptions are not filled, or because patients fail to use the medications as directed. One of the more thorough descriptions of the use of controller medications by inner city children was reported as part of a school- and community-based intervention project.[87] Almost all participating children were from a low-income, single-parent family, and the caregiver was typically uneducated and unemployed. The majority (90%) of these families had insurance or Medicaid; thus, access to care and medication costs were not primary obstacles. Although the children in this study had frequent symptoms and substantial asthma-related morbidity, 20% had no medication or were using only over-the-counter remedies, and only 10% took cromolyn or inhaled steroids. The poor health status of these children resulted from the lack of a competent, familiar health care provider and inadequate engagement of the parent or caretaker in maintenance therapy; an ongoing relationship with a single physician was associated with increased use of antiinflammatory medications, and children were more likely to use these medications if the parent believed that the medications should be taken regularly.

Any effective solution for the inner city asthma epidemic will require the focused allocation of limited resources to produce a health care delivery chain in which all of the essential links are intact—and capable of withstanding the strains that will be produced in treating thousands of disadvantaged children with a chronic disease (Box 37-1).

STRATEGIES FOR INNER CITY ASTHMA INTERVENTIONS

The inability of existing health care practices to stem the rise in inner city asthma morbidity has stimulated research efforts designed to develop interventions that can improve the health of inner city children with asthma. Strategies that have been tested include expanded access to specialty care, structured transitions from acute care sites to appropriate outpatient care, the use of asthma care coordinators and patient tracking, education programs for health care providers, education programs for asthmatic children and their caregivers, school- and community-based outreach programs, and programs to reduce environmental risk factors.[89-100] Some of the general characteristics of selected interventions, with references, are summarized in Table 37-3.

Although these intervention models differ in rationale, goals, and approach, the programs are not mutually exclusive. Each has provided insight and information that can be used to guide the development of integrated programs in the future. From the data and descriptions that have been reported, several observations about inner city asthma interventions can be made. First, it appears that almost any intervention strategy results in improvements in some measure of the health status of inner city children with asthma; thus paying more attention to the problem is likely to produce benefits. Attention focused on solving the individual problems of individual patients and their families improves health status and enhances ongoing patient participation, which is extremely important.[94-96] Frequent contact and consistent follow-up are associated with superior outcomes; education or assistance provided by a single, familiar person is particularly meaningful in this regard. It appears that efforts to educate patients and families about asthma are almost always useful but seldom, if ever, sufficient to deal with all aspects of clinical care for this chronic disease. It remains unclear whether allergen reduction strategies can improve clinical outcomes for inner city children; the challenge of eliminating a mobile and hardy pest like the cockroach from large urban areas appears to be particularly daunting.[97,98]

Efforts to develop interventions that alter patterns of health care utilization or physician practices have met with only modest success. Despite widespread efforts for over a decade, it does not appear that asthma education programs directed solely at health care providers have translated into significant changes in the health of inner city children or the quality of their asthma care. Nonetheless, it does appear that well-structured education programs have the potential to raise the standard of asthma care provided by physicians and to improve what is accomplished during the limited time that is available to primary care physicians for individual patient interactions.[99,100]

Although interventions structured to provide comprehensive, accessible, ongoing specialty care have consistently been shown to improve the health status of patients with asthma, the rationale for many alternative approaches is often based on the premise that direct specialty care interventions are likely to be too expensive to offer to large inner city

---

BOX 37-1	**KEY CONCEPTS**
	Characteristics of Inner City Asthma

- Increases in asthma prevalence, morbidity, and mortality rates during the concluding three decades of the 20th century have been disproportionately great in urban areas, particularly those of the United States.
- The pace and magnitude of these changes have been greatest for inner city dwellers of low socioeconomic status, members of ethnic minorities, and children.
- Deficiencies in the availability or the quality of preventive medical care received by inner city inhabitants have played a major role in the increased asthma *morbidity* experienced by this population.
- Sensitization and subsequent reexposure to high levels of certain allergens commonly found in the inner city (e.g., cockroaches) may contribute to asthma morbidity.
- Although air pollution adversely affects asthma health status, levels of most pollutants have decreased in urban areas during the time period when inner city asthma prevalence and morbidity have increased, and associations between pollutant levels and asthma activity are inconsistent. Exposure to potential immune-modifying pollutants (e.g., diesel particulates, tobacco smoke) may be of etiologic significance.
- Taken together, current evidence suggests that the health status of inner city children with asthma in the United States is a chronicle of inadequate or inappropriate health care superimposed on the social, educational, environmental, and cultural consequences of low socioeconomic status in an urban setting.

TABLE 37-3 Intervention Strategies and Models

Strategic Goal	General Approach	Demonstrated Benefits	References
Enhanced access to specialty care	Provide ongoing access to asthma care specialists. Provide comprehensive care plans in accordance with national asthma care standards.	Reduced acute care visits Reduced hospitalizations Increased preventative care Possible cost reductions	89-92
Structured transition from acute care to outpatient care	Standardize and centralize acute asthma care. Arrange and monitor transition from acute care setting to outpatient settings that provide optimal preventive care.	Reduced length of stay in ED and as inpatient Reduced ED and inpatient readmission rates	93
Patient and family education by specially trained social workers or peer counselors	Educate families, coordinate care activities, assist with allergen reduction efforts, and/or monitor self-management care practices.	Fewer symptomatic days Reduced hospitalizations Possible reduction of acute care visits Improved environmental control measures	94, 95
Community-based social networking and education	Establish informal social networks throughout a community to effect behavior changes, broaden patient education, and improve asthma management practices.	Improved community awareness of asthma	96
Reduction of environmental risk factors	Conduct home visits for environmental evaluation and allergen reduction procedures.	Reduced concentrations of some indoor allergens Reduced acute care visits Improved allergen avoidance practices	97, 98
Educate health care providers	Distribute educational materials and conduct classes targeted to improve physician awareness and compliance with asthma care standards.	Improved use of asthma controller therapy Improved patient education and care practices	99, 100

populations. However, several recent research studies (and our experience with the Breathmobile program in Los Angeles) suggest that specialty care can be provided to inner city populations in a cost-effective fashion.[89-92] Because comprehensive care by asthma specialists has proved to be the most effective and preferred approach for treating asthma in other segments of society, it is logical and reasonable to implement specialty care programs in the inner city, where asthma morbidity is greatest. This approach offers the most promising model to ensure that antiinflammatory medications will consistently be advocated and prescribed. Existing evidence indicates that any intervention strategy that fails to achieve proper use of controller medications (in any setting) will not alter the morbidity of asthma.

Finally, it is important to note that most of these research efforts have evaluated intervention strategies that involve relatively small numbers of patients. The NCICAS Phase II study, which is the largest inner city intervention reported to date, included 515 patients, and the costs to scale and sustain this intervention were not reported. Frequently, there is anticipation that strategies that are effective in controlled trials will translate into changes in health care delivery systems. Although most of the interventions that have been studied have had a positive impact on study participants, they have not translated into widespread, sustained changes in health care services or the health of inner city populations. This may in part reflect the fact that current health care delivery models

are primarily motivated by financial concerns and/or cost efficacy rather than by clinical efficacy. If intervention research is going to have an impact on inner city health care delivery systems, it is important for these efforts to be conducted on a scale and in a manner that evaluates both clinical and cost efficacy.

CONCLUSIONS

One of the most notable aspects of the inner city asthma explosion in the United States relates to its timing. During the past three decades, air pollution has been reduced by more than 90%, the number of people who smoke has declined by 30%, and advances in basic and medical sciences, intensive care practices, and drug development have provided knowledge and tools that would quite reasonably be expected to produce the opposite result, yet almost every parameter of asthma morbidity in the inner cities of the United States has increased by more that 75%. Although efforts to control the problem have increased, gains have been modest; current prevalence data show that asthma continues to be a major health problem for inner city populations, particularly children.

Insight into this paradox, and into the actions that should be taken in the future to effect solutions, has emerged from the many studies of inner city asthma that have been completed. At present, the chronicle of inner city children with asthma is a story about barriers. It is a story about inadequate health care delivery systems superimposed on the consequences of poverty, single-parent households, low literacy and caretaker awareness, and the difficulties of contemporary urban life in the United States. In this setting, children frequently lack access to medical care that is structured to effectively meet the challenges posed by this chronic, but controllable, disease. Families often live in crowded conditions with high levels of exposure to environmental risk factors that are difficult to modify. Transportation difficulties, fears of losing a job, and other challenges of daily living frequently overshadow health care as a routine priority.

It is important to develop comprehensive care and disease management strategies that can improve the health of inner city *populations* in the context of these social, economic, and environmental realities. Efforts dedicated to restructuring the manner in which health care is provided as a means to improving the quality of the medical care that these children receive have been minimal. Instead, research efforts have largely focused on describing the social, cultural, educational, behavioral, and environmental risk factors in an urban environment. Similarly, most inner city asthma interventions have focused on utilizing people who are not professional health care providers to help families in small study cohorts to overcome the consequences of their SES and urban living. Themes such as improving problem solving or communication skills, influencing families to alter their living environment and risk behaviors, or developing supportive social structures have been emphasized. Despite the merits of these goals, health care de-livery has been largely unaffected by the types of intervention studies that have been published in the research literature to date. Entities that pay for and deliver health care have not adopted strategies aimed at modifying social, cultural, and environmental risk factors. Instead, health care delivery models have continued to evolve in response to economic and business pressures that do not regard excellent health outcomes as the single, overriding priority. Other factors such as cost efficacy, scalability, and sustainability become equally important components.

It is important to consider why population-scale, comprehensive care delivery programs have seldom been investigated. Programs of this nature may be too expensive or require an infrastructure too complex to be supported by research grants. However, the large integrated health care enterprises that operate in inner city settings have the substantial infrastructure needed to test and implement comprehensive care programs. Why has this not happened? In large part, this can be explained by the reimbursement patterns that support these institutions. Under current Medicaid reimbursement rules, payments to health care institutions are highest for ED and inpatient care. This provides an unmistakable incentive for these health care institutions to allocate resources to high acuity service areas rather than toward developing comprehensive outpatient disease management programs, which are poorly reimbursed, if at all. Accordingly, the health care delivery systems that have the infrastructure to test comprehensive programs are financially penalized for strategies that shift patient care from ED and

---

BOX 37-2	**THERAPEUTIC PRINCIPLES**

Standards of excellence in medical care should not be compromised.	Asthma care for disadvantaged children should be comprehensive and in full accordance with standards established by the National Asthma Education and Prevention Program (NAEPP).
Care should be provided by a physician with the appropriate knowledge, experience, and level of involvement.	The participation of a concerned asthma specialist is of demonstrated efficacy and offers the most effective and preferred approach.
The proper use of inhaled corticosteroids and other controller medications must be emphasized.	Considerable evidence indicates that any intervention that fails to achieve regular use of controller medications is unlikely to substantially alter asthma morbidity.
Care activities should be accessible, recurrent, and engaging.	Children and family members should have regular contact at a readily accessible site with a stable, familiar team of specially trained health care providers and support personnel.
Adequate time for a meaningful patient-provider interaction is essential.	The time required for appropriate clinical assessment, effective patient education, and assistance with overcoming other barriers to care should be recognized and anticipated in advance.
Teaching is not the same as learning.	Patients and their families must achieve—and demonstrate—a thorough understanding of a written action plan and the purpose and correct use of every medication. This typically requires personal, one-on-one educational efforts that cannot be achieved with pamphlets or video presentations.
Outcomes and patient asthma-related behaviors should be monitored.	An integrated disease management program greatly facilitates patient identification, compliance with appointments and medication use, and targeted efforts to reduce inappropriate utilization of health care resources or detrimental behaviors.

inpatient sites to an outpatient setting. In a sense, the lack of comprehensive asthma care programs in urban health care systems appears to be a logical consequence of current economic incentives, which are not aligned with the health service needs of those with a chronic disease.

To foster the development of comprehensive care programs that are likely to have the greatest impact on inner city asthma, reimbursement incentives should be restructured. The best opportunity to test these strategies for lower socioeconomic populations may reside in the public health sector. With adequate resource allocation, shared risk, and the infrastructure that large health care delivery systems offer, it would be possible to evaluate changes in health status at a population level.

The development of improved health care delivery models is a matter of some urgency. Despite more than a decade of efforts to disseminate information about national and international asthma treatment standards or to educate primary care providers, inner city children continue to receive episodic and inadequate care. During this time span, the majority of children from lower socioeconomic urban backgrounds have also obtained access to health care through Medicaid-sponsored health plans. Although this is an essential component of any solution, improving access to routine care has not affected asthma morbidity among inner city populations. Effective care for chronic conditions is likely to require fundamental changes that allocate resources to regular visits with qualified health care specialists who provide consistent disease-specific education, implement appropriate therapeutic strategies, monitor compliance, and engage families in preventive health care practices. Therapeutic principles for effective asthma care are summarized in Box 37-2.

As noted previously, comprehensive, accessible, ongoing specialty care has consistently been shown to improve the health status of patients with asthma.[75-77,89-93] Despite the proven efficacy of this approach, efforts to develop large-scale, comprehensive asthma care programs to address the inadequacies of health care delivery in urban settings have been thwarted by the widespread belief that comprehensive specialty care would be too expensive to offer to large inner city populations.[94] However, recent data indicate that comprehensive specialty care that improves health status and diminishes acute care needs can be delivered in the context of the social and economic realities of an inner city environment. Furthermore, it has been shown that this is not more expensive than the costs associated with current inadequate practices.[89]

Although a sustainable, integrated health service model for inner city children with asthma may seem implausible, this can be achieved with appropriate financial support and interagency cooperation. In Los Angeles the Southern California Chapter of the Asthma and Allergy Foundation of America, the Los Angeles County Department of Health Services (LAC DHS), and the Los Angeles Unified School District have entered into a partnership to develop a public health model.

During a 6-year period, the program has evolved from a community outreach effort to an integrated disease-management model. Currently, four Breathmobiles serve 85 schools and three county comprehensive health centers across a wide geographic area. More than 4000 patients have been entered into the program, there have been more than 21,000 patient visits, and show rates for follow-up appointment visits at each site have been high, ranging from 70% to 85%. An efficient procedure has been developed to screen children for asthma at their schools and to offer families ongoing care in the program. Clinical information and outcome measures are tracked in a computerized information system. The Pediatric Asthma Disease Management Center provides a reminder before appointments and monitors missed appointments. Care coordination services are provided based on patient need. Computer terminals allow referrals to be sent to the care coordinators from the ED, inpatient wards, and outpatient pediatric clinics of LAC DHS facilities. Performance measures are used to routinely evaluate and modify program operations, and to evaluate program impact. In February 2002, the program became the first disease-specific care program in the United States to be credentialed by the Joint Commission on Accreditation of Healthcare Organizations (JCAHO) after a thorough review process.

This experience clearly demonstrates that, with appropriate financial and infrastructure support, it is possible to develop health service models (Figure 37-1) that provide appropriate, effective care by asthma specialists to a large population of inner city children with asthma (Box 37-3).

BOX 37-3	**KEY CONCEPTS**
	Intervention Strategies and Opportunities

- Effective inner city asthma interventions must incorporate key *therapeutic principles* that can be resourcefully applied within the context of the social, economic, and environmental realities of the contemporary urban setting.

- Intervention strategies designed to educate primary health care providers or to alter existing patterns of health care utilization have not produced significant improvements in the quality or regularity of preventative asthma care received by inner city children or translated into widespread changes in health care delivery systems.

- The best opportunities to develop and establish models of care for inner city populations may lie within large health care delivery systems and public hospitals that already have the necessary infrastructure and network resources.

- Current Medicaid reimbursement policies motivate resource allocation to emergency room and inpatient service areas. As the ultimate purchaser of health care for poor inner city populations, Medicaid reimbursement should be restructured to provide economic incentives for establishing effective outpatient programs that emphasize preventative care.

- Health care models structured to provide ongoing, comprehensive, specialty care are currently feasible and offer an effective approach to improve the health of inner city children with asthma.

- Future efforts toward primary prevention and disease modification may have the greatest impact on asthma health at a population level.

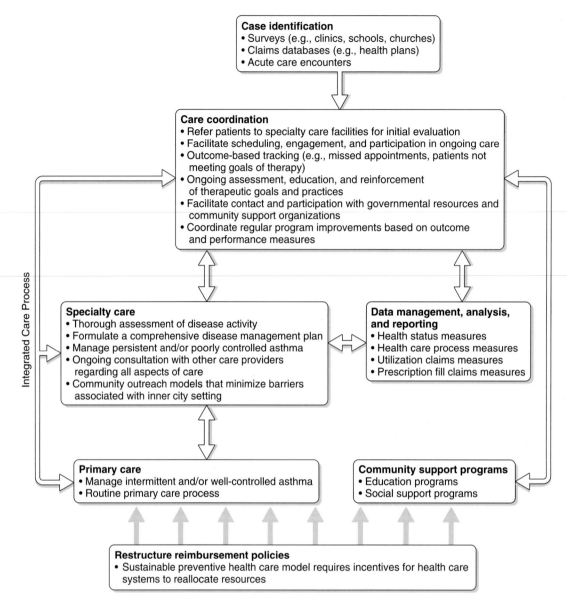

FIGURE 37-1 Algorithm for health service model for inner city asthma care.

An expanded commitment by all components of the health care delivery system to participate in the solution to this problem will be required. When achieving this goal becomes a priority, however, there is reason to be hopeful that the inner city asthma epidemic can be controlled. With continued research, it is possible that the required emphasis on changing health care delivery practices can be augmented with strategies aimed at primary prevention and disease modification.

HELPFUL WEBSITES

The Action Against Asthma website (www.aspe.hhs.gov/sp/asthma/index.htm)
The National Center for Health Statistics, Asthma website (www.cdc.gov/nchs/products/pubs/pubd/hestats/asthma/asthma.htm)

REFERENCES

1. Beasley R, Keil U, von Mutius E, et al: Worldwide variation in prevalence of symptoms of asthma, allergic rhinoconjunctivitis, and atopic eczema: ISAAC, *Lancet* 351:1225-1232, 1998.
2. Mannino DM, Homa DM, Pertowski, CA, et al: Surveillance for Asthma—United States, 1960-1995, *MMWR* 47:1-28, 1998.
3. Bloom B, Tonthat L: Summary health statistics for U.S. children: National Health Interview Survey, 1997, *Vital Health Stat* 10(203), 2002.
4. Strachan DP, Anderson HR, Limb ES, et al: A national survey of asthma prevalence, severity, and treatment in Great Britain, *Arch Dis Child* 70:174-178, 1994.
5. Gergen PJ, Mullally DI, Evans RE III: National survey of prevalence of asthma among children in the United States, 1976 to 1980, *Pediatrics* 81:1-7, 1988.
6. Self-reported asthma prevalence among adults—United States, 2000, *MMWR* 50:682-686, 2001.
7. Weitzman M, Gortmaker SL, Sobol AM, et al: Recent trends in the prevalence and severity of childhood asthma, *JAMA* 268:2673-2677, 1992.

8. Crain EF, Weiss KB, Bijur PE, et al: An estimate of the prevalence of asthma and wheezing among inner-city children, *Pediatrics* 94:356-362, 1994.

9. Christiansen SC, Martin SB, Schleicher NC, et al: Current prevalence of asthma-related symptoms in San Diego's predominantly Hispanic inner city children, *J Asthma* 33:17-26, 1996.

10. Joseph CLM, Foxman B, Leickly FE, et al: Prevalence of possible undiagnosed asthma and associated morbidity among urban schoolchildren, *J Pediatr* 129:735-742, 1996.

11. Grant EN, Daugherty SR, Moy JN, et al: Prevalence and burden of illness for asthma and related symptoms among kindergartners in Chicago public schools, *Ann Allergy Asthma Immunol* 83:113-120, 1999.

12. Persky VW, Slezak J, Contreras A, et al: Relationships of race and socioeconomic status with prevalence, severity, and symptoms of asthma in Chicago school children, *Ann Allergy Asthma Immunol* 81:266-271, 1998.

13. Woolcock AJ: Epidemiologic methods for measuring prevalence of asthma, *Chest* 91:89S-92S, 1987.

14. Action Against Asthma: A Strategic Plan for the Department of Health and Human Services, May 2000. Available on the World Wide Web (accessed November 11, 2002): http://aspe.hhs.gov/sp/asthma/index.htm.

15. Fact sheet. New Asthma Estimates: Tracking Prevalence, Health Care, and Mortality. National Center for Health Statistics National Center for Health Statistics, Center for Disease Control and Prevention, 10/050/01. Available on the World Wide Web (accessed November 11, 2002): http://www.cdc.gov/nchs/products/pubs/pubd/hestats/asthma/asthma.htm.

16. Halfon N, Newacheck PW, Wood DL, et al: Routine emergency department use for sick care by children in the United States, *Pediatrics* 98:28-34, 1996.

17. Rand CS, Butz AM, Kolodner K, et al: Emergency department visits by urban African American children with asthma, *J Allergy Clin Immunol* 105:83-90, 2000.

18. Wissow LS, Gittelsohn AM, Szklo M, et al: Poverty, race and hospitalization for childhood asthma. *Am J Public Health* 78:777-781, 1988.

19. Gergen PJ, Weiss KB: Changing patterns of asthma hospitalization among children: 1979-1987, *JAMA* 264:1688-1692, 1990.

20. Weiss KB, Wagener DK: Changing patterns of asthma mortality: identifying target populations at high risk, *JAMA* 264:1683-1687, 1990.

21. Murphy SL: *Deaths: final data for 1998*, National Vital Statistics Reports, National Center for Health Statistics, Center for Disease Control and Prevention, vol 48, July 24, 2000.

22. Carr W, Zeitel L, Weiss K: Variations in asthma hospitalizations and deaths in New York City, *Am J Public Health* 82:59-65, 1992.

23. Lang DM, Polansky M: Patterns of asthma mortality in Philadelphia from 1969 to 1991, *N Engl J Med* 331:1542-1546, 1994.

24. Targonski PV, Persky VW, Orris P, et al: Trends in asthma mortality among African Americans and whites in Chicago, 1968 through 1991, *Am J Public Health* 84:1830-1833, 1994.

25. Underlying cause of death dataset, 1996. National Center for Health Statistics. Action Against Asthma: A Strategic Plan for the Department of Health and Human Services, May 2000. Available on the World Wide Web (accessed November 11, 2002): http://aspe.hhs.gov/sp/asthma/index.htm.

26. Sly RM: Asthma in the inner city, *Immunol Allergy Clin North Am* 11:103-151, 991.

27. Van Niekerk CH, Weinberg EG, Shore SC, et al: Prevalence of asthma: a comparative study of urban and rural Xhosa children, *Clin Allergy* 9:319-324, 1979.

28. Dalaker J: *U.S. Census Bureau, Current population reports, series P60-214, poverty in the United States: 2000*, Washington, DC, 2001, U.S. Government Printing Office.

29. Schwartz DA: Etiology and pathogenesis of airway disease in children and adults from rural communities, *Environ Health Perspectives* 107:393-401, 1999.

30. von Maffei J, Beckett WS, Belanger K, et al: Risk factors for asthma prevalence among urban and nonurban African American children, *J Asthma* 38:555-564, 2001.

31. Yawn BP, Mainous AG III, Love MM, et al: Do rural and urban children have comparable asthma care utilization? *J Rural Health* 17:32-39, 2001.

32. Arruda KL, Vailes LD, Ferriani VPL, et al: Cockroach allergens and asthma, *J Allergy Clin Immunol* 10:419-428, 2001.

33. Kang B: Study on cockroach antigen as a probable causative agent in bronchial asthma, *J Allergy Clin Immunol* 58:357-365, 1976.

34. Call RS, Smith TF, Morris E, et al: Risk factors for asthma in inner city children, *J Pediatr* 121:862-866, 1992.

35. Rosenstreich DL, Eggleston PA, Kattan M, et al: The role of cockroach allergy and exposure to cockroach allergen in causing morbidity among inner-city children with asthma, *N Engl J Med* 336:1356-1363, 1997.

36. Sarpong SB, Hamilton RG, Eggleston PA, et al: Socioeconomic status and race as risk factors for cockroach allergen exposure and sensitization in children with asthma, *J Allergy Clin Immunol* 97:1393-1401, 1996.

37. Garcia DP, Corbert ML, Sublet JL, et al: Cockroach allergy in Kentucky: a comparison of inner city, suburban, and rural small town populations, *Ann Allergy* 72:203-208, 1994.

38. Arlian LG, Bernstein D, Bernstein IL, et al: Prevalence of dust mites in the homes of people with asthma living in eight different geographic areas of the United States, *J Allergy Clin Immunol* 90:292-300, 1992.

39. Sporik R, Holgate ST, Platts-Mills TAE, et al: Exposure to house-dust mite allergen (Der p I) and the development of asthma in childhood, *N Engl J Med* 323:502-507, 1990.

40. Institute of Medicine: *Clearing the air: asthma and indoor air exposures*, National Academy of Sciences, January 19, 2000. Available on the World Wide Web (accessed November 11, 2002): http://books.nap.edu/catalog/9610.html.

41. Korsgaard J: Mite asthma and residency: a case-control study on the impact of exposure to house-dust mites in dwellings, *Am Rev Respir Dis* 128:231-235, 1983.

42. Murray AB, Ferguson AC: Dust-free bedrooms in the treatment of asthmatic children with house dust or house dust mite allergy: a controlled trial, *Pediatrics* 71:418-422, 1983.

43. Ehnert B, Lau-Schadendorf S, Weber A, et al: Reducing domestic exposure to house dust mite allergen reduces bronchial hyperreactivity in sensitive children with asthma, *J Allergy Clin Immunol* 90:135-138, 1992.

44. Woodcock A, Custovic A: Allergen avoidance: does it work? *Br Med Bull* 56:1071-1086, 2000.

45. Platts-Mills TAE, Carter MC: Asthma and indoor exposure to allergens, *N Engl J Med* 336:1382-1384, 1997.

46. Pearce N, Pekkanen J, Beasley R: How much asthma is really attributable to atopy? *Thorax* 54:268-272, 1999.

47. Pearce N, Douwes J, Beasley R: Is allergen exposure the major primary cause of asthma? *Thorax* 55:424-431, 2000.

48. Kuehni CE, Davis A, Brooke AM, et al: Are all wheezing disorders in very young (preschool) children increasing in prevalence? *Lancet* 357:1821-1825, 2001.

49. Bernton HS, Brown H. Insect allergy—preliminary studies of the cockroach, *J Allergy* 35:506-513, 1964.

50. Teague WG, Bayer CW: Outdoor air pollution. Asthma and other concerns, *Pediatr Clin North Am* 48:1167-1183, 2001.

51. Koenig JQ: Air pollution and asthma, *J Allergy Clin Immunol* 104:717-722, 1999.

52. Strachan DP: The role of environmental factors in asthma, *Br Med Bull* 56:865-882. 2000.

53. Peden DB: Air pollution in asthma: effect of pollutants on airway inflammation, *Ann Allergy Asthma Immunol* 87:12-17, 2001.

54. Martinez FD, Cline M, Burrows B: Increased incidence of asthma in children of smoking mothers, *Pediatrics* 89:21-26, 1992.

55. Chilmonczyk BA, Salmun LM, Megathlin KN, et al: Association between exposure to environmental tobacco smoke and exacerbations of asthma in children, *N Engl J Med* 328:1665-1669, 1993.

56. Evans D, Levison MJ, Feldman CH, et al: The impact of passive smoking on emergency room visits of urban children with asthma, *Am Rev Respir Dis* 135:567-572, 1987.

57. Brownson RC, Jackson-Thompson J, Wilkerson JC, et al: Demographic and socioeconomic differences in beliefs about the health effects of smoking, *Am J Public Health* 82:99-103, 1992.

58. Weiss KB, Gergen PJ, Crain EF: Inner city asthma. The epidemiology of an emerging US public health concern, *Chest* 101:362S-367S, 1992.

59. Coultas DB, Gong H Jr, Grad R, et al: Respiratory diseases in minorities of the United States, *Am J Respir Crit Care Med* 149:S93-S131, 1994.

60. Rona RJ: Asthma and poverty, *Thorax* 55:239-244, 2000.

61. Mielck A, Reitmeir P, Wjst M: Severity of childhood asthma by socioeconomic status, *Int J Epidemiol* 25:388-393, 1996.

62. Malveaux FJ, Houlihan D, Diamond EL: Characteristics of asthma mortality and morbidity in African-Americans, *J Asthma* 30:431-437, 1993.

63. Lozano P, Connell FA, Koepsell TD: Use of health services by African-American children with asthma on Medicaid, *JAMA* 274:469-473, 1995.

64. Nelson DA, Johnson CC, Divine GW, et al: Ethnic differences in the prevalence of asthma in middle class children, *Ann Allergy Asthma Immunol* 78:21-26, 1997.

65. Ray NF, Thamer M, Fadillioglu B, et al: Race, income, urbanicity, and asthma hospitalization in California: a small area analysis, *Chest* 113:1277-1284, 1998.

66. Poma PA: The Hispanic health challenge, *J Natl Med Assoc* 80:1275-1277, 1988.

67. Carter-Pokras OD, Gergen JP: Reported asthma among Puerto Rican, Mexican American, and Cuban children, 1982 through 1984, *Am J Public Health* 83:580-582, 1993.

68. *New asthma estimates: tracking prevalence, health care, and mortality,* National Center for Health Statistics, Asthma, October 2001. Available on the World Wide Web (accessed November 11, 2002): http://www.cdc.gov/nchs/products/pubs/pubd/hestats/asthma/asthma.htm.

69. Recent trends in health insurance coverage among Los Angeles County children. Los Angeles County Department of Health Services, *L.A. Health,* 3(1), October 2000.

70. Beckett WS, Belanger K, Gent JF, et al: Asthma among Puerto Rican Hispanics: a multi-ethnic comparison study of risk factors, *Am J Respir Crit Care Med* 154:894-899, 1996.

71. Zoratti EM, Havstad S, Rodriguez J, et al: Health service use by African Americans and Caucasians with asthma in a managed care setting, *Am Rev Respir Crit Care Med* 158:371-377, 1998.

72. Newacheck PW, Stoddard JJ, Hughes DC, et al: Health insurance and access to primary care for children, *N Engl J Med* 338:513-519, 1998.

73. Andrulis DP: Access to care is the centerpiece in the elimination of socioeconomic disparities in health, *Ann Intern Med* 129:412-416, 1998.

74. Institute of Medicine: *America's children: health insurance and access to care,* Washington, DC, 1998, National Academy Press.

75. Vollmer WM, O'Hollaren M, Ettinger KM, et al: Specialty differences in the management of asthma: a cross-sectional assessment of allergists' patients and generalists' patients in a large HMO, *Arch Intern Med* 157:1201-1208, 1997.

76. Jatulis DE, Meng YY, Elashoff RM, et al: Preventive pharmacologic therapy among asthmatics: five years after publication of guidelines, *Ann Allergy Asthma Immunol* 81:82-88, 1998.

77. Vilar ME, Reddy BM, Silverman BA, et al: Superior clinical outcomes of inner city asthma patients treated in an allergy clinic, *Ann Allergy Asthma Immunol* 84:299-303, 2000.

78. Dales RE, Schweitzer I, Kerr P, et al: Risk factors for recurrent emergency department visits for asthma, *Thorax* 50:520-524, 1995.

79. Crain EF, Kercsmar C, Weiss KB, et al: Reported difficulties in access to quality care for children with asthma in the inner city, *Arch Pediatr Adolesc Med* 152:333-339, 1998.

80. Halfon N, Newacheck PW: Childhood asthma and poverty: differential impacts and utilization of health services, *Pediatrics* 91:56-61, 1993

81. Hanania NA, David-Wang A, Kesten S, et al: Factors associated with emergency department dependence of patients with asthma, *Chest* 111:290-295, 1997.

82. Joseph CLM, Havstad SL, Ownby DR, et al: Racial differences in emergency department use persist despite allergist visits and prescriptions filled for anti-inflammatory medications, *J Allergy Clin Immunol* 101:484-490, 1998.

83. Stern RS, Weissman JS, Epstein AM: The emergency department as a pathway to admission for poor and high-cost patients, *JAMA* 266:2238-2243, 1991.

84. Leickly EF, Wade SL, Crain E, et al: Self reported adherence, management behavior, and barriers to care after an emergency department visit by inner city children with asthma, *Pediatrics* 101:8, 1998.

85. Finkelstein JA, Brown RW, Schneider LC, et al: Quality of care for preschool children with asthma: the role of social factors and practice setting, *Pediatrics* 95:389-394, 1995.

86. Homer CJ, Szilagyi P, Rodewald L, et al: Does quality of care affect rates of hospitalization for childhood asthma? *Pediatrics* 98:18-23, 1996.

87. Eggleston PA, Malveaux FJ, Butz AM, et al: Medications used by children with asthma living in the inner city, *Pediatrics* 101:349-354, 1998.

88. Adams RJ, Fuhlbrigge A, Finkelstein JA, et al: Impact of inhaled anti-inflammatory therapy on hospitalizations and emergency department visits for children with asthma, *Pediatrics* 107:706-711, 2001.

89. Kelly CS, Morrow AL, Shults J, et al: Outcomes evaluation of a comprehensive intervention program for asthmatic children enrolled in Medicaid, *Pediatrics* 105:1029-1035, 2000.

90. Moore CM, Ahmed I, Mouallem R, et al: Care of asthma: allergy clinic versus emergency room, *Ann Allergy Asthma Immunol* 78:373-380, 1997.

91. Sperber K, Ibrahim H, Hoffman B, et al: Effectiveness of a specialized asthma clinic in reducing asthma morbidity in an inner city minority population, *J Asthma* 32:335-343, 1995.

92. Battleman DS, Callahan MA, Silber S, et al: Dedicated asthma center improves the quality of care and resource utilization for pediatric asthma: a multicenter study, *Acad Emerg Med* 8:709-715, 2001.

93. Evans R III, LeBailly S, Gordon KK, et al: Restructuring asthma care in a hospital setting to improve outcomes, *Chest* 116:210S-216S, 1999.

94. Evans R III, Gergen PJ, Mitchell H, et al: A randomized clinical trial to reduce asthma morbidity among inner-city children: results of the National Cooperative Inner-City asthma study, *J Pediatr* 135:332-338, 1999.

95. Persky V, Coover L, Hernandez E, et al: Chicago community-based asthma intervention trial: Feasibility of delivering peer education in an inner-city population, *Chest* 116:216S-223S, 1999.

96. Fisher EB, Strunk RC, Sussman LK, et al: Community organization to reduce acute care for asthma among African American children in low-income neighborhoods: the Neighborhood Asthma Coalition, Manuscript submitted for publication, 2002.

97. Carter MC, Perzanowski MS, Raymond A, et al: Home intervention in the treatment of asthma among inner-city children, *J Allergy Clin Immunol* 108:732-737, 2001.

98. Wood RA, Eggleston PA, Rand C, et al: Cockroach allergen abatement with extermination and sodium hypochlorite cleaning in inner-city homes. *Ann Allergy Asthma Immunol* 87:60-64, 2001.

99. Clark NM, Gong M, Schork MA, et al: Impact of education for physicians on patient outcomes, *Pediatrics* 101:831-836, 1998.

100. Clark NM, Gong M, Schork MA, et al: Long-term effects of asthma education for physicians on patient satisfaction and use of health services, *Eur Respir J* 16:15-21, 2000.

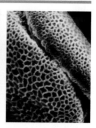

CHAPTER 38

Asthma in Older Children

LEONARD B. BACHARIER ■ ROBERT C. STRUNK

Asthma is the most common chronic disorder of childhood, affecting approximately 7% of children 5 to 14 years of age,[1] with almost 6% of children in this age group reporting an episode of asthma or an asthma attack in the preceding 12 months.[2] However, estimates of wheezing in this age group approach 20% or greater in many industrialized countries, further magnifying the impact of wheezing disease on children. The personal burden of asthma is magnified by the significant impact it exerts upon the daily lives of families. Fortunately, the ability to effectively care for childhood asthma has improved substantially over the past 20 years, and it is now possible for children with asthma to lead fully active lives.

EPIDEMIOLOGY AND ETIOLOGY

Prevalence of Childhood Asthma

The worldwide prevalence of asthma has increased over the past several decades, with asthma prevalence in the United States increasing 74% during 1980 to 1996. Although the rise in asthma prevalence may reflect coding and classification issues, the influence of other factors such as environmental exposures to allergens, infectious agents, endotoxins, and tobacco smoke must also be considered. Place of residence appears to influence asthma prevalence.[3] Furthermore, there appears to be an effect of gender on asthma prevalence, as the male-to-female ratio for asthma is 1.8:1 among children 2 years of age or under, but by puberty, asthma becomes more prevalent among females (M:F ratio of 0.8:1).

Factors Influencing the Etiology of Asthma

A general pattern of factors influencing development of asthma seems to be emerging, including family history/genetics, smoking, diet, obesity, and inactivity, all of which seem to influence the development of asthma and disease outcomes. The following sections detail some of the factors that may play a role in development of asthma (Table 38-1).

Socioeconomic Status

Many clinical or area studies have reported substantially higher rates of asthma prevalence, hospitalization, and mortality in racial and ethnic minorities. However, asthma is also most common among low socioeconomic groups regardless of race. Given that race and socioeconomic status (SES) are highly confounded in the United States, an important question is the extent to which racial/ethnic differences in asthma are caused by poverty. Although black children have higher rates of asthma than white children, most studies have found that black race is not a significant correlate of asthma after controlling for location of residence and SES. The basis for the effects of poverty and urban residence on asthma prevalence is not known and multiple factors could be involved. One potential factor is exposure and sensitization to allergens common in urban environments. Black children in inner-city Atlanta are exposed to high levels of dust mite and cockroach allergen, and a high proportion of the children with asthma was sensitized to these allergens.[4] Litonjua[5] also concluded that a large proportion of racial/ethnic differences in asthma prevalence can be explained by factors related to income, area of residence, and level of education.

Socioeconomic characteristics are powerful determinants of health and disease in general. Level of income and education may impact directly and indirectly on health status. Income is a determinant of access to health care and frequently to the quantity and quality of health care available. Persons who have low income, regardless of race or ethnicity, are more likely to be uninsured, to encounter delays in receiving care or be denied care, to rely on hospital clinics in emergency departments for health services, and to receive substandard care. The usual socioeconomic indicators, education and personal or household income, serve only as surrogates for more complicated correlates of individuals within populations and multiple factors that can impact both on prevalence of asthma and adverse outcomes from the disease.

Genetics

Asthma is clearly a heritable trait, with the tendency for asthma to run in families known for centuries. The genetic basis of heritability has been extensively studied and the studies have yielded some useful information. For example, one feature of asthma is allergy, evidenced by an IgE-mediated response. IgE synthesis is mediated through interleukin (IL)-4 stimulation of B lymphocytes and thus IL-4 serves a disease-modifying role. An association of a sequence variant in the IL-4 gene promoter region at the C589T locus has been made to asthma severity, as indicated by the level of forced expiratory volume in 1 second (FEV_1).[6] The R576 IL-4 receptor α polymorphism has also been associated with asthma severity.[7] There is as yet no set genetic pattern that predicts presence of asthma or defines its severity.

TABLE 38-1 Factors Influencing Disease Development and Severity

Factor	Disease Development	Disease Severity
Atopy	++++	++++
Allergen exposure	++	++++
Rhinitis	++	++
Sinusitis	?	+++
Infection (viral)	+	++++
Gastroesophageal reflux	—	++
Environmental factors		
Intrauterine tobacco smoke	++	?
Passive tobacco smoke	+	++
Air pollution	—	++
Psychologic factors (including stress)	+	++++
Socioeconomic status	++	++++
Adherence	—	++++
Obesity	Adolescent females	++
Diet	?	?
Exercise	?	++*
Drugs (including acetylsalicylic acid/nonsteroidal antiinflammatory drugs)	—	++†

+ Denotes a weak association, ++ denotes a modest association, +++ denotes a strong association, ++++ denotes a very strong association, — denotes no known association, ? denotes uncertain relationship.

*Although exercise is a common precipitant of asthma symptoms, improved physical conditioning can reduce asthma severity.

†Considered in the context of asthma, nasal polyposis, and severe sinus disease.

Allergy

Allergy to aeroallergens has long been known to be associated with the presence of asthma. Studies of the Melbourne, Australia school children by Williams and McNicol[8] have indicated both the increased incidence of asthma and asthma severity with increases in number of positive skin tests and total serum IgE. The relationship between allergy and asthma has more recently been highlighted by the importance of aeroallergen sensitivity in the progression of frequent intermittent wheezing to persistent asthma in young children.[9] Several large epidemiologic studies have clearly indicated the importance of aeroallergen sensitization in asthma development among populations at risk. Sensitization to dust mite and mold was a predictor of asthma in rural Chinese individuals selected on the basis of having at least two siblings with physician-diagnosed asthma.[10] In a similar study, total serum IgE levels and positive skin tests to aeroallergens were correlated with current wheezing.[11] This association was present in children from nonatopic, asymptomatic probands, as well as in the expected atopic asthmatic probands, suggesting that much of the increase in asthma prevalence is associated with specific IgE sensitization and is occurring in persons previously considered to be at low risk for developing asthma or atopy.

Demographic and Environmental Factors

Risk factors of ethnicity and location of residence have been identified and evaluated. Studies from Germany comparing the populations of East and West Germany have shown the prevalence of hay fever and asthma to be significantly higher in West German children, suggesting that environmental factors explain the difference in prevalence in these ethnically similar populations.[12] Several environmental factors have been considered. For example, early exposure to infections (as with being in a day care environment early in life) or exposure to endotoxin (as with growing up on a farm with close exposure to the farm animals) is associated with a decreased prevalence of asthma. In contrast, growing up in an urban environment or generally with an increased standard of living is associated with an increased prevalence of asthma. This latter effect is represented by the increased prevalence of allergic rhinitis and asthma in West Germany compared to East Germany, Sweden compared to Estonia and Poland,[3] and the most recently published North Karelia, Finland compared to Pitkaranta, Russia.[13] Such correlates are also present for atopic diseases other than asthma. In fact, Strachan,[14] who noted that prevalence of hay fever was inversely related to family size, was the first to recognize the importance of early exposures on atopic disease. In the United States asthma is more prevalent in African-Americans and Puerto Ricans. These findings are not explained by the observations on the role of social class in European studies. Given the ethnic differences between African-Americans and whites, these studies may represent gene-by-environment interaction producing varied phenotypic outcomes.

Gene-Environment Interaction

Genetic factors cannot explain the rise in asthma prevalence, morbidity, or mortality.[15] However, a small change in the prevalence of relevant environmental exposures could explain a significant rise in disease prevalence among genetically susceptible individuals. Gene-environment interaction, defined as the co-participation of genetic and environmental factors,[16] is particularly relevant to the etiology of asthma morbidity, particularly in individuals who experience a disproportionate burden of environmental exposures.[17] Relevant exposures include smoking, stress, nutritional factors, infections, allergens, and occupational exposures. In addition, racial/ethnic variability in the distribution of genetic polymorphisms can potentially modify the response to pharmacotherapeutic agents.[18] For example, the prevalence of functional polymorphisms in the β_2-adrenergic receptor gene varies across race.[18]

A genetic polymorphism in the β_2-adrenergic receptor has been found to be associated with asthma severity,[19] as well as with the susceptibility to develop asthma among individuals who smoked (those smokers with the arg/arg polymorphism were 7.7 times as likely to have asthma compared to never-smokers with the gly/gly polymorphism).[20] β_2-Adrenergic receptor polymorphisms are currently being evaluated as disease severity modifiers. Preliminary evidence exists that physical activity, a modifiable risk factor, alters the risk conferred by this polymorphism.[21] Thus interaction between a genetic variant and decreased physical activity, an environmental exposure, may contribute to asthma prevalence.

Stress

The mechanism of the effect of low SES on both prevalence and severity of asthma throughout childhood and adolescence has been studied from a number of different perspectives. Various indicators of stress have been associated with asthma outcomes in childhood. For example, negative family characteristics such as family conflict and family dysfunction discriminated children who died of asthma from children with equally severe asthma who did not die.[22] Parenting difficulties have been associated with a higher risk for the development of asthma early in life.[23] In addition, children with the highest risk of developing early-onset asthma were those in families with both parenting problems and high stress. Recent research has also demonstrated evidence for a stress and asthma link through temporal studies. For example, experiencing an acute negative life event increased children's risk for an asthma attack 4 to 6 weeks after the occurrence of the event.[24] Moreover, the combination of chronic and acute stress plays a role in the temporal association. Experiencing an acute life event among children who had ongoing chronic stress in their lives shortened the time frame in which children were at risk for an asthma attack to within 2 weeks of the acute event.

At the family level, the nature of relationships between parents and children could play a role in asthma and its severity. Children with asthma have been found to have higher rates of clinically significant family stress compared with healthy children.[25] Children whose families are more cohesive are more likely to have controlled, rather than uncontrolled, asthma.[26] Additionally, parenting difficulties early in a child's life, particularly during times of high stress, have been found to predict the onset of asthma in childhood.[23,27]

One psychologic pathway that has been suggested to explain associations of SES with asthma is the differential experiences with stress that low and high SES children face. In healthy children, low SES has been associated with more frequent exposure to stressful life events, and children who live in low SES neighborhoods are more likely to report witnessing violence. Low SES also has been associated with more negative stress appraisals.[28]

Obesity

Results of cross-sectional[29] and longitudinal[30] studies conducted in industrialized countries have shown an association between both increased body mass index (BMI)[29,30] and weight gain[30] and self-reported asthma in adult women. Celadon and colleagues[31] studied adults in China with either physician-diagnosed asthma or airway responsiveness to methacholine. Similar to the results in industrialized countries, they found an association between overweight and presence of asthma or airway hyperresponsiveness. They also found an association between underweight (BMI 16 kg/m^2 or less) and asthma, which could be the result of an effect of asthma symptoms on nutrition or an effect of previous weight loss and development of asthma.

The relationship between obesity and asthma observed in adults has also been observed in adolescent females, but not males. Girls who were overweight or obese at age 11 years were more likely to have current wheezing at ages 11 and 15 years, but not at ages 6 to 8 years. The relationship between obesity and asthma is strongest among females who begin puberty before age 11 years. Females who became overweight or obese between 6 and 11 years are 7 times more likely to develop new asthma symptoms at age 11 and 13.[32] The mechanism of increased asthma with obesity is not clear. The strong gender differences observed by Castro-Rodriguez[32] and others[29] suggest that overweight status itself does not produce the asthma, as an effect directly of weight should be seen in both boys and girls. The results of longitudinal studies[32] suggest that there is a more fundamental relationship as most of the asthma in obese adolescent girls was new-onset asthma. In a study of young adults with asthma,[33] a lower level of physical activity did not explain the association between the incidence of asthma and gain in weight.

Infection

Respiratory infections are a common exacerbating factor of asthma in both younger and older children. Viral respiratory infections are present in up to 85% of children with exacerbated asthma.[34] In addition to simply worsening asthma, a more fundamental relationship between infection and presence of asthma may exist. Such a relationship has been suggested by the finding of a higher-than-expected incidence of bronchial hyperresponsiveness (BHR) in children who had whooping cough, croup, or bronchiolitis in their early years of life.[35]

More recently, the role of infections with *Mycoplasma pneumoniae* or *Chlamydia pneumoniae* in the underlying pathogenesis of asthma has been suggested (see Chapter 35). A conclusive association between development of *C. pneumoniae* or *M. pneumoniae* infection and onset of asthma, or even an association between the presence of the organism and more severe disease, remains to be established in large prospective studies. A relationship may also exist between persistent adenoviral infection and chronic airway obstruction in children[36] (see Chapter 35).

Diet

There is increasing evidence from epidemiologic studies that dietary factors may be involved in the cause of asthma. Although there is much to be learned about this possible risk factor, there have been some studies identifying a relationship between a high dietary intake of vitamins C, A, and E with higher levels of lung function. A longitudinal analysis of decline in FEV$_1$ over a 9-year period in adults found the decline lower among those with a higher average vitamin C intake, but no relationship to magnesium or vitamins A or E.[37] The relationship between diet and atopy is not clearly understood, although there is some evidence for a relationship between concentrations of vitamin E and both allergen skin sensitization and IgE concentrations.[38]

Natural History of Asthma

Progression of Disease into Adulthood

More severe asthma can persist from childhood into adulthood without remission. Another important tendency in the natural history is for symptoms to remit in adolescent only to return again in adulthood. In general, the amount of wheezing in early adolescence seems to be a guide for severity in early adult years, with 73% of those with few symptoms at age 14 years continuing to have little or no asthma at age 28 years.[39] Similarly 68% of those with frequent wheezing at 14 years still suffered from recurrent asthma at age 28 years. Most subjects with frequent wheezing at 21 years continued to have comparable asthma at 28 years. In addition to the importance of symptoms in childhood, childhood degree of bronchial responsiveness in combination with a low FEV_1 were also related to the outcome of asthma in adulthood.[40] Although many children become asymptomatic in adolescence, pulmonary function deficits associated with asthma and wheeze increase throughout childhood,[41] and a significant proportion of children free of symptoms and with normal FEV_1, and even FEV_1/forced vital capacity (FVC) ratios, continue to have increases in bronchial reactivity.[42] This BHR is an independent risk factor for development of a low level of FEV_1 and associated symptoms in early adulthood.[43] What is perhaps most worrisome about the persistence of childhood disease into adulthood is the development of chronic airflow obstruction, with loss of bronchial dilator responsiveness[44] and a decline in FEV_1 over time greater than adults with asthma than asymptomatic peers.[45] These findings suggest that asthma, even uncomplicated by cigarette smoking, may be a precursor of a chronic obstructive pulmonary disease (COPD)—like syndrome in adults. Although it is not known with any certainty, it seems possible that optimal treatment of childhood asthma with careful attention to both symptoms and levels of pulmonary function can improve the outcome of asthma in adulthood and decrease the possibility of development of COPD.

Familial Resemblance of Disease Severity

The Epidemiological Study on Genetics and Environment of Asthma investigated risks of asthma and of severe asthma in first-degree relatives of subjects with asthma. The proportion of asthma in relatives was not related to severity of asthma, but within families with asthma there was a significant resemblance for both clinical severity and levels of FEV_1.[46] Kruzius-Spencer et al[47] found familial correlation in decline of FEV_1 among subjects in the Tucson Epidemiological Study of Airway Obstruction Diseases, with effects most prominent in smokers. Both these studies support the idea that there are genetic factors responsible for changes in pulmonary function over time; however, the role of the environment and gene-environment interactions are candidates as well.

Duration of Disease Is Associated with Degree of Abnormality in Pulmonary Function

Analysis of baseline data from the Childhood Asthma Management Program (CAMP) cohort demonstrated that longer duration of asthma was associated with lower levels of lung function in children with mild to moderate asthma aged 5 to 12 years. This association was independent of levels of atopy, presence of household allergens, and prior use of antiinflammatory medications. Duration of asthma was associated with lower levels of both prebronchodilator and postbronchodilator values for FEV_1 and FEV_1/FVC ratio.[48] The degree of BHR in these children was also related to duration of disease.[49] Because the level of pulmonary function and the degree of BHR are independent predictors of abnormal levels of lung function in adults who had childhood asthma, it is apparent that longer duration of disease in childhood is producing abnormalities of lung function that predispose adults to disease.

Morbidity and Mortality

Asthma causes a significant burden on children and families. Asthma accounted for 14 million missed school days annually in 1996,[2] having increased from 6.2 million in 1980. The percentage of asthmatic children with activity limitation caused by their asthma remained essentially stable in this interval, approximately 25%.[2]

Emergency department visits among children 5 to 14 years of age have increased approximately 25% from 1992 to 1999. Rates among blacks are almost threefold higher than rates for whites. Asthma is the leading admitting diagnosis to children's hospitals,[2] and similar to the emergency department data, blacks have greater than three times more hospitalizations than whites. Rates of hospitalizations in 5- to 14-year-old children have remained stable from 1980 to 1999 and are more than twofold lower than for younger children. A significant proportion of hospitalizations are repeat hospitalizations, with rehospitalization accounting for 20% to 25% of hospitalizations in a single year and up to 43% of hospitalizations in one urban children's hospital within a 5- to 10-year period.[50] A lifetime history of hospitalizations was associated with family impacts (greater family strain and family conflict, greater financial strain), as well as caretaker characteristics of greater personal strain, beliefs about not being able to manage one's child's asthma.[51] Individual characteristics of the caretaker (lower sense of mastery, being less emotionally bothered by asthma) predicted greater likelihood of future asthma hospitalizations.[51]

The rate of deaths due to asthma in 5- to 14-year-old children increased more than twofold from 1980 (1.9 per million) to 1996 (4.6 per million) and then has decreased slightly in 1997 to 1999 (3.6 per million). As with hospitalizations, blacks have many more deaths than whites (in 1999 2.7-fold). Whereas the rate of death in children is relatively small compared to other age groups, physicians find that many, if not most, of these deaths are preventable, with the major reason for death being late arrival at a health care facility associated with poor use of oral corticosteroids.

Efforts should be made to identify patients at risk for death. Although there have been significant efforts toward understanding reasons that fatal and near-fatal asthma episodes occur, the identification of patients at risk for dying remains an art, with no single set of criteria able to identify all patients who die. Prior history of severe events, especially respiratory failure requiring intubation, is an obvious risk factor. However, whereas as many as 25% of patients with a history of respiratory failure die in a 3- to 5-year follow-up, most patients who die have not had respiratory failure.[52] Most studies indicate that a high proportion of patients who have died have had severe asthma, but the number of patients with severe disease is large and only 1% to 3% will die over an extended follow-up period. The importance of psychologic factors in poor outcomes from asthma[22] indicates that patient and family factors resulting in psychologic dysfunction need to be identified as well.

There are certain time intervals when risk is increased. For example, patients may need extra care and communication in periods following hospitalization, as BHR persists after hospitalization much longer than abnormalities in spirometry, and oral steroids are being weaned, further increasing risk. Hospitalizations that occur in spite of optimally prescribed therapy are of special concern.

DIFFERENTIAL DIAGNOSIS

Given the symptoms of asthma, cough, and wheeze, clinicians must be prepared to consider causes other than asthma when a patient presents with lower respiratory tract symptoms. The differential diagnosis of cough and wheeze is reviewed extensively in Chapter 31.

EVALUATION

Figure 38-1 presents an algorithm for evaluation of a school-age or adolescent child who presents with chest symptoms of cough, wheeze, shortness of breath, chest tightness, or chest pain.

History

Historical elements should include specific symptoms, their frequency and severity, triggering factors, and response to therapy. Age of onset of symptoms is important, as 80% of patients with asthma experience symptoms within the first 5 years of life. Thus the adolescent presenting with recent onset of symptoms without a prior history warrants further evaluation of alternative diagnoses. Failure of symptoms to improve with treatment including bronchodilators and corticosteroids should prompt evaluation for other processes, either a nonasthma diagnosis or a comorbid condition complicating underlying asthma.

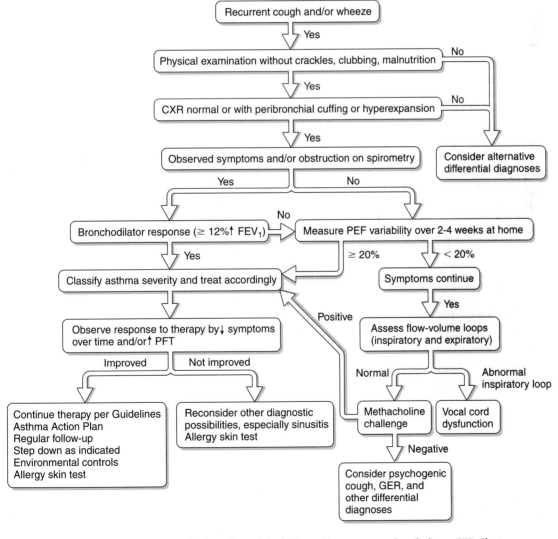

FIGURE 38-1 Algorithm for establishing diagnosis in children with recurrent cough and wheeze. *CXR*, Chest x-ray; *FEV$_1$*, forced expiratory volume in 1 second; *PEF*, peak expiratory flow; *PFT*, pulmonary function test; *GER*, gastroesophageal reflux.

| Numbers 1-7 to be completed by patient/parent at each physician office visit. Please fill in ONE circle for EACH question that BEST describes your/your child's asthma. EXAMPLE: ● |

1. How often have/has you/your child had a cough, wheeze, shortness of breath, or chest tightness during the past MONTH?
○ 2 or fewer times per week ○ 3-6 times per week ○ Daily ○ Continuously

2. How often have/has you/your child awakened from sleep because of coughing, wheezing, shortness of breath, or chest tightness in the past MONTH?
○ 2 or fewer times per month ○ 3-4 times per month ○ 5-9 times per month ○ 10 or more times per month

3. In the past MONTH, how often have/has you/your child had cough, wheeze, shortness of breath, or chest tightness while exercising or playing?
○ 2 or fewer times per month ○ 3-4 times per month ○ 5-9 times per month ○ 10 or more times per month

4. How often does asthma keep you/your child from doing what you/the child want(s)?
○ 2 or fewer times per month ○ 3-4 times per month ○ 5-9 times per month ○ 10 or more times per month

5. Think about all the activities that you/your child did during the past MONTH. How much were/was you/your child bothered by asthma?
○ Not bothered at all ○ Hardly bothered at all ○ Bothered a little ○ Somewhat bothered ○ Quite bothered ○ Very bothered ○ Extremely bothered

6. How many days of school have you/your child missed due to asthma in the last MONTH? ☐☐ days ○ Do not attend school

7. How many days of work have you/your child missed due to asthma in the last MONTH? ☐☐ days ○ Do not work

FIGURE 38-2 Questionnaire to assess asthma-related morbidities.

Figure 38-2 presents a questionnaire completed by patients and/or their parents to provide information on asthma-related morbidity.

Additional history should focus on identification of other comorbid conditions that may worsen asthma severity, including allergen exposure, rhinitis, sinusitis, and gastroesophageal reflux (GER). Furthermore, an assessment of underlying psychosocial factors and adherence to medical regimen may provide valuable clues as to barriers in delivery and receipt of asthma care.

Physical Examination

Findings may include an increased anterior-posterior chest diameter in severe disease and expiratory wheezes and prolongation of the expiratory phase during exacerbation. Presence of nasal polyposis should prompt an evaluation for cystic fibrosis, regardless of the age of the child, as cystic fibrosis remains the leading cause of polyps in childhood. The examination should include careful evaluation to ensure absence of findings suggestive of other diseases, such as the presence of crackles, digital clubbing, and hypoxemia, as well as to uncover factors that worsen disease, including nasal and sinus disease.

Laboratory Evaluation

Peripheral blood eosinophilia and/or elevated serum IgE levels are often found in children with asthma and can be helpful in evaluation of severe disease. Laboratory evaluation is helpful in excluding entities that comprise the differential diagnosis of asthma. Serum immunoglobulin levels (IgG, IgM, and IgA) may be helpful in evaluating for defects in humoral immunity predisposing to recurrent lower respiratory tract illness. Sweat chloride analysis is required to exclude cystic fibrosis. Furthermore, children with bronchiectasis along with chronic otitis media and sinusitis may warrant an evaluation of ciliary structure and function. A purified protein derivative skin test is helpful in excluding mycobacterial infection.

Allergy Skin Testing

Evaluation for allergen-specific IgE should be part of the evaluation of all children with persistent asthma because proper identification of allergic sensitivities and instruction in environmental control measures may provide significant clinical benefit.

Radiology

All children with recurrent episodes of cough and/or wheeze should have a chest radiograph (anteroposterior and lateral views) performed to aid in exclusion of other diagnostic entities. Findings of chronic changes, including bronchiectasis, should lead to further evaluation of alternate diagnoses.

Pulmonary Function Tests

Children as young as 4 to 5 years of age should be capable of performing spirometry. Spirometry measures FVC, FEV_1, the ratio of FEV_1/FVC, as well as other measures of airflow including the forced expiratory flow between 25% and 75% of FVC (FEF_{25-75}). The FEV_1 is the most commonly used and reproducible measure of pulmonary function, whereas the FEF_{25-75} demonstrates much more intrapatient variability. Standards are widely available for most spirometric measures and allow for correction based upon patient age, gender, race, and height. The FEV_1/FVC ratio is an indicator of airflow obstruction and may be more sensitive in identifying airflow abnormalities in asthma than the FEV_1, as most children with asthma have FEV_1 within the normal range, even in the presence of severe disease (see section on classification of asthma severity).

Asthma is characterized by airflow obstruction that is at least partially reversible by bronchodilator. Thus spirometry is often performed before and 20 minutes following administration of a bronchodilator such as albuterol. An increase in the FEV_1 of at least 12% is considered to represent a significant change and exceeds that which is seen in non-asthmatic individuals.

Particular attention should be given to the inspiratory and expiratory flow-volume loops, as they are extremely helpful in excluding other patterns of airway obstruction.[53,54] For example, fixed airway obstruction (abnormalities on both the expiratory and inspiratory loops) can be seen with a mediastinal mass compressing a large airway or variable extrathoracic airway obstructive process (abnormalities just on the inspiratory loop) is seen with vocal cord dysfunction (VCD). Asthma produces variable intrathoracic obstruction (abnormalities on just the expiratory loop). Patients with VCD without asthma do not demonstrate intrathoracic airway obstruction but may show blunting or truncation of the inspiratory loop consistent with variable extrathoracic obstruction. Variability between spirometric trials is not uncommon in patients with VCD, often consisting of normal and abnormal inspiratory loops during a single session.

In addition to spirometry, other tests of pulmonary function may aid in the evaluation of the child with asthma that is difficult to diagnose or control. Patients with asthma generally demonstrate normal total lung capacity (TLC) on lung volume testing by plethysmography, but may demonstrate evidence of air trapping as evidenced by elevated residual volumes (RV) and RV/TLC ratio. Measurement of diffusing capacity of carbon monoxide (DL_{CO}) is normal in patients with asthma, and abnormalities in DL_{CO} should prompt evaluation for interstitial lung diseases.

Challenge Testing

Some children present with atypical features of asthma and may pose greater challenges in confirming an asthma diagnosis. Thus, use of bronchial challenges with agents that provoke bronchoconstriction may be helpful in the diagnosis and management of the child with atypical symptoms, poor response to asthma medications, or lack of a response to bronchodilator during spirometry. Agents used for bronchoprovocation challenges include methacholine, histamine, adenosine, allergen, cold air, and exercise. Challenge studies should be performed in laboratories familiar with such procedures.

Bronchoscopy

Bronchoscopy is rarely indicated in the evaluation and management of children undergoing evaluation for asthma. However, in children with particularly severe disease or with poor response to conventional therapy, direct visualization of the airways along with bronchoalveolar lavage (BAL) may provide important clinical information. Such examinations may reveal the presence of previously undiagnosed foreign body aspiration or other intrinsic airway mass, infection, extrinsic airway compression, and evidence of chronic aspiration, as well as

indicators of airway inflammation (such as eosinophilia or neutrophilia in BAL fluid).

EVALUATION AND MANAGEMENT OF FACTORS THAT INCREASE DISEASE SEVERITY

Overview

Each patient has a unique pattern of exacerbating factors and an understanding of a patient's asthma requires paying careful attention to patterns of symptoms over time. Histories taken from patients with asthma indicate that the most common precipitating factors are respiratory infections and weather changes. Drawing attention to these factors can help patients start increased treatment early in an exacerbation, as they will be looking for increasing symptoms that occur as an infection starts or as weather is changing rapidly. Exercise is also commonly identified as an exacerbating factor. Interestingly, although it is known that exposure to allergens and irritants can worsen asthma (see below), such exposures are much less commonly recognized as important.

Exposure to Inhalant Allergens

Numerous studies have demonstrated the effects of inhalant allergen exposure upon disease severity. Exposure and allergic sensitization to cockroach was associated with a significantly greater risk of asthma hospitalization and greater health care utilization among 476 children aged 4 to 9 years who participated in the National Cooperative Inner-City Asthma Study.[55] Allergic sensitization to the mold Alternaria has been identified as a significant allergen in terms of increasing airway hyperresponsiveness.[56] Furthermore, sensitivity to Alternaria was associated with a nearly 200-fold increased risk of respiratory arrest caused by asthma,[57] emphasizing the importance of determining underlying allergic sensitivities in patients with asthma and providing patients with accurate and practical advice on allergen avoidance techniques.

The Childhood Asthma Management Program, comprised of 1041 children aged 5 to 12 with mild-moderate asthma, found that allergic sensitization to tree pollen, weed pollen, the mold Alternaria, cat dander, dog dander, or indoor molds was associated with greater airway hyperresponsiveness to methacholine.[58] A cross-sectional analysis of a birth cohort of 562 children studied at 11 years of age found that BHR significantly correlated with higher levels of total serum IgE.[59] Burrows and co-workers[60] found a close relationship between total serum IgE and both the severity and persistence of bronchial responsiveness in a longitudinal study of adolescents and adults. In CAMP, whereas sensitivity to tree, weed, Alternaria, cat, dog, and indoor mold allergens were associated with significantly increased sensitivity to methacholine, step-wise regression analysis indicated that only sensitivity to dog and cat dander and the outdoor fungus Alternaria had independent, significant relationships.

A number of studies have followed children with asthma through childhood and adolescence into adulthood. Conclusions from the Melbourne, Australia, study indicate that severity of asthma in adulthood is related to the presence of increased levels of atopy in childhood, with the presence of an atopic condition in childhood shifting the risk of asthma in later life toward more severe outcomes.

There is a clear association between sensitization to pets and current wheezing and BHR.[61,62] Dharmage and co-workers[61] found that a high level of cat allergen in floor dust was associated both with an increased risk of being sensitized to cats and the presence of current asthma. A large prospective population study found that keeping pets at home increased the risk of developing asthma in adulthood.[63] In the CAMP population, children sensitized to dog and exposed to high levels of dog allergen and sensitized to cat and exposed to high levels of cat allergen had a clearly increased risk of nocturnal awakenings.[64]

Two cohort studies provide evidence of a lower risk of asthma among children exposed to pets in early life compared with unexposed children.[65] Other studies find that individuals living with a pet have significantly less asthma or less severe BHR.[66] Studies showing protection from pet ownership are confounded by the likelihood that subjects with less severe asthma can keep the pets, whereas subjects with more severe disease are unable to have pets.

Rhinitis

Rhinitis is common in children with asthma, with estimates of up to 80% of patients with asthma reporting upper airway symptoms. Whereas most rhinitis that worsens asthma is allergic, perennial rhinitis in nonatopic subjects can be a risk factor for more severe asthma.[67] Pharmacologic treatment of rhinitis has been demonstrated to improve several features of asthma. Topical nasal steroid therapy for allergic rhinitis has also been shown to attenuate the increase in BHR during the grass pollen season[68] as well as decrease the risk of emergency department visits[69] or hospitalizations for asthma.[70] Thus treatment plans for patients with asthma and allergic rhinitis should consist of optimal management of concomitant allergic rhinitis (see Chapter 28).

Sinusitis

Sinusitis is often discovered in the search for factors responsible for an overall worsening of asthma unexplained by changes of environment or other obvious historical features. Although many of these patients present with symptoms of upper airway disease along with asthma, some have sinusitis as a significant contributor to difficult-to-control asthma with a paucity of symptoms suggestive of sinusitis.

Radiographic examination of the paranasal sinuses in children hospitalized for acute asthma exacerbations is positive in 30% to 60% of children, partly depending upon the diagnostic technique used (Water's view radiograph or computed tomography of the sinuses). The effect of antibiotic treatment of bacterial sinusitis on asthma control has been examined in several clinical studies, reducing asthma medication use, decreasing asthma symptoms, and improving BHR (see Chapter 35).[71,72] Duration of antibiotic treatment should be individualized but should continue until the patient is symptom-free for at least 7 days.

Gastroesophageal Reflux

GER is common among patients with asthma; in adult asthma patients the estimated prevalence of GER approaches 80%.[73] Studies of prevalence of GER in patients with asthma for the pediatric age group are limited, but include a 64% incidence of a positive pH probe study in a group of 25 children with asthma,[74] suggesting that GER may also be common among children with asthma.

In our experience most young children and even adolescents with GER do not report symptoms classically associated with GER in adults, including heartburn, chest pain, dysphagia, or hoarseness. In fact, children rarely complain of symptoms even in the presence of significant GER demonstrated by pH probe studies. GER can be clinically silent in terms of gastrointestinal symptoms but may contribute to asthma severity and difficult-to-control asthma. Thus a high level of suspicion of underlying GER is necessary in the evaluation of the child with severe asthma, especially uncontrolled asthma associated with nocturnal symptoms. (See Chapter 41 for a more thorough discussion on diagnosis and management of GER.)

Environmental Exposures

Passive exposure to tobacco smoke is a clear exacerbating factor in asthma, with increases in asthma prevalence and asthma severity among children exposed to parental smoking.[75] Cigarette smoking has been reported to be associated with mild airway obstruction and slowed growth of lung function in adolescents without asthma.[76] Furthermore, asthma has been linked to an accelerated rate of decline in FEV_1 over time, and this rate is even greater among asthmatic individuals who smoke.[45]

Many patients report that their asthma is triggered by "weather changes." However, the precise mechanism by which weather changes exacerbate asthma is unclear; weather changes may be accompanied by changes in airborne allergen exposures. However, multiple studies have failed to find a definitive link between airborne outdoor allergen levels (except for an occasional mold) and worsening asthma symptoms. Thus the true link between weather changes and asthma attacks remains unknown. In addition to allergen exposure, epidemiologic studies suggest an association between levels of air pollutants, including ozone, nitrogen oxides, carbon monoxide, and sulfur dioxide, and symptoms or exacerbations of asthma.

Vocal Cord Dysfunction

VCD, a functional respiratory tract disorder resulting from paradoxical adduction of the vocal cords, complicates the diagnosis and management of common respiratory tract problems, including asthma.[77] The recognition of VCD in a patient with atypical or difficult-to-control asthma is critical in minimizing symptoms and potential side effects associated with treatment of severe asthma. The symptoms of VCD are not unique to the disorder and include cough, wheeze, stridor, dyspnea, hoarseness, and choking. Some patients report difficulty swallowing or tightness in the chest or throat. Patients with VCD often report difficulty "getting air in" because of paradoxical adduction of the vocal cords during inspiration, in contrast to difficulty with exhalation as reported by asthma patients. Cough is a common feature of VCD and must be differentiated from cough caused by asthma or from postnasal drainage resulting from rhinosinusitis. Patients with VCD frequently complain of tightness in the throat and/or chest and may speak in a hoarse voice. Nocturnal symptoms are uncommon in uncomplicated VCD, but may occur in patients with both VCD and asthma. Exercise is a frequent precipitant of both VCD and asthma.

Spirometry and inhaled provocation challenges assist in the differentiation between VCD and asthma. Provocation challenges, either pharmacologic (methacholine or histamine) or exercise, are helpful in determining the presence or absence of airways hyperresponsiveness, a feature characteristic of asthma. Exercise challenges frequently reproduce the clinical symptoms and spirometric abnormalities consistent with VCD. These studies are generally sufficient in differentiating between asthma and VCD. However, if this approach fails to establish the diagnosis or if the patient does not respond to appropriate therapy, direct visualization of paradoxical vocal cord movement during symptomatic periods may be helpful in confirming the diagnosis of VCD. Characteristic findings include adduction of the true vocal cords during inspiration with a diamond-shaped opening at the posterior aspect of the glottis. Once the diagnosis of VCD has been established, attention should be focused on patient reassurance and maneuvers directed at laryngeal relaxation (from speech therapy) and discovering underlying stress that is often involved in producing the problem (from psychology). In our experience, combining speech therapy and psychologic evaluation is necessary for successful therapy for VCD. Maintenance therapy for VCD includes minimization of medication use for comorbid conditions frequently confused with VCD (i.e., asthma).

Psychologic Factors

In a group of children with severe asthma, 50% had levels of fitness in the significant abnormal range.[78] Medical characteristics of the patients did not significantly correlate with cardiopulmonary functioning.[78] In contrast, psychologic functioning as determined by structured interviews significantly correlated with cardiopulmonary function.[78] Further emphasizing the relative lack of importance of medical characteristics, 93% of the children studied were able to reach normal fitness levels over short periods of time, indicating that the lack of fitness was not a necessary limitation of their asthma.[79] Similar to the findings in studies of fitness levels, school performance,[80] and gross and fine motor coordination,[81] although generally within a normal range (in contrast to the findings of fitness), overall results correlated with psychologic functioning but not with medical characteristics of asthma.

At the level of characteristics of the individual caretaker, the beliefs that parents hold about their ability to manage their child's asthma and the quality of life that they maintain while caring for a child with asthma may be associated with asthma hospitalizations.[82] A health education intervention study conducted to improve asthma management skills and to build family self-confidence in the ability to manage asthma found that families that participated in the intervention reported better attack management strategies and preventive strategies compared to a control group.[83] Adults with asthma who have greater confidence or trust in the care they receive from their doctor report having better-controlled asthma and are more likely to have mild, as opposed to severe, asthma.[84] Thus parents who believe strongly that they cannot adequately care for their child's asthma may be more likely to bring their child to the hospital repeatedly for acute episodes.

Poor Adherence to Medical Regimen

Numerous studies have reinforced the high rate at which patients do not use their medications as directed. This is often reflected as inadequate asthma control, and often leads to prescription of higher doses or additional controller medications based upon the assumption that the medication prescribed accurately reflects the medication the patient actually takes. However, because most patients miss substantial amounts of medications, even when participating in research studies examining medication adherence,[85] practitioners must focus on patient education regarding the importance of asthma medication use as directed and provision of a written plan of action that is practical for the patient. Complex regimens consisting of several medications given frequently during the day are less likely to be followed than simple regimens with less frequent dosing requirements. When discussing asthma-related information and setting appropriate and achievable short- and long-term goals, excellence in communication between health care providers and patients is essential in establishing the foundation for asthma care and adherence to the recommended treatment approach. The developmental level of the child complicates adherence in the pediatric population. Children's understanding of their asthma and the steps necessary to control the disease evolve over time.

Obesity

Weight reduction in obese patients with asthma has been associated with improvement of lung function and other indicators of lung status.[86] Similar to the importance of monitoring height in children with asthma, both as an indicator of general wellness and effects of medications used to treat asthma, comprehensive care in children with asthma includes monitoring weight acquisition and encouraging weight reduction.

Exercise

Exercise is a common precipitant of asthma symptoms, especially in children and young adults because of their generally active lifestyles. Exercise-induced asthma (EIA) may lead to decreased participation in physical activities because of exertional limitation or fear of symptom development. This may explain the finding that children with asthma are less physically fit than their non-asthmatic peers.[87] Despite these facts, asthma should not be perceived as a limitation on physical fitness, as evidenced by the prevalence of asthma among Olympic athletes approximating twice that of the general population.[88] Increased aerobic fitness decreases EIA, as better-conditioned individuals require less increases in heart rate and ventilation for a given task.[88] Thus, although EIA may still occur, more physical work can be done before it begins (see Chapter 40).

CLASSIFICATION OF ASTHMA SEVERITY

Asthma severity is currently classified as either intermittent or persistent disease (Table 38-2). Although the distinction between intermittent and persistent disease, and even between the various levels of persistent disease, is arbitrary, it serves as a framework for severity classification and ultimately

TABLE 38-2 Classification of Asthma Severity

Severity	Symptoms	Nighttime Symptoms
Intermittent	Symptoms ≤ 2 times/wk	≤ 2 times/mo
	Asymptomatic and normal peak expiratory flow between exacerbations	
	Exacerbations brief (from a few hours to a few days); intensity may vary	
Mild persistent	Symptoms > 2 times/wk but < 1 time/day	3-4 times/mo
	Exacerbations may affect activity	
Moderate persistent	Daily symptoms	5-9 times/mo
	Daily use of inhaled short-acting β_2 agonist	
	Exacerbations affect activity	
	Exacerbations > 2 times/wk; may last days	
Severe persistent	Continual symptoms	≥ 10 times/mo
	Limited physical activity	
	Frequent exacerbations	

Modified from National Asthma Education and Prevention Program: Expert Panel Report II: Pub No. 97-4051A, Bethesda, Md, 1997, US Department of Health and Human Services.

NOTE: Patient is assigned the highest level of severity for which he/she meets any single criterion.

treatment recommendations. Three major features of asthma—daytime symptom frequency, nocturnal symptom frequency, and interference with exercise—further define levels of severity before the institution of controller therapy. Asthma is considered to be persistent if symptoms occur more often than twice a week or if nocturnal symptoms occur more often than twice a month, or if exacerbations begin to affect activity. Nocturnal symptoms are a particularly important marker of more severe disease.[89]

Although most national and international guidelines provide lung function measures that are suggested as those that correspond to each level of asthma severity, these parameters do not appear to be entirely appropriate for the classification of childhood asthma because most children with persistent asthma, even severe asthma, have FEV_1 measures within the normal range (≥ 80% predicted).[90] Thus clinicians and researchers should focus upon symptom frequency and medication use in assigning a level of asthma severity. To maximize the outcome of asthma therapy, goals must be high and be clearly communicated to the child and family. Achievable goals for nearly all children with asthma are outlined in Table 38-3. Routine reassessment of patient attainment of these goals is a critical component of ongoing asthma care. See

Figure 38-2 for a set of questions that can be given to the child/parent while they wait for a visit.

After controller therapy has been initiated, both the level of asthma symptom control and the current level of asthma medication use must be considered in determination of asthma severity (Table 38-4). For example, patients initially defined as having mild persistent asthma who continue to have symptoms more than twice a week or nocturnal symptoms more than twice a month despite treatment appropriate for mild persistent asthma (such as a low-dose inhaled corticosteroid [ICS]) should be considered to have moderate persistent asthma, and their medications should be modified accordingly.

Perception of Bronchoconstriction

Presence of symptoms is an important determinant of severity determinations. Interpretation of symptom histories must be undertaken in the context of overreporting in anxious individuals, underreporting in children who do not want to be bothered by limitations that may be imposed if symptoms are fully reported, and underreporting in children who do not perceive their level of bronchoconstriction, either acutely or chronically. The last of these possibilities is most worrisome because those asthma patients who have difficulty perceiving significant airway obstruction appear to be the most at risk for severe outcomes, such as hospitalization or even death. Review of studies in the literature on this subject do not provide clear guidelines on which patients may be unable to perceive bronchoconstriction, indicating that lung function should be measured at times of regular office visits and the relationship between level of lung function and current symptoms should be discussed. Finding a discrepancy between the level of lung function and current symptoms can be an important part of the education and planning for future exacerbations; a child with no symptoms but with low lung function needs to be aware that any symptoms might mean severe problems were present. Such a child is one who might benefit from regular use of a peak flow meter and should be told to not stop taking measurements when well, as most children tend to do.

TABLE 38-3 Goals of Asthma Treatment

Prevent chronic and troublesome symptoms
Maintain (near) "normal" lung function
Maintain normal activity levels (including exercise)
Prevent recurrent exacerbations of asthma
Eliminate (or minimize) emergency department visits and hospitalizations
Provide optimal pharmacotherapy with minimal or no adverse effects
Meet patients' and families' expectations of and satisfaction with asthma care

Modified from National Asthma Education and Prevention Program: Expert Panel Report II: Pub No. 97-4051A, Bethesda, Md, 1997, US Department of Health and Human Services.

TABLE 38-4 Classification of Asthma Severity by Daily Medication Regimen and Response to Treatment

	Current Treatment Step		
	Step 1: Intermittent	*Step 2: Mild Persistent*	*Step 3: Moderate Persistent*
Patient symptoms on current therapy	**Level of severity**		
Step 1: Intermittent	Intermittent	Mild persistent	Moderate persistent
Symptoms ≤ 2 times per week			
Asymptomatic and normal PEF between exacerbations			
Exacerbations brief (from a few hours to a few days); intensity may vary			
Nocturnal symptoms ≤ 2 times per month			
Step 2: Mild persistent	Mild persistent	Moderate persistent	Severe persistent
Symptoms > 2 times/wk but < 1 time/day			
Exacerbations may affect activity			
Nocturnal symptoms 3-4 times/mo			
Step 3: Moderate persistent	Moderate persistent	Severe persistent	Severe persistent
Daily symptoms			
Daily use of inhaled short-acting β$_2$-agonist			
Exacerbations affect activity			
Exacerbations > 2 times/wk; may last days			
Nocturnal symptoms 5-9 times/mo			
Step 4: Severe persistent	Severe persistent	Severe persistent	Severe persistent
Continual symptoms			
Limited physical activity			
Frequent exacerbations			
Nocturnal symptoms ≥ 10 times/mo			

Modified from National Institutes of Health, National Heart, Lung, and Blood Institute. Global Initiative for Asthma—Global strategy for asthma management and prevention, Bethesda, Md, 2002, NIH Pub No. 02-3659.

TREATMENT OF CHILDHOOD ASTHMA

In addition to the pharmacologic approach to asthma, one must minimize exposure to asthma triggers, including environmental allergens (see Chapter 26) and nonspecific airway irritants (such as tobacco smoke), and treat concomitant medical conditions that influence asthma severity (such as GER and rhinosinusitis). Equally important is providing asthma education and support for the child and family for the process of chronic disease management.

Severity-Based Asthma Management

A central element to any treatment regimen is a written action plan that provides the child and family with a clearly defined approach towards asthma management, including medications for routine daily use and a rescue plan for exacerbations, including medication modifications and signs of asthma symptom progression; the latter should prompt contact with the health care provider or seeking of emergency care.

Pharmacologic Management

Currently, asthma medications are divided into two major categories—those that provide rapid relief of asthma symptoms (quick relievers) and those that serve to decrease airway inflammation and improve asthma on an ongoing basis (long-term controllers). The choice of medications for a given patient depends upon the level of asthma severity (Table 38-5).

Intermittent asthma is managed with as-needed use of short-acting β$_2$ agonists by inhalation. However, all patients with persistent asthma should receive one, or potentially a combination of, controller medications that possess antiinflammatory properties.

Controller Medications

The inflammatory nature of persistent asthma supports the use of medications aimed at decreasing, and ideally eliminating, airway inflammation. Thus agents with antiinflammatory properties are essential in the treatment plan of all children with persistent asthma. Although several agents in this category of medications have been shown to have antiinflammatory properties, the ICSs have been clearly identified as the most effective class of agents currently available for the long-term control of asthma, including the inflammatory component.

Inhaled Corticosteroids

ICSs are the most effective long-term controller medication for asthma in childhood. Studies have demonstrated that ICS therapy leads to significant improvement in asthma control as reflected by reductions in asthma symptom frequency and severity, exacerbation rates, hospitalizations, asthma death, quality of life, and airway hyperresponsiveness. Short-term studies of ICS therapy have reported improvements in measures of lung function and reduction in inflammatory cells and other makers of inflammation within the airways.

CAMP, the largest and longest prospective clinical trial of ICS therapy in children, examined the effect of three treatment strategies in 1041 children with mild-to-moderate asthma.[91] Children received (1) an ICS (budesonide, 200 μg twice daily), (2) a nonsteroidal agent with antiinflammatory

TABLE 38-5 Severity-Based Medication Use

Severity	Preferred Treatment	Alternative Treatments (Listed Alphabetically)	If Needed
Intermittent	No daily medication needed		Severe exacerbations may occur, separated by long periods of no symptoms. A course of systemic corticosteroids is recommended.
Mild persistent	Low-dose inhaled corticosteroid	Cromolyn, leukotriene modifier, nedocromil, OR sustained release theophylline (levels 5-15 μg/ml)	
Moderate persistent	Low-to-medium dose inhaled corticosteroid AND long-acting inhaled β_2 agonists	Increased inhaled corticosteroid within medium dose range, OR Low-to-medium dose inhaled corticosteroid and either leukotriene modifier or theophylline	Particularly in patients with recurring severe exacerbations *Preferred treatment* Increased inhaled corticosteroid within medium dose range and add long-acting inhaled β_2 agonists *Alternative treatment (listed alphabetically)* Increased inhaled corticosteroid within medium-dose range and add either leukotriene modifier or theophylline corticosteroid tablets or syrup (2 mg/kg/day, generally not exceeding 60 mg/day).
Severe persistent	High-dose inhaled corticosteroids and long-acting inhaled β_2 agonists		

Modified from National Institutes of Health, National Heart, Lung, and Blood Institute: Executive summary of the NAEPP Expert Panel Report—Guidelines for the diagnosis and management of asthma—update on selected topics 2002, Bethesda, Md, 2002, NIH Pub No. 02-5075, 2002.
All patients: (1) Short-acting bronchodilator: 2 to 4 puffs short-acting inhaled β_2 agonists as needed for symptoms. (2) Use of short-acting inhaled β_2 agonists on a daily basis, or increasing use, indicates the need to initiate or increase long-term control therapy.

properties (nedocromil sodium, 4 mg twice daily), or (3) a matching placebo for an average of 4.3 years of continuous therapy. All children received albuterol as needed for symptoms, and oral steroids for exacerbations. The primary outcome of the study was the FEV_1 after bronchodilator following a mean of 4.3 years of therapy. Children treated with ICS demonstrated an initial rise in FEV_1 over the first 6 to 12 months of the trial, but upon completion of the trial the ICS group and the placebo group did not differ in terms of FEV_1. The children who received nedocromil were similar to placebo-treated children at all time points. However, children who received ICS therapy experienced numerous clinical benefits not experienced by children who received placebo, including significant improvement in airway hyperresponsiveness, fewer asthma symptoms, less albuterol use, more days without an asthma episode, a longer time until need for oral corticosteroids for an asthma exacerbation, fewer courses of oral corticosteroids, fewer urgent care visits and hospitalizations, and less need for supplemental ICS therapy because of poor asthma control.

Guidelines for asthma management suggest that increasing levels of asthma severity require increasing doses of ICS to achieve disease control. Several studies support a dose-response relationship for ICS. However, this relationship is nonlinear and is complicated by the dose-side effect relationship. Low doses of ICS (as low as 200 μg of budesonide per day[92] or 50 μg of fluticasone propionate twice daily[93]) have been demonstrated to be effective in controlling asthma in children with persistent asthma. Furthermore, each child is likely to demonstrate his or her individual ICS dose-response relationship, as demonstrated in adults.[94] In addition, the rate of improvement of individual measures of asthma control vary, with symptom control and peak flow measures generally responding to low-dose ICS therapy within 2 to 4 weeks,[92] whereas treatment with higher doses for longer periods of time is necessary to maximize effect on airway hyperresponsiveness.[91] Thus ICS dosing must be tailored to the individual patient's needs and response to therapy.

In general, ICS therapy is well tolerated by the majority of patients. However, potential side effects of ICS therapy include the effects of ICS upon skeletal growth and bone density, alteration of the hypothalamic-pituitary-adrenal (HPA) axis, and local side effects including oral candidiasis and hoarseness.

The effect of ICS therapy on growth during childhood has been extensively studied. However, many of the conclusions from these investigations are difficult to fully appreciate because many studies are of short to intermediate durations (generally ranging from 8-12 weeks to 1 year). ICS therapy has been shown to result in short-term reductions in rates of linear growth in children, an effect that is most evident in prepubertal children. These effects are dose and drug dependent, with no significant effect on growth when low doses (100 to 200 μg of fluticasone propionate per day) are used for up to 1 year.[95] When present, these effects appear to be transient reductions in growth velocity early in the treatment course rather than reductions in attained adult height. CAMP demonstrated that children receiving ICS therapy for 4 to 6 years grew 1.1 cm less than those receiving placebo. The growth effect was in the first year of treatment without additional effect as treatment continued. When adult height was predicted using standardized measures based upon current height, current age, bone age, and age at first menses (for females), the ICS-treated children and the placebo-treated children had similar projected final heights.[91] Similar findings have been reported in other populations.[96-98] These results suggest that the effect of low-moderate dose ICS therapy on linear growth is transient and does not predict final adult height.

Additional safety concerns regarding ICS use in children include effects upon the HPA axis and upon bone mineral density (BMD). Numerous studies have examined the effect of ICS therapy on HPA axis function with conflicting results. Although the available evidence suggests that low-moderate dose ICS therapy is generally not associated with alterations in HPA function,[99] the long-term effects of high-dose ICS therapy in growing children remain unclear. The interaction between ICS use and BMD was studied thoroughly in CAMP; 4 years of low-moderate dose ICS therapy did not alter BMD in children 5 to 12 years of age with mild-moderate asthma.[91] The effect of high-dose ICS therapy on BMD in growing children remains uncertain.

There has been some concern that ICS may cause the course of chicken pox to worsen. This concern has come from several case reports of death from chicken pox in individuals on high doses of oral steroids. There has been no case of death with ICS alone, but clinicians caring for children with persistent asthma should ensure varicella immunity, either through prior natural infection or through vaccination, and be prepared to minimize ICS use and add antiviral agents should chicken pox occur in individuals on ICS.

Leukotriene Modifiers

The cysteinyl leukotrienes (LTC4/LTD4/LTE4) are mediators produced by eosinophils and mast cells and trigger many processes central to asthma(mucus secretion, bronchoconstriction, and increased vascular permeability. The clinical effects of agents that modulate leukotriene activity confirm the role of these mediators in the pathophysiology of asthma. Clinical trials have demonstrated the positive effects of leukotriene antagonism on pulmonary function and clinical outcomes in children with asthma.[100,101]

There are currently three leukotriene modifiers (LTMs) available in the United States—two selective leukotriene receptor 1 antagonists (montelukast, zafirlukast), and one that interferes with the function of 5-lipoxygenase, an enzyme critical for the generation of leukotrienes (zileuton). Montelukast improved pulmonary function, reduced rescue albuterol use, improved quality of life, and decreased peripheral blood eosinophil counts over an 8-week period in children 6 to 14 years of age with moderate asthma compared with placebo.[100] In addition, montelukast has been shown to inhibit exercise-induced bronchoconstriction in children with mild-moderate asthma.[101] In addition to having positive effects as monotherapy, LTMs appear to have additive properties when given with ICS.[102]

The inflammatory nature of asthma currently demands that controller medications possess antiinflammatory properties. Although the data regarding the antiinflammatory attributes of LTMs is limited compared to ICS, several studies strongly suggest that these agents decrease markers of allergic airway inflammation, including peripheral blood[100] and sputum eosinophils,[103] nitric oxide in exhaled air,[104,105] and cellular infiltrates in BAL fluid following segmental allergen challenge.[106]

Although the long-term effects of antileukotriene therapy are unknown, these agents possess desirable clinical and biologic properties and deserve consideration in children with all levels of persistent asthma. These agents have excellent safety records in children, and the oral delivery system makes these agents easy to administer to children. There are limited data currently available for LTMs in the treatment of mild persistent asthma in children because most studies reported to date include patients with more severe disease. Furthermore, there are no reported comparative trials of LTMs and ICS in children. However, such trials have been conducted in adults with asthma and consistently show greater improvements in pulmonary function, albuterol use, and symptom control among patients receiving ICS therapy.[107] Caution must be applied in interpreting these results because the trials comparing ICS and LTM therapy in adults generally included patients with moderate-severe asthma. Overall data suggest that LTMs are beneficial for children with mild asthma, and current guidelines support their use as an alternative to ICS as monotherapy in mild persistent asthma. LTMs are also suggested as adjunctive therapy in moderate-severe asthma.

Long-Acting β Agonists

Two long-acting β_2-adrenergic agonists (LABAs), salmeterol and formoterol, have been demonstrated to be safe and effective agents in children, both in terms of bronchodilation and prevention of exercise-induced bronchospasm. Their onsets of action differ, with formoterol having an onset similar to albuterol (3 minutes) whereas salmeterol has a slower onset of action (10 to 20 minutes). Following single-dose administration, both agents demonstrate durations of action of up to 12 hours. Following regular twice-daily administration, bronchodilation remains effective; however, a level of tolerance (or tachyphylaxis) develops, manifested as a loss of bronchoprotective properties to stimuli such as exercise,[108] methacholine, and allergen, although the clinical relevance of these findings is unclear.

The complementary actions of ICS and LABAs suggest that these agents should be effective when used in combination. Extensive data in adults confirm the superiority of the addition of a LABA to patients uncontrolled on ICS compared to increasing the dose of ICS alone.[109,110] However, such data are lacking in the pediatric population. One study found no advantage with the addition of salmeterol to low-dose ICS therapy compared with a doubling of ICS dose in children with mild-moderate asthma.[111] Studies in adults also suggest that LABAs may facilitate ICS reduction in patients whose asthma is controlled on a moderate-to-high dose of ICS.[112] More clinical trials are necessary to fully determine the role of LABAs in the management of persistent asthma in childhood. However, the compelling evidence of the efficacy of ICS and LABA therapy in adults has led to the recommendation for the use of a combination of ICS and LABAs as preferred therapy in children 5 years of age and older with moderate-severe persistent asthma.[113]

Cromolyn and Nedocromil

Cromolyn sodium and nedocromil sodium are inhaled agents that are alternatives to ICS in the management of mild persistent asthma in children. Both drugs have been shown to possess antiinflammatory properties through nonsteroidal mechanisms, although the exact mechanisms for their actions remain unclear. Both agents are effective in the short-term prevention of exercise-induced bronchospasm. Several clinical trials have suggested beneficial effects with regular administration of cromolyn, although a meta-analysis suggests that there is insufficient evidence to support the use of cromolyn as maintenance therapy for asthma.[114] Nedocromil (8 mg/day) therapy for approximately 4 years in children with mild-moderate asthma resulted in a reduction in oral corticosteroid use and urgent-care visits for asthma symptoms compared to placebo/albuterol for symptoms only, but did not affect lung function or rescue albuterol use compared with placebo.[91] These agents are generally well-tolerated, with cough, sore throat, and bronchoconstriction being the most common side effects to cromolyn. Nedocromil is more commonly associated with bad taste, headache, and nausea than cromolyn.

Theophylline

Theophylline has been available as a treatment for asthma since the 1950s. A member of the methylxanthine family, the mechanism of action of theophylline remains uncertain. Theophylline acts as an inhibitor of phosphodiesterase, although at therapeutic serum levels phosphodiesterase inhibition is weak yet bronchodilation occurs. Theophylline also inhibits the effects of adenosine, a molecule known to induce airway narrowing. Several additional mechanisms of action have been reported, including respiratory stimulant properties, improved respiratory muscle strength, and antiinflammatory effects through unclear mechanisms.

Theophylline has been demonstrated to have numerous positive attributes with regard to asthma management.[115] It is more effective than placebo in controlling asthma symptoms and improving pulmonary function, and is particularly effective in preventing nocturnal asthma symptoms. Current guidelines suggest theophylline as an alternative to ICS in children with mild persistent asthma and as add-on therapy with a low-dose ICS in children with moderate-severe asthma.[113] Patients may experience deterioration of asthma control after they stop taking theophylline.[116,117]

Theophylline has the potential for significant toxicity occurring with increasing serum concentrations. Previously, theophylline serum concentrations between 10 to 20 μg/ml were recommended as a target. However, theophylline also has therapeutic effects at levels below 10 μg/ml. The benefits of theophylline may be recognized at lower serum levels than previously recommended, and current guidelines suggest a target range of 5 to 15 μg/ml.[89] Given the narrow therapeutic window, serum drug level monitoring is needed with doses above 12 mg/kg or if side effects occur. Theophylline metabolism is age dependent, with younger children having greater rates of metabolism than older children and adolescents. Close attention must be given to drug interactions that serve to decrease theophylline metabolism, and thus increase serum levels (such as macrolide antibiotics [erythromycin, clarithromycin], cimetidine, ciprofloxacin) and drugs that increase theophylline metabolism, and thus decrease serum levels (such as carbamazepine, phenobarbital, phenytoin, and rifampin).[118] Febrile illnesses may result in decreased theophylline clearance, whereas tobacco and marijuana smoking result in accelerated clearance. Side effects of theophylline are often dose dependent and include anorexia, nausea, emesis, and headache. Less common side effects include tachycardia, palpitations, abdominal discomfort, diarrhea, and rarely gastrointestinal hemorrhage.

Given its relation to other xanthine drugs, such as caffeine, the effects of theophylline on psychomotor functioning and school performance have been examined and have generally shown that there is no significant negative effect of theophylline on learning or behavior.[115,119]

Allergen Immunotherapy

Specific immunotherapy (SIT) is the repetitive parenteral injection of allergen extracts to reduce the manifestations of allergy caused by natural exposure to those allergens. Although there is agreement that SIT offers clinical benefits to patients with allergic rhinitis, the role of SIT in asthma management remains controversial.[120,121] Clinical trials of SIT for asthma pose methodologic challenges, including the need for lengthy study durations, the difficulty of maintaining blinding, and the need for a multi-dimensional assessment of outcome. Nevertheless, a recent Cochrane Database review of randomized, controlled trials of SIT in asthma[122] showed that SIT led to a significant reduction in asthma symptoms and medication requirement as well as improvement in specific and nonspecific bronchial responsiveness. Pulmonary function, however, was not consistently improved. Despite this evidence of efficacy, the benefit of SIT relative to other asthma therapies remains controversial, especially among multiply sensitized asthmatics without prominent allergic rhinitis.[123]

Another dimension of SIT is the recent hypothesis, suggested by limited data to date, that SIT of monosensitized children may prevent the development of both additional sensitivities and asthma.[120] This reduction in the development of future allergic sensitization has been demonstrated in a group of 5- to 8-year-old children with asthma and sensitization to house dust mite.[124] This lends support to the hypothesis that SIT may affect acquisition of new sensitivities by generally shifting lymphocyte phenotype from T helper cell type 2 (Th2) to Th1; proof of this intriguing idea awaits further study. Furthermore, a recent study demonstrated that SIT to pollens in children aged 6 to 14 years with allergic rhinoconjunctivitis without asthma led to fewer asthma symptoms after 3 years of therapy, suggesting that SIT can reduce the development of asthma in children with seasonal allergic rhinoconjuctivitis.[125]

Quick-Reliever Medications

β₂-Adrenergic Agonists. Rapid-acting inhaled β₂-adrenergic receptor agonists are the most effective bronchodilator agents currently available and serve as the preferred treatment for acute symptoms and exacerbations of asthma as well as the prevention of EIA. These agents stimulate the β₂-adrenergic receptors located on bronchial smooth muscle and trigger a signaling cascade culminating in the generation of intracellular cyclic adenosine monophosphate. In addition to relaxation of airway smooth muscle, β₂ agonists stimulate mucociliary transport, modulate the release of mast cell mediators, and decrease edema formation.

β₂ agonists are available for inhalation (by metered-dose inhalers and nebulizers), oral administration (syrup and sustained-release tablets), and parenteral (subcutaneous and intravenous) administration. Inhalation is the preferred route of delivery, as it maximizes efficacy and minimizes side effects. Several different β₂ agonists are currently available and have comparable efficacy and safety properties. Recently, a single isomer preparation of albuterol, called levalbuterol, became available and has the theoretical advantage of possessing bronchodilatory properties (R-isomer of albuterol) without the presence of the nonbronchodilatory isomer (S-albuterol). Clinical trials with this agent demonstrate minimal clinically relevant differences in bronchodilation or side effects related to β_2-adrenergic receptor stimulation, such as tachycardia, tremor, and decreases in serum potassium levels compared to racemic albuterol.[126]

Anticholinergic Agents. Potential mechanisms by which cholinergic pathways contribute to asthma pathophysiology include bonchoconstriction through increased vagal tone, increased reflex bronchoconstriction resulting from stimulation of airway sensory receptors, and increased acetylcholine release induced by inflammatory mediators.[127] Patients with asthma experience lesser degrees of bronchodilation with anticholinergic agents (such as atropine and ipratropium bromide) than with β_2-agonists. There is presently no indication for anticholinergic agents as a component for long-term asthma control. Evidence supports the use of ipratropium bromide in conjunction with inhaled β_2-agonists in the emergency department during acute exacerbations of asthma in children.[128,129] This effect is most evident in patients with very severe exacerbations. Addition of ipratropium has been shown to decrease rates of hospitalization[128] and duration of time in the emergency department.[129]

Systemic Corticosteroids. Systemic steroids are valuable in gaining control of asthma symptoms in patients under poor control. Although the onset of action of systemic corticosteroids is less rapid than that of inhaled bronchodilators, there is evidence that corticosteroids have a more rapid onset of action than that suggested by their primary mechanisms of action, namely inhibiting the function of inflammatory cells and the secretion of cytokines, chemokines, and other pro-inflammatory mediators. Corticosteroids rapidly up-regulate β_2-adrenoreceptor number and improve receptor function, likely leading to clinical improvement within 4 hours of administration.

Systemic corticosteroids hasten the resolution of acute exacerbations of asthma. Corticosteroid administration in the emergency department decreases admission rates for asthma[130] and shortens the length of stay in hospital. Dosing recommendations for acute asthma range from 1 to 2 mg/kg of body weight per day of prednisone. There is no significant difference in the efficacy of oral or parenteral corticosteroids in acute asthma,[131] unless the child is unable to tolerate oral medications because of vomiting. Given the well-described side effect profile of repeated or continuous use of systemic corticosteroids, dosing should always be minimized. Rare patients with severe asthma may require regular steroid therapy to gain or maintain disease control. In these situations, alternate-day dosing is associated with fewer adverse effects, but a very small percentage of patients with severe disease may still require daily steroid administration. Side effects associated with chronic steroid use in severe asthma include hypertension, cushingoid features, decreased morning serum cortisol levels, osteopenia, growth suppression, obesity, hypercholesterolemia, and cataracts.[132] There is no evidence for clinically significant HPA axis suppression following short "bursts" of systemic steroids for acute exacerbations of asthma, and tapering is not required with courses of 10 to 14

days or less in duration. Furthermore, there is no evidence for increased susceptibility to common acute infections.[133]

Management of Acute Asthma Episodes

Most exacerbations, especially those which are mild in nature, can generally be managed without difficulty at home. However, success in outpatient care of acute asthma demands excellent preparation, including a written set of instructions to help guide the patient and family. The Asthma Action Plan is the central component for home asthma management. Patients must be instructed as to the early and accurate recognition of changes in asthma status, as early intervention is likely to lessen the severity and rate of progression of the episode. An algorithm that serves as the basis for the action plan and allows for telephone triage and recommendations is shown in Figure 38-3.

At the onset of asthma symptoms, including cough, chest tightness, wheeze, shortness of breath, or with a decline in peak expiratory flow (PEF) below 80% of personal best, initial therapy should include administration of a rapid-acting bronchodilator such as albuterol, either via metered-dose inhaler (with a spacer device) or nebulizer. This treatment may be repeated up to three times in the first hour, with PEF measured before and after each albuterol administration. Patients who demonstrate rapid improvement following this intervention should be closely followed over the ensuing hours and days for signs of recurrence of symptoms, with particular attention to nocturnal awakenings. Given the potential for progression of symptoms, addition (or increasing the dose) of an ICS is recommended. Increased use is continued until baseline status is achieved and then for an additional 7 to 10 days because of the time needed for resolution of the increased inflammation produced during the exacerbation. Failure of this rescue approach to markedly reduce symptoms and improve PEF to more than 80% personal best should lead to institution of systemic corticosteroids. Several protocols for administration of oral corticosteroids are commonly used. One such approach is to give prednisone, 2 mg/kg/day (up to 60 mg), for 5 days. The approach used in the CAMP trial, 2 mg/kg/day (up to 60 mg) for 2 days followed by 1 mg/kg/day (up to 30 mg) for 2 days,[134] decreases overall steroid exposure and was very effective in resolving exacerbations in patients with mild to moderate asthma. This should be accompanied by frequent reassessment of clinical status and PEF as well as albuterol every 4 to 6 hours, more frequently if needed. Patients who do not improve with this approach are experiencing moderate-severe exacerbation and may need further evaluation and intervention, generally in the physician's office or in the emergency department. Signs of worsening respiratory distress should prompt emergent evaluation and therapy.

CONCLUSIONS

Asthma can significantly impact on the quality of life of both children and their families. Careful attention to details of determination of severity and applying an appropriate therapeutic regimen can bring about control of asthma symptoms in almost all children (Box 38-1). In determining severity and applying the appropriate regimen, it is essential to establish good communication about the goals of therapy and

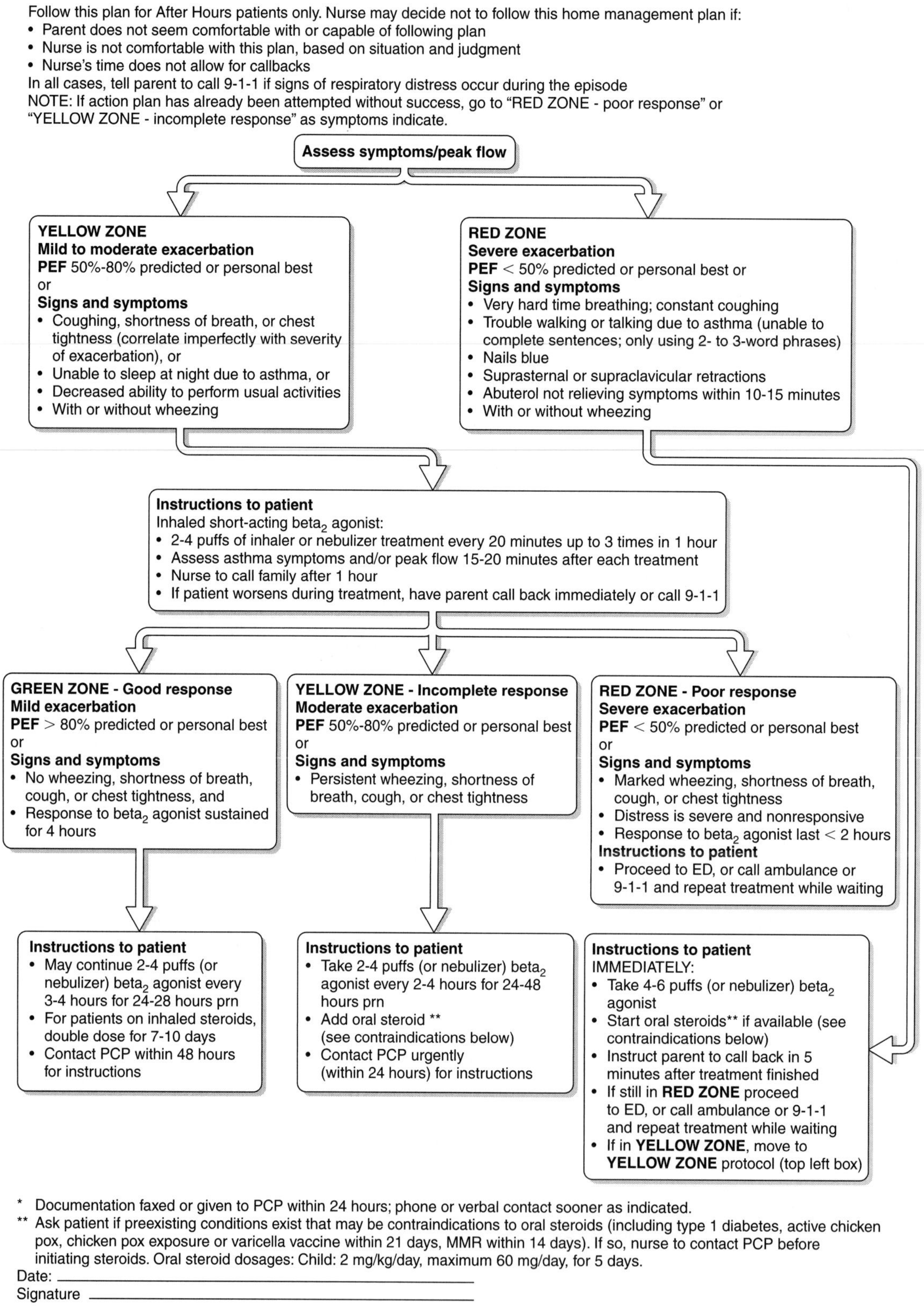

Follow this plan for After Hours patients only. Nurse may decide not to follow this home management plan if:
- Parent does not seem comfortable with or capable of following plan
- Nurse is not comfortable with this plan, based on situation and judgment
- Nurse's time does not allow for callbacks

In all cases, tell parent to call 9-1-1 if signs of respiratory distress occur during the episode

NOTE: If action plan has already been attempted without success, go to "RED ZONE - poor response" or "YELLOW ZONE - incomplete response" as symptoms indicate.

Assess symptoms/peak flow

YELLOW ZONE
Mild to moderate exacerbation
PEF 50%-80% predicted or personal best
or
Signs and symptoms
- Coughing, shortness of breath, or chest tightness (correlate imperfectly with severity of exacerbation), or
- Unable to sleep at night due to asthma, or
- Decreased ability to perform usual activities
- With or without wheezing

RED ZONE
Severe exacerbation
PEF < 50% predicted or personal best or
Signs and symptoms
- Very hard time breathing; constant coughing
- Trouble walking or talking due to asthma (unable to complete sentences; only using 2- to 3-word phrases)
- Nails blue
- Suprasternal or supraclavicular retractions
- Abuterol not relieving symptoms within 10-15 minutes
- With or without wheezing

Instructions to patient
Inhaled short-acting beta$_2$ agonist:
- 2-4 puffs of inhaler or nebulizer treatment every 20 minutes up to 3 times in 1 hour
- Assess asthma symptoms and/or peak flow 15-20 minutes after each treatment
- Nurse to call family after 1 hour
- If patient worsens during treatment, have parent call back immediately or call 9-1-1

GREEN ZONE - Good response
Mild exacerbation
PEF > 80% predicted or personal best
or
Signs and symptoms
- No wheezing, shortness of breath, cough, or chest tightness, and
- Response to beta$_2$ agonist sustained for 4 hours

YELLOW ZONE - Incomplete response
Moderate exacerbation
PEF 50%-80% predicted or personal best
or
Signs and symptoms
- Persistent wheezing, shortness of breath, cough, or chest tightness

RED ZONE - Poor response
Severe exacerbation
PEF < 50% predicted or personal best
or
Signs and symptoms
- Marked wheezing, shortness of breath, cough, or chest tightness
- Distress is severe and nonresponsive
- Response to beta$_2$ agonist last < 2 hours
Instructions to patient
- Proceed to ED, or call ambulance or 9-1-1 and repeat treatment while waiting

Instructions to patient
- May continue 2-4 puffs (or nebulizer) beta$_2$ agonist every 3-4 hours for 24-28 hours prn
- For patients on inhaled steroids, double dose for 7-10 days
- Contact PCP within 48 hours for instructions

Instructions to patient
- Take 2-4 puffs (or nebulizer) beta$_2$ agonist every 2-4 hours for 24-48 hours prn
- Add oral steroid ** (see contraindications below)
- Contact PCP urgently (within 24 hours) for instructions

Instructions to patient
IMMEDIATELY:
- Take 4-6 puffs (or nebulizer) beta$_2$ agonist
- Start oral steroids** if available (see contraindications below)
- Instruct parent to call back in 5 minutes after treatment finished
- If still in **RED ZONE** proceed to ED, or call ambulance or 9-1-1 and repeat treatment while waiting
- If in **YELLOW ZONE**, move to **YELLOW ZONE** protocol (top left box)

*   Documentation faxed or given to PCP within 24 hours; phone or verbal contact sooner as indicated.
** Ask patient if preexisting conditions exist that may be contraindications to oral steroids (including type 1 diabetes, active chicken pox, chicken pox exposure or varicella vaccine within 21 days, MMR within 14 days). If so, nurse to contact PCP before initiating steroids. Oral steroid dosages: Child: 2 mg/kg/day, maximum 60 mg/day, for 5 days.

Date: _____

Signature _____

FIGURE 38-3 Algorithm for treatment of acute asthma symptoms. *PEF,* Peak expiratory flow; *ED,* emergency department; *PCP,* primary care physician. (Courtesy of BJC Health System/Washington University School of Medicine, Community Asthma Program, January 2000.)

understand the family dynamics to ensure that the patient's family can adhere to the therapeutic regimen prescribed. Ongoing evaluation based on communication of current symptoms, with regular assessment of the family's ability to adhere to therapeutic recommendations and the appropriateness of recommendations, is necessary for long-term control of the disease and minimizing the side effects of medications. Review of actions to take during exacerbation, using the Asthma Action Plan as the central mechanism of communication, is part of regular visits for asthma.

BOX 38-1	KEY CONCEPTS

Asthma Management in Older Children

- Failure of symptoms to respond to β agonists and oral steroids should prompt consideration of a process other than asthma causing symptoms.
- Cough that persists despite treatment with bronchodilators and systemic corticosteroids is often not caused by asthma. Consideration of other disorders, particularly sinusitis, is imperative.
- The Asthma Action Plan is the centerpiece of asthma education, focusing the child and parent on early warning signs, when to increase treatment, and when to call for advice during more severe exacerbations. The action plan is relevant directly, focused on action and not theory. An understanding of theory may be helpful when the family can focus on these details.
- Symptoms of gastroesophageal reflux are absent or not recognized in children, especially younger children but even many adolescents.
- Pulmonary function criteria in the Guidelines for Diagnosis and Management of Asthma are not appropriate for children, who can have an FEV_1 in the normal range even with severe disease. The FEV_1/FVC ratio is a much better indicator of severity of disease.
- Simple environmental control measures can make a big difference in disease control. Measures to consider include keeping windows closed for patients with *Alternaria* sensitivity.
- Asthma is controllable in the vast majority of children. Children with even severe asthma can be expected to participate in activities fully. This is an important goal for children and their parents.
- Three questions to gauge asthma severity should be asked at each visit (asthma symptoms on average each week, number of nocturnal awakenings from asthma symptoms per month, and number of interferences with exercise per month). These questions also facilitate communication and focus the child and parent on asthma status and the goals of therapy.
- Asthma severity is often underappreciated by physicians and overtolerated by child and patient (the over-tolerance by the patient and parent result in poor communication with the physician about the status, especially when specific questions are not asked about symptoms present). General questions about status (e.g., "How are you doing?") will lead to underreporting.
- Using more than one canister of albuterol per month is a sign that asthma is uncontrolled.
- Always use the same strength of prednisone or other oral steroid preparation to avoid having to guess what dose of prednisone the patient is taking.
- Asking questions about how the parents administer their child's medications will often reveal that the parent is giving an inhaler without a chamber or using blow-by albuterol via nebulizer, resulting in insufficient medication delivery, and could avoid having to step up therapy.
- Ask the nonthreatening question, "What happens when you skip your medications?" rather than "Do you skip your medications?"

HELPFUL WEBSITES

The Allergy and Asthma Network/Mothers of Asthmatics, Inc. website (www.aanma.org)

The American Academy of Allergy, Asthma and Immunology website (www.aaaai.org)

The American College of Allergy, Asthma and Immunology website (www.allergy.mcg.edu)

The American Lung Association website (www.lungusa. org)

The Asthma and Allergy Foundation of America website (www.aafa.org)

The Childhood Asthma Research and Education Network website (www.asthma-carenet.org)

The National Heart, Lung and Blood Institute Information Center website (www.nhlbisupport.com/asthma/index.html)

REFERENCES

1. Mannino D, Homa D, Pertowski C, et al: Surveillance for Asthma—United States, 1960-1995. CDC Surveillance Summaries, April 24, 1998, *MMWR* 47 (SS-1), 1998.
2. Mannino D, Homa D, Akinbami L, et al: Surveillance for Asthma—United States, 1980-1999. CDC Surveillance Summaries, March 29, 2002, *MMWR* 51:1-15, 2002.
3. von Mutius E, Martinez FD: Epidemiology of childhood asthma. In Murphy S, Kelly H, eds: *Pediatric asthma,* vol 126, New York, 1999, Marcel Dekker.
4. Call RS, Smith TF, Morris E, et al: Risk factors for asthma in inner city children, *J Pediatr* 121:862-866, 1992.
5. Litonjua AA, Carey VJ, Weiss ST, et al: Race, socioeconomic factors, and area of residence are associated with asthma prevalence, *Pediatr Pulmonol* 28:394-401, 1999.
6. Borish L, Mascali J, Klinnert M, et al: SSC polymorphisms in interleukin genes, *Hum Mol Genet* 4:974, 1995.
7. Rosa-Rosa L, Zimmermann N, Bernstein JA, et al: The R576 IL-4 receptor alpha allele correlates with asthma severity, *J Allergy Clin Immunol* 104:1008-1014, 1999.
8. Williams H, McNicol KN: Prevalence, natural history, and relationship of wheezy bronchitis and asthma in children: an epidemiological study, *Br Med J* 4:321-325, 1969.
9. Castro-Rodriguez JA, Holberg CJ, Wright AL, et al: A clinical index to define risk of asthma in young children with recurrent wheezing, *Am J Respir Crit Care Med* 162:1403-1406, 2000.
10. Celedon J, Palmer L, Weiss S, et al: Asthma, rhinitis, and skin test reactivity to aeroallergens in families of asthmatic subjects in Anqing, China, *Am J Respir Crit Care Med* 163:1108-1112, 2001.
11. Christie GL, Helms PJ, Godden DJ, et al: Asthma, wheezy bronchitis, and atopy across two generations, *Am J Respir Crit Care Med* 159:125-129, 1999.
12. von Mutius E, Weiland SK, Fritzsch C, et al: Increasing prevalence of hay fever and atopy among children in Leipzig, East Germany, *Lancet* 351:862-866, 1998.
13. Vartiainen E, Petays T, Haahtela T, et al: Allergic diseases, skin prick test responses, and IgE levels in North Karelia, Finland, and the Republic of Karelia, Russia, *J Allergy Clin Immunol* 109:643-648, 2002.
14. Strachan DP: Hay fever, hygiene, and household size, *Br Med J* 299:1259-1260, 1989.
15. Weiss ST: Gene by environment interaction and asthma, *Clin Exp Allergy* 29:96-99, 1999.
16. Rothman G: *Modern epidemiology,* Philadelphia, 1998, Lippincott-Raven.
17. Sexton K, Gong H Jr, Bailar JC III, et al: Air pollution health risks: do class and race matter? *Toxicol Ind Health* 9:843-878, 1993.
18. Liggett SB: The pharmacogenetics of beta2-adrenergic receptors: relevance to asthma, *J Allergy Clin Immunol* 105:S487-S492, 2000.
19. Reihsaus E, Innis M, MacIntyre N, et al: Mutations in the gene encoding for the beta 2-adrenergic receptor in normal and asthmatic subjects, *Am J Respir Cell Mol Biol* 8:334-339, 1993.
20. Wang Z, Chen C, Niu T, et al: Association of asthma with beta(2)-adrenergic receptor gene polymorphism and cigarette smoking, *Am J Respir Crit Care Med* 163:1404-1409, 2001.

21. Barr RG, Cooper DM, Speizer FE, et al: Beta(2)-adrenoreceptor polymorphism and body mass index are associated with adult-onset asthma in sedentary but not active women, *Chest* 120:1474-1479, 2001.

22. Strunk R, Mrazek D, Fuhrmann G, et al: Physiologic and psychological characteristics associated with deaths due to asthma in childhood: a case-controlled study, *JAMA* 254:1193-1198, 1985.

23. Klinnert MD, Nelson HS, Price MR, et al: Onset and persistence of childhood asthma: predictors from infancy, *Pediatrics* 108:E69, 2001.

24. Sandberg S, Paton JY, Ahola S, et al: The role of acute and chronic stress in asthma attacks in children, *Lancet* 356:982-987, 2000.

25. Bussing R, Burket RC, Kelleher ET: Prevalence of anxiety disorders in a clinic-based sample of pediatric asthma patients, *Psychosomatics* 37:108-115, 1996.

26. Meijer AM, Griffioen RW, van Nierop JC, et al: Intractable or uncontrolled asthma: psychosocial factors, *J Asthma* 32:265-274, 1995.

27. Mrazek DA, Klinnert M, Mrazek PJ, et al: Prediction of early-onset asthma in genetically at-risk children, *Pediatr Pulmonol* 27:85-94, 1999.

28. Chen E, Matthews KA: Cognitive appraisal biases: an approach to understanding the relation between socioeconomic status and cardiovascular reactivity in children, *Ann Behav Med* 23:101-111, 2001.

29. Shaheen SO, Sterne JAC, Montgomery SM, et al: Birth weight, body mass index and asthma in young adults, *Thorax* 54:396-402, 1999.

30. Camargo CA Jr, Weiss ST, Zhang S, et al: Prospective study of body mass index, weight change, and risk of adult-onset asthma in women, *Arch Intern Med* 159:2582-2588, 1999.

31. Celedon JC, Palmer LJ, Litonjua AA, et al: Body mass index and asthma in adults in families of subjects with asthma in Anqing, China, *Am J Respir Crit Care Med* 164:1835-1840, 2001.

32. Castro-Rodriguez JA, Holberg CJ, Morgan WJ, et al: Increased incidence of asthmalike symptoms in girls who become overweight or obese during the school years, *Am J Respir Crit Care Med* 163:1344-1349, 2001.

33. Tobin MJ: Asthma, airway biology, and nasal disorders in AJRCCM 2001, *Am J Respir Crit Care Med* 165:598-618, 2002.

34. Johnston SL, Pattemore PK, Sanderson G, et al: Community study of role of viral infections in exacerbations of asthma in 9- to 11-year-old children, *Br Med J* 310:1225-1229, 1995.

35. Mok JY, Simpson H: Symptoms, atopy, and bronchial reactivity after lower respiratory infection in infancy, *Arch Dis Child* 59:299-305, 1984.

36. Macek V, Sorli J, Kopriva S, et al: Persistent adenoviral infection and chronic airway obstruction in children, *Am J Respir Crit Care Med* 150:7-10, 1994.

37. McKeever TM, Scrivener S, Broadfield E, et al: Prospective study of diet and decline in lung function in a general population, *Am J Respir Crit Care Med* 165:1299-1303, 2002.

38. Fogarty A, Lewis S, Weiss S, et al: Dietary vitamin E, IgE concentrations, and atopy, *Lancet* 356:1573-1574, 2000.

39. Kelly W, Hudson I, Phelan P, et al: Childhood asthma in adult life: a further study at 28 years of age, *Br Med J* 294:1059-1062, 1987.

40. Roorda RJ, Gerritsen J, Van Aalderen WM, et al: Risk factors for the persistence of respiratory symptoms in childhood asthma, *Am Rev Respir Dis* 148:1490-1495, 1993.

41. Gold D, Wypij D, Wang X, et al: Gender- and race-specific effects of asthma and wheeze on level and growth of lung function in children in six U.S. cities, *Am J Respir Crit Care Med* 149:1198-1208, 1994.

42. Blackhall MI: Ventilatory function in subjects with childhood asthma who have become symptom free, *Arch Dis Child* 45:363-366, 1970.

43. Grol MH, Gerritsen J, Vonk JM, et al: Risk factors for growth and decline of lung function in asthmatic individuals up to age 42 years: a 30-year follow-up study, *Am J Respir Crit Care Med* 160:1830-1837, 1999.

44. Oswald H, Phelan PD, Lanigan A, et al: Childhood asthma and lung function in mid-adult life, *Pediatr Pulmonol* 23:14-20, 1997.

45. Lange P, Parner J, Vestbo J, et al: A 15-year follow-up study of ventilatory function in adults with asthma, *N Engl J Med* 339:1194-1200, 1998.

46. Pin I, Siroux V, Cans C, et al: Familial resemblance of asthma severity in the EGEA* study, *Am J Respir Crit Care Med* 165:185-189, 2002.

47. Kurzius-Spencer M, Sherrill DL, Holberg CJ, et al: Familial correlation in the decline of forced expiratory volume in one second, *Am J Respir Crit Care Med* 164:1261-1265, 2001.

48. Zeiger R, Dawson C, Weiss S, et al: Relationships between duration of asthma and asthma severity among children in the Childhood Asthma Management Program (CAMP), *J Allergy Clin Immunol* 103:376-387, 1999.

49. Weiss ST, Van Natta ML, Zeiger RS: Relationship between increased airway responsiveness and asthma severity in the Childhood Asthma Management Program, *Am J Respir Crit Care Med* 162:50-56, 2000.

50. Bloomberg G, Goodman G, Fisher E, et al: The profile of single admissions and readmissions for childhood asthma over a five-year period at St. Louis Children's Hospital, *J Allergy Clin Immunol* 99:S69, 1997.

51. Chen E, Bloomberg G, Fisher EB Jr, et al: Predictors to repeat hospitalizations in children with asthma: the role of psychosocial and socioenvironmental factors, *Health Psychology* 22:12-18, 2003.

52. Strunk RC, Nicklas R, Milgrom H, et al: Risk factors for fatal asthma. In Sheffer A, ed: *Fatal asthma*, vol 115, New York, 1998, Marcel Dekker.

53. Miller RD, Hyatt RE: Evaluation of obstructing lesions of the trachea and larynx by flow-volume loops, *Am Rev Respir Dis* 108:475-481, 1973.

54. Crapo RO: Pulmonary-function testing, *N Engl J Med* 331:25-30, 1994.

55. Rosenstreich DL, Eggleston P, Kattan M, et al: The role of cockroach allergy and exposure to cockroach allergen in causing morbidity among inner-city children with asthma, *N Engl J Med* 336:1356-1363, 1997.

56. Downs SH, Mitakakis TZ, Marks GB, et al: Clinical importance of *Alternaria* exposure in children, *Am J Respir Crit Care Med* 164:455-459, 2001.

57. O'Hollaren M, Yuninger J, Offord K, et al: Exposure to an aeroallergen as a possible precipitating factor in respiratory arrest in young patients with asthma, *N Engl J Med* 324:359-363, 1991.

58. Nelson HS, Szefler SJ, Jacobs J, et al: The relationships among environmental allergen sensitization, allergen exposure, pulmonary function, and bronchial hyperresponsiveness in the Childhood Asthma Management Program, *J Allergy Clin Immunol* 104:775-785, 1999.

59. Sears M, Burrows B, Flannery E, et al: Relation between airway responsiveness and serum IgE in children with asthma and in apparently normal children, *N Engl J Med* 325:1067-1071, 1991.

60. Burrows B, Sears M, Flannery E, et al: Relation of the course of bronchial responsiveness from age 9 to age 15 to allergy, *Am J Respir Crit Care Med* 152:1302-1308, 1995.

61. Dharmage S, Bailey M, Raven J, et al: Current indoor allergen levels of fungi and cats, but not house dust mites, influence allergy and asthma in adults with high dust mite exposure, *Am J Respir Crit Care Med* 164:65-71, 2001.

62. Plaschke P, Janson C, Norrman E, et al: Association between atopic sensitization and asthma and bronchial hyperresponsiveness in Swedish adults: pets, and not mites, are the most important allergens, *J Allergy Clin Immunol* 104:58-65, 1999.

63. Jaakkola JJ, Jaakkola N, Piipari R, et al: Pets, parental atopy, and asthma in adults, *J Allergy Clin Immunol* 109:784-788, 2002.

64. Strunk RC, Sternberg A, Bacharier LB, et al: Nocturnal awakening due to asthma in children with mild to moderate asthma in the Childhood Asthma Management Program, *J Allergy Clin Immunol* 110:395-403, 2002..

65. Nafstad P, Magnus P, Gaarder PI, et al: Exposure to pets and atopy-related diseases in the first 4 years of life, *Allergy* 56:307-312, 2001.

66. Dekker C, Dales R, Bartlett S, et al: Childhood asthma and the indoor environment, *Chest* 100:922-926, 1991.

67. Leynaert B, Bousquet J, Neukirch C, et al: Perennial rhinitis: an independent risk factor for asthma in nonatopic subjects: results from the European Community Respiratory Health Survey, *J Allergy Clin Immunol* 104:301-304, 1999.

68. Foresi A, Pelucchi A, Gherson G, et al: Once-daily intranasal fluticasone propionate (200 micrograms) reduces nasal symptoms and inflammation but also attenuates the increase in bronchial responsiveness during the pollen season in allergic rhinitis, *J Allergy Clin Immunol* 98:274-282, 1996.

69. Adams RJ, Fuhlbrigge AL, Finkelstein JA, et al: Intranasal steroids and the risk of emergency department visits for asthma, *J Allergy Clin Immunol* 109:636-642, 2002.

70. Crystal-Peters J, Neslusan C, Crown WH, et al: Treating allergic rhinitis in patients with comorbid asthma: the risk of asthma-related hospitalizations and emergency department visits, *J Allergy Clin Immunol* 109:57-62, 2002.

71. Rachelefsky GS, Katz RM, Siegel SC: Chronic sinus disease with associated reactive airway disease in children, *Pediatrics* 73:526-529, 1984.

72. Oliveira CA, Sole D, Naspitz CK, et al: Improvement of bronchial hyperresponsiveness in asthmatic children treated for concomitant sinusitis, *Ann Allergy Asthma Immunol* 79:70-74, 1997.

73. Harding SM: Gastroesophageal reflux and asthma: insight into the association, *J Allergy Clin Immunol* 104:251-259, 1999.

74. Martin ME, Grunstein MM, Larsen GL: The relationship of gastroesophageal reflux to nocturnal wheezing in children with asthma, *Ann Allergy* 49:318-322, 1982.

75. Cook DG, Strachan DP: Health effects of passive smoking: summary of effects of parental smoking on the respiratory health of children and implications for research, *Thorax* 54:357-366, 1999.

76. Gold DR, Wang X, Wypij D, et al: Effects of cigarette smoking on lung function in adolescent boys and girls, *N Engl J Med* 335:931-937, 1996.

77. Bacharier LB, Strunk RC: Vocal cord dysfunction: a practical approach, *J Respir Dis Pediatrician* 3:42-48, 2001.

78. Strunk RC, Mrazek DA, Fukuhara JT, et al: Cardiovascular fitness in children with asthma correlates with psychologic functioning of the child, *Pediatrics* 84:460-464, 1989.

79. Ludwick SK, Jones JW, Jones TK, et al: Normalization of cardiopulmonary endurance in severely asthmatic children after bicycle ergometry therapy, *J Pediatr* 109:446-451, 1986.

80. Gutstadt LB, Gillette JW, Mrazek DA, et al: Determinants of school performance in children with chronic asthma, *Am J Dis Child* 143:471-475, 1989.

81. Bender BG, Belleau L, Fukuhara JT, et al: Psychomotor adaptation in children with severe chronic asthma, *Pediatrics* 79:723-727, 1987.

82. Grus CL, Lopez-Hernandez C, Delamater A, et al: Parental self-efficacy and morbidity in pediatric asthma, *J Asthma* 38:99-106, 2001.

83. Clark N, Feldman C, Evans D: The impact of health education on frequency and cost of health care use by low income children with asthma, *J Allergy Clin Immunol* 78:108-114, 1986.

84. Janson S, Reed ML: Patients' perceptions of asthma control and impact on attitudes and self-management, *J Asthma* 37:625-640, 2000.

85. Bender B, Wamboldt FS, O'Connor SL, et al: Measurement of children's asthma medication adherence by self report, mother report, canister weight, and Doser CT, *Ann Allergy Asthma Immunol* 85:416-421, 2000.

86. Hakala K, Stenius-Aarniala B, Sovijarvi A: Effects of weight loss on peak flow variability, airways obstruction, and lung volumes in obese patients with asthma, *Chest* 118:1315-1321, 2000.

87. Strunk RC, Mascia A, Lipkowitz M, et al: Rehabilitation of a patient with asthma in the outpatient setting, *J Allergy Clin Immunol* 87:601-611, 1991.

88. Weiler J, Layton T, Hunt M: Asthma in United States Olympic athletes who participated in the 1996 Summer Games, *J Allergy Clin Immunol* 102:722-726, 1998.

89. National Asthma Education and Prevention Program. Expert Panel Report II: *Guidelines for the diagnosis and management of asthma*, Pub No. 97-4051A, Bethesda, Md, 1997, US Department of Health and Human Services.

90. Bacharier LB, Mauger D, Lemanske RJ, et al: Classifying asthma severity in children—is measuring lung function helpful? *J Allergy Clin Immunol* 109:S266, 2002.

91. Childhood Asthma Management Program Research Group: Long-term effects of budesonide or nedocromil in children with asthma, *N Engl J Med* 343:1054-1063, 2000.

92. Shapiro G, Bronsky EA, LaForce CF, et al: Dose-related efficacy of budesonide administered via a dry powder inhaler in the treatment of children with moderate to severe persistent asthma, *J Pediatr* 132: 976-982, 1998.

93. Peden DB, Berger WE, Noonan MJ, et al: Inhaled fluticasone propionate delivered by means of two different multidose powder inhalers is effective and safe in a large pediatric population with persistent asthma, *J Allergy Clin Immunol* 102:32-38, 1998.

94. Szefler SJ, Martin RJ, King TS, et al: Significant variability in response to inhaled corticosteroids for persistent asthma, *J Allergy Clin Immunol* 109:410-418, 2002.

95. Allen DB, Bronsky EA, LaForce CF, et al: Growth in asthmatic children treated with fluticasone propionate, *J Pediatr* 132:472-477, 1998.

96. Agertoft L, Pedersen S: Effect of long-term treatment with inhaled budesonide on adult height in children with asthma, *N Engl J Med* 343:1064-1069, 2000.

97. Silverstein MD, Yunginger JW, Reed CE, et al: Attained adult height after childhood asthma: effect of glucocorticoid therapy, *J Allergy Clin Immunol* 99:466-474, 1997.

98. Van Bever HP, Desager KN, Lijssens N, et al: Does treatment of asthmatic children with inhaled corticosteroids affect their adult height? *Pediatr Pulmonol* 27:369-375, 1999.

99. Chrousos GP, Harris AG: Hypothalamic-pituitary-adrenal axis suppression and inhaled corticosteroid therapy. 2. Review of the literature, *Neuroimmunomodulation* 5:288-308, 1998.

100. Knorr B, Matz J, Bernstein JA, et al: Montelukast for chronic asthma in 6- to 14-year-old children: a randomized, double-blind trial, *JAMA* 279:1181-1186, 1998.

101. Kemp JP, Dockhorn RJ, Shapiro GG, et al: Montelukast once daily inhibits exercise-induced bronchoconstriction in 6- to 14-year-old children with asthma, *J Pediatr* 133:424-428, 1998.

102. Simons FE, Villa JR, Lee BW, et al: Montelukast added to budesonide in children with persistent asthma: a randomized, double-blind, crossover study, *J Pediatr* 138:694-698, 2001.

103. Pizzichini E, Leff JA, Reiss TF, et al: Montelukast reduces airway eosinophilic inflammation in asthma: a randomized, controlled trial, *Eur Respir J* 14:12-18, 1999.

104. Bisgaard H, Loland L, Oj JA: NO in exhaled air of asthmatic children is reduced by the leukotriene receptor antagonist montelukast, *Am J Respir Crit Care Med* 160:1227-1231, 1999.

105. Bratton DL, Lanz MJ, Miyazawa N, et al: Exhaled nitric oxide before and after montelukast sodium therapy in school-age children with chronic asthma: a preliminary study, *Pediatr Pulmonol* 28:402-407, 1999.

106. Calhoun WJ, Lavins BJ, Minkwitz MC, et al: Effect of zafirlukast (Accolate) on cellular mediators of inflammation: bronchoalveolar lavage fluid findings after segmental antigen challenge, *Am J Respir Crit Care Med* 157:1381-1389, 1998.

107. Busse W, Raphael GD, Galant S, et al: Low-dose fluticasone propionate compared with montelukast for first-line treatment of persistent asthma: a randomized clinical trial, *J Allergy Clin Immunol* 107:461-468, 2001.

108. Simons F: A comparison of beclomethasone, salmeterol, and placebo in children with asthma, *New Engl J Med* 337:1659-1665, 1997.

109. Greening AP, Ind PW, Northfield M, et al: Added salmeterol versus higher-dose corticosteroid in asthma patients with symptoms on existing inhaled corticosteroid, *Lancet* 344:219-224, 1994.

110. Shrewsbury S, Pyke S, Britton M: Meta-analysis of increased dose of inhaled steroid or addition of salmeterol in symptomatic asthma (MIASMA), *Br Med J* 320:1368-1373, 2000.

111. Verberne AA, Frost C, Duiverman EJ, et al: Addition of salmeterol versus doubling the dose of beclomethasone in children with asthma, *Am J Respir Crit Care Med* 158:213-219, 1998.

112. Fowler SJ, Currie GP, Lipworth BJ: Step-down therapy with low-dose fluticasone-salmeterol combination or medium-dose hydrofluoroalkane 134a-beclomethasone alone, *J Allergy Clin Immunol* 109: 929-935, 2002.

113. National Institutes of Health, National Heart, Lung, and Blood Institute: *Executive Summary of the NAEPP Expert Panel Report—Guidelines for the Diagnosis and Management of Asthma—Update on Selected Topics 2002*, Bethesda, Md, 2002, NIH Pub No. 02-5075.

114. Tasche MJ, Uijen JH, Bernsen RM, et al: Inhaled disodium cromoglycate (DSCG) as maintenance therapy in children with asthma: a systematic review, *Thorax* 55:913-920, 2000.

115. Blake K: Theophylline. In Murphy S, Kelly H, eds: *Pediatric asthma*, vol 126, New York, 1999, Marcel Dekker.

116. Brenner M, Berkowitz R, Marshall N, et al: Need for theophylline in severe steroid-requiring asthmatics, *Clin Allergy* 18:143-150, 1988.

117. Baba K, Sakakibara A, Yagi T, et al: Effects of theophylline withdrawal in well-controlled asthmatics treated with inhaled corticosteroid, *J Asthma* 38:615-624, 2001.

118. Weinberger M, Hendeles L: Theophylline in asthma, *N Engl J Med* 334:1380-1388, 1996.

119. Bender BG, Ikle DN, DuHamel T, et al: Neuropsychological and behavioral changes in asthmatic children treated with beclomethasone dipropionate versus theophylline, *Pediatrics* 101:355-360, 1998.

120. Bousquet J: Pro: immunotherapy is clinically indicated in the management of allergic asthma, *Am J Respir Crit Care Med* 164:2139-2140, 2001.

121. Adkinson NF Jr: Immunotherapy is not clinically indicated in the management of allergic asthma, *Am J Respir Crit Care Med* 164:2140-2141, 2001.

122. Abramson MJ, Puy RM, Weiner JM: Allergen immunotherapy for asthma, *Cochrane Database Syst Rev* CD001186, 2000.

123. Adkinson NF Jr, Eggleston PA, Eney D, et al: A controlled trial of immunotherapy for asthma in allergic children, *N Engl J Med* 336:324-331, 1997.

124. Pajno GB, Barberio G, De Luca F, et al: Prevention of new sensitizations in asthmatic children monosensitized to house dust mite by specific immunotherapy. A six-year follow-up study, *Clin Exp Allergy* 31: 1392-1397, 2001.

125. Moller C, Dreborg S, Ferdousi HA, et al: Pollen immunotherapy reduces the development of asthma in children with seasonal rhinoconjunctivitis (the PAT-study), *J Allergy Clin Immunol* 109:251-256, 2002.

126. Gawchik SM, Saccar CL, Noonan M, et al: The safety and efficacy of nebulized levalbuterol compared with racemic albuterol and placebo in the treatment of asthma in pediatric patients, *J Allergy Clin Immunol* 103:615-621, 1999.

127. Martinati LC, Boner AL: Anticholinergic antimuscarinic agents in the treatment of airways bronchoconstriction in children, *Allergy* 51:2-7, 1996.

128. Qureshi F, Pestian J, Davis P, et al: Effect of nebulized ipratropium on the hospitalization rates of children with asthma, *N Engl J Med* 339:1030-1035, 1998.

129. Zorc JJ, Pusic MV, Ogborn CJ, et al: Ipratropium bromide added to asthma treatment in the pediatric emergency department, *Pediatrics* 103:748-752, 1999.

130. Scarfone RJ, Fuchs SM, Nager AL, et al: Controlled trial of oral prednisone in the emergency department treatment of children with acute asthma, *Pediatrics* 92:513-518, 1993.

131. Becker JM, Arora A, Scarfone RJ, et al: Oral versus intravenous corticosteroids in children hospitalized with asthma, *J Allergy Clin Immunol* 103:586-590, 1999.

132. Covar RA, Leung DY, McCormick D, et al: Risk factors associated with glucocorticoid-induced adverse effects in children with severe asthma, *J Allergy Clin Immunol* 106:651-659, 2000.

133. Grant CC, Duggan AK, Santosham M, et al: Oral prednisone as a risk factor for infections in children with asthma, *Arch Pediatr Adolesc Med* 150:58-63, 1996.

134. Childhood Asthma Management Program Research Group: The Childhood Asthma Management Program (CAMP): design, rationale, and methods, *Control Clin Trials* 20:91-120, 1999.

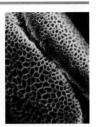

CHAPTER **39**

Asthma Education Programs for Children

SANDRA R. WILSON ■ HAROLD J. FARBER

Asthma control is not intuitive. Quick-relief medicine does not control the underlying problem, and long-term control medicine may not "feel" as though it is effective. Patients commonly fail to adhere to recommendations for asthma control and self-monitoring.[1-4]

Controlling persistent asthma in children and coping successfully with the condition require complex changes in lifestyle and behavior: reducing asthma triggers; monitoring lung function; following an asthma management plan; taking asthma control medication daily; recognizing an asthma flare promptly and escalating therapy appropriately; effectively using the health care system and other resources; ensuring effective communication among the child's adult caregivers; and promoting positive adjustment of the child as well as positive adjustment of other family members to the child's condition and resultant needs while not neglecting their own needs.[5]

Patient education is an essential component of guidelines for the medical management of asthma. For more than a decade, consensus guidelines have emphasized that patient education and a sound partnership between clinician and patient (or parent) are essential, both for optimal disease outcome and for preventing asthma crises.[6] However skillful a clinician may be in other respects, failure to effectively educate patients and families can thwart the other components of medical management (Box 39-1).

In the revised 1997 National Asthma Education and Prevention Program (NAEPP) guidelines[7] and in the related guide *Pediatric Asthma: Promoting Best Practice*, prepared by the American Academy of Allergy, Asthma, and Immunology and the American Academy of Pediatrics,[8] the primary asthma caregiver is given responsibility for ensuring adequate patient education. In these guidelines, failure to provide patients with basic education about the nature and management of their condition from time of diagnosis through all subsequent clinical contact is considered inconsistent with current standards of asthma care. When necessary, families also should be provided or referred to sources of supplementary education, which may be provided in a format and setting matched to institutional and community resources.

Delivery of education should be documented in the patient record. To facilitate documentation and to ensure that critical elements are included, it may be helpful to adopt a special form (Figure 39-1) to place in the patient's health record. Documentation should also indicate how a patient's (or parent's) understanding and competence was assessed. This documentation should provide evidence not only that the education was delivered but also that it was received and understood.

Patient and parent understanding of and adherence to asthma control practices still may not be sufficient, by itself, to ensure adequate asthma control. Day care and school personnel may need to administer quick-relief or long-term control medication, or both. They must be able to recognize an asthma flare and to take appropriate action. School environments also may be important sources of asthma triggers.[9]

Communities may have substantial air pollution[10,11]; exposure to environmental tobacco smoke may be unavoidable in public facilities (e.g., restaurants, public bathrooms, shopping malls, entertainment venues); and homes (particularly in inner city areas) may be contaminated with mold, infested with cockroaches, or require the use of a gas stove for heat—all of which are conditions associated with increased asthma prevalence, severity, or both.[12-15]

Because schools and communities play an important role in the health of a child, education of school personnel and of the community as a whole about asthma, its management, and the conditions that exacerbate asthma plays an important role in creation of an asthma-friendly community.

GOALS OF ASTHMA EDUCATION FOR PATIENTS AND PARENTS

The goal of asthma education for children and their families is to help them make the behavioral, lifestyle, and environmental changes necessary to control asthma. Research in three areas—effective and ineffective actions of parents and children in managing asthma,[5,16] factors associated with nonad-

BOX 39-1	KEY CONCEPTS
	Role of Asthma Education

- Asthma education is a critical part of asthma care.
- Effective patient education does more than provide knowledge—it facilitates the behavioral, lifestyle, and environmental changes necessary to control asthma.
- Effective care of chronic asthma involves partnership among patient, family, and physician. Effective asthma education is the foundation of this partnership.

ASTHMA EDUCATION DOCUMENTATION FORM

LEARNING/TEACHING CONTENT	HEALTH CARE PROVIDER ACTION		PATIENT/SIGNIFICANT OTHER ACTION/RESPONSE	
	Information Provided	Task Demonstrated	Verbalizes Understanding	Task Demonstrated
A. Basic Facts about Asthma				
• What asthma is				
• Difference between normal and asthmatic lungs				
• What happens to airway during asthma attack				
B. Role of Medications				
• Short-acting rescue drugs				
• Preventive and control drugs				
• Flare-reversing drugs				
C. Skills				
• How to use an inhaler				
• How to measure peak flow				
D. Environmental Control Measures				
• Triggers				
E. Adverse Reactions				
• When to call M.D.				
F. Use of Self-Management Plan				
G. Referral to Outpatient Asthma Coordinator				
H. Written Information Provided				
I. Educational Videos Shown				

FIGURE 39-1 Form for documenting (in medical chart) provision of asthma education and response of parent or child to the education.

herence,[17,18] and analysis of the knowledge and skills required to carry out these complex tasks—suggests that parents and children need specific skills and understanding. The NAEPP Expert Panel Report has recommended that five key educational messages be integrated into every step of clinical asthma care[7] (Figure 39-2).

1. Basic facts about asthma
   • The contrast between asthmatic and normal airways
   • What happens to the airway during an asthma attack
2. Role of medication
   • The difference between long-term control and quick-relief medication

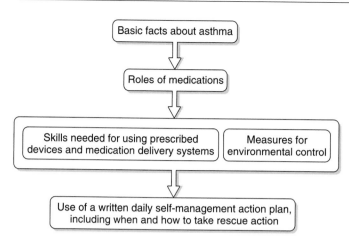

FIGURE 39-2 Focus asthma education on key messages. (Modified from National Heart, Lung, and Blood Institute, National Asthma Education and Prevention Program: Expert panel Report 2: guidelines for the diagnosis and management of asthma, Bethesda, Md, 1997, National Institutes of Health, National Heart, Lung, and Blood Institute, NIH Pub No. 97-4051. Also available on the World Wide Web [accessed April 10, 2002]: http://www.nhlbi.nih.gov/guidelines/asthma/asthgdln.pdf.)

3. Skills
   - Proper inhaler use, taught by demonstration and coaching
   - How to use a spacer and holding chamber
   - How to monitor symptoms and peak flow and how to recognize early signs of health deterioration
4. Measures for environmental control
   - How to identify and avoid environmental precipitants or exposure
5. When and how to take rescue action
   - Use of a written daily self-management and action plan

Epidemiologic research has substantiated the importance of patients and their parents understanding the role of long-term control medication. The Asthma Care Quality Assessment in Medicaid Managed Care study surveyed parents of children with persistent asthma and reported that regular use of inhaled antiinflammatory asthma control medication was much lower if a parent of a child with persistent asthma misunderstood the role of the child's asthma control medication as being for treatment of symptoms (i.e., *after* they begin) rather than for prevention of symptoms (i.e., *before* they begin).[17]

Written asthma management plans are important for conveying key messages to patients. Books on asthma in the popular press have stated that "Good doctors give written instructions,"[19,20] and U.S. and international asthma care guidelines recommend written asthma management plans.[7,21] Having a written asthma management plan is associated with decreased risk of hospitalization and emergency department visits as well as with improved adherence to regular use of asthma control medication.[22,23]

The goal of asthma education is not simply to disseminate information or even to develop skills. Attitudes and motivation also are critical for implementing an effective asthma regimen. These attitudes are not fixed characteristics of particular individuals but can be affected by education and by whether a strong partnership exists between a clinician and a patient's family. Effective asthma education is the foundation for developing this partnership: True partnership cannot exist if a parent or patient lacks essential information and skills or if a clinician fails to elicit essential information about a patient's concerns, preferences, and any barriers faced in implementing therapy. Many experts believe in the importance of jointly developing treatment goals to promote patient adherence.[7,19,24] If crisis care is a patient's goal, then developing adherence to long-term control strategies may be difficult. And unless a treatment plan meets the patient's real goals, the plan is unlikely to be implemented on an ongoing basis.

Opposition or reluctance to giving a child any medication regularly (or particular fears regarding use of corticosteroid agents) may, in a parent's mind, override any benefit a physician claims for asthma control medications. Without guidance or assistance, a patient may be unable to surmount barriers to complying with recommendations. Out-of-pocket costs for medication, health care, and environmental control may also serve as barriers to adherence. Parents addicted to tobacco may be unable and unwilling to avoid passive exposure of their child to this environmental pollutant and consequently may discount its relation to asthma symptoms. Even parents who do wish to avoid exposing the child to environmental tobacco smoke may misunderstand what are effective and ineffective strategies for avoiding this exposure. Mothers may also have difficulty eliminating this exposure if they and their children are dependent on a smoker (e.g., a spouse/partner or their own parent) for housing or for other necessities.[25] And many other factors, such as complex dosing schedules, unpleasant taste, and unpleasant side effects (real or anticipated), can contribute to nonadherence—as can unmet patient expectations, failure to address health beliefs, and failure to address patient preferences.[26-29] Mental health comorbidity is associated with nonadherence[30] and with worsened asthma control.[31]

Ongoing follow-up is important not only for assessing disease status but also for encouraging the development of effective asthma self-management by patients or their parents. Desired changes often are not made at the first clinic visit, and both progress and success must be monitored and reinforced. Without substantial follow-up, single-session educational programs in the acute care setting appear not to achieve substantial behavior change,[32] whereas greater success appears to have been achieved with programs consisting of multiple small-group sessions with time between sessions for families to practice, evaluate, and make further change.

ACHIEVING BEHAVIOR CHANGE THROUGH EDUCATION

Effective Patient-Provider Communication

Clark and Gong[33] cited 10 techniques for effective communication that are based on studies of the physician-patient relationship and can improve patient self-management of asthma (Table 39-1). Such communication techniques can improve clinician-patient communication. In addition, in a controlled trial, teaching physicians to use these strategies was associated with better patient outcomes and greater satisfaction with care during a 22-month follow-up period.[34,35] Physicians who attended a seminar on improving patient communication used these strategies more often yet spent no more time with patients than clinicians who did not attend the seminar.[34,35] The seminar included brief lectures by asthma specialists, a

TABLE 39-1 Ten Principles of Effective Communication Applicable to Education of Asthmatic Patients and Their Parents about the Condition and Its Treatment

Attend to patient and parent.
  Make eye contact.
  Sit rather than stand when conversing with the patient.
  Move closer to the patient.
  Lean slightly forward to attend to the discussion.
Elicit underlying concerns about the condition.
  Construct reassuring messages that alleviate fears.
  Reduce fear as a distraction (this enables parent/patient to focus on what you are saying).
Address any immediate concerns that are expressed.
  This enables patients to refocus their attention toward the information being provided.
  Adherence suffers if concerns, beliefs, and goals are not identified.
Engage parent and patient in interactive conversation.
  Use open-ended questions.
  Use simple language.
  Use analogies to teach important concepts.
Use appropriate encouragement when patient reports using correct disease management strategies.
  Provide a pat on the shoulder.
  Nod in agreement.
  Give verbal praise.
Elicit patient's immediate objective for controlling the disease; reach an agreement on a short-term goal.
  Choose objectives that both provider and patient will strive to reach and that are important to the patient.
Tailor and simplify treatment regimen by eliciting and addressing potential problems with timing, dose, or side effects of drugs recommended and with environmental control recommendations.
  Minimize number of medications.
  Fit dosing schedule and frequency to patient's routine.
  Consider patient's ability to afford medications.
  Consider barriers to implementing environmental control measures.
  Consider interpersonal conflicts over medications and environmental control.
Provide tools (e.g., simple written and pictorial materials to help patients implement recommended actions and skills).
  Provide daily management and asthma action plans in written form.
  Provide instructions for inhaler, nebulizer, and peak flow meter use.
  Provide a formal prescription for avoiding child's exposure to environmental tobacco smoke.
  Provide materials on how to recognize asthma symptoms and assess their severity.
Review long-term plan for treatment by considering the following.
  What to expect over time
  Situations under which the physician will modify treatment
  Criteria for judging the success of the treatment plan, as follows:
    Freedom from symptoms during day and at night
    Optimal lung function and normal development
    Normal performance level in physical and social activities
    Minimal need for urgent-care visits; no hospitalization
    Minimal use of asthma rescue medication
    As few side effects as possible
    Patient/parent satisfaction with the asthma care provided
Help patient plan ahead for decision-making.
  Use diary information or guidelines for handling potential problems.
  Explore contingencies in managing the disease.

Modified from Clark NM, Gong M: *Br Med J* 320:572-575, 2000.

videotape on the 10 effective communication techniques, discussion of case studies of troublesome clinical problems, a protocol for self-assessment of each clinician's communication, and review of basic messages that must be communicated to patients as well as tools and materials to use for patient teaching.

The effectiveness and efficiency of patient education in changing patient behavior appear to depend on whether health care practitioners have a well thought out plan for patient education, have appropriate patient education tools readily available, and focus their messages on patients. One

proposed technique focuses on "three lines of defense,"[19] as follows.

- Manage the environment (control asthma triggers).
- Manage the breathing tubes (regular use of long-acting control medicines to make the breathing tubes less sensitive).
- Manage asthma flares (early recognition followed by appropriate action).

Consideration of a "stages of self-regulation" model[36] may also help clinicians focus asthma control messages, especially if those messages are planned to be appropriate to a family's current stage of asthma self-management and to the goal of moving them to a higher stage.

Stage 1: Asthma avoidance—Asthma is viewed by the family as a child's episodic problem.

Stage 2: Asthma acceptance—The family acknowledges that the child has asthma symptoms between attacks; however, the family takes action only when the child is symptomatic.

Stage 3: Asthma adherence—The family adheres to a preventive medication regimen but perceives that fluctuation in asthma status represents treatment failure.

Stage 4: Asthma control—The family applies an action plan when symptoms change and discusses efficacy of the treatment plan during regular consultation with their child's physician.[36]

IMPORTANCE OF MATERIALS WRITTEN AT LOW LITERACY LEVEL

Written materials are essential tools for asthma education and self-management. However, these materials should not simply be handed to a patient or parent to be read on their own and cannot be relied on as a substitute for education by a clinician. Provision of a written asthma self-management plan is associated with improved adherence to regular use of inhaled anti-inflammatory medication[23] and reduction in risk for asthma hospitalization and emergency department visits.[22] Parents often prefer simple management plan forms with pictorial/graphic material in color to more complex text-based forms.[37] Many models of such plans exist, both in published asthma education programs and as downloadable documents from noncommercial websites.[38]

Written materials must be comprehensible and written in a language understood by patients. Many people in the United States have low literacy skills and even lower comprehension of quantitative information. Studies from public university hospitals have found mean literacy skills among adults to be at the seventh- or eighth-grade level.[39] A survey of parents accompanying children with asthma to an inner-city emergency department found that 20% of parents could read only at the sixth-grade level or below and that 49% could read only at the eighth-grade level or below.[40] Self-reported parental education attainment is not an accurate predictor of reading ability. A study of patients seen at a public university hospital in northeastern Louisiana found that although 95% of these patients had graduated from high school, two thirds were reading below the ninth-grade level and one third were reading below the seventh-grade level.[39]

Practical and more reliable means of assessing literacy in the clinical setting are available. The Rapid Estimate of Adult Literacy in Medicine is a validated instrument that can be easily administered within 2 to 3 minutes in a clinical setting to determine literacy level.[41] This instrument uses recognition of medical and health-related words and has been found to correlate highly with the more time-consuming Test of Functional Health Literacy in Adults, which directly evaluates reading comprehension.[42]

Despite these commonly limited capabilities among patients, surveys of patient education materials used in pediatric practice have found that close to three fourths of the materials had readability levels of ninth grade or higher.[43,44] Even the asthma care management plan forms included as part of the NAEPP Expert Panel Report II required a reading grade level of 7.5 to 9.[43] For patients with extremely low reading levels, alternatives to printed text may be needed.[45] For example, the videotape for parents and the pictorial materials designed for use with children aged 4 to 6 years from the *Wee Wheezers* educational program[46] have been translated and adapted for use with non–English-speaking Hmong families, translated into Spanish, and adapted for use by nurses in home visits with low-income African American families in Atlanta, Georgia.[47] The need continues for good-quality asthma education materials that can be understood by people with low or marginal literacy or who do not speak or read English.

APPROACHES TO ASTHMA EDUCATION AND BEHAVIOR CHANGE

Individual Education in the Course of Clinical Care

As discussed, asthma education in the course of a typical patient visit can use approaches that have been shown to effectively change patient behavior. Such education can be made more efficient and effective by careful attention to the 10 principles of effective communication[33] and by incorporating carefully developed asthma action plans, diaries, peak flow meters (and other aids to self-monitoring), and other available asthma education materials and patient management tools. Many of the most powerful strategies for changing behavior are used most effectively in a small-group setting with patients who are somewhat similar in age and circumstance.[48] Nevertheless, much can be done during relatively brief encounters between a clinician and individual patient or parent if educational messages and strategies are carefully planned.

Video Games

Because asthma education delivered by a health care practitioner or health educator can be labor intensive, alternative methods of teaching asthma care skills have been explored. Interactive computer games may allow opportunity for active engagement, for return demonstration, for feedback, and for problem-solving, assuming that the educational content is appropriate to the developmental level of the child.

Shegog et al[49] found that children with asthma who played the *Watch, Discover, Think, and Act* computer game improved their knowledge about self-regulation, prevention, and treatment. These children also had higher scores on measures of self-efficacy. Homer et al[50] compared education delivered by a computer game *(Asthma Control)* with asthma education delivered by a research assistant and found that these methods similarly improved asthma control. However, the children who played the *Asthma Control* interactive computer game showed greater improvement in their knowledge about asthma than did children educated by the research assistant.[50]

Interactive computer games hold promise as asthma education aids. Use of these games may be particularly valuable in settings where health care practitioners lack sufficient time or skills to effectively deliver asthma education to children.[51] The effectiveness of computer games in parental asthma education remains to be determined.

TABLE 39-2 Outline of Parent Sessions of the *Wee Wheezers: An Educational Program for Parents of Children with Asthma Under the Age of Seven*

Session 1
  I. Introductions and Overview of Program (10 minutes)
    A. Introduction of participants
    B. Introduction of program
  II. Basic Concepts of Asthma (30 minutes)
    A. Asthma facts and figures
    B. Asthma physiology
    C. Video 1—*Asthma: What happens in the Lungs*
    D. Diagnosis of asthma
  III. Coping in a Crisis (25 minutes)
    Video 2—*Fears and Anxieties*
  IV. Action Plan for Asthma Management (25 minutes)
    A. Recognizing early warning signs of asthma
    B. Getting your child to recognize his or her own early warning signs
    C. Use of peak flow meter
    D. Preparing your action plan
  V. Homework Assignment and Wrap-up (10 minutes)

Session 2
  I. Discussion of Homework (5 minutes)
  II. Continuing asthma action plan (30 minutes)
    A. Understanding asthma medications
    B. Non-medication techniques for managing asthma symptoms
  III. Symptoms of an Acute Episode (45 minutes)
    A. Treating early symptoms
      Video 3—*Asthma: The Symptoms*
      Video 4—*Symptoms Quiz*
    B. Signs of a more severe asthma episode
    C. Seeking medical assistance
  IV. Homework Assignment and Wrap-up (5 minutes)

Session 3
  I. Discussion of Homework and Medication Questions (10 minutes)
  II. Considering How You Feel about Your Child Having a Chronic Health Problem (20 minutes)
    Video 5—*Living with a Chronic Illness*
  III. Symptom Prevention (50 minutes)
    A. Trigger identification (5 minutes)
    B. Control of nonenvironmental triggers (10 minutes)
    C. Environmental control (15 minutes)
    D. Homework (5 minutes)
    E. Using preventive medications (10 minutes)
    F. Using premedication (5 minutes)
  IV. Wrap-up (10 minutes)

Session 4
  I. Review of Homework (10 minutes)
  II. Communicating About Asthma (60 minutes)
    With teachers and childcare workers (20 minutes)
    With your physician (20 minutes)
      Video 6—*Communicating with the Doctor*
    Within your family (20 minutes)
      Video 7—*Communicating with Family and Friends*
  III. Preview of Follow-up Sessions and Wrap-up (10 minutes)

From Wilson SR, Fish L, Page A, et al: *Wee Wheezers: an educational program for children with asthma under seven years of age,* rev ed, Palo Alto, Calif, 1999, Palo Alto Medical Foundation Research Institute (complete program available in English and Spanish; videos and handouts available in Hmong).

Small-Group Asthma Education Programs

Education delivered to patients or parents in small groups led by a trained facilitator has been associated, in controlled trials, with improved asthma outcomes.[33] Such programs have been delivered in clinical settings as well as in schools, in other community settings (e.g., voluntary health associations), and at asthma camps. A small-group asthma education program for adults was directly compared with (1) one-on-one sessions by comparably trained asthma educators delivering the same educational content and using the same visual aids and handouts and (2) a self-study workbook containing the same content and other materials. The small-group program showed substantially better outcomes and required less time per person educated than the intervention delivered individually.[48] Presumably, the reason for its greater success is that the small-group format permits use of more powerful behavioral change methods, which are not as easily used either in a one-on-one encounter or in written materials alone; such methods include role playing and modeling, social comparison, and social support.[52]

Among the most widely disseminated small-group pediatric asthma education programs in the United States are the *Open Airways* program,[53] *Air Power,*[54] *Open Airways for Schools,*[55] and *ACT—Asthma Care Training for Kids*[56]—all of which are intended for delivery to school-aged children and have been shown, in controlled trials, to improve asthma management behaviors, disease outcomes, or both. These programs may provide some education to parents as well (e.g., *Air Power*) or may reach parents through their children, as in the case of the *Open Airways for Schools* program.[57] Some programs are specifically designed for use in a school setting; others may be used in a variety of clinical and community settings.

Sesame Street's *A is for Asthma,*[58] developed for the American Lung Association, is directed at parents, their preschool-aged children, and child care providers. The *Wee Wheezers* program is essentially the only published asthma education program specifically directed to children under the age of 7 years that has been evaluated in a controlled trial. The program necessarily directs education primarily to parents. The *Wee Wheezers* program also includes basic asthma education for children aged 4 to 6 years.[46] The educational objectives and strategies that this program uses to encourage behavior change were based on research that identified both the effective and the ineffective asthma management practices of parents of very young children with asthma.[5] The resultant comprehensive asthma education program (Table 39-2)[59] illustrates what can and may need to be provided to some families to supplement the education provided during clinical care.

With the exception of the Sesame Street *A is for Asthma* program, all of the cited programs were evaluated under controlled conditions and were associated with improvement in one or more asthma management behaviors, with improved disease outcomes, or with both of these results.

Asthma Case Management

For many patients, severity of asthma, complexity of medical and psychosocial needs, or all these factors may necessitate not only supplementary asthma education but also engagement of other resources to address broader issues. This use of other resources typically requires more time and focused attention than can be devoted within the time constraints of a typical clinical visit and also requires somewhat different skills from those of a physician. Moreover, when first identified, such patients may be receiving most of their care from urgent or emergency services and hence from multiple providers instead of from a single primary care practitioner or asthma specialist. For these reasons, other models have been developed for addressing these patients' educational and other needs and for providing the basic asthma education that may be lacking in the medical care these patients receive.

Many health care systems are now targeting for special intervention those patients with high-risk asthma profiles as determined on the basis of these patients' emergency department visits, hospitalizations, high levels of use of quick-relief medication, and multiple asthma care providers.[60] Case management is a particularly powerful way to improve asthma self-care for persons with moderate persistent to severe persistent asthma. Case management involves an allied health professional (a specially trained nurse, respiratory therapist, or clinical pharmacist) who provides education and ongoing follow-up for a patient and family. The case manager identifies and addresses the patient's and family's educational needs, reinforces the asthma action plan, and acts as an advocate with the physician if the plan does not seem to be working. The case manager also provides telephone support. Home health visits may be conducted, and support services (educational materials, spacers, peak flow meters) may be provided.[61]

In a randomized controlled clinical trial conducted by Harvard Pilgrim Health Care,[62] 57 children with poorly controlled asthma were recruited both from hospital admission lists and from physician referral. Greater reduction in emergency department visits, number of hospital admissions, and out-of-plan costs was seen in the outreach intervention group.[62] A randomized controlled clinical trial[63] of a multifaceted, individually tailored case management intervention run by social workers for inner-city children with asthma showed a reduction in the number of asthma symptom days and a tendency toward less hospitalization for asthma in the intervention group (14.8% vs. 18.9%, $P = 0.07$). In addition to addressing asthma issues, investigators found that, to be effective, they needed to address more general problem-solving skills and psychosocial issues in relation to the lives of these children and their parents.[63]

In clinical practice, accumulated experience with asthma care management has been positive. At Tripler Army Medical Center, Oahu, Hawaii, 79 children hospitalized for asthma (mean age, 5.82 years; SD, 3.93 years) were enrolled in a program of asthma care management. The rehospitalization rate was only 10% for patients in this care management program, and the overall asthma admission rate for the service population decreased.[64] The Kaiser Permanente Napa-Solano Service Area observed a 72% reduction in emergency department visits in the year after enrollment among patients participating in asthma care management (H.J. Farber, unpublished data, 1998). Experience with asthma care management in a sample of adult members of ConnectiCare, Inc. (a regional health maintenance organization) who overused beta agonist medication found that repeated telephone contact resulted in more appropriate use of inhaled corticosteroid medications compared with a single telephone contact.[65] Both groups were mailed an asthma information packet and were invited to an asthma class.

Change in Health Care Systems with Regard to Asthma Care

Health care systems can either facilitate or impair behavioral change that patients need to make to control their asthma. Among the key determinants of change are whether the asthma care efforts of the health care system focus on chronic or acute care, whether financial incentives for patients and clinicians promote or discourage asthma follow-up, whether appropriate asthma education materials are readily available, and whether physicians prescribe appropriate treatment.

Clinical pathways are often used to coordinate care and to reduce variation in clinical practice when treating hospitalized patients with common diagnoses. Studies of asthma clinical pathways have focused on acute care as well as reduction in length of hospital stay.[66,67] However, hospitalization for asthma often indicates unmet needs for chronic care and may provide a "captive audience" for addressing those needs at the moment when a patient may be most receptive to asthma education.

An asthma clinical pathway should not only address the need for acute care but also improve long-term outcomes by ensuring that the need for chronic care is met. Ideally, in addition to accommodating the need for acute care, an asthma clinical pathway should provide asthma education, identify and offer strategies for reducing asthma-triggering conditions (including environmental tobacco smoke), assess severity of chronic disease, initiate appropriate use of long-acting control medication, provide a written asthma self-care plan, and ensure smooth transition to follow-up outpatient care with an identified personal health care practitioner.[68]

CHANGING SPECIFIC SKILLS AND BEHAVIOR

Considerable evidence (some of which is reviewed earlier in this chapter) shows that asthma education programs can effectively improve clinical outcomes for children with asthma. Some evidence shows the effectiveness of programs that specifically focus on increasing adherence to preventive medication regimens, on using an asthma action plan to adjust medication according to symptoms, or on using both a preventive medication regimen and an action plan. However, most educational programs strive to address multiple self-management behaviors in addition to medication adherence and symptom management. Consequently, much remains to be learned. What, for example, are the most effective educational approaches for promoting specific self-management behaviors? Which behavioral changes lead to the greatest reduction in morbidity? Among specific behavioral changes of interest are improved technique in use of metered-dose inhalers (MDIs) and dry-powder inhalers and improved environmental control practices.

Metered-Dose/Dry-Powder Inhaler and Peak Flow Meter Technique

Many patients and health care practitioners have ineffective or suboptimal technique for using inhaled medication and for measuring peak flow rate.[69-73] Poor technique is common regardless of type of inhalation system.[74,75] Children and their parents often overestimate the quality of the child's inhaler technique.[76] Ineffective inhaler technique is a common reason for poorly controlled asthma.[77]

Observing a patient's inhaler technique instead of simply demonstrating or verbally describing correct technique can allow clinicians to detect important problems.[78] Periodically reevaluating inhaler technique can help to ensure that effective inhaler skills are being maintained. Nonadherence to correct inhaler technique may result from something as simple as inadequate skill or knowledge, but a patient's technique may consciously be chosen to address a problem the patient or parent has experienced. The spacer used with the MDI may be difficult to carry, may be unattractive, may seem childish, or may reflect a combination of these factors. Actuating the MDI multiple times before inhalation may seem an easier way to take multiple puffs. Administering nebulized medication via "blow-by" technique instead of via close-fitting mask may seem more comfortable and acceptable to a child. Part of optimal inhaler use involves discovering the patient's likes and dislikes and attempting to match choice of inhaled medication delivery system to the patient.

Monitoring peak expiratory flow rate is also a useful tool for pediatric asthma self-management, although its role and importance are still somewhat uncertain. Ineffective technique can lead to erroneous results, which then can lead to inappropriate actions. Accurate results depend on maximal exhalation effort after complete inhalation. An erroneously low measurement can result from submaximal effort, submaximal inspiration, or an incomplete seal between the patient's lips and the mouthpiece of the meter. An erroneously high measurement can result from building up pressure in the mouth before releasing it as a blast into the meter (the "chipmunk maneuver"). Demonstration by the clinician and return demonstration by the patient are important for ensuring that a patient is able to obtain accurate readings.

Environmental Control

Nearly all comprehensive, rigorously evaluated small-group asthma education programs have attempted to improve control of environmental triggers of asthma symptoms. However, despite careful design of such randomized controlled trials, relatively little attention has been given to assessing the effectiveness of education in reducing children's exposure to allergens and irritants or even in increasing parents' attempts to reduce this environmental exposure. As a result, relatively little is known about whether education can generate clinically meaningful changes in exposure.[79] The National Cooperative Inner-City Asthma Program reported some success in temporarily reducing the concentration of cockroach allergen by providing professional extermination services as well as directed education. However, concentrations returned to clinically significant baseline levels within 12 months.[80]

An interventional study of environmental control in low-income, inner-city families with children with asthma in Atlanta, Georgia, provided home visits and either sham or real allergen-proof mattresses and pillowcases with instructions to wash bedding weekly in hot or cold water.[81] Study subjects were compared with each other and with subjects who did not have a home visit or home assessment. The number of clinic visits for acute asthma was reduced among subjects who received home visits and among those who were sensitized to dust mite allergen and had reduced dust mite allergen in the home during the study. Exposure and medical utilization decreased similarly among both intervention and sham home visit groups. This study thus suggests that the fact of the home visit may have been the most important part of the intervention.[81]

Environmental tobacco smoke exposure is associated with exacerbation of pediatric asthma.[82-84] Education and counseling have yielded preliminary results that, with further refinement, may reduce exposure to environmental tobacco smoke.[25,85,86] Although research on effective educational interventions to decrease asthma-triggering conditions in the home is still in its infancy, most experts recommend that education about environmental control be included as part of routine asthma care.[6,21,87,88] Reducing indoor and outdoor environmental exposure that exacerbates asthma remains an important technical, public policy, and educational challenge.

CONCLUSIONS

Optimal management of persistent asthma requires behavioral and lifestyle changes on the part of patients and their families. An effective asthma education and management program facilitates these changes. Programs that are effective in facilitating these changes improve asthma outcomes (Box 39-2).

Carefully developed and evaluated asthma education programs and materials exist that can be adopted or adapted for use in a wide range of settings. Initial research and experience with case management for patients at highest risk are promising. Continued research is needed to determine the most effective and efficient asthma management strategies for diverse communities.

Acknowledgment

The Kaiser Foundation Hospitals, Inc, Medical Editing Department provided editorial assistance.

REFERENCES

1. Kleiger JH, Dirks JF: Medication compliance in chronic asthmatic patients, *J Asthma Res* 16:93-96, 1979.
2. Dekker FW, Dieleman FE, Kaptein AA, et al: Compliance with pulmonary medication in general practice, *Eur Respir J* 6:886-890, 1993.

BOX 39-2

THERAPEUTIC PRINCIPLES
Patient Education and Behavior Change

Keep messages simple and focused.

Use simple written materials to reinforce verbal messages. Many patients and parents require educational materials written at lower literacy levels.

Review, reinforcement, and return demonstration of skills are important.

Identify readiness to change and barriers to change.

Identify the patient's and family's concerns and goals for asthma treatment.

More intensive intervention (e.g., multisession small-group asthma education classes, asthma case management, or some combination) may benefit patients who have more severe disease and those whose families have difficulty accomplishing behavioral and lifestyle changes.

3. Rand CS, Wise RA: Measuring adherence to asthma medication regimens, *Am J Respir Crit Care Med* 149:S69-S76, discussion S77-S78, 1994.

4. Apter AJ, Reisine ST, Affleck G, et al: Adherence with twice-daily dosing of inhaled steroids: socioeconomic and health-belief differences, *Am J Respir Crit Care Med* 157:1810-1817, 1998.

5. Wilson SR, Mitchell JH, Rolnick S, et al: Effective and ineffective management behaviors of parents of infants and young children with asthma, *J Pediatr Psychol* 18:63-81, 1993.

6. National Asthma Education Program: *Guidelines for the diagnosis and management of asthma,* Bethesda, Md, 1991, National Institutes of Health, Pub No. 91-3042.

7. National Heart, Lung and Blood Institute, National Asthma Education and Prevention Program: *Expert Panel Report 2: guidelines for the diagnosis and management of asthma,* Bethesda, Md, 1997, National Institutes of Health, National Heart, Lung and Blood Institute, Pub No. 97-4051. Also available on the World Wide Web (accessed April 10, 2002): http://www.nhlbi.nih.gov/guidelines/asthma/asthgdln.pdf.

8. American Academy of Allergy, Asthma and Immunology: *Pediatric asthma: promoting best practice (guide for managing asthma in children),* Milwaukee, Wisc, 1999, The Academy.

9. U.S. Environmental Protection Administration: *Indoor air quality (IAQ) tools for schools kit.* Available on the World Wide Web (accessed April 20, 2002): http://www.epa.gov/iaq/schools/tools4s2.html.

10. McConnell R, Berhane K, Gilliland F, et al: Asthma in exercising children exposed to ozone: a cohort study, *Lancet* 359:386-391, 2002.

11. Kim YK, Baek D, Koh YI, et al: Outdoor air pollutants derived from industrial processes may be causally related to the development of asthma in children, *Ann Allergy Asthma Immunol* 86:456-460, 2001.

12. Rosenstreich DL, Eggleston P, Kattan M, et al: The role of cockroach allergy and exposure to cockroach allergen in causing morbidity among inner-city children with asthma, *N Engl J Med* 336:1356-1363, 1997.

13. Dales RE, Burnett R, Zwanenburg H: Adverse health effects among adults exposed to home dampness and molds, *Am Rev Respir Dis* 143:505-509, 1991.

14. Brunekreef B, Dockery DW, Speizer FE, et al: Home dampness and respiratory morbidity in children, *Am Rev Respir Dis* 140:1363-1367, 1989.

15. Lanphear BP, Aligne CA, Auinger P, et al: Residential exposures associated with asthma in US children, *Pediatrics* 107:505-511, 2001.

16. McNabb WL, Wilson-Pessano SR, Jacobs AM: Critical self-management competencies for children with asthma, *J Pediatr Psychol* 11:103-117, 1986.

17. Farber HJ, Capra AM, Lozano P, et al: Misunderstanding of asthma medications: effects on adherence, *J Asthma* (in press).

18. Rubin DH, Bauman LJ, Lauby JL: The relationship between knowledge and reported behavior in childhood asthma, *J Dev Behav Pediatr* 10:307-312, 1989.

19. Farber HJ, Boyette M: *Control your child's asthma: a breakthrough program for the treatment and management of childhood asthma,* New York, 2001, Henry Holt.

20. Plaut TF: *Children with asthma: a manual for parents,* ed 2, Amherst, Mass, 1995, Pedipress.

21. Global Initiative for Asthma: Global Strategy for Asthma Management and Prevention, [Revised 2002]. 2002, National Institutes of Health, National Heart, Lung, and Blood Institute. (NIH Pub No. 02-3659). Available on the World Wide Web (accessed April 20, 2002): http://www.ginasthma.com.

22. Lieu TA, Quesenberry CP Jr, Capra AM, et al: Outpatient management practices associated with reduced risk of pediatric asthma hospitalization and emergency department visits, *Pediatrics* 100:334-341, 1997.

23. Finkelstein JA, Lozano P, Farber HL, et al: Under-use of controller medications among Medicaid-insured children with asthma, *Arch Pediatr Adolesc Med* 156:562-567, 2002.

24. Hanson JE: Patient education in pediatric asthma. In Murphy S, Kelly HW, eds: *Pediatric asthma,* Monticello, NY, 1999, Marcel Dekker.

25. Wilson SR, Yamada EG, Sudhakar R, et al: A controlled trial of an environmental tobacco smoke reduction intervention in low-income children with asthma, *Chest* 120:1709-1722, 2001.

26. Francis V, Korsch BM, Morris MJ: Gaps in doctor-patient communication. Patients' response to medical advice, *N Engl J Med* 280:535-540, 1969.

27. Clark GM, Troop RC. One-tablet combination drug therapy in the treatment of hypertension, *J Chronic Dis* 25:57-64, 1972.

28. Mann M, Eliasson O, Patel K, et al: A comparison of the effects of bid and qid dosing on compliance with inhaled flunisolide, *Chest* 101:496-499, 1992.

29. Hyland ME: Rationale for once-daily therapy in asthma: compliance issues, *Drugs* 58:1-6, discussion 51, 1999.

30. Christiaanse ME, Lavigne JV, Lerner CV: Psychosocial aspects of compliance in children and adolescents with asthma, *J Dev Behav Pediatr* 10:75-80, 1989.

31. Weil CM, Wade SL, Bauman LJ, et al: The relationship between psychosocial factors and asthma morbidity in inner-city children with asthma, *Pediatrics* 104:1274-1280, 1999.

32. Farber HJ, Oliveria L: Can provision of patient education and a written management plan as part of an Emergency Room (ER) visit improve outcomes for inner city children with asthma? [abstract], *Am J Respir Crit Care Med* 163:A542, 2001.

33. Clark NM, Gong M: Management of chronic disease by practitioners and patients: are we teaching the wrong things? *Br Med J* 320:572-575, 2000.

34. Clark NM, Gong M, Schork MA, et al: Impact of education for physicians on patient outcomes, *Pediatrics* 101:831-836, 1998.

35. Clark NM, Gong M, Schork MA, et al: Long-term effects of asthma education for physicians on patient satisfaction and use of health services, *Eur Respir J* 16:15-21, 2000.

36. Zimmerman BJ, Bonner S, Evans D, et al: Self-regulating childhood asthma: a developmental model of family change, *Health Educ Behav* 26:55-71, 1999.

37. Farber HJ, Smith-Wong K, Nichols L, et al: Patients prefer simple, visual asthma self management plan forms, *Permanente J* 5:35-37, 2001.

38. The Regional Asthma Management and Prevention Initiative (RAMP): Asthma Resources for Providers. Available on the World Wide Web (accessed May 14, 2002): http://www.rampasthma.org/resources.htm.

39. Davis TC, Mayeaux EJ, Fredrickson D, et al: Reading ability of parents compared with reading level of pediatric patient education materials, *Pediatrics* 93:460-468, 1994.

40. Farber HJ, Johnson C, Beckerman RC: Young inner-city children visiting the emergency room (ER) for asthma: risk factors and chronic care behaviors, *J Asthma* 35:547-552, 1998.

41. Davis TC, Long SW, Jackson RH, et al: Rapid estimate of adult literacy in medicine: a shortened screening instrument, *Fam Med* 25:391-395, 1993.

42. Parker RM, Baker DW, Williams MV, et al: The test of functional health literacy in adults: a new instrument for measuring patients' literacy skills, *J Gen Intern Med* 10:537-541, 1995.

43. Forbis SG, Aligne CA: Poor readability of written asthma management plans found in national guidelines of asthma, 109:e52, 2002.

44. Klingbeil C, Speece MW, Schubiner H: Readability of pediatric patient education materials. Current perspectives on an old problem, *Clin Pediatr (Phila)* 34:96-102, 1995.

45. Davis TC, Michielutte R, Askov EN, et al: Practical assessment of adult literacy in health care, *Health Educ Behav* 25:613-624, 1998.

46. Wilson SR, Latini DM, Starr NJ, et al: Education of parents of infants and very young children with asthma: a developmental evaluation of the Wee Wheezers program, *J Asthma* 33:239-254, 1996.

47. Brown JV, Bakeman R, Celano MP, et al: Home-based asthma education of young low-income children and their families, *J Pediatr Psychol* 27:677-688, 2002.

48. Wilson SR, Scamagas P, German DF, et al: A controlled trial of two forms of self-management education for adults with asthma, *Am J Med* 94:564-576, 1993.

49. Shegog R, Bartholomew LK, Parcel GS, et al: Impact of a computer-assisted education program on factors related to asthma self-management behavior, *J Am Med Inform Assoc* 8:49-61, 2001.

50. Homer C, Susskind O, Alpert HR, et al: An evaluation of an innovative multimedia educational software program for asthma management: report of a randomized, controlled trial, *Pediatrics* 106:210-215, 2000.

51. McPherson A, Glazebrook C, Smyth A: Double click for health: the role of multimedia in asthma education, *Arch Dis Child* 85:447-449, 2001.

52. Bandura A: *Social foundations of thought and action: a social cognitive theory,* New York, 1986, Prentice-Hall.

53. Clark NM, Feldman CH, Evans D, et al: Managing better: children, parents, and asthma, *Patient Educ Couns* 8:27-38, 1986.

54. Wilson-Pessano SR, McNabb WL: The role of patient education in the management of childhood asthma, *Prev Med* 14:670-687, 1985.

55. Evans D, Clark NM, Feldman CH, et al: A school health education program for children with asthma aged 8-11 years, *Health Educ Q* 14:267-279, 1987.

56. Lewis CE, Rachelefsky G, Lewis MA, et al: A randomized trial of A.C.T. (asthma care training) for kids, *Pediatrics* 74:478-486, 1984.

57. Evans D, Clark NM, Levison MJ, et al: Can children teach their parents about asthma? *Health Educ Behav* 28:500-511, 2001.

58. American Lung Association: Bilingual multimedia asthma awareness project targets preschoolers [press release], April 21, 1998. Available on the World Wide Web (accessed May 14, 2002): http://www.lungusa.org/press/association/asnsesame.html.

59. Wilson SR, Fish L, Page A, et al: *Wee Wheezers: an educational program for children with asthma under seven years of age,* rev ed, Palo Alto, Calif, 1999, Palo Alto Medical Foundation Research Institute (complete program available in English and Spanish; video and handouts available in Hmong).

60. Lieu TA, Quesenberry CP, Sorel ME, et al: Computer-based models to identify high-risk children with asthma, *Am J Respir Crit Care Med* 157:1173-1180, 1998.

61. Rieve JA: Asthma case management outcomes, *Case Manager* 10:26-27, 1999.

62. Greineder DK, Loane KC, Parks P: A randomized controlled trial of a pediatric asthma outreach program, *J Allergy Clin Immunol* 103:436-440, 1999.

63. Evans R 3rd, Gergen PJ, Mitchell H, et al: A randomized clinical trial to reduce asthma morbidity among inner-city children: results of the National Cooperative Inner-City Asthma Study, *J Pediatr* 135:332-338, 1999.

64. Chan DS, Callahan CW, Moreno C: Multidisciplinary education and management program for children with asthma, *Am J Health Syst Pharm* 58:1413-1417, 2001.

65. Delaronde S: Using case management to increase antiinflammatory medication use among a managed care population with asthma, *J Asthma* 39:55-63, 2002.

66. Johnson KB, Blaisdell CJ, Walker A, et al: Effectiveness of a clinical pathway for inpatient asthma management, *Pediatrics* 106:1006-1012, 2000.

67. Wazeka A, Valacer DJ, Cooper M, et al: Impact of a pediatric asthma clinical pathway on hospital cost and length of stay, *Pediatr Pulmonol* 32: 211-216, 2001.

68. Glauber JH, Farber HJ, Homer CJ: Asthma clinical pathways: toward what end? *Pediatrics* 107:590-592, 2001.

69. Cochrane MG, Bala MV, Downs KE, et al: Inhaled corticosteroids for asthma therapy: patient compliance, devices, and inhalation technique, *Chest* 117:542-550, 2000.

70. Scarfone RJ, Capraro GA, Zorc JJ, et al: Demonstrated use of metered-dose inhalers and peak flow meters by children and adolescents with acute asthma exacerbations, *Arch Pediatr Adolesc Med* 156:378-383, 2002.

71. Resnick DJ, Gold RL, Lee-Wong M, et al: Physicians' metered dose inhaler technique after a single teaching session, *Ann Allergy Asthma Immunol* 76:145-148, 1996.

72. Amirav I, Goren A, Pawlowski NA: What do pediatricians in training know about the correct use of inhalers and spacer devices? *J Allergy Clin Immunol* 94:669-675, 1994.

73. Hanania NA, Wittman R, Kesten S, et al: Medical personnel's knowledge of and ability to use inhaling devices. Metered-dose inhalers, spacing chambers, and breath-actuated dry powder inhalers, *Chest* 105:111-116, 1994.

74. van Beerendonk I, Mesters I, Mudde AN, et al: Assessment of the inhalation technique in outpatients with asthma or chronic obstructive pulmonary disease using a metered-dose inhaler or dry powder device, *J Asthma* 35:273-279, 1998.

75. Kamps AW, van Ewijk B, Roorda RJ, et al: Poor inhalation technique, even after inhalation instructions, in children with asthma, *Pediatr Pulmonol* 29:39-42, 2000.

76. Child F, Davies S, Clayton S, et al: Inhaler devices for asthma: do we follow the guidelines? *Arch Dis Child* 86:176-179, 2002.

77. Chapman KR: Asthma unresponsive to usual therapy. In Fitzgerald JM, Ernst P, Boulet L-P, et al, eds: *Evidence based asthma management,* Hamilton, Ontario, Canada, 2001, BC Decker.

78. Chiang AA, Lee JC: Misunderstandings about inhalers, *N Engl J Med* 330:1690-1691, 1994.

79. Institute of Medicine, Committee on the Assessment of Asthma and Indoor Air: *Clearing the air: asthma and indoor air exposures,* Washington, DC, 2000, National Academy Press.

80. Gergen PJ, Mortimer KM, Eggleston PA, et al: Results of the National Cooperative Inner-City Asthma Study (NCICAS) environmental intervention to reduce cockroach allergen exposure in inner-city homes, *J Allergy Clin Immunol* 103:501-506, 1999.

81. Carter MC, Perzanowski MS, Raymond A, et al: Home intervention in the treatment of asthma among inner-city children, *J Allergy Clin Immunol* 108:732-737, 2001.

82. U.S. Environmental Protection Agency, Office of Health and Environmental Assessment: *Respiratory health effects of passive smoking: lung cancer and other disorders,* Washington, DC, 1992, The Agency, report No. EPA/600/6-90/006F.

83. California Environmental Protection Agency, Office of Environmental Health Hazard Assessment: *Health effects of exposure to environmental tobacco smoke: final report,* Sacramento, Calif, 1997, Office of Environmental Health Hazard Assessment, The Agency.

84. Cook DG, Strachan DP: Health effects of passive smoking-10. Summary of effects of parental smoking on the respiratory health of children and implications for research, *Thorax* 54:357-366, 1999.

85. Hovell MF, Meltzer SB, Zakarian JM, et al: Reduction of environmental tobacco smoke exposure among asthmatic children: a controlled trial, *Chest* 106:439-446, 1994.

86. Wahlgren DR, Hovell MF, Meltzer SB, et al: Reduction of environmental tobacco smoke exposure in asthmatic children. A 2-year follow-up, *Chest* 111:81-88, 1997.

87. Platts-Mills TA, Vaughan JW, Carter MC, et al: The role of intervention in established allergy: avoidance of indoor allergens in the treatment of chronic allergic disease, *J Allergy Clin Immunol* 106:787-804, 2000.

88. Lara M, Rosenbaum S, Rachelefsky G, et al: Improving childhood asthma outcomes in the United States: a blueprint for policy action, *Pediatrics* 109:919-930, 2002.

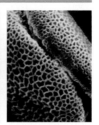

CHAPTER 40

Asthma and the Athlete

DAVID A. STEMPEL

Asthma and the Athlete is meant to be an inclusive title that moves beyond the terms of exercise-induced bronchospasm, exercise-induced asthma (EIA), and exercise-induced airway narrowing. The focus is on the limitations on exercise caused by childhood asthma. In a book dedicated to the health of children, it recognizes that all children should have the potential to be an athlete, unencumbered by the restrictions of illness. The goal applies even to the children banished to "right field." The impact of asthma on normal daily activity of all children, whether for an elite athlete or the majority of children at all other levels of skill, is the topic of this chapter.

The Global Initiative for Asthma (GINA) released in 2002 states that EIA is "one expression of airway hyperresponsiveness, not a special form of asthma. EIA often indicates that the patient's asthma is not adequately controlled; therefore appropriate antiinflammatory therapy generally results in the reduction of exercise-related symptoms."[1] Exercise is occasionally the only apparent trigger of asthma. The GINA document states that one goal of asthma management is to "enable most patients to participate in any activity they choose without experiencing symptoms."[1] This expert panel further recommends in addition to pharmacotherapy that physical activity be part of the therapeutic approach to EIA. This is an evolution from the laboratory concept of exercise-induced bronchospasm to the clinical reality of the effect of asthma on daily physical activity. EIA may be formally defined as a "transient narrowing of the airways that follows vigorous exercise."[2] *Exercise-induced asthma* is the common term used to describe this form of asthma, but *activity-induced asthma* (AIA) is a more descriptive definition for children who wheeze with any type of exertion. *Exercise* is too limiting a term for the pediatric population because it focuses attention on formal exertion and not the frequent limitations imposed by asthma on a child's daily activities, which include bursts of physical exertion, competition in athletic events, and informal playground activities. Therapy for children needs to reflect the frequency of physical activity and on-demand need for bronchoprotection. AIA may occur in children with varying exercise levels, much of which are not considered vigorous. EIA is the term used in this chapter because it is the present standard in the literature.

EIA is defined from a physiologic point of view as intermittent airflow obstruction of the airways measured by a decline in forced expiratory volume in 1 second (FEV_1) or peak expiratory flow rate (PEFR). Exercise is a common, if not nearly universal, trigger of asthma for children and adolescents. Asthma even in the absence of symptoms is associated with inflammation. Inflammation may even be a component of asthma in remission.[3] Although most triggers of asthma induce significant increases in airway inflammation, the role of inflammation in acute EIA is not well defined. Because EIA occurs in children with persistent asthma, inflammation is frequently found in the child with incompletely controlled disease. Activity by itself is rarely the only trigger of asthma, and isolated EIA may suggest the need to search for an alternative diagnosis. Whether EIA can exist in isolation is not clear. The literature discusses the treatment of EIA in the absence of persistent asthma but does not describe whether these patients lack the inflammatory changes noted with the chronic forms of the disease (Box 40-1).

The symptoms of EIA may include any of the following associated with increased activity: shortness of breath, cough, wheeze, chest tightness, or difficulty breathing. Less commonly reported as symptoms of EIA are lack of endurance and impairment in quality of life (Table 40-1). Similar to other forms of asthma, EIA is underrecognized by the patient and parent, underdiagnosed by the health care professional, and therefore undertreated. For many children and adolescents, the only symptom may be the perception that they are out of shape or lack the interest to participate in exertional activity. Bronchial hyperresponsiveness (BHR) correlates with decreasing activity level in children with asthma.[4] It is unclear whether increasing disease severity further restricts a child's activity level or whether a more sedentary lifestyle has a further negative impact on BHR. Poor perception of the symptoms of EIA is common. Different activities will produce different degrees of airway narrowing. Godfrey et al[5] established a rank order exercise leading to EIA from the largest to the smallest effect on reduction in PEFR: free range running,

---

BOX 40-1   **KEY CONCEPTS**
Exercise-Induced Asthma

- Exercise-induced asthma (EIA) occurs in most children and adolescents with persistent asthma.
- From 10% to 14% of children have EIA.
- The treatment of EIA begins with the treatment of persistent asthma.

TABLE 40-1 Subjective and Objective Findings in Exercise-Induced Asthma

Subjective findings with exertion
Wheezing
Cough
Shortness of breath
Perception of poor physical conditioning
Lack of interest in physical activities

Objective findings with exertion
Fall in lung function of 10% to 15%
Protection against a 15% fall in forced expiratory volume in 1 second
Protection with bronchodilators

treadmill, bicycle ergometer, swimming, and walking. Ambient temperature and humidity also are discussed in this chapter, as are additional variables on the effect size of EIA.

This chapter is divided into three sections: the definition, epidemiology, and differential of EIA; studies of the mechanism of disease; and the treatment of EIA.

DEFINITION AND PREVALENCE

All children with asthma should be assessed in the history for the impact of asthma on their activity level. As many as 90% of children with asthma are thought to have symptoms of EIA. In addition, all children with isolated EIA should be assessed for the presence of persistent asthma. The reporting of EIA may vary depending on the type of exertion, the effort of the child, the duration of the activity, and the ambient climate at the time of the activity. These and other variables are important when one compares the reported incidence of EIA[6] (Table 40-2). For the child with asthma, exercise with concurrent allergen exposure or viral infection may further increase the degree of airway narrowing.

EIA is found in virtually all children with a diagnosis of asthma.[7] Godfrey,[7] in his classic review article, describes the prevalence rate with testing and retesting. A fall of 10% to 15% in FEV_1 and a 15% fall in PEFR are usually used as the standards for the diagnosis of EIA. False-positive test results in normal subjects without atopic backgrounds are uncommon. In children, a history of previous wheeze, a family history of asthma, and a diagnosis of allergic rhinitis all appear to be risk factors for greater bronchial reactivity with or without clinical EIA. The therapeutic implication of children with allergic rhinitis who manifest a 15% fall in FEV_1 in the absence of any clinical symptoms or physical limitations raises the following

TABLE 40-2 Variables in Exercise-Induced Asthma

Type of exercise
Duration of exercise
Ambient temperature
Ambient humidity
Associated triggers
Controller asthma medications
Bronchoprotective treatments

important but unanswered questions. Would these children benefit from therapy? Are these children more likely to have later adult-onset asthma?

The appropriate diagnosis of EIA starts with the proper identification of children with chronic asthma (Table 40-3). A detailed history, including prior response to inhaled short-acting beta-agonists and measurement of lung function in children over 5 years of age, is helpful. Baseline FEV_1 in children with persistent asthma may be normal even in the presence of active disease.[8] Children with asthma, if appropriately questioned, will usually respond that they have physical activity limitations imposed by exercise. What is more important and more difficult to do is to assess the undiagnosed asthmatic population for the presence of EIA.

The formal diagnosis of EIA is usually made after a 10% to 15% fall in FEV_1. The lower value is selected for laboratory studies and the higher value for field testing.[2] The average decline in FEV_1 after exertion for normal individuals is 5%. In healthy school children, 92% have less than a 10% fall in PEFR and 98% have less than a 15% fall in PEFR.[9] Response to treatment is frequently defined as protection against a fall of greater than 10% to 15% after exercise challenge. The literature does not stipulate what the baseline fall in FEV_1 needs to be in studies designed to demonstrate efficacy other than children must demonstrate a 10% to 15% fall with exertion for diagnostic purposes. It is difficult to compare various studies of children with EIA because of the variability of these baseline parameters. Furthermore, when discussing the addition of a second controller medication, there are no established baseline lung function parameters or objective symptoms to use to classify patients. Godfrey[9] described the classic response of lung function to an exercise challenge. During the initial minutes of the exercise challenge, there is a small increase in PEFR, followed by a more significant fall in PEFR and a gradual return to normal lung function with rest over a 1-hour period (Figure 40-1). This pattern may not be applicable to a large number of children who start with their FEV_1 reduced below their personal best. Unfortunately, these data are not well documented in the literature.

The prevalence of EIA varies in reports from 45% to 94%.[10] Godfrey's[9] review reported that up to 86% of children with asthma demonstrated EIA on testing. These data suggest that exercise is the most universal trigger of asthma for children and adolescents. McFadden[11] reported in a survey of more than 400 consecutive patients with asthma that 94% indicated that they had airflow limitation associated with exercise. Children who no longer demonstrate active symptoms of asthma appear to retain some of their airway lability associated with exercise.[10] This may be related to the persistent finding of inflammation and increased submucosal collagen deposition found in this group of former childhood asthmatics.[3]

Even 2.8% to 17% of elite world-class athletes may have a diagnosis of EIA. Weiler et al[12] conducted a questionnaire of athletes competing for the United States in the 1996 summer

TABLE 40-3 Assessment for Exercise-Induced Asthma

History
Baseline spirometry
Exercise challenge

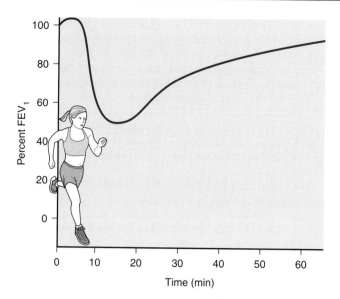

FIGURE 40-1 Change in forced expiratory volume in 1 second *(FEV₁)* after a 6-minute exercise challenge in a child with persistent asthma.

Olympic games. Of the athletes responding to the survey, 15.3% answered "yes" to whether they had been told in the past that they had asthma or EIA.[12] When both history of asthma and previous use of asthma medications were combined, the rate increased to 16.7%. This was a 50% increase from the 1984 games, although the criteria were somewhat different in the earlier survey. The prevalence of EIA appeared to be higher with exercise at extremely high activity levels and in cold environments.[13] In this study 10.4% of the athletes had need for medications at the time of the 1996 Olympic games. More females (19.9%) than males (14.3%) had a positive history of asthma or need for asthma medications. This is higher than the approximately 10% lifetime prevalence of asthma for the U.S. population recently reported.[14]

Hammerman et al[15] reported on an assessment of high school athletes for asthma. They investigated 801 student athletes with a questionnaire, measurement of PEFR, and finally a free run challenge (a 15% drop in PEFR after an 8-minute run). Of the athletes responding to the questionnaire, 5.7% stated that they had asthma or EIA. All of these students had a positive exercise challenge. Of the known asthmatics, 85% had a positive exercise challenge despite using their prescribed medications. An additional 6.1% of these athletes had a positive exercise challenge and were identified as having undiagnosed asthma. Of these students who did not consider themselves as having asthma, 55% were identified by the questionnaire as having EIA. The prevalence of EIA was 16% of females and 9% of males.

Rupp et al[16] demonstrated that baseline spirometry and questionnaire had significant false-positive and -negative rates when used as a screening tool for EIA in a group of 166 high school athletes. Exercise challenge was then used as the definitive test. Forty-eight students were considered at risk for EIA by history and screening spirometry. Twenty-two of the entire group of students had positive exercise challenges, for a rate of 13%. Of these students, 14, or 64%, were not identified by the screening tools, suggesting the potential need for testing all athletes. There are several explanations for the high rate of

inaccuracy of screening. First, high school athletes are more likely to have higher than normal baseline lung function, false-negative results for the presence of EIA. There also is the possibility that there is a denial factor in the response to the questionnaire, also leading to false-negative results.

A British Columbia study used a "free running asthma screening test" and a questionnaire to assess EIA. This study screened 830 teenage volunteers.[17] Unlike the previous study, these were not restricted to just the athletes in the high school. Of the students, 13.2% were identified by the exercise test with a 15% fall in PEFR after 6 minutes of activity that doubled their resting heart rate. The questionnaire failed to identify 34% of the students with EIA-positive tests even though they participated in a 15-minute workshop on asthma before filling out the survey. Performed in populations with diverse ethnic backgrounds, these two studies demonstrate the lack of specificity of questionnaires.

A large study was undertaken in Barcelona to look at the prevalence of asthma by history and to correlate bronchial responsiveness to exercise in 3000 school-age children aged 13 to 14 years. As in the previous studies, approximately 11% of children were noted to have positive exercise tests. In contrast, only 4% were noted to have "current asthma" as defined by positive responses to the International Study of Asthma and Allergies in Childood questionnaire and a history of bronchial responsiveness.[18] Present wheezing and treatment for respiratory symptoms in the past 12 months were the most predictive for positive exercise challenges. This discordance between positive challenge and the presence of active asthma symptoms raises further questions of testing.

DIFFERENTIAL DIAGNOSIS

For the child who volunteers the history of EIA (wheeze, cough, dyspnea with activity), it is important to document the type of exercise, the duration of the activity, and the limitations placed by the associated respiratory difficulty. Response to various treatments is also important. More difficult to diagnosis is the child with a sedentary lifestyle or the child with a preference for sedentary activities. Is this preference or a response to the inability to breathe comfortably with exertion? Frequently the child's response to a question regarding activity level is that he or she is not in "good shape." In addition, there are a group of children with EIA who have a significant fall in FEV₁ without symptoms. On the other side of the issue is the highly skilled nonasthmatic athlete who experiences more rapid breathing with exertion that may be the normal physiologic response to activity and whose child, family, or physician is concerned that the diagnosis may be asthma.

The previous studies of the prevalence of EIA in high school students indicate that approximately 11% to 13% of adolescents with symptoms of cough and dyspnea associated with exercise have this diagnosis. Empiric therapy usually starts with a trial of a short-acting inhaled beta-agonist. When that therapy succeeds, one has presumptive confirmation of the diagnosis. When the treatment fails, one needs to consider other diagnoses. Exercise-induced hyperventilation needs to be included in the differential. Hammo and Weinberger[19] report a study of 32 children with uncertain diagnosis of EIA who had an exercise challenge consisting of treadmill running and monitoring of O_2 saturation and end-tidal CO_2. Four of the children had a classic asthma response to the challenge, and 17 had no significant change in any of the three study parameters. Of interest were the 11 children who experienced chest tightness with no significant fall in the FEV_1 or change in the O_2 saturation. These children had the largest fall: 23.2% in end-tidal CO_2. As a group they appeared to be highly competitive athletically and usually complained of dyspnea during times of peak performance.

Vocal cord dysfunction (VCD) needs to be included in the differential of children with atypical EIA. EIA and VCD may occur concurrently. Patients with VCD may appear to be refractory to normal treatment for EIA. VCD differs from EIA in that the symptoms appear and resolve abruptly. VCD is associated with inspiratory wheeze and is more likely to occur during the day. In a report by Landwehr et al,[20] the majority of the children studied had concurrent psychologic difficulties. Abnormal movement of the arytenoid region during exercise has also been identified as a cause of exertional dyspnea associated with exercise. In this case it was associated with bronchial hyperreactivity and was responsive to speech therapy.[21] In the differential one needs to exclude fixed central airway obstruction and muscle disorders. EIA is distinguished from these illnesses by its more classic concave pattern of obstructive airways disease noted on the flow-volume curve. Finally, cardiac disease and other restrictive and obstructive respiratory disorders need to be considered (Table 40-4).

What is the gold standard for the diagnosis of EIA? This is the child with a positive history of EIA that is confirmed by an exercise challenge with a fall of 15%. Does the child with a 15% fall in FEV_1 without symptoms have EIA? What if this change in lung function is noted in a child with seasonal allergic rhinitis? Is this underappreciated disease in a child with persistent asthma, or just evidence of increased BHR that deserves no active treatment? There is no definitive answer, although one might propose a therapeutic trial with either pretreatment with a short-acting beta-agonist or use of inhaled corticosteroids as controller therapy, as discussed later. Methacholine hyperreactivity is present in most patients with a positive exercise test, but BHR is also found in the absence of EIA. Of interest is the fact that treatment of EIA produces protection against the symptoms of exercise before there is improvement in exercise challenge, and this occurs before protection against nonspecific BHR.[22] Although there is a strong association of these two challenges, nonspecific bronchial hyperreactivity may lead to a high rate of false-positive values if it is used as a surrogate marker of EIA.

MECHANISM OF DISEASE

There are presently two main theories to explain the pathophysiology of EIA. The "thermal hypothesis"[11] states that the transfer of heat from the airway mucosa to the airways and back to the mucosa during hyperpnea is the primary feature of the disease. In this theory, hyperventilation and exercise that ensures control of ambient temperature and humidity demonstrate the same degree of airway obstruction. The "osmotic theory"[23] stresses that the exercising person has evaporation from the airway surface that leads to an osmotic gradient resulting in cell volume loss. This process then leads to bronchial smooth muscle contraction. Whether heat loss or water loss is the primary etiology of EIA, it is clear that breathing cold, dry air produces airway narrowing in the asthmatic patient.

The importance of inflammatory mediators in the pathophysiology of EIA has been controversial. Hallstrand et al[24] exercise-challenged a group of 13 mild atopic asthmatics. Venous blood samples after exercise showed an increase in T helper cell type 2 lymphocyte activation with increased numbers of CD23+ B cells and CD25+ T cells. This study proposes an inflammatory mechanism for EIA. The variable attenuation of EIA by both a leukotriene receptor antagonist (LTRA) and histamine suggests a partial, varying, or incomplete involvement of these mediators in the pathophysiology of EIA. Prostaglandins have also been demonstrated to have a significant role in EIA.[25] In the osmotic hypothesis, it is suggested that the osmotic gradient caused by the water loss induces cells to release mediators that are implicated in the inflammatory process.

EIA occurs most commonly in the presence of persistent asthma. Airway inflammation is a universal characteristic of persistent asthma whether the disease is active or asymptomatic. In addition, individuals demonstrating increased bronchial hyperreactivity to exercise and challenge (methacholine or histamine) have evidence of active airway inflammation. Patients with EIA have significantly higher levels of eosinophils and eosinophilic cationic protein in their sputum than asthmatics without EIA and with normal subjects. Furthermore, the severity of the EIA correlates with the percent of sputum eosinophils.[26]

TREATMENT

The vast majority of pediatric patients with EIA have underlying persistent asthma, with exercise as one of many triggers of their disease. One can possibly make the argument that EIA does not occur in the absence of persistent asthma. The initial component of treatment is controller therapy for persistent asthma as recommended by both National Heart, Lung, and Blood Institute and GINA guidelines. The recognition of the importance of inflammation in the pathophysiology of asthma has led to the early introduction of inhaled corticosteroids as the most effective controller therapy for persistent asthma and therefore needs to be considered as the primary treatment for EIA in the presence of persistent asthma. The list of potential controller medications that may be beneficial in treating the underlying asthma includes inhaled corticosteroids, cromolyn, nedocromil, theophylline, salmeterol, and LTRAs. The short-acting beta-agonists cromolyn and ipratropium have also been studied as bronchoprotective pretreatments for EIA. Unfortunately, there are very few comparative trials of these different agents (Figure 40-2).

In an attempt to present the evidence from the literature in a uniform fashion, the baseline maximum fall in FEV_1 and the percent protection reported are the variables presented in this

---

TABLE 40-4 Differential for Exercise-Induced Asthma

Exercise-induced hyperventilation
Vocal cord dysfunction
Central airway obstruction
Cardiac disease
Other restrictive or obstructive pulmonary disease
Muscle disorders

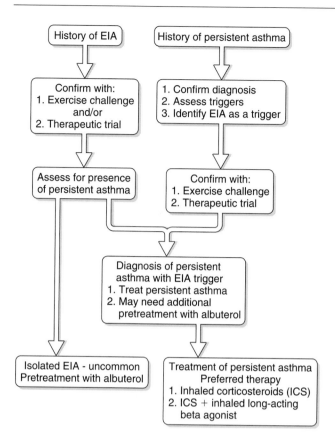

FIGURE 40-2 Clinical algorithm for exercise-induced asthma *(EIA)*.

TABLE 40-5 Treatment Options for Exercise-Induced Asthma

Aerobic conditioning
Warm-up exercise
Treatment of persistent asthma
Pretreatment with or without persistent medications

review. Area under the curve FEV_1 is reported in some studies, but because the traditional variable is percent maximal fall or percent protection of FEV_1, these will be the standard data presented. The studies vary by challenge, the testing environment, and baseline characteristics of the study subjects. Some investigators have used protection against a 15% fall in FEV_1 as the standard for efficacy of a therapeutic agent. Other authors have reported the percent change. The heterogeneity of the baseline fall in lung function makes it difficult to compare studies. The baseline severity differs with baseline falls in FEV_1 of 15% to 20% in some studies and others have greater than 30%. Another variable reported in some recent studies has been the time to recovery from EIA.

EIA can be attenuated with physical conditioning alone or in the presence of active pharmacologic therapy. Aerobic conditioning has been demonstrated to improve aerobic fitness, reduce the dyspnea associated with exertion, and improve the ventilatory capacity in patients with EIA.[27] Patients with EIA appear to have less difficulty if they perform warm-up exercise before exertion. Endogenous production of prostaglandin-2 may relax airway smooth muscle during this initial phase of activity[28] (Table 40-5).

The first step in the pharmacologic treatment of EIA is to gain control of the underlying airway inflammation in the child with persistent asthma. As mentioned in the beginning of this chapter, EIA occurs most often in children with persistent asthma for whom controller therapy is appropriate. Table 40-6 lists the studies in children of controller therapy and their impact on EIA. Inhaled corticosteroids are the most effective controller treatment for persistent asthma. This class of medication is associated with the greatest decrease in airway

inflammation and the largest improvement in BHR, a surrogate marker for inflammation. Several decades ago studies were done with inhaled corticosteroids to determine whether single doses of these medications used immediately before exercise had an effect in protecting against EIA. The results were uniformly negative. The following studies were done with chronic treatment. In a 4-week trial, Henriksen and Dahl[29] studied the effect of inhaled budesonide 200 μg twice daily and terbutaline alone and in combination in a group of children. The inhaled corticosteroid produced a significant, pre-exercise improvement in FEV_1 (19%) after 1 week of therapy. Terbutaline, budesonide, and the combination of the two therapies reduced the fall in FEV_1 by 30%, 51%, and 84%. The combination was thought to be additive and not synergistic. In addition, the authors found that the protection afforded by inhaled corticosteroids was related to their effect on BHR and not simply the improvement in lung function.

Another study investigated whether there was a dose-response protective effect of 100, 200, and 400 μg/day of budesonide against exercise challenge. Children with moderate to severe asthma who were naïve to inhaled corticosteroids were studied and received increasing doses of budesonide every 4 weeks. There was a dose-dependent increase in FEV_1 between the three doses of budesonide, but the diary recordings of day and night PEFR, day symptoms, and night symptoms improved after the use of budesonide for 4 weeks but did not differ among the three doses. In contrast, there was a dose-dependent protection against EIA. The maximum protection against the fall in FEV_1 after exercise for 100, 200, and 400 μg/day of budesonide was 54%, 64%, and 82%, respectively.[30] As in the previous study, greater improvement in FEV_1 appeared to be associated with greater bronchoprotection.

Jónasson et al[31] studied a group of children with mild asthma and EIA. Their baseline FEV_1 was 100% of predicted. The children were placed on one of three doses of budesonide 100 or 200 μg once daily, 100 μg twice daily, or placebo. Budesonide improved both daily symptoms and protected against EIA. The protection with the three doses was similar and ranged from 58% to 74%.

Hofstra et al[22] addressed the issue of whether the effect of inhaled corticosteroids on EIA was dose dependent or varied by the duration of the treatment. In this study, children were treated with either fluticasone propionate (FP) at doses of 100 or 250 μg twice daily or placebo for 6 months. The fall in FEV_1 after exercise was reduced by 71% to 79% and did not differ significantly with the dose or from week 3 to week 24. In contrast, the PD_{20} methacholine increased significantly over time during the 6 months ($P = 0.04$) of the trial. The higher doses of inhaled corticosteroids correlated with greater protection ($P = 0.06$) that approached statistical significance. The implication of this greater protection against methacholine noted with the higher dose of inhaled corticosteroid in the absence

TABLE 40-6 Pediatric Trials for the Treatment of Exercise-Induced Asthma

Reference	Treatment	N	Maximum Fall in FEV_1 (%)	Protection (%)
Kemp et al[33] (CO)	Placebo	25	26	
	Montelukast	25	18	31
Pearlman et al[35] (CO)	Placebo	39	16.7	
	Zafirlukast 5 mg	20	8.9	47
	Zafirlukast 10 mg	19	11.1	34
	Zafirlukast 20 mg	20	8.5	49
	Zafirlukast 40 mg	19	10.2	6.5
Hofstra et al[22] (PG)	Placebo	12	27.1	
	Fluticasone 100 μg	11	9.9	63
	Fluticasone 250 μg	14	7.6	72
Jónasson et al[31] (PG)	Placebo	14	16	21
	Budesonide 100 μg	14	7	73
	Budesonide 200 μg	14	7.5	70
	Budesonide 100 μg twice daily	15	7	56
Pederson and Hansen[30] (CO)	Budesonide 100 μg	19	25.7	54
	Budesonide 200 μg	19	20.1	64
	Budesonide 400 μg	19	9.9	83
Vidal et al[39] (CO)	Baseline	20	24	
	Budesonide 400 μg twice daily	20	6	75
	Montelukast 10 mg	20	12	50
Simons et al[46] (CO)	Budesonide (AM)	14	16	
	Salmeterol (AM)	14	4	75
	Budesonide (PM)	14	10	
	Salmeterol (PM)	14	15	33

FEV_1, Forced expiratory volume in 1 second; *CO*, crossover study; *PG*, parallel group.

of greater clinical effect on bronchoprotection is difficult to explain. Sont et al[32] also demonstrated a dose-response effect to inhaled corticosteroids when the dose is varied to reflect BHR. In that report there was greater protection against mild asthma exacerbations as BHR improved. Interesting in the study by Hofstra et al[22] is that there is no greater improvement in exercise challenge to correlate with the greater improvement in BHR.

Two pediatric studies looked at the effect of LTRA on EIA. The first study by Kemp et al[33] evaluated 27 children with EIA treated with montelukast 5 mg for 2 days in a crossover fashion. The challenges were then performed at 20 to 24 hours postdose. The percent maximum fall in FEV_1 was 26% for placebo and 18% for montelukast. There was a 31% inhibition of EIA with the active medication. The recovery time after the fall in lung function post-EIA was also reduced 38% for the montelukast-treated patients. These results are comparable to a 12-week study in adults by Leff et al.[34] At the challenge at 12 weeks, the patients had a 31.6% inhibition of EIA and a recovery time that was reduced by 27%.

In another study, Pearlman et al[35] assessed the effects of zafirlukast. The study subjects were controller naive. There were two groups of patients, with each completing a three-way crossover. Group 1 was treated with 5 mg and 20 mg of zafirlukast and placebo. Group 2 was given 10 and 40 mg of zafirlukast, and there was a placebo arm. Study medications were given 4 hours before exercise challenge. Baseline FEV_1 was 88% to 91% of predicted. Maximum fall in FEV_1 with placebo was 16.3% to 17.1%, and with 5, 10, 20, and 40 mg of zafirlukast was 8.9%, 11.1%, 8.7%, and 10.2%, respectively.[35] The protection afforded by zafirlukast did not appear to be

dose related. Overall, there was a 42% protective effect with this LTRA.

Two studies from the adult literature have compared 8-week treatment of EIA with either montelukast or salmeterol as controller therapy. In the article by Edelman et al,[36] patients were not allowed to use inhaled corticosteroids, and in the study by Villaran et al,[37] only 6% and 14% of patients were on inhaled steroids in addition to salmeterol and montelukast, respectively. These studies performed exercise challenge only at the approximate end of the dosing period, 9 and 21 hours for salmeterol and montelukast, respectively. In both studies, the percent protection was greater for montelukast. In the Edelman et al study,[36] montelukast did not appear to prevent a mean 15% fall in FEV_1 with exercise. As noted by Nelson et al,[38] the bronchoprotective effect in EIA of salmeterol decreases between 9 and 12 hours posttherapy. But more important, the GINA and National Heart, Lung, and Blood Institute guidelines do not recommend the use of salmeterol as monotherapy for asthma. Salmeterol for asthma is recommended as add-on therapy only.

There is one study reported in the literature that compares the use of inhaled corticosteroids and an LTRA in the treatment of EIA. In this crossover study of 20 asthmatics with a median age of 17 years, patients are treated with either budesonide 400 μg twice daily or montelukast 10 mg daily. The baseline FEV_1 was 100% to 101% for both groups with no change in baseline spirometry from either therapy before the exercise challenge. Both medications provided protection against EIA. Budesonide was more effective in 80% of the patients, with a mean protection in EIA of 75% versus 50% for montelukast.[39] Although budesonide was more effective in a greater number of patients, both treatments had significant heterogeneity in their bronchoprotection, from 0% to 100%.

The role of dual controler therapy in protecting against pediatric EIA is not supported or negated by the evidence from the literature. Although adult studies have demonstrated greater improvement in lung function and symptom control with the addition of a long-acting bronchodilator to an inhaled corticosteroid than with an LTRA, these studies have not been replicated in children and adolescents.[38,40]

The use of salmeterol in children as a bronchoprotective medication demonstrates its effectiveness over time 12 hours compared with placebo and albuterol. Blake et al[41] studied the use of albuterol, two doses of salmeterol (25 μg and 50 μg), and placebo in a four-way crossover study. In this study, albuterol and salmeterol prevented a fall in FEV_1 from the predose lung function after a standard treadmill exercise. At 6 and 12 hours, salmeterol, but neither albuterol nor placebo, protected significantly against the fall in FEV_1 after challenge. Bronsky et al[42] used a dose of 50 μg of salmeterol to replicate the results of this study. Their report demonstrated that salmeterol at 6 and 12 hours increased baseline lung function before challenge and minimized the fall in FEV_1.

The literature does raise some cautions concerning the chronic use of salmeterol. With single dosing of this medication, it appears that the duration of protection of salmeterol extends to 12 hours. With chronic use, it appears that the duration of effect is 9 hours. In a study of 20 adults, Nelson et al[43] demonstrated that the evening protection against EIA for patients treated with salmeterol decreased from day 1 to 14 with no further decrease over time. This effect was not noted in the morning bronchoprotection but only after 9 hours after dosing. Salmeterol did offer increased lung function throughout the 4-week study, and the FEV_1 postchallenge was similar to the preexercise FEV_1 of the placebo-treated patients. Although protection against EIA may be reduced between 9 and 12 hours, there is continued protection against methacholine-induced bronchoconstriction of one doubling dose out to 24 weeks. These challenges were conducted 10 to 14 hours postdose.[44] In children, the overall response to the bronchodilator effect of salmeterol persisted over a 12-week study.[45] It is important to remember, however, that salmeterol is recommended as controller therapy only in patients with persistent asthma who are taking concurrent inhaled corticosteroids.

The study by Simons et al[46] demonstrated a statistically significant bronchoprotective effect after 4 weeks of treatment with salmeterol at 1 but not 9 hours. In this study of 14 children on inhaled beclomethasone, 100 to 200 μg twice daily, with baseline FEV_1 of 98% to 106%, the fall in FEV_1 at 9 hours was 9% with salmeterol and 15% with placebo. The patients on inhaled corticosteroids alone have demonstrated some degree of protection against EIA, and the limited effect of salmeterol may be due to the small fall in lung function with exercise challenge in the placebo-treated patients. The difference between salmeterol and placebo was not statistically different but, by definition, salmeterol prevented a 15% fall in FEV_1. Two children on placebo exited the study because of worsening asthma.

A recent study investigated patients with persistent asthma and EIA with incomplete control of their EIA on FP 250 μg twice daily or the equivalent. These patients still had a greater than 20% decline in FEV_1 with exercise despite using inhaled corticosteroids. Patients were randomized for 4 weeks to either FP 250 μg or FP 250 μg and salmeterol 50 μg combination (FSC) twice daily. They were exercise challenged on day 1 and at week 4 and at 1 and 8.5 hours postmedication dosing. The study revealed that at all time points the combination FSC produced greater protection and no loss of bronchoprotection over the 4-week trial ($P < 0.016$).[47] At the 8.5-hour challenge on week 4, the FP monotherapy patients had an approximately 20% and the FSC patients had a 12% decline in FEV_1 with exercise challenge. These data are consistent with the data from the Simons et al study,[46] but with the larger sample of nearly 100 patients in each cohort, a clinical and statistically different 40% greater protection is shown.

The use of antihistamines has been proposed as a potential treatment for EIA, although they have limited use in the treatment of persistent asthma. Badier et al[48] investigated the effect of terfenadine 120 mg twice daily (2 times the recommended dose) and demonstrated an attenuation of hyperventilation-induced bronchospasm. Baki and Orhan[49] treated 11 children with 10 mg of loratadine and demonstrated a 42% reduction in EIA with the medication at 5 minutes postchallenge. The authors caution that loratadine failed to prevent a 15% fall in FEV_1, the accepted standard used to define protection against EIA. Dahlén et al[50] presented data on the use of zafirlukast 80 mg twice daily (4 times the recommended dosage), loratadine 10 mg twice daily (2 times the recommended dosage), the combination of the two medications, and placebo in a four-way crossover trial. Subjects used these medications for 7 days before the exercise challenge. Their mean FEV_1 at baseline was 90% predicted with a mean fall of 25.7% postexercise. Patients on placebo had a mean fall in FEV_1 with exercise of 21.6%; loratadine, 22.8%; zafirlukast, 13.9%; and the combination of the two active therapies, 10.3%. In this trial, there was no benefit from loratadine in preventing EIA either alone or in addition to zafirlukast. In general, the data with antihistamines remain inconclusive and do not support their role in the treatment of EIA.

The use of medications immediately before exertion has been the classic strategy for the treatment of EIA. It can be used in the presence of controller therapy as demonstrated in the trial by Henriksen and Dahl or as an isolated treatment for patients with just EIA. Further research is needed to establish the prevalence or existence of isolated EIA. For pretreatment of EIA, inhaled beta-agonists are the most effective therapy. Two inhalations of a short-acting inhaled corticosteroid 15 minutes before exercise provides most subjects with significant improvement for 1 to 2 hours. Long-acting bronchodilators such as salmeterol and formoterol may provide 8 to 10 hours of protection if used intermittently to protect against EIA. Neither of these medications should be used as a single controller therapy. Cromolyn and nedocromil have also been used as bronchoprotective therapy with less efficacy than albuterol. The benefit from oral bronchodilators and inhaled anticholinergics is limited.[11]

Two nonpharmacologic therapies have been suggested for EIA. One is to start a program of physical training. First, there are multiple physical and social reasons to have people exercise regularly. This can be initially achieved with the use of traditional asthma medications. The effect of physical training on blunting EIA has shown variable results. Warm-up exercise can attenuate EIA in some cases, but the effect has only a 30- to 40-minute duration of action. Second, there have been attempts to design devices that warm and humidify the air to

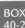

BOX 40-2

THERAPEUTIC PRINCIPLES

Appropriate diagnosis

   Recognize exercise-induced asthma (EIA) as a component of most persistent asthma.

   Assess for persistent asthma if history of isolated EIA.

   Rule out other causes of exertional dyspnea.

Ensure normal or near-normal physical activity level.

Treat persistent asthma with "stepwise approach."[51]

   Inhaled corticosteroids (low dose)

   ICS (low dose) + inhaled long-acting β_2 agonists

Pretreatment if needed with inhaled short-acting β_2 agonists

alveolar conditions. These have shown some benefit but are generally not acceptable to the athletes.

CONCLUSIONS

EIA occurs in 10% to 14% of children. It is the most common trigger of persistent childhood asthma. The history for EIA can be complicated by the lack of perception of significant airway obstruction during exercise. One must carefully identify those children with EIA from the group of children who report low level of activity because of lack of interest or because they are "out of shape." Baseline spirometry of children with persistent asthma is frequently normal. Spirometry, however, is important to identify those children with EIA who under-recognize their disease but should not be used as evidence of absence of disease if normal. Formal exercise testing should be considered when the diagnosis is unclear or if there appears to be a lack of bronchoprotection with inhaled albuterol.

The goal of treatment of EIA should be the attainment of normal activity level for children and adolescents. Identification of the limits imposed by EIA and establishment of goals of therapy with the child and family should be the initial action. Inactivity in the presence of this diagnosis should not be accepted. Therapy for EIA starts with control of the underlying persistent asthma (Box 40-2). Inhaled corticosteroids are the most effective initial treatment of both EIA and persistent asthma in children and adolescents. The addition of long-acting bronchodilators appears to afford further protection when used as a dual controller therapy. These are the preferred treatments for mild to moderate persistent asthma as stated in the National Asthma Education and Prevention Program 2002 update for children.[51] The roles of LTRA and cromones appear as less effective treatment options for primary controller therapy. There are no studies at present on the use of LTRA and inhaled corticosteroids. EIA is a common aspect of a prevalent disease that warrants proper diagnosis and treatment.

REFERENCES

1. Global Initiative for Asthma: *Global strategy for asthma management*, Washington, DC, February 2002, U.S. Department of Health and Human Services. NIH Pub No. 02-3659.
2. Anderson SD, Holzer K: Exercise-induced asthma: is it the right diagnosis in the elite athlete? *J Allergy Clin Immunol* 106:419-428, 2000.
3. Van Den Toorn LM, Overbeck SE, De Jongste JC, et al: Airway inflammation is present during clinical remission of atopic asthma, *Am J Respir Crit Care Med* 164:2107-2113, 2001.
4. Nystad W, Stigum H, Carlsen KH: Increase level of bronchial responsiveness in inactive children with asthma, *Respir Med* 95:806-810, 2001.
5. Godfrey S, Silverman M, Anderson SD: Problems of interpreting exercise-induced asthma, *J Allergy Clin Immunol* 52:199-209, 1973.
6. McFadden ER, Gilbert IA: Exercise-induced asthma. *N Engl J Med* 330:1362-1367, 1994.
7. Godfrey S: Exercise-induced asthma–clinical, physiological, and therapeutic implications, *J Allergy Clin Immunol* 56:1-17, 1975.
8. Childhood Asthma Management Program Research Group: Long-term effects of budesonide or nedocromil in children with asthma, *N Engl J Med* 343:1054-1063, 2000.
9. Godfrey S: Exercise-induced asthma–clinical, physiological and therapeutic implications, *J Allergy Clin Immunol* 56:1-17, 1975.
10. Spector SL, Nicklas RA, eds: Exercise-induced asthma in practice parameters for the diagnosis and treatment of asthma, *J Allergy Clin Immunol* 96:831-835, 1995.
11. McFadden ER: Exercise-induced airway narrowing. In Middleton E, Reed CE, Ellis EF, et al, eds: *Allergy: principles and practice*, ed 5, St Louis, 1998, Mosby.
12. Weiler JM, Layton T, Hunt M: Asthma in the United States Olympic athletes who participated in the 1996 Summer games, *J Allergy Clin Immunol* 102:722-726, 1998.
13. Becker A: Controversies and challenges of exercise-induced bronchoconstriction and their implications for children, *Pediatr Pulmonol* 21S: S38-S45, 2001.
14. Mannino DM, Homa DM, Akinbami LJ, et al: Surveillance for asthma–United States, 1980-1999, *MMWR* 5:1-14, 2002.
15. Hammerman SI, Becker JM, Rogers J, et al: Asthma screening for high school athletes: identifying the undiagnosed and poorly controlled, *Ann Allergy Asthma Immunol* 88:380-384, 2002.
16. Rupp NT, Brudno S, Guill MF: The value of screening for risk of exercise-induced asthma in high school athletes, *Ann Allergy* 70:339-342, 1993.
17. Vacek L: Incidence of exercise-induced asthma in high school population in British Columbia, *Allergy Asthma Proc* 18:89-91, 1997.
18. Busquets RM, Antó JM, Sunyer J, et al: Prevalence of asthma-related symptoms and bronchial responsiveness to exercise in children aged 13-14 yrs in Barcelona, Spain, *Eur Respir J* 9.2094-2098, 1996.
19. Hammo AH, Weinberger MW: Exercise-induced hyperventilation: a pseudoasthma syndrome, *Ann Allergy Asthma Immunol* 82:574-578, 1999.
20. Landwehr LP, Wood RP II, Blager FB, et al: Vocal cord dysfunction mimicking exercise-induced bronchospasm in adolescents, *Pediatrics* 98: 971-974, 1996.
21. Bittleman DB, Smith RJH, Weiler JM: Abnormal movement of the arytenoid region during exercise presenting as exercise-induced asthma in an adolescent athlete, *Chest* 106:615-616, 1994.
22. Hofstra WB, Neijems HJ, Duiverman EJ, et al: Dose-responses over time to inhaled fluticasone propionate treatment of exercise- and methacholine-induced bronchoconstriction in children, *Pediatr Pulmonol* 29:415-423, 2000.
23. Anderson SA, Daviskas E: The mechanism of exercise-induced asthma is. . . , *J Allergy Clin Immunol* 106:453-459, 2000.
24. Hallstrand TS, Ault KA, Bates PW, et al: Peripheral blood manifestations of T(H)2 lymphocyte activation in stable atopic asthma and during exercise-induced bronchospasm, *Ann Allergy Asthma Immunol* 80:424-432, 1998.
25. Anderson SA, Brannan JD: Exercise-induced asthma: is there still a case for histamine, *J Allergy Clin Immunol* 109:771-773, 2002.
26. Yoshikawa T, Shoji S, Fujii T, et al: Severity of exercise-induced bronchoconstriction is related to airway eosinophilic inflammation in patients with asthma, *Eur Respir J* 12:879-884, 1998.
27. Hallstrand TS, Bates PW, Schoene RB: Aerobic conditioning in mild asthma decreases the hyperpnea of exercise and impoves exercise and ventilatory capacity, *Chest* 118:1460-1469, 2000.
28. Becker A: Controversies and challenges of exercise-induced bronchoconstriction and their implications for children, *Pediatr Pulmonol* 21:38-45, 2001.
29. Henriksen JM, Dahl R: Effects of inhaled budesonide alone and in combination with low-dose terbutaline in children with asthma, *Am Rev Respir Dis* 128.993-997, 1983.
30. Pederson S, Hansen OR: Budesonide treatment of moderate and severe asthma in children: a dose response effect, *J Allergy Clin Immunol* 95: 29-33, 1995.

31. Jónasson G, Carlsen K-H, Hultquist C: Low-dose budesonide improves exercise-induced bronchospasm in schoolchildren, *Pediatr Allergy Immunol* 11:120-125, 2000.

32. Sont JK, Willems LNA, Bel EH, et al: Clinical control and histopathological outcome of asthma when using airway hyperresponsiveness as an additional guide to long-term treatment, *Am J Respir Crit Care Med* 159:1043-1051, 1999.

33. Kemp JP, Dockhorn RJ, Shapiro GG, et al: Montelukast once daily inhibits exercise-induced bronchoconstriction in 6- to 14-year-old children with asthma, *J Pediatr* 133:424-428, 1998.

34. Leff JA, Busse WW, Perlman D, et al: Montelukast, a leukotriene-receptor antagonist, for the treatment of mild asthma and exercise-induced asthma, *N Engl J Med* 339:147-152, 1998.

35. Pearlman DS, Ostrom NK, Bronsky EA, et al: The leukotriene D$_4$-receptor antagonist zafirlukast attenuates exercise-induced bronchoconstriction in children, *J Pediatr* 134:273-279, 1999.

36. Edelman JM, Turpin JA, Bronsky EA, et al: Oral montelukast compared with inhaled salmeterol to prevent exercise-induced bronchoconstriction, *Ann Intern Med* 132:97-104, 2000.

37. Villaren C, O'Neill SJ, Helbling A, et al: Montelukast versus salmeterol in patient with asthma and exercise-induced bronchoconstriction, *J Allergy Clin Immunol* 104:547-553, 1999.

38. Nelson HS, Busse WW, Kerwin E, et al: Fluticasone propionate/salmeterol combination provides more effective asthma control that low-dose inhaled corticosteroid plus montelukast, *J Allergy Clin Immunol* 106:1088-1095, 2000.

39. Vidal C, Fernández-Ovide E, Piñeiro J, et al: Comparison of montelukast versus budesonide in the treatment of exercise-induced bronchoconstriction, *Ann Allergy Asthma Immunol* 86:655-658, 2001.

40. Fish JE, Murray JJ, Boone EA, et al: Salmeterol powder provides significantly better benefit than montelukast in asthmatic patients receiving concomitant inhaled corticosteroid therapy, *Chest* 120:423-430, 2001.

41. Blake K, Perlman DS, Scott C, et al: Prevention of exercise-induced bronchospasm in pediatric asthma patients: a comparison of salmeterol powder with albuterol, *Ann Allergy Asthma Immnol* 82:205-211, 1999.

42. Bronsky EA, Perlman DS, Pobiner BF, et al: Prevention of exercise-induced bronchospasm in pediatric asthma patients: a comparison of two salmeterol powder delivery devices, *Pediatrics* 104:501-506, 1999.

43. Nelson JA, Strauss L, Sakowronski M, et al: Effect of long-term salmeterol treatment on exercise-induced asthma, *N Engl J Med* 339:141-146, 1998.

44. Rosenthal RR, Busse WW, Kemp JP, et al: Effect of long-term salmeterol therapy with as-needed albuterol use on airway hyperresponsiveness, *Chest* 116:595-602, 1999.

45. Weinsterin SF, Pearlman DS, Bronsky EA, et al: Efficacy of salmeterol xinafoate powder in children with chronic persistent asthma, *Ann Allergy Asthma Immunol* 81:51-58, 1998.

46. Simons FER, Gerstner TV, Cheang MS: Tolerance to the bronchoprotective effect of salmeterol in adolescents with exercise-induced asthma using concurrent inhaled glucocorticoid treatment, *Pediatrics* 99:655-659, 1997.

47. Dorinsky P, Kalberg C, Jones S, et al: Sustained protection against activity induced bronchospasm (AIB) during chronic treatment with the fluticasone propionate/salmeterol combination (FSC), *Am J Respir Crit Care Med* 165:A568, 2002.

48. Badier M, Beaumont D, Orehek J: Attenuation of hyperventilation-induced bronchospasm by terfenadine: a new antihistamine, *J Allergy Clin Immunol* 81:437-440, 1988.

49. Baki A, Orhan F: The effect of loratadine in exercise-induced asthma, *Arch Dis Child* 86:38-39, 2002.

50. Dahlén B, Roquet A, Inman MD: Influence of zafirlukast and loratadine on exercise-induced bronchospasm, *J Allergy Clin Immunol* 109:789-793, 2002.

51. Executive summary of the Expert Panel report: *Guidelines for the diagnosis and management of Asthma: update on selected topics 2002,* Bethesda, Md, June 2002, NAEPP, NIH Pub No. 02-5075.

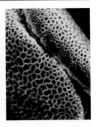

CHAPTER **41**

Refractory Childhood Asthma: New Insight into the Pathogenesis, Diagnosis, and Management

JOSEPH D. SPAHN ■ DONNA L. BRATTON

Asthma is a chronic respiratory disease characterized by reversible airflow limitation and airway hyperresponsiveness to a variety of stimuli. Our understanding of the pathogenesis of asthma has evolved from that of a purely bronchospastic disease to one in which airway inflammation plays a central role.[1,2] Glucocorticoids (GC) have broad antiinflammatory effects, and as such have become first-line agents for both the acute (systemic) and chronic (inhaled) manifestations of this disease.[3-5] Although the majority of patients with asthma have mild to moderate disease, approximately 5% to 10% have severe disease that is often recalcitrant to the available treatment modalities.[6] Severe or "refractory" asthma, although uncommon, accounts for a significant proportion of the health care costs of asthma.[7,8] In addition, those with refractory asthma are most likely to have the greatest morbidity, not only from their disease but also from the medications used to treat the disease. At the extreme end of refractory asthma is a group of asthma patients who no longer respond favorably to GC therapy. These patients have been termed *GC insensitive* or *GC resistant*.

This chapter addresses the complexity and heterogeneity of refractory asthma. In addition, it highlights several new immunologic assays and pharmacotherapy that may help in understanding the pathogenesis of asthma and provide an advance in the management of refractory asthma.

DEFINITION

The child with refractory asthma displays evidence of ongoing disease activity despite receiving optimal pharmacologic therapy. First, one must distinguish between asthma severity and control. Asthma control and asthma severity, although related, are often confused with each other (Table 41-1). Severity appears to be reflective of the natural history of the disease and is less likely to vary over the long term, whereas control is reflective of disease activity based on levels of symptoms over a recent period of time. For example, one can have severe but well-controlled asthma. These subjects will often require high-dose inhaled GC therapy to maintain good control. In contrast, a patient with moderate asthma may have frequent daytime and nocturnal symptoms requiring frequently administered beta agonists. This subject has poorly controlled asthma and is likely to be inadequately treated with controller therapy. Once a controller agent is instituted, the patient's

asthma control improves significantly. In an attempt to differentiate control from severity, it has been suggested that the need for daily inhaled GC requirements be used as the measure of an individual's disease severity, whereas frequency of symptoms (day and night) be used as a measure of control.

A recent study sought to determine the relationships between disease severity and level of asthma control and frequency of emergency room (ER) visits and hospitalizations in a cohort of 1251 asthma patients from a database of 496 family practitioners.[9] Asthma control was ascertained by questionnaire in 1130 subjects with 42% reporting moderate or poor control based on frequency of symptoms. During the 12-month study period, 14.8% reported at least one ER visit or hospitalization with a significant correlation between asthma control and hospital contact noted ($P < 0.001$). The odds ratio for a hospital contact for an individual with good

---

TABLE 41-1 Measures of Asthma Severity Versus Asthma Control

Measures of asthma severity (long-term)
Need for and dose of inhaled glucocorticoid:
    Mild intermittent: no inhaled glucocorticoid
    Mild persistent: 100-400 µg/day budesonide or equivalent
    Moderate persistent: 400-800 µg/day budesonide or equivalent
    Severe persistent: > 800 µg/day budesonide or equivalent
Frequency, dose, duration, and magnitude of response to a short course of systemic glucocorticoid therapy to optimize asthma control
Need for, and number of, previous hospitalizations, emergency department visits, and unscheduled physician visits
History of life-threatening events
    Cyanosis
    Seizures
    Need for intubation/mechanical ventilation
    Intensive care unit admission

Measures of asthma control (short-term)
Frequency of daytime and nighttime symptoms
Exercise tolerance, with or without pretreatment with beta agonists
Need for and frequency of inhaled beta agonist use
Degree of diurnal variability in peak expiratory flow rate or forced expiratory volume in 1 second

control was 0.5 versus an odds ratio of 2.2 in patients with poor asthma control. Of importance, this association was seen independent of inhaled GC use and dose required (the surrogate marker of disease severity) before entry into the study. Patients with poor control were six times more likely to report a hospital contact than patients with good control and three times more likely than patients with moderate control.

Second, the National Heart, Lung, and Blood Institute (NHLBI) Guidelines on asthma severity[3] are based on symptoms and lung function in patients not already on controller therapy. Once a child is on controller therapy, levels of severity are no longer applicable. Third, the lung function values the NHLBI guidelines used to judge asthma severity (i.e., forced expiratory volume in 1 second [FEV_1] > 85% for mild persistent, between 60% and 85% for moderate, and < 60% of predicted for severe persistent asthma) are likely to underestimate disease severity based on symptoms. This point has recently been demonstrated by Bacharier et al,[10] who found children with asthma on controller therapy of all levels of asthma severity based on symptoms to have FEV_1 values that are higher (i.e., better) than the guidelines recommend when assessing severity. We recently reported similar findings in children referred to National Jewish Hospital.[11] The NHLBI recently convened a workshop on severe asthma.[6] They concluded that a refractory asthmatic should have at least three of the following clinical criteria: (1) history of referral to an asthma specialist; (2) receiving maximal usual asthma therapy, including high-dose inhaled and often even oral glucocorticoid therapy; (3) lung function abnormalities with FEV_1 values consistently less than 70% of those predicted; (4) persistent symptoms and decreased quality of life; or (5) a history of a previous respiratory failure/intubation, or near-fatal episode. An FEV_1 of less than 70% of those predicted may be "setting the bar too low" to define refractory asthma in childhood, as many of these children have values greater than 70% of those predicted. In fact, a recently published study from Fuhlbrigge[12] evaluated the lung function of over 3000 asthmatic children performed over a 15-year period. These investigators found only 0.7% of the FEV_1 values obtained from this data set to be less than 60% of those predicted. In addition, 5.5% of the observations had FEV_1 values between 60% and 80%, 51% with values between 80% and 100%, and 43% with values greater than 100% of those predicted! These data suggest that pediatric predictive values may require reevaluation.

CLINICAL CHARACTERISTICS

A recent prospective study of children with severe asthma referred for treatment to a multidisciplinary day program revealed that they were 44% female, 17% minority, and 25% of lower socioeconomic status.[8] Onset of age of asthma was a median of 2 years (slightly less than 12 months for preschool children); 81% were classified as atopic by skin testing and 65% were living with a cat or dog in the home at the time of admission. Comorbidity was frequent: rhinosinusitis (90%), gastroesophageal reflux disease (GERD) (57%), and atopic dermatitis (21%). Although these characteristics do not distinguish this population from children who have milder asthma, other measures of severity and poor control set them apart. The median lifetime hospital admissions numbered 6.5/patient. A significant percentage had experienced cyanotic episodes (64%), loss of consciousness (30%), and intubation for respiratory arrest (25%). Reported symptom frequency at admission was on average weekly for preschoolers and school-aged children, and daily for adolescents; 66% of patients were taking oral corticosteroids on admission with a median dose of 10 mg/day for adolescents, 6.3 mg/day for school-age children, and 0.6 mg/day for preschoolers. Steroid side effects were reported in 79%. Nearly half the cohort was morbidly obese (body mass index [BMI] ≥ 95%) or at risk of obesity (BMI ≥ 85%), a comorbid condition receiving recent attention in the literature.[13-15] The children showed marked physical deconditioning with a median functional endurance of 8% of predicted for age. BMI was significantly correlated with corticosteroid dose at admission (0.42; $P < 0.0001$) and inversely correlated with functional endurance (0.66; $P < 0.0001$). Perhaps surprisingly, given the frequency of symptoms, duration and severity of illness, median FEV_1 was 80% of predicted before beta agonist use and 90% afterwards. Median absence from school because of asthma for the previous school year was 26.5 days; 81% had identified difficulty in one or more psychosocial arenas with adolescents showing frequent evidence for depression (60%) and anxiety (55%).

Significantly, patients with refractory asthma will often display evidence of ongoing disease activity despite receiving optimal pharmacologic therapy. As a result, a retrospective review of 164 consecutive pediatric admissions to National Jewish Hospital for refractory asthma was undertaken to examine response to optimized therapy.[16] The cohort studied were mainly adolescents with a long duration of asthma (median age 14.0 years, median duration of asthma 11.9 years). Over 50% required chronically administered oral GC (15 mg/day median) on admission and all were on high-dose inhaled GC (1500 μg/day median) therapy. Despite high-dose inhaled GC therapy, the group had moderate airflow obstruction and airtrapping with a median FEV_1 77% of predicted, and residual volume 204% of that predicted. In addition, the majority of children were atopic, with 73% having at least one positive prick skin test to an aeroallergen.

Of interest, 50% of the study cohort required an oral GC burst secondary to poor asthma control at some point during their evaluation at National Jewish Hospital. Of those who required a prednisone burst, nearly one quarter (24%) failed to respond with a greater than 15% improvement in their morning prebronchodilator FEV_1 reading. These children, by definition, had GC-insensitive asthma. Risk factors associated with GC insensitivity included need for oral GCs at an earlier age, need for higher-maintenance oral GC, and African American ethnicity. Furthermore, two distinct spirometric patterns were noted. Those with a "chaotic" pattern displayed wide swings in lung function with no improvement in baseline lung function during the prednisone burst. In contrast, the "nonchaotic" subjects displayed little in the way of diurnal variability while demonstrating no improvement in baseline lung function. In summary, the prevalence of GC-insensitive asthma in this population of children with refractory asthma was higher than that anticipated. Those with GC-insensitive asthma appeared to have a more aggressive form of the disease, as evidenced by their need for GC at a much earlier age. Lastly, African-Americans were more likely to have GC-insensitive asthma than Caucasians.

PATHOGENESIS

The vast majority of studies evaluating the role airway inflammation in asthma have utilized adults with mild to moderate asthma in the absence of inhaled GC therapy who underwent bronchoscopy with bronchoalveolar lavage with or without endobronchial biopsies. These studies in GC-naive subjects have uniformly demonstrated airway epithelial desquamation with varying degrees of inflammatory cell infiltration consisting primarily of eosinophils, mast cells, and activated T lymphocytes. Whether the pathology of patients with refractory asthma already receiving high-dose antiinflammatory therapy was similar to mild asthma was until recently unknown.

Vrugt and colleagues[17] performed bronchoscopy with biopsy in 15 severe, GC-dependent asthmatics (median dose of prednisolone 40 mg/day; inhaled GC dose 2400 µg/day), 10 mild asthmatics, and 10 nonasthmatic controls. Of note, there were significantly fewer airway eosinophils noted among the patients with GC-dependent asthma compared to those with mild asthma. In contrast, the GC-dependent asthmatics had significantly greater numbers of activated T cells than both the nonasthmatic controls and those with mild asthma. Associated with the increase in activated T cells were greater numbers of cells expressing interleukin (IL)-5, an important cytokine for eosinophil recruitment and activation. Of note, the authors found no differences in the number of neutrophils among the three groups studied, nor were there differences in the total number of CD3- or CD4-positive cells.

Wenzel et al[18] performed bronchoscopy with endobronchial biopsies on 34 severe and GC-dependent, 11 moderate, and 10 mild asthmatics, plus 11 nonasthmatic controls. The investigators found the patients with severe asthma could be separated into those with airway eosinophilia (eosinophil positive) and those without airway eosinophilia (eosinophil negative). The eosinophil-positive group was also noted to have elevated numbers of T lymphocytes (CD3-, CD4-, and CD8-positive cells), mast cells, and macrophages. In addition, the sub–basement membrane thickness was greater among the eosinophil-positive compared to the eosinophil-negative group. Eosinophil-positive refractory asthma patients were also more likely to have required intubation secondary to respiratory failure, despite the fact that the eosinophil-negative group had a lower baseline FEV_1. Lastly, airway neutrophilia was a prominent feature in all of the GC-dependent asthmatics independent of their eosinophil status.

In one of the only bronchoscopic studies performed to date in children with refractory asthma, Payne et al[19] studied the relationship between exhaled nitric oxide (eNO) and airway eosinophilia in 31 children with refractory asthma following a 2-week course of prednisolone. In general, there was little evidence of active airway inflammation in the majority of children following the 2-week course of prednisolone therapy. The investigators found a significant correlation between levels of eNO and tissue eosinophils ($R = 0.54$; $P = 0.03$), with the strongest relationship found among the small number ($N = 4$) of children who remained symptomatic following the prednisolone course. In these subjects, an eNO level of greater than 7 ppb was associated with an elevated number of tissue eosinophils. There was no difference in the median eosinophil scores between the children with severe asthma postprednisone therapy and nonasthmatic children. These data suggest that persistent eosinophilia occurs in a minority of refractory asthmatic children who remain symptomatic following a prednisolone burst. In addition, airway eosinophilia was associated with elevated eNO levels.

EVALUATION

In evaluating patients with difficult-to-control asthma (Box 41-1) and obtaining a thorough history including the patient's past history, current symptoms, medication use, physical examination, spirometry, and complete pulmonary function studies, the following questions should be addressed.

Does the Patient Have Asthma?

There are many "masqueraders" of asthma that can confound the clinical picture and therapeutic response (Table 41-2). A history of acute and reversible episodes of cough, wheezing, or shortness of breath with clearly defined triggers and precipitants supports the diagnosis of asthma as does a history of bronchial hyperresponsiveness (BHR).[3] BHR is manifested clinically by a circadian variation in pulmonary function, with the lowest values in early-morning peak expiratory flow rate (PEFR) or FEV_1 compared with other times during the day, and bronchoconstriction induced by exercise or cold air.[20] A child with refractory asthma can have an FEV_1 value within the normal range. As such a more sensitive measure of airflow obstruction is the FEV_1/forced vital capacity (FVC) ratio.

BOX 41-1

THERAPEUTIC PRINCIPLES
Evaluation Algorithm for Refractory Asthma

PULMONARY FUNCTION STUDIES

Regularly performed spirometry in the clinic with home peak expiratory flow monitoring

Body box plethysmography to evaluate lung volumes

Methacholine challenge to quantitate degree of bronchial hyperresponsiveness to rule out confounding factors such as vocal cord dysfunction

Occasionally performed studies:
Pressure-volume relationship study
Hypoxic/hypercarbic drive study

IMMUNOLOGIC/PHARMACOLOGIC STUDIES

Total eosinophil count, morning cortisol, quantitative IgE level

Prick skin testing to common allergens

Prednisone/methylprednisolone pharmacokinetic studies, especially if patient displays few glucocorticoid-associated adverse effects

Markers of allergic inflammation/immune activation (sputum eosinophils, exhaled nitric oxide if available)

Glucocorticoid-lymphocyte stimulation assay

RADIOLOGIC STUDIES

Baseline chest radiograph

Screening sinus computed tomography scan

High-resolution chest computed tomography scan (if clinically indicated)

OTHER STUDIES

24-Hour esophageal pH probe study and barium swallow

Rhinolaryngoscopy to assess nasal anatomy and to evaluate for vocal cord dysfunction if suspected

TABLE 41-2 Masqueraders of Asthma

Aspiration syndromes (especially in young children)
Foreign body aspiration
Tracheomalacia, bronchomalacia
Vocal cord dysfunction (especially in older children)
Bronchiectasis (secondary to humoral immunodeficiency, ciliary
    dyskinesia)
Bronchiolitis
Cystic fibrosis
Tracheal ± bronchial compression syndromes
Tuberculosis
Allergic bronchopulmonary aspergillosis

Are Other Medical Conditions Contributing to Refractory Asthma?

Because most children with refractory asthma are atopic, the question of ongoing allergen exposure is paramount for many patients. Special consideration is also given to the conditions of gastroesophageal reflux and sinusitis because they are frequently encountered in this population and can contribute significantly to exacerbations of asthma. Finally, vocal cord dysfunction (VCD), a masquerader of asthma, can also accompany asthma. Because VCD does not generally respond to medications for asthma, it can be misperceived as refractory asthma by both the patient and physician, thereby leading to inappropriate escalation of medical treatment.

Ongoing Allergen Exposure

Chronic allergen exposure may significantly contribute to the pathogenesis and persistence of airway inflammation in atopic asthma patients. Thus strict allergen avoidance can, by lessening the allergen load within the airway, result in decreased airway inflammation and improved asthma control, which in turn can lessen the need for chronic glucocorticoid therapy.[21,22] Environmental control is addressed thoroughly in Chapter 26. Where effective avoidance is impossible, immunotherapy can be considered (see Chapter 27), recognizing that immunotherapy in refractory childhood asthma is incompletely studied and less likely to be effective than in milder disease.[23,24] Immunotherapy is contraindicated in many such patients because of disease lability.[23-25]

Gastroesophageal Reflux Disease

Recent studies show a general prevalence of 47% to 75% of GERD in children with asthma, including severe asthma,[8,26-29] which is similar to adults with asthma and about two to four times the prevalence in the general population. Field et al found that 41% of adult asthmatics noted reflux-associated respiratory symptoms, prompting 28% to use their inhalers.[30] Similarly, Harding[31] noted that 79% of respiratory symptoms were temporally associated with esophageal acidification during 24-hour esophageal pH testing. Additionally, an increasing cognizance of extrapulmonary and atypical manifestations of GERD should raise suspicion of its presence.[32-37] Nonetheless, sobering data has suggested that GERD can be silent in as many as 33% of adults with asthma[31,38] and 44% of infants with daily wheezing.[28] Indeed, a recent study by Harding et al[39] suggests that even these estimates may be low in that 62% of asthmatic adults were shown to have abnormal 24-hour

esophageal pH probe studies in spite of being asymptomatic for GERD. As such, GERD must always be considered, even in the absence of symptoms, in the treatment of any patient with asthma, and particularly with severe asthma and escalating need for medications.

Although there is a clear association of asthma and GERD, there is debate as to the importance of GERD in asthma control. Disparity in methods of diagnosis, measurement of outcomes, and stratification by disease severity (both GERD and/or asthma) among studies may be at the heart of conflicting results. Several studies support the hypothesis that the degree of esophageal damage may be an important determinant in the possible relationship between GERD and asthma; nocturnal reflux is more damaging to the esophagus than upright reflux because of prolonged acid contact time. Several studies in children suggest that severe nocturnal asthma is more likely to be associated with GERD than daytime asthma.[40,41] In a recent study of adult nocturnal asthma patients with moderate to severe GERD by Cuttitta et al,[42] reflux was significantly and temporally associated with enhanced lower airways resistance.

Determining the significance of GERD in asthma is further complicated by the fact that physiologic alterations often seen in asthma, particularly severe asthma, can clearly promote GERD.[32] These include an increase in transient lower esophageal sphincter (LES) relaxation, LES hypotonia, and esophageal dysmotility, which may be increased because of autonomic dysfunction in asthma.[43] Additionally, asthma medications (particularly theophylline and oral beta agonists) may increase LES dysfunction. Furthermore, the LES pressure augmented by the crural diaphragm normally prevents GERD, but this augmentation is prevented by hyperinflation and hiatal hernia, or LES pressure is overcome by increased negative intrathoracic pressures (e.g., in bronchospasm, cough, upper-airway resistance syndrome, and obstructive apnea), increased intraabdominal pressures (e.g., in obesity) and steroid-induced myopathy.[8,32]

On the other hand, recent studies shed light on four mechanisms by which GERD can affect airway function.[32,44] Vagally mediated reflexive alterations of respiratory function (respiratory rate, minute ventilation, resistance, and the sensation of dyspnea) have been demonstrated during acid infusion into the esophagus. Second, esophageal acidification has been associated with heightened nonspecific hyperresponsivity of the airways to bronchochonstrictors, thus "priming" the airway to other triggers. Third, animal models suggest that esophageal acidification can lead to the release of substance P and other tachykinins into the airway, which results in neurogenic inflammation of the airway.[45] Finally, microaspiration occurs in a minority of patients, although it may be more common in young children than older individuals. Jack et al[46] simultaneously monitored proximal esophageal and tracheal pH (via a probe inserted percutaneously into the trachea) in a small number of patients with severe asthma. Of 37 documented episodes of prolonged (i.e., > 5 minutes) proximal acid reflux, 5 were associated with tracheal acidification and significant deterioration in pulmonary function; episodes that did not result in tracheal acidification had much less effect on pulmonary function.

Thus asthma, particularly severe asthma, can predispose to GERD just as GERD can contribute to asthma severity in a seemingly vicious cycle. Importantly, treatment of GERD, particularly with the vastly superior proton pump inhibitors

(PPIs) now available, leads to improvement in asthma symptoms[47-49] and/or function.[48,50,51] Although diagnostic testing may not be required before empiric PPI treatment for symptomatic patients,[32,44] confirmation of the diagnosis where desired and/or verification of acid suppression following a 3-month course of PPI therapy requires 24-hour esophageal pH probe monitoring. Even though this test is the current gold standard for determining the presence of pathologic GER, a recent study using two consecutive 24-hour periods suggested less than optimal reproducibility, with a false-negative rate of 19% for the first day.[52] Importantly, scoring criteria developed to estimate the potential for development of esophagitis (e.g., the Johnson and Demeester scoring system[53]) is not necessarily applicable to other diseases, and there is no consensus on criteria and predictive values for asthma.[32,39,54] Other testing such as barium swallow and endoscopy provide important data but are neither sensitive nor specific for the diagnosis of GERD.[29,32]

Response among asthmatics to PPI therapy is heterogeneous and lack of response may result from nonsuppression of acid production on conventional PPI dosing, demonstrated in up to 30% of subjects,[51] accompanied by poor healing of the esophagus.[50] For severe GERD or refractory asthma with GERD, twice-daily dosing of a PPI for 3 months is recommended (e.g., lansoprazole 30 mg twice daily in adolescents and approximately 0.7 to 1 mg/kg twice daily up to this dose for younger children using either the sachet or opened capsule delivered in a variety of vehicles, such as applesauce).[55] Longer-term maintenance PPI treatment (often given as half the dose above once a day) is required in many patients. In addition to PPI therapy, recommendations are to elevate the head of the bed by 6 inches, abstain from eating 2 hours before bedtime, and avoiding spicy, fatty foods and caffeinated and carbonated beverages. Some adult patients have been shown to require the addition of H_2 blockers for acid suppression at night,[56] and prokinetic agents (e.g., metaclopramide) are employed if regurgitation is prominent.

The medical and surgical antireflux and asthma treatment outcomes literature has recently been reviewed by Field.[30,47] Both surgery and medical antireflux therapy (although only four studies using PPIs were published at the time of the review) appear to result in improvement in approximately 70% of asthma patients. To date no trials have compared surgery with PPI therapy. Predictors of response to either form of therapy are identified as presence of regurgitation, proximal esophageal acid acidification, esophagitis healing on medical therapy, and noted association of reflux with respiratory symptoms and obesity.[44,57] At this time, with obvious gaps in our information, we recommend surgery for those patients with severe asthma in whom persistent, documented GERD improves with PPIs but requires very protracted therapy, for those with documented GERD unwilling or unable to comply with medical therapy, and for those in whom life-threatening disease warrants definite treatment.

Sinusitis

Radiographic evidence for sinus disease is also commonly seen in asthma. Mounting data link the physiology of the upper and lower airways and support the hypothesis that the same pathology underlies both sinusitis and asthma[58,59] (see Chapter 30). Studies demonstrate that inflammation of the nose and sinuses is associated with lower-airway hyperre-

sponsiveness,[60,61] and that nasal allergen challenge results in airway hyperresponsiveness,[62] and adhesion molecule expression and eosinophilia of both the upper and lower airways.[63]

Importantly, treatment of the upper airway, generally with nasal corticosteroids, has in several studies led to amelioration of lower-airway hyperreactivity.[64-68] There are also reports of significant improvement in control in asthmatics with successfully managed sinus disease, following medical (topical GC, and/or antibiotics) and occasionally surgical intervention.[69-71] A screening computed tomography scan of the sinuses provides greater resolution and thus greater sensitivity than[72] conventional sinus radiographs and thus should be utilized when evaluating for sinusitis[73] (see Chapter 30).

Vocal Cord Dysfunction

Since the first descriptions of VCD, defined as inappropriate or paradoxical adduction of the vocal cords during inspiration, it has emerged as a frequent masquerader of asthma[74-76] (Table 41-3). Approximately 10% to 20% of severe asthma patients referred to our tertiary referral center are diagnosed with VCD rather than asthma (unpublished data). At the same time, there has been a growing appreciation that VCD can also occur *with* asthma.[77] It was identified in 10% of pediatric patients (approximately 20% of adolescents) with severe asthma treated at National Jewish Hospital.[8] In either case, frequent or unremitting symptoms can be misinterpreted as refractory asthma and can lead to overtreatment.[78-83] (See discussion of VCD diagnosis and management in Chapters 31 and 38.)

TABLE 41-3 Immunologic Abnormalities in and Etiology of Glucocorticoid-Resistant Asthma

Cellular abnormalities
Immunologic abnormalities
Diminished ability of glucocorticoids to inhibit PHA-induced lymphocyte proliferation
Increased numbers of circulating T cells bearing surface activation markers (HLA-DR, CD25) and elevated serum levels of interleukin (IL)-2R
Diminished ability of glucocorticoids to inhibit mitogen-stimulated IL-2 and interferon-β
Increased mRNA expression of IL-2 and IL-4 from bronchoalveolar lavage lymphocytes
Failure of glucocorticoids to inhibit mRNA IL-4 expression from bronchoalveolar lavage lymphocytes
Blunted eosinopenic response following the administration of glucocorticoids

Etiology
Molecular abnormalities of the glucocorticoid receptor
Diminished ligand-binding affinity
Diminished DNA-binding affinity
Diminished glucocorticoid receptor numbers
Up-regulation of glucocorticoid receptor β, a functionally inactive glucocorticoid receptor

Other etiologies for apparent glucocorticoid resistance
Poor adherence to glucocorticoid therapy
Glucocorticoid pharmacokinetic abnormalities (poor absorption or rapid clearance)

A number of modalities for treatment (e.g., speech therapy, hypnosis, heliox, topical anesthetics) have been used successfully to abort acute episodes, to help patients learn to distinguish VCD from asthma, and for long-term control.[84-86] Psychosocial evaluation is recommended if symptoms persist. Accurate assessment of lower-airways symptoms, function, and degree of reactivity (in natural circumstances or in the challenge laboratory setting) is often not possible until VCD is controlled.

What is the Level of Asthma Severity and Control?

To assess this question, one must inquire as to the frequency of spontaneous severe exacerbations, history of previous ER visits, and hospitalizations, whether there have been life-threatening episodes such as loss of consciousness, seizures, or the need for intubation secondary to respiratory failure or arrest. In addition, one must inquire as to the interventions required during exacerbations and chronically to maintain adequate control. In particular, questions should be asked regarding the dose and duration of systemic GC required for improvement in symptoms and lung function, and the dose of inhaled GC required to maintain long-term control. Questions designed to address asthma control should include the frequency of nocturnal awakenings with asthma symptoms, the severity of exercise-induced bronchospasm (with or without inhaled beta agonist pretreatment), variability in lung function, and the frequency with which the patient requires rescue therapy (i.e., inhaled beta agonist). Need for frequent beta agonist is clearly a red flag and must be addressed, especially in light of reports that have implicated overuse of beta agonist therapy as contributing to asthma morbidity and mortality.[87-89] Whether increased use of beta agonist therapy is responsible for poor asthma control or whether it is a marker of poorly controlled asthma remains to be determined. Nevertheless, in our experience, the greater the need for rescue therapy, the greater the need for better asthma control, which may involve a combination of antiinflammatory agents and long-acting β_2-adrenergic agonists (LABAs).

Is the Patient's Current Asthma Medication Regimen Sufficient for Asthma Control?

Optimal control of a child's asthma should allow normal or near-normal daily activities including participation in gym class and other athletic activities, normal sleep with no need for nocturnally administered beta agonists, little need for short-acting beta agonists for rescue of symptoms, and few severe exacerbations requiring oral rescue GCs, ER visits, or hospitalizations. With increasing asthma severity, inhaled GC doses are increased and combination therapy with LABAs, leukotriene receptor antagonists (LTRAs), or theophylline is recommended. The combination of a LABA and an inhaled GC provides better symptom control and lung function and results in fewer exacerbations.[90-93] As such, patients whose symptoms are suboptimally controlled on an inhaled GC would likely benefit from the addition of a LABA to the inhaled GC.

Rescue agents such as the short-acting inhaled β-agonists are used for acute episodes of wheezing and in preventing exercise-induced bronchospasm. When these medications are

used and adherence has been demonstrated to be good, optimal control of the disease is achievable in most children with asthma. Even with well-controlled asthma, acute exacerbations will occur and in this case, short courses of oral GCs during the acute exacerbation are recommended. Unfortunately, a minority of refractory asthma patients will require chronically administered oral glucocorticoid therapy to maintain symptom control. In these "GC-dependent" asthma patients the goal of therapy is directed at administering the lowest possible dose while maintaining sufficient control of asthma symptoms. Alternate-day dosing is preferable to daily dosing because the incidence of long-term steroid-associated adverse effects can be minimized with this strategy. Short courses of high-dose oral/parenteral therapy should be used as needed for severe exacerbations in the steroid-dependent asthma patient and tapered based on clinical response and objective measures of pulmonary function.

Is Inhaler Technique Adequate and Is Poor Adherence a Factor?

Technique with Inhaled Medications

In addition to investigating for poor compliance, one must evaluate the patient's inhaled medication technique. The proper use of inhaled GC therapy has allowed a significant number of patients with severe asthma to reduce their oral steroid requirement.[94,95] To maximize effectiveness while decreasing the potential for local and systemic effects, all metered-dose inhaled GC formulations should be administered with a spacer device.[96-98] The newer dry powder devices do not require a spacer device, nor do the inhaled GCs dissolved in 1,1,1,2-tetrafluoroethane such as Qvar (3-M). Rinsing the mouth and spitting out orally deposited corticosteroid is recommended to prevent undesirable local and systemic absorption.

Medication Adherence

Not surprisingly, poor compliance with GC therapy is often a significant contributing factor for poor response (see Chapter 42), yet it is often difficult to substantiate.[99-101] A number of recently published studies have documented poor adherence with inhaled GC therapy in both children and adults with asthma.[102,103] An important study by Rand et al[99] evaluated adherence with a metered-dose inhaler (MDI) and found that although 75% of the study participants reported using their MDIs as directed, only 15% of the participants actually used the MDI as instructed. We noted a similar pattern with reported oral GC use in patients with poorly controlled asthma.[104] Even under the best of circumstances, adherence with inhaled GCs remains unacceptably low.

Does the Child Have GC-Insensitive Asthma?

If these conditions are recognized and adequately treated and the patient continues to display evidence of poorly controlled asthma, further evaluation as described later should be undertaken (see Table 41-3).

Definition of GC-Insensitive Asthma

GC-insensitive asthma patients constitute a subgroup of patients with refractory asthma who do not adequately respond to systemically administered GC. These children are characterized by persistent respiratory symptoms, nocturnal exacerbations, and chronic airflow limitation. More importantly, these individuals will fail to clinically respond to a short course of high-dose oral GC therapy. Specifically, these individuals' lung function will fail to improve following a 7- to 14-day course of high-dose ($\geq$ 40 mg/day) oral GC therapy as measured by a less than 15% improvement in morning prebronchodilator FEV_1. If the child's FEV_1 fails to improve by at least 15% following the GC course, the diagnosis is substantiated.

What Is the Etiology of the Patient's Steroid Resistance?

Once the diagnosis of GC-insensitive asthma has been established and all other contributing factors adequately addressed, an attempt should be made to identify causes for this apparent resistance (see Table 41-4). Poor adherence to the prescribed medical regimen, especially inhaled and oral GC therapy, is the most likely factor.

Is a Pharmacokinetic Abnormality Contributing to Poor Responsiveness to GCs?

Abnormal GC pharmacokinetics can be a contributing factor in children with refractory asthma who display fewer than expected GC-associated adverse effects.[105] A highly sensitive and specific high-pressure liquid chromatography methodology[106] allows for plasma concentrations of cortisol and synthetic GCs to be determined. For prednisone, three blood samples are obtained (0-, 2-, and 6-hour) following the administration of prednisone (40 mg/m^2). The predose (0-hour) sample is evaluated for cortisol and prednisolone, the active metabolite of prednisone, and provides information regarding the extent of adrenal suppression and also ensures that the predose prednisolone concentration is undetectable. The second sample is obtained at the theoretically maximum prednisolone concentration and provides information regarding the rate and extent of absorption of the oral dose. The third sample is used in estimating prednisolone clearance.[105] A more extensive sampling procedure is required for methylprednisolone with samples drawn 0, 0.5, 1.5, 2, 3, 4, 6, 8, 10, and 12 hours postdose. Clearance is then calculated by determining the area under the plasma concentration-time curve and dividing it by the dose administered. Rapid oral GC clearance may be related to poor absorption, rapid elimination, or failure to convert prednisone to prednisolone. Rapid elimination may result from drug interaction or rapid metabolism from increased metabolic activity related to undefined factors, such as genetic control.

Poor absorption (i.e., peak prednisolone level < 400 ng/ml following the administration of a standardized dose of 40 mg/1.73 m^2 of prednisone) is relatively uncommon and requires an intravenous study to differentiate rapid clearance as a contributing factor. In patients with defined poor absorption of prednisone or methylprednisolone, one must assess the possibility of a drug interaction with adsorbents such as antacids. If a patient has impaired absorption of prednisone or methylprednisolone tablets, a liquid prednisone or liquid prednisolone formulation should be used because poor absorption of liquid prednisone is highly unlikely.

Drug interactions, especially the anticonvulsants phenobarbital, phenytoin, and carbamazepin[107] and the anti-

tuberculosis agent rifampin[108] can result in rapid GC clearance. In addition to drug-induced accelerated clearance, diseases such as hyperthyroidism and cystic fibrosis can increase GC clearance.[107] Lastly, a group of patients have been identified as having inherently rapid clearance.[105] If rapid clearance is associated with a drug interaction, one can attempt to discontinue the medication responsible for rapid clearance (if possible) or one can alter either the formulation (i.e., methylprednisolone in place of prednisone or vice versa), dose, or frequency of GC administration. Of note, methylprednisolone is much more susceptible to enzyme induction by anticonvulsants than prednisolone is[107] and should be avoided with these drugs, with prednisone used as an alternative. In some cases we have identified rapid clearance of methylprednisolone and normal clearance of prednisolone and vice versa.

Does the Child Have an Abnormality in Glucocorticoid Receptor Binding, Number, or Function?

Studies in patients with refractory asthma suggest that abnormalities in glucocorticoid receptor (GCR) number, GCR binding (ligand and/or DNA binding), and up-regulation of an alternatively spliced and inactive form of the GCR, termed $GR\beta$, likely account for the poor response to GC therapy noted in SR asthma. These defects appear to be functional rather than genetic in that chemical mutational analyses of the GCR from SR asthma patients failed to reveal mutations that would explain the phenomenon.[109]

Ligand Binding and GCR Number Abnormalities

Two distinct GCR abnormalities have been identified in the peripheral blood mononuclear cells of patients with GC-insensitive asthma.[110] The first abnormality (type 1) involves a significant reduction in GCR-binding affinity whereas the second abnormality (type 2) manifests as a relative deficiency of GC receptor sites per cell. The type 1 GCR defect is the most commonly identified abnormality. The binding defect appears to be localized to inflammatory cells, reverses when the cells are cultured in the absence of cytokines, and can be sustained by the co-culture of the cells with the combination of IL-2 and IL-4.[111] Of interest, airway cells from subjects with GC-insensitive asthma express elevated levels of IL-2 and IL-4 mRNA compared to steroid sensitive (SS) asthmatics. In addition, the expression of these cytokines does not fall following a GC course as they do in SS asthma patients.[112] IL-13, a cytokine with properties similar to IL-4, can induce diminished GCR-binding affinity in monocytes, rendering these cells less sensitive to the suppressive effects of GC.[113] The type 2 GCR defect is much less commonly identified, and may be an irreversible abnormality affecting all cell types; it is associated with low numbers of GCRs.[110] These individuals fail to derive benefit from GC while developing few steroid adverse effects despite long histories of chronic oral steroid use.

DNA-Binding Defects

In addition to ligand binding defects, abnormalities in DNA binding have also been described.[114,115] Adcock et al[115] found dexamethasone ineffective in increasing DNA binding in patients with GC-insensitive asthma, whereas dexamethasone induced significant increases in DNA binding in GC-sensitive asthmatics and nonasthmatic controls. A follow-up article by the same group found patients with GC-insensitive asthma to have increased basal expression of the transcription factor AP-1, suggesting that increased levels of AP-1 inhibited GCR-DNA binding.[114]

Up-regulation of GRβ

Leung et al[116] have recently described increased expression of an alternatively spliced form of the GCR termed *GCRβ* in the peripheral blood and bronchoalveolar lavage cells of GC-insensitive asthmatics. Of significance, expression of this inactive form of the GCR is up-regulated following exposure to the combination of IL-2 and IL-4 *in vitro*. GRβ is an alternatively spliced form of the GCR that does not bind to GCs and appears to antagonize the transactivating effects of the functional GCR.[117] Thus up-regulation of GRβ results could also play an important role in the pathogenesis of GC-insensitive asthma, namely by inhibiting the GC-GCR complex from modulating the transcription of proinflammatory molecules.

MANAGEMENT

Nonpharmacologic Interventions

Successful management of any refractory asthmatic patient begins with frequent clinic visits and objective measures of pulmonary function performed daily at home and during clinic visits. Twice-daily home monitoring of peak expiratory flow before and following inhaled bronchodilator therapy can help to identify a breakdown in asthma control and assess the effect of various interventions. Spirometry provides valuable information regarding the child's level of pulmonary function[118] and other disorders such as VCD can be identified.[119] Yearly evaluation of lung volumes performed by body box plethysmography are also important as this can provide information regarding the degree of hyperinflation, air trapping, and airway resistance/conductance. Other measures of pulmonary function that are occasionally used during the evaluation of the suspected steroid-resistant asthmatic include pressure volume curves, methacholine challenges, and hypoxic/hypercarbic drive studies. We and others have observed that many difficult-to-control asthmatics have pressure volume curves that are shifted upward and to the left, suggestive of a loss of elastic recoil.[120,121] Whether this observed abnormality is an acquired and reversible finding and whether this apparent loss of elastic recoil has clinical relevance are at present under investigation.

A multidisciplinary approach may be required. The management of the refractory asthmatic presents several challenges. A comprehensive approach that incorporates all aspects of disease management as previously discussed is essential for these challenging patients. Finally, for some patients, a tertiary referral to a center of excellence may be necessary. We have taken such a global approach to patients with refractory asthma through a multidisciplinary outpatient program that facilitates collaborative assessment and treatment by medical, nursing, psychosocial, and rehabilitation care providers. Two-year outcome data from a recent cohort of 98 children enrolled in this program have recently been published.[8] Sustained improvements were seen in corticosteroid use, asthma functional severity, perceived competence in asthma management, and quality of life for both caregiver and child. Importantly, emergency department visits and hospital days were significantly reduced in the 2-year follow-up period compared to the year before participation in the program. Significantly, median total medical encounter cost per patient for the year before participation, estimated at $16,250, was reduced to $1902 at 1-year and $690 at 2-year follow-up.

Pharmacotherapy

The pharmacologic goals of the difficult-to-control asthma patient are similar to those of all asthmatics. These goals include using bronchodilators as needed to relieve airflow obstruction, protecting the airway from irritating stimuli and subsequent airway inflammation, and utilizing antiinflammatory medications to treat ongoing airway inflammation, which will aid in the reduction of airway hyperresponsiveness.[122]

Systemic Glucocorticoid Therapy

Significant improvements in symptoms and pulmonary function are noted in the vast majority of asthmatics following institution of inhaled GC therapy. Unfortunately, a small percentage of asthmatics require chronically administered oral GC therapy in addition to high-dose inhaled GC therapy for adequate symptom control. Although effective, chronic use of oral GCs in combination with high-dose inhaled GCs is often associated with a number of debilitating adverse effects such as adrenal suppression, growth suppression, osteoporosis, cataracts, hypertension, diabetes mellitus, myopathy, obesity, and cushingoid features as recently documented by Covar et al.[123] As a result, every effort should be made to determine the minimal effective oral GC dose. To determine the child's "threshold" oral GC dose, a gradual oral GC taper should be attempted, with close monitoring of the patient's symptoms and pulmonary function. The daily oral GC dose should be tapered by 5 mg/wk until 20 mg on alternate days is reached or until breakthrough asthma symptoms or declining pulmonary function is observed. Because most of subjects will be adrenally suppressed, the taper is then slowed with weekly reductions in the oral GC dose by 2.5 mg every other week with periodic measurement of morning cortisol levels to assess adrenal recovery. If during the glucocorticoid taper the patient develops increasing asthma symptoms and/or diminished pulmonary function, the threshold dose is defined. It should be emphasized that the threshold requirement is dynamic and likely to change over time depending on time of year (viral exacerbations in the winter and aeroallergen exposure during the spring, summer, and fall), changes in intrinsic disease severity, and increasing age. If the child's threshold dose is greater than 20 mg of prednisone (or its equivalent) on alternate days, consideration of alternative asthma medications is warranted.

High-Dose "Second-Generation" Inhaled Glucocorticoid Therapy

High-dose second-generation inhaled GC therapy has been shown to result in significant oral GC dose reduction in adults with GC-dependent asthma. This is likely because these GCs display greater topical to systemic potencies compared with the other available inhaled GCs, with the end result being a better therapeutic index. The superior therapeutic index is the result of increased antiinflammatory potency of these compounds on a microgram to microgram basis, and reduced oral bioavailability because of extensive first-pass metabolism.[124] Over 80% of the adult asthmatics randomized to high-dose fluticasone propionate (FP) therapy (2000 μg/day) were able to be completely tapered off oral GC therapy.[125] In addition, those on high-dose FP had a significant improvement in their lung function despite the significant oral steroid dose reduction. Budesonide has been shown to display significant, albeit less striking oral GC-sparing effects in adults with oral GC-dependent asthma as reported by Nelson et al.[126] Most recently, high-dose mometasone furoate (MF), which has yet to be approved for use in the United States, permitted a significant reduction in oral glucocorticoid requirement in patients with steroid-dependent asthma.[127] The ability of the second-generation inhaled GCs FP, budesonide, and MF to result in significant oral steroid-sparing effects appears to be unique to these compounds in that similar effects have not been noted with the other available inhaled GCs.[128] Although useful in reducing the need for oral GCs, high doses alone have been associated with significant GC-induced side effects in some patients.

Leukotriene Antagonists
The leukotriene antagonists (synthesis inhibitors and receptor antagonists) represent an entirely new class of asthma medications that are being used with increasing frequency. Studies in subjects with moderate asthma have found these medications to be less effective than inhaled GCs in improving lung function.[129] A recently published study found montelukast to result in a modest, yet statistically significant inhaled GC-sparing effect in patients with moderate to severe asthma on high-dose inhaled GC therapy.[130] Robinson et al,[131] in one of the few published studies that attempted to determine whether the addition of an LTRA would improve symptoms and/or lung function in refractory asthmatics already on inhaled GCs and long-acting beta agonists, did not find montelukast to offer any added benefit compared to placebo. It should be noted that the mean age of the population studied was 52.3 years. Whether the addition of a leukotriene-modifying agent will offer benefit in children already on inhaled GCs, LABAs, and oral GCs remains to be determined. An LTRA can be added in combination with inhaled GC and LABAs in children with refractory symptoms and patients can be observed for improvement in asthma control over a period of 2 months.

Theophylline
Although theophylline is not used as frequently as it once was because of fears regarding its potential toxicity, it is still an effective asthma therapy. Theophylline, when used chronically can reduce symptoms as well as the need for supplemental beta agonist use.[132] Theophylline may also have some steroid-sparing effects in individuals with steroid dependent asthma.[133] Thus theophylline therapy should be attempted in all individuals with severe or steroid-dependent asthma. Long-acting theophylline preparations are also useful for patients with a significant nocturnal component to their asthma. Theophylline has a narrow therapeutic window, and consequently, levels need to be routinely monitored, especially if the child has a viral illness associated with a fever or is placed on

a medication known to delay theophylline clearance, such as macrolide antibiotics (erythromycin and clarithromycin), cimetidine, antifungal agents, oral contraceptives, and ciprofloxacin.[134]

Alternative Asthma Therapies
Methotrexate. Methotrexate has been extensively studied in refractory asthma with several randomized, placebo-controlled studies performed to evaluate its role as an oral GC-sparing agent. Unfortunately, these studies have been performed primarily in adults, and they have yielded contrasting results, making it difficult to determine its effectiveness.[135,136] A recent meta-analysis of all controlled studies that evaluating the effectiveness of methotrexate in GC-dependent asthma found it to display a mild steroid-sparing effect (mean reduction: 3.3 mg/day reduction).[137] As with all alternative medications, reductions in oral GC dose are not sustained after the therapy is discontinued. Methotrexate at the doses used to treat asthma is relatively safe, with a low frequency of adverse effects. Serious but rare adverse effects include serious infection, pulmonary fibrosis, and liver toxicity. No studies have evaluated methotrexate in GC-insensitive asthma specifically.

Cyclosporine A. Cyclosporine A (CyA) is a potent immunosuppressive agent. When used in low doses CyA therapy is effective in several autoimmune diseases. Alexander et al[138] were among the first to study CyA in 33 adults with refractory asthma enrolled into a 12-week crossover study of CyA or placebo. CyA therapy was effective in improving lung function and reducing the frequency of asthma exacerbations. Of note, a wide range of responses was seen, from no response to significant improvement. CyA therapy in asthma does not result in sustained remissions once discontinued. In contrast, Nizankowska et al[139] failed to find CyA to be effective in improving lung function or reducing the oral GC dose requirement in an equally severe cohort of adults with GC-dependent asthma. CyA has several potential serious adverse effects, including nephrotoxicity, hypertension, and immunosuppression.[113] Although CyA appears to be ideally suited for the treatment of refractory asthma, the potential for severe and potentially irreversible nephrotoxicity has limited its use in children with refractory asthma. In fact, there are no published control studies evaluating the safety or effectiveness of CyA in children with refractory asthma. Tacrolimus (FK506) is a macrolide immunosuppressive agent with actions similar to those of cyclosporine. A dermatologic formulation is approved for use in moderate to severe atopic dermatitis. Given its potent antiinflammatory effects and its demonstrated efficacy in patients with severe atopic dermatitis, an inhaled formulation for use in asthma is undergoing Phase II clinical trials.

Intravenous Immunoglobulin. Intravenous immunoglobulin (IVIG) has recently been shown to be effective in several immune-mediated diseases. Mazer and Gelfand[140] evaluated the effectiveness of monthly high-dose IVIG therapy in steroid-dependent children and reported a threefold reduction in oral GC dose, reduction in symptoms, and improved PEFRs. In addition, the total IgE level fell from 324 IU before therapy to 133 IU and was associated with a reduction in skin test reactivity to allergens. The investigators noted improvements in parameters studied within the first one or two infusions, but noted deterioration in these same parameters 8 to 12 weeks after cessation of therapy.

Despite its use as a steroid-sparing agent, little is known regarding its mechanism(s) of GC dose reduction. *In vitro* studies have demonstrated the effects of IVIG on suppressing lymphocyte stimulation in the presence and absence of added dexamethasone.[141] Eleven subjects with severe steroid-dependent asthma were enrolled into a 6-month open-label trial where they received 2 g/kg of IVIG every 4 weeks. IVIG therapy resulted in a significant reduction in oral GC requirement, number of oral GC bursts, and hospitalizations compared to the 6-month period before enrollment into the study. In addition, IVIG acted synergistically with dexamethasone in suppressing lymphocyte stimulation *in vitro*. Specifically, when IVIG (10 mg/ml) was co-cultured with dexamethasone, the lymphocytes became much more sensitive to the suppressive effects of dexamethasone than those cultured with dexamethasone alone. This study found a synergistic effect with the two compounds. It is of significance that many of the patients enrolled in this study had documented GC-insensitive asthma; IVIG was as effective in this subgroup of patients as in those with steroid-dependent yet sensitive asthma.

Salmun et al[142] recently published the results of a randomized, placebo-controlled study on the effectiveness of IVIG on oral GC dose reduction in patients with severe GC-dependent asthma. Twenty-eight patients received placebo or 400 mg/kg IVIG every 3 weeks for 9 months following a 3-month run-in period. The mean age of the study participants was 17.3 years and the mean oral GC dose was 14.5 mg/day. Both placebo and IVIG resulted in significant reductions in oral GC requirement during the study, with IVIG resulting in a greater reduction (starting dose 10.5 mg with a reduction to 3.5 mg/day) versus placebo (starting dose 9.3 with a reduction to 8.8 mg/day). It was notable that IVIG was more effective than placebo in subjects requiring more than 2000 mg of oral GC in the 12 months before the study (mean dose reduction from 16.4 to 3 mg/day for IVIG vs. 10.4 to 10.2 mg/day for placebo). Despite a significant reduction in oral GC dose, all lung function parameters remained stable. In contrast, Kishiyama et al[143] found high-dose IVIG (1 or 2 mg/kg) to be no more effective than placebo in oral GC dose reduction, or any other variable in a group of older patients and those with less severe asthma (mean age 39.7 years, mean FEV_1 82.8% of predicted). The investigators also found an unacceptably high rate of adverse reactions in the 2 g/kg IVIG group, with 3 of 16 subjects developing aseptic meningitis.

In summary, there are conflicting reports regarding the efficacy and safety of IVIG therapy in severe asthma. We are still awaiting definitive studies, that is, large randomized, placebo-controlled trials, before its true efficacy is known. Patients with the most severe asthma who have the greatest oral GC requirement appear to derive the most benefit from IVIG therapy. Thus IVIG can be an effective and relatively safe alternative medication in highly selected patient populations. Although the safety profile of IVIG is acceptable, adverse effects can occur and include anaphylaxis, headache, and rarely aseptic meningitis. In addition, its use is often cost prohibitive and it carries the remote potential for blood-borne infection.

Anti-IgE. Anti-IgE is a humanized murine monoclonal antibody to IgE that inhibits IgE binding to the IgE receptor on mast cells and basophils. Phase I and II studies have found anti-IgE to significantly reduce the amount of circulating free IgE and to inhibit both the early- and late-phase asthmatic responses following an allergen challenge.[144] Milgrom et al[145] studied 317 asthmatics with moderate to severe asthma, all of whom were on inhaled GC with 10% also requiring chronic oral GC therapy. The subjects received high- or low-dose anti-IgE or placebo every 2 weeks for 20 weeks. The inhaled and oral GC doses were held stable during the first 12 weeks and then tapered as tolerated in the ensuing 8 weeks of the trial. High-dose anti-IgE was associated with improved symptom scores, fewer asthma exacerbations, and oral GC dose reduction compared to placebo. Anti-IgE has also recently been shown to be both safe and effective in reducing the inhaled GC requirement of children with moderate asthma.[145] Once available, studies utilizing anti-IgE in patients with refractory asthma should be performed to determine what role, if any, this compound has in the management of these patients.

Miscellaneous Alternative Agents. Oral gold (auranofin) has been used in the treatment of rheumatoid arthritis for several years. A few randomized, placebo-controlled trials have been performed in adults with GC-dependent asthma.[146] In general, they have shown auranofin to have modest GC-sparing effects. There is little published data on the safety and efficacy of oral gold in children with severe asthma. The most common reported adverse effect with oral gold is diarrhea. Nebulized lidocaine has also been reported to display GC-sparing effects. Two open-label studies,[147,148] one in children and the other in adults, found nebulized lidocaine permitted the majority of GC-dependent asthma patients to be completely tapered off of prednisone (5 of 6 children and 13 of 20 adults). The most common adverse effect of nebulized lidocaine is bronchospasm. As a result, a low dose should be administered under supervision when initiating this form of therapy. Lastly, there have yet to be any placebo-controlled studies demonstrating efficacy of nebulized lidocaine in the treatment of refractory asthma.

CONCLUSIONS

A subpopulation of asthma patients exists that, despite optimal pharmacologic therapy, displays evidence of ongoing disease. These patients with refractory asthma often require frequent systemic courses of GCs and a minority will require chronically administered oral GC to marginally control their disease. As a result, they often experience substantial morbidity from GC-associated adverse effects in addition to the morbidity associated with their disease. At the extreme end of refractory asthma are the GC-insensitive asthma patients who fail to adequately respond to aggressive courses of high-dose oral and inhaled GC therapy. Persistent immune activation and airway inflammation that is resistant to GC therapy appear to define the immunologic abnormality underlying refractory asthma. Although much insight into the pathogenesis of refractory asthma has been gained, several issues remain unresolved. First, ongoing airway inflammation is thought to contribute to refractory asthma, but at present there is no noninvasive way to determine the extent of airway inflammation. Second, significant airway remodeling can occur in children as young as 7 years of age. Structural changes to the airway may also significantly contribute to ongoing respiratory symptoms, persistent BHR, and diminished

14. Gennuso J, Epstein LH, Paluch RA, et al: The relationship between asthma and obesity in urban minority children and adolescents, *Arch Pediatr Adolesc Med* 152:1197-1200, 1998.

15. von Kries R, Hermann M, Grunert VP, et al: Is obesity a risk factor for childhood asthma? *Allergy* 56:318-322, 2001.

16. Chan MT, Leung DY, Szefler SJ, et al: Difficult-to-control asthma: clinical characteristics of steroid-insensitive asthma, *J Allergy Clin Immunol* 101:594-601, 1998.

17. Vrugt B, Wilson S, Underwood J, et al: Mucosal inflammation in severe glucocorticoid-dependent asthma, *Eur Respir J* 13:1245-1252, 1999.

18. Wenzel SE, Schwartz LB, Langmack EL, et al: Evidence that severe asthma can be divided pathologically into two inflammatory subtypes with distinct physiologic and clinical characteristics, *Am J Respir Crit Care Med* 160:1001-1008, 1999.

19. Payne DN, Adcock IM, Wilson NM, et al: Relationship between exhaled nitric oxide and mucosal eosinophilic inflammation in children with difficult asthma, after treatment with oral prednisolone, *Am J Respir Crit Care Med* 164:1376-1381, 2001.

20. Standards for the diagnosis and care of patients with chronic obstructive pulmonary disease (COPD) and asthma. This official statement of the American Thoracic Society was adopted by the ATS Board of Directors, November 1986, *Am Rev Respir Dis* 136:225-244, 1987.

21. Platts-Mills TA, Tovey ER, Mitchell EB, et al: Reduction of bronchial hyperreactivity during prolonged allergen avoidance, *Lancet* 2:675-678, 1982.

22. Simon HU, Grotzer M, Nikolaizik WH, et al: High altitude climate therapy reduces peripheral blood T lymphocyte activation, eosinophilia, and bronchial obstruction in children with house-dust mite allergic asthma, *Pediatr Pulmonol* 17:304-311, 1994.

23. Bousquet J, Michel FB: Specific immunotherapy in asthma: is it effective? *J Allergy Clin Immunol* 94:1-11, 1994.

24. Creticos PS: The consideration of immunotherapy in the treatment of allergic asthma, *J Allergy Clin Immunol* 105:S559-S574, 2000.

25. Reid MJ, Lockey RF, Turkeltaub PC, et al: Survey of fatalities from skin testing and immunotherapy 1985-1989, *J Allergy Clin Immunol* 92:6-15, 1993.

26. Tucci F, Resti M, Fontana R, et al: Gastroesophageal reflux and bronchial asthma: prevalence and effect of cisapride therapy, *J Pediatr Gastroenterol Nutr* 17:265-270, 1993.

27. Shapiro GG, Christie DL: Gastroesophageal reflux in steroid-dependent asthmatic youths, *Pediatrics* 63:207-212, 1979.

28. Sheikh S, Stephen T, Howell L, et al: Gastroesophageal reflux in infants with wheezing, *Pediatr Pulmonol* 28:181-186, 1999.

29. Balson BM, Kravitz EK, McGeady SJ: Diagnosis and treatment of gastroesophageal reflux in children and adolescents with severe asthma, *Ann Allergy Asthma Immunol* 81:159-164, 1998.

30. Field SK, Underwood M, Brant R, et al: Prevalence of gastroesophageal reflux symptoms in asthma, *Chest* 109:316-322, 1996.

31. Harding SM, Guzzo MR, Richter JE: 24-h esophageal pH testing in asthmatics: respiratory symptom correlation with esophageal acid events, *Chest* 115:654-659, 1999.

32. Bratton DL, Hanna PD: Gastroesophageal reflux in severe asthma. In Leung DYM, Szefler S, eds: *Severe asthma*, New York, 2001, Marcel Dekker.

33. Theodoropoulos DS, Ledford DK, Lockey RF, et al: Prevalence of upper respiratory symptoms in patients with symptomatic gastroesophageal reflux disease, *Am J Respir Crit Care Med* 164:72-76, 2001.

34. Jailwala JA, Shaker R: Oral and pharyngeal complications of gastroesophageal reflux disease: globus, dental erosions, and chronic sinusitis, *J Clin Gastroenterol* 30:S35-S38, 2000.

35. Ulualp SO, Toohill RJ, Hoffmann R, et al: Possible relationship of gastroesophagopharyngeal acid reflux with pathogenesis of chronic sinusitis, *Am J Rhinol* 13:197-202, 1999.

36. Halstead LA: Role of gastroesophageal reflux in pediatric upper airway disorders, *Otolaryngol Head Neck Surg* 120:208-214, 1999.

37. Stein MR, Baker J: Prevalence of gastroesophageal reflux (GER) in rhinitis: part II, *J Allergy Clin Immunol* 105:S198, 2000.

38. Irwin RS, Curley FJ, French CL: Difficult-to-control asthma: contributing factors and outcome of a systematic management protocol, *Chest* 103:1662-1669, 1993.

39. Harding SM, Guzzo MR, Richter JE: The prevalence of gastroesophageal reflux in asthma patients without reflux symptoms, *Am J Respir Crit Care Med* 162:34-39, 2000.

40. Gustafsson PM, Kjellman NI, Tibbling L: Oesophageal function and symptoms in moderate and severe asthma, *Acta Paediatr Scand* 75:729-736, 1986.

BOX 41-2

KEY CONCEPTS

Evaluation of the Child with Suspected Refractory Asthma

When evaluating any child with suspected refractory asthma, the following questions must be addressed:

- Does the patient have asthma?
- Are there medical conditions contributing to refractory asthma?
- What is the level of asthma severity and control?
- Is the current asthma medication regimen sufficient for control?
- Is inhaler technique adequate and is poor adherence a factor?
- Does the child have glucocorticoid-insensitive asthma?

---

lung function despite aggressive treatment with antiinflammatory agents; indeed, there may be GC-independent mechanisms involved in the pathogenesis of severe asthma that have yet to be identified. More information is needed on the pathology of refractory asthma to determine whether ultrastructural abnormalities are present that may be irreversible. In this regard it is possible that aggressive courses of antiinflammatory or immunomodulator therapy can suppress acute inflammation, but airway remodeling may predispose the patient to residual symptoms and the development of irreversible airway disease. What is clear is that more effort must be made to understand the cause of refractory asthma in children to guide pharmacotherapy for this challenging group of patients (Box 41-2).

REFERENCES

1. Robinson DS, Hamid Q, Ying S, et al: Predominant TH2-like bronchoalveolar T-lymphocyte population in atopic asthma, *N Engl J Med* 326:298-304, 1992.

2. Bousquet J, Chanez P, Lacoste JY, et al: Eosinophilic inflammation in asthma, *N Engl J Med* 323:1033-1039, 1990.

3. Expert Panel Report II: Guidelines for the Diagnosis and Management of Asthma, 1997.

4. International Consensus Report on Diagnosis and Treatment of Asthma, Pub No. 92-3091, 1992.

5. Szefler SJ: Glucocorticoid therapy for asthma: clinical pharmacology, *J Allergy Clin Immunol* 88:147-165, 1991.

6. Busse WW, Banks-Schlegel S, Wenzel SE: Pathophysiology of severe asthma, *J Allergy Clin Immunol* 106:1033-1042, 2000.

7. Billings J, Kretz SE, Rose R, et al: National Asthma Education and Prevention Program working group report on the financing of asthma care, *Am J Respir Crit Care Med* 154:S119-S130, 1996.

8. Bratton DL, Price M, Gavin L, et al: Impact of a multidisciplinary day program on disease and healthcare costs in children and adolescents with severe asthma: a two-year follow-up study, *Pediatr Pulmonol* 31:177-189, 2001.

9. Van Ganse E, Boissel JP, Gormand F, et al: Level of control and hospital contacts in persistent asthma, *J Asthma* 38:637-643, 2001.

10. Bacharier LB, Mauger DT, Lemanske RF, et al: Classifying asthma severity in children: is measuring lung function helpful? *J Allergy Clin Immunol* 109:S266, 2002.

11. Jenkins HA, Szefler SJ, Covar R, et al: New insight into the clinical characteristics of adults vs. children with severe asthma, *J Allergy Clin Immunol* 109: S353, 2002.

12. Fuhlbrigge AL, Kitch BT, Paltiel D, et al: FEV_1 is associated with risk of asthma attacks in a pediatric population, *J Allergy Clin Immunol* 107:61-67, 2001.

13. Beckett WS, Jacobs DR Jr, Yu X, et al: Asthma is associated with weight gain in females but not males, independent of physical activity, *Am J Respir Crit Care Med* 164:2045-2050, 2001.

41. Martin ME, Grunstein MM, Larsen GL: The relationship of gastro-esophageal reflux to nocturnal wheezing in children with asthma, *Ann Allergy* 49:318-322, 1982.

42. Cuttitta G, Cibella F, Visconti A, et al: Spontaneous gastroesophageal reflux and airway patency during the night in adult asthmatics, *Am J Respir Crit Care Med* 161:177-181, 2000.

43. Lodi U, Harding SM, Coghlan HC, et al: Autonomic regulation in asthmatics with gastroesophageal reflux, *Chest* 111:65-70, 1997.

44. Harding SM: Gastroesophageal reflux and asthma: insight into the association, *J Allergy Clin Immunol* 104:251-259, 1999.

45. Hamamoto J, Kohrogi H, Kawano O, et al: Esophageal stimulation by hydrochloric acid causes neurogenic inflammation in the airways in guinea pigs, *J Appl Physiol* 82:738-745, 1997.

46. Jack CIA, Calverley PMA, Donnelly RJ, et al: Simultaneous tracheal and oesophageal pH measurements in asthmatic patients with gastro-oesophageal reflux, *Thorax* 50:201-204, 1995.

47. Field SK, Sutherland LR: Does medical antireflux therapy improve asthma in asthmatics with gastroesophageal reflux? A critical review of the literature, *Chest* 114:275-283, 1998.

48. Levin TR, Sperling RM, McQuaid KR: Omeprazole improves peak expiratory flow rate and quality of life in asthmatics with gastroesophageal reflux, *Am J Gastroenterol* 93:1060-1063, 1998.

49. Kiljander TO, Salomaa ER, Hietanen EK, et al: Gastroesophageal reflux in asthmatics: a double-blind, placebo-controlled crossover study with omeprazole, *Chest* 116:1257-1264, 1999.

50. Meier JH, McNally PR, Punja M, et al: Does omeprazole (Prilosec) improve respiratory function in asthmatics with gastroesophageal reflux? A double-blind, placebo-controlled crossover study, *Dig Dis Sci* 39:2127-2133, 1994.

51. Harding SM, Richter JE, Guzzo MR, et al: Asthma and gastroesophageal reflux: acid suppressive therapy improves asthma outcome, *Am J Med* 100:395-405, 1996.

52. Mahajan L, Wyllie R, Oliva L, et al: Reproducibility of 24-hour intra-esophageal pH monitoring in pediatric patients, *Pediatrics* 101:260-263, 1998.

53. Johnson LF, Demeester TR: Twenty-four-hour pH monitoring of the distal esophagusL a quantitative measure of gastroesophageal reflux, *Am J Gastroenterol* 62:325-332, 1974.

54. Richter JE, Bradley LA, DeMeester TR, et al: Normal 24-hr ambulatory esophageal pH values: influence of study center, pH electrode, age, and gender, *Dig Dis Sci* 37:849-856, 1992.

55. Chun AH, Erdman K, Zhang Y, et al: Effect on bioavailability of admixing the contents of lansoprazole capsules with selected soft foods, *Clin Ther* 22:231-236, 2000.

56. Peghini PL, Katz PO, Bracy NA, et al: Nocturnal recovery of gastric acid secretion with twice-daily dosing of proton pump inhibitors, *Am J Gastroenterol* 93:763-767, 1998.

57. Kiljander T, Salomaa ER, Hietanen E, et al: Asthma and gastro-oesophageal reflux: can the response to anti-reflux therapy be predicted? *Respir Med* 95:387-392, 2001.

58. Togias AG: Systemic immunologic and inflammatory aspects of allergic rhinitis, *J Allergy Clin Immunol* 106:S247-S250, 2000.

59. Christodoulopoulos P, Cameron L, Durham S, et al: Molecular pathology of allergic disease. II: Upper airway disease, *J Allergy Clin Immunol* 105:211-223, 2000.

60. Leone C, Teodoro C, Pelucchi A, et al: Bronchial responsiveness and airway inflammation in patients with nonallergic rhinitis with eosinophilia syndrome, *J Allergy Clin Immunol* 100:775-780, 1997.

61. Bucca C, Rolla G, Scappaticci E, et al: Extrathoracic and intrathoracic airway responsiveness in sinusitis, *J Allergy Clin Immunol* 95:52-59, 1995.

62. Corren J, Adinoff AD, Irvin CG: Changes in bronchial responsiveness following nasal provocation with allergen, *J Allergy Clin Immunol* 89:611-618, 1992.

63. Braunstahl GJ, Overbeek SE, Kleinjan A, et al: Nasal allergen provocation induces adhesion molecule expression and tissue eosinophilia in upper and lower airways, *J Allergy Clin Immunol* 107:469-476, 2001.

64. Watson WTA, Becker AB, Simons FE: Treatment of allergic rhinitis with intranasal corticosteroids in patients with mild asthma: effect on lower airway responsiveness, *J Allergy Clin Immunol* 91:97-101, 1993.

65. Foresi A, Teodoro C, Leone C, et al: Eosinophil apoptosis in induced sputum from patients with seasonal allergic rhinitis and with asymptomatic and symptomatic asthma, *Ann Allergy Asthma Immunol* 84:411-416, 2000.

66. Corren J, Adinoff AD, Buchmeier AD, et al: Nasal beclomethasone prevents the seasonal increase in bronchial responsiveness in patients with allergic rhinitis and asthma, *J Allergy Clin Immunol* 90:250-256, 1992.

67. Aubier M, Levy J, Clerici C, et al: Different effects of nasal and bronchial glucocorticosteroid administration on bronchial hyperresponsiveness in patients with allergic rhinitis, *Am Rev Respir Dis* 146:122-126, 1992.

68. Welsh PW, Stricker WE, Chu C-P, et al: Efficacy of beclomethasone nasal solution, flunisolide, and cromolyn in relieving symptoms of ragweed allergy, *Mayo Clin Proc* 62:125-134, 1987.

69. Berquist WE, Rachelefsky GS, Kadden M: Gastroesophageal reflux-associated recurrent pneumonia and chronic asthma in children, *Pediatrics* 68:29-35, 1981.

70. Rachelefsky GS, Katz RM, Siegel SC: Chronic sinus disease with associated reactive airway disease in children, *Pediatrics* 73:526-529, 1984.

71. Rachelefsky CS, Goldberg M, Katz RM, et al: Sinus disease in children with respiratory allergy, *J Allergy Clin Immunol* 61:310-314, 1978.

72. Foresi A, Pelucchi A, Gherson G, et al: Once-daily intranasal fluticasone propionate (200 micrograms) reduces nasal symptoms and inflammation but also attenuates the increase in bronchial responsiveness during the pollen season in allergic rhinitis, *J Allergy Clin Immunol* 98:274-282, 1996.

73. McAlister WH, Lusk R, Muntz HR: Comparison of plain radiographs and coronal CT scans in infants and children with recurrent sinusitis, *Am J Roentgenol* 153:1259-1264, 1989.

74. Christopher KL, Wood RP II, Eckert RC, et al: Vocal-cord dysfunction presenting as asthma, *N Engl J Med* 308:1566-1570, 1983.

75. Corren J, Newman KB: Vocal cord dysfunction mimicking bronchial asthma, *Postgrad Med* 92:153-156, 1992.

76. Thomas PS, Geddes DM, Barnes PJ: Pseudo-steroid resistant asthma, *Thorax* 54:352-356, 1999.

77. Brugman SM, Howell JH, Mahler JL, et al: The spectrum of pediatric vocal cord dysfunction, *Am Rev Respir Dis* 149:A353, 1994.

78. Newman KB, Mason UG III, Schmaling KB: Clinical features of vocal cord dysfunction, *Am J Respir Crit Care Med* 152:1382-1386, 1995.

79. Elshami AA, Tino G: Coexistent asthma and functional upper airway obstruction. Case reports and review of the literature, *Chest* 110:1358-1361, 1996.

80. Martin SJ, Finucane DM, Amarante-Mendes GP, et al: Phosphatidylserine externalization during CD95-induced apoptosis of cells and cytoplasts requires ICE/CED-3 protease activity, *J Biol Chem* 271:28753-28756, 1996.

81. Meltzer EO, Orgel HA, Kemp JP, et al: Vocal cord dysfunction in a child with asthma, *J Asthma* 28:141-145, 1991.

82. Wood RP II, Jafek BW, Cherniack RM: Laryngeal dysfunction and pulmonary disorder, *Otolaryngol Head Neck Surg* 94:374-378, 1986.

83. Barnes PJ, Woolcock AJ: Difficult asthma, *Eur Respir J* 12:1209-1218, 1998.

84. Anbar RD, Hehir DA: Hypnosis as a diagnostic modality for vocal cord dysfunction, *Pediatrics* 106:E81, 2000.

85. Archer GJ, Hoyle JL, McCluskey A, et al: Inspiratory vocal cord dysfunction: a new approach in treatment, *Eur Respir J* 15:617-618, 2000.

86. Weir M: Vocal cord dysfunction mimics asthma and may respond to heliox, *Clin Pediatr (Phila)* 41:37-41, 2002.

87. Martin RJ: Managing the patient with intractable asthma, *Hosp Pract* 31:61-64, 69-74, 79-80, 1996.

88. Sears MR, Taylor DR, Print CG, et al: Regular inhaled β-agonist treatment in bronchial asthma, *Lancet* 336:1391-1396, 1990.

89. Spitzer WO, Suissa S, Ernst P, et al: The use of β-agonists and the risk of death and near death from asthma, *N Engl J Med* 326:501-506, 1992.

90. Greening AP, Ind PW, Northfield M, et al: Added salmeterol versus higher-dose corticosteroid in asthma patients with symptoms on existing inhaled corticosteroid. Allen & Hanburys Limited UK Study Group, *Lancet* 344:219-224, 1994.

91. Woolcock A, Lundback B, Ringdal N, et al: Comparison of addition of salmeterol to inhaled steroids with doubling of the dose of inhaled steroids, *Am J Respir Crit Care Med* 153:1481-1488, 1996.

92. Kavuru M, Melamed J, Gross G, et al: Salmeterol and fluticasone propionate combined in a new powder inhalation device for the treatment of asthma: a randomized, double- blind, placebo-controlled trial, *J Allergy Clin Immunol* 105:1108-1116, 2000.

93. O'Byrne PM, Barnes PJ, Rodriguez-Roisin R, et al: Low-dose inhaled budesonide and formoterol in mild persistent asthma: the OPTIMA randomized trial, *Am J Respir Crit Care Med* 164:1392-1397, 2001.

94. Cameron SJ, Cooper EJ, Crompton GK, et al: Substitution of beclomethasone aerosol for oral prednisolone in the treatment of chronic asthma, *Br Med J* 4:205-207, 1973.

95. Tarlo SM, Broder I, Davies GM, et al: Six-month double-blind, controlled trial of high-dose, concentrated beclomethasone dipropionate in the treatment of severe chronic asthma, *Chest* 93:998-1002, 1988.

96. Whelan AM, Hahn NW: Optimizing drug delivery from metered-dose inhalers, *DICP* 25:638-645, 1991.

97. Newman SP: Therapeutic aerosols. In Clarke SW, Pavia D, eds: *Aerosols and the lung: clinical and experimental aspects,* London, 1984, Butterworths.

98. Toogood JH, Jennings B, Baskerville J, et al: Clinical use of spacer systems for corticosteroid inhalation therapy: a preliminary analysis, *Eur J Respir Dis Suppl* 122:100-107, 1982.

99. Rand CS, Wise RA, Nides M, et al: Metered-dose inhaler adherence in a clinical trial, *Am Rev Respir Dis* 146:1559-1564, 1992.

100. Anderson RJ, Kirk LM: Methods of improving patient compliance in chronic disease states, *Arch Intern Med* 142:1673-1675, 1982.

101. Mellins RB, Evans D, Zimmerman B, et al: Patient compliance. Are we wasting our time and don't know it? *Am Rev Respir Dis* 146:1376-1377, 1992.

102. Kelloway JS, Wyatt RA, Adlis SA: Comparison of patients' compliance with prescribed oral and inhaled asthma medications, *Arch Intern Med* 154:1349-1352, 1994.

103. Milgrom H, Bender B, Ackerson L, et al: Noncompliance and treatment failure in children with asthma, *J Allergy Clin Immunol* 98:1051-1057, 1996.

104. Spahn JD, Leung DYM, Surs W, et al: Reduced glucocorticoid binding affinity in asthma is related to ongoing allergic inflammation, *Am J Respir Crit Care Med* 151:1709-1714, 1995.

105. Hill MR, Szefler SJ, Ball BD, et al: Monitoring glucocorticoid therapy: a pharmacokinetic approach, *Clin Pharmacol Ther* 48:390-398, 1990.

106. Ebling WF, Szefler SJ, Jusko WJ: Analysis of cortisol, methylprednisolone, and methylprednisolone hemisuccinate: absence of effects of troleandomycin on ester hydrolysis, *J Chromatogr* 305:271-280, 1984.

107. Bartoszek M, Brenner AM, Szefler SJ: Prednisolone and methylprednisolone kinetics in children receiving anticonvulsant therapy, *Clin Pharmacol Ther* 42:424-432, 1987.

108. Udwadia ZF, Sridhar G, Beveridge CJ, et al: Catastrophic deterioration in asthma induced by rifampicin in steroid-dependent asthma, *Respir Med* 87:629, 1993.

109. Lane SJ, Arm JP, Staynov DZ, et al: Chemical mutational analysis of the human glucocorticoid receptor cDNA in glucocorticoid-resistant bronchial asthma, *Am J Respir Cell Mol Biol* 11:42-48, 1994.

110. Sher ER, Leung DYM, Surs W, et al: Steroid-resistant asthma: cellular mechanisms contributing to inadequate response to glucocorticoid therapy, *J Clin Invest* 93:33-39, 1994.

111. Kam JC, Szefler SJ, Surs W, et al: Combination IL-2 and IL-4 reduces glucocorticoid receptor-binding affinity and T cell response to glucocorticoids, *J Immunol* 151:1-7, 1993.

112. Leung DYM, Martin RJ, Szefler SJ, et al: Dysregulation of interleukin 4, interleukin 5, and interferon gamma gene expression in steroid-resistant asthma, *J Exp Med* 181:33-40, 1995.

113. Spahn JD, Szefler SJ, Surs W, et al: A novel action of IL-13: induction of diminished monocyte glucocorticoid receptor-binding affinity, *J Immunol* 157:2654-2659, 1996.

114. Adcock IM, Lane SJ, Brown CR, et al: Abnormal glucocorticoid receptor-activator protein 1 interaction in steroid-resistant asthma, *J Exp Med* 182:1951-1958, 1995.

115. Adcock IM, Lane SJ, Brown CR, et al: Differences in binding of glucocorticoid receptor to DNA in steroid-resistant asthma, *J Immunol* 154:3500-3505, 1995.

116. Leung DYM, Hamid Q, Vottero A, et al: Association of glucocorticoid insensitivity with increased expression of glucocorticoid receptor beta, *J Exp Med* 186:1567-1574, 1997.

117. Bamberger CM, Bamberger AM, de Castro M, et al: Glucocorticoid receptor beta, a potential endogenous inhibitor of glucocorticoid action in humans, *J Clin Invest* 95:2435-2441, 1995.

118. Bye MR, Kerstein D, Barsh E: The importance of spirometry in the assessment of childhood asthma, *Am J Dis Child* 146:977-978, 1992.

119. Martin RJ, Blager FB, Gay M, et al: Paradoxic vocal cord motion in presumed asthmatics, *Semin Respir Med* 8:332-337, 1987.

120. Liu AH, Brugman SM, Schaeffer EB, et al: Reduced lung elasticity may characterize children with severe asthma, *Am Rev Respir Dis* 141:A906, 1990.

121. Gelb AF, Licuanan J, Shinar CM, et al: Unsuspected loss of lung elastic recoil in chronic persistent asthma, *Chest* 121:715-721, 2002.

122. Szefler SJ: Alternative therapy in severe asthma: rationale and guidelines for applications, *Allergy Principles and Practice Update* 11:1991.

123. Covar RA, Leung DY, McCormick D, et al: Risk factors associated with glucocorticoid-induced adverse effects in children with severe asthma, *J Allergy Clin Immunol* 106:651-659, 2000.

124. Lipworth BJ: New perspectives on inhaled drug delivery and systemic bioactivity, *Thorax* 50:105-110, 1995.

125. Noonan M, Chervinsky P, Busse WW, et al: Fluticasone propionate reduces oral prednisone use while it improves asthma control and quality of life, *Am J Respir Crit Care Med* 152:1467-1473, 1995.

126. Nelson HS, Bernstein IL, Fink J, et al: Oral glucocorticosteroid-sparing effect of budesonide administered by Turbuhaler: a double-blind, placebo-controlled study in adults with moderate-to-severe chronic asthma. Pulmicort Turbuhaler Study Group, *Chest* 113:1264-1271, 1998.

127. Fish JE, Karpel JP, Craig TJ, et al: Inhaled mometasone furoate reduces oral prednisone requirements while improving respiratory function and health-related quality of life in patients with severe persistent asthma, *J Allergy Clin Immunol* 106:852-860, 2000.

128. Hummel S, Lehtonen L: Comparison of oral-steroid sparing by high-dose and low-dose inhaled steroid in maintenance treatment of severe asthma, *Lancet* 340:1483-1487, 1992.

129. Malmstrom K, Rodriguez-Gomez G, Guerra J, et al: Oral montelukast, inhaled beclomethasone, and placebo for chronic asthma. A randomized, controlled trial. Montelukast/Beclomethasone Study Group, *Ann Intern Med* 130:487-495, 1999.

130. Lofdahl CG, Reiss TF, Leff JA, et al: Randomised, placebo-controlled trial of effect of a leukotriene receptor antagonist, montelukast, on tapering inhaled corticosteroids in asthmatic patients, *Br Med J* 319:87-90, 1999.

131. Robinson DS, Campbell D, Barnes PJ: Addition of leukotriene antagonists to therapy in chronic persistent asthma: a randomised double-blind placebo-controlled trial, *Lancet* 357:2007-2011, 2001.

132. Weinberger M: The value of theophylline for asthma, *Ann Allergy* 63:1-3, 1989.

133. Brenner M, Berkowitz R, Marshall N, et al: Need for theophylline in severe steroid-requiring asthmatics, *Clin Allergy* 18:143-150, 1988.

134. Hendeles L, Weinberger M, Szefler S, et al: Safety and efficacy of theophylline in children with asthma, *J Pediatr* 120:177-183, 1992.

135. Mullarkey MF, Blumenstein BA, Andrade WP, et al: Methotrexate in the treatment of corticosteroid-dependent asthma. A double-blind crossover study, *N Engl J Med* 318:603-607, 1988.

136. Erzurum SC, Leff JA, Cochran JE, et al: Lack of benefit of methotrexate in severe, steroid-dependent asthma. A double-blind, placebo-controlled study, *Ann Intern Med* 114:353-360, 1991.

137. Aaron SD, Dales RE, Pham B: Management of steroid-dependent asthma with methotrexate: a meta-analysis of randomized clinical trials, *Respir Med* 92:1059-1065, 1998.

138. Alexander AG, Barnes NC, Kay AB: Trial of cyclosporin in corticosteroid-dependent chronic severe asthma, *Lancet* 339:324-328, 1992.

139. Nizankowska E, Soja J, Pinis G, et al: Treatment of steroid-dependent bronchial asthma with cyclosporin, *Eur Respir J* 8:1091-1099, 1995.

140. Mazer BD, Gelfand EW: An open-label study of high-dose intravenous immunoglobulin in severe childhood asthma, *J Allergy Clin Immunol* 87:976-983, 1991.

141. Spahn JD, Leung DY, Chan MT, et al: Mechanisms of glucocorticoid reduction in asthmatic subjects treated with intravenous immunoglobulin, *J Allergy Clin Immunol* 103:421-426, 1999.

142. Salmun LM, Barlan I, Wolf HM, et al: Effect of intravenous immunoglobulin on steroid consumption in patients with severe asthma: a double-blind, placebo-controlled, randomized trial, *J Allergy Clin Immunol* 103:810-815, 1999.

143. Kishiyama JL, Valacer D, Cunningham-Rundles C, et al: A multicenter, randomized, double-blind, placebo-controlled trial of high-dose intravenous immunoglobulin for oral corticosteroid-dependent asthma, *Clin Immunol* 91:126-133, 1999.

144. Fahy JV, Fleming HE, Wong HH, et al: The effect of an anti-IgE monoclonal antibody on the early- and late-phase responses to allergen inhalation in asthmatic subjects, *Am J Respir Crit Care Med* 155:1828-1834, 1997.

145. Milgrom H, Berger W, Nayak A, et al: Treatment of childhood asthma with anti-immunoglobulin E antibody (omalizumab), *Pediatrics* 108:E36, 2001.

146. Bernstein IL, Bernstein DI, Dubb JW, et al: A placebo-controlled multicenter study of auranofin in the treatment of patients with corticosteroid-dependent asthma. Auranofin Multicenter Drug Trial, *J Allergy Clin Immunol* 98:317-324, 1996.

147. Decco ML, Neeno TA, Hunt LW, et al: Nebulized lidocaine in the treatment of severe asthma in children: a pilot study, *Ann Allergy Asthma Immunol* 82:29-32, 1999.

148. Hunt LW, Swedlund HA, Gleich GJ: Effect of nebulized lidocaine on severe glucocorticoid-dependent asthma, *Mayo Clin Proc* 71:361-368, 1996.

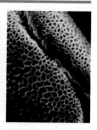

CHAPTER 42

Promoting Adherence and Effective Self-Management in Patients with Asthma

BRUCE G. BENDER ■ THOMAS L. CREER

Treatment adherence with asthma regimens, as with virtually all chronic medical conditions, is often poor. The term *adherence* is most frequently reserved to reflect medication use. However, even *medication use* consists of several behaviors: filling prescriptions, using correct inhalation techniques, and taking the correct dose at correct time intervals. In the case of beta-agonist medication, the behaviors required of the patient may also include making judgments about inhalation frequency and interval in relationship to perceived symptoms and peak flow measurements. Effective asthma self-management also involves other behaviors, including recording peak flow measurements, avoiding potential triggers of attacks, observing optimal inhalation techniques, recognizing symptom changes, and communicating appropriately with the health caregiver.

For the most part the term *adherence* is used in the recent literature to reflect the degree to which patients with asthma take their medication as prescribed. Most studies have focused on daily controller medication regimens. Adherence to such treatments averages about 50% or less for chronic conditions in general,[1] including patients with asthma[2,3]; this definition of adherence means that about half of the prescribed medication was taken, although it does not necessarily signify that it was taken in the appropriate manner. In addition, the report of 50% medication adherence reflects the average of groups of patients studied but does not translate into a uniform pattern of taking every other dose of medication. Individual adherence patterns include widely varying behaviors, with some patients taking close to all their medications at the appropriate time and others taking almost no medication.[3] Individual adherence fluctuates greatly over time, often with periods of drug "holidays" during which patients take no medication for varying periods, sometimes several days at a time.[4]

HOW MUCH ADHERENCE IS SUFFICIENT?

Medication adherence sufficient to establish consistent asthma control occurs only in 26% to 52% of adult patients.[5] Depending on the duration of action and the drug side effects profile, drug holidays may have several potential consequences, including waning drug action, hazardous rebound effects when administration stops abruptly, and overdose effects when administration of full-strength drugs suddenly resumes.[4] In studies of metered-dose inhaler (MDI) use among children with asthma, inhalers were not used on 48% of study days and abandonment of medication typically occurred for several consecutive days.[6] The consequences of such start-and-stop adherence patterns are unknown. Time to onset of the effectiveness of inhaled corticosteroids in the treatment of mild-to-moderate asthma is about 3 weeks, with faster impact (3 days) reflected on morning peak expiratory flow values in patients with severe asthma.[7] It remains to be determined how varying patterns of adherence translate into asthma control and whether, for example, control in patients with relatively high adherence who fail to use their medication for 1 week or longer is poorer than in patients who use less total medication but with better regularity.[8]

WHAT HAPPENS WHEN PATIENTS ARE NONADHERENT?

While the assumption that underuse of asthma controller medication can result in less control over the disorder is accurate, conclusions about the amount of medication required by any individual patient are difficult to establish largely because of individual variations in disease characteristics, medication requirements, and drug metabolism rates. The prevailing standard, as reflected by the Expert Panel guidelines for the diagnosis and management of asthma, is that increased medication administration is the correct response to inadequate symptom control.[9] The potential benefit of medication escalation on the part of the physician is realized only if the patient responds by adhering to the new regimen. Although some studies have defined nonadherence as greater than 75% of medication taken, it is impossible to establish a minimum level of adherence that is sufficient for all patients. Evidence exists that inhaled cortocosteroids (ICSs) are highly effective in controlling asthma, that some benefit exists even at relatively low dosing frequency, and that a dose-response relationship exists between degree of adherence and degree of benefit. Suissa et al,[10] for example, conducted a nested case-control study of patients with severe asthma and found that decreasing number of ICS pharmacy refills was associated with increasing risk of death from asthma. As few as three ICS canisters per year reduced risk by one half, with increasing protection gained as refills increased up to a full adherence level of 12 canisters per year. Clearly, as adherence levels drop, asthma becomes less controlled. For example, in a 3-month study, children with a median ICS adherence of 14% had asthma exacerbations requiring urgent office visits and oral steroid bursts, whereas those with adherence levels of 68% remained medically stable.[11] Nonadherent adults with asthma had more airway obstruction than adherent patients.[12] Children who did not adhere to their asthma treatment regimen had poorer asthma control and required more urgent-care visits, steroid bursts, and hospitalizations.[11,13] Tragically, nonadherence has been associated with asthma-related deaths in children, particularly where psychologic dysfunction was observed in the patient or the patient's family.[14]

WHAT CAN BE DONE ABOUT THIS PROBLEM?

The problem of treatment nonadherence has been well recognized and documented; in turn, numerous efforts have been directed at changing patient behavior, often through the development and implementation of patient education programs. However, changing patient adherence behavior through patient education has not been easy. Two meta-analyses combining multiple reports about patient education programs reached opposing conclusions, with one finding that systematic asthma education can change clinical outcomes[15] and the other analysis concluding that asthma education did not.[16] One group found that patient education improved adherence and clinical outcome in their original report[17] but because of factors to be described were unable to replicate their findings in a second study.[18] Patient scores on asthma knowledge questionnaires do not correlate well with medication adherence.[19] Although a lack of knowledge about asthma predicts poor adherence, the relationship between knowledge and appropriate behaviors is nonlinear. Asthma knowledge is a necessary but insufficient factor in adherence. Once asthma knowledge is acquired, for example, the translation of knowledge into performance becomes necessary.[20] Clearly, educating and motivating patients to manage their asthma effectively involve more than simply imparting information. For patients to have sufficient knowledge, skill, and motivation to perform the daily tasks necessary to control their disease, they must receive sufficient self-management training. The Expert Panel guidelines recognize and address this with the following recommendations[9]: (1) patient education beginning at the time of diagnosis and integrated into every step of asthma care; (2) patient education provided by all members of the team, including behavioral scientists; (3) teaching asthma self-management skills by tailoring information and treatment to fit the needs of each patient; (4) teaching and reinforcing at every opportunity such behavioral skills as inhaler use, self-monitoring, and environmental control; (5) joint development of treatment plans by team members and patients; (6) encouragement of an active partnership by providing written self-management and individualized asthma action strategies to patients; (7) encouraging adherence to the treatment plan jointly developed by the interdisciplinary team and patients encouragement; and (8) referral to a psychologist, psychiatrist, social worker, or other mental health professional when the existence of a psychologic problem prevents successful treatment.

ROLE OF PHYSICIANS AND OTHER HEALTH CARE PROVIDERS IN TRAINING PATIENTS TO MANAGE THEIR ASTHMA

Effective asthma self-management training cannot occur without commitment help from the health caregiving team. However, not all physicians provide asthma care consistent with the Expert Panel guidelines, and even those who do may be unaware of or unwilling to address the significant problem of treatment nonadherence.[21] Many patients with asthma are unwilling to participate in an asthma self-management training program, and many health care systems are reluctant to absorb the costs of such programs; thus, for the majority of patients, the sole opportunity for education and motivation must be found in the health caregiver's office. The Expert Panel guidelines[9] recognize that the patient-physician relationship is essential to treatment success and emphasize the development of a partnership between patient and physician within which discussion about treatment goals and progress will occur. In such a relationship, the caregiver bears responsibility both to provide appropriate treatment and to impress on patients the importance of adherence to prescribed treatments.

Unfortunately, many patients with asthma receive inadequate treatment. Of 433 children admitted to the emergency department (ED) of a Philadelphia hospital, less than half received asthma care consistent with the Expert Panel guidelines that included daily antiinflammatory therapy (38%), use of a peak flow meter (34%), and a written action plan (29%).[22] In a group of 80 Medicaid asthma patients who were repeat users of the ED or overnight hospitalization, only 46% had been prescribed inhaled steroids and only 43% had a written action plan.[23] Less than half of Tennessee Medicaid children had an oral corticosteroid prescription filled following an ED visit or a hospitalization for asthma.[24] Many physicians have insufficient familiarity with the Expert Panel guidelines,[25] and others disagree with or are unwilling to follow them.[26]

When physicians are uncertain about the appropriate treatment for asthma, it is unlikely that they convey a message of confidence in the drug they are prescribing, and consequently it is unlikely that the patient will adhere to the treatment. Patients are more likely to follow a treatment plan if they have sufficient faith in the physician and the treatment.[27] There is evidence that training programs can improve physician adherence to treatment guidelines and, secondarily, may improve patient medication adherence and consequently treatment outcomes. A total of 777 continuing medical education programs for physicians were, on aggregate, effective in improving physician adherence to appropriate standards of preventive medicine.[28] Even a brief verbal presentation to ED residents on state-of-the-art therapies improved the frequency of prescribing appropriate asthma medications.[29] A tutorial directed at helping the physician recognize and address nonadherence resulted in greater blood pressure control relative to patients whose physicians did not receive the tutorial.[30]

It is easier to change how physicians prescribe drugs than to affect how they communicate with and motivate patients. A comprehensive comparison of physician education programs arrived at two important conclusions.[28] First, changes in physicians' clinical management and patient counseling skills were more difficult to achieve than changes in prescribing practices. Second, changes in patient outcomes, including improved disease control and reduced health care costs, were more likely to result from programs that included workshops providing case discussion and rehearsal of practice behaviors than from didactic programs. One study demonstrated change in physician behavior by randomizing 69 primary care physicians to either a communication skills training group or a control group. Patients of physicians who received the intervention, consisting of training in recognizing and addressing patient distress, demonstrated a greater reduction in psychologic distress and a short-term reduction in health care utilization.[31] A program aimed at physicians who treat diabetes reported that patients of residents who were randomized to an intervention (which included focused seminars conducted by specialists, small groups discussions, and emphasis toward patient attitudes, beliefs, skills, and clinical support systems) had improved fasting plasma glucose relative to control patients.[32] The disease control improvements were even greater when physician education was combined with programmatic patient education.[32]

Studies of patients with asthma have revealed significantly improved outcomes when teaching and communication skills were taught to physicians.[33-35] Seventy-four general practitioners in Ann Arbor, Michigan, and New York City were randomized to an intervention or control condition.[33] Those in the intervention condition received training to improve ability to communicate effectively, understand patient behavior, create a supportive atmosphere, and educate patients in problem solving and asthma management. In contrast to the control group, patients of physicians in the intervention group received more oral and written information directing them in modifying their therapy even though the average amount of time spent per patient was no greater than in the control group. Patients in this group were also more likely to receive a prescription for inhaled antiinflammatory medication, which resulted in a significant decrease in office visits, ED visits, and hospitalizations during the 2-year follow up.[33]

How Can Health Care Providers Educate and Motivate Patients to Manage Their Asthma?

Successful self-management of asthma occurs when patients are well informed about their asthma, understand their own behaviors will determine successful outcomes, and are motivated to perform these behaviors. Three processes are involved; they must occur in order for effective self-management to improve disease control: preparation, acquisition and performance of asthma self-management, and maintenance of self-management skills.

Preparation

Before health care providers and patients can mutually agree on steps that should be performed to manage the patient's asthma, several preparatory steps are required. First, patient-provider communication must be established. By doing so, the expectations of both health care providers and patients can be clearly spelled out. For the most part, physicians who regularly treat asthma are apt to follow treatment guidelines promulgated by the National Institutes of Health.[9,36] These health care providers actively encourage a partnership with patients by promoting open communication, individualizing treatment plans, and emphasizing goals and outcomes of treatment. These expectations may be foreign to patients who, as in the treatment of an acute condition, may anticipate relying on medical care only to manage and alleviate their asthma.

Second, health care providers must be certain patients possess knowledge of both asthma and the role of asthma medications, including both controller and relief drugs; and have appropriate skills necessary to avoid and to manage asthma exacerbations. It is here where individual differences between patients become apparent. For example, one group of investigators found that in attempting to replicate an earlier study, the baseline of existing asthma knowledge was much higher (e.g., the patients were more knowledgeable about asthma and its management) when they attempted to replicate an earlier study.[18] Although intervention resulted in less robust outcomes, it revealed the equally impressive finding that patients had already learned about asthma and its treatment before entering the study and were therefore better prepared for acquiring and performing asthma self-management skills. On the other hand, another group of investigators found that while studying factors related to the use of urgent-care services for asthma, 49% of 409 patients disagreed with the statement that "asthma is a lifelong condition with no cure."[37] Taken together, the two studies illustrate the range of patient knowledge regarding asthma and its treatment before self-management training. Physicians or other health care providers may wish patients to attend formal educational programs, if available, before introducing them to asthma self-management. In many cases, however, formal patient education programs may be unavailable, in which case physicians and other health care providers must teach patients the knowledge about asthma they need and the self-management skills they must perform to become effective partners in the management of asthma.

Third, patients with an acute disorder expect the total alleviation of problems such as influenza or a broken bone. Such expectations are unrealistic with asthma. Despite the combined effort of health care providers and patients, there remains a possibility that a particular treatment will not work or that physiologic or environmental changes may necessitate revamping a treatment regimen.

Fourth, there must be open and honest exchange of information regarding how the patient perceives and treats his or her asthma. Knowledge of the patient's perception of asthma severity, frequency of nocturnal asthma, medication use, and number of hospitalizations or ED visits for asthma is invaluable in developing treatment plans. Knowledge regarding a patient's reliance on an ED for management of an asthma attack is particularly useful in that while the patient's behavior has often been reinforced by quick relief from asthma, the practice of ED use is both costly and amenable to behavioral change.[38]

Finally, setting common goals involves looking at the comprehensive picture of a patient's asthma. Relying solely on medications to manage the asthma, for example, may prove both expensive and ineffective. All the ramifications of establishing control over asthma must be considered, including the avoidance of attacks by removing or escaping from environmental triggers.

Acquisition and Performance of Asthma Self-Management

Several processes are involved in the self-management of chronic conditions, including asthma.[39] These processes include (1) goal selection, (2) information collection, (3) information processing and evaluation, (4) decision-making, (5) action, and (6) self-reaction. These processes, as well as the psychologic and behavioral skills entailed in each process, provide the framework for our discussion.

Goal Selection. Goal selection takes place only after the preparatory steps described above. It is imperative that patients have a solid knowledge of asthma and how it can be managed; they cannot be equal partners in the treatment and control of their asthma if they cannot personally contribute to goal selection. By possessing such knowledge, patients can also actively help develop a self-management program that is tailored specifically for their asthma and its management.

Once goals for asthma treatment have been jointly set by patients and health care providers, they should be precisely described in writing. What results is an asthma action plan, a blueprint for treatment of asthma that can be followed by patients, their families, and health care providers. The written plan explicitly defines not only goals but also the processes by which they will be achieved. It can be consulted over time and serve as a prompt to guide future actions. Three additional consequences can emerge from establishing and spelling out treatment goals.[39] First, they establish what is considered as the optimal degree of treatment of a patient's asthma that can be achieved with a minimal amount of medications and environmental change. Knowledge of the patient's asthma, by both the patient and the patient's physician, permits a precise tailoring of outcome preferences. Second, treatment goals increase the commitment of both health care providers and patients toward performing goal-relevant self-management skills. Health care providers become committed because they have applied their knowledge of asthma and of the idiosyncratic features of the patient's condition to tailor the best possible treatment program for that individual. Patients, on their part, are committed because they contributed their knowledge and experience to developing their own treatment plan. Finally, goal selection establishes common expectancies for health care providers and patients. Health care providers expect certain outcomes to result when they and their patients pursue common goals. Patients in turn recognize what actions they must take to achieve the goals they have jointly set with their health care provider.

The process of goal selection may be the only activity where there is true collaboration between health care providers and their patients; hence, it is important that both parties be satisfied with the goals they have established and the respective responsibilities of each party. This means both that health care providers believe that individual patients can achieve goals they have helped set and that patients recognize that they can assume primary responsibility for achieving the goals.

Information Collection. *Information collection* is self-monitoring or the self-observation and self-recording of information on oneself. It is a key ingredient in self-management. In setting goals of asthma management, health care providers need to identify explicitly the information they want each patient to gather about his or her asthma. Topics usually covered are those spelled out in a patient's asthma plan and include (1) data on any symptoms experienced, including nocturnal awakenings caused by asthma; (2) all asthma medications taken, including both controller and relief drugs; (3) the highest of three peak flow values obtained in the morning and evening (if this criterion is set by a patient and his or her physician); and (4) any asthma exacerbations, including information on what antecedent stimuli may have triggered the attack, behaviors performed to control it, and the consequences of these actions (the ABCs of attack management).

Three points need to be stressed with respect to self-monitoring. First, individuals should attend only to phenomena that can be operationally defined as target responses by physicians and their patients. A way to prompt the collection of accurate data is to develop a recording form with categories where information can be readily entered daily and where the categories are clearly defined in simple language. Second, the information that is gathered should be the result of a joint agreement between patients and physicians. The latter may wish patients to use a peak flow meter regularly; such a meter provides a relatively objective measure of airway obstruction. Other health care providers, however, may wish the patient to concentrate on gathering data on symptoms and adherence to a medication schedule. Whatever phenomena are observed and recorded should be tailored for the needs of the individual patient. Finally, gathering and recording of information should occur on a regular basis, usually daily. However, it is wise to gather this information for only specified periods of time because most patients are not motivated to do so over prolonged periods of time.[39]

Information Processing and Evaluation. Individual patients must learn to process and evaluate the information they collect about themselves and their asthma. In some cases, this step involves detecting signs of an impending attack, such as chest tightness, difficulty in breathing, etc. These signs in turn may prompt the patient to take corrective action such as using a relief inhaler. At other times, the patient may determine that there has been a slowly decreasing rate of peak flow values recorded over the past few days; the decreasing trend may prompt the patient to consider the possibility of an impending attack and, if possible, prevent it. Or, a lower peak flow value may be associated with physical signs, such as a change in breathing. Whatever sign is observed, whether subjective or objective, it is important that the patient discriminate the change in breathing and initiate appropriate action.

Equally important is patient consideration of the context within which an attack occurs, as there are multidirectional interactions between the context and the interpretation of breathing changes. If the patient is awakened by an attack, for example, he or she is apt to use a relief inhaler and, with luck, fall back to sleep. In other settings, however, the context of the attack may be less clear. For example, the patient may not distinguish a change in asthma symptoms from feelings of anxiety, particularly in a setting where the patient tends to feel anxious. Attack context, such as experiencing panic or fear during a recent attack, was shown to be an important mediator between psychologic status and asthma outcomes.[40] The investigators in this study suggested that strong cognitive/affective responses to attacks may represent a window of opportunity for patients to seek and perform self-management. Because asthma attacks do not occur in a vacuum, it is important that patients always analyze events that occur antecedent to breathing changes to appropriately treat an attack or, if the breathing change is not indicative of an asthma exacerbation, take other actions (e.g., relax in the face of anxiety-provoking stimuli).

Decision-making. After patients collect, process, and evaluate data they have gathered about themselves and their asthma, they need to make appropriate decisions based on the information. Despite an increasing amount of data regarding medical decision-making, there is a paucity of data as to how individual patients make decisions regarding their asthma. In many cases, patient decisions are idiosyncratic to themselves and to the context in which they make decisions. However, with experience at making appropriate decisions, both patients and physicians exceptionally skilled at asthma management show remarkably similar strategies in making decisions.[41] These strategies include (1) relying on past experience in asthma treatment but treating each attack as a separate event that may require a unique approach to treatment; (2) generating a number of treatment options and then selecting what appears to be the best option for a given attack; (3) treating the attack in a stepwise manner; (4) considering potential outcomes in terms of probability (e.g., "my approach will likely work, but if it doesn't, I'll try something else"); and (5) not relying on memory.

Action. The asthma action plan outlines the steps the patient should take to control an exacerbation. Action on the plan entails the performance of whatever self-management skills are needed to achieve the goal. Self-instruction underlies whatever action is taken by patients during an asthma attack; the steps include prompting, directing, and maintaining of the performance of required self-management skills. Self-instruction is integral to the successful self-management of asthma for two other reasons.[39] First, establishing control over an asthma episode requires that patients perform, usually in a stepwise fashion, the tactics they have worked out and outlined in the asthma action plan. For example, the physician and a patient may decide that, if possible, the patient escapes from the stimulus that is triggering his or her asthma. If the action does not restore normal breathing, the next step may be that the patient uses an inhaled quick-acting beta-agonist relief medication. Whatever steps are needed to abort the episode must be considered and, if necessary, performed by the patient. Second, it is important that the patient use self-instruction to guide him or her in performing whatever steps are needed to control an attack. Although the patient and his or her physician jointly established the goals of attack management, including what action to take to achieve these goals, it is solely up to the patient to perform whatever actions are needed to establish control over the episode.

Self-Reaction. *Self-reaction* refers to the patient's response to evaluating his or her overall self-management performance.[42] On the basis of their personal evaluation, patients may establish realistic expectations regarding the outcome of their performance. They may also decide if they need more training and expertise. With respect to the latter, patients may feel that the successful management of their asthma requires that they again sit down with their health care provider and review the goals of treatment. In some cases, particularly if the patient is skilled at avoiding unnecessary attacks by behavioral action, a medication regimen may be changed in response to fewer attacks. Perhaps the physician will decide that the patient no longer needs a controller drug. On the other hand, if the patient's best efforts have failed to establish what the patient and his or her physician have agreed is optimal asthma

control, a more powerful treatment regimen, including use of a controller drug, may be warranted. It is the self-reaction of the patient that alerts his or her physician to the need for any changes in treatment goals or the action needed to achieve the goals. By monitoring their progress or lack thereof, patients can discuss with their physicians whatever steps may be required to establish asthma control. The entire approach to asthma self-management thus becomes an ongoing viable strategy that can be adjusted to fit the needs of the patient. Patients and health care providers can adjust or refine the blueprint of treatment they have written and implemented. Only patients can adjust their behavior to perform the self-management skills needed to achieve the goal of controlling their asthma.

Maintenance of Self-Management Skills

There is evidence that training in self-management, which involves self-monitoring by peak expiratory flow or symptoms coupled with regular medical review and a written action plan, appears to improve adherence and health outcomes for adults with asthma.[43] Similar findings have been reported with children.[44] These reviews of adults and children cogently describe methods and procedures involved in teaching self-management skills to patients and, in the case of children, their families.

Although the acquisition of asthma self-management skills has been well described in the literature, short-term outcome data gathered 1 year or so after conclusion of formal training have usually been presented to support the performance of these skills. Consequently, we know much about the acquisition of asthma self-management but far less about *relapse*—defined as falling back into a former state after apparent improvement—or maintenance of self-management skills. Because asthma has no cure, is often of long duration, and has an uncertain course of progression, information on relapse and maintenance of self-management skills by asthma patients is essential.[45] Maintenance data constitute the most significant information collected about asthma self-management, particularly with respect to determining the effectiveness and costs of self-management training. If the approach is not cost-effective, for example, why should such efforts to teach and perform self-management skills be supported?

Although there is a lack of data available on the long-term outcomes of self-management performance with other chronic conditions, a few studies have described long-term follow-up data with asthma patients.[45-47] While presenting but a sketch of information, the long-term data suggest two major trends. First, to one degree or another, all participants continue to perform self-management skills they perceive as necessary to manage their asthma. Thus, although one group of investigators reported benefits were less at 2 years than at 6 years, they also noted that emergency visits to physicians had significantly decreased from 41% at baseline to 18% at the 6-year follow-up.[47] In another study, 20 patients were classified as relapsers according to established criteria for relapse, and the remaining 33 patients as maintainers of self-management performance.[45] Although an unexpectedly high percentage (50%) of those classified as relapsers reported they no longer needed to perform asthma self-management because their asthma was in remission, all participants reported that they continued to use self-management as needed 7 years after acquiring these skills. The trend suggests that while patients may not manage their asthma so that it is optimally controlled from a medical standpoint, they have established their own criteria of what they perceive as adequate control. Therefore they do what they must to achieve and maintain their self-set standard.

Second, the ongoing performance of asthma self-management is motivated by self-efficacy. Bandura[48] described perceived self-efficacy as "beliefs in one's capabilities to organize and execute the course of action required to produce given attainments." In other words, self-efficacy is the belief that one can do what is necessary to produce certain outcomes. Self-efficacy and outcome expectations were likely the forces that maintained patient self-management behaviors for 6 to 7 years after training.[45,47] Continued reinforcement of self-management skills, occurring when physicians provide ongoing assessment and encouragement during office visits, will generate more enduring benefits.[47]

CONCLUSIONS

Nonadherence to asthma treatment regimens may result from a number of factors, including inadequate knowledge and skill on the part of the patient and inadequate awareness of the problem or skill to address it on the part of the physician (Box 42-1). Patients must have a basic understanding of their illness and its treatment for clinicians to expect even minimal treatment adherence. Achievement of adherence requires much more from both the patient and caregiver. To perform the daily behaviors necessary for successful asthma control, patients must be well motivated and convinced that their own behaviors will result in better health. Simply giving information to patients is unlikely to change behavior. Health care providers must understand the psychologic principles that underlie self-management training and comprehend that motivating patients requires more than imparting brief information to the patient about the prescription that has just been written. At the core of these principles is the need to establish treatment goals that can be embraced by both physicians and patients in a partnership that requires regular and reciprocal communication (Box 42-2). Patients will not perform the work necessary to achieve goals they do not understand or do not view as necessary and important. Once such goals are established, most patients require assistance in determining how to evaluate their changing symptoms and use their written action plan to make effective decisions about appropriate daily self-management behaviors.

Programs designed to train physicians to communicate with and to motivate their patients have resulted in improved treatment outcomes. Physicians who believe neither that their patients are seriously nonadherent nor that they lack the skills necessary to educate and motivate their patients are unlikely to accept or use training in communication or behavior change skills. It is perhaps for this reason that successful physician training in behavioral principles appears to have focused primarily on young physicians who may be most open to new learning.

The Cochrane group completed a recent review of the published literature describing studies that attempted to use interventions to change patient adherence behaviors across numerous diseases.[49] Of the 19 adherence-intervention studies reviewed, 17 reported changes in adherence behaviors but only 9 led to improvements in outcomes such as disease exacerbation and health care utilization. Apparently, small and temporary behavior change in the remaining 8 studies was insufficient to alter illness outcomes. Numerous and sometimes innovative interventions were represented, including (1) counseling; (2) simplification of dosing; (3) automated, telephone-based, computer-assisted patient monitoring or patient-physician contacts; (4) pill packaging with electronic reminders; (5) reinforcements and reward for adherence; and (6) support groups. The Cochrane group concluded that

---

BOX 42-1

KEY CONCEPTS

Motivating Patient Adherence

- Medication adherence sufficient to establish consistent asthma control occurs in only 26% to 52% of patients.
- Poorly controlled asthma is often the consequence of nonadherence yet is frequently addressed by increasing the treatment regimen.
- Medications that are easier to take invite better adherence, but no medication provides sufficient symptom control when adherence is poor.
- Health caregivers can significantly influence treatment adherence.
- Expert Panel guidelines recognize that the patient-physician relationship is essential to treatment success and emphasize the development of a partnership between patient and physician within which discussion about treatment goals and progress will occur.
- Patient education from the health caregiver should begin at the time of diagnosis and be integrated into sequential visits.

BOX 42-2

THERAPEUTIC PRINCIPLES

Patient and Physician Requisites to Establishing Treatment Adherence

Patient requisites for improved adherence

Basic understanding of asthma

Thorough understanding of the role of each medication prescribed

Understanding of and commitment to a negotiated treatment goal

Sufficient skill to make self-management decisions

Belief in one's own ability to manage the illness

Trust in the physician

Physician requisites to enhance adherence

Thorough understanding of asthma and its treatment

Willingness to communicate with the patient

Willingness to negotiate a shared treatment goal with the patient

Willingness to change the prescribed treatment to improve adherence

Acceptance of the fact that most patients do not take all of the medication

studies which included many of these elements in sometimes complex interventions produced changes that in many instances were not cost effective; that is, the small amount of adherence behavior change was not justified by the large cost of implementing the programs.[49] Additional criticisms of the studies included inadequate sample size, excessive cost, and inadequate measurement of outcomes most typically seen in studies that relied on patient reports of behavior and health care utilization. The group concluded that, in the absence of compelling evidence for large-scale programs, several basic principles should be observed. First, patients who see a physician regularly are more likely to take at least some of their medication. Infrequent patient-physician contacts, particularly in patients without a personal physician or who frequently change physicians, may use less of their medication. Second, patients who fail to attend a scheduled visit should be contacted. This may be as simple as having a staff member call the patient, express concern that the patient did not attend the visit, and reschedule. This low-cost intervention may have the greatest relative benefit. Only when the patient attends a visit is there opportunity to communicate, educate, and motivate. Finally, despite great strides in developing medications for asthma both in the recent past and in the future, no drug is apt to successfully control asthma unless patients comply with their treatment regimens. In this respect, developing new ways to improve medication adherence in patients is possibly the most important innovation that can occur in asthma.

REFERENCES

1. Valenti WM: Treatment adherence improves outcomes and manages costs, *IDS Read* 11:77-80, 2001.
2. Baum D, Creer TL: Medication compliance in children with asthma, *J Asthma* 23:49-59, 1986.
3. Bender B, Milgrom H, Rand C, et al: Psychological factors associated with medication nonadherence in asthmatic children, *J Asthma* 35:347-353, 1998.
4. Urquhart J: Role of patient compliance in clinical pharmacokinetics, *Clin Pharmacokinet* 27:202-215, 1994.
5. Tashkin DP, Rand C, Nides M, et al: A nebulizer chronolog to monitor compliance with inhaler use, *Am J Med* 91:4S-36S, 1991.
6. Bender BG, Wamboldt FS, O'Connor SL, et al: Measurement of children's asthma medication adherence by self-report, mother report, canister weight, and Doser CT, *Ann Allergy Asthma Immunol* 85:416-421, 2000.
7. Szefler S, Boushey H, Pearlman D: Time to onset of effect of fluticasone propionate in patients with asthma, *Allergy Clin Immunol* 103:780-788, 1999.
8. Bender B: *Psychosocial factors mediating asthma treatment outcomes,* London, 2001, Martin Dunitz Ltd.
9. National Heart, Lung, and Blood Institute: *Expert Panel report 2: guidelines for the diagnosis and management of asthma,* Washington, DC, 1997, U.S. Department of Health and Human Services.
10. Suissa S, Ernst P, Benayoun S, et al: Low-dose inhaled corticosteroids and the prevention of death from asthma, *N Engl J Med* 343:332-336, 2000.
11. Milgrom H, Bender B, Ackerson L, et al: Non-compliance and treatment failure in children with asthma, *J Allergy Clin Immunol* 98:1051-1057, 1996.
12. Horn C, Clar T, Cochrane G: Compliance with inhaled therapy and morbidity from asthma, *Respir Med* 84:67-70, 1990.
13. Bender B, Milgrom H, Rand C: Nonadherence in asthmatic patients: is there a solution to the problem? *Ann Allergy Asthma Immunol* 79:177-186, 1997.
14. Strunk RC: Asthma deaths in childhood: Identification of patients at risk and intervention, *J Allergy Clin Immunol* 80:472-477, 1987.
15. Devine EC: Meta-analysis of the effects of psychoeducational care in adults with asthma, *Res Nursing Health* 19:367-376, 1996.
16. Bernard-Bonnin A, Stachenko S, Bonin D, et al: Self-management teaching programs and morbidity of pediatric asthma: a meta-analysis, *J Allergy Clin Immunol* 95:34-41, 1995.
17. Bailey W, Richards J, Brooks C, et al: A randomized trial to improve self-management practices in adults with asthma, *Arch Intern Med* 150:1664-1668, 1990.
18. Bailey WC, Kohler CL, Richards JM Jr, et al: Asthma self-management. Do patient education programs always have an impact, *Arch Intern Med* 159:2422-2428, 1999.
19. Ho J, Bender B, Gavin LA, et al: The relationships between asthma knowledge, treatment adherence, and outcome, *J Allergy Clin Immunol* 2002, in press.
20. Mühlhauser I, Richter B, Kraut D, et al: Evaluation of a structured treatment and teaching programme on asthma, *J Intern Med* 230:157-164, 1991.
21. Milgrom H, Bender B, Wamboldt F: Assessing adherence with asthma medication: making the counts count, *Ann Allergy Asthma Immunol* 88:429-431, 2002.
22. Scarfone RJ, Zorc JJ, Capraro GA: Patient self-management of acute asthma: adherence to national guidelines a decade later, *Pediatrics* 108:1332-1338, 2001.
23. Apter AJ, Van Hoof TJ, Sherwin TE, et al: Assessing the quality of asthma care provided to Medicaid patients enrolled in managed care organizations in Connecticut, *Ann Allergy Asthma Immunol* 86:211-218, 2001.
24. Cooper WO, Hickson GB: Corticosteroid prescription filling for children covered by Medicaid following an emergency department visit or hospitalization for asthma, *Arch Pediatr Adolesc Med* 155:1111-1115, 2001.
25. Doerschug KC, Peterson MW, Dayton CS, et al: Asthma guidelines: an assessment of physician understanding and practice, *Am J Respir Crit Care Med* 159:1735-1741, 1999.
26. Cabana MD, Rand CS, Powe NR, et al: Why don't physicians follow clinical practice guidelines? A framework for improvement, *JAMA* 282:1458-1465, 1999.
27. Spilker B: Methods of assessing and improving patient compliance in clinical trials. In Cramer J, Spilker B, editors: *Patient compliance in medical practice and clinical trials,* New York, 1991, Raven Press.
28. Davis D, Thomson M, Oxman A, et al: Evidence for the effectiveness of CME: a review of 50 randomized controlled trials, *JAMA* 268:1111-1117, 1992.
29. Duke T, Kellermann A, Ellis R, et al: Asthma in the emergency department: impact of a protocol on optimizing therapy, *Am J Emerg Med* 9:432-435, 1991.
30. Inui TS, Yourtee EL, Williamson JW: Improved outcomes in hypertension after physician tutorials, *Ann Intern Med* 84:646-651, 1976.
31. Roter D, Hall J, Kern D: Improving physicians' interviewing skills and reducing patients' emotional distress: a randomized clinical trial, *Arch Intern Med* 155:1877-1884, 1995.
32. Vinicor F, Cohen SJ, Mazzuca SA, et al: DIABEDS: a randomized trial of the effects of physician and/or patient education on diabetes patient outcomes, *J Chronic Dis* 40:345-356, 1987.
33. Clark N, Gong M, Schork M, et al: Impact of education for physicians on patient outcomes, *Pediatrics* 101:831-836, 1998.
34. Clark NM, Gong M, Schork MA, et al: Long-term effects of asthma education for physicians on patient satisfaction and use of health services, *Eur Respir J* 16:15-21, 2000.
35. Evans D, Mellins R, Lobach K, et al: Improving care for minority children with asthma: professional education in public health clinics, *Pediatrics* 99:157-164, 1997.
36. National Heart, Lung, and Blood Institute: *Executive summary: guidelines for the diagnosis and management of asthma,* Washington, DC, 1991, U.S. Department of Health and Human Services.
37. Joyce DP, McIvor RA: Use of inhaled medications and urgent care services. Study of Canadian asthma patients, *Can Family Physician* 45:1707-1713, 1999.
38. Creer TL: *Asthma therapy: a behavioral health care system for respiratory disorders,* New York, 1979, Springer.
39. Creer T, Bender B: Asthma. In Gatchel R, Blanchard E, editors: *Psychophysiological disorders: research and clinical applications,* Washington, DC, 1993, American Psychological Association.
40. Greaves CJ, Eiser C, Seamark D, et al: Attack context: an important mediator of the relationship between psychological status and asthma outcomes, *Thorax* 57:217-221, 2002.
41. Creer TL: Assessment of decision-making in asthma maintenance and relapse, American Thoracic Society, 97th Annual Meeting. San Francisco, CA, May 22, 2001.
42. Creer TL, Holroyd KA: Self-management. In Baum A, McManus C, Newman S, et al, editors: *Cambridge handbook of psychology, health, and medicine,* Cambridge, 1997, Cambridge University Press.

43. Gibson PG, Coughlan J, Wilson AJ, et al: *Self-management education and regular practitioner review for adults with asthma (Cochrane Review)*, The Cochrane Library, ed 4, Oxford, 2002, Update Software Ltd.

44. Wigal JK, Creer TL, Kotses H, et al: A critique of 19 self-management programs for childhood asthma. Part I. The development and evaluation of the programs, *Pediatr Asthma Allergy Immunol* 4:17-39, 1990.

45. Caplin DL, Creer TL: A self-management program for adult asthma. Part III. Maintenance and relapse of skills, *J Asthma* 38:343-356, 2001.

46. Creer TL, Backial M, Burns KL, et al: Living with asthma: Part I. Genesis and development of a self-management program for childhood asthma, *J Asthma* 25:335-362, 1988.

47. D'Souza WJ, Slater T, Fox C, et al: Asthma morbidity 6 years after an effective asthma self-management programme in a Maori community, *Eur Respir J* 15:464-469, 2000.

48. Bandura A: *Self-efficacy: the exercise of control*, New York, 1997, WH Freeman.

49. Haynes RB, McDonald H, Garg AX, et al: Interventions for helping patients to follow prescriptions for medications, *Cochrane Database Syst Rev* 2:CD000011, 2002.

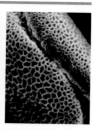

CHAPTER 43

New Directions in Asthma Management

STANLEY J. SZEFLER

Recent statistics indicate that the concerted effort to halt the trend of increasing asthma mortality and morbidity has been successful because both those areas have reached a plateau.[1] A strategy to establish a decline in morbidity and mortality would be to recognize patients at risk for persistent asthma and to intervene early. This review will highlight new information available on asthma pathogenesis and treatment that will help shape a new direction in managing childhood asthma.

At this time, asthma is characterized as a chronic inflammatory disease. Inhaled glucocorticoids, the most potent anti-inflammatory asthma medications, have emerged as the cornerstone for the management of persistent asthma. Since the early 1980s substantial gains have been made in understanding the pathogenesis of asthma.[2] This effort has resulted in the introduction of new medications and delivery systems, as well as new initiatives to improve medication labeling for young children to facilitate early intervention. Consequently, new opportunities have emerged to improve the overall management of childhood asthma.

New directions include recognizing asthma in its early stages and taking steps to intervene earlier with environmental control and long-term control therapy. This movement will continue to lead to better methods to diagnose asthma and a critical analysis of the role of early intervention in altering the natural history of asthma. Although inhaled glucocorticoid therapy has played a major role in stabilizing the rise in asthma morbidity and mortality, there is still much to learn regarding its efficacy in preventing progression of asthma and thus altering the natural history of the disease.[3]

This review will begin by briefly summarizing the recommended principles of asthma management as a stepping stone to discussing methods that could strengthen the areas of weakness. To advance to a level where we can speak of a "cure" for asthma, we must be able to take a proactive approach and recognize the disease early and intervene appropriately (Box 43-1).

PHASE OF RAPID EVOLUTION

Principles of inhaled glucocorticoid therapy dosing emerged in the late 1970s along with clear evidence of efficacy in the management of asthma for both adults and children.[4] In the mid-1990s several important new classes of medications were introduced. Long-acting β_2-adrenergic agonists salmeterol and formoterol, with a 12-hour duration of action, were introduced. To limit the adverse effects of short-acting β agonists, the stereoisomer of albuterol, levalbuterol, was developed and introduced. In addition, the class of leukotriene modifiers was introduced. One of the oral leukotriene antagonists, montelukast, has emerged as a popular first-line long-term control therapy in children with asthma because of the availability of dosage guidelines and the demonstration of its safety in children as young as 2 years of age. In addition, renewed interest has developed for the combination of medications in one formulation, such as an inhaled steroid and a long-acting β-adrenergic agonist, based on evidence of additive effects, convenience for the patient, and the potential to further reduce the risk for significant exacerbations.[5] With the availability of numerous choices for medication selection, it is important to organize the approach to a treatment plan.

CURRENT MANAGEMENT OF CHILDHOOD ASTHMA

Current guidelines emphasize environmental control, objective monitoring, cooperative management, and pharmacotherapy as the core elements of asthma management. Asthma is now classified as *intermittent, mild persistent, moderate persistent,* and *severe persistent* based on symptoms,

BOX 43-1	KEY CONCEPTS
	New Directions in Asthma Management

- Early recognition and effective intervention hold the key to altering the natural history of persistent asthma.
- Young children with frequent wheezing episodes and risk factors for persistent asthma should be considered candidates for early intervention with either environmental control or inhaled glucocorticoids.
- Response to intervention with inhaled glucocorticoids is highly individualized and requires careful monitoring for each feature of asthma control.
- Continuing investigation regarding patient characteristics and genetics associated with the development of an asthma phenotype and response to medications holds promise to advance the management of asthma.

nighttime episodes, and pulmonary function. The most recent guidelines have consisted of updated versions of the Global Initiative for Asthma and the National Heart, Lung, and Blood Institute (NHLBI) Guidelines for the Diagnosis and Management of Asthma.[6-8]

The updated National Asthma Education and Prevention Program (NAEPP) guidelines include an attempt to address the needs of childhood asthma with evidence-based reviews.[8] The evidence for various steps in asthma management for children less than 5 years of age has been weak because of the paucity of studies in this age group and many assumptions continue to be based on adult studies and ultimately relegated to expert opinion. Studies are in progress to fill some of these gaps as investigators and the pharmaceutical industry realize the need for improved dosing guidelines as well as new medications for this age group.

The updated version of the NAEPP guidelines establish inhaled glucocorticoids as the preferred first-line treatment in both children and adults.[8] The preferred additive therapy for inadequate control with a low-medium dose of inhaled glucocorticoid is a long-acting β-adrenergic agonist. Leukotriene antagonists are considered alternative first-line therapy and alternative additive therapy once inhaled glucocorticoids have been initiated. Two major areas that require ongoing research include the appropriate time to initiate long-term control therapy and the management of severe persistent asthma in children. Currently, several medications are now labeled for use in young children, specifically nebulized budesonide for children as young as a year old and montelukast for children as young as 2 years of age. There is a need for an easily administered, long-acting β-adrenergic agonist with specific labeling for use in children under 5 years of age.

SPECIAL PROBLEMS FOR MANAGING ASTHMA IN YOUNG CHILDREN

Current therapy is based on the belief that chronic inflammation is a major feature of asthma. Because persistent asthma can occur early in life, attention is moving toward early recognition and early intervention. It is assumed but not yet proven that early recognition and early treatment with antiinflammatory therapy could modify the disease process and the natural history of asthma.[9] Prospective randomized control studies are needed to verify whether long-term outcome can be significantly altered by this approach.[8]

Although the approach to asthma control in young children is similar to that in older children and adults, there are limitations to the evaluation of asthma in young children. Assessment is primarily based on symptoms because pulmonary function cannot be measured reliably in young children. Environmental control measures can be applied if allergen sensitivity is defined and exposure confirmed. In addition, limiting exposure to viral respiratory infections could also reduce the frequency of significant acute exacerbations but this is difficult to achieve in day care settings and schools. Pharmacotherapy can also be a challenge because the route of administration for inhaled medication administration must be adjusted to patient cooperation. First-line therapy may begin with low-dose inhaled glucocorticoid via nebulizer or a spacer/holding chamber and facemask.[8]

Current global guidelines and recent revisions to the United States guidelines recommend an inhaled glucocorticoid by facemask and nebulized administration, respectively, as first-line therapy in young children with persistent asthma. Comparative studies are needed to determine whether the inhaled glucocorticoid by spacer/facemask or nebulized administration is the preferred route of administration. In the United States no inhaled glucocorticoid in the dry powder or metered-dose inhaler formulation is approved for use in children younger than 4 years of age. Because it is not feasible to administer a dry powder formulation to young children based on the necessary inspiratory flow rate, it will be important to evaluate the new hydrofluoroalkane preparations for use in young children.

For moderate persistent asthma, it is now recommended that a medium dose of inhaled glucocorticoid be administered or that a long-acting β-adrenergic agonist be added.[8] The latter recommendation is primarily based on conclusions derived from adult studies. Unfortunately, there is no long-acting β-adrenergic agonist approved for use in children younger than 5 years of age. Therefore, the application is a non-approved use of an approved medication if administered via a metered-dose inhaled along with a spacer. It would also be useful to develop a nebulized form of a long-acting β-adrenergic agonist for those patients unable to adhere to the metered-dose inhaler and spacer.

Alternatively, a leukotriene antagonist could be added to an inhaled glucocorticoid. For more severe asthma, high-dose inhaled glucocorticoids are recommended, and if needed, systemic glucocorticoid with adjustment to the lowest dose either daily or on alternate days sufficient to stabilize symptoms should be used. This algorithm will continue to be refined as more information is obtained on the efficacy of the available approved medications for young children.

NEW INSIGHTS

Several recent studies provide important insight for the management of persistent asthma. These studies solidify the role of inhaled glucocorticoids as first-line therapy in the management of persistent asthma and also point to some limitations in the efficacy of inhaled glucocorticoids. These concepts should now be considered in the individualized management of asthma. It is also important that new treatment strategies address the limitations of inhaled glucocorticoids in altering the natural history of asthma and reversing pulmonary function in long-standing, poorly controlled asthma.

Outcomes Following Long-Term Inhaled Glucocorticoid Administration

The recent series of publications from the Childhood Asthma Management Program (CAMP) Research Group provide many new insights into the efficacy of long-term control therapy.[10-14] The major outcome report in particular generates a number of questions to be considered in future studies.[14] This trial was initiated in 1991 in order to evaluate whether continuous long-term treatment with either an inhaled glucocorticoid (budesonide) or an inhaled nonsteroid (nedocromil) control medication could improve lung growth safely over a 4- to 6-year treatment period compared to treatment based on the frequency and severity of symptoms (albuterol as needed).

Post-bronchodilator FEV_1% predicted was selected as the primary outcome and the parameter to assess lung growth

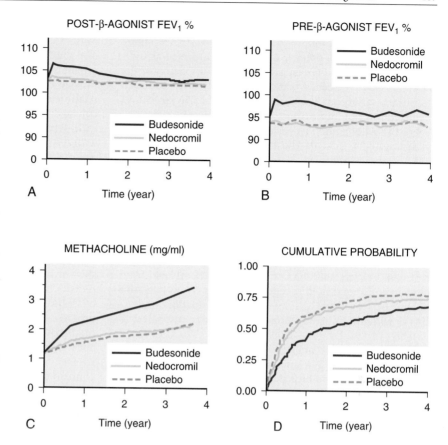

FIGURE 43-1 Results of the Childhood Asthma Management Program (CAMP) Study. **A,** Description of the change in post-bronchodilator forced expiratory volume in 1 second *(FEV₁)* during the duration of the study. There was an initial improvement in post-bronchodilator FEV_1 in patients receiving budesonide, but by the end of the study there were no differences between the three treatment groups. **B,** Description of the change in pre-bronchodilator therapy. Budesonide resulted in a modest yet statistically significant improvement in pre-bronchodilator FEV_1 throughout the treatment period compared with placebo. **C,** Description of the change in methacholine responsiveness over time. Note that all subjects had improvement in bronchial hyperresponsiveness (BHR), as indicated by the increase in methacholine PC_{20} values over the 4 to 6 years of the trial. Patients randomized to budesonide had a significantly greater reduction in BHR than the placebo-treated patients. **D,** A Kaplan-Meier curve describing the cumulative probability of a first course of prednisone during 4 years of follow-up in the budesonide-, nedocromil-, and placebo-treated children. (From Childhood Asthma Management Program Research Group: *N Engl J Med* 343:1054-1063, 2000.)

because it is a measure of maximal lung capacity. This technique minimizes the effects of factors that influence airway constriction and has less variability over time than the pre-bronchodilator measurements applied in previous studies. The results of the CAMP trial showed that budesonide treatment improved post-bronchodilator FEV_1% predicted from a mean 103.2% predicted to 106.8% predicted within 2 months, but this measurement gradually diminished to 103.8% predicted by the end of the treatment period (Figure 43-1, *A*). At the end of the treatment period the post-bronchodilator FEV_1% predicted in the budesonide group was not significantly different from that in the placebo group. The nedocromil group was similar to the placebo group in this measure throughout the study period.

The finding that neither budesonide nor nedocromil improved lung function, as measured by the percent predicted value for FEV_1 after the administration of a bronchodilator, was not expected based on a previous report of inhaled glucocorticoid effect in asthmatic children.[9] However, that study did not examine post-bronchodilator FEV_1 measurements. In fact, there are few studies in childhood asthma that utilize post-bronchodilator FEV_1 as an outcome measure. Because a decline in FEV_1% predicted has been interpreted as an indication of airway remodeling, the CAMP study results raise questions about whether airway remodeling is occurring in this population of mild to moderate persistent asthma and whether inhaled glucocorticoids have any effect on preventing this change in airway pathology. The CAMP results indicate that FEV_1% predicted did not decline in either the placebo group or the inhaled nedocromil group. Furthermore, the

temporary increase in post-bronchodilator FEV_1% predicted after initiating treatment was not sustained over the treatment period and was comparable to the placebo group at the end of the study. Therefore this decline in post-bronchodilator FEV_1% predicted in the budesonide treatment arm might reflect progression of disease despite inhaled glucocorticoid therapy. Another explanation is that perhaps these patients were nonadherent to the treatment and this will be examined in ongoing analysis.

Based on the observed absence of decline in post-bronchodilator FEV_1% predicted one can only speculate on the potential impact on the concept of airway remodeling in this patient population. First, FEV_1% predicted may not be sufficiently sensitive to serve as an indicator of airway remodeling. Second, by the fact that the study design limited enrollment to patients with mild to moderate persistent asthma, patients susceptible to airway remodeling or a progressive loss in FEV_1% predicted may have been screened out. Third, the mean duration of asthma in the study population was 5 years. It is possible that the most significant effect on FEV_1 or airway remodeling occurred before the patients were enrolled in the study.[15,16] If the latter is true, then emphasis should be placed on early recognition and early intervention.

Other measures of post-bronchodilator spirometry including FEV_1 (liters), FEV_1/FVC, FVC% predicted, FEV_1/FVC were not significantly different upon completion of the treatment phase. For pre-bronchodilator measurements of pulmonary function, several parameters in the treatment group differed from placebo. At the end of the treatment period the difference in pre-bronchodilator FEV_1% predicted following inhaled budesonide treatment compared to baseline exceeded that in the placebo group (2.9 vs. 0.9, $P = 0.02$; see Figure 43-1, B). The $FEV_1\%$ predicted could be interpreted as indicating that functional airway caliber upon completion of the treatment phase exceeded that of the placebo arm. Although statistically significant, the total difference of 2.0% for $FEV_1\%$ predicted was not impressive.

Pre-bronchodilator $FEV_1\%$ predicted for inhaled budesonide was higher than placebo and inhaled nedocromil for the first 2 years of treatment. However, the inhaled nedocromil group did not differ from placebo during any point of the treatment phase, indicating there was no detectable effect of this treatment arm on pre-bronchodilator $FEV_1\%$ predicted. For change in FEV_1/FVC, the difference attributed to inhaled budesonide was less than that following placebo (-0.2 vs. -1.8, $P < 0.001$). This indicates that the decline in FEV_1/FVC, another measure of airway obstruction, over the course of treatment was less with inhaled budesonide. Because FEV_1 in liters demonstrated no difference among the treatments, this difference is probably the result of the reduction in FVC (liters) with the inhaled steroid treatment as compared to placebo (1.29 vs. 1.35, $P = 0.001$).

For inhaled nedocromil the only difference in pre- and post-bronchodilator spirometry as compared with placebo was observed with pre-bronchodilator FEV_1 (liters). The end result indicated the difference at the end of treatment from the baseline value was less for inhaled nedocromil than placebo (0.6 vs. 2.4, $P = 0.02$). Furthermore, all values of pre- and post-bronchodilator spirometry were comparable for the three treatment groups following the 4-month discontinuation of active study medication, indicating that any beneficial effect observed on a pulmonary function parameter was lost within 4 months of discontinuing treatment. This is an important observation because it suggests that inhaled glucocorticoids do not have a sustaining effect on the natural history of asthma.

The most distinct effect observed on a measure of pulmonary function was the significant and consistent effect of inhaled budesonide on reducing airway hyperresponsiveness (see Figure 43-1, C). By the end of treatment the PC_{20} ratio as compared with baseline was 3 for inhaled budesonide compared to 1.9 for placebo ($P < 0.001$). Once again, there was no difference in a comparison of inhaled nedocromil to placebo throughout the treatment period. Another surprising observation was that all three groups were comparable for methacholine PC_{20} following the 4-month washout phase. Therefore, this additional surrogate marker of airway remodeling is not permanently affected by inhaled glucocorticoid therapy as compared to the other two treatment options.

During the overall treatment course the most consistent effects on changes in the total panel of clinical outcomes was observed with the inhaled glucocorticoid treatment arm as compared to placebo. For inhaled budesonide hospitalizations, urgent care visits, and prednisone courses were significantly lower than the placebo arm by approximately 45%. Other measures showing a difference with inhaled budesonide as compared with placebo included lower symptom score, higher number of episode-free days per month, and less albuterol inhalations per week. Treatment with inhaled nedocromil demonstrated effects only on reduction of urgent care visits and prednisone courses as compared to placebo.

Two additional measures of asthma control over the course of the treatment period included the time to the first significant exacerbation requiring prednisone therapy and the time for intervention with inhaled beclomethasone dipropionate. Inhaled budesonide was distinctly different than placebo in relation to the proportion of courses and the time for the first course of prednisone (see Figure 43-1, D). Similarly, the time for intervention with inhaled beclomethasone therapy along with the proportion of patients necessitating this intervention was much lower in the inhaled budesonide group. For both of these measures inhaled nedocromil was comparable to placebo.

The CAMP results challenge conclusions that have been derived in short-term studies, especially those related to pulmonary function and body development measures. The study alleviated growing concerns regarding the long-term effect of inhaled glucocorticoid therapy on body development by showing that the only detectable adverse effect was a transient reduction in growth velocity limited to 1 cm in the first year of treatment. This effect on growth was persistent but did not progress. Based on bone age measurements and projection of final growth, it was estimated that there would be no difference in growth among the three treatments when the children reached final adult stature. Studies by Agertoft and Pedersen[17] confirm this projection by showing in a long-term follow-up study that final height is not reduced in young adults who received inhaled glucocorticoid therapy during childhood.

It is also clear that the medications used in CAMP did not completely eliminate the morbidity associated with asthma, and there is certainly room for improvement. The rich CAMP database will continue to be evaluated as the ongoing CAMP Continuation Study progresses. This cohort study enables follow-up for an additional 5 years for those who were managed intensively for the 4- to 6-year treatment phase. The CAMP Continuation Study is specifically designed to evaluate the long-term effects of long-term treatment on lung development and growth. The CAMP subjects will be followed into late adolescence and early adulthood in an attempt to define maximal lung and body growth parameters.

Early Recognition

Reports from the Tucson Children's Respiratory Study show that children who wheezed during lower respiratory tract illnesses in the first 3 years of life and were still wheezing at age 6 ("persistent wheezers") had slightly but not significantly lower levels of lung function than children who never wheezed before age 6. By age 6, however, persistent wheezers had significant deficits in lung function. The lowest levels of infant lung function were observed among children who wheezed before age 3 and were not current wheezers at age 6 ("transient wheezers").[15,18]

Information was derived on the risk factors for persistent asthma based on the natural history observed in this series of participants.[19] An Asthma Predictive Index was established from this investigation that suggests that frequent wheezing during the first 3 years of life and either one major risk factor (parental history of asthma or eczema) or two of three minor risk factors (eosinophilia $> 4\%$, wheezing without colds, and allergic rhinitis) could predict the persistence of asthma. It has been proposed that early intervention with inhaled glucocorticoid therapy can be effective in preventing

THERAPEUTIC PRINCIPLES
Early Intervention

Young children presenting with wheezing episodes must be assessed carefully for signs of persistent asthma and signs of progression, for example, increasing symptoms and loss of pulmonary function.

Environmental control and inhaled glucocorticoids are the preferred forms of initial intervention.

Uncontrolled asthma carries the risk for progressive loss in pulmonary function, especially within the first years of disease onset.

Response to treatment varies and must be carefully monitored.

---

the progression of the disease and the risk for irreversible changes in the airways that could contribute to the persistence of symptoms (Box 43-2).

Variable Response to Inhaled Glucocorticoid Therapy

A recently published study conducted by the NHLBI Asthma Clinical Research Network described the significant variability in response to inhaled glucocorticoids in adults with persistent asthma and reduced pulmonary function.[20] This study examined 30 adult subjects with persistent asthma with FEV_1 between 55% and 85% and predicted and reported the effect of increasing doses of inhaled glucocorticoids. Multiple parameters of response were examined.

This study reported several key observations. First, near maximal FEV_1 and methacholine PC_{20} effects occurred with low-medium dose for both inhaled glucocorticoids used in this study, namely inhaled fluticasone propionate and inhaled beclomethasone dipropionate administered via metered-dose inhaler with a spacer device. High-dose inhaled glucocorticoid therapy did not significantly increase the efficacy measures that were evaluated, but increased the systemic effect measure of overnight plasma cortisol. Second, significant intersubject variability in response occurred with both inhaled glucocorticoids. The investigators cautioned that perhaps higher doses of inhaled glucocorticoids may be necessary to manage more severe patients or to achieve goals of therapy not evaluated in this study, such as prevention of significant asthma exacerbations.

Of interest, approximately one third of the subjects had a good response (> 15%) as determined by improvement in FEV_1 over the baseline, whereas another third had a marginal response (5% to 15%) and the final third failed to respond (> 5%). The same pattern was observed with methacholine PC_{20} improvement. The FEV_1 improvement did not correlate to the PC_{20} improvement in this group of subjects. However, certain biomarkers, such as exhaled nitric oxide and sputum eosinophils, and asthma characteristics, such as duration of asthma and bronchodilator response, were associated with the two response parameters.[20] The NHLBI Asthma Clinical Research Network will conduct additional studies to understand the nature of poor response to inhaled glucocorticoid therapy as well as the association of poor response to inhaled

glucocorticoids with the frequency of significant asthma exacerbations.

In addition, studies are being conducted in the NHLBI Childhood Asthma Research and Education Network to determine if this refractoriness to inhaled glucocorticoid therapy is present in children and whether the high proportion of poor responders identified in the adult population is similar in children. The study will also characterize the concomitant response to a leukotriene antagonist in these patients to determine if the response to a leukotriene antagonist is proportional to the response to an inhaled glucocorticoid or whether there are patients who respond to one medication but not the other or who fail to respond to either medication. This assessment, combined with careful phenotypic and genotypic analyses, could provide insight into the identification of predictors of response to these two medications in children with mild to moderate persistent asthma.

Difficult-to-Control Asthma

Unfortunately, there has been only limited activity in the area of understanding and managing severe persistent asthma in children. A review by Payne and Balfour-Lynn[21] provides a summary of the current understanding of this concerning patient population. Payne and Balfour-Lynn[21] developed an algorithmic approach to the evaluation of children presenting with a history of difficult-to-control asthma (Figure 43-2). Once the features of diagnosis, behavior, and environmental control are addressed, the remaining issues center around appropriate medication use. Considerations must be given to the appropriate combination of bronchodilator and antiinflammatory therapy along with decisions about dose, delivery device for inhaled medications, and timing of treatment (chronotherapy). Interestingly, these researchers propose that tools to measure airway inflammation such as exhaled nitric oxide, induced sputum, bronchoalveolar lavage, and biopsy be utilized to assist in decisions about pursuing more aggressive forms of antiinflammatory therapy (methotrexate, cyclosporin, intravenous gamma globulin, etc.) or bronchodilator therapy (subcutaneous terbutaline); however, there is little evidence in either children or adults that these measures can be reliably applied in the clinical arena.

Nevertheless, a report by Sont et al[22] indicates that a treatment approach for the use of inhaled glucocorticoids that is guided by measures of airway hyperresponsiveness leads to better overall asthma control, as indicated by improved pulmonary function and reduced symptoms. The additional benefit could also be a reduction in airway collagen deposition. The previously discussed report by Szefler et al[20] adds a note of caution for this approach because certain patients may be refractory to improvements in FEV_1 or reduction in airway hyperresponsiveness despite the administration of high-dose inhaled glucocorticoid therapy. These patients may have persistent inflammation or may have structural airway changes that are refractory to treatment. These patients are candidates for alternative forms of treatment. Unfortunately, there is limited information on guiding the direction of treatment to overcome losses in pulmonary function that are poorly responsive to conventional therapy.

Another interesting observation in this patient population of severe asthma is the variable pattern of pulmonary function that can persist despite optimal management. Chan et al[23]

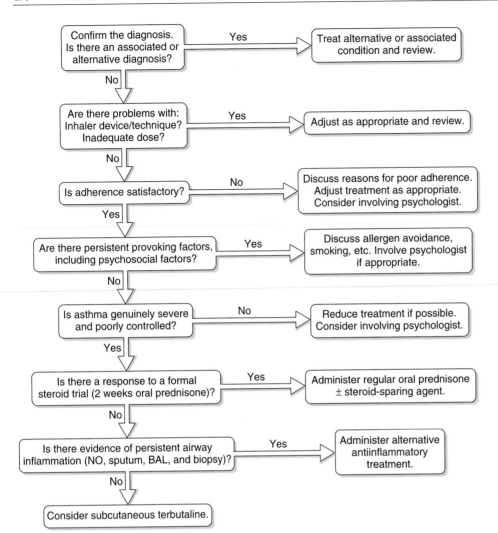

FIGURE 43-2 Algorithm for the management of a child with difficult asthma. (From Payne DNR, Balfour-Lynn IM: *J Asthma* 38:189-203, 2001.)

found that there were basically two patterns of pulmonary function in the population of patients classified as having steroid-resistant asthma, that is, those who failed to improve pulmonary function despite high-dose daily oral glucocorticoid therapy. There was one group of patients who maintained an FEV_1 below 70% and failed to improve, whereas another group had a pattern of variable pulmonary function throughout the day with periodic measurements below an FEV_1 of 70% predicted. Also, African-Americans had a 38% prevalence of steroid-resistant asthma as compared to 12% in Caucasians. Further investigation is under way to understand the underlying mechanisms for these two patterns of steroid resistance and the predisposition for the high rate of steroid resistance in African-Americans. This information could lead to innovative approaches to management for these patients who are refractory to treatment with steroids.

New Medications

The insight gained through ongoing research that incorporates bronchoscopy, bronchoalveolar lavage, biopsy, molecular biology, and noninvasive measures of airway inflammation has stimulated questions regarding the judicious use of available medications and the potential for the development of new medications. Identification of predominant mediators associated with airway inflammation, especially those associated with allergic inflammation, such as interleukin (IL)-4, IL-5, IL-13 and interferon gamma, have resulted in development of pharmaceutical agents to counteract the activity of these pathways of inflammation.[24] To date, these approaches have provided only limited success. An additional approach is to develop DNA vaccine therapy with antisense oligonucleotides that could block the inflammatory response through a variety of approaches.[25]

Although most of the early attempts at selective therapy have been disappointing, continuous assessment regarding the trial design is needed to link the treatment with the population most likely to see a benefit. The medication closest to approval appears to be anti-IgE. In addition, promising medications such as inhibitors of phosphodiesterase 4 are undergoing early clinical trials and other agents are at the Phase 1 level of testing.

Pharmacogenetics

A new area of genetics has emerged, namely pharmacogenetics, that is designed to understand the relationship of genetics to medication response.[26-28] It is becoming increasingly important to define risk factors for patients who are likely to develop persistent asthma, patients predisposed to severe life-threatening exacerbations, patients with severe persistent asthma requiring extensive therapy, and patients with steroid-insensitive asthma. Advances in genetic associations could help define relevant asthma phenotypes associated with response to medications and pave the way for individualized treatment approaches based on the identification of an asthma phenotype.

The response to these medications could be related to genetic polymorphisms altering the site of action such as the drug receptor, or the availability of the drug at the site of action such as in relation to cytochrome P_{450}-dependent metabolic pathways. Genetic analysis can now be directed to genes directly related to the response for asthma medications, such as the β-adrenergic agonist receptor, enzymes controlling leukotriene synthesis, the leukotriene receptor, and the glucocorticoid receptor.[28]

In addition, genes related to asthma-associated disease features could affect the response to these medications. For example, one predominant feature of asthma is allergy, an IgE-mediated response. IgE synthesis is mediated through IL-4 stimulation of B lymphocytes and thus IL-4 serves a disease-modifying role. Genetic features of IL-4-mediated IgE synthesis could be related to at least two polymorphisms, increased IL-4 synthesis (C589T) or increased sensitivity to IL-4 at the IL-4 receptor level (R576 IL-4 receptor α).[29-35] An association of a sequence variant in the IL-4 gene promoter region at the C589T locus has been made to asthma severity, as indicated by the level of FEV_1.[32] The R576 IL-4 receptor α polymorphism has also been associated with asthma severity.[34] Because IL-13 also acts at the IL-4 receptor level and has been demonstrated to contribute to corticosteroid resistance in monocytes, polymorphisms at the IL-13 level are also of interest.[35,36]

Therefore the benefit of a medication could be tied to an active disease pathway influenced by a specific drug, for example, leukotriene synthesis and leukotriene antagonists as well as cytokine synthesis and an alteration of the glucocorticoid receptor.[28,37,38] Failure to respond to treatment could be caused by excessive activity of this pathway or possibly alternative pathways involved in the disease. This area is in its infancy but holds promising opportunities for understanding the variability in response to treatment as well as insights into developing individualized treatment programs.

CONCLUSIONS

We now have answers to many questions regarding the effect of continuous long-term use of three treatment options available for managing childhood asthma through the results of the CAMP clinical trial. Additional studies are in progress to evaluate earlier intervention and the effect of other medications, such as leukotriene receptor antagonists, on clinical outcomes and the natural history of asthma. It is possible that early indicators of asthma, such as increased symptoms or altered lung growth in children could prompt early intervention. With the right intervention it is possible that the disease could be controlled and thus in a sense a remission or relative "cure" could be maintained. Current interest regarding early pharmacologic intervention options centers around the comparative effects of inhaled glucocorticoids and leukotriene antagonists; however, neither of these agents may be sufficient to control asthma progression (Box 43-3; see Box 43-2).

On the other extreme, patients with severe asthma have low and irreversible pulmonary function. Their disease often has its onset in early childhood. Does this information suggest that children who manifest low pulmonary function and

BOX 43-3

THERAPEUTIC PRINCIPLES
Persistent Asthma

Establish follow-up after an initial wheezing episode.

With each wheezing episode, assess risk criteria for persistent asthma.

If the patient demonstrates frequent wheezing episodes and fits the high-risk profile, assess for allergen sensitivity and exposure.

If environmental control is inadequate, begin intervention with low-dose inhaled glucocorticoids.

Follow response by assessing both clinical control and pulmonary function.

Increase dose of inhaled glucocorticoids or add long-acting β-adrenergic agonist if asthma control is inadequate or pulmonary function is compromised.

Titrate therapy after control is established and pulmonary function maximized.

persistent symptoms in the presence of antiinflammatory therapy are at increased risk for further disease progression? If so, it will be important to recognize these patients and provide more effective interventions at critical stages of their disease progression. Furthermore, it would then be important to measure persistent inflammation and use this as another gauge to adjust therapy.

Once persistent asthma is established, it may be necessary to measure the response to treatment by evaluating the individual parameters of response, for example, symptoms, pulmonary function, and progression. Recent studies have clearly demonstrated that certain patients may respond to conventional treatment, such as inhaled glucocorticoids, in one category, for example, improvement in FEV_1, but not another, such as reduction in airways hyperresponsiveness.[20] Recognizing this deficiency in selective responses could prompt direction of treatment to improving individual response categories.

This review has concentrated on the current understanding of the therapeutic intervention and the possibilities it provides for improving asthma management and potentially inducing a remission or cure for the disease. However, none of this is possible without an integrated approach to patient care. There are serious deficiencies in the health care system that influence access to health care. The recent observation of an arrest in the rise in asthma mortality and morbidity is encouraging but offers a challenge to determine whether a reduction in morbidity and mortality is achievable.[1] Concerted efforts are now being directed toward understanding this phenomenon and recommendations have been made to integrate the various national resources available to improve outcomes of asthma care for children in the United States.[39]

REFERENCES

1. Mannino DM, Homa DM, Akinbami LJ, et al: Surveillance for asthma—United States, 1980-1999, *MMWR* 51:1-13, 2002.
2. Hamid QA, Minshall EM: Molecular pathology of allergic disease: I: lower airway disease, *J Allergy Clin Immunol* 105:20-36, 2000.
3. Suissa S, Ernst P: Inhaled corticosteroids: impact on asthma morbidity and mortality, *J Allergy Clin Immunol* 107:937-944, 2001.
4. Spahn JD, Szefler SJ: Inhaled glucocorticoids from combination therapy for asthma and COPD. In Martin RJ, Kraft M, eds: *Lung biology in health and diseases series*, New York, 2000, Marcel Dekker.

5. Matz J, Emmett A, Rickard K, et al: Addition of salmeterol to low-dose fluticasone versus higher-dose fluticasone: an analysis of asthma exacerbations, *J Allergy Clin Immunol* 107:783-789, 2001.

6. National Institutes of Health, National Heart, Lung, and Blood Institute: *Global Initiative for Asthma—Global strategy for asthma management and prevention,* NHLBI/NIH workshop report, 2002.

7. National Asthma Education and Prevention Program Expert Panel Report: Guidelines for the diagnosis and management of asthma update on selected topics 2002, *J Allergy Clin Immunol* 110:1A-8A, S141-S219, 2002.

8. National Asthma Education and Prevention Program: *Guidelines for the Diagnosis and Management of Asthma Update on Selected Topics 2002,* National Institutes of Health, National Heart, Lung, and Blood Institute, www.nhlbi.nih.gov.

9. Agertoft L, Pedersen S: Effects of long-term treatment with an inhaled corticosteroid on growth and pulmonary function in asthmatic children, *Respir Med* 88:373-381, 1994.

10. Zeiger RS, Dawson C, Weiss S: Relationships between duration of asthma and asthma severity among children in the Childhood Asthma Management Program (CAMP), *J Allergy Clin Immunol* 103:376-387, 1999.

11. Nelson HS, Szefler SJ, Jacobs J, et al: The relationships among environmental allergen sensitization, allergen exposure, pulmonary function, and bronchial hyperresponsiveness in the Childhood Asthma Management Program, *J Allergy Clin Immunol* 104:775-785, 1999.

12. Bender BG, Annett RD, Iklé D, et al: Relationship between disease and psychological adaptation in children in the Childhood Asthma Management Program and their families: CAMP Research Group, *Arch Pediatr Adolesc Med* 154:706-713, 2000.

13. Annett RD, Aylward EH, Lapidus J, et al: Neurocognitive functioning in children with mild and moderate asthma in the Childhood Asthma Management Program. The Childhood Asthma Management Program (CAMP) Research Group, *J Allergy Clin Immunol* 105:717-724, 2000.

14. The Childhood Asthma Management Program Research Group: Long-term effects of budesonide or nedocromil in children with asthma, *N Engl J Med* 343:1054-1063, 2000.

15. Martinez FD, Wright AL, Taussig LM, et al: Asthma and wheezing in the first six years of life, *N Engl J Med* 332:133-138, 1995.

16. Phelan PD, Robertson CF, Olinsky A: The Melbourne Asthma Study: 1964-1999, *J Allergy Clin Immunol* 109:189-194, 2002.

17. Agertoft L, Pedersen S: Effect of long-term treatment with inhaled budesonide on adult height in children with asthma, *N Engl J Med* 343:1064-1069, 2000.

18. Martinez FD: Development of wheezing disorders and asthma in preschool children, *Pediatrics* 109:362-367, 2002.

19. Castro-Rodriguez JA, Holberg CJ, Wright AL, et al: A clinical index to define risk of asthma in young children with recurrent wheezing, *Am J Respir Crit Care Med* 162:1403-1406, 2000.

20. Szefler SJ, Martin RJ, King TS, et al for the Asthma Clinical Research Network of the National Heart, Lung, and Blood Institute: Significant variability in response to inhaled corticosteroids for persistent asthma, *J Allergy Clin Immunol* 109:410-418, 2002.

21. Payne DNR, Balfour-Lynn IM: Children with difficult asthma: a practical approach, *J Asthma* 38:189-203, 2001.

22. Sont JK, Willems LNA, Bel EH, et al and the AMPUL Study Group: Clinical control and histopathologic outcome of asthma when using airway hyperresponsiveness as an additional guide to long-term treatment, *Am J Respir Crit Care Med* 159:1043-1051, 1999.

23. Chan MT, Leung DYM, Szefler SJ, et al: Difficult-to-control asthma: clinical characteristics of steroid-insensitive asthma, *J Allergy Clin Immunol* 101:594-601, 1998.

24. Barnes P: New targets for future asthma therapy. In Yeadon M, Diamont Z, eds: *New and exploratory therapeutic agents for asthma, lung biology in health and disease,* vol 139, New York, 2000, Marcel Dekker.

25. Kline JN: DNA therapy for asthma, *Curr Opin Allergy Immunol* 2:69-73, 2002.

26. Ober C, Moffatt ME: Contributing factors to the pathobiology: the genetics of asthma, *Clin Chest Med* 21:245-261, 2000.

27. Fenech A, Hall IP: Pharmacogenetics of asthma, *Br J Clin Pharmacol* 53: 2-15, 2002.

28. Palmer LJ, Silverman ES, Weiss ST, et al: Pharmacogenetics of asthma, *Am J Respir Crit Care Med* 165:861-866, 2002.

29. Marsh DG, Neely JD, Breazeale DR, et al: Linkage analysis of IL4 and other chromosome 5q31.1 markers and total serum immunoglobulin E concentrations, *Science* 264:1152-1156, 1994.

30. Borish L, Mascali JJ, Klinnert M, et al: SSC polymorphisms in interleukin genes, *Hum Mol Genet* 4:974, 1995.

31. Rosenwasser LJ, Klemm DJ, Dresback JK, et al: Promoter polymorphisms in the chromosome 5 gene cluster in asthma and atopy, *Clin Exp Allergy* 25:74-78, 1995.

32. Burchard EG, Silverman EK, Rosenwasser LJ, et al: Association between a sequence variant in the IL-4 gene promoter and FEV_1 in asthma, *Am J Respir Crit Care Med* 160:919-922, 1999.

33. Hershey GK, Friedrich MF, Esswein LA, et al: The association of atopy with a gain-of-function mutation in the alpha subunit of the interleukin-4 receptor, *N Engl J Med* 337:1720-1725, 1997.

34. Rosa-Rosa L, Zimmermann N, Bernstein JA, et al: The R576 IL-4 receptor alpha allele correlates with asthma severity, *J Allergy Clin Immunol* 104:1008-1014, 1999.

35. Martinez FD: Maturation of immune responses at the beginning of asthma, *J Allergy Clin Immunol* 103:355-361, 1999.

36. Spahn JD, Szefler SJ, Surs W, et al: A novel action of IL-13: induction of diminished monocyte glucocorticoid receptor-binding affinity, *J Immunol* 157:2654-2659, 1996.

37. Kam JC, Szefler SJ, Surs W, et al: Combination IL-2 and IL-4 reduces glucocorticoid receptor binding affinity and T cell response to glucocorticoids, *J Immunol* 151:3460-3466, 1993.

38. Sher ER, Leung DYM, Surs W, et al: Steroid-resistant asthma: cellular mechanisms contributing to inadequate response to glucocorticoid therapy, *J Clin Invest* 93:33-39, 1994.

39. Lara M, Rosenbaum S, Rachelefsky G, et al: Improving childhood asthma outcomes in the United States: a blueprint for policy action, *Pediatrics* 109:919-930, 2002.

CHAPTER **44**

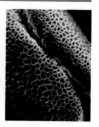

Mucosal Immunity: An Overview

LLOYD D. MAYER

The nature of a food-allergic response is similar to that of any immune response: it requires an antigenic stimulus, an appropriate genetic background of the host, and the input of the microenvironment. Specific antigens drive the response, but it is the microenvironment in which the antigen is recognized by cells of the immune system that truly dictates the nature of the reaction. With food antigens the microenvironment is the gastrointestinal (GI) tract, which is unique in its responses. This uniqueness is dictated by unusual challenges to what is the largest lymphoid organ in the body. The surface area of the entire GI tract could cover two tennis courts. Within that expansive surface is a rich supply of immunocompetent cells (T cells, B cells, macrophages, and dendritic cells). These cells are exposed to antigen (dietary, bacterial) at a level that is several orders of magnitude greater than that seen by cells of the systemic immune system. Coexistence with the external environment is key to the normal homeostasis of the gut; without such peaceful coexistence, inflammation would run rampant throughout the GI tract. Regulated immune responses are the norm in the intestine and deviation from such regulation has dire consequences.

ORGANIZATION OF GUT-ASSOCIATED LYMPHOID TISSUE

The mucosal immune system in the GI tract is unique largely because of its proximity to an enormous antigenic load (dietary, viral, and bacterial antigens). The organization of the gut-associated lymphoid tissue (GALT) is critical to a peaceful coexistence. Components of both innate and adaptive immunity come together to promote tolerance to nonpathogens and active immunity to true pathogens. The physical barrier of mucin glycoproteins produced by goblet cells and trefoil factors produced by the underlying epithelium promote nonimmune exclusion of antigens (trapped in the mucus) and barrier repair (trefoil factors) when breeches in epithelial integrity occur.[1-5] The epithelium itself serves as a physical barrier to many antigens. Tight junctions between epithelial cells composed of claudins, JAM, occludens, and ZO-1 and ZO-2 proteins make paracellular trafficking of antigens almost impossible.[6,7] The apical epithelial membrane actively excludes particulate antigens and noninvasive viruses and bacteria. Specialized epithelium in the crypts produce defensins, natural antibacterial products that eliminate potential pathogens in the lumen.[6-9]

Underlying the epithelium is a loose connective tissue stroma called the *lamina propria*. Within the lamina propria there is an abundance of activated T cells, B cells, macrophages, dendritic cells, and plasma cells. When activated under normal conditions they remain in a state of what has been termed *controlled* or *physiologic inflammation*.[10-12] It is clear that the lamina propria can act as an effector site, being the home for IgA plasma cells.[13-15] Secretory IgA (sIgA) gains entry into the lumen via a specialized transport system through the epithelium (polymeric Ig receptor [pIgR] or secretory component [SC]).[16-18] What is less clear is whether the lamina propria can serve as an inductive site as well.

The only organized lymphoid tissue in the GALT is the Peyer's patch (PP).[19] Like peripheral lymph nodes, these have both T cell and B cell areas. The unique features of the PP are that it is the inductive site for IgA production and always underlies a specialized epithelium called *M cells* or *follicle-associated epithelium*.[20-22] Selected antigens from the lumen can pass through the M cell unprocessed and be taken up by differentiated cells (DCs) and macrophages in the subepithelial M cell pocket. Antigens taken up in this manner are brought into the patch, where they elicit an IgA response. IgA-committed B cells migrate out of the patch into the draining mesenteric lymph nodes (MLNs) and then into the thoracic duct (the large lymphatic draining the GI tract) and into the vena cava. Once in the systemic circulation these cells migrate to other mucosal sites where they can mediate protection (sIgA secretion) against the offending pathogen more broadly.[23-25] This dissemination of IgA-committed B cells has been termed the *common mucosal immune system*. Mucosal homing receptors (e.g., α4β7) are induced on mucosally primed T and B cells, which allows them to migrate to different mucosal sites (lung, genitourinary tract, mammary gland).[23-25] Because the most likely sites of pathogen exposure are mucosal, this process makes sense. More recently, however, investigators have demonstrated more compartmentalization of the mucosa-associated lymphoid tissue (MALT). For example, nasal exposure provides protective immunity in the lung and genitourinary tract.[26-29] Exposure in the small bowel may result in cells that migrate to the mammary gland but not the respiratory tract. Although the mechanism underlying this segmentation is not clear, it may reflect the nature of the antigen and how the exposure occurred (e.g., invasive vs. noninvasive).

M cells are not uniformly distributed throughout the GI tract. They occur predominantly in the small bowel, although the rectal mucosa is enriched in M cells.[22] Thus, this mechanism of antigen sampling may be limited and site specific. A potential colonic equivalent of PPs has been reported by Ishikawa et al.[30] These smaller lymphoid aggregates have been termed *cryptopatches*. Their role in regulating colonic mucosal immune responses has not been clearly elucidated.

Immunoregulation in the Intestine

Every immune response needs to be regulated. Responses to pathogenic organisms shut down once the infection is cleared and autoreactive responses are tightly controlled. This process is magnified several billion times in the GI tract. Classic immune responses in the gut are characterized by one major theme: suppression. Several linked immunologic phenomenon in the GALT speak to this suppressed state. The first is the phenomenon of oral tolerance, which is the active non-response to an antigen administered via the oral route.[31-36] It is generally accepted that this is the mechanism whereby there is a failure to generate immune responses to dietary antigens. There are several factors involved in the development of oral tolerance (Table 44-1); with regard to food allergy and pediatrics, age is a factor. Neonates fail to tolerize when given antigen orally.[37] This has been worked out in murine and rat systems but is basically unexplained in humans. At the time of weaning, "gut closure" occurs and immunologic maturity ensues with the development of tolerance. The concept of gut closure relates to intestinal permeability. It is recognized that the normally tight junctions between epithelial cells are less tight in the newborn, thereby allowing for paracellular transport of antigens.[38] Such events may allow antigens to bypass normal regulatory inducing pathways and allow for exposure

to antigens that may normally be excluded by physical and immunologic barriers.

A second key factor in tolerance induction is the nature of the antigen, and in most models the best tolerogens are proteins.[39] The majority of dietary proteins induce tolerance and these comprise the bulk of antigens in most diets. The form of the antigen is also crucial to its ability to induce tolerance. Soluble antigens are more tolerogenic than particulate antigens.[40,41] For example, soluble ovalbumin, if administered, will induce tolerance but aggregated ovalbumin will not. The process of digestion (in the stomach and upper small bowel) degrades many particulate antigens into soluble ones.

The dose of the antigen administered is also critical to the type of tolerance generated. Low doses of antigen appear to elicit the activation of regulatory T cells whereas high doses of antigen induce either clonal deletion or anergy. This may be important in terms of attempting to generate antigen-specific suppression of an undesired response (i.e., low doses of autoantigen suppressing an autoreactive response). Several groups have utilized this strategy in mouse models of autoimmunity; in humans, similar studies have been less successful. The genetics of the host also plays a role in tolerance induction. In murine systems Balb/c mice are most easily tolerized whereas other strains are not capable of generating oral tolerance.[42] There are no studies available in genetically outbred mice although oral tolerance has been reported in man.

Lastly, oral tolerance is influenced by the nature of the antigen-presenting cell (APC). Professional APCs in the intestine are different than their counterparts in the systemic immune system. Intestinal macrophages, while activated, have downregulated many properties ascribed to peripheral macrophages, including a loss of lipopolysaccharide responsiveness, a lack of CD14 expression, and an inability to adhere to plastic.[43,44] Less information is available regarding intestinal DCs except that distinct DC subpopulations migrate to specific sites in the GI tract (dome epithelium, PP, interfollicular spaces, and subepithelial compartment).[45] Recent data suggest that DCs can express tight junction proteins in their dendrites and, as such, are capable of extending these processes between the epithelium and into the lumen, where they might presumably sample luminal antigens.[46] DCs in the PP have been reported to secrete transforming growth factor-β, which is critical for IgA regulation but potently immunosuppressive for other isotypes and T cell responses.[47,48] Treatment of mice with Flt 3 ligand, an activator of DCs, not only increases DC migration to the GI tract but also enhances oral tolerance.[49,50] The mechanism whereby this occurs has not been explained. Lastly, intestinal epithelial cells (IECs) have been reported to function as nonprofessional APCs. These cells constitutively express class I and class II molecules as well as a number of nonclassic class I (class Ib) molecules such as CD1d, MICA/B TL, and HLA-E.[51-54] Epithelial cells take up soluble protein antigens and can activate both CD4 and CD8+ T cell expansion. CD8+ T cells activated in these systems exhibit suppressor activity.[55,56] There are no data to support a role for these cells in oral tolerance induction, but they may be crucial for the maintenance of controlled/physiologic inflammation.

The role of the different cell types and structures has been addressed recently in a number of animal models. Mice treated with lymphotoxin β-Ig fusion proteins at birth fail to develop PP or MLNs and fail to develop oral tolerance.[57] This would suggest that PPs are important for tolerance induction.

TABLE 44-1 Factors Influencing Induction of Oral Tolerance

1. Nature of the antigen: soluble >> particulate; protein >> carbohydrate
2. Genetics of host
3. Age: neonates are not tolerized
4. Dose of antigen: low dose—regulatory T cell activation/ high dose—clonal anergy or deletion
5. Antigen-presenting cell: epithelium versus macrophage versus dendritic cell

However, these animals have defects in the splenic architecture as well, so systemic immune responses may be defective and so contribute to the lack of tolerance.

Because B cells appear to be important in the development of M cells (and therefore PPs),[20,58] the ability to induce oral tolerance was tested in mice deficient in B cells.[59] Oral tolerance was achieved in this model although it was not tolerance associated with regulatory T cells (low-dose tolerance) but rather tolerance associated with deletion of antigen-reactive cells. More recently, using a segregated ileal loop model, investigators were able to document that tolerance could be achieved to either degraded antigen or immunogenic peptides in loops that were devoid of M cells/PPs as well as in loops containing these cells/structures. These data suggest that there may be multiple pathways to achieving tolerance in the GI tract and support the concept that the epithelial cell may be involved.

Controlled/Physiologic Inflammation

A phenomenon linked to oral tolerance is that of controlled/physiologic inflammation. Broadly defined, this is the state of activation of cells within the lamina propria at any given time. Barring invasion with a known pathogen or some breach in the mucosal barrier, this inflammatory state remains constant. It does not change with diet, antibiotic use, or time of day. The key term here is *controlled*, meaning that some process is regulating this response. The activated state goes so far and no further. Disruption of the barrier or entry of a pathogen results in an increase in the inflammatory response but processes are rapidly brought into play to restore the level of controlled inflammation. There are diseases where this regulation has gone awry and simple triggers (e.g., infections, nonsteroidal antiinflammatory drugs) can result in aggressive uncontrolled inflammation.[11] These diseases underscore the crucial importance of the normally immunosuppressed tone of the GALT.

Controlled inflammation does not arise *de novo*. In mice reared in a germ-free environment, infiltration of the lamina propria with activated lymphocytes and macrophages is limited or absent. Clearly diet has nothing to do with physiologic inflammation because these mice from a germ-free environment are eating normal (irradiated) mouse chow. Furthermore, dead bacteria are not stimulus for physiologic inflammation because these exist in abundance in the same mouse chow. However, if one reintroduces defined nonpathogenic normal flora, there is a rapid recruitment of activated cells to the lamina propria. Luminal bacteria thus not only drive the influx of cells but must also be involved in triggering cells that control the process as well.

Role of Bacterial Flora in Mucosal Responses

This latter observation has opened up a new area of research related to mucosal immunity; the role of the flora in shaping mucosal immune responses and in driving mucosal homeostasis. The sheer numbers of bacteria per gram of colonic tissue (10^{12} to 10^{14}) far outweigh the number of cells in the human body. There is a clear symbiotic relationship that has been established. Luminal bacteria aid in digestion, produce vitamins, and communicate with the epithelium to promote a program of growth and differentiation.[60] The numbers of these commensal organisms either attached to the epithelium or in the unstirred mucus layer prevent colonization by many potential pathogens. They can create a hostile environment for such bacteria by competing for nutrients as well as physically blocking access to the epithelium.

There is also a growing appreciation of a group of bacteria, called *probiotics*, which not only enhance this competition with pathogens but may also stimulate the production of cytokines involved in suppression of inflammation (e.g., interleukin-10).[61,62] Probiotics are now being tested in a number of intestinal disorders including irritable bowel disease, pouchitis, bacterial overgrowth, recurrent *Clostridium difficile* toxin-induced colitis, and irritable bowel syndrome.[61,63,64] The potential role of probiotics in food allergy has not been tested, but if in fact these bacteria can alter the immunologic repertoire of the GI tract (as well as the systemic immune system), this would be a worthwhile study. With regard to the repertoire, one additional intriguing observation has been made. Mice reared in a germ-free environment are relatively immunodeficient, failing to generate optimal responses to antigens administered systemically. The repertoire is restored once normal flora are reintroduced. These data suggest that luminal flora plays a role in shaping the repertoire of the systemic immune system. One's own flora is difficult to alter, affected by the natural colonization that occurs during exposure to bacteria via maternal interactions and the local environment. Genetics plays a role as well, regulating the attachment of distinct bacteria to the epithelium by the expression of specific blood group substances.[65] Although it is difficult to actually characterize the normal flora of a given individual (because of the number of bacteria and the various culture conditions required for the growth of these fastidious organisms), the studies performed to date suggest that even after bowel cleansing a similar flora is restored. Newer technology utilizing species-specific 16S RNA primers has allowed for better characterization of the normal flora but the task remains a daunting one.

Secretory IgA System

The only truly positive aspect of the GALT is the production of a unique antibody, sIgA. IgA is produced along the length of the MALT by lamina propria plasma cells. Given the surface area of the GI tract, the number of IgA plasma cells and IgA molecules far outweighs any other antibody in the body.[13,15,17] In the MALT, IgA is secreted as a dimer bound by J chain (same as that used for IgM). Dimeric IgA secreted into the lamina propria binds to an epithelial cell-derived glycoprotein called *SC* or the *pIgR*.[14,16,18] This receptor has two functions: it actively transports IgA across the epithelium and into the lumen and provides a level of protection of the dimer against degradation by luminal proteases.[65] Once in the lumen the protected sIgA (dimeric IgA bound to SC) can bind to bacteria or viruses, either preventing them from attaching to the epithelium or trapping them in the mucus layer that gets passed out with the stool. sIgA does not activate the classic complement pathway, so its actions are generally noninflammatory. sIgA provided in breast milk survives gastric proteases in the newborn's stomach and provides passive immunity to environmental pathogens. IgA deficiency is the most common primary immunodeficiency with an incidence of between 1/300 to 1/750 individuals. Selective IgA deficiency is not typically associated with disease and it is assumed that IgM, which is produced in the lamina propria and capable of binding SC, can compensate for the absence of IgA.

The transport of other immunoglobulins into the lumen is regulated differently. Although initial studies had suggested that there was no IgG or IgE in mucosal secretions, this has been shown not to be the case. Both antibodies exist in the lumen although they do not appear to protected from luminal protease-mediated degradation. Some recent evidence suggests that the neonatal Fcε receptor (FcR$_N$) can promote bidirectional transport of both monomeric and complexed IgG.[66,67] Others have reported that under specific circumstances the low-affinity Fcε receptor can be expressed by epithelial cells.[68,69] How these function *in vivo* is unclear and whether they play a role in food allergy has not been completely explored.

Antigen Sampling in the Gastrointestinal Tract

As in any immune response the primary stimulus is antigen. How and who processes antigen in the systemic immune system is critical to the type of immune response generated. This may be more the case in the GALT. The section on oral tolerance has already described the various cells thought to be involved in antigen sampling. This section will explore the nature of the antigens sampled by the different pathways and the nature of the immune response generated.

M cells appear to be important in aiding in the generation of protective immune responses in the gut. M cells have the capacity to take up large particulate antigens (bacteria, viruses) and deliver them to the PP where a protective sIgA response is generated.[70] Given the number of M cells in comparison to the normal absorptive epithelium, there is an inherent limitation in their function. However, the dome epithelium overlying PP physically extends into the lumen, thereby providing access to luminal antigens. However, not all antigens are equally sampled by the M cells. There are glycoconjugates expressed on the M cell surface that allow for selective binding of reovirus, polio, and others.[71,72] Soluble proteins are not efficiently taken up by these same cells. This is of interest because soluble proteins are the best tolerogens. Because M cells have been partly linked to tolerance induction, other mechanisms for sampling of this group of antigens must exist.

IECs do take up soluble proteins and can elicit the activation of CD8+ suppressor T cells *in vitro*.[55,56] *In vivo* support of this phenomenon has not been generated although the ileal loop model just described suggests that IECs can be involved in tolerance induction.

IECs, however, may play a role in food allergy. Recent studies have documented that IECs are induced to express the low-affinity IgE receptor (CD23-FcεR) and that this receptor can rapidly transport IgE/antigen immune complexes across the epithelium and hand off the antigen to the high-affinity FcεR expressing mucosal mast cells.[68,69] This series of events leads to the induction of secretion of chloride ions by IECs into the lumen. Food allergens transported in this fashion can not only elicit local intestinal symptoms but may allow for dissemination of these cells to other mucosal sites. Such a series of events could explain the more disseminated responses seen upon food allergen reexposure.

CONCLUSIONS

This chapter has sought to define the unique concepts of the MALT both in the normal state as well as in disease (Box 44-1). Given the surface area of the mucosa and its exposure

---

BOX 44-1   KEY CONCEPTS

Specific Aspects of Mucosal Immunity

- The mucosal immune system is regulated different from the systemic immune system.
- The dominant immune response in the intestine is one of suppression. Examples of this suppressed state include oral tolerance and controlled/physiologic inflammation.
- Oral tolerance is governed by multiple factors including genetics of the host, age of the host, dose of the antigen, and form of the antigen.
- Secretory IgA is an immunologic barrier to infection and potentially prevents immune responses to nonpathogens.
- Antigens are sampled differently in the gastrointestinal tract. This includes novel forms of antigen-presenting cells.
- Epithelial cells can function as antigen-presenting cells and may play a role in mediating food-allergic responses.

---

to the external environment as well as introduced antigens (food), the potential for pathologic responses is high. However, mechanisms of tight regulation allow us to generally coexist peacefully with this external environment. Defects in this regulatory process, induced or genetically programmed, may result in inflammatory or allergic disease.

Acknowledgments

Supported by PHS grants AI-23504, AI-24671, and AI-44236.

REFERENCES

1. Podolsky DK, Lynch-Devaney JL, Stow P, et al: Identification of human intestinal trefoil factor: goblet cell-specific expression of a peptide targeted for apical secretion, *J Biol Chem* 268:669-702, 1993.
2. Wright NA, Poulsom G, Stamp S, et al: Trefoil peptide gene expression in gastrointestinal epithelial cells in inflammatory bowel disease, *Gastroenterology* 104:12-20, 1993.
3. Wright NA: Trefoil peptides and the gut, *Gut* 34:577-579, 1993.
4. Podolsky DK, Lynch-Devaney JL, Stow P, et al: Identification of human intestinal trefoil factor: goblet cell-specific expression of a peptide targeted for apical secretion, *J Biol Chem* 268:12230, 1993.
5. Thim L: Trefoil peptides: a new family of gastrointestinal molecules, *Digestion* 55:353-360, 1994.
6. Muresan Z, Paul DL, Goodenough DA: Occludin 1B, a variant of the tight junction protein occludin, *Mol Biol Cell* 11:627-634, 2000.
7. Itoh M, Furuse K, Morita K, et al: Direct binding of three tight junction-associated MAGUKs, ZO-1, ZO-2, and ZO-3, with the COOH termini of claudins, *J Cell Biol* 147:1351-1363, 1999.
8. Ayabe T, Satchell DP, Pesendorfer P, et al: Activation of Paneth cell alpha-defensins in mouse small intestine, *J Biol Chem* 277:5219-5228, 2002.
9. Ayabe T, Satchell DP, Wilson CL, et al: Secretion of microbicidal alpha-defensins by intestinal Paneth cells in response to bacteria, *Nat Immunol* 1:113-118, 2000.
10. Mayer L: Mucosal immunity and gastrointestinal antigen processing, *J Pediatr Gastroenterol Nutr* 30:S4-S12, 2000.
11. Sartor RB: Current concepts of the etiology and pathogenesis of ulcerative colitis and Crohn's disease, *Gastroenterol Clin North Am* 24:475-507, 1995.
12. Geboes K: From inflammation to lesion, *Acta Gastroenterol Belg* 57:273-284, 1994.
13. Keren DF: Intestinal mucosal immune defense mechanisms, *Am J Surg Pathol* 12:100-105, 1988.
14. Mestecky J, Lue C, Russell MW: Selective transport of IgA: cellular and molecular aspects, *Gastroenterol Clin North Am* 20:441-471, 1991.

15. Farstad IN, Carlsen H, Morten HC, et al: Immunoglobulin A cell distribution in the human small intestine: phenotypic and functional characteristics, *Immunology* 101:354-363, 2000.

16. Mostov KE: Transepithelial transport of immunoglobulins, *Annu Rev Immunol* 12:63-84, 1994.

17. Godding V, Vaerman JP, Sibille Y: Secretory mucosal immune mechanisms, *Acta Otorhinolaryngol Belg* 54:255-261, 2000.

18. Kaetzel CS, Robinson JK, Lamm ME: Epithelial transcytosis of monomeric IgA and IgG cross-linked through antigen to polymeric IgA: a role for monomeric antibodies in the mucosal immune system, *J Immunol* 152:72-76, 1994.

19. Brandtzaeg P, Bjerke K: Human Peyer's patches: lympho-epithelial relationships and characteristics of immunoglobulin-producing cells, *Immunol Invest* 18:29-45, 1989.

20. Kraehenbuhl JP, Pringault E, Neutra MR: Review article: intestinal epithelia and barrier functions, *Aliment Pharmacol Ther* 11:3-9, 1997.

21. Neutra MR: Interactions of viruses and microparticles with apical plasma membranes of M cells: implications for human immunodeficiency virus transmission, *J Infect Dis* 179:S441-S443, 1999.

22. Neutra MR, Phillips TL, Mayer EL, et al: Transport of membrane-bound macromolecules by M cells in follicle-associated epithelium of rabbit Peyer's patch, *Cell Tissue Res* 247:537-546, 1987.

23. Shaw SK, Brenner MB: The beta 7 integrins in mucosal homing and retention, *Semin Immunol* 7:335-342, 1995.

24. Tsuzuki Y, Miura S, Suematsu M, et al: Alpha 4 integrin plays a critical role in early stages of T lymphocyte migration in Peyer's patches of rats, *Int Immunol* 8:287-295, 1996.

25. Viney JL, Jones S, Chiu H, et al: Mucosal addressin cell adhesion molecule-1: a structural and functional analysis demarcates the integrin-binding motif, *J Immunol* 157:2488-2497, 1996.

26. Hordnes K, Tynning T, Brown A, et al: Nasal immunization with group B streptococci can induce high levels of specific IgA antibodies in cervico-vaginal secretions of mice, *Vaccine* 15:1244-1251, 1997.

27. Wu HY, Russell MW: Induction of mucosal and systemic immune responses by intranasal immunization using recombinant cholera toxin B subunit as an adjuvant, *Vaccine* 16:286-292, 1998.

28. Ugozzoli M, O'Hagan DT, Ott GS: Intranasal immunization of mice with herpes simplex virus type 2 recombinant gD2: the effect of adjuvants on mucosal and serum antibody responses, *Immunology* 93:563-571, 1998.

29. Parr EL, Parr MB: Immune responses and protection against vaginal infection after nasal or vaginal immunization with attenuated herpes simplex virus type-2, *Immunology* 98:639-645, 1999.

30. Ishikawa H, Saito H, Suzuki K, et al: New gut-associated lymphoid tissue "cryptopatches" breed murine intestinal intraepithelial T cell precursors, *Immunol Res* 20:243-250, 1999.

31. Weiner HL, Mayer LF: Oral tolerance: mechanisms and applications: introduction, *Ann N Y Acad Sci* 778:xiii-xviii, 1996.

32. Weiner HL, Friedman A, Miller A, et al: Oral tolerance: immunologic mechanisms and treatment of animal and human organ-specific autoimmune diseases by oral administration of autoantigens, *Annu Rev Immunol* 12:809-837, 1994.

33. Titus RG, Chiller JM: Orally induced tolerance. Definition at the cellular level, *Int Arch Allergy Appl Immunol* 65:323-338, 1981.

34. Strober W, Kelsall B, Marth T: Oral tolerance, *J Clin Immunol* 18:1-30, 1998.

35. Mowat AM, Steel M, Worthey EA, et al: Inactivation of Th1 and Th2 cells by feeding ovalbumin, *Ann N Y Acad Sci* 778:122-132, 1996.

36. MacDonald TT: T cell immunity to oral allergens, *Curr Opin Immunol* 10:620-627, 1998.

37. Strobel S: Neonatal oral tolerance, *Ann N Y Acad Sci* 778:88-102, 1996.

38. Peng HJ, Turner MW, Strobel S: Failure to induce oral tolerance to protein antigens in neonatal mice can be corrected by transfer of adult spleen cells, *Pediatr Res* 26:486-490, 1989.

39. Alpan O: Oral tolerance and gut-oriented immune response to dietary proteins, *Curr Allergy Asthma Rep* 1:572-577, 2001.

40. Mayer L, Sperber K, Chan L, et al: Oral tolerance to protein antigens, *Allergy* 56:12-15, 2001.

41. Mayer L: Oral tolerance: new approaches, new problems, *Clin Immunol* 94:1-8, 2000.

42. Stokes CR, Swarbrick ET, Soothill JF: Genetic differences in immune exclusion and partial tolerance to ingested antigens, *Clin Exp Immunol* 52:678-684, 1983.

43. Smith PD, Janoff EN, Mosteller-Barnum M, et al: Isolation and purification of CD14-negative mucosal macrophages from normal human small intestine, *J Immunol Methods* 202:1-11, 1997.

44. Smith PD, Smythies LE, Mosteller-Barnum M, et al: Intestinal macrophages lack CD14 and CD89 and consequently are down-regulated for LPS- and IgA-mediated activities, *J Immunol* 167:2651-2656, 2001.

45. Kelsall BL, Strober W: Distinct populations of dendritic cells are present in the subepithelial dome and T cell regions of the murine Peyer's patch, *J Exp Med* 183:237-247, 1996.

46. Rescigno M, Urbano M, Valzasina B, et al: Dendritic cells express tight junction proteins and penetrate gut epithelial monolayers to sample bacteria, *Nat Immunol* 2:361-367, 2001.

47. Spalding DM, Koopman MJ, Edridge JH, et al: Accessory cells in murine Peyer's patch. I. Identification and enrichment of a functional dendritic cell, *J Exp Med* 157:1646-1659, 1983.

48. Spalding DM, Williamson SI, Koopman WJ, et al: Preferential induction of polyclonal IgA secretion by murine Peyer's patch dendritic cell-T cell mixtures, *J Exp Med* 160:941-966, 1984.

49. Williamson E, Westrich GM, Viney JL: Modulating dendritic cells to optimize mucosal immunization protocols, *J Immunol* 63:3668-3675, 1999.

50. Viney JL, Mowat AM, O'Malley JM, et al: Expanding dendritic cells *in vivo* enhances the induction of oral tolerance, *J Immunol* 160:5815-5825, 1998.

51. Hershberg R, Eghtesady P, Sydora B, et al: Expression of the thymus leukemia antigen in mouse intestinal epithelium, *Proc Natl Acad Sci U S A* 87:9727-9731, 1990.

52. Salter-Cid L, Nonaka M, Flajnik MF: Expression of MHC class Ia and class Ib during ontogeny: high expression in epithelia and coregulation of class Ia and lmp7 genes, *J Immunol* 160:2853-2861, 1998.

53. Blumberg RS, Balk SP: Intraepithelial lymphocytes and their recognition of non-classical MHC molecules, *Int Rev Immunol* 11:15-30, 1994.

54. Balk SP, Burke S, Polischuk JE, et al: Beta 2-microglobulin-independent MHC class Ib molecule expressed by human intestinal epithelium, *Science* 265:259-262, 1994.

55. Mayer L, Shlien R: Evidence for function of Ia molecules on gut epithelial cells in man, *J Exp Med* 166:1471-1483, 1987.

56. Bland PW, Warren LG: Antigen presentation by epithelial cells of the rat small intestine. II. Selective induction of suppressor T cells, *Immunology* 58:9-14, 1986.

57. Fujihashi K, Dohi T, Rennert PD, et al: Peyer's patches are required for oral tolerance to proteins, *Proc Natl Acad Sci U S A* 98:3310-3315, 2001.

58. Kerneis S, Bogdanova A, Kraehenbuhl JP, et al: Conversion by Peyer's patch lymphocytes of human enterocytes into M cells that transport bacteria, *Science* 277:949-952, 1997.

59. Gonnella PA, Waldner HP, Weiner HL: B cell-deficient mice have alterations in the cytokine microenvironment of the gut-associated lymphoid tissue (GALT) and a defect in the low-dose mechanism of oral tolerance, *J Immunol* 166:4456-4464, 2001.

60. Bry L, Falk PG, Midtvedt T, et al: A model of host-microbial interactions in an open mammalian ecosystem, *Science* 273:1380-1383, 1996.

61. Madsen KL: The use of probiotics in gastrointestinal disease, *Can J Gastroenterol* 15:817-822, 2001.

62. Madsen KL: Inflammatory bowel disease: lessons from the IL-10 gene-deficient mouse, *Clin Invest Med* 24:250-257, 2001.

63. Dunlop SP, Spiller RC: Nutritional issues in irritable bowel syndrome, *Curr Opin Clin Nutr Metab Care* 4:537-540, 2001.

64. Kennedy RJ, Kirk SJ, Gardiner KR: Probiotics in IBD, *Gut* 49:873, 2001.

65. Holgersson J, Jovall PA, Breimer ME: Glycosphingolipids of human large intestine: detailed structural characterization with special reference to blood group compounds and bacterial receptor structures, *J Biochem (Tokyo)* 110:120-131, 1991.

66. Blumberg RS, Balk SP: Intraepithelial lymphocytes and their recognition of non-classical MHC molecules, *Int Rev Immunol* 11:15-30, 1994.

67. Ishikawa H, Saito H, Suzuki T, et al: New gut-associated lymphoid tissue "cryptopatches" breed murine intestinal intraepithelial T cell precursors, *Immunol Res* 20:243-250, 1999.

68. Berin MC, Kiliaan AJ, Yang PC, et al: Rapid transepithelial antigen transport in rat jejunum: impact of sensitization and the hypersensitivity reaction, *Gastroenterology* 113:856-864, 1997.

69. Berin MC, Yang PC, Ciok L, et al: Role for IL-4 in macromolecular transport across human intestinal epithelium, *Am J Physiol* 276:C1046-C1052, 1999.

70. Kraehenbuhl JP, Pringault E, Neutra MR: Review article: intestinal epithelia and barrier functions, *Aliment Pharmacol Ther* 11:3-8, 1997.

71. Giannasca KT, Giannasca PJ, Neutra MR: Adherence of *Salmonella typhimurium* to Caco-2 cells: identification of a glycoconjugate receptor, *Infect Immunol* 64:135-145, 1996.

72. Giannasca PJ, Giannasca KT, Leichtner AM, et al: Human intestinal M cells display the sialyl Lewis A antigen, *Infect Immunol* 67:946-953, 1999.

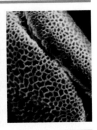

CHAPTER 45

Evaluation of Food Allergy

S. ALLAN BOCK ■ HUGH A. SAMPSON

The understanding of food allergy/hypersensitivity has progressed substantially since 1950, when Loveless[1] first suggested using masked food challenges to objectively determine the veracity of patients' histories of food allergy. May[2] codified this approach and established the double-blind, placebo-controlled food challenge (DBPCFC) as the gold standard for the investigation and accurate diagnosis of adverse reactions to food. The definition of the term *allergy* has been replete with misunderstanding when applied to foods. This chapter restricts the use of the term *allergy* to those adverse food reactions that have been shown to have an immunologic basis or strong immunologic association. Food allergy or hypersensitivity will be differentiated from other forms of adverse food reaction, and an approach will be outlined that may be used to determine whether an individual truly has an immunologically based adverse reaction to food.

The European Academy of Allergy and Clinical Immunology[3] has proposed definitions for food reactions based on the mechanisms thought to be involved. *Adverse reaction* is a useful generic term to describe any untoward reaction following the ingestion of a food or food constituent. These may be divided into *toxic* and *nontoxic* adverse reactions. Toxic reactions (e.g., food poisoning) may occur in any individual if a sufficient dose of the toxin is ingested. Nontoxic reactions are more individual and may depend on immune reactions (allergy/hypersensitivity) or nonimmune (*intolerance*) reactions (carbohydrate malabsorption). The two broad groups of immune reactions are *IgE mediated* and *non–IgE mediated*. The IgE-mediated reactions are usually divided into immediate-onset reactions (immediate in time) and immediate plus late phase (in which the immediate-onset symptoms are followed by prolonged, in time, or ongoing symptoms). The former have been well characterized in many studies, whereas the latter are under intense scrutiny to determine their mechanisms and unravel the role of the immune system. Non–IgE-mediated reactions (believed to be T cell–mediated) are typically delayed in onset (i.e., 4 to 48 hours) and most frequently involve the gastrointestinal tract.

EPIDEMIOLOGY/ETIOLOGY

Epidemiologic studies of food hypersensitivity have involved a number of different approaches, all designed to answer commonly raised questions about the frequency of these conditions in different populations. It is instructive to review this subject from both the "public perception" and the scientific inquiries that have been published. As noted in several sources, the general public regards food allergy or adverse reactions to food as a very common problem. An article in a widely read popular magazine reported a survey, which suggested that about 25% of the population believed that at least one family member had "food allergy."[4] Another estimate based on a questionnaire concluded that 15% of households contained at least one individual affected by food allergy.[5] A French study used a scientifically validated questionnaire on a representative sample and found a prevalence of approximately 3%.[6] In the United Kingdom 7500 households were surveyed, and 20% reported "food intolerance." In this population, 19% had their symptoms confirmed by DBPCFC. Analysis of this group suggests a prevalence of adverse food reactions of about 1.5%.[7] In another European study, a Dutch group[8] found that 10% of a randomly selected adult population described adverse reactions to food, but the results of blinded food challenges in this group indicated that only 2% of these adults truly had confirmed food reactions.

Prevalence studies on populations of children are less readily available. A study of 480 consecutive children born into a single pediatric practice recorded complaints of adverse food reactions in 28% of the infants. However, only 8% of these children were shown to be food related following reintroduction into the diet and very few could be shown to be IgE mediated. The foods most commonly incriminated were fruits. These reactions resolved and were no longer reported by age 3.[9] Similarly, Eggesbo et al[10] reported a population-based pediatric study. The children were younger than 2 years of age and included 3623 youngsters. Data were collected by questionnaire and involved assessment of prevalence, incidence, and cumulative incidences for multiple foods. The authors estimated that the cumulative incidence of adverse reactions to food was 35% by age 2. Fruit, milk, and vegetables accounted for about two thirds of the reactions. Interestingly the duration of the reactions was brief, with about two thirds not reported at the next questionnaire about 6 months later, very similar to the findings in the study mentioned earlier.[9] A number of studies have been conducted to establish the prevalence of reactions to specific foods. Cow's milk allergy has been assessed in a number of different nations. A study[11] of 1386 Dutch infants found that 2.8% exhibited cow's milk allergy. In 1759 Danish infants the prevalence of cow's milk allergy was 2.2% in the first year of life.[12] In a well-defined population of infants being studied on the Isle of Wight, the prevalence of cow's milk allergy was also found to be about 2%.[13] Taken together, these studies, from multiple nations, suggest that the prevalence of cow's milk allergy in infants and young children is about 2%. Recently a series of studies[14-16] were published suggesting that reactions to different conformations of the allergenic epitopes may differentiate children who quickly lose their reactivity to cow's milk from those who do not. A study of egg hypersensitivity in children in Germany reported a prevalence of about 1.3%, slightly lower than the prevalence of milk allergy.[17] Using a random digit dial survey, Sicherer et al[18] found that about 0.5% of pediatric patients are allergic to peanuts.

Children with atopic disorders are more likely to have food allergy. Burks et al[19] found that about one third of children with atopic dermatitis attending a university's allergy and dermatology clinics had DBPCFC documented food hypersensitivity. Eigenmann et al[20] found similar results (37%) in children with moderate to severe atopic dermatitis referred to a university dermatology clinic. Both studies found relatively few foods responsible for cutaneous symptoms (egg, milk, wheat, peanut, soy, tree nuts). A study by Guillet and Guillet[21] concluded that the more severe the degree of skin disease, the more likely it is that food hypersensitivity is involved. Consequently, the more severe the atopic dermatitis and the more difficult it is to manage, the more likely that an allergy evaluation and dietary intervention will be helpful.

Children with asthma also are more likely to have food allergy, especially if they have atopic dermatitis or a history of atopic dermatitis, gastroesophageal reflux, a history of feeding difficulties as an infant, and/or refractory asthma. Onorato et al[22] studied 300 consecutive asthmatic subjects from 7 months to 80 years from a respiratory diseases clinic for food allergy. Of the 300 asthmatics, 25 were thought to have food hypersensitivity triggering asthma, but only six (2% of the population) actually had positive DBPCFCs. Of note, the subjects experiencing positive food challenges were six children ranging in age from four to seventeen years. One half of these youngsters had a reaction to at least one food in which wheezing was the only symptom, whereas the other half had additional symptoms involving the gastrointestinal tract or skin. Novembre et al[23] studied 140 children presenting with histories of food-induced asthma. Wheezing was reproduced by DBPCFC in 8 (6%) of the children and their ages were 2 to 9 years. Only one of these subjects had wheezing as the sole symptom of the food reaction. In a population of 100 milk-allergic infants, Hill et al[24] described three different patterns of reactions based on the timing of the occurrence of symptoms. In the group having immediate reactions (< 4 hours), 29% had lower airway symptoms; in the group having intermediate-onset symptoms (4 to 24 hours), 4% had lower airway symptoms; and in the most delayed-onset group (> 24 hours), 50% had lower airway symptoms. This study has not been replicated in a similar group of children, so the general applicability of these results is not certain. Another study examined 410 selected children with asthma referred to a pulmonary center; 279 (68%) presented a history of one or more foods triggering asthma. All underwent DBPCFCs and 168 (60%) developed one or more symptoms (gastrointestinal, cutaneous, respiratory). Of the 168 reacting, 67 (40%) experienced wheezing as one of the symptoms. Most of the subjects had other respiratory symptoms as well. Only five (3% of 168) subjects had wheezing as the only symptom.[25]

Food allergy clearly has a genetic component. Sicherer et al[26] has shown that concordance for peanut allergy is much higher in monozygotic as contrasted with dizygotic twins. Monozygotic twins had a pairwise concordance of 64%, whereas the dizygotic group was only 7%. Despite the importance of genetics in food allergy, this study clearly demonstrates a crucial role for environmental factors, that is, food proteins.[27] In a review of 220 families under study for food allergy or atopic dermatitis, Sampson found two or more children with food hypersensitivity in 20 families. Eighteen sibling pairs were found to be allergic to the same food(s) (H.A. Sampson, unpublished observations).

In children, few foods account for about 90% of food hypersensitivity reactions. Food allergens are glycoproteins that are water soluble and range from 5 to 70 kD in molecular weight. They are usually stable to heat, acid, and proteases.[27] An increasing number of these allergens have been identified, isolated, sequenced, and cloned. The identification of the IgE-, IgG-, and T cell epitopes are leading to the promise of specific treatments that will modify the immune response without the potential for triggering allergic symptoms.[28-32]

Most reported series of "oral allergy syndrome" (food-pollen allergy syndrome) have been in adults. However, this "syndrome," which provokes oral pruritus and minimal oral swelling, is also observed in children. In addition, reports of adverse reactions to fruits in young infants are common, but most of these are rapidly "outgrown."[9]

DIFFERENTIAL DIAGNOSIS

The European classification of adverse food reactions provides a useful approach for evaluating food allergy (Table 45-1). Toxic food reactions are fairly common and need to be considered as the history is acquired. Children may be less likely than adults to experience food poisoning, but one must consider this possibility during the evaluation. Although scrombroid fish poisoning has not been reported in children,

TABLE 45-1 Differential Diagnosis of Adverse Reactions to Foods

Toxic reactions
  Toxic reactions (food poisoning, for example, scrombroid fish poisoning)
Nontoxic reactions
  Intolerances
    Carbohydrate malabsorption (e.g., lactase deficiency, sucrase-isomaltase deficiency)
  Psychologic reactions (strongly held beliefs)
  Immune
    IgE mediated
      Immediate (gastrointestinal, respiratory, cutaneous, ocular, cardiovascular, anaphylactic)
      Immediate and late phase (atopic dermatitis, allergic gastrointestinal disorders)
    Non–IgE immune mediated
      Gluten-sensitive enteropathy (celiac disease, dermatitis herpetiformis)
      Food protein–induced gastrointestinal illnesses
        Allergic eosinophilic esophagitis and gastroenteritis
        Allergic proctocolitis
      Heiner's syndrome (food-induced pulmonary hemosiderosis)

it certainly might occur. Nontoxic reactions may be the result of "intolerance" (nonimmune) or hypersensitivity (immune) reactions. In youngsters, carbohydrate malabsorption is probably the most common cause of an adverse food reaction. Lactose intolerance is often secondary to infection-induced gastroenteritis with lactase activity requiring some time to return to adequate levels to digest this milk sugar. This may result in a period of persistent bloating and diarrhea that has been confused with food hypersensitivity. Carbohydrate malabsorption of the complex sugars in fruit juices has been reported to be a very common cause of diarrhea in young children.[33] When young children are referred for an allergy evaluation for chronic diarrhea, it may be most useful to eliminate these possibilities by using a brief elimination diet before embarking on a more complete allergen elimination diet.

Parental perceptions of their child's food allergy can be very convincing and must be considered in the differential. Most children do not believe that they have food allergy unless they have had reactions that have made them ill, and then they develop aversions to the foods in question. Children have been frequently placed on very restricted and potentially nutritionally inadequate diets because of parental beliefs.[34] The extension of some of these situations has resulted in Munchausen's disease by proxy. (There have even been a few well-reported fatalities described in the media.) Less extreme but equally perplexing are the diets that parents have used in an attempt to modify their children's behavior. There is a long lineage of these diets, starting early in the twentieth century and continuing unabated but now based on more sophisticated "pseudoscience."

The hypersensitivity food reactions include all of those that have been shown to be or are thought to be immune mediated. The most well characterized reactions are those IgE-mediated immediate hypersensitivity responses. The major systems involved include the skin, respiratory system, gastrointestinal tract, and cardiovascular system. Most familiar are the immediate-onset cutaneous symptoms. Acute urticaria with a sudden onset and brief duration (hours) is commonly because of food hypersensitivity. More difficult are the youngsters with prolonged urticaria lasting weeks to months. Allergists are frequently asked to evaluate youngsters with chronic urticaria with or without angioedema, but these are rarely because of food allergy. Occasionally children may become allergic to a food ingested on a daily basis. These rare reactions are most likely to be identified by the use of a strict oligoantigenic food diet that excludes most foods commonly found in the youngster's diet. Food additives have been reported to cause chronic urticaria in adults.[35] Angioedema without urticaria does occur in children and adolescents but is very rare in infants and toddlers. When it occurs, the child must be evaluated for hereditary angioedema with appropriate testing for C4 and the level and function of C1 esterase inhibitor.

Atopic dermatitis exacerbated by food hypersensitivity has now been well characterized in controlled DBPCFCs in multiple centers.[19,20,36] Food hypersensitivity provokes cutaneous symptoms in about one third of youngsters with moderate to severe atopic dermatitis. The lesion produced during the food challenge is usually a pruritic morbiliform rash. Less typically, children may react initially with erythema of the skin and some urticaria and then the eczematous rash becomes more prominent hours later. During challenges under observation, children may be noted to exhibit discomfort, irritability, and pruritus some time before the recognizable lesions appear.

Immediate gastrointestinal symptoms elicited during DBPCFCs include nausea, abdominal pain, and diarrhea. The immediate symptoms may be explosive and impressive. Equally impressive is the rapid resolution of all discomfort that may occur after emesis, which completely empties the stomach, and the child's appetite returns. This observation, when reported historically by parents or patients, strongly supports the search for a food allergen proximate to the onset of gastrointestinal symptoms. IgE-mediated diarrhea is more difficult to characterize but does occur in a constellation with the other gastrointestinal symptoms and usually within an hour or two of the time the food is ingested. Two additional areas for which there is controversial support for the role of IgE-mediated food allergy are colic and chronic constipation. Controlled challenges lend credence to the notion that in some children these problems are food related and that the immune system is playing some role.[37-43]

Respiratory symptoms caused by food hypersensitivity are often seen concurrently with cutaneous or gastrointestinal manifestations. Sneezing, rhinorrhea, and eye symptoms (included with respiratory manifestations during this discussion) are frequently noted as minor but significant accompaniments to symptoms within the other two systems mentioned. Cough, wheezing, and laryngospasm are also noted during allergic reactions to foods. When these lower respiratory symptoms occur, they are often quite impressive and require immediate therapeutic intervention. Asthma as the sole manifestation of food allergy is less common and is discussed in more detail in Chapter 50.

Cardiovascular collapse during a food allergic reaction is the most catastrophic manifestation and may result in death. It is crucial to appreciate that cardiovascular collapse may occur in the absence of any other signs or symptoms of anaphylaxis and consequently may not be recognized promptly. In the differential diagnosis of conditions that may cause sudden, unexpected death in children, anaphylaxis should be considered high on the list of possibilities. A universally accepted definition of anaphylaxis is not currently available. However, severe allergic reactions, whatever the definition, must be identified and may include any of the symptoms noted earlier. When evaluating histories of potential allergic reactions, most authors would agree that they are severe if they involve the cardiovascular system (fall in blood pressure), respiratory symptoms that compromise breathing, and swelling in respiratory structures. Whether isolated urticaria and/or angioedema constitutes anaphylaxis may be moot, because they frequently serve as a harbinger of more severe symptoms.

EVALUATION AND MANAGEMENT

History

The acquisition of the history achieves two goals: (1) to make an accurate diagnosis based on the history and (2) to ascertain relevant information to be used to reproduce the reported signs and symptoms by food challenge (Table 45-2). To accomplish the second goal, a detailed description of the signs and symptoms must be obtained from the patient/parent. Important information includes the time from ingestion of the food to the onset of symptoms, the number of occasions on which the reaction has occurred, the quantity of food required to elicit the reaction (the smallest and largest quantities previously observed), the most recent occurrence, and the association of additional factors such as exercise and possibly concurrent medication ingestion (more common in adults). If the history suggests anaphylaxis, then an attempt to determine the quantity

Description of symptoms and signs
Timing from ingestion to onset of symptoms
Frequency with which reactions have occurred
Time of most recent occurrence
Quantity of food required to evoke reaction
Associated factors (activity, medication)

of food responsible for these severe reactions will be most useful in counseling the patient/parent about avoidance and possible future reactions occurring after accidental ingestion. A history of an *isolated* ingestion of the suspected allergen or a specific food ingested on several occasions leading to a reaction accompanied by evidence of IgE to the suspected food (positive skin test or *in vitro* test) is considered diagnostic.[44] One must be certain that the offending allergen is correctly identified because an error in identification would expose the patient to future anaphylaxis with the potential for dire consequences. If the identity of the offending allergen is not clear, a food challenge must be performed. In cases where idiopathic anaphylaxis is suspected, more detailed diagnostic efforts must be performed.

Diet diaries are variably helpful in the evaluation of food hypersensitivity. Sometimes parents will present the physician with months of carefully detailed notes about foods the child has eaten each day, and it will not be possible to identify any offender. Parents suspect most culprits producing prompt onset of symptoms; therefore, diet diaries are not helpful. In more chronic situations, they may be helpful, but the use of an oligoantigenic diet for a few days may be more revealing (e.g., the child's atopic dermatitis suddenly becomes more easily managed). Diet diaries may be helpful when a "suspect" food is identified, but allergic symptoms persist. A detailed diary of all foods ingested for a few days may detect the ingestion of a food that contains the offending allergen not detected by the parents. This may explain apparent inconsistencies in the history and alleviate any concern that new food allergies have developed.

Physical Examination

The physical examination is directed toward the respiratory, cutaneous, and gastrointestinal systems, seeking to identify atopic features. If the child exhibits growth failure or signs of a nonallergic disorder, a detailed evaluation for those problems must be pursued. Asthmatic patients require a detailed evaluation as described elsewhere in this volume. As noted earlier, it is rare for food allergy to trigger only chronic asthma. However, there are rare situations in which a strict elimination diet might be worthwhile to "rule out" the chance that a food or foods in the daily diet is responsible for severe asthma.

Laboratory Studies

If the history suggests an immediate hypersensitivity reaction, evidence of food-specific IgE should be sought.

Skin Testing

Several skin testing techniques have been used to evaluate IgE-mediated food reactions including the prick skin test (PST), scratch testing, and intradermal skin testing. Glycerinated food extracts using 1:10 or 1:20 weight per volume dilutions are placed on the skin and accompanied by appropriate negative (diluent) and positive (histamine) controls. The skin is pricked or punctured with an appropriate needle, and food allergens eliciting wheal diameters at least 3 mm larger than those produced by the negative control are interpreted as positive, whereas smaller responses are considered negative. Using this technique, the negative predictive accuracies for the common food allergens are greater than 95%, so a negative PST essentially excludes IgE-mediated food hypersensitivity. The converse is not true. The positive predictive accuracy of a positive skin test for many foods is less than 50%, thus indicating the presence of IgE antibody but not confirming a diagnosis of symptomatic food hypersensitivity.[45-48] When there is a history of a severe or anaphylactic reaction to an isolated food and the skin test is positive, a positive skin test to the implicated food may be viewed as diagnostic.

For children less than 3 years of age, the negative predictive accuracy of PST is not quite as high (80% to 85%). In this age group, the level of sensitization or reactivity of cutaneous mast cells may be too low to detect by skin testing. Hill and others[49,50] have reported that PST wheals of 8 mm or larger are diagnostic of reactivity in infants and children 2 years of age or younger. However, skin test results are quite variable because the outcome is dependent on the reagents utilized (which are not standardized) and the personnel applying and interpreting the test.

The choice of appropriate food extracts to use is based on the history. It is recommended that only food allergens suspected of provoking symptoms, rather than a "panel" of foods, be used in the evaluation. This prevents the common situation of finding numerous positive skin tests in highly atopic children, who tolerate many of the foods to which they are skin test positive.

A number of variables must be considered when performing PSTs: (1) commercially prepared extracts frequently lack the labile proteins responsible for IgE-mediated sensitivity to many fruits and vegetables (apples, oranges, bananas, pears, melons, potatoes, carrots, celery, etc.)[51-53]; (2) skin testing on skin surfaces that have been treated with topical steroids for atopic dermatitis may induce smaller wheals than tests performed on untreated surfaces; (3) negative PSTs with commercially prepared extracts that do not support convincing histories of food allergic reactions should be repeated with the fresh food before concluding that food allergen–specific IgE is absent[54] and a challenge performed under observation to be certain that the food can be safely returned to the diet; and (4) long-term high-dose systemic corticosteroid therapy may reduce allergen-induced wheal size.

Intradermal skin testing is not recommended for the evaluation of food allergy. Studies indicate that intradermal skin tests provide no significant increase in sensitivity or predictive value when compared to DBPCFC,[45] and fatalities have been reported after intradermal skin testing for foods.[55]

Fresh fruits and vegetables may be used with the "prick by prick" technique, that is, pricking the food to be tested and then pricking the skin of the patient being evaluated.[56] Similar data may be obtained using Finn Chambers.[57] It is essential that at least one other person (not likely to be sensitized) be used as a negative control to rule out nonspecific irritation. This same technique may be used for other substances when no commercial extracts are available. Spices are a prominent example. Several spices have been confirmed as the allergens provoking anaphylaxis in a number of subjects,[58-60] but the evaluation of such histories is hampered by the absence of commercially available and validated testing materials. Extracts of spices may be prepared using a mortar and pestle to grind the material into a powder and then extracting it with the diluent used for skin testing. In this situation a positive result is helpful (with a negative control subject) and a negative response to the test is not informative and should not be regarded as proving that sensitization is not present.

In Vitro Testing

The most useful *in vitro* measurements used for the diagnosis of immediate food hypersensitivity is the determination of specific IgE to food allergens. Radioallergosorbent tests (RASTs) and the enzyme-linked immunosorbent assay are used to screen patients suspected of IgE-mediated food allergies. These tests have been considered less sensitive than skin tests, but one study comparing Phadebas RAST with DBPCFCs found PSTs and RASTs to have similar sensitivities and specificities when RAST scores of 3 or greater were considered positive.[61] The RAST may be preferred in some clinical settings: (1) patients with significant dermatographism, (2) patients with severe skin disease (e.g., atopic dermatitis) and limited surface area for testing, and (3) patients who cannot discontinue antihistamines. In two studies using the CAP-RAST Fluorescent Enzyme Immunoassay in children, Sampson and Ho[62,63] used receiver operating characteristic curves and demonstrated that quantification of food-specific IgE provided increased positive predictive accuracies for egg, milk, peanut, and fish hypersensitivity compared with PSTs.[62-65] Individuals with serum food allergen–specific IgE levels in excess of the 95% predictive value may be considered reactive, and the need for an oral food challenge would be obviated. A patient with a food allergen–specific IgE less than the 95% predictive value may be reactive and would require a food challenge to confirm the diagnosis (Table 45-3). In addition, recent data suggest that monitoring the allergen-specific IgE values may be useful in predicting when follow-up challenges are likely to be negative (i.e., when patients "outgrow" their food allergies).[66] Based on these data, the patient evaluation may begin with the history, progress to skin testing for the suspected foods, and then provide quantification of the level of serum food-specific IgE to determine the probability that a reaction will occur.

Basophil histamine release assays and intestinal mast cell histamine release assays have been investigated in research settings but have not yet been shown to have clinical advantage over skin testing or RAST. Monitoring "spontaneous" basophil histamine release and measuring the generation of "histamine-releasing factor" have been shown to be highly predictive of IgE-mediated food allergy and ongoing ingestion of the responsible food allergen; however, the measurement has not proved to be practical in the clinical setting at this time.[67,68]

Investigation of lymphocyte stimulation tests have been reported to be useful in identifying subjects with food hypersensitivity[69,70]; however, Hoffman et al[71] was not able to reproduce these results, and clinical applicability of this approach remains to be proved. At this time there are no rigorously controlled studies demonstrating that IgG RASTs have any clinical validity. In fact, most individuals make some IgG antibodies to foods they ingest, and an absence of food-specific IgG might suggest that a child has immunodeficiency. Serum food-specific IgG levels may be elevated in disorders affecting protein absorption, such as celiac disease and inflammatory bowel disease.[72]

TABLE 45-3 Diagnostic Food-Specific IgE Values (CAP-System Fluorescent Enzyme Immunoassay) of Greater than 95% Positive Predictive Value

Food	Serum IgE Value (kU$_A$/L)	Rechallenge Value
Egg	≥ 7.0	≤ 1.5
≤ 2 yr old	≥ 2.0*	
Milk	≥ 15.0	≤ 7.0
≤ 2 yr old	≥ 5.0†	
Peanut	≥ 14.0	≤ 5.0‡
Fish	≥ 20.0	
Tree nuts	≥ 15.0	

From Sampson HA: *J Allergy Clin Immunol* 107:891-896, 2001.
Note: Patients with food-specific IgE values less than the listed diagnostic values may experience an allergic reaction following challenge. Unless history strongly suggests tolerance, a physician-supervised food challenge should be performed to determine if the child can ingest the food safely.
*Boyano-Martinez T, Garcia-Ara C, Diaz-Pena JM, et al: *Clin Exp Allergy* 31:1464-1469, 2001.
†Garcia-Ara C, Boyano-Martinez T, Diaz-Pena JM, et al: *J Allergy Clin Immunol* 107:185-190, 2001.
‡If no reactions after third birthday.

Oral/Labial Testing

Rance and Dutau,[73] in France, have been studying the efficacy of diagnosing food hypersensitivity by applying food extracts to the inner lip of the oral mucosa. If the positive predictive accuracy of this approach is shown to be high enough to eliminate the need for standard oral food challenges, it may gain wider application. A potential limitation of the technique is that some individuals may not react to foods if they are coated with other foods but the symptoms occur when the food is absorbed. Conversely, challenges in capsules that bypass the oral mucosa may not elicit symptoms that are manifested only during contact with oropharyngeal structures. Thus the clinical applicability of this test remains to be determined.

Atopy Patch Testing

The atopy patch test has been studied in combination with the PST to determine if the combination is more sensitive and specific for diagnosing food allergy in atopic dermatitis and some gastrointestinal hypersensitivities.[74-77] It has been touted as being useful in the diagnosis of non–IgE-mediated food reactions. Further studies are necessary to determine its place in the diagnostic armamentarium for food hypersensitivity.

Food Challenges

The oral food challenge is recognized as the gold standard against which all other tests must be assessed. It provides investigators with a technique that may be varied to fit most situations if proper facilities are available and sufficient rigor is applied. As noted earlier, the use of food challenges has demonstrated that an *in vitro* test may replace the food challenge for detection of hypersensitivity to some foods. New therapies that are being developed need a gold standard by which to make the diagnosis and then confirm that the treatment is effective. In fact, it may be argued that this standard allows for precision in diagnosis and assessment of treatment that is superior to techniques currently available for the study of aeroallergens.

Open Food Challenges

Open food challenges are very useful in circumstances in which it is unlikely that the patient will react to one or more foods of concern. They may occasionally be performed at home rather than in a medical facility, whereas in other situations they must be administered under medical supervision, but generally in situations that require less rigor than that needed for blinded challenges. Physicians often find themselves confronted with a young milk- or egg-allergic child who during skin testing is found to have a positive test for peanuts. Such children often have never knowingly consumed peanuts. These children should be challenged openly under observation so that in the unlikely event of symptoms occurring, they may be treated promptly. In other cases, children may have a vague history of an adverse reaction to a food, but the history or a food diary suggests that the food has been ingested in another food regularly consumed in the diet. Open food challenges under medical observation may be very helpful with these subjects to refute the history.

Single-Blind Food Challenge

Single-blind food challenges (SBFCs) are very useful in daily clinical allergy practice. They are less time consuming than DBPCFCs and often provide an excellent diagnostic aid in confirming or refuting histories of food hypersensitivity reactions. In circumstances in which patient opinions or concerns may influence the outcome, the SBFC offers an alternative that will be convincing to most patients and physicians. The nurse providing the challenge material should be trained in techniques that do not "telegraph" the challenge substance (suspected food or placebo) to the subject being challenged. For immediate symptoms, the challenge is administered in a graded fashion over a period of 1 to 2 hours (see later) and then the individual is observed for an additional 2 to 4 hours, depending on the occurrence of symptoms. The SBFC is especially helpful in shortening a long list of suspicions that are not amenable to open challenge, leaving the DBPCFC for investigating reactions that are more difficult to confirm or refute.

Double-Blind, Placebo-Controlled Food Challenge

The DBPCFC is the gold standard for detecting any suspected permutation of adverse food reactions if the challenge is organized correctly.[2,78-83] The food challenge is designed to reproduce the individual's history, as determined during the acquisition of the history. There are several protocols that are used for the administration of food challenges. One approach is to have a single day for the active food challenge and a separate day for the placebo challenge. Unfortunately, time constraints have rendered this approach less practical for suspected immediate reactions than in the past, but for some research questions it remains essential. Often one challenge (active or placebo) is dispensed in the morning while the other is given in the afternoon (at least a few hours after the end of the morning challenge). Time constraints have resulted in both challenges being administered on the same day. The potential limitations of this approach are that slow or delayed onset symptoms could be missed or produce confusion rendering interpretation of the results difficult. Should this outcome transpire, the challenge must be repeated using separate active

food and placebo days. When multiple foods are being challenged, some placebo challenges may be omitted if it is found that another suspect food does not elicit symptoms. In some cases it may be acceptable to challenge two foods on the same day: one in the morning and one in the afternoon. However, if both elicit symptoms, then interpreting the results may be confusing. When evaluating subjective symptoms it may be useful to interchange the active and placebo doses. The process may begin with the first one or two doses being placebo. Interchanging the doses may be done in a random fashion, but the entire challenge is consumed on the same day. Thus the subject will be ingesting different quantities of food at different times in an apparently random manner. This will add to the blinding of the procedure. If capsules are being used to blind the challenge material, some investigators feel that all challenges must contain the same number of capsules; therefore, they have started with the placebo and then gradually replaced some placebo capsules with food capsules. In some instances the physician may want to alter the challenge following certain doses, depending on the response. In this situation, the investigator sends the challenge to the study unit to be administered by a nurse. This procedure may be useful when studying subjective or vague complaints that are reported to begin promptly after ingestion of the incriminating food. For example, when studying children with headache, abdominal pain, or behavioral changes, the ability to change the challenge from suspected food to placebo and back, during a single challenge day, has proved to be most helpful.

As noted earlier, the quantity and timing of the challenge doses are determined by the patient history. Some authors recommend that the starting dose be about one half of the amount that is thought to be the minimum amount likely to elicit the immediate onset of symptoms. Other investigators use a more specific dosing protocol so that every subject receives the same dose at set intervals. Hourihane et al[84] used a threshold challenge protocol in studying peanut allergy, starting with a very low dose that has never elicited a response in any subject tested. A number of different approaches may prove useful depending on the nature of the investigation. The timing of challenges must be arranged so that the interval between each challenge dose is long enough to allow symptoms to occur. This interval is determined from the history. The doses may be doubled at the chosen interval or some other increase in dosage may be chosen. When the challenge is negative with up to 8 to 10 g of dried food in a single dose or 60 to 100 g of wet food in a single dose, the challenge is terminated and the results are presented to the patient and/or parents. However, a negative challenge is not considered complete until the food under study is consumed under observation in usual portions without eliciting symptoms. The ability of the child to ingest the incriminating food without developing symptoms eliminates any concern about the effect of preparation, digestion, and other variables inherent in the blinded food challenge. Administering an insufficient quantity of food during the oral challenge is the most likely variable to result in a reaction after a negative blinded challenge.[85-87] Oral symptoms may not be provoked during open feedings if the challenge vehicle prevents sufficient allergen contact with oral tissues. Positive subjective symptoms after a negative blinded challenge also may be the result of the subject's strongly held belief that the food will cause symptoms. This is rarely a problem when challenging children.

The procedures described earlier have been very successful and relatively straightforward when used to evaluate children with immediate hypersensitivity. Few delayed-onset reactions have been confirmed in children except for those eliciting gastrointestinal symptoms. The DBPCFC also is quite useful in evaluating delayed-onset symptoms. Children may present with one of two symptom/timing patterns. In some cases, a single dose of food provokes symptoms hours to days after ingestion. In this situation the food is administered under observation in the morning. The subject is then asked to return when the symptoms appear. In other cases, repeated doses of the food are purportedly necessary to provoke symptoms. In such cases, the challenge is administered on several consecutive mornings, in the office or clinic, to settle the issue of the child requiring daily ingestion with the symptoms occurring at the end of prolonged exposure. Use of the placebo is crucial and the challenge procedure should be "crossed-over" two or three times to ensure that the challenge is reproducible.

When the history suggests that the food must be ingested multiple times per day over multiple days, then the only optimal means for administration of a true DBPCFC is in a setting where the administration of all the doses are supervised and symptoms can be observed. In this era, the resources to accomplish this goal are usually unavailable. However, the child can be challenged at home if the food is administered in a form that is difficult for the patient/parents to discern. This may be accomplished with very cooperative subjects having no strongly held bias. If the result is negative and the food returned to the diet, a substantial service has been provided to the family.

At the present time many different vehicles are used for administering food challenges (Table 45-4). Many of these mask the challenge food rather than completely blinding it; however, for research purposes, the subjects must not be able to discern the contents of the challenge or the results may not be valid. Fortunately, children are often not able to detect the hidden material and are easily distracted from attempting to do so. The original challenge vehicle used by May[2] in 1976 was opaque capsules used for both challenge food and placebo. The capsule approach was very effective at hiding nearly any food; however, it was often difficult to administer adequate quantities of food with this method. The use of dehydrated foods circumvented this problem for many substances. Now it is possible to hide large quantities of food in various vehicles without the active ingredient being detected. As the table shows, the list is quite long and varied, allowing nearly any food to be hidden or masked in an effective vehicle. The placebo portion of the challenge must be another food of a texture similar to the challenge food and known to be tolerated by the individual. When capsules are used, dextrose is often an excellent placebo. For substances such as chocolate that make the capsule dark, carob is an effective choice.

Certain procedures are required for administering challenges. Families are educated about the nature of the procedure, the reason for doing the challenge, and the possible outcomes. Whenever possible, food challenges are performed with children having discontinued all medication before initiation of the challenge. This is not always possible because some children with severe asthma are unable to discontinue their maintenance medications. In a few instances, challenges have been performed with children consuming antihistamines. Challenges in these circumstances have demonstrated that despite taking asthma medications and antihistamines, some children have positive challenges. This demonstrates that these mediations are not likely to be sufficient to prevent allergic reactions to foods.

TREATMENT

The treatments of specific disorders are discussed in chapters pertaining to those illnesses. However, a few general concepts are helpful to remember. The most important aspect of current management of food hypersensitivity is avoidance with proper education. The education component cannot be overemphasized because it is the improper avoidance of known food allergens that leads to death.[88,89] In contrast, inadequately diagnosing the correct food allergen often leads to the avoidance of excessive numbers of foods. This leads to frustration, accidents, and intentional "cheating" on the elimination diet by youngsters who do not believe that they need to avoid a long list of foods. To obviate this problem, periodic challenges should be performed. For milk and egg, challenge intervals of a year have been associated with identification of children who have "outgrown" their reactivity. The determination of specific IgE to these foods may help determine the challenge interval noted earlier. In the case of foods for which there is not yet an in vitro test to provide this information, challenge intervals of 6 to 24 months may be appropriate, depending on the age of the child, the severity of the previous reaction, any accidental or cross-contact ingestions, and family preference. Recent studies suggest that some children appear to lose their reactivity to peanuts.[90,91]

Children with known anaphylaxis to foods must always carry epinephrine and their caretakers must be educated about the appropriate management of accidental ingestion. For the practitioner caring for children with food anaphylaxis, the Food Allergy and Anaphylaxis Network (800-929-4040 or www.foodallergy.org) provides excellent materials for the education of families, community members, restaurants, schools, camps, and so on.

Specific medication treatment of food reactions or anaphylaxis because of food follows the usual principles and guidelines for treating allergic reactions and is covered in Chapter 52. Future treatments based on immunotherapy with modified food allergens also hold great promise.

CONCLUSIONS

The evaluation of food allergy should follow an orderly approach. The history may not allow the practitioner to accurately make the diagnosis, but it can be used to formulate a plan that will include skin testing, determination of food-specific serum IgE, diagnostic laboratory or endoscopic studies, the use of limited or oligoantigenic food elimination diets, and ultimately the decision of whether to perform food challenges (Figure 45-1). The rigor of challenge used is dictated by

TABLE 45-4 Vehicles Used in Food Challenges	
Capsules	Hamburger
Infant formula	Tuna fish
Applesauce	Ice cream (grape)
Popsicles	Lentil soup
Milkshakes	Mashed potatoes
Chocolate pudding	Amino acid–based formulas
Tapioca–fruit mixture cereal	Grape juice

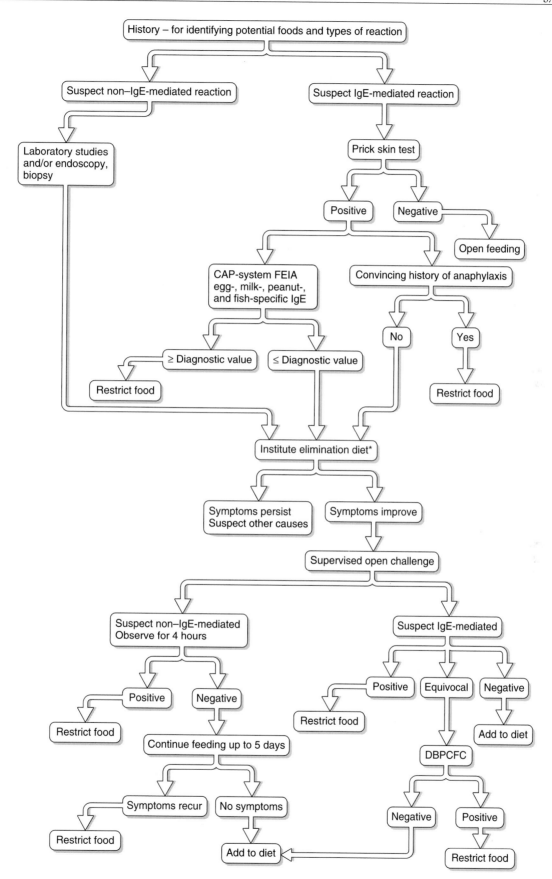

* Up to 2 weeks for IgE-mediated reactions; up to 8 weeks for non–IgE-mediated food hypersensitivity.

FIGURE 45-1 Algorithm diagnosing food hypersensitivity. *IgE,* Immunoglobulin E; *DBPCFC,* double-blind, placebo-controlled food challenge.

BOX
45-1

KEY CONCEPTS
Evaluation of Food Allergy

- In evaluating adverse food reactions, the work-up depends on differentiating food intolerance from food hypersensitivity and whether the food hypersensitivity is IgE or non–IgE mediated.
- IgE-mediated food hypersensitivities typically provoke symptoms within minutes to hours, whereas non–IgE-mediated hypersensitivities induce symptoms from hours to days.
- The patient history not only suggests the type of food hypersensitivity and causative food allergen but also provides information necessary to design an appropriate food challenge for confirming the diagnosis.
- Relatively few foods account for about 90% of food allergy (milk, egg, peanuts, nuts, soy, wheat, and fish).
- Although negative prick skin tests are an excellent means of excluding IgE-mediated food allergy, the majority of children with positive skin tests to foods will not experience allergic symptoms when ingesting that food.
- Some form of oral food challenge is usually necessary to establish the diagnosis of food hypersensitivity.
- Prescribing a food elimination diet is no different than prescribing any medication and must be based on a firm diagnosis of specific food allergy.

the nature of the problem and the setting in which the challenges are to be performed, recognizing that families can be greatly aided without having to involve a tertiary medical center. Clinicians should not feel overwhelmed or confused about how to approach this subject and how to solve the problems presented. It has become one of the more straightforward areas of allergy diagnosis and treatment if the steps outlined in this section are followed (Box 45-1). Future treatments offer great hope for the amelioration and eventual elimination of mild to severe food hypersensitivity in children.

HELPFUL WEBSITE

The Food Allergy and Anaphylaxis Network website (www.foodallergy.org)

REFERENCES

1. Loveless M: Milk allergy: a survey of its incidence: experiments with a masked ingestion test, *J Allergy* 21:489-500, 1950.
2. May CD: Objective clinical and laboratory studies of immediate hypersensitivity reactions to food in asthmatic children, *J Allergy Clin Immunol* 58:500-515, 1976.
3. Bruijnzeel-Koomen C, Ortolani C, Aas K, et al: Adverse reactions to food (position paper), *Allergy* 50:623-635, 1995.
4. Sloan AE, Powers ME: A perspective on popular perceptions of adverse reactions to foods, *J Allergy Clin Immunol* 78:127-133, 1986.
5. Altman DR, Chiaramonte LT: Public perception of food allergy, *J Allergy Clin Immunol* 97:1247-1251, 1996.
6. Kanny G, Moneret-Vautrin D-A, Flabbee J, et al: Population study of food allergy in France, *J Allergy Clin Immunol* 108:133-140, 2001.
7. Young E, Stoneham MD, Petruckevitch A, et al: A population study of food intolerance, *Lancet* 343:1127-1130, 1994.
8. Niestijl Jansen JJ, Kardinaal AFM, Huijbers GH, et al: Prevalence of food allergy and intolerance in the adult Dutch population, *J Allergy Clin Immunol* 93:446-456, 1994.
9. Bock SA: Prospective appraisal of complaints of adverse reactions to foods in children during the first 3 years of life, *Pediatrics* 79:683-688, 1987.
10. Eggesbo M, Halvorsen R, Tambs K, et al: Prevalence of parentally perceived adverse reaction to food in young children, *Pediatr Allergy Immunol* 10:122-132, 1999.
11. Schrander JJP, van den Bogart JPH, Forget PP, et al: Cow's milk protein intolerance in infants under 1 year of age: a prospective epidemiological study, *Eur J Pediatr* 152:640-644, 1993.
12. Host A, Halken S: A prospective study of cow's milk allergy in Danish infants during the first 3 years of life, *Allergy* 45:587-596, 1990.
13. Hide DW, Guyer BM: Cow milk intolerance in Isle of Wight infants, *Br J Clin Pract* 37:285-287, 1983.
14. Sicherer SH, Sampson HA: Cow's milk protein-specific IgE concentrations in two age groups of milk-allergic children and in children achieving clinical tolerance, *Clin Exp Allergy* 29:507-512, 1999.
15. Chatchatee P, Jarvinen K-M, Bardina L, et al: Identification of IgE-and IgG binding epitopes on α_{s1}-casein: differences in patients with persistent and transient cow's milk allergy, *J Allergy Clin Immunol* 107:379-383, 2001.
16. Vila L, Beyer K, Jarvinen K-M, et al: Role of conformational and linear epitopes in the achievement of tolerance in cow's milk allergy, *Clin Exp Allergy* 31:1599-1606, 2001.
17. Nickel R, Kulig M, Forster J, et al: Sensitization to hen's egg at the age of twelve months if predictive for allergic sensitization to common indoor and outdoor allergens at the age of 3 yrs, *J Allergy Clin Immunol* 99:613-617, 1997.
18. Sicherer SH, Munoz-Furlong A, Burks AW, et al: Prevalence of peanut and tree nut allergy in the United States of America, *J Allergy Clin Immunol* 103:559-562, 1999.
19. Burks AW, Mallory SB, Williams L, et al: Atopic dermatitis: clinical relevance of food hypersensitivity reactions, *J Pediatr* 113:447-451, 1988.
20. Eigenmann PA, Sicherer SH, Borkowski TA, et al: Prevalence of IgE mediated food allergy among children with atopic dermatitis, *Pediatrics* 101:3, 1998. Accessed at URL:http://www.pediatrics.org/cgi/content/full/101/3/e8 electronic pgs.
21. Guillet B, Guillet MH: Natural history of sensitization in atopic dermatitis, *Arch Dermatol* 128:187-192, 1992.
22. Onorato J, Merland N, Terral C, et al: Placebo-controlled double-blind food challenge in asthma, *J Allergy Clin Immunol* 78:1139-1146, 1986.
23. Novembre E, de Martino J, Vierucci A: Foods and respiratory allergy, *J Allergy Clin Immunol* 81:1059-1065, 1988.
24. Hill DJ, Firer MA, Shelton MJ, et al: Manifestations of milk allergy in infancy: clinical and immunological findings, *J Pediatr* 109:270-276, 1986.
25. Bock SA: Respiratory reactions induced by food challenges in children with pulmonary disease, *Pediatr Allergy Immunol* 3:188-194, 1992.
26. Sicherer SH, Furlong TJ, Maes HH, et al: Genetics of peanut allergy: a twin study, *J Allergy Clin Immunol* 106:53-56, 2000.
27. Sampson HA: Food allergy. Part 1: Immunopathogenesis and clinical disorders, *J Allergy Clin Immunol* 103:717-729, 1999.
28. Cooke SK, Sampson HA: Allergenic properties of ovomucoid, *J Immunol* 159:2026-2032, 1997.
29. Burks AW, Shin D, Cockrell G, et al: Mapping and mutational analysis of the IgE-binding epitopes on Ara h 1, a legume vicilin protein and a major allergen in peanut hypersensitivity, *Eur J Biochem* 245:334-339, 1997.
30. Burks AW, Cockrell G, Connaughton C, et al: Epitope specificity of the major peanut allergen, Ara h II, *J Allergy Clin Immunol* 95:607-611, 1995.
31. Rabjohn P, Helm EM, Stanley JS, et al: Molecular cloning and epitope analysis of the peanut allergen Ara h 3, *J Clin Invest* 103:535-542, 1999.
32. Sampson HA: Immunological approaches to the treatment of food allergy, *Pediatr Allergy Immunol* 12:91-96. 2001.
33. Hyams JS, Etienne NL, Leichter AM, et al: Carbohydrate malabsorption following fruit juice ingestion in young children, *Pediatrics* 88:64-68, 1988.
34. Roesler TA, Barry PC, Bock SA: Factitious food allergy and failure to thrive, *Arch Pediatr Adolesc Med* 148:1150-1155, 1994.
35. Goodman DL, McDonnell JT, Nelson HS, et al: Chronic urticaria exacerbated by the antioxidant food preservatives, butylated hydroxyanisole (BHA) and butylated hydroxytoluene (BHT), *J Allergy Clin Immunol* 86:570-575, 1990.
36. Sampson HA, McCaskill CM: Food hypersensitivity and atopic dermatitis: evaluation of 113 patients, *J Pediatr* 107:669-675, 1985.
37. Jakobsson I, Lindberg T: Cow's milk proteins cause infantile colic in breast-fed infants: a double-blind crossover study, *Pediatrics* 71:268-271, 1983.
38. Lothe L, Lindberg T: Cow's milk whey protein elicits symptoms of intractable colic in colicky formula-fed infants: a double-blind crossover study, *Pediatrics* 83:262-266, 1989.

39. Forsythe BWC: Colic and the effect of changing formulas: a double-blind multiple crossover study, *J Pediatr* 115:521-526, 1989.

40. Sampson HA. Infantile colic and food allergy: fact or fiction? *J Pediatr* 115:583-584, 1989.

41. Hill DJ, Hudson IL, Sheffield L, et al: A low allergen diet is a significant intervention in infantile colic: results of a community-based study, *J Allergy Clin Immunol* 96:886-892, 1995.

42. Lucassen PLBJ, Assendelft WJJ, Bubbels JW, et al: Infantile colic crying time reduction with a whey hydrolysate: a double-blind randomized placebo-controlled trial, *Pediatrics* 106:1349-1354, 2000.

43. Iacono G, Cavataio F, Montalto G, et al: Intolerance of cow's milk and chronic constipation in children, *N Engl J Med* 339:1100-1104, 1998.

44. Sampson HA: Food allergy, part 2: diagnosis and management, *J Allergy Clin Immunol* 103:981-989, 1999.

45. Bock SA, Buckley J, Holst A, et al: Proper use of skin tests with food extracts in diagnosis of hypersensitivity to food in children, *Clin Allergy* 7:375, 1977.

46. Bock SA, Lee W-Y, Remigo LK, et al: Appraisal of skin tests with food extracts for diagnosis of food hypersensitivity, *Clin Allergy* 8:559, 1978.

47. Sampson HA, Albergo R: Comparison of results of skin tests, RAST and double-blind, placebo-controlled food challenges in children with atopic dermatitis, *J Allergy Clin Immunol* 74:26-33, 1984.

48. Burks AW, James JM, Hiegel A, et al: Atopic dermatitis and food hypersensitivity, *J. Pediatr* 132:132-136, 1998.

49. Sporik R, Hill DJ, Hosking CS: Specificity of allergen skin testing in predicting positive open food challenges to milk, egg and peanut in children, *Clin Exp Allergy* 30:1540-1546, 2000.

50. Hill DJ, Hosking CS, Reyes-Benito MLV: Reducing the need for food allergen challenges in young children: comparison of *in vitro* with *in vivo* tests, *Clin Exp Allergy* 31:1031-1035, 2001.

51. Ortolani C, Ispano M, Pastorello EA, et al: Comparison of results of skin prick tests (with fresh foods and commercial food extracts) and RAST in 100 patients with oral allergy syndrome, *J Allergy Clin Immunol* 83: 683-690, 1989.

52. Pastorello E, Ortolani C, Farioli L, et al: Allergenic cross-reactivity among peach, apricot, plum, and cherry in patients with oral allergy syndrome: an *in vivo* and *in vitro* study, *J Allergy Clin Immunol* 94:699-707, 1994.

53. Rance F, Juchet A, Bremont F, et al: Correlations between skin prick tests using commercial extracts and fresh foods, specific IgE, and food challenges, *Allergy* 52:1031-1035, 1997.

54. Rosen J, Selcow J, Mendelson, L, et al: Skin testing with natural foods in patients suspected of having food allergies: is it necessary? *J Allergy Clin Immunol* 93:1068-1070, 1994.

55. Lockey RF: Adverse reactions associated with skin testing and immunotherapy, *Allergy Proc* 16:293-296, 1995.

56. Dreborg S, Foucard T: Allergy to apple, carrot and potato in children with birch pollen allergy, *Allergy* 38:167-172, 1983.

57. Hannuksela M, Lahti A: Immediate reactions to fruits and vegetables, *Contact Dermatitis* 3:79-84, 1977.

58. Bock SA: Anaphylaxis to coriander: a sleuthing story, *J Allergy Clin Immunol* 92:1232-1233, 1993.

59. Boxer M, Roberts M, Grammer L: Cumin anaphylaxis: a case report, *J Allergy Clin Immunol* 99:722-723, 1997.

60. Kanny G, Fremont S, Talhouarne G, et al: Anaphylaxis to mustard as a masked allergen in "chicken dips," *Ann Allergy* 75:340-342, 1995.

61. Sampson HA, Albergo R: Comparison of results of skin tests, RAST, and double-blind, placebo-controlled food challenges in children with atopic dermatitis, *J Allergy Clin Immunol* 74:26, 1984.

62. Sampson HA, Ho DG: Relationship between food-specific IgE concentrations and the risk of positive food challenges in children and adolescents, *J Allergy Clin Immunol* 100:444-451, 1997.

63. Sampson HA: Utility of food-specific IgE concentrations in predicting symptomatic food allergy, *J Allergy Clin Immunol* 107:891-896, 2001.

64. Boyano-Martinez T, Garcia-Ara C, Diaz-Pena JM, et al: Validity of specific IgE antibodies in children with egg allergy, *Clin Exp Allergy* 31: 1464-1469, 2001.

65. Garcia-Ara C, Boyano-Martinez T, Diaz-Pena JM, et al: Specific IgE levels in the diagnosis of immediate hypersensitivity to cows' milk protein in the infant, *J Allergy Clin Immunol* 107:185-190, 2001.

66. Sicherer SH, Sampson HA: Cow's milk protein-specific IgE concentrations in two age groups of milk-allergic children and in children achieving clinical tolerance, *Clin Exp Allergy* 29:507-512, 1999.

67. May CD: High spontaneous release of histamine *in vitro* from leukocytes of persons hypersensitive to food, *J Allergy Clin Immunol* 58:432-437, 1976.

68. Sampson HA, Broadbent KR, Bernhisel-Broadbent J: Spontaneous release of histamine from basophils and histamine-releasing factor in patients with atopic dermatitis and food hypersensitivity, *N Engl J Med* 321:228-232, 1989.

69. Agata H, Kondo N, Fukutomi O, et al: Effect of elimination diets on food-specific IgE antibodies and lymphocyte proliferation responses to food antigens in atopic dermatitis patients exhibiting sensitivity to food allergens, *J Allergy Clin Immunol* 91:668-679, 1993.

70. Kondo N, Fukutomi O, Agata H, et al: The role of T lymphocytes in patients with food-sensitive atopic dermatitis, *J Allergy Clin Immunol* 91:658-668, 1993.

71. Hoffman KM, Ho DG, Sampson HA: Evaluation of the usefulness of lymphocyte proliferation assays in the diagnosis of allergy to cow's milk, *J Allergy Clin Immunol* 99:360-366, 1997.

72. Sheffer AL, Lieberman PL, Aaronson DW, et al: Measurement of circulating IgG and IgE food immune complexes, *J Allergy Clin Immunol* 81: 758-759, 1988.

73. Rance F, Dutau G: Labial food challenge in children with food allergy, *Pediatr Allergy Immunol* 8:41-44, 1997.

74. Niggemann B, Reibel, S, Wahn U: The atopy patch test (APT): a useful tool for the diagnosis of food allergy in children with atopic dermatitis, *Allergy* 55:281-285, 2000.

75. Niggeman B: Atopy patch test (APT): its role in diagnosis of food allergy in atopic dermatitis. *Indian J Pediatr* 69:57-59, 2002.

76. Spergel JM, Beausoliel JL, Mascarenhas M, et al: The use of skin prick tests and patch tests to identify causative foods in eosinophilic esophagitis, *J Allergy Clin Immunol* 109:363-368, 2002.

77. Roehr CC, Reibel S, Ziegert M, et al: Atopy patch tests, together with determination of specific IgE levels, reduce the need for oral food challenges in children with atopic dermatitis, *J Allergy Clin Immunol* 107:548-553, 2001.

78. Bock SA, Sampson HA, Atkins FM, et al: Double blind placebo controlled food challenge (DBPCFC) as an office procedure: a manual, *J Allergy Clin Immunol* 82:986-997, 1988.

79. Sicherer SH, Morrow EH, Sampson HA: Dose response in double blind placebo controlled oral food challenges in children with atopic dermatitis, *J Allergy Clin Immunol* 105:582-586, 2000.

80. Sicherer SH: Food allergy: when and how to perform oral food challenges, *Pediatr Allergy Immunol* 10:226-234, 1999.

81. Niggemann B, Sielaff B, Beyer K, et al: Outcome of DBPCFC tests in 107 children with atopic dermatitis, *Clin Exp Allergy* 29:91-96, 1999.

82. Metcalfe D, Sampson H: Workshop on experimental methodology for clinical studies of adverse reactions to foods and food additives, *J Allergy Clin Immunol* 86:421-442, 1990.

83. Reibel S, Rohr C, Ziegert M, et al: What safety measures need to be taken in oral food challenges in children? *Allergy* 55:940-944, 2000.

84. Hourihane JO, Kilburn SA, Nordlee JA, et al: An evaluation of the sensitivity of subjects with peanut allergy to very low doses of peanut protein: a randomized, double-blind, placebo-controlled food challenge study, *J Allergy Clin Immunol* 100:596-600, 1997.

85. Bock SA, Atkins FM: Patterns of food hypersensitivity during 16 years of double-blind placebo-controlled food challenges, *J Pediatr* 117:561-567, 1990.

86. Caffarelli C, Petroccione T: False-negative food challenges in children with suspect food allergy, *Lancet* 358:1871-1872, 2001.

87. Sampson HA: Use of food-challenge tests in children, *Lancet* 358: 1832-1833, 2001.

88. Sampson HA, Mendelson L, Rosen JP: Fatal and near-fatal anaphylactic reaction to food in children and adolescents, *N Engl J Med* 327:380-384, 1992.

89. Bock SA, Munoz-Furlong A, Sampson HA: Fatalities because of anaphylactic reactions to foods, *J Allergy Clin Immunol* 107:101-103, 2001.

90. Vander Leek TK, Liu AH, Stefanski K, et al: The natural history of peanut allergy in young children and its association with serum peanut-specific IgE, *J Pediatr* 137:749-755, 2000.

91. Skolnick H, Barnes-Koerner C, Walker MKC, et al: The natural history of peanut allergy, *J Allergy Clin Immunol* 107:367-374, 2001.

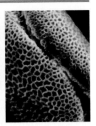

Approach to Feeding Problems in the Infant and Young Child

ARNE HØST ■ SUSANNE HALKEN

For the past two to three decades, an increasing awareness of food allergy has emerged in Western industrialized societies. However, the public perceives food allergy different from physicians. About one in four of American households change their dietary habits because at least one member of the family is perceived to have food allergy.[1] Given the public's frequent misperception that various mild symptoms are caused by food-induced allergic reactions, it is very important to perform careful evaluation and correct diagnostic procedures to avoid overdiagnosis, which may lead to malnutrition, eating disorders, and psychosocial problems as well as family disruption. In contrast, underdiagnosis may result in unnecessary symptoms, growth failure, and physical impairment.

Much of the controversy about food allergy may be ascribed to different nomenclature. According to the European Academy of Allergy and Clinical Immunology,[2] *adverse reactions* to foods are defined as any abnormal reaction that occurs after the ingestion of a food or food additive.

Recently, a revised nomenclature for allergic and related reactions that can be used independently of target organ or patient age group was published.[3] In this position paper, the term *hypersensitivity* was defined as "objective, reproducible symptoms or signs, initiated by exposure to a defined stimulus at a dose tolerated by normal subjects." Allergy is a hypersensitivity reaction initiated by immunologic mechanisms (defined or strongly suspected), whereas the term *nonallergic hypersensitivity* has been proposed when immunologic mechanisms cannot be proved. Allergy can be antibody or cell mediated. In most patients, the antibody typically responsible for an allergic reaction belongs to the IgE isotype, and these patients may be said to have IgE-mediated allergy. In non–IgE-mediated allergy, different mechanisms may be responsible (IgG, immune complexes, cell mediated). The classifications of food hypersensitivity and food are shown in Figure 46-1.

True food allergies (i.e., immune-mediated reactions) are most often IgE-mediated reactions, the classic type I, which is the most thoroughly investigated type of food allergy. However, recent evidence indicates that non–IgE-mediated reactions type III (immune complexes) and, in particular, type IV (cell-mediated reactions) may play a major role in delayed reactions. It is evident that a correct classification of an adverse reaction to foods will depend on the extent and the quality of the diagnostic tests and procedures performed. For nonscien-

tific purposes, the diagnosis of an adverse reaction to food will often be based solely on the result of elimination and challenge procedures.

No single laboratory test is diagnostic of food allergy. Therefore the diagnosis has to be based on strict well-defined food elimination and challenge procedures, preferably double-blind placebo-controlled food challenges (DBPCFCs) in children older than 1 to 2 years of age.[4] In infants, open controlled challenges have been shown to be reliable when performed under professional observation in a hospital setting or a clinic.[5]

Food allergy is primarily a problem in infancy and early childhood. Most often the infants develop food allergies in the same order as that in which the foods have been introduced into the diet. Thus the prevalence of reactions to different foods depends in part on the eating habits of a given population.

This review concentrates on gastrointestinal symptoms, which may cause suspicion of food allergy in early childhood, focusing on indications for food allergy evaluation. Specific disease entities, such as enterocolitis, proctocolitis, enteropathies, and allergic eosinophilic esophagitis (gastroesophageal reflux [GER])/gastroenterocolitis, are discussed in other chapters (see Chapters 48 and 49).

FREQUENCY

In prospective studies, the incidence of cow's milk protein allergy (CMPA) during the first year of life has been estimated to be about 2% to 3% based on strict diagnostic criteria, as reviewed by Høst.[6] Other common food allergens in children are egg, fish, nuts, soy, and cereals. The total cumulated incidence of food protein allergy during the first 3 years of life has been found to be about 7% to 8%.[7]

Adverse reactions to *food additives* have been demonstrated in school children to affect less than 1% of unselected children when using DBPCFCs.[8] The most common positive reaction was worsening of atopic eczema and urticaria in atopic children. Among children with atopic symptoms referred to hospital allergy clinics,[9] 23% of 335 were suspected of food additive intolerance. However, only 7% reacted to food additive on open challenge and only 2% had reproducible reactions when DBPCFCs were performed.

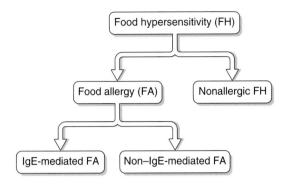

FIGURE 46-1 Algorithm for food allergy classification. (Data from Johansson SG, Hourihan JO, Bousquet J, et al: *Allergy* 56:813-824, 2001.)

In children with symptoms suggestive of food allergy, it has been possible to confirm the diagnosis in only about one third by means of controlled elimination/challenge procedures.[6,7]

Age at Onset of Symptoms

The age at which symptoms start depends on the time of introduction of the foods; infants will develop food allergies in the same order as that in which the foods have been introduced into the diet. Many prospective studies as reviewed by Høst[6] have demonstrated that symptoms in CMPA develop in early infancy, rarely after 12 months of age. The onset of disease is in most cases closely related to the time of introduction of cow's milk–based formula. Allergies against fruit and juice often have a later age of onset.[7] In a Spanish study[10] of 355 children (mean age, 5.4 years), allergy to milk, egg, and fish began predominantly before the second year, demonstrating a clear relationship with the introduction of these foods into the child's diet, whereas allergy to vegetables began after the second year (Table 46-1).

CLINICAL FEATURES

The clinical features of food allergy in childhood are shown in Table 46-2. In early infancy the most common food allergy is allergy to cow's milk protein. Most infants develop symptoms before 1 month of age, often within 1 week after introduction of cow's milk–based formula. Similar to other food allergies, the majority have at least two symptoms and symptoms that affect at least two organs. About 50% to 70% have cutaneous symptoms; 50% to 60%, gastrointestinal symptoms; and about 20% to 30%, respiratory symptoms.[5] Also, exclusively

TABLE 46-1 Age at Onset of Food Allergy Against Different Foods

Age (yr)	Food
0-1	Milk, egg*
1-2	Fish*
> 2	Fruits, legumes, vegetables*
> 3	Pollen-related cross-reactivities (oral allergy syndrome)†

From Crespo JF, Pascual C, Burks AW, et al: *Pediatr Allergy Immunol* 6:39-43, 1995.
*N = 355 with food allergy; mean age, 5.4 years.
†From Bruijnzeel-Koomen C, Ortolani C, Aas K, et al: *Allergy* 50:623-635, 1995.

TABLE 46-2 Clinical Features of Food Protein Allergy/Intolerance in Children

Cutaneous reactions

IgE mediated	Atopic dermatitis
	Urticaria, acute or chronic (rare)
	Angioedema
Non–IgE mediated	Contact rash (e.g., perioral flare due to benzoic acid in citrus fruits)
	Atopic dermatitis (some forms?)

Gastrointestinal reactions

IgE mediated	Immediate gastrointestinal hypersensitivity (e.g., nausea, vomiting, diarrhea)
	Oral allergy syndrome
	Colic
Non–IgE mediated	Allergic eosinophilic esophagitis, gastritis, or gastroenterocolitis
	Enterocolitis syndrome
	Dietary protein colitis
	Dietary protein enteropathy

Respiratory reactions

IgE mediated	Rhinoconjunctivitis
	Asthma (wheezing, cough)
	Laryngeal edema
	Food-dependent exercise-induced asthma
Non–IgE mediated	Pulmonary hemosiderosis (Heiner's syndrome [rare])

Systemic anaphylaxis

Other reactions	Otitis media (secondary to allergic rhinitis and eustachian tube dysfunction or an allergic middle ear inflammation)
Unknown mechanisms	Migraine (rare), arthritis (rare), Henoch-Schönlein purpura (rare)

breast-fed infants may react to food protein in their mother's milk, around 0.5%,[6] and in these infants severe atopic eczema is the predominant symptom. CMPA onset after 1 year of age is extremely rare. Symptoms occurring within a few minutes to 2 hours after food exposure (i.e., "immediate reactions") are mostly IgE mediated, whereas symptoms occurring more than 2 hours after food intake are classified as delayed reactions. Late reactions may occur after many hours even up to a few days, such as allergic eosinophilic gastroenteritis. Most often delayed reactions are non–IgE mediated. Anaphylaxis has been reported with varying frequencies, reflecting differences in patient selection. It is clear that patterns of reactions to foods may vary due to different exposure levels and different time intervals between exposures as well as different thresholds of reaction.

Immediate IgE-mediated reactions to foods often involve two or more target organs, such as the gastrointestinal tract, the skin, and the lungs, and may result in a variety of symptoms, including life-threatening reactions such as exacerbations of asthma, laryngeal edema, and anaphylaxis with cardiovascular collapse. An exception is the food-pollen allergy, or *oral allergy syndrome* (OAS), a mucosal equivalent of urticaria. After the ingestion of specific foods (fresh fruits and vegetables), itching and swelling in the mouth and oropharynx occur, and these symptoms may lead to refusal of the offending food by the child. OAS is associated with allergic

TABLE 46-3 Common Cross-Reactivities: Food-Pollen Allergy Syndrome (Oral Allergy Syndrome)

Pollen	Fruit/Vegetable
Birch	Apple, hazelnut, carrot, potato, kiwi, celery, cherry, pear, others
Mugwort (artemissia)	Celery, carrot, fennel, parsley, others
Ragweed	Melon, banana
Grass	Potato, tomato, watermelon, kiwi, peanuts?

From Bruijnzeel-Koomen C, Ortolani C, Aas K, et al: *Allergy* 50:623-635, 1995.

rhinoconjunctivitis and allergy to pollen, especially to birch, grass, ragweed, and mugwort. Cross-reactivity occurs when two or more allergens share epitopes and therefore are bound by the same IgE antibodies. Thus patients sensitized to one of the allergens may also react to the other without previous exposure and sensitization. The most often reported cross-reactivities among pollen, fruits, and vegetables are shown in Table 46-3. Other cross-reactivities are between natural rubber latex and, for example, banana, avocado, peach, kiwi, apricot, grape, passion fruit, pineapple, and chestnut. The diagnosis of OAS is based on a typical history and the demonstration of a positive skin prick test or specific IgE antibodies.[2]

The age of onset of "oral allergy syndrome" is beyond infancy but often before school age. The symptoms include oral manifestations such as burning, swelling, itching, and erythema.

GASTROINTESTINAL PROBLEMS IN EARLY CHILDHOOD

Gastrointestinal manifestations of food allergy can be classified as a continuum from clearly IgE mediated to mixed reactions dominated by eosinophilic granulocytes as effector cells to clearly non–IgE-mediated reactions.[11] Immediate gastrointestinal hypersensitivity and oral allergy symptoms are mainly IgE mediated; allergic eosinophilic esophagitis, allergic eosinophilic gastritis, and allergic eosinophilic gastroenterocolitis are mixed–IgE- and non–IgE-mediated reactions, and dietary protein enterocolitis, dietary protein proctitis, dietary enteropathy, and celiac disease are non–IgE mediated. The most frequent adverse reactions to food in the infant and young child are immediate IgE-mediated reactions with manifestations like nausea, abdominal pain (colic), and vomiting within 1 to 2 hours after food intake and diarrhea within 1 to 6 hours. The frequency of presenting gastrointestinal symptoms in infants with CMPA is shown in Table 46-4.

Among mixed–IgE- and non–IgE-mediated disorders, dietary protein enterocolitis and dietary protein proctitis have their onset in early infancy up to 6 to 12 months of age. Allergic eosinophilic gastritis and allergic eosinophilic gastroenterocolitis may have their debut between early infancy and adolescence. Dietary protein enteropathy and celiac disease occur in early childhood depending on the age of exposure to the antigen involved. The mixed–IgE- and non–IgE-mediated disorders are discussed in detail in other chapters (see Chapters 48 and 49).

The symptoms caused by immediate gastrointestinal allergy typically develop within minutes to 2 hours after food intake. None of the symptoms are pathognomonic for allergy and may be caused by many other factors or diseases. Symptoms like colic, vomiting, and diarrhea may be chronic or intermittent. Frequently, the children have poor appetite, poor weight gain, and intermittent abdominal pain and show failure to thrive. Children who show concomitant symptoms in other organ systems like urticaria or atopic dermatitis or respiratory symptoms may easily be suspected of food allergy. When symptoms from other organ systems are lacking, the cause of the symptoms may remain undiagnosed for prolonged periods. A family history of atopic disease in such cases should give a clue to the diagnosis of possible food allergy. A

TABLE 46-4 Presenting Gastrointestinal Symptoms in Infants with Cow's Milk Protein Allergy

	Selected Patient Samples (%)			Unselected, Prospectively Followed Patients from Birth Cohorts (%)		
Symptom	Goldman et al,[29] 1963[a] (N = 89)	Gerrard et al,[30] 1967[b] (N = 150)	Hill et al,[22] 1986[c] (N = 100)	Gerrard et al,[31] 1973[d] (N = 59)	Jakobsson and Lindberg,[32] 1979[e] (N = 20)	Høst and Halken,[5] 1990[f] (N = 39)
Colic	28	19	14	20	35	46
Vomiting	33	34	34	22	50	38
Diarrhea	37	47	48	41	25	8
Failure to thrive	NG	NG	22	NG	10	8
Diarrhea with blood	NG	NG	4	NG	NG	0
Gastroesophageal reflux	NG	NG	6	NG	NG	NG

NG, Not given.

[a]Age at investigation: Group A median, 6 mo (2 wk to 6 yr). Group B median, 10 mo (6 wk to 13 yr).

[b]Age at investigation: not given.

[c]Age at investigation: mean, 16 mo (3 to 66 mo).

[d]Age at investigation: not given, but infants followed 0 to 2 yr.

[e]Age at investigation: median, 4 mo (3 wk to 1 yr)

[f]Age at investigation: median, 3.5 mo (1 to 11 mo), infants followed 0 to 3 yr.

variety of feeding problems in young infants may be associated with food allergy.

Infantile Colic

Infantile colic has often been related to food allergy, especially CMPA, and high frequencies up to 71% of food allergy in children with colic have been reported.[12] In that study and another study,[13] the infants with colic due to cow's milk protein only rarely showed other features of CMPA. Although infantile colic is a common symptom of CMPA, it is almost always seen in combination with other features of CMPA.[5,6]

Spitting Up/Vomiting

Symptoms of spitting up and vomiting may be very normal in young infants. The most common cause of vomiting is overfeeding, or hypernutrition. Such infants show a normal growth and development in contrast to infants with underlying gastrointestinal disease.

Diarrhea

Diarrhea is often reported as a symptom due to food allergy in young infancy. On the other hand, diarrhea is also a very common symptom due to "normal reactions" caused by inappropriate or excessive intake of certain foods, such as raisins, carrots, legumes, and other fruit—toddlers' diarrhea. Transient or secondary lactose deficiency may occur in response to gastrointestinal infections, which are very common in infancy. This intolerance to lactose often lasts only a few days, after which there is a complete recovery.

Failure to Thrive

Failure to thrive may be caused by immediate gastrointestinal food allergy but is more often due to mixed–IgE- and non–IgE-mediated disorders in the gastrointestinal tract causing malabsorption, severe vomiting, or diarrhea.

Constipation

Constipation is a common clinical problem affecting up to 10% of infants and children.[14] It may cause blood in the stools as well as symptoms of colitis and recurrent abdominal pain in older children. Recent reports[15-17] describe chronic constipation as a manifestation of CMPA. Thus CMPA should be considered in severe cases of chronic constipation, but constipation does not appear to be a common manifestation of CMPA.

Gastroesophageal Reflux

It has been reported that nearly half of the cases of GER in infants less than 1 year of age are not only CMPA associated but also CMPA induced.[18,19] GER is a common disease, affecting up to 10% of infants in the first year of life. It is related to esophagitis but may be present without visible or histologic inflammation of the esophagus. Typical symptoms of GER include vomiting with weight loss and symptoms of esophagitis (dysphagia, vomiting, abdominal pain, sleep disturbance), as

TABLE 46-5 Symptoms of Gastroesophageal Reflux

Regurgitation	**Respiratory symptoms**
Failure to thrive	Wheezing
Esophagitis	Recurrent pneumonia
Feeding problems	Apnea, cyanotic episodes
Signs of pain in particular with meals	Laryngospasm
Anemia, hematemesis	**Neurologic symptoms**
Stricture symptoms	Sandifer's syndrome

well as respiratory symptoms (Table 46-5). Proteins other than cow's milk have been implicated in allergic eosinophilic esophagitis, such as wheat, soy, peanut, and egg, often multiple antigens. Most cases resolve in less than 1 year. Thus some studies suggest that a portion of patients have both CMPA and GER and that food allergy, especially CMPA, may play a causal role (see Chapter 49). Because of possible selection bias in previously reported studies, more population-based studies on this subject are warranted to evaluate the significance of this possible causal relationship.

DIFFERENTIAL DIAGNOSIS

The differential diagnostic considerations of possible food-related symptoms are extremely age dependent and include, for example, chronic gastrointestinal infections, nonspecific diarrhea of childhood, irritable bowel syndrome, and recurrent abdominal pain, as described in Table 46-6. Some differential diagnoses to food allergy are mainly related to the upper gastrointestinal tract such as colic, recurrent abdominal pain, gastroesophageal reflux, pyloric stenosis, hiatal hernia, and tracheoesophageal fistula, whereas others are associated with diseases in the lower gastrointestinal tract, such as enzyme deficiencies, malabsorption diseases, constipation, and Hirschsprung's disease.

Nonenteral Infections

Commonly seen in all ages, although most frequent in early infancy, are the nonenteral infections that may cause gastrointestinal upset, regardless of the focus of the infection: "secondary dyspepsia." Such sequelae after acute or chronic gastrointestinal infection should always be ruled out before evaluation of food allergy.

Lactose Intolerance

Lactase deficiency is an important differential diagnosis to food allergy, especially cow's milk allergy. Lactose constitutes the majority of the carbohydrate content of human and cow's milk and is an important part of the energy supply for infants in particular. Lactose is degraded in the gastrointestinal mucosa by the enzyme lactase. Lactose intolerance in the newborn is extremely rare and is caused by congenital deficiency of lactase. Acquired or adult-type lactase deficiency usually appears at the age of 3 to 5 years. Adult-type lactase deficiency is very common in those of African and Asian ancestries. It is

TABLE 46-6 Differential Diagnosis of Food Allergy

Infant
Upper gastrointestinal symptoms
    Infection
    Colic*
    Gastroesophageal reflux*
    Pyloric stenosis (defined age group)
    Hiatal hernia
    Tracheoesophageal fistula
Lower gastrointestinal symptoms
    Enzyme deficiency
    Disaccharidase deficiencies (lactase, sucrose-isomaltase, glucose-galactose)
    Galactosemia
    Phenylketonuria
    Infection
    Constipation*
    Hirschsprung's disease

Toddler
Infection
Toddler's diarrhea
Gastroesophageal reflux*
Constipation*
Lactose intolerance
Malabsorption (celiac disease, cystic fibrosis)
Bizarre diets

School-age child
Infection
Recurrent abdominal pain
Lactose intolerance
Malabsorption (celiac disease, cystic fibrosis, Schwachman syndrome)
Inflammatory bowel disease
Eosinophilic gastroenteritis*
Other causes (immunodeficiency, Henoch-Schönlein disease)

*Could be caused by food allergy.

less common in whites, especially in some groups, such as the Scandinavian populations; in Denmark, only 3% of adults are affected.

Secondary lactase deficiency is temporary and may occur in response to malnutrition or gastrointestinal infections, which cause a temporary damage of the villi of the small intestine, where the enzyme lactase is produced. This sensitivity to lactose often lasts only a few days, followed by complete recovery.

Lactose intolerance may be diagnosed by oral lactose challenge tests and measurements of increased H_2 in breath tests, by glucose measurements, or by direct enzyme measurements within a duodenal biopsy.

Adult-type or primary lactase deficiencies are lifelong conditions. The treatment of lactose intolerance is to diminish the amount of milk and dairy products with lactose. Avoidance does not need to be complete, such as for children with CMPA. A firm diagnosis of lactose intolerance and the threshold for development of symptoms should be established because the sensitivity to lactose is variable. In many lactose-intolerant individuals, considerable amounts of lactose may be ingested before symptoms develop. Usually the amount of milk product corresponding to one glass of milk during a meal may be ingested without adverse reactions.[20]

Irritable Bowel Syndrome

Irritable bowel syndrome (IBS) or recurrent abdominal pain in children is a clinical syndrome with a variable pathogenic background, including psychosomatic reactions, lactose intolerance, food allergy, and inflammatory conditions such as gastritis or inflammatory bowel disease. Conflicting data have been published on the role of food allergy/intolerance in IBS. It has been concluded that food reactions are unlikely to be major determinants in the pathogenesis of IBS and that double-blind placebo-controlled food challenges are mandatory for investigation of this possible causal relationship.[21]

Toddlers' Diarrhea

To avoid unnecessary investigations for food allergy, it is important to pay attention to this very common "disorder." Many infants and young children have a high intake of dietary fiber from enormous amounts of fruits, legumes, vegetables, and raisins and great volumes of fruit juice (instead of water). This is a normal cause of loose stools and diarrhea often resulting in referrals to allergists for investigation of food allergy. There is no reason for such investigations when children have normal growth and development. Laypersons, especially parents, need more information and knowledge about "normal" reactions to foods in children. The simple advice is to reduce the intake of such foods to normalize the bowel function.

Münchhausen's Syndrome by Proxy

During the past decade, many infants and young children have been investigated for allergy, and especially food allergy, without convincing indication for such often comprehensive diagnostic procedures. In cases where there is a lack of obvious possible allergic symptoms, physicians should abstain from unnecessary and potentially harmful investigations of healthy children with parent-, often mother-, induced or imaginary symptoms.

EVALUATION AND MANAGEMENT

In infants and young children, food allergy should be suspected in cases of persistent severe symptoms, especially if there is more than one symptom and if relevant differential diagnoses are excluded (Boxes 46-1 and 46-2).

Gastrointestinal symptoms in food allergy are often chronic or acute vomiting, diarrhea, and colic. Colic appears to be a common symptom,[22] but nearly always in combination with other symptoms.[5,6,22] Because most of these gastrointestinal symptoms are nonspecific and may be caused by other conditions, a careful evaluation for other causes in the differential diagnoses, such as lactose intolerance and coincidental infections, is important at an early stage.

None of the symptoms related to immunologically or non-immunologically mediated adverse reactions to foods are pathognomonic, although some characteristics should be suggestive of food allergy (Box 46-1).

BOX 46-1

KEY CONCEPTS
Characteristics of Food Allergy

- Persistent symptoms
- Symptoms related to food intake
- Allergic predisposition
- Two or more different symptoms
- Symptoms in two or more different organs

No laboratory test is diagnostic of food allergy.[2,23] Therefore, the diagnosis has to be based on a careful case history and on strict, well-defined food elimination and challenge procedures establishing a causal relation between the ingestion of a particular food (or food protein) and a subsequent obvious clinical reaction.[2,4,6,24-28]

Possible helpful diagnostic tests include skin prick tests or determinations of specific serum IgE to relevant food allergens and basophil histamine release test.

Importantly, it should be born in mind that no laboratory tests/skin prick tests are diagnostic of food allergy, although they may be useful in choosing the elimination diet and the challenge procedure for the classification of the disorder and for determining the prognosis.

CONCLUSIONS

Food allergy is primarily a problem in infancy and early childhood. Children with food allergy may experience a variety of

BOX 46-2

THERAPEUTIC PRINCIPLES
General Approach to Evaluation of Food Allergy in Children with Gastrointestinal Problems

CONSIDER EVALUATION IN CASE OF

Persistent symptoms in infancy/early childhood with vomiting, diarrhea, colic, or failure to thrive and

Other common differential diagnoses are excluded, especially gastroenteritis and lactose intolerance

Particularly in case of
History of symptoms exacerbated by particular foods or

Other coexisting atopic manifestations, especially

    Atopic eczema/urticaria

    Allergic rhinitis

INITIAL SCREEN

Careful case history and physical examination

Skin prick test/specific IgE to implicated foods

    Extra suspicion for "history-positive" foods

    Extra suspicion for common food allergens (milk, hen's egg, wheat, soy, peanut, tree nut, fish, shellfish)

Consider elimination diet for a sufficient period to eliminate symptoms

Consider controlled challenges to exclude/confirm food allergy

symptoms affecting different organ systems. The disease manifestations often are localized to the gastrointestinal tract, but food allergy/intolerance may also cause local symptoms in the skin and the respiratory tract. About 50% to 70% of allergic infants show cutaneous symptoms; 50% to 60%, gastrointestinal symptoms; and about 20% to 30%, respiratory symptoms. Among young children with cow's milk allergy, the majority has two or more symptoms, and symptoms generally affect two or more organ systems. Mostly, the symptoms occur within a few minutes after food exposure (immediate reactions), but delayed reactions involving the skin, the gastrointestinal tract, and the lungs may also occur. Many children who experience these symptoms will not have food allergy. Among children presenting with symptoms suggestive of food allergy/intolerance, the diagnosis can be confirmed by controlled elimination/challenge procedures in only about one third of individuals.

To avoid unnecessary diets and stigmatization, it is important to rule out "normal reactions" to foods and relevant differential diagnoses before specific comprehensive diagnostic procedures for food allergy. To avoid unnecessary diets and the risk of malnutrition, it is important to make the proper diagnosis in case of suspected food allergy.

REFERENCES

1. Sloan AE, Powers ME: A perspective on popular perceptions of adverse reactions to foods, *J Allergy Clin Immunol* 78:127-133, 1986.
2. Bruijnzeel-Koomen C, Ortolani C, Aas K, et al: Adverse reactions to food. European Academy of Allergology and Clinical Immunology Subcommittee, *Allergy* 50:623-635, 1995.
3. Johansson SG, Hourihane JO, Bousquet J, et al: A revised nomenclature for allergy. An EAACI position statement from the EAACI Nomenclature Task Force, *Allergy* 56:813-824, 2001.
4. Bock SA, Sampson HA, Atkins FM, et al: Double-blind, placebo-controlled food challenge (DBPCFC) as an office procedure: a manual, *J Allergy Clin Immunol* 82:986-997, 1988.
5. Høst A, Halken S: A prospective study of cow milk allergy in Danish infants during the first 3 years of life. Clinical course in relation to clinical and immunological type of hypersensitivity reaction, *Allergy* 45:587-596, 1990.
6. Høst A: Cow's milk protein allergy and intolerance in infancy. Some clinical, epidemiological and immunological aspects, *Pediatr Allergy Immunol* 5:1-36, 1994.
7. Bock SA: Prospective appraisal of complaints of adverse reactions to foods in children during the first 3 years of life, *Pediatrics* 79:683-688, 1987.
8. Fuglsang G, Madsen C, Saval P, et al: Prevalence of intolerance to food additives among Danish school children, *Pediatr Allergy Immunol* 4:123-129, 1993.
9. Fuglsang G, Madsen G, Halken S, et al: Adverse reactions to food additives in children with atopic symptoms, *Allergy* 49:31-37, 1994.
10. Crespo JF, Pascual C, Burks AW, et al: Frequency of food allergy in a pediatric population from Spain, *Pediatr Allergy Immunol* 6:39-43, 1995.
11. Sampson HA, Anderson JA: Summary and recommendations: classification of gastrointestinal manifestations due to immunologic reactions to foods in infants and young children, *J Pediatr Gastroenterol Nutr* 30:S87-S94, 2000.
12. Iacono G, Carroccio A, Montalto G, et al: Severe infantile colic and food intolerance: a long-term prospective study, *J Pediatr Gastroenterol Nutr* 12:332-335, 1991.
13. Lothe L, Lindberg T, Jakobsson I: Cow's milk formula as a cause of infantile colic: a double-blind study, *Pediatrics* 70:7-10, 1982.
14. Clayden GS, Lawson JO: Investigation and management of long-standing chronic constipation in childhood, *Arch Dis Child* 51:918-923, 1976.
15. Daher S, Tahan S, Sole D, et al: Cow's milk protein intolerance and chronic constipation in children, *Pediatr Allergy Immunol* 12:339-342, 2001.
16. Iacono G, Cavataio F, Montalto G, et al: Intolerance of cow's milk and chronic constipation in children, *N Engl J Med* 339:1100-1104, 1998.

17. Shah N, Lindley K, Milla P: Cow's milk and chronic constipation in children, *N Engl J Med* 340:891-892, 1999.

18. Cavataio F, Iacono G, Montalto G, et al: Clinical and pH-metric characteristics of gastro-oesophageal reflux secondary to cows' milk protein allergy, *Arch Dis Child* 75:51-56, 1996.

19. Iacono G, Carroccio A, Cavataio F, et al: Gastroesophageal reflux and cow's milk allergy in infants: a prospective study, *J Allergy Clin Immunol* 97:822-827, 1996.

20. Srinivasan LR, Minocha A: When to suspect lactose intolerance. Symptomatic, ethnic and laboratory clues, *Postgrad Med* 104:109-123, 1998.

21. Ortolani C, Bruijnzeel-Koomen C, Bengtsson U, et al: Controversial aspects of adverse reactions to food. European Academy of Allergology and Clinical Immunology (EAACI) Reactions to Food Subcommittee, *Allergy* 54:27-45, 1999.

22. Hill DJ, Firer MA, Shelton MJ, et al: Manifestations of milk allergy in infancy: clinical and immunologic findings, *J Pediatr* 109:270-276, 1986.

23. Bindslev-Jensen C: Food allergy, *Br Med J* 316:1299-1302, 1998.

24. Bindslev-Jensen C, Poulsen LK: *In vitro* diagnostic methods in the diagnosis of food hypersensitivity. In Metcalfe DD, Sampson H, Simon R, eds: *Food allergy: adverse reactions to foods and food additives,* ed 2, Oxford, 1996, Blackwell Science.

25. Høst A, Koletzko B, Breborg S, et al: Dietary products used in infants for treatment and prevention of food allergy. Joint statement of the European Society of Paediatric Allergology and Clinical Immunology (ESPACI) Committee of Hypoallergeneic Formulas and the European Society for Paediatric Gastroenterology, Hepatology and Nutrition (ESPGHAN) Committee on Nutrition, *Arch Dis Child* 8:80-84, 1999.

26. Zeiger RS, Sampson HA, Bock SA, et al: Soy allergy in infants and children with IgE-associated cow's milk allergy, *J Pediatr* 134:614-622, 1999.

27. Metcalfe DD, Sampson HA: Workshop on experimental methodology for clinical studies of adverse reactions to foods and food additives, *J Allergy Clin Immunol* 86:421-442, 1990.

28. Niggemann B, Wahn U, Sampson HA: Proposals for standardization of oral food challenge tests in infants and children, *Pediatr Allergy Immunol* 5:11-13, 1994.

29. Goldman AS, Anderson DW Jr, Sellers WA, et al: Allergy. I. Oral challenges with milk and isolated milk proteins in allergic children, *Pediatrics* 32:425-443, 1963.

30. Gerrard JW, Lubos MC, Hardy LW, et al: Milk allergy: clinical picture and familial incidence, *Can Med Assoc J* 97:780-785, 1967.

31. Gerrard JW, MacKenzie JW, Goluboff N, et al: Cow's milk allergy: prevalence and manifestations in an unselected series of newborns, *Acta Paediatr Scand Suppl* 234:1-21, 1973.

32. Jakobsson I, Lindberg T: A prospective study of cow's milk protein intolerance in Swedish infants, *Acta Paediatr Scand* 68:853-859, 1979.

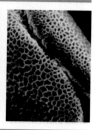

CHAPTER 47

Prevention and Natural History of Food Allergy

NOAH J. FRIEDMAN ■ ROBERT S. ZEIGER

Although much funding and media attention is focused on new modalities to treat allergic disease, an increasing amount of research is examining ways of preventing allergies. The prevention of food allergy in particular remains a vexing problem and a great opportunity in light of the fact that IgE-mediated sensitivity to ingested substances frequently occurs early in life and is often a harbinger of future atopic disease. Infancy represents a time when an allergic phenotype may be determined. An infant's immune system can either have a T helper cell type 2 (Th2) dominance with more secretion of interleukin (IL)-4 or a Th1 dominance with a cytokine balance toward interferon gamma (IFN-γ) production. Therefore interventions to prevent food allergies and the development of the atopic phenotype are best made early in life. Numerous factors may be involved in this phenotype determination (Figure 47-1) and are the subject of much current research.

Allergy prevention has traditionally been categorized as follows:

1. Primary prevention: prevention of allergy before any IgE-mediated disease has occurred.
2. Secondary prevention: prevention of further sensitivities once IgE-mediated disease has developed.
3. Tertiary prevention: prevention of manifestations of allergic disease once IgE-mediated sensitivity has occurred.

The focus of primary prevention of allergic disease has changed over the last several years. Recently, the Nutritional Committee from the American Academy of Pediatrics (AAP) and a joint Nutritional Committee of the European Society for Paediatric Allergology and Clinical Immunology (ESPACI) and the European Society for Paediatric Gastroenterology, Hepatology and Nutrition (ESPGHAN) have separately published guidelines for the primary prophylaxis of allergic disease through dietary manipulation of infant-mother pairs. The recommendations of both these groups are to be considered works in progress and based on the best data currently available. There are similarities and differences between the recommendations of the two groups and these will be discussed throughout this chapter.

Although lifestyle and dietary manipulation have been at the center of research over the past few decades, with varying degrees of success more and more resources are being expended on immunomodulation as a way of altering the Th1/Th2 balance of young children. Because of the logistical barriers inherent in insisting on prolonged breast-feeding with maternal avoidance diets, the use of hypoallergenic formulas, and environmental control, hope for a truly "user-friendly" form of primary prevention of food allergy and hence atopic disease in general seems to lie in immunomodulatory measures.

IMMUNOMODULATION

Immunomodulatory Role of Breast Milk

The results of studies regarding the effects of breast-feeding and the prevention of allergy remain inconclusive. Even if maternal diets are devoid of allergenic foods, prevention of food allergy in infancy appears to be transient at best. There is now an increasing body of literature to suggest that the reason for this inability to determine a conclusive role for breast-feeding in the prevention of atopy is the complex nature of breast milk itself and its immunostimulatory and immunosuppressive effects on the infant's intestinal milieu (Table 47-1).

A recent review[1] suggests that food allergens themselves, passing from the breast milk to the infant, may have either sensitizing or tolerizing effects on the infant's immune system. Secretory IgA has long been known to be passed to the infant through breast milk, possibly conferring passive protection to the infant's immune system. Past studies have suggested that low levels of colostral S-IgA might be associated with an increased risk of cow's milk allergy in infants.[2] More recent studies report that whereas lower levels of S-IgA to ovalbumin but not to β-lactoglobulin or cat were found in the colostrum and mature milk of allergic as opposed to nonallergic mothers,[3] the presence of these antibodies was not predictive for the development of atopic disease in the infants.[4]

There is some suggestion that cytokine concentration in breast milk differs between allergic and nonallergic mothers, with IL-4, IL-5, and IL-13 being present in higher concentrations in the breast milk of atopic women. These are cytokines known to be intimately involved with IgE production and induction of eosinophils. However, transforming growth factor (TGF)-β and IL-6 are the predominant cytokines in human breast milk.[5] TGF-β has been shown to increase the ability of the infant to produce its own IgA against β-lactoglobulin, casein, ovalbumin, and gliadin.[6] The soluble form of CD14, a cytokine that is thought to be central in the induction of a Th1

It is thus clear that breast milk has properties that allow it to be immunostimulatory and immunoprotective. This interplay of factors begins to explain the difficulty in developing a unifying theory of whether breast-feeding is an effective way to prevent food allergies in high-risk infants.

As much of the current thinking in preventing allergic disease leads researchers to develop new ways to induce a Th1 phenotype, it becomes logical to look toward the intestinal microflora. These 1 to 10 billion organisms most likely represent the major source of microbial stimulation of the immune system in the newborn by stimulating the maturation of the reticuloendothelial system. Furthermore, the use of these species is being investigated as a tool in both primary and secondary prevention of food allergy because lactobacilli have long been known to protect the gut against colonization with pathogens, to be completely nonpathogenic themselves, and to enhance immune responses; these strains have been dubbed *probiotics*. Studies since the late 1990s have demonstrated a decrease in the severity of atopic dermatitis in children if they are given probiotics,[10] including demonstration of a significant decrease in atopic dermatitis severity SCORAD scores in a double-blind, placebo-controlled study of probiotic supplemented whey hydrolysate formula.[11] Immunologically, probiotics have been shown to (1) decrease soluble CD4 in the serum and eosinophil protein X in the urine of children,[11] (2) decrease effects of bovine casein on lymphocyte proliferation and anti-CD3 antibody induced IL-4 production *in vitro,* and (3) suppress naturally fed antigen-specific IgE production by stimulation of IL-12 production in mice.[12]

Recently Kalliomaki et al[13] reported that infants whose mothers had been given probiotics 4 weeks prepartum and were either given probiotic-supplemented formula or their mothers were given probiotics during breast-feeding had significantly less atopic dermatitis during the first 2 years of life. This was not correlated with a decrease in total serum or food specific IgE. Further research will need to be done to determine the future of this intervention in the prevention of food

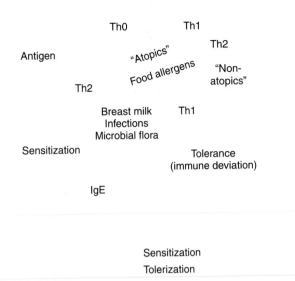

Several factors modify the primary immune response encountered early in life involving the T cell response. (Modified from Middleton E Jr, Reed CD, Ellis EE, et al, eds: *Allergy principles and practice,* ed 5, St Louis, 1998, Mosby.)

response by bacterial antigens,[7] is found in very high concentrations in human breast milk,[8] suggesting that this cytokine may play a role in the protective effect of breast-feeding on the development of allergy.

The composition of polyunsaturated long-chain fatty acids in human breast milk has also been shown to influence the development of atopy in infant. A high arachidonic acid to eicosapentaenoic acid ratio in human breast milk has been shown to increase the risk of allergic disease in the recipient.[3]

In Belgium, Dandrifosse and colleagues[9] have proposed that polyamines (including spermine and spermidine) present in breast milk decrease the permeability of the intestinal mucosa and thus are protective against the development of allergic disease in infants. Their data have come from studies in both suckling rats and humans.[9]

Factors in Breast Milk that Either Induce or Protect against Food Allergies

Factors	Inducing	Protective
Antigens	Sensitizing allergens	Tolerizing allergens
Cytokines	IL-4	TGF-β
	IL-5	sCD14
	IL-13	
Immunoglobulins		s-IgA to ovalbumin
Polyunsaturated fatty acids	Arachidonic acid	Eicosapentaenoic acid
	C22:4n-6	Docosapentaenoic acid
	C22:5n-6	Docosatetraenoic acid
		α-Linoleic acid
		n-3 Polyunsaturated fatty acids
Chemokines	RANTES	
	IL-8	
Polyamines		Spermine
		Spermidine

IL, Interleukin; *TGF-β,* transforming growth factor-beta; *RANTES,* regulated on activation, normal T cell expressed and secreted.

allergies. A follow-up study[14] reported a significant increase in the level of TGF-β2 in the breast milk of mothers who had been given probiotics.

Exposure to Infection

Although beyond the scope of this chapter because it does not address the prevention of food allergy specifically but rather the prevention of asthma, the "hygiene hypothesis" suggests that exposure to common respiratory infections early in infancy may actually decrease the risk of allergic diseases such as asthma by preferentially selecting a Th1-predominant immune system rather than a Th2-predominant atopic immune system. Therefore the reader is referred to several excellent reviews on this topic[15-17] as well as to the first two chapters of this book. Briefly, although for years it has been noted that certain early infections such as respiratory syncytial virus may predispose infants to develop asthma later in childhood, much data has been accumulating that children who are either placed in daycare early or have older siblings have higher rates of wheezing during early infancy but lower rates of asthma after age 6.[15,18] It has been suggested that intracellular microorganisms have a particularly strong immunomodulatory effect in that they are able to induce a strongly polarized Th1 response and a long-lived memory immunity.[16] There is also an association of frequent use of antibiotics in infancy with an increased odds ratio for the development of subsequent asthma.[19] In a similar vein, bacterial endotoxin may also have a protective effect against the development of allergies, but may sensitize people who are already atopic.[20]

This hypothesis is appealing because it may help to explain the increasing incidence of asthma over the past few decades. Unfortunately, because much of the tertiary prevention of asthma, that is, preventing asthma attacks in children, involves limiting exposure to infection, it is unclear how to incorporate such information into a comprehensive allergy-prevention program.

PRINCIPLES OF TRADITIONAL ALLERGY PREVENTION

Primary Prevention

Prediction of Allergy
The first question that needs to be asked when evaluating the practicality of primary prevention of food allergy is which children should be the targets of any intervention or manipulation of diet or lifestyle. Several factors have been investigated as predictors of the development of atopic disease, including family history of allergy and cord blood IgE. In part through the work of the human genome project, numerous genes have been uncovered that can predict allergy in some populations. Although it appears unlikely that a true "allergy gene" exists, these genes may prove to have more and more utility in predicting which patients may be candidates for certain interventions, including which infants might be candidates for immunomodulation or dietary manipulation to prevent food allergy.

"Allergy Genes"

By linking an atopic phenotype to certain polymorphic genetic markers, numerous genes have been shown to be associated with allergy.[21] Some loci appear to show linkage with allergy in certain ethnic groups whereas other loci appear to be more universal susceptibility markers. These regions include 11q13, which encodes the beta chain of the high-affinity IgE receptor[22,23]; 5q31-33, which contains a cytokine gene cluster; and the genes for the β-adrenergic and steroid receptors CD14 and fibroblast growth factor,[24] 12q, which contains the gene for IFN-γ and 6p21, which contains the HLA-D region. Although linkages between these regions and allergies have been well documented, the usefulness of this knowledge in determining which children might be candidates for intervention to prevent food allergy is not yet clear.

Family History and Cord Blood IgE as Predictors of Allergy

Although a genetic test for allergy risk remains elusive, family history remains in practice the most clinically useful determinant of risk of atopy in a child. Prospective studies of allergic families, with a variety of methodologic limitations, performed since the 1970s have estimated the risk of atopy to be between 38% to 58% in an offspring with one allergic parent and as high as 60% to 80% in a child born to two allergic parents. A child with a negative family history has about a 5% chance of developing allergy.[25] Swedish studies by Kjellman, however, have calculated the sensitivity of family history in the prediction of food allergy to be 45%, whereas the specificity was 74%. Cord blood IgE, a less practical indicator to obtain, was only 26% sensitive in determining the risk of atopy, whereas it was 74% specific. Combining these two factors, sensitivity rose to 56%. More recent studies have attempted to demonstrate a role for measuring cord blood IgE.[26] For example, a Canadian study[27] of 397 high-risk infants (defined by a maternal history of asthma or two first-degree relatives with other IgE-mediated disease), showed a significant increase in the incidence of "urticaria caused by food allergy" in infants with high cord blood IgE. However, the definition of urticaria with food allergy was wheals within 30 minutes of ingesting a particular food. There is neither mention of correlation to measurement of specific IgE to that particular food nor controlled food challenges to document true allergy. There remains therefore only limited usefulness for the measurement of cord blood IgE in the prediction of allergy.

DIETARY MANIPULATION DURING PREGNANCY, LACTATION, AND EARLY INFANCY

Dietary Manipulation during Pregnancy

Although in 1980 Michel et al[29] reported specific IgE sensitization to food during gestation,[28] more recent evidence suggests that this is a rare event, occurring in less than 0.3% of monitored pregnancies. In addition, studies that have examined the prophylactic effect of maternal avoidance of highly allergenic foods such as milk and egg[30,31] during pregnancy in high-risk groups showed no beneficial effects in the development of food allergy if the infant was otherwise maintained on a hypoallergenic diet after birth. It is therefore now widely accepted that maternal avoidance diets during pregnancy should not be recommended as a way to prevent allergic disease in children and may be potentially harmful in light of the increased risk of maternal malnutrition. However, because peanut is a major allergen and not an essential food, there would be no harm in recommending peanut avoidance during pregnancy, particularly as a way to acclimate the mother to a diet without peanuts that might be recommended during lactation.

Breast-Feeding

There is little controversy that breast-feeding is the best nourishment for infants. It offers the young child numerous nutritional, immunologic, and psychologic benefits that cannot be duplicated by formula. The AAP is unequivocal in its advocacy of breast-feeding in the newborn.[32] However, it is also clear that there is a potential immunologic downside to exposing a child at risk of atopy to highly allergenic foodstuffs through breast milk. It has long been known that β-lactoglobulin, casein, and bovine gammaglobulin,[33] three common milk antigens, have been measured in nanogram concentrations in lactating women who are not specifically avoiding milk during that time. Similarly, egg[34] and wheat[35] antigens have also been detected in breast milk. These substances can be measured as little as 2 to 6 hours after ingestion and can be detected up to 1 to 4 days later. The presence of peanut protein in the breast milk of women 1 to 2 hours after ingestion of peanut has recently been documented by sandwich enzyme-linked immunosorbent assay (ELISA).[36] The same authors also report the detection of two major peanut proteins, Ara h 1 and Ara h 2, in breast milk via immunoblot analysis.

Therefore the effect of breast-feeding on the development of food allergies has been the source of vigorous debate over the past few decades. Starting with Grulee and Sanford[37] in 1939, who noted in a nonrandomized study of over 20,000 infants that breast-feeding reduced the incidence of eczema sevenfold, numerous studies with a variety of strengths and weaknesses have filled the literature with evidence of both the protective and the sensitizing effects of breast-feeding *vis-a-vis* food allergy. Methodologic flaws that make it difficult to directly compare one study to another and draw long-term, clinically relevant conclusions include insufficient sample size, nonrandomization of study groups (e.g., of socioeconomic status, parental smoking, and time of introduction of solid foods), and lack of definitive documentation of food allergy by double-blind, placebo-controlled food challenge. These flaws are present in studies that demonstrate a positive effect of breast-feeding on the prevention of allergies as well as in those that do not support a protective effect. Nevertheless, many important observations have been made.

Studies performed since the 1980s have demonstrated that infants who were exclusively breast-fed had (1) lower serum IgE in early infancy,[38] (2) less atopic dermatitis,[39,40] and (3) fewer episodes of asthma[39] compared to infants who were given cow's milk formula. The effect on atopic dermatitis was shown in infants with or without high cord blood IgE in one study[39] but the protective effect of breast-feeding on atopic dermatitis was seen only in patients with an elevated serum IgE level at 5 days of age in another.[40] A 17-year follow-up study of one of these cohorts[41] suggests a protective effect against respiratory allergies later in adolescence as well.

Conversely, other studies performed in the 1980s showed that breast-feeding had no protective effect on the development of food allergy as compared to formula feeding.[42-45] Only three of these studies[42,43,45] reported supporting immunologic data.

More recent studies have even demonstrated an increased risk of the development of allergic disease in breast-fed children. For example, in a prospective but nonrandomized study, Wetzig et al[46] demonstrated that an increased number of infants with high cord blood IgE became sensitized to egg if they were exclusively breast-fed for greater than 5 months. Moreover, children with a family history of allergy and elevated cord blood IgE were noted to have a greater incidence of atopic dermatitis at 1 year of age if they had been exclusively breast-fed for greater than 5 months, as opposed to those with the same risk factors who had been nursed for a shorter period.

None of these studies either supporting or negating the protective effects of breast-feeding with regard to the development of allergy were randomized, prospective studies. However in 1990 Lucas at al[47] did perform such a study, comparing the effects of banked human breast milk versus preterm cow's milk formula for use as the diet for 446 premature neonates. This group of infants would already be considered at high risk for allergic sensitization to food antigens because of their delayed gut maturity. Within the cohort taken as a whole there was no statistically significant difference between the two groups by 18 months of age with regard to the development of allergy, but within the group of children with an atopic family history, the infants fed cow's milk formula had a 41% chance of developing an allergic reaction (especially atopic dermatitis) compared to 16% of the breast-fed infants. No skin testing or other confirmatory immunologic data was presented.

Recently a meta-analysis of prospective studies of breast feeding and its effect on the development of atopic dermatitis from 1966 to 2000 was published.[48] Studies were chosen based on strict criteria including blinding of the investigators, defined diagnostic criteria (but not immunologic confirmation of atopy), separate assessment of children with high risk of atopy), duration of breast-feeding for at least 3 months, and exclusivity of breast-feeding. Statistical analysis of these studies revealed a significant protective effect against the development of atopic dermatitis by breast-feeding. The overall odds ratio for this protective effect was 0.68 in all studies combined with an even greater protective effect, an odds ratio 0.58, in children at risk for atopy. No protective effect was noted in the meta-analysis of the few studies that looked at children with no increase risk for atopy. In a related meta-analysis,[49] the same group demonstrated that exclusive breast-feeding for at least the first 3 months of life also led to a decreased rate of childhood asthma if a positive family history of allergies was present. The protective effect was negligible in children with no family history of atopy.

Based on the above data, both the AAP and ESPACI/ESPGHAN committees strongly endorse exclusive breast-feeding as the hallmark for allergy prevention. They differ slightly in their recommendations with regard to the duration of nursing: the AAP recommends at least 6 months of breast-feeding whereas the European committee recommends 4 to 6 months. In addition, the AAP recommends continued but not exclusive breast-feeding until 12 months of age for all infants, whether at risk for atopy or not.[50] The safety of exclusive breast-feeding for 6 months has recently been confirmed by meta-analysis.[51] Furthermore, increasing breast-feeding can reduce community-wide infant illness[52] and reduce the cost of health services for the breast-fed infant.[53]

Maternal Avoidance Diets during Lactation

A possible explanation for the tremendous discrepancy found in the results of these studies examining the role of breast-feeding in the prevention of allergies is that maternal diet was not controlled. Milk, egg, and peanut allergens have been measured in breast milk and would therefore be expected to be passed on to the young recipient. Whether these food proteins sensitize or act as protective immunomodulators is unclear at this time. Several studies have attempted to determine whether sensitization to highly allergenic foodstuffs could be prevented in high-risk infants if lactating mothers avoid these foods; these studies are summarized in Table 47-2.

In 1989 Hattevig et al[54] reported the results of a study comparing two groups of high-risk infants. Both groups of infants were fed breast milk and supplemented with hypoallergenic diets including casein hydrolysate formulas. The mothers of the infants in the study group avoided egg, cow's milk, and fish during the first 3 months of lactation; the mothers of infants in the control group had no such restrictions on their diets. The control group infants had significantly more atopic dermatitis at 3 and 6 months than the children in the study group. No difference was found in the levels of IgE to milk or egg in the two groups after 6 months of age, which was thought to be because of eventual introduction of these foods into the infants' diet. It was also noted that the development of IgG antibodies to ovalbumin in some of the infants did not lead to decreased production of IgE antibodies to egg protein, suggesting that IgG antibodies do not have a protective effect against allergic sensitization. Follow-up at 10 years showed no long-lasting protective effect in the prevention of allergy in the group whose mothers had ingested a hypoallergenic diet during lactation.[55]

Similar clinical findings were noted in a prospective, randomized controlled Canadian study that same year,[56] in which the incidence of atopic dermatitis was found to be 22% by 18 months of age in infants whose mothers avoided milk, egg, fish, peanut, and soy during lactation as compared to 48% in infants of mothers on an unrestricted diet. No immunologic confirmation was reported.

In 1996 two studies were published, one a nonrandomized but well-controlled prospective investigation[57] and the other a nonrandomized nested case control study,[58] that contradicted these findings. The former study demonstrated no protective effects on the development of allergic disease in infants if egg and cow's milk were avoided by the mother during 3 months of lactation and solid foods were not introduced until the infant was 3 months old. The latter study actually showed that significantly more eczema and food allergy sensitization was found in the infants whose mothers avoided highly allergenic foods during lactation. A recent Cochrane meta-analysis[59] suggested a protective effect of maternal allergen avoidance on the incidence of atopic dermatitis during the first 12 to 18 months of life, but noted that the number of studies was too small to consider the findings definitive.

Particularly in light of contradictory evidence as to the beneficial effect of avoidance diets during lactation, care must be taken to make sure that the mother's food intake remains balanced during such a diet to prevent maternal malnutrition. A reassuring Finnish study[60] demonstrated that bone mineral density measured at the second postpartum bleed in 24 mothers on elimination diets (some using and some not using calcium supplementation) was no lower than that of 25 lactating women who were not on elimination diets.

Based on the results of the meta-analysis, the AAP currently recommends that mothers should eliminate peanuts and nuts (and consider avoiding eggs, cow's milk, and fish) during lactation. However, the guidelines of the ESCAPI/ESPGHAN committee recommend no special maternal lactation diet because of the methodologic shortcomings of the positive studies and the two negative ones. Because of these contradictory recommendations, maternal avoidance diets during lactation should be instituted on a case-by-case basis only after evaluating the degree of risk for atopy and the motivation of the family. Peanut avoidance is safe to recommend in that peanut is not an essential food and can easily be removed from the diet without any risk to maternal or infant well-being. On the other hand, if cow's milk is avoided, one must take care to ensure that the mother is ingesting sufficient calcium, up to 1500 mg of elemental calcium daily.

Soy Formula and Prevention of Allergic Disease

Although there was a suggestion in the early 1950s, via the results of a retrospective study, that children at high risk of atopy might have less allergic disease if fed a soy-based formula as opposed to cow's milk formula,[61-63] studies in the 1960s[64] and 1970s[65] have shown this not to be the case. The latter study, in particular, which was well designed, controlled, randomized, and immunologically supported, showed no difference in the occurrence of atopy in infants fed either soy or cow's milk formula. There is even some evidence that up to 10% to 15% of children with cow's milk allergy have IgE antibodies to soy. A recent study of 93 infants with cow's milk allergy (documented by either double-blind, placebo-controlled food challenge or by documentation of cow's milk IgE coupled with a compelling history of anaphylaxis) demonstrated that soy allergy (documented by double-blind, placebo-controlled food challenge) occurred in 13%.[66] Therefore, despite the existence of a large soy milk industry and although soy formula is certainly nutritious and not deleterious to nonallergic infants, soy formula cannot be recommended for primary prevention of allergic disease. It can, however, be recommended as a safe alternative to cow's milk formula in the majority of infants with cow's milk allergy after screening documents indicate no coexisting soy allergy.

Protein Hydrolysate Formula and Prevention of Allergic Disease

The ideal protein hydrolysate formula should not contain peptides larger than 1.5 kD, should contain no intact proteins, should demonstrate no anaphylaxis in animals, and should reveal protein determinant equivalents less than 1/1,000,000 of the original protein.[67] Most importantly, the formula must be demonstrated safe in milk-allergic infants by both double-blind placebo-controlled food challenge and by open challenge.

These formulas were first developed in the early 1940s and have been extremely effective for feeding infants with milk intolerance, milk allergy, and malabsorbtion. Over the

TABLE 47-2 Prospective, Randomized, Controlled Studies of the Effects of Maternal Food Allergen Avoidance during Pregnancy and Lactation on the Prevention of Atopy in Infants of Atopic Parents

Study and Reference	Intervention (N)	Pregnancy Diet	Lactation Diet	Infant Diet	F/U	SPT/RAST	DBPCFC	Atopic Disease	Comments
Falth-Magnusson, Kjellman[31]	3rd trimester (no egg, CM) vs. no restriction (N = 197)	Yes	No	Breast +/or casein hydrolysate (3 mo); solids (> 4 mo); CM (> 6 mo); egg/fish (> 9 mo)	5 yr	NS	No	NS	Pregnancy diet had no effect on infant atopy, SPT, or IgE
Lilja et al[30]	3rd trimester (no egg, CM) vs. no restrictions (N = 162)	Yes	No	Exclusive breast (5-6 mo) vs. no restrictions	1.5 yr	NS	No	NS	Pregnancy diet had no effect on infant atopy, SPT, or IgE
Hattevig et al[54,55]	1st 3 mo of lactation (no egg, CM, fish) vs. no restrictions (N = 115)	No	Yes	Breast ± casein hydrolysate (6 mo); CM/solids (> 6 mo); egg/fish (> 9 mo)	10 yr	Reduced number of CM ± egg-IgE tests at 3 mo†	No	Reduced AD at 3†, 6*, and 48† but not at 18 or 120 mo	Groups assigned by hospital rather than by true randomization
Chandra, Puri, Hamed[56]	Entire lactation (no egg, CM, peanuts, soy, fish) vs. no restrictions (N = 97)	No	Yes	Exclusive breast (~ 6 mo), solids (~ 6 mo)	1.5 yr	Not determined	No	Reduced AD by 1.5 yr*	No immunologic or food challenge confirmation

F/U, Follow-up; *SPT/RAST*, skin prick test/radioallergosorbent test; *DBPCFC*, double-blind, placebo-controlled food challenge; *CM*, cow's milk; *NS*, not significant; *AD*, atopic dermatitis.

*P < 0.05.

†P < 0.01.

Comments: Nutramigen (N), Pregestimil, and Profylac are extensive or ultrafiltrated PH; Good Start = NanHA = partial PH.

decades new formulations have come on the market with attempts made to decrease allergenicity via the use of small peptides while maintaining palatability and a reasonable cost.

Acceptable hypoallergenic formulas need to be extensively hydrolyzed in order to be composed of small enough peptides to be considered truly safe in children with milk allergy. Three casein hydrolysate formulas, Pregestimil (Mead Johnson Nutritionals, Evansville, IN), Nutramigen (Mead Johnson Nutritionals, Evansville, IN), and Alimentum (Ross Products, Abbott Laboratories, Columbus, OH), are widely available in the United States, fit these criteria, and are considered hypoallergenic.[68] Profylac (ALK, Denmark) is a less extensively hydrolyzed ultrafiltrated formula, unavailable in the United States, which has also been shown to be hypoallergenic.[15] However, although truly hypoallergenic, these formulas are not completely nonallergenic and allergic reactions can occur.[69,70] Nutramigen has been shown to be hypoimmunogenic by its ability to inhibit the IgG β-lactoglobulin response by an order of more than one log in high risk[25] and normal infants[71] up to 1 year of age. The residual allergenicity of partially and extensively hydrolyzed formulas has recently been evaluated by ELISA inhibition assays with polyclonal antibodies against milk proteins.[72]

Neocate (SHS International, Rockville, MD) and EleCare (Ross Products, Abbott Laboratories, Columbus, OH), both amino acid–derived elemental formulas, may be safe in most patients who cannot tolerate the protein hydrolysate formulas and are excellent alternatives.[73] Good Start (Nestle, Vevey, Switzerland; called NanHA outside the United States), a partial whey hydrolysate that was developed in the 1980s as a hypoallergenic formula, has numerous peptides of more than 4 kD and can cause allergic reactions in 40% to 60% of children with IgE-mediated cow's milk allergy and can therefore not be considered a safe alternative for these patients.[74]

The rationale for using extensively hydrolyzed protein hydrolysate formulas to prevent the development of food allergy in high-risk infants stems from the fact that these formulas are hypoimmunogenic, hypoallergenic, nutritious, and well tolerated. Moreover, the concentration of β-lactoglobulin in extensively hydrolyzed protein hydrolysate formulas is similar in range to its level in human breast milk.[75]

Numerous prospective controlled studies to determine the role of protein hydrolysate formulas as either a single intervention (summarized in Table 47-3)[76-80] or as part of a combined regimen, including a combined maternal/infant avoidance regimen (see Table 47-2), have been performed.

In a particularly well-controlled study, Halken et al[81] demonstrated a degree of cow's milk allergy in infants exclusively fed extensively hydrolyzed protein hydrolysate formula similar to that of infants who were breast-fed. Exclusive feeding with protein hydrolysate formula appears to be particularly effective if instituted before 6 months of age, even if the infant has been maintained on breast milk and follows a hypoallergenic regimen before that age.[82]

Decreased atopic dermatitis, cow's milk allergy, milk-specific IgE, and asthma have been reported in infants who have been fed extensively and partially hydrolyzed formulas, as compared with cow's milk or soy formula-fed babies. A greater protective effect was seen, however, with the extensively hydrolyzed formulas. Two recent prospective, randomized, controlled studies from Scandinavia compared extensive protein hydrolysate formulas versus partial protein hydroly-

sates in primary allergy prevention. In the Swedish study in which mothers and infants avoided cow's milk, egg, and fish, infants fed extensively hydrolyzed formula for 9 months had a significantly lower cumulative incidence of atopic symptoms, eczema, and positive egg skin tests at 9 months as compared to those infants who were fed partial hydrolysate formula.[83] The Danish study reported that cow's milk allergy, both by parental report as well as documented by food challenge, was significantly reduced from birth to 18 months in children whose breast-feeding was supplemented with an extensively hydrolyzed formula up to 4 months as compared to those infants who received a partially hydrolyzed formula for the same period of time.[84]

Both the AAP and ESPACI/ESPGHAN committees recommend the use of protein hydrolysate formulas in the primary prevention of allergy in high-risk infants who are bottle-fed. The AAP recommends extensively hydrolyzed formulas or possibly partially hydrolyzed formula whereas the European committee suggests a formula with confirmed reduced allergenicity. The AAP recommendations take into account the higher cost and lower palatability of extensively hydrolyzed formulas that limit their usefulness if solely for the purpose of preventing atopy. On the other hand, partially hydrolyzed formulas, which are less expensive and better tasting, are less effective in food allergy prevention. The lower palatability of the extensively hydrolyzed protein hydrolysate formulas may be overcome, however, by their early introduction to infants, before the child has developed a taste for other formulas. Therefore, if cost is not an issue, an extensively hydrolyzed formula should be used in infants at high risk for atopy if they are to be exclusively bottle-fed or if breast-feeding is to be supplemented.

Delayed Introduction of Solid Foods

In a prospective, unselected birth cohort study initially published in 1983[85] with follow-up in 1990,[86] Fergusson et al demonstrated that children who had been exposed to numerous solid foods during the first 4 months of life had higher rates of eczema at 2 years and 10 years of age. Also in 1983, a Finnish prospective, nonrandomized study demonstrated that in 115 infants with atopic family histories, those who exclusively breast-fed for 6 months had a 14% rate of eczema at 1 year as compared to 35% of those infants whose diets were supplemented with solid food.[87] Although not conclusive, these studies suggest that early introduction of solid foods might lead to an increased risk of eczema. The AAP recommends that in children with a high risk of allergy, "solid foods should not be introduced until 6 months of age, with dairy products delayed until 1 year, eggs until 2 years, and peanuts, nuts, and fish until 3 years of age."[32] On the other hand, the European guidelines are much less restrictive, recommending only that solid foods be introduced after 5 months of age. The latter group decided on general rather than specific recommendations because data regarding the introduction of specific foods at given ages is incomplete and inconclusive at this time.

Combined Infant and Maternal Avoidance of Allergenic Foods

Since the late 1980s two studies[25,88-90] have examined whether food atopy can be prevented by controlling the intake of highly allergenic foods by a high-risk infant from a variety of

TABLE 47-3 Prospective, Randomized, Controlled Studies of the Effects of Protein Hydrolysate Formulas on the Prevention of Cow's Milk Allergy in Infants of Atopic Parents

Study and Reference	Intervention (N)	Pregnancy Diet	Lactation Diet	Infant Diet	F/U	SPT/RAST	DBPCFC	Atopic Disease	Comments
Chandra, Singh, Shridhara	Nutramigen vs. CM vs. soy (N = 124)	None	None	Exclusive formula × 6 mo (diet ad lib ≥ 6 mo)	1.5 yr	Not determined	No	1. Reduced AD prevalence† and severity* by 1.5 yr with casein PH: N = 21%, soy = 63%, CM = 70%	1. No immune work-up or food challenges 2. AD prevalence exceptionally high
Chandra[77]	Good Start (PPH) vs. CM vs. soy vs. BM (N = 288)	None	None	Exclusive formula or BM × 6 mo (egg or fish > 18 mo; peanut > 3 yr)	5 yr	CM-IgE at ≤ 6 mo in PPH vs. CM*	DBPCFC	1. CMA: PPH (6%) < CM (21%)* ≤ 1yr 2. Cum AD reduced with PPH vs. CM† or soy* 3. Cum asthma < 18-60 mo with PPH vs. CM† or soy† 1. CMA at < 6† and 12* mo with PPH	1. Multiple comparison statistics not used 2. No aeroallergen sensitization determined 3. Relationship of asthma to atopic sensitization not determined
Vandenplas et al[78]	Good Start (PPH) vs. CM (N = 67)	None	None	Exclusive formula × 6 mo (diet ad lib ≥ 6 mo)	5 yr	CM-IgE at ≤ 6 mo: PPH < CM†	DBPCFC	1. CMPA/CMPI prevalence at 6 mo especially high (34%) in controls 2. Period prevalence of atopy after 1 yr similar in PPH and CM 3. PPH preventive effect specific for CMA; no effect on wheezing
Mallet, Henocq[79]	Pregestimil vs. CM (N = 165)	None	None	Formula ± BM × 4 mo (diet ad lib ≥ 4 mo)	4 yr	Determined on small subgroup only (3/27 with CM-IgE)	No	1. PH: lower eczema: 4 mo (P = 0.07), 2 yr† and 4 yr† but not 1 yr 2. No effect on asthma 1. CMA similar in	1. Dropout 25% at 1 yr 2. No control for confounding 3. CMA too low (0.6%) to determine preventive effect of PH on CMA

Study	Intervention		Maternal diet	Infant diet	Follow-up	IgE	Challenge	Comments
Halken et al[81]	Nutramigen vs. Profylac vs. BM (N = 141)	None	None	Exclusive formula ± BM × 6 mo (diet ad lib ≥ 6 mo; no CM × 6 mo)	1.5 yr	CM-IgE in 4/5 with CMPA/CMPI	Open challenge	1. CMPA/CMPI = 3.6% vs. 20% in 1985 cohort with no allergy prevention
Marini et al[80]	Good Start (PPH) vs. CM (N = 84)	None	None	Exclusive formula × 5 mo; CM > 5 mo; egg, fish > 1 yr; nuts > 2 yr	3 yr	CM-IgE: PPH (1/43) vs. CM (5/40) (NS)	No	1. CMA not determined 2. Cum AD reduced at 1 yr in PPH by multivariate analysis; OR = 0.3 (95% CI = 0.1-0.9) but not in univariate analysis 3. Asthma and AR unaffected
Odelram et al[82]	Profylac vs CM (N = 91)	None	Entire lactation (no egg, CM, fish)	Formula on weaning (median 6 mo) vs. BM solely > 9 mo (no egg, CM, or fish × 12 mo)	1.5 yr	CM-IgE ~ in groups; sIgE levels > median in CM > Profylac*	Single-blind challenge	1. CMA only in CM (3/39) 2. Atopic disease ~ between groups
Oldaeus et al[83]	Nutramigen vs. partial whey/casein PH vs. CM (N = 141*)	None	Entire lactation (no egg, CM, fish)	BM + formula at mean 3.5 mo (no CM × 9 mo; no egg, fish × 1 yr; no solids × 4 mo)	1.5 yr	CM-IgE same; egg SPT + at 9 mo: 10% N vs. 33% PPH†	DBPCFC	1. Cum atopy 6-18 mo: N < CM* 2. Cum atopy 6-9 mo: N < PPH*
Halken et al[84]	Nutramigen vs. Profylac vs. partial PH (N = 246)	None	None	BM + formula at median 1 mo (no CM or solids × 4 mo)	1.5 yr	Not reported	Open plus DBPCFC for ± reactions	1. Cum CMA 0-18 mo: N/Profylac < PPH (0.6% vs. 4.7%)*

SPT/RAST, Skin prick test/radioallergosorbent test; *DBPCFC*, double-blind, placebo-controlled food challenge; *CM*, cow's milk; *AD*, atopic dermatitis; *PH*, protein hydrolysate; *PPH*, partially hydrolyzed PH; *BM*, breast milk; *CMA*, CM allergy = CMPA + CMPI; *Cum*, cumulative prevalence; *CMPI*, CM protein intolerance; *NS*, not significant; *OR*, odds ratio; *CI*, confidence interval; *AR*, allergic rhinitis.

*$P < 0.05$.

†$P < 0.01$.

Comments: Nutramigen (N), Pregestimil, and Profylac are extensive and/or ultrafiltrated PH; Good Start = NanHA = partial PH (PHH).

sources, that is, both direct ingestion and indirect ingestion through the breast milk. Both studies were done before it became clear that allergen avoidance during pregnancy does not have an effect on subsequent allergic disease in the offspring.

In 1986 Chandra et al[88] reported that in a prospective, randomized, unblinded study of 71 infants with atopic siblings, severity of eczema was significantly reduced and its incidence marginally reduced if mothers excluded milk, egg, peanut, fish, and beef throughout pregnancy and lactation. No supporting immunologic data or double-blind placebo-controlled food challenges were presented.

In a prenatally randomized, physician-blinded, parallel-controlled study the effect of multiple food allergen avoidance in both the lactating mothers and their infants was compared to standard feeding practices in children with a positive family history of allergy.[91] This study found that children whose intake of allergenic foods from a variety of sources was restricted showed (1) a significantly lower incidence of allergic diseases such as atopic dermatitis at 1 year of age because of a lower incidence of food allergy and (2) lower specific IgE and IgG to cow's milk up to 2 years of age compared with acceptable infants. There was no effect on the occurrence of respiratory allergy or sensitization to environmental allergens from birth to 7 years.[25,86,90]

These studies suggest that, whereas food allergies can be avoided in the first 1 to 2 years of life by carefully limiting dietary intake of highly allergenic foods for more than 6 months, this is not followed by a reduction in allergic disease later in childhood. Because many food allergies spontaneously remit, there may be value in this transient reduction of food allergy if these restrictive measures are carried out by highly motivated families. Because of the difficulty and potential danger to maternal health, decisions to recommend to families with atopic histories a complicated regimen of maternal and infant food allergen avoidance in an attempt to prevent food allergy must be made individually.

Combined Maternal and Infant Food Allergen and House Dust Mite Avoidance

In addition to these measures, a group from the Isle of Wight also attempted a prospective, randomized, controlled study including dust mite control measures (plastic encasing of mattress and pillows and acaricide treatment of household carpets and furniture) with postpartum infant and maternal avoidance diets in the prevention of both food allergies and respiratory allergy.[92,93] Results showed that there was a significant decrease in atopy in general, eczema and asthma at 1 year of age, and food or aeroallergen sensitization by 4 years of age as well. They found that an unrestricted diet during infancy, low socioeconomic status, parental smoking, and maternal atopy were all risk factors for the development of allergic diseases.

Secondary Prevention

The success of primary prevention of allergy rests, in part, on overcoming several obstacles. Highly motivated patients and physicians are needed to carry out inconvenient intervention in a healthy infant solely on the basis of family history or cord blood IgE levels. However, once a child is determined to be atopic by either clinical observation and or immunologic confirmation, secondary prevention can be carried out to prevent progression of the "atopic march."[94] Currently, there is much research being conducted to determine if there is any way to halt the inexorable atopic march through medical intervention. Ketofen has been shown to reduce the frequency of asthma by over 60% over 1[95] and 3[96] years in two double-blind, placebo-controlled studies of high-risk infants with atopic dermatitis. There was no concomitant effect on total or allergen-specific IgE, suggesting that symptoms may have been ameliorated rather than the disease actually prevented. The Early Treatment of the Atopic Child[97] network in Europe has presented data that cetirizine prevented asthma secondary to mite and grass pollen exposure. Recent publications suggest that immunotherapy may be effective in secondary allergy prevention.[98] The Childhood Asthma Research and Education network in the United States is currently actively involved in research dealing with the prevention of early asthma in high-risk children.

Tertiary Prevention

Tertiary prevention remains the most widely practiced and least controversial of all forms of food allergy prevention. There is little doubt that avoidance of any offending food is the mainstay of tertiary food allergy prevention. Patient support and education groups such as the Food Allergy and Anaphylaxis Network (FAAN) can be helpful for many patients. Because it is clear that allergen avoidance alone will not prevent the manifestations of atopic dermatitis, appropriate use of antiinflammatory medications, emollients, antihistamines, and antimicrobials remains an integral part of treating this illness and is discussed in depth elsewhere in this book. It is also incumbent upon physicians to provide patients who have life-threatening food allergies with an action plan that includes the appropriate use of epinephrine in case of accidental ingestion of the offending allergen.

If the "atopic march" proceeds and patients develop respiratory allergy, appropriate education should be provided to the patient and/or his or her family regarding environmental control and the proper use of allergy medications. In particular, preventive medicines should be encouraged where deemed appropriate. Although early upper respiratory infections (URIs) may decrease the risk of the development of atopic disease in later childhood, avoidance of URIs, when possible, still appears to be the most prudent option for preventing asthma flares in children with known disease. Influenza vaccination should be recommended annually (note: flu vaccine contains egg protein).

Natural History of Food Allergy

Food allergy is most commonly acquired during the first year of life, with peak incidence of 6% to 8% occurring at 1 year of age. The prevalence falls until late childhood, where it plateaus at 1% to 2% through adulthood. The prevalence of perceived, but unconfirmed, food allergy or food intolerance is as high as 25%.[99]

In a Danish study by Host and Halken[100] 1749 children were followed prospectively from birth to age 3. Milk allergy was suspected in 117 children (6.7%) and confirmed by milk elimination and oral challenge in 39 (2.2%), with more than half having documented IgE-mediated disease. In a study from the Isle of Wight[101] all children born over a 1-year period (N = 1456) were followed for the development of peanut and tree nut allergy until 4 years of age. Fifteen (1.2%) of the 981 skin-tested children were found to be sensitized to peanuts or tree nuts. In a large German study published in 1997,[102] RASTs were performed yearly to age 6 on a birth cohort of 4082 children. Prevalence of sensitization to foods peaked at 10% at 1 year, declining to 3% at 6 years of age. Egg and milk RASTs were the most common positives, followed by wheat and soy; no clinical confirmation of food allergy was reported.

It has long been established that whereas milk and egg allergies are most frequently outgrown by a child's third birthday, peanut allergy most commonly remains a lifelong issue. Tree nut, fish, and shellfish allergy are also much more likely to continue into adulthood than are egg and cow's milk allergy. More light has been shed on predicting which patients may "outgrow" their food allergies and in whom allergies will persist.

Sampson and Scanlon[103] have reported that 85% of children with milk allergy will be able to tolerate milk by age 3. Several studies since the early 1990s have examined ways to predict which children will outgrow their milk allergy by 3 years of age. Total[104] and specific[105] IgE to cow's milk, IgE levels specific to casein and β-lactoglobulin, and IgE:IgG ratio[106] were all significantly higher in those children with persistent cow's milk allergy. Recently, Vila et al[107] demonstrated that the specific cow's milk IgE from patients with persistent cow's milk allergy is more likely to bind to the linear (sequential) epitopes of α1- and β-casein as compared to higher levels of IgE to the conformational (native) epitopes in children who had lost their clinical sensitivity to cow's milk as documented by food challenge. These data may yield insight not only into predicting which milk-allergic children will more likely be able to ultimately tolerate cow's milk but also why some people with milk or egg allergy are able to tolerate small amounts of cooked milk or egg but cannot tolerate these foods in raw, or native, states.[108,109]

The natural history of peanut allergy has also been the subject of extensive study. In 1989 Bock and Atkins[70] reported that among 32 patients contacted 2 to 14 years after positive double-blind, placebo-controlled food challenge to peanut, 16 had had a clinical reaction to peanut in the year before contact, 8 had a reaction 1 to 5 years before contact, and 8 had not knowingly ingested peanut. These data suggest that it is rare to lose clinical sensitivity to peanut in children with true IgE-mediated disease. In 2000 Vanderleek et al[110] reported that 75% of peanut-allergic patients followed for up to 10 years after being diagnosed had adverse reactions to accidental peanut exposure. Although patients with lower concentrations of peanut-specific IgE were more likely to have dermatologic symptoms only, there was no clear cutoff in IgE concentration below which a patient would be considered at low risk for systemic allergic symptoms. More recently, by performing oral peanut challenge on patients with a history of peanut allergy who had no recollection of peanut reaction in the past year and with peanut-specific IgE levels less than 20 kU/L, Skolnick et al[111] determined that peanut allergy may be "outgrown" in 21.5% of patients. Hourihane et al[112] showed in a study of 30 patients with a history of peanut allergy that the 15 patients with resolved peanut allergy were less likely to be allergic to other foods and were less likely to have a prick skin test with more than 6 mm wheal than were those patients with persistent peanut allergy. In this study peanut-specific IgE was found to be no different in those patients who outgrew their peanut allergy as compared to those in whom it was persistent.

In reviewing these data it appears that although it is clear that a peanut challenge can be extremely useful in identifying patients in whom peanut allergy has resolved, there is no clear consensus of what indications should be used to determine in whom such a challenge would be considered safe. The utility of quantitating food-specific IgE fluorescent enzyme-linked immunosorbent assay (CAP-FEIA) in the diagnosis of food allergy and in determining which children do not need food challenges to confirm a sensitivity is discussed in Chapter 45.

Although it has generally been thought that once food allergies have resolved they are unlikely to recur, some recent abstracts have reported the unsettling recurrence of peanut[113] and fish[114] allergy in patients with previously negative food challenges following a history of earlier allergy. Further studies are needed to determine how great a threat this is to patients whose diets have been liberalized based on negative food challenges.

CONCLUSIONS

A reliable, consistently effective method of preventing food allergies in high-risk children that is also easy to adhere to remains elusive. Whereas immunomodulatory measures are promising as the future of food allergy prevention, they must still be considered experimental and cannot be routinely recommended at this time other than as part of controlled studies. Currently, dietary manipulation remains the best intervention for motivated families, although this is clearly suboptimal. Parental compliance with such measures is a major obstacle and, despite recommendations that have been in place for many decades, food allergy continues to rise. The Nutrition Committees of the AAP and ESCAPI/ESPGHAN have published somewhat differing recommendations for primary prevention of allergy in children (Table 47-4) because of the incomplete and somewhat contradictory data available. The authors of this chapter offer an approach to prevention of food allergy in children that reconciles the reasoned guidelines of both of these organizations (Table 47-5).

Once food allergies have been diagnosed, skin test and/or CAP-FEIA should be monitored to see if sensitivity has disappeared, particularly in patients with milk and egg allergy. More sophisticated tests, such as epitope recognition, might also play a role in determining who is most likely to "outgrow" their food allergies. Food challenges should be performed when appropriate (Box 47-1).

HELPFUL WEBSITE

The Food Allergy and Anaphylaxis Network website (www.foodallergy.org)

TABLE 47-4 Summary of Recommendations for Prophylaxis (Primary Prevention) of Food Allergy by the Committees on Nutrition of the AAP and ESPACI/ESPGHAN

Parameter	AAP, 2000[5]	ESPACI/ESPGHAN, 1999[6]	Comments
High-risk infants	Yes: biparental; parent and sibling	Yes: affected parent or sibling	Prevention appears limited to high-risk infants.
Maternal pregnancy diet	Not recommended, with possible exception of peanut	Not recommended	Studies fail to show benefit from prenatal CM and egg avoidance (potential for affecting maternal and infant weights adversely). Peanut is not an essential food, avoidance will not lead to nutritional deficits, and its avoidance may better prepare for postpartum avoidance.
Exclusive breast-feeding	6 mo	4-6 mo	Studies confirm at least 4-6 mo may be adequate for beneficial preventive effect.
Maternal lactation diet	Eliminate peanuts and nuts (consider eliminating eggs, CM, fish)	Not recommended	Contradictory because conflicting studies exist and issue is not resolved; some believe such a diet should be investigational at this time; others believe efforts should be limited to peanuts.
Supplemental calcium and vitamins during restricted lactation diets	Yes	Not discussed	Need to prevent nutritional deficiencies with nutritional supplementation.
Avoid soy formulas	Yes	Yes	Most studies failed to show a benefit with soy formulas in primary prevention.
Hypoallergenic formula for bottle-fed high-risk infants	Yes: use a hypoallergenic (extensive) or possibly partial hydrolysate when not breast-feeding	Yes: use formula with confirmed reduced allergenicity	There is greater support for extensively hydrolyzed products at this time, but their greater expense may limit their use and lead to use of partially hydrolyzed products.
Hypoallergenic formula for supplementation	Yes: use extensive or possibly partial hydrolysate	Yes: use formula with confirmed reduced allergenicity	There is greater support for extensively hydrolyzed products at this time, but their greater expense may limit their use and lead to use of hypoallergenic formula for supplementation.
Delayed introduction of solid foods to infant	Start least allergenic at 6 mo; CM at 12 mo; eggs at 24 mo; peanuts, nuts, and fish at 36 mo	Start at 5 mo	The less restrictive ESPACI recommendations are based on studies in which CM allergy was prevented even when CM was introduced at 5 mo. The AAP recommendation is based on consensus rather than direct evidence.

From Zeiger RS: *Pediatrics* (in press) 2003.
AAP, American Academy of Pediatrics; *ESPACI*, European Society for Paediatric Allergology and Clinical Immunology; *ESPGHAN*, European Society for Paediatric Gastroenterology, Hepatology and Nutrition; *CM*, cow's milk.

TABLE 47-5 Authors' Approach to Primary Prevention of Food Allergy, Incorporating Current Guidelines of the AAP and ESCAPI/ESPGHAN

Interventions	Recommendations
Immunomodulation	Still experimental; cannot be recommended at this time
Pregnancy diet	Not recommended; avoiding peanut would not be harmful
Breast-feeding	Exclusive breast-feeding strongly recommended for at least 6 mo and continued breast-feeding recommended up to 1 yr
Lactation diet	Peanut avoidance can clearly be encouraged; milk and egg avoidance is not routinely recommended but may be offered on a case-by-case basis to highly motivated families; if instituted, mother must take supplemental calcium
Soy formula	Not recommended
Protein hydrolysate formula	An extensively hydrolyzed protein hydrolysate formula is strongly recommended if infant is to be bottle-fed or as a supplement to breast milk
Delayed introduction of solid foods	Solid food may be added at 6 mo; avoid cow's milk until 1 yr; in motivated families, egg may be avoided until 2 yr and peanuts, tree nuts, and fish until 3 yr

AAP, American Academy of Pediatrics; *ESCAPI*, European Society for Paediatric Allergology and Clinical Immunology; *ESPGHAN*, European Society for Paediatric Gastroenterology, Hepatology and Nutrition.

KEY CONCEPTS
Prevention and Natural History of Food Allergy

Primary Prevention

Immunomodulation

- Breast milk may be both immunoprotective and immunostimulatory via complex interplay of cytokines and allergen content.
- Probiotics are still experimental with regard to prevention of food allergy.

Dietary manipulation

- Dietary manipulation during pregnancy is of little benefit.
- Exclusive breast-feeding during first 6 months of life, with continued breast-feeding for the first year, is recommended.
- Mothers should consider avoiding peanuts and tree nuts and possibly eggs, cow's milk, and fish while lactating.
- Soy formula is not recommended in the primary prevention of allergic disease.
- Fully hydrolyzed, hypoallergenic protein hydrolysate formulas are recommended in the primary prevention of food allergy.
- Similarities and differences exist between European and American Committees on Nutrition.

Secondary Prevention

- Much current research is ongoing to prevent the progression of the "atopic march."

Tertiary Prevention

- Allergen avoidance, emergency action plans, and medications remain the mainstay.

Natural History of Food Allergy

- Peak incidence of food allergy reaches 6% to 8% at 1 year of age.
- Prevalence plateaus of 1% to 2% occur during adulthood.
- Egg and cow's milk allergy are frequently "outgrown," with 85% of children with milk allergy able to tolerate milk by 3 years of age.
- Peanut allergy persists in 75% to 80% of cases.

REFERENCES

1. Hoppu U, Kalliomaki M, Laiho K, et al: Breast milk: immunomodulatory signals against allergic diseases, *Allergy* 56:23-26, 2001.
2. Taylor B, Wadsworth J, Golding J, et al: Breast feeding, eczema, asthma, and hayfever, *J Epidemiol Community Health* 37:95-99, 1983.
3. Casas R, Bottcher MF, Duchen K, et al: Detection of IgA antibodies to cat, beta-lactoglobulin, and ovalbumin allergens in human milk, *J Allergy Clin Immunol* 105:1236-1240, 2000.
4. Duchen K, Casas R, Fageras-Bottcher M, et al: Human milk polyunsaturated long-chain fatty acids and secretory immunoglobulin A antibodies and early childhood allergy, *Pediatr Allergy Immunol* 11:29-39, 2000.
5. Bottcher MF, Jenmalm MC, Garofalo RP, et al: Cytokines in breast milk from allergic and nonallergic mothers, *Pediatr Res* 47:157-162, 2000.
6. Kalliomaki M, Ouwehand A, Arvilommi H, et al: Transforming growth factor-beta in breast milk: a potential regulator of atopic disease at an early age, *J Allergy Clin Immunol* 104:1251-1257, 1999.
7. Baldini M, Lohman IC, Halonen M, et al: A polymorphism* in the 5' flanking region of the CD14 gene is associated with circulating soluble CD14 levels and with total serum immunoglobulin E, *Am J Respir Cell Mol Biol* 20:976-983, 1999.
8. Labeta MO, Vidal K, Nores JE, et al: Innate recognition of bacteria in human milk is mediated by a milk-derived highly expressed pattern recognition receptor, soluble CD14, *J Exp Med* 191:1807-1812, 2000.
9. Dandrifosse G, Peulen O, El Khefif N, et al: Are milk polyamines preventive agents against food allergy? *Proc Nutr Soc* 59:81-86, 2000.
10. Majamaa H, Isolauri E: Probiotics: a novel approach in the management of food allergy, *J Allergy Clin Immunol* 99:179-185, 1997.
11. Isolauri E, Arvola T, Sutas Y, et al: Probiotics in the management of atopic eczema, *Clin Exp Allergy* 30:1604-1610, 2000.
12. Murosaki S, Yamamoto Y, Ito K, et al: Heat-killed Lactobacillus plantarum L-137 suppresses naturally fed antigen-specific IgE production by stimulation of IL-12 production in mice, *J Allergy Clin Immunol* 102:57-64, 1998.
13. Kalliomaki M, Salminen S, Arvilommi H, et al: Probiotics in primary prevention of atopic disease: a randomised placebo-controlled trial, *Lancet* 357:1076-1079, 2001.
14. Rautava S, Kalliomaki M, Isolauri E: Probiotics during pregnancy and breast-feeding might confer immunomodulatory protection against atopic disease in the infant, *J Allergy Clin Immunol* 109:119-121, 2002.
15. Openshaw PJ, Hewitt C: Protective and harmful effects of viral infections in childhood on wheezing disorders and asthma, *Am J Respir Crit Care Med* 162:S40-S43, 2000.
16. von Hertzen LC: Puzzling associations between childhood infections and the later occurrence of asthma and atopy, *Ann Med* 32:397-400, 2000.
17. Strannegard O, Strannegard IL: The causes of the increasing prevalence of allergy: is atopy a microbial deprivation disorder? *Allergy* 56:91-102, 2001.
18. Ball TM, Castro-Rodriguez JA, Griffith KA, et al: Siblings, day-care attendance, and the risk of asthma and wheezing during childhood, *N Engl J Med* 343:538-543, 2000.
19. Wickens K, Pearce N, Crane J, et al: Antibiotic use in early childhood and the development of asthma, *Clin Exp Allergy* 29:766-771, 1999.
20. Liu AH, Leung DY: Modulating the early allergic response with endotoxin, *Clin Exp Allergy* 30:1536-1539, 2000.
21. Barnes KC: Atopy and asthma genes—where do we stand? *Allergy* 55:803-817, 2000.
22. Daniels SE, Bhattacharrya S, James A, et al: A genome-wide search for quantitative trait loci underlying asthma, *Nature* 383:247-250, 1996.
23. Shirakawa T, Li A, Dubowitz M, et al: Association between atopy and variants of the beta subunit of the high-affinity immunoglobulin E receptor, *Nat Genet* 7:125-129, 1994.
24. Shek LP, Tay AH, Chew FT, et al: Genetic susceptibility to asthma and atopy among Chinese in Singapore—linkage to markers on chromosome 5q31-33, *Allergy* 56:749-753, 2001.
25. Zeiger RS, Heller S, Mellon MH, et al: Genetic and environmental factors affecting the development of atopy through age 4 in children of atopic parents: a prospective randomized study of food allergen avoidance, *Pediatr Allergy Immunol* 3:110-127, 1992.
26. Kjellman NI: Prediction and prevention of atopic allergy, *Allergy* 53:67-71, 1998.
27. Kaan A, Dimich-Ward H, Manfreda J, et al: Cord blood IgE: its determinants and prediction of development of asthma and other allergic disorders at 12 months, *Ann Allergy Asthma Immunol* 84:37-42, 2000.
28. Michel FB, Bousquet J, Greillier P, et al: Comparison of cord blood immunoglobulin E concentrations and maternal allergy for the prediction of atopic diseases in infancy, *J Allergy Clin Immunol* 65:422-430, 1980.
29. Zeiger RS: Prevention of food allergy in infancy, *Ann Allergy* 65:430-442, 1990.
30. Lilja G, Dannaeus A, Foucard T, et al: Effects of maternal diet during late pregnancy and lactation on the development of atopic diseases in infants up to 18 months of age—*in vivo* results, *Clin Exp Allergy* 19:473-479, 1989.
31. Falth-Magnusson K, Kjellman NI: Development of atopic disease in babies whose mothers were receiving exclusion diet during pregnancy: a randomized study, *J Allergy Clin Immunol* 80:868-875, 1987.
32. American Academy of Pediatrics Committee on Nutrition: Hypoallergenic infant formulas, *Pediatrics* 106:346-349, 2000.
33. Stuart CA, Twiselton R, Nicholas MK, et al: Passage of cows' milk protein in breast milk, *Clin Allergy* 14:533-535, 1984.
34. Cant A, Marsden RA, Kilshaw PJ: Egg and cows' milk hypersensitivity in exclusively breast fed infants with eczema, and detection of egg protein in breast milk, *Br Med J (Clin Res Ed)* 291:932-935, 1985.
35. Troncone R, Scarcella A, Donatiello A, et al: Passage of gliadin into human breast milk, *Acta Paediatr Scand* 76:453-456, 1987.

36. Vadas P, Wai Y, Burks W, et al: Detection of peanut allergens in breast milk of lactating women, *JAMA* 285:1746-1748, 2001.

37. Grulee CG, Sanford HN: The influence of breast and artificial feeding on infantile eczema, *J Pediatr* 9:223-225, 1930.

38. Saarinen UM, Kajosaari M, Backman A, et al: Prolonged breast-feeding as prophylaxis for atopic disease, *Lancet* 2:163-166, 1979.

39. Chandra RK, Puri S, Cheema PS: Predictive value of cord blood IgE in the development of atopic disease and role of breast-feeding in its prevention, *Clin Allergy* 15:517-522, 1985.

40. Duchateau J, Casimir G: Neonatal serum IgE concentration as predictor of atopy, *Lancet* 1:413-414, 1983.

41. Saarinen UM, Kajosaari M: Breastfeeding as prophylaxis against atopic disease: prospective follow-up study until 17 years old, *Lancet* 346: 1065-1069, 1995.

42. Gordon RR, Noble DA, Ward AM, et al: Immunoglobulin E and the eczema-asthma syndrome in early childhood, *Lancet* 1:72-74, 1982.

43. Van Asperen PP, Kemp AS, Mellis CM: Immediate food hypersensitivity reactions on the first known exposure to the food, *Arch Dis Child* 58:253-256, 1983.

44. Hide DW, Guyer BM: Clinical manifestations of allergy related to breast and cow's milk feeding, *Pediatrics* 76:973-975, 1985.

45. Rowntree S, Cogswell JJ, Platts-Mills TA, et al: Development of IgE and IgG antibodies to food and inhalant allergens in children at risk of allergic disease, *Arch Dis Child* 60:727-735, 1985.

46. Wetzig H, Schulz R, Diez U, et al: Associations between duration of breast-feeding, sensitization to hens' eggs and eczema infantum in one- and two-year-old children at high risk of atopy, *Int J Hyg Environ Health* 203:17-21, 2000.

47. Lucas A, Brooke OG, Morley R, et al: Early diet of preterm infants and development of allergic or atopic disease: randomised prospective study, *Br Med J* 300:837-840, 1990.

48. Gdalevich M, Mimouni D, David M, et al: Breast-feeding and the onset of atopic dermatitis in childhood: a systematic review and meta-analysis of prospective studies, *J Am Acad Dermatol* 45:520-527, 2001.

49. Gdalevich M, Mimouni D, Mimouni M: Breast-feeding and the risk of bronchial asthma in childhood: a systematic review with meta-analysis of prospective studies, *J Pediatr* 139:261-266, 2001.

50. Breastfeeding and the use of human milk: American Academy of Pediatrics Work Group on Breastfeeding, *Pediatrics* 100:1035-1039, 1997.

51. Kramer MS, Kakuma R: Optimal duration of exclusive breastfeeding (Cochrane Review), Cochrane Database Syst Rev CD003517, 2002.

52. Wright AL, Bauer M, Naylor A, et al: Increasing breastfeeding rates to reduce infant illness at the community level, *Pediatrics* 101:837-844, 1998.

53. Ball TM, Wright AL: Health care costs of formula-feeding in the first year of life, *Pediatrics* 103:870-876, 1999.

54. Hattevig G, Kjellman B, Sigurs N, et al: Effect of maternal avoidance of eggs, cow's milk and fish during lactation upon allergic manifestations in infants, *Clin Exp Allergy* 19:27-32, 1989.

55. Hattevig G, Sigurs N, Kjellman B: Effects of maternal dietary avoidance during lactation on allergy in children at 10 years of age, *Acta Paediatr* 88:7-12, 1999.

56. Chandra RK, Puri S, Hamed A: Influence of maternal diet during lactation and use of formula feeds on development of atopic eczema in high-risk infants, *Br Med J* 299:228-230, 1989.

57. Herrmann ME, Dannemann A, Gruters A, et al: Prospective study of the atopy-preventive effect of maternal avoidance of milk and eggs during pregnancy and lactation, *Eur J Pediatr* 155:770-774, 1996.

58. Pollard C, Phil M, Bevin S. Influence of maternal diet during lactation upon allergic manifestation in infants: tolerization or sensitization, *J Allergy Clin Immunol* 97:240, 1996.

59. Kramer MS: Maternal antigen avoidance during lactation for preventing atopic disease in infants of women at high risk, Cochrane Database Syst Rev CD000132, 2000.

60. Holmberg-Marttila D, Sievanen H, Sarkkinen E, et al: Do combined elimination diet and prolonged breastfeeding of an atopic infant jeopardise maternal bone health? *Clin Exp Allergy* 31:88-94, 2001.

61. Glaser J, Johnstone DE: Soybean milk as a substitute for mammalian milk in early infancy: with special reference to preventiuon of allergy to cow's milk, *Ann Allergy* 10:433, 1952.

62. Glaser J, Johnstone DE: Prophylaxis of allergic disease in newborn, *JAMA* 153:620, 1953.

63. Johnstone DE, Glaser J: Use of soybean milk as an aid in prophylaxis of allergic disease in children, *J Allergy* 24:434-436, 1953.

64. Johnstone DE, Dutton A: The value of hyposensitization therapy for bronchial asthma in children: a 14-year study, *Pediatrics* 42:793-802, 1968.

65. Kjellman NI, Johansson SG: Soy versus cow's milk in infants with a biparental history of atopic disease: development of atopic disease and immunoglobulins from birth to 4 years of age, *Clin Allergy* 9:347-358, 1979.

66. Zeiger RS, Sampson HA, Bock SA, et al: Soy allergy in infants and children with IgE-associated cow's milk allergy, *J Pediatr* 134:614-622, 1999.

67. Oldaeus G, Bradley CK, Bjorksten B, et al: Allergenicity screening of "hypoallergenic" milk-based formulas, *J Allergy Clin Immunol* 90:133-135, 1992.

68. Sampson HA, Bernhisel-Broadbent J, Yang E, et al: Safety of casein hydrolysate formula in children with cow milk allergy, *J Pediatr* 118: 520-525, 1991.

69. Lifschitz CH, Hawkins HK, Guerra C, et al: Anaphylactic shock due to cow's milk protein hypersensitivity in a breast-fed infant, *J Pediatr Gastroenterol Nutr* 7:141-144, 1988.

70. Bock SA, Atkins FM: The natural history of peanut allergy, *J Allergy Clin Immunol* 83:900-904, 1989.

71. Vaarala O, Saukkonen T, Savilahti E, et al: Development of immune response to cow's milk proteins in infants receiving cow's milk or hydrolyzed formula, *J Allergy Clin Immunol* 96:917-923, 1995.

72. Plebani A, Restani P, Naselli A, et al: Monoclonal and polyclonal antibodies against casein components of cow milk for evaluation of residual antigenic activity in 'hypoallergenic' infant formulas, *Clin Exp Allergy* 27:949-956, 1997.

73. Sampson HA, James JM, Bernhisel-Broadbent J: Safety of an amino acid-derived infant formula in children allergic to cow milk, *Pediatrics* 90:463-465, 1992.

74. Businco L, Cantani A, Longhi MA, et al: Anaphylactic reactions to a cow's milk whey protein hydrolysate (Alfa- Re, Nestle) in infants with cow's milk allergy, *Ann Allergy* 62:333-335, 1989.

75. Host A, Husby S, Hansen LG, et al: Bovine beta-lactoglobulin in human milk from atopic and non-atopic mothers: relationship to maternal intake of homogenized and unhomogenized milk, *Clin Exp Allergy* 20:383-387, 1990.

76. Chandra RK, Singh G, Shridhara B: Effect of feeding whey hydrolysate, soy and conventional cow milk formulas on incidence of atopic disease in high-risk infants, *Ann Allergy* 63:102-106, 1989.

77. Chandra RK: Five-year follow-up of high-risk infants with family history of allergy who were exclusively breast-fed or fed partial whey hydrolysate, soy, and conventional cow's milk formulas, *J Pediatr Gastroenterol Nutr* 24:380-388, 1997.

78. Vandenplas Y, Hauser B, Van den BC, et al: The long-term effect of a partial whey hydrolysate formula on the prophylaxis of atopic disease, *Eur J Pediatr* 154:488-494, 1995.

79. Mallet E, Henocq A: Long-term prevention of allergic diseases by using protein hydrolysate formula in at-risk infants, *J Pediatr* 121:S95-S100, 1992.

80. Marini A, Agosti M, Motta G, et al: Effects of a dietary and environmental prevention programme on the incidence of allergic symptoms in high atopic risk infants: three years' follow-up, *Acta Paediatr Suppl* 414:1-21, 1996.

81. Halken S, Host A, Hansen LG, et al: Preventive effect of feeding high-risk infants a casein hydrolysate formula or an ultrafiltrated whey hydrolysate formula: a prospective, randomized, comparative clinical study, *Pediatr Allergy Immunol* 4:173-181, 1993.

82. Odelram H, Vanto T, Jacobsen L, et al: Whey hydrolysate compared with cow's milk-based formula for weaning at about 6 months of age in high allergy-risk infants: effects on atopic disease and sensitization, *Allergy* 51:192-195, 1996.

83. Oldaeus G, Anjou K, Bjorksten B, et al: Extensively and partially hydrolysed infant formulas for allergy prophylaxis, *Arch Dis Child* 77:4-10, 1997.

84. Halken S, Hansen KS, Jacobsen HP, et al: Comparison of a partially hydrolyzed infant formula with two extensively hydrolyzed formulas for allergy prevention: a prospective, randomized study, *Pediatr Allergy Immunol* 11:149-161, 2000.

85. Fergusson DM, Horwood LJ, Shannon FT: Asthma and infant diet, *Arch Dis Child* 58:48-51, 1983.

86. Fergusson DM, Horwood LJ, Shannon FT: Early solid feeding and recurrent childhood eczema: a 10-year longitudinal study, *Pediatrics* 86:541-546, 1990.

87. Kajosaari M, Saarinen UM: Prophylaxis of atopic disease by six months' total solid food elimination: evaluation of 135 exclusively breast-fed infants of atopic families, *Acta Paediatr Scand* 72:411-414, 1983.

88. Chandra RK, Puri S, Suraiya C, et al: Influence of maternal food antigen avoidance during pregnancy and lactation on incidence of atopic eczema in infants, *Clin Allergy* 16:563-569, 1986.

89. Zeiger RS, Heller S: The development and prediction of atopy in high-risk children: follow-up at age seven years in a prospective randomized study of combined maternal and infant food allergen avoidance, *J Allergy Clin Immunol* 95:1179-1190, 1995.

90. Zeiger RS, Heller S, Mellon MH, et al: Effect of combined maternal and infant food-allergen avoidance on development of atopy in early infancy: a randomized study, *J Allergy Clin Immunol* 84:72-89, 1989.

91. Zeiger RS: Development and prevention of allergic disease in childhood. In Middleton EJ, Reed CE, Ellis EE, et al, eds: *Allergy principles and practice*, ed 3, St Louis, 1993, Mosby.

92. Arshad SH, Matthews S, Gant C, et al: Effect of allergen avoidance on development of allergic disorders in infancy, *Lancet* 339:1493-1497, 1992.

93. Hide DW, Matthews S, Tariq S, et al: Allergen avoidance in infancy and allergy at 4 years of age, *Allergy* 51:89-93, 1996.

94. Zeiger RS: Secondary prevention of allergic disease: an adjunct to primary prevention, *Pediatr Allergy Immunol* 6:127-138, 1995.

95. Iikura Y, Naspitz CK, Mikawa H, et al: Prevention of asthma by ketotifen in infants with atopic dermatitis, *Ann Allergy* 68:233-236, 1992.

96. Bustos GJ, Bustos D, Bustos GJ, et al: Prevention of asthma with ketotifen in preasthmatic children: a three-year follow-up study, *Clin Exp Allergy* 25:568-573, 1995.

97. Allergic factors associated with the development of asthma and the influence of cetirizine in a double-blind, randomised, placebo-controlled trial: first results of Early Treatment of the Atopic Child, *Pediatr Allergy Immunol* 9:116-124, 1998.

98. Des RA, Paradis L, Menardo JL, et al: Immunotherapy with a standardized *Dermatophagoides pteronyssinus* extract. VI. Specific immunotherapy prevents the onset of new sensitizations in children, *J Allergy Clin Immunol* 99:450-453, 1997.

99. Wood RA: The natural history of food allergy, *Pediatrics* (in press) 2003.

100. Host A, Halken S: A prospective study of cow milk allergy in Danish infants during the first 3 years of life: clinical course in relation to clinical and immunological type of hypersensitivity reaction, *Allergy* 45:587-596, 1990.

101. Tariq SM, Stevens M, Matthews S, et al: Cohort study of peanut and tree nut sensitisation by age of 4 years, *Br Med J* 313:514-517, 1996.

102. Kulig M, Bergmann R, Klettke U, et al: Natural course of sensitization to food and inhalant allergens during the first 6 years of life, *J Allergy Clin Immunol* 103:1173-1179, 1999.

103. Sampson HA, Scanlon SM: Natural history of food hypersensitivity in children with atopic dermatitis, *J Pediatr* 115:23-27, 1989.

104. Schrander JJ, Oudsen S, Forget PP, et al: Follow up study of cow's milk protein intolerant infants, *Eur J Pediatr* 151:783-785, 1992.

105. Hill DJ, Firer MA, Ball G, et al: Natural history of cows' milk allergy in children: immunological outcome over 2 years, *Clin Exp Allergy* 23:124-131, 1993.

106. James JM, Sampson HA: Immunologic changes associated with the development of tolerance in children with cow milk allergy, *J Pediatr* 121:371-377, 1992.

107. Vila L, Beyer K, Jarvinen KM, et al: Role of conformational and linear epitopes in the achievement of tolerance in cow's milk allergy, *Clin Exp Allergy* 31:1599-1606, 2001.

108. Eigenmann PA: Anaphylactic reactions to raw eggs after negative challenges with cooked eggs, *J Allergy Clin Immunol* 105:587-588, 2000.

109. Urisu A, Ando H, Morita Y, et al: Allergenic activity of heated and ovomucoid-depleted egg white, *J Allergy Clin Immunol* 100:171-176, 1997.

110. Vander Leek TK, Liu AH, Stefanski K, et al: The natural history of peanut allergy in young children and its association with serum peanut-specific IgE, *J Pediatr* 137:749-755, 2000.

111. Skolnick HS, Conover-Walker MK, Koerner CB, et al: The natural history of peanut allergy, *J Allergy Clin Immunol* 107:367-374, 2001.

112. Hourihane JO, Dean TP, Warner JO: Peanut allergy in relation to heredity, maternal diet, and other atopic diseases: results of a questionnaire survey, skin prick testing, and food challenges, *Br Med J* 313:518-521, 1996.

113. Busse PJ, Noone SA, Nowak-Wegrzyn AH: Recurrence of peanut allergy, *J Allergy Clin Immunol* 109:S92, 2002.

114. De Frutos C, Zapatero L, Martinez I: Re-sensitization to fish in allergic children after a temporary tolerance period: two case reports, *J Allergy Clin Immunol* 109:S306, 2002.

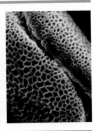

CHAPTER **48**

Enterocolitis, Proctocolitis, and Enteropathy

SCOTT H. SICHERER

Food hypersensitivity disorders are defined by an adverse immune response to benign dietary proteins. They are categorized by immunopathophysiology, among disorders with an acute onset after ingestion that are associated with food-specific IgE antibody (e.g., oral allergy syndrome), those that are chronic in nature and sometimes associated with IgE antibody (e.g., eosinophilic gastroenteropathies), and those that are cell mediated and not associated with detectable IgE antibody. Four of the non–IgE-mediated food hypersensitivity disorders are the focus of this chapter: food protein–induced proctocolitis, enterocolitis, enteropathy, and celiac disease.[1] These disorders have overlapping symptoms but are distinguishable clinically and have distinct patterns of symptoms and clinical course.

EPIDEMIOLOGY/ETIOLOGY

Dietary Protein Proctocolitis

This disorder of infancy is characterized by the presence of mucousy, bloody stools in an otherwise well-appearing infant caused by an immune response directed, most commonly, against cow's milk protein. The mean age at diagnosis is approximately 60 days, with a range of 1 day to 6 months.[2,3] The bleeding is often mistakenly attributed to perirectal fissures. Occasionally there is associated colic or increased frequency of bowel movements, but failure to thrive is absent. Up to 60% of cases occur in breast-fed infants, where the immune response results from maternal ingestion of the food allergen, usually cow's milk, which is passed in immunologically recognizable form into the breast milk. Similarly, in infants fed commercial formula, the reaction is associated with cow's milk or, less commonly, soy.[4-9] The disorder has rarely been described in infants fed protein hydrolysate formulas[10]; such formulas contain only minute quantities of allergenic protein. Additional observations in some series include a mild peripheral blood eosinophilia and sometimes mild hypoalbuminemia.[2,8] Anemia develops in a minority of infants.[3,4] Markers of atopy such as atopic dermatitis or positive family history for atopy are not significantly increased compared with the general population.[2,4]

Endoscopic examination is usually not needed for diagnostic purposes but, when performed, shows patchy erythema, friability, and a loss of vascularity generally limited to the rectum but sometimes extending throughout the colon.[5] Histologically, high numbers of eosinophils (5 to 20 per high-power field) or eosinophilic abscesses are seen in the lamina propria,

crypt epithelium, and muscularis mucosa.[2,9,11,12] The eosinophils are frequently associated with lymphoid nodules (lymphonodular hyperplasia).[2] However, lymphonodular hyperplasia is not unique to this condition.[2,9] Aggregates of small, dark granules, "nuclear dust," are sometimes observed and represent the remains of apoptotic epithelial cells.[13] The specific immunologic mechanisms responsible are unknown. Because the disorder is confined to the lower colon and the disorder is most prominent in breast-fed infants, it has been hypothesized that dietary antigens complexed to breast milk IgA may play a part in the activation of eosinophils and the distribution of the inflammatory process.[14] Although peripheral eosinophilia and positive radioallergosorbent tests (RASTs) to milk have been reported, they are unusual findings.[5-7,11]

Dietary Protein Enteropathy

This disorder is characterized by protracted diarrhea, vomiting, malabsorption, and failure to thrive. Additional features may include abdominal distention, early satiety, edema, hypoproteinemia, and protein-losing enteropathy. Symptoms usually begin in the first several months of life, depending on the time of exposure to the causal proteins.[15-19] The disorder is most commonly caused by an immune response to cow's milk protein, but soy, cereal grains, egg, and seafood have all been implicated. This disorder appears to occur more commonly in infants taking formula, rather than breast-feeding, particularly when such formulas were not commercially processed. A decrease in prevalence has been documented in Finland[20] and Spain[21] and attributed to a rise in breast-feeding and/or the use of adapted infant formula. The disorder sometimes follows viral gastroenteritis and may then represent either an unmasking of a hypersensitivity response or a new adverse immune response that develops during a window period of altered immunity.[22,23]

Biopsy reveals variable small bowel villus injury, increased crypt length, intraepithelial lymphocytes, and few eosinophils. The immune mechanisms appear to involve T cell responses[24] and are not associated with IgE antibodies. Cytokine profiles determined from evaluation of lamina propria lymphocytes in affected infants reveal increased interferon (IFN)-γ and interleukin (IL)-4 and less IL-10 production than controls. In addition, IFN-γ–secreting cells were more numerous, indicating an overall predominance of T helper cell type 1–type responses. Kokkonen et al[25] identified an increased density of gamma-delta–positive intraepithelial T cells in children with cow's milk enteropathy compared with controls (but the density was lower than that seen in celiac disease). In some studies, immunohistochemical stains of the mucosa reveal deposition of eosinophil products.[26] Unlike gluten-sensitive enteropathy (celiac disease [discussed later]), this enteropathy generally resolves in 1 to 2 years, and there is no increased threat of future malignancy.[17]

Dietary Protein Enterocolitis

Dietary protein enterocolitis (also termed *food protein–induced enterocolitis syndrome* [FPIES]) describes a symptom complex of profuse vomiting and diarrhea usually diagnosed in the first months of life and most commonly attributable to an immune response to cow's milk or soy. Both the small and large bowels are involved in the inflammatory process. When the causal protein remains in the diet, chronic symptoms can include bloody diarrhea, poor growth, anemia, hypoalbuminemia, and fecal leukocytes, and the illness may progress to dehydration and hypotension. Removal of the causal protein leads to resolution of symptoms. Powell[27] initially characterized the syndrome. She described nine infants with severe, protracted diarrhea and vomiting. The symptoms developed at 4 to 27 days after birth (mean, 11 days) in infants on a cow's milk–based formula. Switching to a soy-based formula resulted in transient improvement, but symptoms generally recurred in 7 days. Seven of the nine infants were below birth weight, and eight of nine presented with dehydration. Eight of the infants appeared acutely ill and underwent sepsis evaluations that were negative. All infants were noted to have low serum albumin, elevated peripheral blood polymorphonuclear leukocyte counts, and stools that were positive for heme and reducing substances. The hospital course usually involved improvement while on intravenous fluids followed by recurrence of dramatic symptoms with reintroduction of soy- or cow's milk–based formula, including the development of shock in several infants. Follow-up with oral challenges was carried out with cow's milk and soybean formulas at a mean age of 5.5 months, and 14 of the 18 challenges were positive. Ten of 14 challenges resulted in vomiting (onset, 1 to 2.5 hours after ingestion; mean, 2.1 hours) and all experienced diarrhea (onset, 2 to 10 hours; mean, 5 hours) with blood, polymorphonuclear leukocytes and eosinophils, and increased carbohydrate in the stool. There was a rise in peripheral blood polymorphonuclear cell counts in all positive challenges peaking at 6 hours after ingestion, with a mean rise of 9900 cells/mm³ (range, 5500 to 16,800 cells/mm³). Only isolated gastrointestinal symptoms were reported.

The results of these studies led Powell[27,28] to propose criteria for a positive oral challenge to diagnose food protein–induced enterocolitis of infancy.[29] Confirmation of the allergy included a negative search for other causes, improvement when not ingesting the causal protein, and a positive oral challenge resulting in vomiting/diarrhea, evidence of gastrointestinal inflammation through stool examination, and a rise in the peripheral polymorphonuclear leukocyte count over 3500 cells/ml. Infants with symptoms consistent with severe enterocolitis who fulfilled, or are highly likely to have fulfilled, these criteria are included in many reports of milk or soy allergy of infancy.[15,30-36]

Because infantile FPIES is a diagnosis that can be made clinically, there are no large series in which biopsies are performed solely in patients fulfilling Powell's criteria. Thus specific descriptions of the histologic findings are lacking, and only assumptions can be drawn by considering descriptions from case reports or series that likely included these patients. Colonic biopsy results in symptomatic patients reveal crypt abscesses and a diffuse inflammatory cell infiltrate with prominent plasma cells; small bowel biopsies reveal edema, acute inflammation, and mild villous injury.[5,11,37-39] In some cases, focal erosive gastritis and esophagitis are found, with prominent eosinophilia and villous atrophy.[38,40,41]

An understanding of the immunologic basis of the syndrome is emerging with an appreciation for the role of T cell–derived cytokines. Heyman et al[34] demonstrated that tumor necrosis factor alpha (TNF-α) secreted by circulating milk protein–specific T cells increased intestinal permeability. Benlounes et al[35,42] showed that significantly lower doses of intact cow's milk protein stimulated TNF-α secretion from peripheral blood mononuclear cells of patients with FPIES compared with either patients whose sensitivity resolved or those with skin, rather than intestinal, manifestations of cow's milk hypersensitivity. Fecal TNF-α was increased after positive milk challenge in enterocolitis patients.[43] Conversely, transforming growth factor (TGF)-β1 is a cytokine that protects the epithelial barrier of the gut.[44] Immunohistochemical staining of duodenal biopsy specimens in infants with FPIES revealed a depression of TGF-β1 expression and a decreased expression of the type 1 TGF-β receptor.[45]

Celiac Disease

Celiac disease, also termed *Celiac sprue* or *gluten-sensitive enteropathy,* is caused by an immune response triggered by wheat gluten or related rye and barley proteins that results in inflammatory injury to the small intestinal mucosa.[46,47] The classic presentation occurs in infants after weaning, at the time when cereals are introduced into the diet. Exclusion of gluten from the diet results in amelioration of clinical disease. Symptoms partly reflect malabsorption, with patients exhibiting failure to thrive, anemia, and muscle wasting. Additional symptoms are varied and include diarrhea, abdominal pain, vomiting, bone pain, and aphthous stomatitis. Subclinical or minimal disease is possible, delaying diagnosis into adulthood. Chronic ingestion of gluten-containing grains in celiac patients is associated with increased risk of enteropathy-associated T cell lymphoma.[48] Celiac disease is most common among Europeans and those of European descent. Serologic studies in the United Kingdom indicate a prevalence of 1:300.[49] Celiac disease is associated with autoimmune disorders and IgA deficiency. Another associated disorder is *Dermatitis herpetiformis*,[50,51] a gluten-responsive dermatitis characterized by pruritic, erythematous papules and/or vesicles distributed symmetrically on the extensor surfaces of the elbows and knees and on the face, buttocks, neck, and trunk. Immunohistologic examination of the skin reveals a deposition of granular IgA at the dermal papillary tips and the disorder is usually (> 85%) associated with celiac disease.

Endoscopy of the small bowel in active celiac disease typically reveals total villous atrophy and extensive cellular infiltrate. The disorder is caused by gliadin-specific T cell responses enhanced by deamidated gliadin produced by tissue transglutaminase.[46,52] Antigen presentation appears to be a central issue in immunopathology because more than 95% of

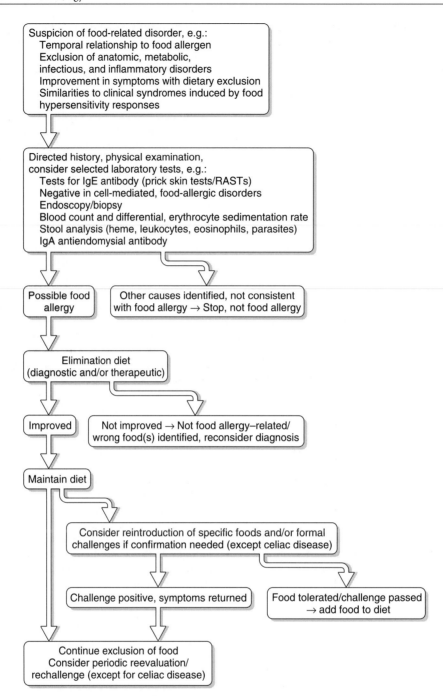

FIGURE 48-1 The evaluation of food allergy requires a simultaneous consideration for alternative diagnoses (infection, anatomic, metabolic, etc.) and disorders caused by food allergy including those described in this chapter and others (i.e., oral allergy syndrome, anaphylaxis, eosinophilic gastroenteropathies, food-related reflux disease) and nonimmune adverse reactions to foods (lactose intolerance). Laboratory tests and decisions for elimination and challenge are based on specific elements of the history and an appreciation of the clinical manifestations and course of the various disorders (see text). *RAST,* Radioallergosorbent test.

patients are HLA DQ2.[53] Gliadin is one of the few substrates for tissue transglutaminase, which deamidates specific glutamines within gliadin, creating epitopes that bind efficiently to DQ2 gut-derived T cells.[54,55] The activation of DQ2-restricted T cells initiates the inflammatory response.[56] Histopathologic studies reveal that lymphocytes, predominantly of the CD8+ cytotoxic/suppressor phenotype, are prominent in the intraepithelial space, and γ/δ T cells are increased in the jejunal mucosa as well as the peripheral blood.[57] Elimination of gliadin from the diet results in a down-regulation of the T cell–induced inflammatory process and normalizing of the mucosal histology.

DIFFERENTIAL DIAGNOSIS

Dietary protein–induced proctocolitis, enteropathy, enterocolitis, and celiac disease have in common the pathophysiologic mechanisms of cell-mediated adverse reactions to dietary proteins with symptoms primarily affecting the gastrointestinal tract. Because the gastrointestinal tract has a limited number of responses to inflammatory damage, there is overlap in the symptoms observed with these disorders. Differentiating them from each other requires consideration of key distinct clinical features and directed laboratory examinations. Moreover, numerous medical disorders must be considered in the evaluation of patients presenting with gastrointestinal complaints. Some of these disorders include other food hypersensitivities, but food intolerance (nonimmune disorders such as lactase deficiency) and toxic reactions (e.g., bacterial poisoning) are potential considerations.

In a broad sense, the differential diagnosis is vast and can encompass virtually any cause of abdominal complaint, including the following categories: infection (viral, bacterial, parasitic), anatomy (pyloric stenosis, anal fissures, motility disorders, lymphangiectasia, Hirschsprung's disease, reflux, intussusception), inflammatory disorders (inflammatory bowel disease), metabolism (disaccharidase deficiencies), malignancy, immunodeficiency, and others. Depending on the constellation of findings, various diagnostic strategies are used that are beyond the scope of this chapter. However, the presence of a number of clinical elements may underscore the possibility of a food allergic disorder. The general approach to the diagnosis of food-allergic disorders affecting the gut is outlined in Figure 48-1. Various features may suggest a differentiation of the disorders described in this chapter from those related to IgE antibody–mediated gastrointestinal allergies (oral allergy, gastrointestinal anaphylaxis) and those that are sometimes associated with IgE antibody (eosinophilic gastroenteropathies and reflux). The chronicity following ingestion of the causal food (acute in IgE antibody–mediated disease), symptoms (isolated vomiting in gastroesophageal reflux disease), and selected test results (biopsy revealing an eosinophilic infiltrate in allergic eosinophilic gastroenteropathy) differentiate these food allergy disorders. The food-related disorders must also be distinguished from a host of disorders that have similar clinical findings but alternative etiologies. Table 48-1 delineates the disorders that may most closely overlap the cell-mediated food allergy disorders.

The distinguishing clinical features of dietary protein–induced proctocolitis, enteropathy, enterocolitis, and celiac disease are listed in Table 48-2. Although they may represent a spectrum of disorders with similar etiologies, the treatment and natural course of the diseases vary, making a specific diagnosis imperative. The causal foods, symptoms, and family history usually indicate the likely disorder. In some cases, the diagnosis requires initial confirmation of reactivity/association determined by (1) resolution of symptoms with an elimination diet and (2) recurrence of symptoms after oral challenge. In

TABLE 48-1 Examples of Clinical Disease that May Overlap Symptoms of Cell-Mediated, Dietary Protein–Induced Disease

Clinical Disease	Symptoms
Proctocolitis	Anal fissure
	Infection
	Perianal dermatitis
	Necrotizing enterocolitis
	Volvulus
	Hirschsprung's disease
	Intussusception
	Coagulation disorders
Enterocolitis	Sepsis
	Necrotizing enterocolitis
	Intussusception
	Volvulus
Enteropathy	Infection
	Eosinophilic gastroenteropathy
	Bowel ischemia
	Inflammatory bowel disease
	Lymphangiectasia
	Autoimmune enteropathy
	Immune deficiency
	Tropical sprue
	Collagenous sprue
	Malignancy

some cases, specific tests are needed (e.g., serologic tests for IgA endomysial or tissue transglutaminase antibody and small bowel biopsy). The disorders are not IgE antibody mediated, but if there has been immediate onset of symptoms following ingestion or an association of gastrointestinal allergy with other features of IgE antibody–mediated food allergy (e.g., atopic dermatitis, asthma), screening tests for food-specific IgE antibody (prick skin tests, RAST) may be helpful in defining the process causing the reactions. A number of tests are of unproved use for the diagnosis of food allergy and should not be used. These include measurement of IgG_4 antibody, provocation-neutralization (drops placed under the tongue or injected to diagnose and treat various symptoms), and applied kinesiology (muscle strength testing).[58]

EVALUATION AND MANAGEMENT

Dietary Protein Proctocolitis

The diagnosis of dietary protein proctocolitis should be entertained in an infant who is otherwise well and presents with mucousy, bloody stools; an absence of symptoms indicating a

TABLE 48-2 Clinical Features Helpful to Distinguish Dietary Protein-Induced Proctocolitis, Enteropathy, Enterocolitis, and Celiac Disease

	Vomiting	Diarrhea	Growth	Foods	Other	Onset
Proctocolitis	Absent	Minimal, bloody	Normal	Breast/milk/soy		Days to 6 mo
Enterocolitis	Prominent	Prominent	Poor	Milk/soy	Reexposure: severe, subacute symptoms	Days to 1 yr
Enteropathy	Variable	Moderate	Poor	Milk/soy	Edema	2 to 24 mo
Celiac disease	Variable	Variable	Poor	Gluten	HLA DQ2–associated	> 4 mo

systemic disease; coagulation defect; or another source of bleeding. The definitive diagnosis requires withdrawal of the presumed allergen with monitoring for resolution of symptoms. This dietary trial is usually sufficient to make the diagnosis. In cow's milk– or soy formula–fed infants, substitution with a protein hydrolysate formula generally leads to cessation of obvious bleeding within 72 hours, although it is unknown how long occult bleeding continues. The majority of infants who develop this condition while ingesting protein hydrolysate formulas will experience resolution of bleeding with the substitution of an amino acid–based formula.[10,59] Management in breast-fed infants is more difficult. Restriction of cow's milk (most common), soy, or egg from the mother's diet usually results in resolution of symptoms.[4] In cases where there is no response to maternal dietary manipulation, no data are currently available to know whether breast-feeding may be safely continued in an otherwise healthy-appearing infant. If bleeding is dramatic, monitoring of the red blood cell count is prudent. Progressive bleeding despite dietary restriction should prompt reevaluation with consideration for proctocolonoscopy and biopsy.[12] The majority of infants will tolerate cow's milk and soy products by 1 to 2 years of age. Because there is generally no risk of a severe reaction, the foods can be gradually reintroduced into the diet at the appropriate age. If there was a suspicion of mild enterocolitis (e.g., vomiting in addition to hematochezia) or a history to suggest IgE-mediated reactions, dietary advancement may require caution (supervised oral food challenge).

Enterocolitis

As noted earlier, the diagnosis of dietary protein enterocolitis syndrome rests on clinical and challenge criteria. In most cases many patients would not undergo a formal challenge during infancy because the diagnosis becomes self-evident after elimination of the causal protein, and frequently patients experience inadvertent reexposure, proving their sensitivity before a physician-made diagnosis. It must be appreciated that chronic ingestion or reexposure to the causal food can result in a clinical picture that is severe and may mimic sepsis. In a review of 17 infants hospitalized with this disorder, Murray and Christie[60] reported 6 infants who presented with acidemia (mean pH 7.03) and methemoglobinemia. Several other clinical features have emerged.[36,61] Approximately half of the infants react to both cow's milk and soy. Sensitivity to milk was lost in 60% and to soy in 25% of the patients after 2 years from the time of presentation. In addition, some patients maintain their allergy beyond age 6 years,[62] and a widening variety of foods have been implicated including oat,[63] rice, and poultry.[61,64,65]

Because there is a high percentage of patients with sensitivity to both cow's milk and soy, switching directly to a casein hydrolysate is recommended. For the rare patients reactive to hydrolysate, an amino acid–based formula is appropriate.[66] Families must be instructed about the careful avoidance of cow's milk and/or soy. Follow-up challenges should be performed at intervals to determine tolerance (approximately every 12 to 24 months, depending on the clinical severity). These challenges should be performed under physician supervision with emergency medications immediately available because dramatic reactions, including shock, can occur. Reevaluation for the development of antigen-specific IgE antibody before challenge may be helpful because a few children may convert to IgE-mediated reactions over time.[61] In the experience of the author and his colleagues,[61] about half of positive challenges require treatment (usually intravenous fluids). In view of the presumed pathophysiology, corticosteroids have been administered for severe reactions. The role of epinephrine for treatment is not known, but it should be available for severe cardiovascular reactions. Considering the risk for hypotension, the challenge is best performed under physician supervision with an intravenous access. Food challenges for this non–IgE-mediated syndrome are typically performed with 0.15 to 0.6 g/kg of the causal protein. The challenge protocol and definition of a positive response are shown in Table 48-3.

Dietary Protein Enteropathy and Celiac Disease

There are no specific diagnostic tests for dietary protein–induced enteropathy; therefore, the diagnosis depends on exclusion of alternative diagnoses, biopsy evidence of enteropathy, and proof of sensitivity through dietary elimination and

---

TABLE 48-3 Oral Food Challenges for Food Protein–Induced Enterocolitis Syndrome

Diagnostic Step	Procedures and Assessment
Preparation for challenge	Verify normal weight gain, no gastrointestinal symptoms while off causal protein Obtain baseline stool sample and peripheral blood polymorphonuclear leukocyte count Intravenous line in place Medications ready to treat reaction
Administration of challenge	Administer challenge (typically 0.15-0.6 g/kg) Observe for symptoms (usual onset 1-4 hr) Repeat peripheral blood polymorphonuclear leukocyte count 6 hr after ingestion Collect subsequent stools for 24 hr
Evaluation of positive challenge	Symptoms (vomiting, diarrhea) Fecal blood (gross or occult) Fecal leukocytes Fecal eosinophils Rise in peripheral polymorphonuclear leukocyte count (> 3500 cells/mm^3) Positive challenge: three of five criteria positive Equivocal: two of five criteria positive

From Powell G: *Comp Ther* 12:28-37, 1986; Sicherer SH, Eigenmann PA, Sampson HA: *J Pediatr* 133:214-219, 1998.

rechallenge. Because the symptoms are not as dramatic as enterocolitis syndrome, observation during dietary ingestion and exclusion of the causal protein must be undertaken to verify the diagnosis. Unlike dietary protein enteropathy, celiac disease can be evaluated in part through specific *in vitro* tests. Tests for IgA antiendomysial antibody (using tissue transglutaminase) are sensitive (85% to 98%) and specific (94% to 100%), with excellent positive (91% to 100%) and negative (80% to 98%) predictive values.[46] If celiac disease is suspected based on a suspicious cadre of findings (family history, steatorrhea, anemia, failure to thrive), serologic tests for IgA endomysial antibody and small bowel biopsy should be undertaken.[46] If there is enteropathy but negative serology, alternative diagnoses (see Tables 48-1 and 48-2) should be reconsidered. If the tests are positive and histology normal, the biopsy should be repeated; repeated biopsies are no longer routinely performed if the serology is positive. However, some recommend repeated biopsy after several months on a gluten-free diet to confirm resolution and response.[46,47] If the diagnosis is not strongly suspected, the *in vitro* tests can be undertaken, and if negative the diagnosis is generally excluded, but a positive test would warrant confirmation with a biopsy. A gluten-free diet is necessary to treat celiac disease and must be maintained indefinitely. However, enteropathy induced by milk generally resolves in 1 to 2 years, at which time rechallenge is warranted (Box 48-1).

BOX 48-1

KEY CONCEPTS

Evaluation and Management of Dietary Protein–Induced, Cell-Mediated Disorders

- The differential diagnosis of cell-mediated (non–IgE-mediated) gastrointestinal food allergic disorders includes other types of food hypersensitivity (IgE-mediated, eosinophilic gastroenteropathy), nonimmune reactions to foods, and disorders with similar manifestations (infection, anatomic disorders, metabolic disease).
- Diagnosis requires a history, physical examination, exclusion of alternative diagnoses, and selected diagnostic procedures including dietary elimination and oral challenge, biopsy, and selected laboratory evaluations.
- Proctocolitis occurs in infants and consists of mucousy, bloody stools. It is usually attributed to cow's milk protein passed in maternal breast milk and usually resolves by age 1 year.
- Enteropathy occurs in infancy and has symptoms related to protein malabsorption. It is most commonly caused by cow's milk protein and generally resolves by age 1 to 3 years.
- Enterocolitis occurs in infancy and has symptoms that include prominent vomiting, diarrhea, and growth failure with possible progression to a sepsis-like clinical picture. It is usually attributed to cow's milk and/or soy protein and usually resolves by age 2 to 3 years.
- Celiac disease often presents at weaning due to an immunologic response to gluten. The disease may present at any age. Classic symptoms include vomiting, anemia, poor growth, and steatorrhea. The diagnosis is assisted through serology for IgA antiendomysial antibodies and is a lifelong disorder requiring elimination of gluten.

TREATMENT

There are no curative therapies for dietary protein–induced proctocolitis, enteropathy, enterocolitis, or celiac disease; treatment is based solely on dietary elimination. Only patients with dietary protein enterocolitis or some individuals with celiac disease who experience "celiac crisis" experience severe reactions, so these patients must also be instructed on how to proceed in the event of an accidental exposure. Such patients should report to an emergency department in the event that fluid resuscitation is needed.

Although symptoms may respond to oral steroids, the cornerstone of therapy for these disorders is dietary elimination. Education concerning dietary management is reviewed elsewhere (Chapter 52). It must be emphasized that education about the details of avoidance is crucial so that dietary elimination trials and therapeutic interventions are accurately undertaken. Often, recurrence of symptoms is caused by poor adherence, possibly from an underappreciation for the difficulty that strict avoidance poses. Issues of cross-contamination, label reading, restaurant dining, and even the use of medications that may contain causal food proteins make avoidance of major dietary proteins of milk, soy, and gluten very difficult. With celiac disease, oat appears not to be toxic,[67-69] but contamination of oat flour with gluten remains a problem. Support groups and the advice of a knowledgeable dietitian are crucial adjuncts for patients undertaking these nutritionally and socially limiting diets.

Even without performing adjunctive laboratory tests or challenges to confirm a specific disorder, switching from among milk, soy, and casein-hydrolysate formulas is commonly undertaken by pediatricians and families as a test of intolerance or allergy. There are no specific guidelines concerning these formula changes. It is helpful to know that only a small proportion of infants with IgE-mediated cow's milk allergy (14%) will react to soy.[70] In contrast, those with non–IgE-mediated cow's milk allergy are frequently (> 50%) reactive to soy protein (see review[71]). For these infants, a switch to extensively hydrolyzed cow's milk–based formula is the treatment of choice.[72] For the few infants with symptoms that persist while taking a casein hydrolysate, amino acid–based formula may be required.[10,72,73] Breast-feeding is usually preferred over commercial formula as the source for infant nutrition and is also cost-effective,[74] but maternally ingested protein can elicit allergic symptoms in the breast-fed infant.[75] Therefore, maternal dietary manipulation (e.g., avoidance of milk protein) can be undertaken for treatment in breast-fed infants, but with infants who have multiple food allergies it may be difficult to do, and substitution with infant formulas may be needed in some cases.[76]

Except for celiac disease, resolution of the allergy is expected, so a review of the diet, any accidental exposures, and tests as indicated are undertaken on a yearly basis with the expectation that proctocolitis will resolve in 1 year and protein-induced enteropathy and enterocolitis would resolve in general in 1 to 3 years. Unfortunately, some patients maintain sensitivity with the latter two disorders later into childhood. It has been hypothesized that some adults with isolated gastrointestinal responses to foods (usually seafood) may also represent patients with a stable form of mild enterocolitis.

CONCLUSION

Dietary protein–induced proctocolitis, enterocolitis, and enteropathy (including celiac disease) represent well-characterized immunologic responses to dietary proteins. Although distinct in their clinical presentation, they represent cell-mediated hypersensitivity disorders that are not based on IgE antibody–mediated mechanisms. The symptoms of these disorders generally present in infancy or early childhood and must be differentiated from disorders with similar symptoms and from each other. A careful clinical history, limited laboratory studies, and directed elimination and challenge can readily disclose the type of disorder and causal foods. Knowledge of the course of these disorders assists in making a plan for long-term therapy: either reintroduction of the food to determine if tolerance has occurred or prolonged dietary elimination. The immunologic mechanisms of these disorders are being elucidated, and these advances are likely to permit improved diagnostic and therapeutic strategies in the future.

REFERENCES

1. Sampson HA, Anderson JA: Summary and recommendations: classification of gastrointestinal manifestations due to immunologic reactions to foods in infants and young children, *J Pediatr Gastroenterol Nutr* 30: S87-S94, 2001.
2. Odze RD, Bines J, Leichtner AM, et al: Allergic proctocolitis in infants: a prospective clinicopathologic biopsy study, *Hum Pathol* 24:668-674, 1993.
3. Wilson NW, Self TW, Hamburger RN: Severe cow's milk induced colitis in an exclusively breast-fed neonate. Case report and clinical review of cow's milk allergy, *Clin Pediatr Phila* 29:77-80, 1990.
4. Lake AM, Whitington PF, Hamilton SR: Dietary protein-induced colitis in breast-fed infants, *J Pediatr* 101:906-910, 1982.
5. Jenkins HR, Pincott JR, Soothill JF, et al: Food allergy: the major cause of infantile colitis, *Arch Dis Child* 59:326-329, 1984.
6. Anveden HL, Finkel Y, Sandstedt B, et al: Proctocolitis in exclusively breast-fed infants, *Eur J Pediatr* 155:464-467, 1996.
7. Pittschieler K: Cow's milk protein-induced colitis in the breast-fed infant, *J Pediatr Gastroenterol Nutr* 10:548-549, 1990.
8. Machida H, Smith A, Gall D, et al: Allergic colitis in infancy: clinical and pathologic aspects, *J Pediatr Gastroenterol Nutr* 19:22-26, 1994.
9. Winter HS, Antonioli DA, Fukagawa N, et al: Allergy-related proctocolitis in infants: diagnostic usefulness of rectal biopsy, *Mod Pathol* 3:5-10, 1990.
10. Vanderhoof JA, Murray ND, Kaufman SS, et al: Intolerance to protein hydrolysate infant formulas: an underrecognized cause of gastrointestinal symptoms in infants, *J Pediatr* 131:741-744, 1997.
11. Goldman H, Proujansky R: Allergic proctitis and gastroenteritis in children. Clinical and mucosal biopsy features in 53 cases, *Am J Surg Pathol* 10:75-86, 1986.
12. Pumberger W, Pomberger G, Geissler W: Proctocolitis in breast fed infants: a contribution to differential diagnosis of haematochezia in early childhood, *Postgrad Med J* 77:252-254, 2001.
13. Kumagai H, Masuda T, Maisawa S, et al: Apoptotic epithelial cells in biopsy specimens from infants with streaked rectal bleeding, *J Pediatr Gastroenterol Nutr* 32:428-433, 2001.
14. Lake AM: Food-induced eosinophilic proctocolitis, *J Pediatr Gastroenterol Nutr* 30:S58-S60, 2000.
15. Kuitunen P, Visakorpi J, Savilahti E, et al: Malabsorption syndrome with cow's milk intolerance: clinical findings and course in 54 cases, *Arch Dis Child* 50:351-356, 1975.
16. Iyngkaran N, Yadav M, Boey C, et al: Severity and extent of upper small bowel mucosal damage in cow's milk protein-sensitive enteropathy, *J Pediatr Gastroenterol Nutr* 8:667-674, 1988.
17. Walker-Smith JA: Cow milk-sensitive enteropathy: predisposing factors and treatment, *J Pediatr* 121:S111-S115, 1992.
18. Iyngkaran N, Robinson MJ, Prathap K, et al: Cows' milk protein-sensitive enteropathy. Combined clinical and histological criteria for diagnosis, *Arch Dis Child* 53:20-26, 1978.
19. Yssing M, Jensen H, Jarnum S: Dietary treatment of protein-losing enteropathy, *Acta Paediatr Scand* 56:173-181, 1967.
20. Verkasalo M, Kuitunen P, Savilahti E, et al: Changing pattern of cow's milk intolerance. An analysis of the occurrence and clinical course in the 60s and mid-70s, *Acta Paediatr Scand* 70:289-295, 1981.
21. Vitoria JC, Sojo A, Rodriguez-Soriano J: Changing pattern of cow's milk protein intolerance, *Acta Paediatr Scand* 79:566-567, 1990.
22. Walker-Smith JA: Cow's milk intolerance as a cause of postenteritis diarrhoea, *J Pediatr Gastroenterol Nutr* 1:163-173, 1982.
23. Kleinman RE: Milk protein enteropathy after acute infectious gastroenteritis: experimental and clinical observations, *J Pediatr* 118:S111-S115, 1991.
24. Hauer AC, Breese EJ, Walker-Smith JA, et al: The frequency of cells secreting interferon-gamma and interleukin-4, -5, and -10 in the blood and duodenal mucosa of children with cow's milk hypersensitivity, *Pediatr Res* 42:629-638, 1997.
25. Kokkonen J, Haapalahti M, Laurila K, et al: Cow's milk protein-sensitive enteropathy at school age, *J Pediatr* 139:797-803, 2001.
26. Chung HL, Hwang JB, Kwon YD, et al: Deposition of eosinophil-granule major basic protein and expression of intercellular adhesion molecule-1 and vascular cell adhesion molecule-1 in the mucosa of the small intestine in infants with cow's milk-sensitive enteropathy, *J Allergy Clin Immunol* 103:1195-1201, 1999.
27. Powell GK: Milk- and soy-induced enterocolitis of infancy, *J Pediatr* 93:553-560, 1978.
28. Powell GK: Enterocolitis in low-birth-weight infants associated with milk and soy protein intolerance, *J Pediatr* 88:840-844, 1976.
29. Powell G: Food protein-induced enterocolitis of infancy: differential diagnosis and management, *Comp Ther* 12:28-37, 1986.
30. Hill DJ, Firer MA, Shelton MJ, et al: Manifestations of milk allergy in infancy: clinical and immunological findings, *J Pediatr* 109:270-276, 1986.
31. Fontaine J, Navarro J: Small intestinal biopsy in cow's milk protein allergy in infancy, *Arch Dis Child* 50:357-362, 1975.
32. Hill DJ, Firer MA, Ball G, et al: Natural history of cows' milk allergy in children: immunological outcome over 2 years, *Clin Exp Allergy* 23:124-131, 1993.
33. Perkkio M, Savilahti E, Kuitunen P: Morphometric and immunohistochemical study of jejunal biopsies from children with intestinal soy allergy, *Eur J Pediatr* 137:63-69, 1981.
34. Heyman M, Darmon N, Dupont C, et al: Mononuclear cells from infants allergic to cow's milk secrete tumor necrosis factor alpha, altering intestinal function, *Gastroenterology* 106:1514-1523, 1994.
35. Benlounes N, Dupont C, Candalh C, et al: The threshold for immune cell reactivity to milk antigens decreases in cow's milk allergy with intestinal symptoms, *J Allergy Clin Immunol* 98:781-789, 1996.
36. Burks AW, Casteel HB, Fiedorek SC, et al: Prospective oral food challenge study of two soybean protein isolates in patients with possible milk or soy protein enterocolitis, *Pediatr Allergy Immunol* 5:40-45, 1994.
37. Gryboski J: Gastrointestinal milk allergy in infancy, *Pediatrics* 40:354-362, 1967.
38. Lake AM: Food protein-induced colitis and gastroenteropathy in infants and children. In Metcalfe DD, Sampson HA, Simon RA, eds: *Food allergy: adverse reactions to foods and food additives*, Boston, 1997, Blackwell Scientific Publications.
39. Halpin TC, Byrne WJ, Ament ME: Colitis, persistent diarrhea, and soy protein intolerance, *J Pediatr* 91:404-407, 1977.
40. Forget PP, Arenda JW: Cow's milk protein allergy and gastroesophageal reflux, *Eur J Pediatr* 144:298-300, 1985.
41. Coello-Ranurez P, Larrosa-Haro A: Gastrointestinal occult hemorrhage and gastroduodenitis in cow's milk protein intolerance, *J Pediatr Gastroenterol Nutr* 3:215-218, 1984.
42. Benlounes N, Candalh C, Matarazzo P, et al: The time-course of milk antigen-induced TNF-alpha secretion differs according to the clinical symptoms in children with cow's milk allergy, *J Allergy Clin Immunol* 104:863-869, 1999.
43. Majamaa H, Miettinen A, Laine S, et al: Intestinal inflammation in children with atopic eczema: faecal eosinophil cationic protein and tumour necrosis factor-alpha as non-invasive indicators of food allergy, *Clin Exp Allergy* 26:181-187, 1996.
44. Planchon S, Martins C, Guerrant R, et al: Regulation of intestinal epithelial barrier function by TGF-beta 1, *J Immunol* 153:5730-5739, 1994.
45. Chung HL, Hwang JB, Park JJ, et al: Expression of transforming growth factor beta1, transforming growth factor type I and II receptors, and TNF-alpha in the mucosa of the small intestine in infants with food pro-

tein-induced enterocolitis syndrome, *J Allergy Clin Immunol* 109: 150-154, 2002.

46. Farrell RJ, Kelly CP: Celiac sprue, *N Engl J Med* 346:180-188, 2002.
47. Ciclitira PJ, King AL, Fraser JS: AGA technical review on celiac sprue. American Gastroenterological Association, *Gastroenterology* 120:1526-1540, 2001.
48. Holmes G, Prior P, Lane M, et al: Malignancy in coeliac disease: effect of a gluten-free diet, *Gut* 30:333-338, 1989.
49. Hin H, Bird G, Fisher P, et al: Coeliac disease in primary care: case finding study, *Br Med J* 318:164-167, 1999.
50. Egan CA, Smith EP, Taylor TB, et al: Linear IgA bullous dermatosis responsive to a gluten-free diet, *Am J Gastroenterol* 96:1927-1929, 2001.
51. Egan CA, O'Loughlin S, Gormally S, et al: Dermatitis herpetiformis: a review of fifty-four patients, *Ir J Med Sci* 166:241-244, 1997.
52. Molberg O, McAdam S, Lundin KE,, et al: T cells from celiac disease lesions recognize gliadin epitopes deamidated *in situ* by endogenous tissue transglutaminase, *Eur J Immunol* 31:1317-1323, 2001.
53. Sollid LM, Markussen G, Ek J, et al: Evidence for a primary association of celiac disease to a particular HLA-DQ alpha/beta heterodimer, *J Exp Med* 169:345-350, 1989.
54. Sakaguchi M, Nakayama T, Inouye S: Food allergy to gelatin in children with systemic immediate-type reactions, including anaphylaxis, to vaccines, *J Allergy Clin Immunol* 98:1058-1061, 1996.
55. Anderson RP, Degano P, Godkin AJ, et al: *In vivo* antigen challenge in celiac disease identifies a single transglutaminase-modified peptide as the dominant A-gliadin T-cell epitope, *Nat Med* 6:337-342, 2000.
56. Lundin KE, Scott H, Hansen T, et al: Gliadin-specific, HLA-DQalpha 1*0501,beta 1*0201. restricted T cells isolated from the small intestinal mucosa of celiac disease patients, *J Exp Med* 178:187-196, 1993.
57. Klemola T, Tarkkanen J, Ormala T, et al: Peripheral gamma/delta cell receptor-bearing lymphocytes are increased in children with celiac disease, *J Pediatr Gastroenterol Nutr* 18:435-439, 1994.
58. Terr AI, Salvaggio JE: Controversial concepts in alergy and clinical imunology. In Bierman CW, Pearlman DS, Shapiro GG, et al, eds: *Allergy, asthma, and immunology from infancy to adulthood,* Philadelphia, 1996, WB Saunders.
59. Wyllie R: Cow's milk protein allergy and hypoallergenic formulas [editorial], *Clin Pediatr Phila* 35:497-500, 1996.
60. Murray K, Christie D: Dietary protein intolerance in infants with transient methemoglobinemia and diarrhea, *J Pediatr* 122:90-92, 1993.

61. Sicherer SH, Eigenmann PA, Sampson HA: Clinical features of food protein-induced enterocolitis syndrome, *J Pediatr* 133:214-219, 1998.
62. Busse P, Sampson HA, Sicherer SH: Non-reolution of infantile food protein-induced enterocolitis syndrome (FPIES) (abstract), *J Allergy Clin Immunol* 105:S129, 2000.
63. Nowak-Wegrzyn AH, Sampson HA, Wood RA, et al: Food protein-induced enterocolitis syndrome caused by oat (abstract), *J Allergy Clin Immunol* 107:S195, 2001.
64. Vandenplas Y, Edelman R, Sacre L: Chicken-induced anaphylactoid reaction and colitis, *J Pediatr Gastroenterol Nutr* 19:240-241, 1994.
65. Vitoria JC, Camarero C, Sojo A, et al: Enteropathy related to fish, rice and chicken, *Arch Dis Child* 57:44-48, 1982.
66. Kelso JM, Sampson HA: Food protein-induced enterocolitis to casein hydrolysate formulas, *J Allergy Clin Immunol* 92:909-910, 1993.
67. Janatuinen EK, Pikkarainen PH, Kemppainen TA, et al: A comparison of diets with and without oats in adults with celiac disease, *N Engl J Med* 333:1033-1037, 1995.
68. Hardman CM, Garioch JJ, Leonard JN, et al: Absence of toxicity of oats in patients with dermatitis herpetiformis, *N Engl J Med* 337:1884-1887, 1997.
69. Hoffenberg EJ, Haas J, Drescher A, et al: A trial of oats in children with newly diagnosed celiac disease, *J Pediatr* 137:361-366, 2000.
70. Zeiger RS, Sampson HA, Bock SA, et al: Soy allergy in infants and children with IgE-associated cow's milk allergy, *J Pediatr* 134:614-622, 1999.
71. Zoppi G, Guandalini S: The story of soy formula feeding in infants: a road paved with good intentions, *J Pediatr Gastroenterol Nutr* 28:541-543, 1999.
72. Isolauri E, Sutas Y, Makinen KS, et al: Efficacy and safety of hydrolyzed cow milk and amino acid-derived formulas in infants with cow milk allergy, *J Pediatr* 127:550-557, 1995.
73. de Boijjieu D, Matarazzo P, Dupont C: Allergy to extensively hydrolyzed cow milk proteins in infants: Identification and treatment with an amino acid-based formula, *J Pediatr* 131:744-747, 1997.
74. Ball TM, Wright AL: Health care costs of formula-feeding in the first year of life, *Pediatrics* 103:870-876, 1999.
75. Jarvinen KM, Makinen-Kiljunen S, Suomalainen H: Cow's milk challenge through human milk evokes immune responses in infants with cow's milk allergy, *J Pediatr* 135:506-512, 1999.
76. Isolauri E, Tahvanainen A, Peltola T, et al: Breast-feeding of allergic infants, *J Pediatr* 134:27-32, 1999.

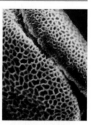

CHAPTER 49

Eosinophilic Esophagitis, Gastroenteritis, and Proctocolitis

CHRIS A. LIACOURAS ■ JONATHAN E. MARKOWITZ

The eosinophilic gastroenteropathies are an interesting, yet somewhat poorly defined, set of disorders that by definition include the infiltration of at least one layer of the gastrointestinal (GI) tract with eosinophils. First reported more than 50 years ago, the clinical spectrum of these disorders was defined solely by various case reports. As these reports became more frequent, various aspects of the disease became better described and stratified. Additional insight into the role of the eosinophil in health and disease has allowed further description of these disorders with respect to the underlying defect that drives the inflammatory response in those afflicted. Perhaps most important to the definition of these disorders has been the understanding of the heterogeneity of the sites affected within the GI tract.

Much as another inflammatory disorder of the GI tract, inflammatory bowel disease (IBD), has been stratified into Crohn's disease and ulcerative colitis based on clinical features including sites of the GI tract affected, the eosinophilic gastroenteropathies can be classified in a similar manner. Within the broad definition of these disorders lie at least three clinical entities that are defined in large part by the presence of abnormal numbers of eosinophils in various GI sites: eosinophilic proctocolitis (EoP), eosinophilic gastroenteritis (EoG), and eosinophilic esophagitis (EoE). In this chapter, we attempt to define these disorders, highlighting their similarities as well as their differences.

EOSINOPHILIC PROCTOCOLITIS

EoP, also known as allergic proctocolitis or milk-protein proctocolitis, has been recognized as one of the most common causes of rectal bleeding in infants.[1,2] This disorder is characterized by the onset of rectal bleeding, generally in children younger than 2 months of age.

Epidemiology/Etiology

The GI tract plays a major role in the development of oral tolerance to foods. Through the process of endocytosis by the enterocyte, food antigens are generally degraded into nonantigenic proteins.[3,4] Although the GI tract serves as an efficient barrier to ingested food antigens, this barrier may not be mature for the first few months of life.[5] As a result, ingested antigens may have an increased propensity for being presented intact to the immune system. These intact antigens have the potential for stimulating the immune system and driving an inappropriate response directed at the GI tract. Because the major component of the young infant's diet is milk or formula, it stands to reason that the inciting antigens in EoP are derived from the proteins found in them.

Commercially available infant formulas most commonly utilize cow's milk as the protein source. There are at least 25 known immunogenic proteins within cow's milk, with beta-lactoglobulin and casein serving as the most antigenic.[6] It is thought that up to 7.5% of the population in developed countries exhibit cow's milk allergy, although there is wide variation in the reported data.[7-9] Soy protein allergy is thought to be less common than cow's milk allergy, with a reported prevalence of approximately 0.5%.[6] However, soy protein intolerance becomes more prominent in individuals who have developed milk protein allergy, with prevalence from 15% to 50% or more in milk protein–sensitized individuals.[10] For this reason, substitution of a soy protein–based formula for a milk protein–based formula in patients with suspected milk protein proctocolitis is often unsuccessful.

Maternal breast milk represents a different challenge to the immune system. Up to 50% of the cases of EoP occur in breast-fed infants, but, rather than developing an allergy to human milk protein, it is thought that the infants are manifesting allergy to antigens ingested by the mother and transferred via the breast milk. The transfer of maternal dietary protein via breast milk was first demonstrated in 1921.[11] Recently, the presence of cow's milk antigens in breast milk has been established.[12-14]

When a problem with antigen handling occurs, whether secondary to increased absorption through an immature GI tract or though a damaged epithelium secondary to gastroenteritis, sensitization of the immune system results. Once sensitized, the inflammatory response is perpetuated with continued exposure to the inciting antigen. This may explain the reported relationship between early exposures to cow's milk protein or viral gastroenteritis and the development of allergy.[15-17]

Clinical Features

Diarrhea, rectal bleeding, and increased mucus production are the typical symptoms seen in patients who present with EoP.[2,18] In a well-appearing infant, rectal bleeding often begins gradually, initially appearing as small flecks of blood. Usually, increased stool frequency occurs accompanied by water loss or mucus streaks. The development of irritability or straining with stools is also common and can falsely lead to the initial diagnosis of anal fissuring. Atopic symptoms, such as eczema and reactive airway disease, may be associated. Continued exposure to the inciting antigen causes increased bleeding and may, on rare occasions, cause anemia or poor weight gain. Despite the progression of symptoms, the infants are generally well appearing and rarely appear ill. Other manifestations of GI tract inflammation, such as vomiting, abdominal distention, or weight loss, almost never occur.

Differential Diagnosis

EoP is primarily a clinical diagnosis, although several laboratory parameters and diagnostic procedures may be useful. Initial assessment should be directed at the overall health of the child. A toxic-appearing infant is not consistent with the diagnosis of EoP and should prompt evaluation for other causes of GI bleeding. A complete blood count is useful because the majority of infants with EoP have a normal or, at worst, borderline low hemoglobin count. An elevated serum eosinophil count may be present. Stool studies for bacterial pathogens such as *Salmonella* and *Shigella* should be performed in the setting of rectal bleeding. An assay for *Clostridium difficile* toxins A and B should also be considered, although infants may be asymptomatically colonized with this organism.[19,20] A stool specimen may be analyzed for the presence of white blood cells and specifically for eosinophils. However, the sensitivity of these tests is not well documented, and the absence of a positive finding on these tests does not exclude the diagnosis.[21]

Although not always necessary, flexible sigmoidoscopy may be useful to demonstrate the presence of colitis. Visually, one may find erythema, friability, or frank ulceration of the colonic mucosa. Alternatively, the mucosa may appear normal or show evidence of lymphoid hyperplasia.[22,23] Histologic findings typically include increased eosinophils within the lamina propria, with generally preserved crypt architecture. Findings may be patchy, so care should be taken to examine many levels of each biopsy specimen if necessary.[24,25]

Treatment

In a well-appearing patient with a history consistent with EoP, it is acceptable to make an empiric change in the protein source of the formula. Because of the propensity of milk-sensitized infants to develop sensitivity to other whole proteins, such as soy, a protein-hydrolysate formula is often the best choice.[16] Resolution of symptoms begins almost immediately after the elimination of the problematic food. Although symptoms may linger for several days to weeks, continued improvement is the rule. If symptoms do not quickly improve or persist beyond 4 to 6 weeks, other antigens should be considered, as well as other potential causes of rectal bleeding. In breastfed infants, dietary restriction of milk and soy-containing products for the mother may result in improve-ment; however, care should be taken to ensure that the mother maintains adequate protein and calcium intake from other sources.

EOSINOPHILIC GASTROENTERITIS

EoG is a general term that describes a constellation of symptoms attributable to the GI tract, in combination with pathologic infiltration by eosinophils. Shaped in large part by case reports and series over the years, there are no strict diagnostic criteria for this disorder. Rather, a combination of GI complaints with supportive histologic findings is sufficient to make the diagnosis. EoG was originally described by Kaijser in 1937.[26] It is a disorder characterized by tissue eosinophilia that can affect different layers of the bowel wall, anywhere from the mouth to anus. The gastric antrum and small bowel are frequently affected. In 1970 Klein et al[27] classified EoG into three categories: mucosal, muscular, and serosal forms.

Epidemiology/Etiology

EoG affects patients of all ages, with a slight male predominance. Most commonly, eosinophils infiltrate only the mucosa, leading to symptoms associated with malabsorption, such as growth failure, weight loss, diarrhea, and hypoalbuminemia. Mucosal EoG may affect any portion of the GI tract. A review of the biopsy findings in 38 children with EoG revealed that all patients examined had mucosal eosinophilia of the gastric antrum.[2] Of the patients studied, 79% also demonstrated eosinophilia of the proximal small intestine, with 60% having esophageal involvement and 52% having involvement of the gastric corpus. Those with colonic involvement tended to be under 6 months of age and were ultimately classified as having EoP.

The exact cause of EoG remains unknown. In the past, both IgE- and non–IgE-mediated sensitivities were thought to be responsible.[28] The association between IgE-mediated inflammatory response (typical allergy) and EoG is supported by the increased likelihood of other allergic disorders such as atopic disease, food allergies, and seasonal allergies.[29,30] Specific foods have been implicated in the cause of EoG.[31,32] In contrast, the role of non–IgE-mediated immune dysfunction, in particular the interplay between lymphocyte-produced cytokines and eosinophils, has also received attention.

Recently, interleukin (IL)-5, a chemoattractant responsible for tissue eosinophilia, has been implicated.[33] Desreumaux et al[34] found that among patients with EoG, the levels of IL-3, IL-5, and granulocyte-macrophage colony-stimulating factor were significantly increased compared with control patients. Once recruited to the tissue, eosinophils may further recruit similar cells through their own production of IL-3 and IL-5, as well as production of leukotrienes.[35] Finally, new evidence by Beyer et al[36] suggests that the release of T helper cell type 2 cytokines from patients with milk allergy enteritis occurs on stimulation of milk-sensitive T cells. This mixed type of immune dysregulation in EoG has implications for the way this disorder is diagnosed, as well as the way it is treated.

Clinical Features

The most common symptoms of EoG include colicky abdominal pain, bloating, diarrhea, weight loss, dysphagia, and vomiting.[37,38] In addition, up to 50% have a past or family history of atopy.[2] Other features of severe disease include GI bleeding, iron deficiency anemia, protein-losing enteropathy (hypoalbuminemia), and growth failure.[37] Approximately 75% of affected patients have an elevated blood eosinophilia.[39] Males are more commonly affected than females. Rarely, ascites occurs.[39,40]

Differential Diagnosis

EoG should be considered in any patient with a history of chronic symptoms, including vomiting, abdominal pain, diarrhea, anemia, hypoalbuminemia, or poor weight gain in combination with the presence of eosinophils in the GI tract. As identified in Table 49-1, other causes of eosinophilic infiltration of the GI tract include the other disorders of the eosinophilic gastroenteropathy spectrum (EoP, EoE), as well as parasitic infection, IBD, neoplasm, chronic granulomatous disease, collagen vascular disease, and the hypereosinophilic syndrome.[41-45]

In an infant, EoG may present in a manner similar to hypertrophic pyloric stenosis, with progressive vomiting, dehydration, electrolyte abnormalities, and thickening of the gastric outlet.[46,47] When an infant presents with this constellation of symptoms in addition to atopic symptoms such as eczema and reactive airway disease, an elevated eosinophil count, and a strong family history of atopic disease, EoG should be considered in the diagnosis before surgical intervention if possible.

Uncommon presentations of EoG include acute abdomen[48] or colonic obstruction.[49] There also have been reports of serosal infiltration with eosinophils, with associated complaints of abdominal distention, eosinophilic ascites, and bowel perforation.[40,50-54]

Evaluation

When EoG is suspected, there are a number of tests that may aid in the diagnosis, but no single test is pathognomonic. Before EoG can be truly entertained as a diagnosis, the presence of eosinophils in the GI tract must be documented. This is most readily done with biopsies of either the upper GI tract through esophagogastroduodenoscopy or of the lower GI tract through flexible sigmoidoscopy or colonoscopy. A history of atopy is supportive of the diagnosis but is not a necessary feature. Blood evaluation may demonstrate an elevated peripheral eosinophil count or IgE level in approximately 70% of affected individuals.[55] Measures of absorptive activity such as the *d*-xylose absorption test and lactose hydrogen breath testing may reveal evidence of malabsorption, reflecting small intestine damage. Radiographic contrast studies may demonstrate mucosal irregularities or edema, wall thickening, ulceration, or luminal narrowing. A lacy mucosal pattern of the gastric antrum known as *areae gastricae* is a unique finding that may be present in patients with EoG.[56]

Evaluation of other causes of eosinophilia should be undertaken, including stool analysis for ova and parasites. Signs of intestinal obstruction warrant abdominal imaging. The value of radioallergosorbent test (RAST) studies, as well as skin testing for environmental antigens, is limited. Skin testing using both traditional prick tests and patch tests may increase the sensitivity for identifying foods responsible for EoG by evaluating both IgE-mediated and T cell–mediated sensitivities.[57]

TABLE 49-1 Causes of Gastrointestinal Eosinophilia

Esophagus
Eosinophilic esophagitis
Gastroesophageal reflux
Food allergy

Stomach
Eosinophilic gastroenteritis
Menetrier's disease
Chronic granulomatous disease
Vasculitis
Oral gold therapy
Hyper-IgE syndrome
Idiopathic hypereosinophilic syndrome

Small intestine
Eosinophilic gastroenteritis
Inflammatory bowel disease (Crohn's disease)
Infection (parasites)
Food allergy
Vasculitis
Oral gold therapy
Hyper-IgE syndrome
Idiopathic hypereosinophilic syndrome

Colon
Food allergy
Eosinophilic gastroenteritis
Inflammatory bowel disease (ulcerative colitis)
Infection (parasites)
Vasculitis

Treatment

There is as much ambiguity in the treatment of EoG as there is in its diagnosis. This is in large part because the entity of EoG was defined mainly by case series, each of which used their own modes of treatment. Because EoG is a difficult disease to diagnose, randomized trials for its treatment are uncommon, leading to considerable debate as to which treatment is best.

Food allergy is considered one of the underlying causes of EoG, and elimination of pathogenic foods, as identified by any form of allergy testing or by random removal of the most likely antigens, should be a first line treatment. Unfortunately, this approach results in improvement in only a limited number of patients. In severe cases or when other treatment options have failed, the administration of a strict diet, using an elemental formula, has been shown to be successful.[30,58] In these cases, formulas such as Neocate 1+ or Elecare provided as the sole source of nutrition have been reported to be effective in the resolution of clinical symptoms and tissue eosinophilia.

When the use of a restricted diet fails, corticosteroids are often used due to their high likelihood of success in attaining remission.[38] However, when weaned, the duration of remission is variable and can be short lived, leading to the need for repeated courses or continuous low doses of steroids. In addition, the chronic use of corticosteroids carries an increased likelihood of undesirable side effects, including cosmetic problems (cushingoid facies, hirsutism, acne), decreased bone density, impaired growth, and personality changes. A response to these side effects has been to look for substitutes that may act as steroid-sparing agents while still allowing for control of symptoms.

Orally administered cromolyn sodium has been used with some success,[38,59-61] and recent reports have detailed the efficacy of other oral antiinflammatory medications. Montelukast, a selective leukotriene receptor antagonist used to treat asthma, has been reported to successfully treat two patients with EoG.[62,63] Treatment of EoG with inhibition of leukotriene D_4, a potent chemotactic factor for eosinophils, relies on the theory that the inflammatory response in EoG is perpetuated by the presence of the eosinophils already present in the mucosa. By interrupting the chemotactic cascade, it is thought that the inflammatory cycle can be broken. Suplatast tosilate, another suppressor of cytokine production, has also been reported as a treatment for EoG.[64]

Given the varied possibilities for treatment of EoG, the combination of therapies incorporating the best chance of success with the smallest likelihood of side effects should be used. When particular food antigens that may be causing disease can be identified, elimination of those antigens should be first-line therapy. When testing fails to identify potentially pathogenic foods, a systematic elimination of the most commonly involved foods[65] can be made. If this approach fails, total elimination diet with an amino acid–based formula should be considered. Trials of nonsteroidal antiinflammatory drugs such as sodium cromolyn, montelukast, and suplatast are a reasonable option, although some might prefer to wait for more definitive studies.

When other treatments fail, corticosteroids remain a reliable treatment for EoG, with attempts at limiting the total dose or the number of treatment courses where possible. Because of the diffuse and inconsistent nature of symptoms in this disease, serial endoscopy with biopsy is a useful and important modality for monitoring disease progression.

EOSINOPHILIC ESOPHAGITIS

Recently, EoE has come to the forefront in individuals previously suspected as having severe, chronic gastroesophageal reflux disease (GERD). EoE is a disease of children and adults characterized by an isolated, severe eosinophilic infiltration of the esophagus manifested by gastroesophageal reflux–like symptoms, such as regurgitation, epigastric and chest pain, vomiting, heartburn, feeding difficulties, and dysphagia unresponsive to acid suppression therapy.

History

In 1977 Dobbins et al[66] reported one of the first cases of dysphagia associated with EoE. They described a case of a 51-year-old man with asthma and environmental allergies who presented with dysphagia and chest pain. An upper endoscopy demonstrated a severe EoE combined with increased eosinophils in the duodenum. They suggested that the esophageal eosinophilia was part of the larger disease process of EoG. In 1983 Matzinger and Daneman[67] reported dysphagia associated with a significant esophageal eosinophilia in an adolescent. Their patient not only had dysphagia but also displayed food allergies, a peripheral serum eosinophilia, and histologic evidence of eosinophils in his esophagus and stomach. Shortly thereafter, Lee[68] reported on a series of 11 patients

with documented EoE consisting of greater than 10 eosinophils per ×40 high-power microscopic field (HPF). These patients were initially studied because all 11 presented with dysphagia, symptoms of gastroesophageal reflux, vomiting, and strictures. Although 1 patient improved on antireflux medication, another became asymptomatic after being treated with systemic steroids. No follow-up was conducted for the remaining 9 patients. An allergic disorder was entertained as the cause in many of these patients.

In 1993 Attwood et al[69] were the first to compare patients with EoE with those with GERD. They studied 12 patients who presented with dysphagia and had more than 20 eosinophils per ×40 HPF found by biopsy. These patients had an average of 56 eosinophils per HPF, and their symptoms were unresponsive to acid blockade. Eleven had normal pH probe monitoring; 7 had evidence of systemic allergy including rhinitis, asthma, and eczema; and only 1 had increased antral eosinophils. This group was compared with a group of 90 patients with GERD documented by an abnormal pH probe. All of the patients diagnosed with reflux were responsive to acid blockade, and only 43 had evidence of an esophageal eosinophilia, with a mean number of 3.3 eosinophils per HPF. The patients with severe esophageal eosinophilia did not respond to acid blockade. Vitellas et al[70] reported on a series of 13 male patients with isolated EoE. Twelve patients demonstrated dysphagia and an increased peripheral eosinophilia, whereas 10 had atopic symptoms and esophageal strictures requiring repeated dilatation. All except 1 patient responded to systemic corticosteroids, and in these patients, esophageal dilatation was no longer required.

Role of Esophageal Eosinophils

Eosinophils in the GI tract have long been associated with intestinal inflammatory disorders such as EoG, IBD, parasitic infections, and acid-related disorders. In normal, healthy volunteers, eosinophils are commonly visualized in almost all portions of the GI tract (except the esophagus), which often makes the diagnosis of a pathologic process secondary to eosinophilia difficult. In 1996 Bischoff et al[71] suggested that eosinophils released mediators (cationic proteins, leukotrienes, prostaglandins, platelet-activating factor) that promote tissue inflammation. They also believed that these cells exert cytotoxic effects by producing oxygen free radicals and peroxidase. Mast cells were thought to be involved in tissue repair.

In 1982 Winter et al[72] suggested that esophageal intraepithelial eosinophils may be related to tissue injury secondary to gastroesophageal reflux. They postulated that these eosinophils could be used as a new diagnostic criterion for reflux esophagitis. The authors evaluated 46 patients, aged 3 months to 19 years, who had recurrent vomiting, epigastric pain, and other symptoms of GERD including dysphagia, abdominal pain, and regurgitation. Diagnostic testing was performed with pH probes, manometry, and upper endoscopy. These patients were compared with a group of nine asymptomatic control patients. The control group had normal pH probe results, normal esophageal manometry, and no esophageal eosinophils by biopsy. In contrast, in the study group, 18 patients demonstrated esophageal eosinophils on biopsy, with a mean of two eosinophils per HPF. The majority of these patients also had abnormal pH probes and other histologic features of reflux, including basal zone thickening and papillary lengthening. Winter concluded that the presence of intraepithelial eosinophils correlated with delayed esophageal acid clearance. This study was followed by reports from Brown et al[73] and Tummala et al,[74] who performed similar studies in adults and found comparable results. Since then, the finding of intraepithelial esophageal eosinophils has become an accepted feature of gastroesophageal reflux.

Etiology

For more than 10 years, the esophageal eosinophil was used as a pathognomonic marker for gastroesophageal reflux. However, in 1995, Kelly et al[75] established that patients with an isolated, severe esophageal eosinophilia unresponsive to measures attempting to control acid instead responded to a strict elemental diet. They suggested that the cause was specific food allergens. For the next few years, an argument existed among pediatric gastroenterologists and pathologists regarding the etiology of a severe, isolated esophageal eosinophilia.[76-78] The discussion centered on the small numbers of patients who were identified with EoE (most likely because of the belief that esophageal eosinophilia was only considered to be diagnostic of reflux disease) and the lack of controlled trials demonstrating a response of a severe esophageal eosinophilia to the removal of foods. Recently, with the improved knowledge of EoE, including several published reports, EoE is now considered an important cause of esophageal disease.[79-85]

EoE appears to be caused by an abnormal immunologic response to specific food antigens. Although several studies have documented resolution of EoE with the strict avoidance of food antigens, in 1995, Kelly et al[75] published the classic paper on EoE. Because the suspected etiology was an abnormal immunologic response to specific unidentifiable food antigens, each patient was treated with a strict elimination diet that included an amino acid–based formula (Neocate). Patients were also allowed clear liquids, corn, and apples. Seventeen patients were initially offered a dietary elimination trial, with 10 patients adhering to the protocol. The initial trial was determined by a history of anaphylaxis to specific foods and abnormal skin testing. These patients were subsequently placed on a strict diet consisting of an amino acid–based formula for a median of 17 weeks. Symptomatic improvement was seen within an average of 3 weeks after the introduction of the elemental diet (resolution in eight patients, improvement in two). In addition, all 10 patients demonstrated a significant improvement in esophageal eosinophilia. Subsequently, all patients reverted to previous symptoms on reintroduction of foods. Predietary and postdietary trial evaluations demonstrated a significant improvement in clinical symptoms and almost complete resolution in esophageal eosinophilia, from a mean of 41 eosinophils per HPF to less than 1 per HPF. Open food challenges were then conducted, with a demonstration of a return of symptoms with challenges to milk (7 patients), soy (4), wheat (2), peanuts (2), and egg (1).

Although an exact cause was not determined, Kelly[75] suggested an immunologic basis secondary to a delayed hypersensitivity or a cell-mediated hypersensitivity response as the cause for EoE. A recent report by Spergel et al[57] demonstrated that foods that cause EoE are often not based on an immediate hypersensitivity reaction. By using a combination of traditional skin testing and a newer technique of atopy "patch testing," he established that a delayed cell-mediated allergic response may be responsible for many cases of EoE. Recently, CD8 lymphocytes have been identified as the predominant T cell within the squamous epithelium of patients diagnosed with EoE.[80] Finally, although other causes of EoE have been suggested, such as aeroallergens or infectious agents, only food antigens have thus far been implicated.[28,79-81,86,87]

Clinical Presentation

EoE occurs in children and adults. The presentation of EoE in children is similar to the symptoms associated with gastroesophageal reflux (Table 49-2). Boys appear to develop EoE more frequently than do girls. The typical symptoms include nausea, vomiting, regurgitation, epigastric abdominal pain, and poor eating. Young children may demonstrate food refusal, whereas adolescents often experience dysphagia. Adults present with similar symptoms, but dysphagia occurs much more commonly and can be associated with esophageal strictures. Uncommon symptoms include growth failure,

TABLE 49-2 Comparison between Eosinophilic Esophagitis and Reflux Esophagitis

	Eosinophilic Esophagitis	Reflux Esophagitis
Symptoms	Nausea, vomiting, epigastric pain, dysphagia	Nausea, dysphagia, vomiting, epigastric pain
Endoscopic findings	Esophageal furrows, rings	Esophageal erythema, ulceration
Histologic findings	Usually > 20 eosinophils per HPF	Usually < 5 eosinophils per HPF
Esophageal strictures	Midesophageal strictures	Distal esophageal strictures
pH probe results	Normal, except for increased frequency of episodes	Usually abnormal
Peripheral eosinophils	Usually increased	Usually normal
Serum IgE level	Usually increased	Usually normal
Allergic history	Increased incidence of asthma, rhinitis, eczema	Not increased
Family history	Increased incidence of asthma, rhinitis, eczema	Not increased
Acid blockade		
Symptoms	Minimally improved	Significantly improved
Histology	No change in histology	Significantly improved
Fundoplication	Not effective	Effective in severe cases
Corticosteroids	Effective; however, disease recurs when discontinued	Unknown
Dietary therapy	Effective	Not effective

HPF, High-power field.

hematemesis, globus, and water brash. The clinical features of EoE may evolve over years. Symptoms such as abdominal pain and heartburn occur regularly; however, patients with vomiting or dysphagia may display these symptoms sporadically, complaining only once or twice a month. Although the use of acid suppression medication often improves the patient's symptoms, it does not eliminate the symptoms or change the abnormal esophageal histology. Approximately 50% of affected children also exhibit other allergic signs and symptoms, including bronchospasm, allergic rhinitis, and eczema. Frequently, there is a strong family history of food allergies or other allergic disorders.

Diagnosis

Presently, the diagnosis of EoE can be made only by esophageal biopsy. In 1999 Ruchelli et al[88] studied 102 patients who presented with symptoms of GERD and who had evidence of esophagitis documented by at least one intraepithelial eosinophil by endoscopy. Once the diagnosis of probable reflux was made, these patients were treated with H_2 blockers and prokinetic agents. If the patients' symptoms persisted after 3 months of therapy with H_2 blockers, a proton pump inhibitor was begun, and the patients were reevaluated 3 months later by endoscopy with biopsy. The treatment response was classified into three categories: clinical improvement (1.1 eosinophils per HPF), relapse of clinical symptoms (6.4 eosinophils per HPF), and failure of medical treatment (24.5 eosinophils per HPF). All except two patients had isolated esophageal involvement. He concluded that the number of esophageal eosinophils predicted whether the patient could be successfully treated with acid suppression medication or whether another cause (allergic disease) was possible.

Although an isolated, severe, esophageal eosinophilia unresponsive to acid blockade is necessary for the diagnosis of EoE, several reports have suggested that the diagnosis of EoE may be made endoscopically without biopsy. Orenstein et al[81,89] reported on series of children with probable EoE and suggested that the endoscopic appearance (Figure 49-1) revealed a granular, subtle, furrowed, ringed appearance. In addition, a recent report by Teitlebaum et al[80] suggested that in patients successfully treated for EoE, a furrowed, ringed appearance may persist despite normal biopsy results. However, a ringed esophageal appearance can also be appreciated in patients who have other causes of severe esophagitis.[90-92] Other methods for diagnosis have been attempted, including endoscopic ultrasound.[79,93] Although ultrasound demonstrated that the mucosa-to-submucosa ratio and muscularis propria thickness were greater in EoE patients than a control group, no comparison was made with patients who had esophagitis secondary to other disorders. Finally, EoE can occur in both the mid- and distal portions of the esophagus. Several previous reports in adults have demonstrated midesophageal involvement associated with stricture formation.[66,67,94] Most adults with EoE have been reported to have a significant number of eosinophils in the midesophagus; however, many of these patients did not have their distal esophagus biopsied. In contrast, Liacouras et al[95] established that even in those cases of proximal esophageal involvement, the distal esophagus was also involved. Moreover, peripheral eosinophilia and increased IgE levels have been reported in 20% to 60% of patients with EoE.[75,80,81,83]

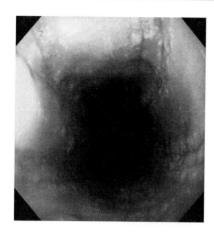

FIGURE 49-1 Endoscopic photograph of the midesophagus in a 12-year-old patient with eosinophilic esophagitis. Linear furrows and circumferential rings in the mucosa are prominent.

The definitive diagnosis of EoE is made endoscopically in patients who have reflux-like symptoms, who have normal (or borderline normal) pH probes, and who are unresponsive to acid inhibition. This fact underscores the importance of obtaining esophageal biopsy samples whenever questions arise regarding the disease process. The performance of esophageal pH monitoring is also important because significant acid reflux disease can be excluded. In EoE, pH probe findings often reveal frequent, brief reflux episodes but normal esophageal acid clearance and a normal reflux index.[83] The number of esophageal eosinophils per HPF is used to make the diagnosis. A review of recent studies suggests that the vast majority of patients with EoE present with more than 20 eosinophils per HPF.[75,79,81-83,87,88]

Evaluation

Patients with chronic symptoms of vomiting, regurgitation, epigastric abdominal pain, or dysphagia or patients with symptoms of gastroesophageal reflux unresponsive to medical therapy should be evaluated for EoE (Table 49-3). For accurate diagnosis, every evaluation should include a radiographic upper GI series to rule out anatomic abnormalities, a 24-hour pH probe, and an upper endoscopy with biopsy. In a patient with normal anatomy, the presence of an isolated, severe esophageal eosinophilia (> 20 eosinophils per HPF), obtained while the patient is receiving adequate gastric acid blockade with a proton pump inhibitor, strongly suggests the diagnosis of EoE (Figure 49-2). Acid disease is excluded with the performance of a 24-hour pH probe. The pH probe should be completed while the patient is off of all acid-suppressing medications. Although the pH probe may reveal frequent, brief reflux episodes (three episodes per hour), the probe should demonstrate normal esophageal acid clearance and a normal reflux index. Patients with severely abnormal pH probe findings should undergo further evaluation for GERD. The diagnosis of EoE is confirmed on repeat endoscopy with biopsy after treatment (Figure 49-3).

Treatment

The identification and removal of allergic dietary antigens is the mainstay of treatment for EoE. The removal of the offending

TABLE 49-3 Evaluation of Patients with Eosinophilic Esophagitis

Patients suspected of having eosinophilic esophagitis

Patients with chronic gastroesophageal reflux symptoms unresponsive to acid blockade

Patients with dysphagia or isolated esophageal strictures

Patients with past medical or family history of allergic disorders and gastrointestinal symptoms of unknown etiology

Diagnostic testing for eosinophilic esophagitis

Radiographic upper gastrointestinal series to the ligament of Treitz (anatomic causes)

Clinical history (including past medical and family history) and physical examination attempting to identify stigmata of allergic disease

Laboratory studies including complete blood count (differential); comprehensive chemistry panel; quantitative IgE level, sedimentation rate

Upper endoscopy with biopsy of esophagus (middle and distal); antrum and duodenum (with patient on proton pump inhibitor if reflux symptoms exist)

24-Hour pH probe (performed off of acid blockade) to determine if acid reflux is the cause of problem

In patients with EoE

The reflux index should be normal ($< 6.0\%$ of study)

The esophageal acid clearance should be normal (longest reflux episode < 15 minutes; < 0.3 episode/hr of episodes lasting more than 5 minutes).

While the total number of reflux episodes may be increased (normal < 2 episodes/hr), these episodes are brief and all other pH parameters are normal.

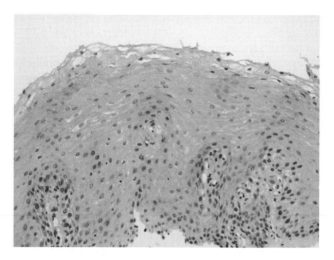

FIGURE 49-3 Histologic biopsy of squamous esophageal mucosa taken from the distal esophagus of a 10-year-old patient with eosinophilic esophagitis after treatment with a strict elemental diet. Normal stratified epithelium is visualized after treatment.

foods reverses the disease process in patients with EoE, but in many cases, the identification of these foods is extremely difficult. Often, patients with EoE cannot correlate their GI symptoms with the ingestion of a specific food. This occurs because the cause of EoE is most likely based on a delayed hypersensitivity response. Several reports have demonstrated that it takes several days for symptoms to recur on ingestion of antigens that cause EoE.[75,83] Furthermore, allergy testing using skin tests and

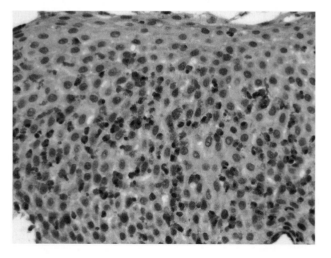

FIGURE 49-2 Histologic biopsy of squamous esophageal mucosa taken from the distal esophagus of a 10-year-old patient diagnosed with eosinophilic esophagitis before treatment. Numerous eosinophils can be appreciated as well as hyperplasia of the basal layer.

RAST studies provide limited value in the vast majority of patients with EoE.[57] Even when a particular food causing EoE has been isolated, it may take days or weeks for the symptoms to resolve. In addition, although one food may be identified, there may be several other foods (not easily identified) that could also be contributing to EoE. Upper endoscopy with biopsy is the only diagnostic test that has been shown to document resolution of the disease.

Although attempts should be made to identify and eliminate potential food allergens through a careful history and the use of allergy testing, because it may be difficult to determine the responsible allergic foods, the administration of a strict diet, using an amino acid–based formula, is often necessary. As established by Kelly et al[75] and Markowitz et al,[96] the use of an elemental diet rapidly improves both clinical symptoms and histology in patients with EoE. Because of poor palatability, the elemental formula is most often provided by continuous nasogastric feeding. The diet may be supplanted by water, one fruit (e.g., apples, grapes), and the corresponding pure fruit juice. The use of this diet not only proves the diagnosis of EoE but also heals the inflamed mucosa. Reversal of symptoms typically occurs within 10 days, with histologic improvement in 4 weeks.[83] Although the strict use of an amino acid–based formula (typically provided by nasogastric tube feeding) may be difficult for patients (and parents) to comprehend, its benefits outweigh the risks of other treatments. First, only food allergens have thus far been implicated in the etiology of EoE and removal of these allergens cures the disease. In contrast, while the use of other medications, such as corticosteroids, may improve the disease and its symptoms, on their discontinuation, if the offending antigen has not been identified and removed, the disease recurs. Once the esophagus is healed, if allergy testing has not determined the causative foods, foods are reintroduced systematically (Table 49-4). Endoscopy should be used to document an improvement in esophageal histology.

Treatment of EoE with aggressive acid blockade, including medical and surgical therapy, has not been proven to be effective. Several published reports have demonstrated that the

TABLE 49-4 Guidelines for Food Reintroduction in Patients with Eosinophilic Esophagitis or Gastroenteritis

Before food reintroduction
    Diagnosis of eosinophilic esophagitis or gastroenteritis is confirmed by biopsy.
    Food allergens are identified by skin or patch testing.
If foods identified by allergy testing:
    Remove offending foods.
        As determined by allergy testing or clinical history.
        Alternative option, if no foods identified, is to remove most likely food allergens (milk, soy, eggs, wheat, nuts).
    Repeat esophageal biopsy in 4 to 6 weeks.
    If biopsy normal, reintroduce foods (one at a time) every 5 to 7 days.
        If symptoms develop, withdraw food; otherwise add two or three additional foods.
        If no symptoms, a repeat biopsy is necessary to document continued resolution of disease.
    If biopsy abnormal, begin elemental diet (using Neocate 1+).
        Repeat endoscopic biopsy after 4 weeks to look for disease resolution.
        After resolution, reintroduce one new food every 5 to 7 days (see food chart).
        If symptoms do not develop, repeat endoscopic biopsy after reintroduction of groups of five foods.
    If positive biopsies recur, remove last introduced foods.
NOTES:
1. If food has a history of IgE-mediated reaction, initial food reintroduction should be performed as a formal food challenge in a hospital setting.
2. Positive foods, identified by biopsy, allergy testing, or history (and confirmed by biopsy), should be avoided for at least 2 years.

FOOD CHART (Begin with foods from column A and move to column D and from top to bottom)

A	B	C	D
Vegetables	Citrus fruits	Legumes	Corn
Noncitrus fruits	Tropical fruits	Grains	Peas
	Melons	Meats	Wheat
	Berries	Fish/shellfish	Beef
		Tree nuts	Peanuts
			Soy
			Eggs
			Milk

failure of H_2 blocker and proton-pump therapy in patients with EoE.[80,82,88] Although acid blockade may improve clinical symptoms by improving acid reflux that occurs secondary to the underlying inflamed esophageal mucosa, it does not reverse the esophageal histologic abnormality. Furthermore, Liacouras[97] published findings on two patients found to have an isolated eosinophilic infiltration of the esophagus who failed medical therapy and underwent Nissen fundoplication. In both cases, the patients continued to have clinical symptoms and continued evidence of an isolated esophageal eosinophilia by biopsy after fundoplication. Subsequently, each responded to oral corticosteroids with resolution of their clinical symptoms and a return to normal of their esophageal mucosa. In one patient, symptoms recurred on discontinuation of corticosteroids; however, the patient later responded to the introduction of an elemental diet. Similarly, four patients reported by Kelly et al[75] had undergone Nissen fundoplication and continued to have clinical symptoms.

Before 1997, reports suggested that systemic corticosteroids improved the symptoms of EoE in adults identified with a severe EoE.[68,70] In 1997 Liacouras et al[82] were the first to publish the use of oral corticosteroids in 20 children diagnosed with EoE. These patients were treated with oral methylprednisolone (average dosage, 1.5 mg/kg/day; maximum dosage, 48 mg/day) for 1 month. Symptoms were significantly improved in 19 of 20 patients by an average of 8 days. A repeat endoscopy with biopsy, 4 weeks after the initiation of therapy, demonstrated a significant reduction of esophageal eosinophils, from 34 to 1.5 eosinophils per HPF. However, on discontinuation of corticosteroids, 90% have had recurrence of symptoms.

In 1999 Faubion et al[84] reported that swallowing a metered dose of inhaled corticosteroids was also effective in treating the symptoms of EoE in children. Four patients diagnosed with EoE manifested by epigastric pain, dysphagia, and a severe esophageal eosinophilia unresponsive to aggressive acid blockade were given fluticasone four puffs twice a day. Patients were instructed to use inhaled corticosteroids but to immediately swallow after inhalation to deliver the medication to the esophagus. Histologic improvement was not determined. Within 2 months, all four patients responded with an improvement in symptoms. Two patients required repeat use of inhalation therapy. This therapy was recently confirmed.[80] Although this therapy can improve EoE, the side effects can include esophageal candidiasis and growth failure.[98,99] In addition, often symptoms recur in patients on discontinuation of the therapy.[80]

The mast cell–stabilizing agent cromolyn sodium has also been used to treat children with EoE.[38,100,101] In a fashion similar to its use for children with EoG, oral cromolyn has been given to patients with a severe esophageal eosinophilia in conjunction with other systemic signs and symptoms of allergic disease. However, no controlled reports have been performed, and efficacy for oral cromolyn in children with EoE has not been established. Finally, the use of montelukast has been reported to provide an improvement in symptoms in patients with eosinophilic disorders of the GI tract.[62]

CONCLUSIONS

Eosinophilic disorders of the GI tract are becoming increasingly recognized. Although EoG is rare and difficult to diagnose, EoP and EoE are much more common and easily diagnosed by endoscopic biopsy. EoP is a well-accepted entity, but the diagnosis of EoE has recently been receiving a great deal of attention. Argument still exists regarding the etiology and treatment of EoE. Further studies are needed to effectively differentiate patients with EoE from those with reflux esophagitis (Boxes 49-1 and 49-2). It appears that significant esophageal eosinophilia (> 20 per HPF) suggests a diagnosis of EoE, whereas esophageal eosinophilia (< 15 per HPF) and an improvement with acid blockade suggests GERD. The diagnosis is equivocal when an esophageal biopsy reveals 5 to 20 eosinophils per HPF, thus leading to the question: What is the best way to diagnose and treat patients with EoE?

Future research should focus on clarifying the prevalence and natural history (e.g., the potential development of strictures) and optimizing the diagnostic approach and treatment options of all GI eosinophilic disorders. Many unanswered questions remain. Why have EoG and EoE been reported in some parts of the United States and not at all in others? Can the diagnosis be made using less invasive techniques than endoscopy with biopsy? How can we better identify offending food antigens and allergens other than elemental formulas with a strict protein elimination diet? Do environmental or infectious agents play a role in the disease process? Are there medications that can cure the disease? In addition, biochemical studies need to be pursued so that we can determine a cause of these disorders. Is the eosinophil dysregulation due to an immunologic defect or an allergy? These and other research questions reinforce the limitations of our current understanding of GI eosinophilic disease.

BOX 49-1	**KEY CONCEPTS** *Eosinophilic Disorders*

- Eosinophilic disorders of the gastrointestinal (GI) tract should be considered in any child who has chronic GI symptoms including abdominal pain, vomiting, nausea, diarrhea, GI bleeding, and failure to thrive.
- These disorders are often difficult to diagnose because they mimic many other GI disorders.
- GI mucosal biopsies are mandatory for the diagnosis of these disorders. Biopsies should be obtained (colonic for eosinophilic proctocolitis and gastroenteritis; esophagus, stomach, and duodenum for eosinophilic esophagitis and gastroenteritis) even when the visual inspection of the mucosa is normal.
- Eosinophilic proctocolitis is typically a disease that occurs in the first year of life and is related to specific food allergies. It usually resolves by age 2.
- Eosinophilic esophagitis is often mistaken for gastroesophageal reflux disease. Endoscopic biopsy is critical to make the diagnosis. Foods are the causative agent.
- Eosinophilic gastroenteritis is the least understood and most difficult to treat eosinophilic disorder. The cause appears to be an alteration in immunologic function. Treatment options include elemental diets and immunosuppressive medications.

BOX 49-2	**THERAPEUTIC PRINCIPLES** Eosinophilic Disorders

CONTINUE STEPWISE PROGRESSION IF NO IMPROVEMENT IN DISEASE

Eosinophilic proctocolitis (EoP)

Step 1. Remove milk/soy from diet (and from mother's diet if breastfeeding). Use protein hydrolysate formula.

Step 2. Remove all foods from diet. Use amino acid–based formula.

After resolution of EoP (on above therapy), foods may be reintroduced at 1 year of age. Challenge should be performed in an office setting when the history of symptoms is mild and in a hospital setting if anaphylaxis is a possibility.

Eosinophilic gastroenteritis (EoG)

Step 1. Administer strict elemental diet using amino acid–based formula.

Step 2. Administer a trial of corticosteroids and cromolyn sodium.

Step 3. Consider other immunosuppressive agents (6-MP, imuran).

Eosinophilic esophagitis (EoE)

Step 1. Perform endoscopy with biopsy on aggressive acid blockade (omeprazole).

Step 2. Consult allergist; remove suspected foods; repeat endoscopy with biopsy in 4 to 6 weeks.

Step 3. Administer strict amino acid–based formula for 4 weeks followed by repeat endoscopy with biopsy.

Step 4. Reintroduce foods one at a time every 4 to 5 days. Consider repeat endoscopy after every five foods reintroduced unless symptomatic response occurs.

Allergic foods should be avoided.

Corticosteroids should be used only in severe cases to alleviate symptoms until diet restriction can be initiated.

HELPFUL WEBSITES

The American Partnership for Eosinophilic Disorders website (www.apfed.org)
The Food Allergy and Anaphylaxis Network website (www.foodallergy.org)

REFERENCES

1. Jenkins HR, Pincott JR, Soothill JF, et al: Food allergy: the major cause of infantile colitis, *Arch Dis Child* 59:326-329, 1984.
2. Goldman H, Proujansky R: Allergic proctitis and gastroenteritis in children. Clinical and mucosal biopsy features in 53 cases, *Am J Surg Pathol* 10:75-86, 1986.
3. Heyman M, Grasset E, Ducroc R, et al: Antigen absorption by the jejunal epithelium of children with cow's milk allergy, *Pediatr Res* 24:197-202, 1988.
4. Husby S, Host A, Teisner B, et al: Infants and children with cow milk allergy/intolerance. Investigation of the uptake of cow milk protein and activation of the complement system, *Allergy* 45:547-551, 1990.
5. Kerner JA Jr: Formula allergy and intolerance, *Gastroenterol Clin North Am* 24:1-25, 1995.
6. Simpser E: Gastrointestinal Allergy. In Altschuler SM, Liacouras CA, eds: *Clinical pediatric gastroenterology*, Philadelphia, 1998, Churchill Livingstone.
7. Gerrard JW, MacKenzie JW, Goluboff N, et al: Cow's milk allergy: prevalence and manifestations in an unselected series of newborns, *Acta Paediatr Scand Suppl* 234:1-21, 1973.

8. Host A, Halken S: A prospective study of cow milk allergy in Danish infants during the first 3 years of life. Clinical course in relation to clinical and immunological type of hypersensitivity reaction, *Allergy* 45:587-596, 1990.

9. Strobel S: Epidemiology of food sensitivity in childhood—with special reference to cow's milk allergy in infancy, *Monogr Allergy* 31:119-130, 1993.

10. Eastham EJ: Soy protein allergy. In Taylor RH, ed: *Allergology, immunology, and gastroenterology,* New York, 1989, Raven Press.

11. Shannon WR: Demonstration of food proteins in human breast milk by anaphylactic experiments in guinea pig, *Am J Dis Child* 22:223-225, 1921.

12. Makinen-Kiljunen S, Palosuo T: A sensitive enzyme-linked immunosorbent assay for determination of bovine beta-lactoglobulin in infant feeding formulas and in human milk, *Allergy* 47:347-352, 1992.

13. Axelsson I, Jakobsson I, Lindberg T, et al: Bovine beta-lactoglobulin in the human milk. A longitudinal study during the whole lactation period, *Acta Paediatr Scand* 75:702-707, 1986.

14. Pittschieler K: Cow's milk protein-induced colitis in the breast-fed infant, *J Pediatr Gastroenterol Nutr* 10:548-549, 1990.

15. Vandenplas Y, Hauser B, Van den Borre C, et al: Effect of a whey hydrolysate prophylaxis of atopic disease, *Ann Allergy* 68:419-424, 1992.

16. Juvonen P, Mansson M, Jakobsson I: Does early diet have an effect on subsequent macromolecular absorption and serum IgE? *J Pediatr Gastroenterol Nutr* 18:344-349, 1994.

17. Kaczmarski M, Kurzatkowska B: The contribution of some environmental factors to the development of cow's milk and gluten intolerance in children, *Rocz Akad Med Bialymst* 33-34:151-165, 1988.

18. Katz AJ, Twarog FJ, Zeiger RS, et al: Milk-sensitive and eosinophilic gastroenteropathy: similar clinical features with contrasting mechanisms and clinical course, *J Allergy Clin Immunol* 74:72-78, 1984.

19. Donta ST, Myers MG: Clostridium difficile toxin in asymptomatic neonates, *J Pediatr* 100:431-434, 1982.

20. Cooperstock MS, Steffen E, Yolken R, et al: Clostridium difficile in normal infants and sudden infant death syndrome: an association with infant formula feeding, *Pediatrics* 70:91-95, 1982.

21. Hirano K, Shimojo N, Katsuki T, et al: [Eosinophils in stool smear in normal and milk-allergic infants], *Arerugi* 46:594-601, 1997.

22. Anveden-Hertzberg L, Finkel Y, Sandstedt B, et al: Proctocolitis in exclusively breast-fed infants, *Eur J Pediatr* 155:464-467, 1996.

23. Odze RD, Bines J, Leichtner AM, et al: Allergic proctocolitis in infants: a prospective clinicopathologic biopsy study, *Hum Pathol* 24:668-674, 1993.

24. Machida HM, Catto Smith AG, Gall DG, et al: Allergic colitis in infancy: clinical and pathologic aspects, *J Pediatr Gastroenterol Nutr* 19:22-26, 1994.

25. Goldman H. Allergic disorders. In Ming S-C, Goldman H, eds: *Pathology of the gastrointestinal tract,* Philadelphia, 1992, WB Saunders.

26. Kaijser R: Zur Kenntnis der allergischen Affektioner desima Verdeanungaskanal von Standpunkt desmia Chirurgen aus, *Arch Klin Chir* 188:36-64, 1937.

27. Klein NC, Hargrove RL, Sleisenger MH, et al: Eosinophilic gastroenteritis, *Medicine (Balt)* 49:299-319, 1970.

28. Spergel JM, Pawlowski NA: Food allergy: mechanisms, diagnosis, and management in children, *Pediatr Clin North Am* 49:73-96, vi, 2002.

29. Park HS, Kim HS, Jang HJ: Eosinophilic gastroenteritis associated with food allergy and bronchial asthma, *J Korean Med Sci* 10:216-219, 1995.

30. Justinich C, Katz A, Gurbindo C, et al: Elemental diet improves steroid-dependent eosinophilic gastroenteritis and reverses growth failure, *J Pediatr Gastroenterol Nutr* 23:81-85, 1996.

31. Leinbach GE, Rubin CE: Eosinophilic gastroenteritis: a simple reaction to food allergens? *Gastroenterology* 59:874-889, 1970.

32. Caldwell JH, Sharma HM, Hurtubise PE, et al: Eosinophilic gastroenteritis in extreme allergy. Immunopathological comparison with nonallergic gastrointestinal disease, *Gastroenterology* 77:560-564, 1979.

33. Kelso A: Cytokines: structure, function and synthesis, *Curr Opin Immunol* 2:215-225, 1989.

34. Desreumaux P, Bloget F, Seguy D, et al: Interleukin 3, granulocyte-macrophage colony-stimulating factor, and interleukin 5 in eosinophilic gastroenteritis, *Gastroenterology* 110:768-774, 1996.

35. Takafuji S, Bischoff SC, De Weck AL, et al: IL-3 and IL-5 prime normal human eosinophils to produce leukotriene C4 in response to soluble agonists, *J Immunol* 147:3855-3861, 1991.

36. Beyer K, Castro R, Birnbaum A, et al: Human milk-specific mucosal lymphocytes of the gastrointestinal tract display a TH2 cytokine profile, *J Allergy Clin Immunol* 109:707-713, 2002.

37. Kelly KJ: Eosinophilic gastroenteritis, *J Pediatr Gastroenterol Nutr* 30:S28-S35, 2000.

38. Whitington PF, Whitington GL: Eosinophilic gastroenteropathy in childhood, *J Pediatr Gastroenterol Nutr* 7:379-385, 1988.

39. Talley NJ, Shorter RG, Phillips SF, et al: Eosinophilic gastroenteritis: a clinicopathological study of patients with disease of the mucosa, muscle layer, and subserosal tissues, *Gut* 31:54-58, 1990.

40. Santos J, Junquera F, de Torres I, et al: Eosinophilic gastroenteritis presenting as ascites and splenomegaly, *Eur J Gastroenterol Hepatol* 7:675-678, 1995.

41. DeSchryver-Kecskemeti K, Clouse RE: A previously unrecognized subgroup of "eosinophilic gastroenteritis." Association with connective tissue diseases, *Am J Surg Pathol* 8:171-180, 1984.

42. Dubucquoi S, Janin A, Klein O, et al: Activated eosinophils and interleukin 5 expression in early recurrence of Crohn's disease, *Gut* 37:242-246, 1995.

43. Levy AM, Yamazaki K, Van Keulen VP, et al: Increased eosinophil infiltration and degranulation in colonic tissue from patients with collagenous colitis, *Am J Gastroenterol* 96:1522-1528, 2001.

44. Griscom NT, Kirkpatrick JA, Jr., Girdany BR, et al: Gastric antral narrowing in chronic granulomatous disease of childhood, *Pediatrics* 54:456-460, 1974.

45. Harris BH, Boles ET Jr: Intestinal lesions in chronic granulomatous disease of childhood, *J Pediatr Surg* 8:955-956, 1973.

46. Aquino A, Domini M, Rossi C, et al: Pyloric stenosis due to eosinophilic gastroenteritis: presentation of two cases in mono-ovular twins, *Eur J Pediatr* 158:172-173, 1999.

47. Khan S, Orenstein SR: Eosinophilic gastroenteritis masquerading as pyloric stenosis, *Clin Pediatr (Phila)* 39:55-57, 2000.

48. Redondo-Cerezo E, Cabello MJ, Gonzalez Y, et al: Eosinophilic gastroenteritis: our recent experience: one-year experience of atypical onset of an uncommon disease, *Scand J Gastroenterol* 36:1358-1360, 2001.

49. Shweiki E, West JC, Klena JW, et al: Eosinophilic gastroenteritis presenting as an obstructing cecal mass: a case report and review of the literature, *Am J Gastroenterol* 94:3644-3645, 1999.

50. Huang FC, Ko SF, Huang SC, et al: Eosinophilic gastroenteritis with perforation mimicking intussusception, *J Pediatr Gastroenterol Nutr* 33:613-615, 2001.

51. Deslandres C, Russo P, Gould P, et al: Perforated duodenal ulcer in a pediatric patient with eosinophilic gastroenteritis, *Can J Gastroenterol* 11:208-212, 1997.

52. Wang CS, Hsueh S, Shih LY, et al: Repeated bowel resections for eosinophilic gastroenteritis with obstruction and perforation. Case report, *Acta Chir Scand* 156:333-336, 1990.

53. Hoefer RA, Ziegler MM, Koop CE, et al: Surgical manifestations of eosinophilic gastroenteritis in the pediatric patient, *J Pediatr Surg* 12:955-962, 1977.

54. Lerza P: A further case of eosinophilic gastroenteritis with ascites, *Eur J Gastroenterol Hepatol* 8:407, 1996.

55. Caldwell JH, Tennenbaum JI, Bronstein HA: Serum IgE in eosinophilic gastroenteritis. Response to intestinal challenge in two cases, *N Engl J Med* 292:1388-1390, 1975.

56. Teele RL, Katz AJ, Goldman H, et al: Radiographic features of eosinophilic gastroenteritis (allergic gastroenteropathy) of childhood, *AJR Am J Roentgenol* 132:575-580, 1979.

57. Spergel JM, Beausoleil JL, Mascarenhas M, et al: The use of skin prick tests and patch tests to identify causative foods in eosinophilic esophagitis, *J Allergy Clin Immunol* 109:363-368, 2002.

58. Vandenplas Y, Quenon M, Renders F, et al: Milk-sensitive eosinophilic gastroenteritis in a 10-day-old boy, *Eur J Pediatr* 149:244-245, 1990.

59. Van Dellen RG, Lewis JC: Oral administration of cromolyn in a patient with protein-losing enteropathy, food allergy, and eosinophilic gastroenteritis, *Mayo Clin Proc* 69:441-444, 1994.

60. Moots RJ, Prouse P, Gumpel JM: Near fatal eosinophilic gastroenteritis responding to oral sodium chromoglycate, *Gut* 29:1282-1285, 1988.

61. Di Gioacchino M, Pizzicannella G, Fini N, et al: Sodium cromoglycate in the treatment of eosinophilic gastroenteritis, *Allergy* 45:161-166, 1990.

62. Schwartz DA, Pardi DS, Murray JA: Use of montelukast as steroid-sparing agent for recurrent eosinophilic gastroenteritis, *Dig Dis Sci* 46:1787-1790, 2001.

63. Neustrom MR, Friesen C: Treatment of eosinophilic gastroenteritis with montelukast, *J Allergy Clin Immunol* 104:506, 1999.

64. Shirai T, Hashimoto D, Suzuki K, et al: Successful treatment of eosinophilic gastroenteritis with suplatast tosilate, *J Allergy Clin Immunol* 107:924-925, 2001.

65. Bengtsson U, Hanson LA, Ahlstedt S: Survey of gastrointestinal reactions to foods in adults in relation to atopy, presence of mucus in the stools, swelling of joints and arthralgia in patients with gastrointestinal reactions to foods, *Clin Exp Allergy* 26:1387-1394, 1996.

66. Dobbins JW, Sheahan DG, Behar J: Eosinophilic gastroenteritis with esophageal involvement, *Gastroenterology* 72:1312-1316, 1977.

67. Matzinger MA, Daneman A: Esophageal involvement in eosinophilic gastroenteritis, *Pediatr Radiol* 13:35-38, 1983.

68. Lee RG: Marked eosinophilia in esophageal mucosal biopsies, *Am J Surg Pathol* 9:475-479, 1985.

69. Attwood SE, Smyrk TC, Demeester TR, et al: Esophageal eosinophilia with dysphagia: a distinct clinicopathologic syndrome, *Dig Dis Sci* 38:109-116, 1993.

70. Vitellas KM, Bennett WF, Bova JG, et al: Idiopathic eosinophilic esophagitis, *Radiology* 186:789-793, 1993.

71. Bischoff SC, Herrmann A, Manns MP: Prevalence of adverse reactions to food in patients with gastrointestinal disease, *Allergy* 51:811-818, 1996.

72. Winter HS, Madara JL, Stafford RJ, et al: Intraepithelial eosinophils: a new diagnostic criterion for reflux esophagitis, *Gastroenterology* 83: 818-823, 1982.

73. Brown LF, Goldman H, Antonioli DA: Intraepithelial eosinophils in endoscopic biopsies of adults with reflux esophagitis, *Am J Surg Pathol* 8:899-905, 1984.

74. Tummala V, Barwick KW, Sontag SJ, et al: The significance of intraepithelial eosinophils in the histologic diagnosis of gastroesophageal reflux, *Am J Clin Pathol* 87:43-48, 1987.

75. Kelly KJ, Lazenby AJ, Rowe PC, et al: Eosinophilic esophagitis attributed to gastroesophageal reflux: improvement with an amino acid-based formula, *Gastroenterology* 109:1503-1512, 1995.

76. Sondheimer JM: What are the roles of eosinophils in esophagitis? *J Pediatr Gastroenterol Nutr* 27:118-119, 1998.

77. Hassall E: Macroscopic versus microscopic diagnosis of reflux esophagitis: erosions or eosinophils? *J Pediatr Gastroenterol Nutr* 22:321-325, 1996.

78. Levine MS, Saul SH: Idiopathic eosinophilic esophagitis: how common is it? *Radiology* 186:631-632, 1993.

79. Walsh SV, Antonioli DA, Goldman H, et al: Allergic esophagitis in children: a clinicopathological entity, *Am J Surg Pathol* 23:390-396, 1999.

80. Teitelbaum JE, Fox VL, Twarog FJ, et al: Eosinophilic esophagitis in children: immunopathological analysis and response to fluticasone propionate, *Gastroenterology* 122:1216-1225, 2002.

81. Orenstein SR, Shalaby TM, Di Lorenzo C, et al: The spectrum of pediatric eosinophilic esophagitis beyond infancy: a clinical series of 30 children, *Am J Gastroenterol* 95:1422-1430, 2000.

82. Liacouras CA, Wenner WJ, Brown K, et al: Primary eosinophilic esophagitis in children: successful treatment with oral corticosteroids, *J Pediatr Gastroenterol Nutr* 26:380-385, 1998.

83. Liacouras CA, Markowitz JE: Eosinophilic esophagitis: A subset of eosinophilic gastroenteritis, *Curr Gastroenterol Rep* 1:253-258, 1999.

84. Faubion WA Jr, Perrault J, Burgart LJ, et al: Treatment of eosinophilic esophagitis with inhaled corticosteroids, *J Pediatr Gastroenterol Nutr* 27:90-93, 1998.

85. Ahmad M, Soetikno RM, Ahmed A: The differential diagnosis of eosinophilic esophagitis, *J Clin Gastroenterol* 30:242-244, 2000.

86. Vieth M, Stolte M: [Eosinophilic esophagitis: a largely unknown entity?], *Z Gastroenterol* 38:447-448, 2000.

87. Furuta GT: Eosinophilic esophagitis: an emerging clinicopathologic entity, *Curr Allergy Asthma Rep* 2:67-72, 2002.

88. Ruchelli E, Wenner W, Voytek T, et al: Severity of esophageal eosinophilia predicts response to conventional gastroesophageal reflux therapy, *Pediatr Dev Pathol* 2:15-18, 1999.

89. Siafakas CG, Ryan CK, Brown MR, et al: Multiple esophageal rings: an association with eosinophilic esophagitis: case report and review of the literature, *Am J Gastroenterol* 95:1572-1575, 2000.

90. Bousvaros A, Antonioli DA, Winter HS: Ringed esophagus: an association with esophagitis, *Am J Gastroenterol* 87:1187-1190, 1992.

91. Gupta SK, Fitzgerald JF, Chong SK, et al: Vertical lines in distal esophageal mucosa (VLEM): a true endoscopic manifestation of esophagitis in children? *Gastrointest Endosc* 45:485-489, 1997.

92. McKinley MJ, Eisner TD, Fisher ML, et al: Multiple rings of the esophagus associated with gastroesophageal reflux [case report], *Am J Gastroenterol* 91:574-576, 1996.

93. Stevoff C, Rao S, Parsons W, et al: EUS and histopathologic correlates in eosinophilic esophagitis, *Gastrointest Endosc* 54:373-377, 2001.

94. Vitellas KM, Bennett WF, Bova JG, et al: Radiographic manifestations of eosinophilic gastroenteritis, *Abdom Imaging* 20:406-413, 1995.

95. Liacouras C, Markowitz JE, Spergel JM: Eosinophilic esophagitis in children: a 5 year review (abstract), *J Pediatr Gastroenterol Nutr* 33:418, 2001.

96. Markowitz JE, Spergel JM, Ruchelli E, et al: Elemental diet is an effective treatment for eosinophilic esophagitis in children and adolescents, *Am J Gastroenterol* 2003 (in press).

97. Liacouras CA: Failed Nissen fundoplication in two patients who had persistent vomiting and eosinophilic esophagitis, *J Pediatr Surg* 32: 1504-1506, 1997.

98. Simon MR, Houser WL, Smith KA, et al: Esophageal candidiasis as a complication of inhaled corticosteroids, *Ann Allergy Asthma Immunol* 79:333-338, 1997.

99. Sharek PJ, Bergman DA: The effect of inhaled steroids on the linear growth of children with asthma: a meta-analysis, *Pediatrics* 106:E8, 2000.

100. Dahl R: Disodium cromoglycate and food allergy. The effect of oral and inhaled disodium cromoglycate in a food allergic patient, *Allergy* 33:120-124, 1978.

101. Businco L, Cantani A: Food allergy in children: diagnosis and treatment with sodium cromoglycate, *Allergol Immunopathol (Madr)* 18:339-348, 1990.

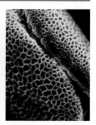

CHAPTER 50

Food Allergy, Respiratory Disease, and Anaphylaxis

JOHN M. JAMES

Food allergy may result in respiratory tract symptoms with different clinical manifestations that generally involve IgE-mediated responses. Skin and intestinal tract symptoms are commonly involved with these respiratory symptoms, which rarely occur in isolation.[1] Specific respiratory symptoms that have been attributed to food allergy include nasal congestion, rhinorrhea, sneezing, itching of the nose and throat, coughing, and/or wheezing. Exposure is usually through ingestion, but in some cases inhalation of food may also trigger reactions. Food allergy in early childhood is actually a marker for later respiratory allergy. Upper and lower respiratory reactions are often a significant aspect of systemic anaphylactic reactions, but chronic and isolated asthma or rhinitis caused only by food allergy is unusual. The role of food allergy in otitis media is controversial and probably is extremely rare. Asthmatic reactions to food additives can occur but are uncommon. Studies have demonstrated that foods can elicit airway hyperreactivity and asthmatic responses, so evaluation for food allergy should be considered among patients with recalcitrant or otherwise unexplained acute, severe asthma exacerbations, asthma triggered following ingestion of particular foods, and asthma and other manifestations of food allergy (e.g., anaphylaxis, moderate-to-severe atopic dermatitis).

EPIDEMIOLOGY/ETIOLOGY

Overview

Adverse reactions to foods encompass a wide spectrum of clinical signs and symptoms ranging from cutaneous findings to systemic anaphylactic reactions. These food reactions consist of any abnormal clinical responses following the ingestion of a food or food additive and can be further divided into two major categories.[1] The vast majority of adverse food reactions can be categorized as adverse physiologic reactions or food intolerance, which are not mediated by specific immunologic mechanisms. For example, an exaggerated physiologic reaction following the ingestion of monosodium glutamate (MSG), including headache, flushing, muscle tightness, and generalized weakness, is a classic example of a food intolerance. In contrast, food allergy is an immunologic-mediated food reaction unrelated to any physiologic effect of the food or additive. A typical example of food allergy is an IgE-mediated reaction to an ingested peanut resulting in laryngeal edema, coughing, and/or wheezing. Understanding this terminology and basic

classification of adverse food reactions will aid in the interpretation of the scientific studies implicating food allergy in respiratory tract symptoms and anaphylaxis.

Prevalence

The true prevalence of respiratory tract symptoms induced by food allergy has been very difficult to ascertain and establish. For example, there is an elevated public perception of food allergy-induced asthma.[2] These public perceptions, however, have not always been substantiated when careful objective investigations, including food challenges, have been undertaken to confirm patient histories.[3,4] When the specific focus has been on the role of food allergy and respiratory tract manifestations, the incidence has been estimated to be between 2% and 8% in children and adults with asthma.[5,6]

A French population study of food allergy was recently completed to determine the prevalence, clinical features, specific allergens, and risk factors of food allergy.[7] During this investigation 33,110 persons completed a questionnaire addressing various issues related to food allergy. The overall prevalence of food allergy was estimated to be 3.24%. Of the respiratory reactions reported, rhinitis and asthma were documented in 6.5% and 5.7% of cases, respectively. In addition, the clinical expression of food allergy was dependent on the existence of sensitization to pollens and was typically expressed in the form of rhinitis, asthma, or angioedema. Another survey found that 17% of 669 adult respondents in Australia reported food-induced respiratory symptoms.[8] Although the patients with asthma did not report food-related illness more frequently than those respondents without asthma, those reporting respiratory symptoms following food ingestion were more likely to be atopic.

Investigators from the Isle of Wight have reported that egg allergy in infancy predicts respiratory allergic disease by 4 years of age.[9] A cohort of 1218 consecutive births was recruited and followed until 4 years of age. Of these, 29 (2.4%) developed egg allergy by 4 years of age. Increased respiratory allergy (e.g., rhinitis, asthma) was associated with egg allergy (odds ratio [OR]: 5.0, 95% confidence interval [CI]: 1.1-22.3; $P < 0.05$) with a positive predictive value of 55%. Furthermore, the addition of the diagnosis of eczema to egg allergy increased the positive predictive value to 80%. The investigators concluded that egg allergy in infancy, especially when associated with eczema, increases respiratory allergic symptoms in early childhood. In addition, Rhodes et al[10] conducted a prospective cohort study of subjects at risk of asthma and atopy in England. Of the 100 babies of atopic parents who were recruited at birth, 73 were followed up at 5 years, 67 at 11 years, and 63 at 22 years. Skin sensitivity to hen's egg, cow milk, or both in the first 5 years of life was predictive of asthma (OR: 10.7, 95% CI: 2.1-55.1; $P = 0.001$; sensitivity 57%; specificity 89%).

An investigation by Sicherer and colleagues summarized data from a voluntary registry of 5149 individuals (median age 5 years) with peanut and/or tree nut allergy.[11] The primary objective was to characterize clinical features including respiratory reactions in the registrants. Respiratory reactions, including wheezing, throat tightness, and nasal congestion, were reported in 42% and 56% of respondents as part of their initial reactions to peanuts and tree nuts, respectively. One half of the reactions involved more than one system and more than 75% required some form of medical treatment. Interestingly, registrants with asthma were significantly more likely than those without asthma to have severe reactions (33% vs. 21%; $P < 0.0001$).

Pathogenesis

Immune responses mediated by specific IgE antibodies to food allergens are the most widely recognized mechanisms for food-induced respiratory tract symptoms.[12] Atopic patients produce IgE antibodies to specific epitopes in the food allergen. These antibodies bind to high-affinity IgE receptors on basophils and tissue mast cells throughout the body, including the upper and lower respiratory tract. The establishment of IgE-bearing cells in the nasal or bronchial mucosa during the allergic sensitization process enables their activation during subsequent allergen exposure.[13] When antigen binds to multiple adjacent IgE antibodies on a mast cell or basophil, these cells become activated, degranulate, and release proinflammatory mediators such as histamine, tryptase, leukotrienes, and prostaglandins. These mediators are responsible for the immediate allergic reaction characterized by vasodilatation, smooth muscle contraction, and mucus secretion, which in turn leads to the different clinical symptoms observed in the respiratory tract.

These specific mediators can also contribute to late-phase allergic reactions that occur 4 to 8 hours after an immediate allergic response. Mast cell–derived mediators can cause endothelial cells to increase expression of adhesion molecules for eosinophils, basophils, and lymphocytes. In addition, tryptase may activate endothelial cells, increasing vascular permeability. Leukocytes are then drawn to the airways during a relatively symptom-free recruitment phase, where they release cytokines and tissue-damaging proteases that contribute to the late-phase response, including congestion in allergic rhinitis and bronchoconstriction in asthma. Chronic inflammation may eventually cause an increase in airway hyperresponsiveness. Specific T cells also generate a memory response, which may contribute to the exacerbation of asthma symptoms on reexposure to relevant stimuli.

Allergens

A short list of specific foods has been implicated in respiratory reactions and subsequently confirmed in well-controlled, blinded food challenges.[3,14-16] These foods include chicken egg, cow's milk, peanuts, fish, shellfish, and tree nuts (Table 50-1). Certainly other foods have been implicated in respiratory reactions secondary to food allergy, but this short list of more common foods should be considered a part of any evaluation of patients with these presenting clinical histories. Finally, investigations of patients experiencing near-fatal and/or fatal anaphylactic reactions following food ingestion have mainly been secondary to peanuts, tree nuts, and shellfish.[17-19]

In addition, a high percentage of patients with asthma perceive that food additives contribute to worsening of their respiratory symptoms.[20] Several different food additives, including MSG, sulfites, and aspartame, have been implicated in adverse respiratory reactions.[21] Well-controlled investigations in this area, however, have reported a prevalence rate of less than 5%.[5,14]

There is conflicting evidence that some people with asthma are more likely to have adverse effects from MSG compared with the general population. Woods and co-workers[22] designed a randomized, double-blind, placebo-controlled MSG-challenge protocol for identifying early and late asthmatic reactions. They were unable to demonstrate MSG-induced immediate or late asthmatic reactions in a group of 12 adult asthma patients who perceived that this food additive negatively affected their overall asthma control. In addition, these investigators observed no significant changes in bronchial hyperresponsiveness or soluble inflammatory markers (e.g., eosinophil cationic protein, tryptase) during this investigation protocol. In addition, another recent investigation performed double-blind, placebo-controlled oral challenges with MSG in subjects who had histories of adverse reactions to this food additive.[23] Although the participants experienced no specific upper or lower respiratory complaints, 22 (36.1%) of the 61 enrolled subjects had confirmed adverse reactions to MSG including headache, muscle tightness, numbness, general weakness, and flushing.

ROUTE OF EXPOSURE AND SUBSEQUENT RESPIRATORY SYMPTOMS

Oral Ingestion of Food Allergens

Oral ingestion is the primary route of exposure to food that can cause or exacerbate respiratory symptoms (e.g., asthma). The vast majority of published reports, which are highlighted in this chapter, focus on respiratory tract symptoms following the ingestion of food allergens. These reactions will be discussed in more detail throughout this chapter.

TABLE 50-1   Common Food Allergens Implicated in Respiratory Disease

All Respiratory Reactions	Near-Fatal and Fatal Anaphylaxis
Chicken egg	Peanuts
Cow's milk	Tree nuts
Peanuts	Shellfish
Fish	
Shellfish	
Tree nuts	

Inhalation of Food Allergens

Several investigations have highlighted cases of respiratory allergy disease that have been precipitated by the inhalation exposure to airborne food allergens. One report focused on three patients who developed asthma and rhinitis caused by exposure to raw, but not cooked, green beans and chards in a non-occupational environment.[24] Minor differences were observed in IgE reactivity between nitrocellulose-blotted raw and boiled green bean extracts. In addition, highly allergic persons may react when exposed to clinically relevant levels of allergenic food in a seafood restaurant or when fish, shellfish, or eggs are cooked in a confined area.[12] Another report highlighted allergic reactions associated with airborne fish particles in patients with fish allergy.[25] These investigators evaluated children who reported allergic reactions upon incidental inhalation of fish odors or fumes. Of the 21 patients evaluated, 9 had wheezing or rhinitis alone and 3 had respiratory and cutaneous symptoms together. Methods of exposure included boiling or frying fish and simple exposure to fish. Finally, Sicherer and colleagues recently reported that peanut-allergic patients might experience adverse respiratory reactions when they are exposed to peanut dust on airline flights serving peanut snacks.[26]

Occupational exposures to airborne food allergens can also result in chronic asthma. For example, Baker's asthma is caused by occupational exposure to airborne cereal grain dust.[27] Patients with this disorder experience cough and shortness of breath following the inhalation of wheat proteins while baking. Affected patients usually have positive skin tests to extracted wheat proteins.[27] Another report highlighted an observation that inhalation of lupine flour may be an important cause of allergic sensitization in exposed workers and may actually give rise to occupational asthma and food allergy.[28] Three patients reported work-related symptoms immediately after being exposed to lupine. Skin prick test results with an extract of lupine seed flour were positive in all patients; lupine-specific IgE antibodies were detected in two subjects. Interestingly, one patient underwent a bronchial provocation with lupine seed flour extract and experienced an immediate fall (25%) in forced expiratory volume in 1 second (FEV_1). In summary, lupine seed flour may be a potential sensitizing agent by inhalation in exposed workers and may give rise to occupational asthma and food allergy.

These data clearly illustrate that respiratory allergic disease can be precipitated by the inhalation exposure of airborne food allergens. Children with food allergy and their caregivers should be educated about the potential for these types of reactions, which can occur following the incidental inhalation of fumes or vapors from relevant food allergens. These anticipatory guidance measures can be helpful in the prevention of these allergic reactions.

DIFFERENTIAL DIAGNOSIS OF FOOD-INDUCED RESPIRATORY SYNDROMES

In the overall evaluation of patients with respiratory tract symptoms, one must consider numerous etiologies in the differential diagnosis (Figure 50-1). As compared to viral upper respiratory tract infections, allergic rhinitis, and sinusitis, food allergy as a specific etiology for respiratory tract symptoms is less common and has been less well defined.

Rhinitis Induced by Food Allergy

Adverse nasal symptoms have been attributed to food ingestion. For example, nasal symptoms, especially rhinitis, can certainly be observed during positive blinded oral food challenges. Rhinitis accounted for 70% of the overall respiratory symptoms observed in a large group of children undergoing double-blind, placebo-controlled food challenges (DBPCFCs).[29] These symptoms typically occur in association with other clinical manifestations (i.e., cutaneous and/or gastrointestinal symptoms) during allergic reactions to foods and rarely occur in isolation.[14,29]

Although many patients associate the ingestion of cow's milk and other dairy products with an increase in the production and thickness of nasal secretions, this cannot always be attributed to a specific allergic reaction. Pinnock and

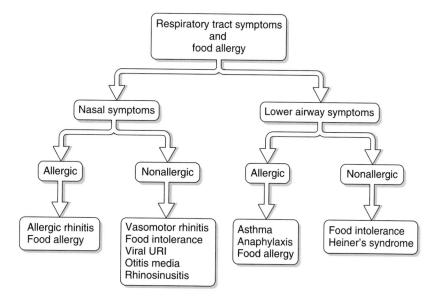

FIGURE 50-1 Respiratory tract symptoms and food allergy: differential diagnosis. *URI*, Upper respiratory tract infection.

co-workers[30] investigated the relationship between milk intake and mucus production in adult volunteers challenged with rhinovirus-2. Milk and dairy product intake was not associated with an increase in upper or lower respiratory tract symptoms of congestion or nasal secretion weight. Overall, no statistically significant association was detected between milk and dairy product intake and symptoms of mucus production in healthy adults, either asymptomatic or symptomatic, with rhinovirus infection. Another investigation used a randomized, crossover, double-blind, placebo-controlled trial to examine the effects of dairy products in patients who perceived that their asthma worsened with the ingestion of these products.[31] For both FEV_1 and peak expiratory flow rate, there was no statistically significant differences in the group mean between active challenges and placebo challenges, between sequences of administration, or between perceptions. The investigators concluded that it is unlikely that dairy products have a specific bronchoconstrictor effect in most patients with asthma, regardless of their perception.

Gustatory rhinitis is a form of food intolerance that can also provoke nasal symptoms.[32] In one questionnaire, greater than 60% of those surveyed reported rhinorrhea following the ingestion of very spicy foods such as hot chili peppers, horseradish, and hot and sour soup. Unlike typical rhinitis, affected individuals do not develop sneezing, congestion, or pruritus. The spicy food elicits rhinorrhea within a few minutes of ingesting the food and resolves almost immediately after the spicy food is eaten. The reaction results from the stimulation of atropine-inhibitable muscarinic receptors.[32]

Serous Otitis Media Induced by Food Allergy

Serous otitis media has multiple etiologies, of which the most common is viral upper respiratory tract infections. Allergic inflammation in the nasal mucosa may cause eustachian tube dysfunction and subsequent otitis media with effusion. The role of food allergy in recurrent serous otitis media has been proposed; however, this association has been overestimated and is controversial.[33] One report cautiously suggests that in a subset of infants with recurrent otitis media, IgG complexes with food antigens, particularly cow milk proteins, may contribute to the middle ear inflammation in this disorder.[34] Respiratory atopy (e.g., allergic rhinitis, allergic asthma) may be a more important predisposing factor than food allergy alone.[35] More scientific data obtained from well-controlled investigations are needed before general recommendations can be made regarding this association.

Food-Induced Pulmonary Hemosiderosis (Heiner's Syndrome)

In 1960 Heiner[36] reported a syndrome in infants consisting of recurrent episodes of pneumonia associated with chronic rhinitis, pulmonary infiltrates and hemosiderosis, gastrointestinal blood loss, iron-deficiency anemia, and failure to thrive. This rare syndrome is most often associated with a non–IgE-mediated hypersensitivity to cow's milk proteins, but reactivity to egg and pork have also been reported.[37] Whereas peripheral blood eosinophilia and multiple serum precipitins to cow's milk are commonly observed, the specific immunologic mechanisms responsible for this disorder are not known. The diagnosis is suggested when elimination of the precipitating allergen leads to subsequent resolution of symptoms. The presence of characteristic laboratory data including precipitating antibodies to cow's milk is also considered necessary to make the diagnosis. Avoidance of the precipitating allergen leads to resolution of symptoms, but the natural history of this disorder is not known.

Asthma Induced by Food Allergy

The majority of information regarding food allergy and respiratory tract symptoms focuses on asthma. In one investigation, 300 consecutive patients with asthma (age range: 7 months to 80 years) were evaluated in a pulmonary clinic.[5] Twenty-five (12%) patients had a history of food allergy suggested by clinical symptoms and/or positive tests of food-specific IgE antibodies. Food-induced wheezing was documented in 6 (2%) of the cases; all were children aged 4 to 17 years. In another investigation, 140 children, aged 2 through 9 years, with asthma were screened by clinical history, and testing for food-specific IgE antibodies.[38] Of these children, 32 patients were able to undergo blinded food challenges: 13 (9.2%) had food-induced respiratory symptoms, and 8 (5.7%) had specific asthmatic reactions documented during food challenges; only 1 patient had asthma as the sole symptom during a positive food challenge. Interestingly, the patients with food allergy and asthma were generally younger and had a past medical history of atopic dermatitis.

Continuing with this theme, Oehling and co-workers[39] reported that food-induced bronchospasm was present in 8.5% of 284 asthmatic children evaluated. The majority of the allergic sensitization occurred in the first year of life and was caused by a single food, especially egg. In addition, Businco and colleagues[40] evaluated 42 children (age range: 10 to 76 months) with atopic dermatitis and milk allergy. Of these patients, 11 (27%) developed asthmatic symptoms during a positive food challenge. Finally, an investigation from Turkey confirmed that food allergy can elicit asthma in children younger than 6 years; the incidence was 4%. The most common food allergens implicated were egg and cow's milk.[41]

The prevalence of food-related wheezing does appear to be highest in younger patients with atopic disease. Published investigations from Australia have reported 100 children (mean age: 16 months) who had clinical histories of adverse reactions to cow's milk.[42] The children were separated into three distinct groups based on symptoms. The first group consisted of 27 infants who reacted acutely to cow's milk ingestion (29% had lower airway responses on oral challenges) and had cow's milk–specific IgE antibodies. A second group consisted of 53 infants with primarily non–IgE-mediated gastrointestinal reactions to cow's milk challenges; only 4% in this group experienced lower airway symptoms. The third group included 20 patients characterized by late-onset reactions to oral challenges with cow's milk. The majority of these patients had chronic asthma or atopic dermatitis and 50% had wheezing after the milk challenges.

Respiratory reactions induced by food challenges in children with pulmonary disease at National Jewish Center for Immunology and Respiratory Medicine have been reported by Bock.[43] Of the 410 children with a history of asthma, 279 (68%) had a history of food-induced asthma. There were positive food challenges in 168 (60%) of the 279 patients. This investigation documented that 67 (24%) of the 279 children with a history of food-induced asthma had a positive blinded food challenge that included wheezing. The most common foods that were responsible for these reactions included: peanuts, 19; cow's milk, 18; egg, 13; and tree nuts, 10. Interestingly, only 5 (2%) of these patients had wheezing as their only objective adverse symptom.

A total of 320 children with atopic dermatitis undergoing blinded food challenges at Johns Hopkins Hospital were monitored for respiratory reactions.[29] The patients, ages 6 months to 30 years, were highly atopic and had multiple allergic sensitivities to foods, and over one half had a prior diagnosis of asthma. Food allergy was confirmed by blinded challenges in 205 (64%) of these patients; almost two thirds of these patients experienced respiratory reactions during their positive food challenges (e.g., nasal 70%, laryngeal 48%, pulmonary 27%). Overall, 34 (17%) of 205 children with positive food challenges developed wheezing as part of their reaction. Furthermore, 88 of these patients were monitored with pulmonary function testing during positive and negative food challenges. Thirteen (15%) developed lower respiratory symptoms, including wheezing; however, only six patients had a more than 20% decrease in FEV_1. As documented in the investigations cited earlier, wheezing as the only manifestation of the respiratory reaction was a rare observation.

In summary, these results suggest that respiratory symptoms may be provoked in a subset of patients with asthma. Table 50-2 provides a comparison of the prevalence of food allergy–induced asthmatic reactions in different patient populations.

Airway Hyperresponsiveness Induced by Food Allergy

In a select subset of pediatric patients the chronic ingestion of a food to which the patient is allergic may result in increased airway hyperreactivity despite the absence of acute symptoms following ingestion. In one investigation 26 children with asthma and food allergy were evaluated using methacholine inhalation challenges for changes in their airway hyperreactivity before and after blinded food challenges.[44] Of the 22 positive blinded food challenges, 12 involved chest symptoms (cough, laryngeal reactions, and/or wheezing). Another 10 positive food challenges included laryngeal, gastrointestinal, and/or skin symptoms without any chest symptoms. Significant increases in airway hyperreactivity were documented several hours after positive food challenges in 7 of the 12 patients who experienced chest symptoms during these challenges. During the actual food challenges decreases in FEV_1 were not generally observed in these 7 patients, which suggests that significant changes in airway hyperreactivity can occur without

demonstrable pulmonary function changes in a preceding food challenge. These data indicate that food-induced allergic reactions may increase airway reactivity in a subset of patients with moderate to severe asthma, and may do so without inducing acute asthma symptoms.

In contrast, a different investigation concluded that food allergy is an unlikely cause of increased airway reactivity.[45] Eleven adults with asthma, a history of food-induced wheezing, and positive prick skin tests to the suspected foods were evaluated. An equal number of patients had increased airway reactivity, as determined by methacholine inhalation challenges, after blinded food challenges to either food allergen or placebo. Unfortunately, the small number of patients investigated and the lack of environmental controls prior to the repeat methacholine challenges limit their conclusions.

Food-Induced Anaphylactic Reactions

Anaphylactic reactions including respiratory symptoms can occur after the oral ingestion of a food allergen. Patients with underlying asthma who experience an anaphylactic reaction following food ingestion constitute a high-risk group because these patients have been frequently reported in series of fatal and near-fatal reactions following food ingestion.[17-19] These symptoms typically include pruritus in the oropharynx, angioedema (e.g., laryngeal edema), stridor, cough, dyspnea, wheezing, and dysphonia. In a survey of six fatal and seven near-fatal anaphylactic reactions following food ingestion, all patients had asthma and respiratory symptoms as part of their clinical presentations.[18] The foods responsible for these serious reactions were peanut, tree nuts, egg, and cow milk. Another report summarized acute allergic reactions to peanut and/or tree nuts in 122 atopic children. In this group 52% had lower respiratory tract symptoms as part of their overall reactions.[46] A recent Italian investigation summarized the clinical characteristics and treatment of 113 episodes of acute anaphylaxis triggered by different agents including medications (49%), Hymenoptera venom (29%), and food allergens (8%).[47] Most of the events occurred at home (63%) and the most frequent symptoms were respiratory and cutaneous, 90% and 78%, respectively. Of note, initial symptoms never involved the cardiovascular system. Specific foods identified as triggers included mustard, mussels, shrimp, soy, peanut, and fish. In summary, the presence of asthma and a short list of common food allergens are significant risk factors for serious and even fatal cases of food-induced anaphylaxis.[17,48] Box 50-1 summarizes the major considerations for implicating the specific role of food allergy in respiratory tract symptoms.

EVALUATION/MANAGEMENT

Medical History

A comprehensive medical history should be obtained in patients suspected of having food allergy–induced respiratory tract symptoms or anaphylaxis.[12] The history should include questions about the timing of the reaction in relation to food ingestion, the minimum quantity of food required to cause symptoms, specific upper and lower respiratory signs and symptoms, and the reproducibility of the symptoms. A family history positive for allergy and/or asthma can be a useful historical point. When there is a history of an unexplained sudden asthma exacerbation, details about preceding food

TABLE 50-2 Estimated Prevalence of Food Allergy–Induced Asthmatic Reactions	
Clinical Population	**Estimated Prevalence**
Infants with cow's milk allergy	29%
Food-induced wheezing	2%-24%
Food additive–induced wheezing	< 5%
Patients with atopic dermatitis	17%-27%

- Food-induced respiratory tract symptoms are typically accompanied by either cutaneous or gastrointestinal symptoms.
- Food allergy–induced respiratory symptoms rarely occur in isolation.
- Egg, cow milk, peanut, soy, fish, shellfish, and tree nuts are the most common food allergens confirmed to elicit respiratory reactions.
- Allergic sensitization or clinical reactions to foods in infancy predict the later development of respiratory allergies and asthma.
- Food-induced asthma is more common in young pediatric patients than in older children and adults.
- Children with atopic dermatitis, especially those with food allergy confirmed during blinded food challenges, are at increased risk for food-induced asthma.
- Food-induced allergic reactions may increase airway reactivity in some patients with moderate to severe asthma and may do so without inducing acute asthma symptoms.
- Asthmatic reactions induced by food allergy are considered risk factors for fatal and near-fatal anaphylactic reactions.

ingestion should be elicited. A history of a severe or anaphylactic reaction following the ingestion of a food may be sufficient to indicate a causal relationship. Finally, documentation of the specific treatment received and its response should be documented.

Diet diaries rarely identify an unrecognized association between a food and a patient's respiratory symptoms. Moreover, elimination diets, which are typically implemented for 7 to 14 days, are rarely diagnostic of food allergy, particularly in chronic disorders such as atopic dermatitis or asthma. Their success depends on identifying the correct allergen and completely eliminating it in all forms from the diet. All efforts should be made to prevent complications from unnecessary dietary restrictions such as poor weight gain and failure to thrive.[49]

Investigations previously highlighted in this chapter have helped to identify which patients with nasal symptoms and/or asthma to consider for a food allergy evaluation. First, patients with recalcitrant or otherwise unexplained acute, severe asthma exacerbations should be considered for evaluation. Second, patients with asthma triggered following ingestion of particular foods should be evaluated. Third, patients with asthma and other manifestations of food allergy (e.g., moderate to severe atopic dermatitis, anaphylaxis) should be considered for an evaluation of food allergy. Finally, patients with a history of difficult-to-manage gastroesophageal reflux and/or a history of feeding problems in infancy should be considered for this evaluation.

Physical Examination

In evaluating patients with respiratory system complaints that may be induced by food allergy, the physical examination can be useful. Findings here are helpful in assessing overall nutri-

tional status, growth parameters, and any signs of allergic disease, especially atopic dermatitis. Moreover, this examination will help to rule out other conditions that may mimic food allergy.

Skin Testing for Food Allergy

Skin tests (i.e., prick, puncture) are used to screen for IgE-mediated food allergies and can be performed even in infants in the first few months after birth.[50] When used in conjunction with standard criteria of interpretation, these tests give reliable clinical information in a short period of time (i.e., 15 to 20 minutes). If high-quality extracts are used, the skin testing is an excellent method of excluding IgE-mediated food allergies; the negative predictive accuracy is greater than 95%. Conversely, the positive predictive accuracy is generally less than 50%, which limits the clinical interpretation of positive skin tests. This emphasizes the need to confirm the clinical history and positive skin test with a food challenge, if the history is not convincing for anaphylaxis. Intradermal skin testing with foods has questionable diagnostic benefit and should never be performed before a standard prick or puncture skin test is conducted. This method of skin testing increases the risk of inducing a systemic reaction and is less specific when compared to prick skin testing.[50,51]

In summary, skin testing provides reliable clinical information in the overall work-up of a patient with suspected food allergy-induced respiratory tract reactions. The routine use of skin testing to foods in patients presenting with asthma, however, is not practical. Of children evaluated in a tertiary care hospital emergency room, 97 patients with asthma or bronchiolitis were skin tested to common foods and aeroallergens and compared to similar testing in 60 control patients without any respiratory disease.[52] Most specific IgE antibody responses among wheezing children were to aeroallergens; the prevalence of specific IgE antibodies to food allergens was low.

Other Testing

Laboratory assessment of food allergy may include the measurement of food-specific IgE in the serum (e.g., IgE radioallergosorbent testing). When highly sensitive assays are used, the sensitivity and specificity are similar to those of skin tests.[50,53-55] In contrast, basophil histamine release assays, which are mainly limited to research settings, have not been shown conclusively to be reproducible, diagnostic tests for food allergy.[56] Finally, the diagnostic values of the following tests are not currently supported by objective scientific evidence: food-specific IgG or IgG subclass antibody concentrations, food antigen–antibody complexes, cytotoxic food tests, and subcutaneous provocation and neutralization.[57,58]

Food Challenges

When there is a clinical suspicion of a food-induced respiratory tract reaction and the test for specific IgE antibody to the food is positive, an elimination diet may be implemented to see if there is a resolution of clinical symptoms. Confirming this association, however, can be very difficult. Food challenges can be very useful and reliable in the diagnostic evaluation of a patient with food-induced respiratory symptoms. An excellent publication has reviewed the combined clinical experience of six centers doing food challenges.[59] Of these procedures, the DBPCFC is the best method to diagnose and confirm food allergy and other adverse food reactions.[12,50] These challenges should be conducted in a clinic or hospital setting with available personnel and equipment for treating systemic anaphylaxis. If the clinical history does not suggest a high risk of a severe reaction, an oral food challenge can be performed in the office setting. A recent publication summarizes the major considerations in performing supervised food challenges[12] (Table 50-3). In summary, a practical algorithm for diagnosis of food-induced allergic rhinitis and/or asthma is illustrated in Figure 50-2.

TREATMENT

Once a food allergy has been confirmed as a cause for respiratory tract symptoms, strict avoidance of the offending food is necessary.[14,50,56] A properly managed elimination diet can lead to resolution of clinical symptoms, such as chronic asthma.

TABLE 50-3 Evaluation of Food Allergy and Respiratory Symptoms

1. The medical history supplemented with appropriate laboratory testing and well-designed food challenges can provide useful information in the workup of patients with respiratory symptoms that may be induced by food allergy.
2. A diagnosis based solely on history or skin test/RAST is not acceptable.
3. If no specific foods are implicated in the history and if skin tests to foods are negative, further workup for IgE-mediated allergy is not generally indicated.
4. With positive skin tests and/or respiratory symptoms associated with specific foods, an elimination diet may be instituted for 7 to 14 days.
5. If symptoms persist, food is not likely to be the problem, except in some cases of atopic dermatitis or chronic asthma.
6. Symptoms recurring after a regular diet is resumed should be evaluated with a properly designed food challenge.

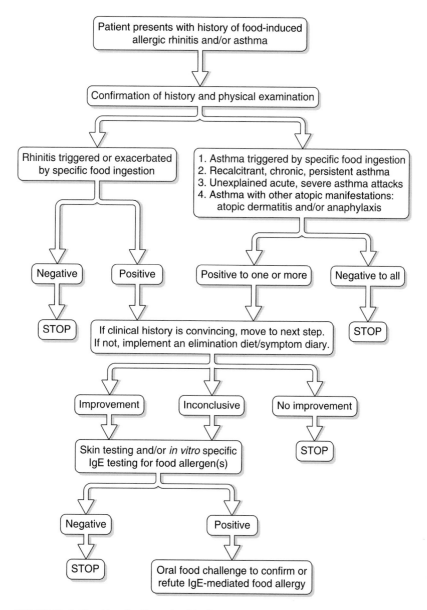

FIGURE 50-2 Algorithm for diagnosis of food-induced allergic rhinitis or asthma.

Appropriate nutritional counseling is important to ensure that an elimination diet is well balanced, to provide appropriate substitutes for foods that are eliminated from the diet, and to avoid any anticipated nutritional deficiencies, such as calcium deficiency.[60-62] Growth parameters should be closely monitored, especially in infants and children on elimination diets. Woods and co-workers[22] were unable to prove that the ingestion of dairy products induced bronchoconstriction in a group of adults with asthma. They recommended that patients with asthma should not be unnecessarily restricting their dairy product intakes, which could lead to the development of nutritional deficiencies. Therefore restriction diets should exclude only those foods proven to provoke food allergy.[14,50]

Implementing an elimination diet may sound simple, but the complete removal of any given food allergen requires diligence and careful attention to detail. For example, in a cow's milk–free diet, patients must be educated to not only avoid all milk products but also to read food ingredient labels for key words that may indicate the presence of cow's milk proteins (e.g., casein, whey, lactalbumin, lactoglobulin, and caramel color). This process will help the patient avoid accidentally ingesting hidden ingredients.[63,64] As highlighted previously, patients with asthma and food allergies appear to be at a higher risk for suffering a severe allergic reaction or anaphylaxis if they ingest a given food allergen.[17,18]

Organizations such as the Food Allergy Network (Fairfax, Va.; phone: 800-929-4040; www.foodallergy.org) and the International Food Informational Council (Washington, D.C.; phone: 202-296-6540, www.ific.org) are excellent resources for patients with food allergies, their families, physicians, and other caretakers. Moreover, the Food Allergy Network provides a special service to alert families when contamination or mislabeling occurs in commercial food products.

An emergency plan should be written to help patients manage any clinical symptoms caused by accidental ingestion of a relevant food allergen.[50] For children, the written plan should be given to the appropriate school personnel. Self-injectable epinephrine and antihistamines must be on hand to treat allergic reactions in case of accidental ingestions. Epinephrine is the drug of choice to treat acute, severe reactions and to allow time to seek immediate medical attention.

CONCLUSIONS

In summary, previous investigations have clearly established the pathogenic role of food allergy in respiratory tract symptoms. These symptoms are typically accompanied by skin and gastrointestinal manifestations and rarely occur in isolation. Specific foods have been implicated in these reactions. Allergic sensitization to foods in infancy predicts the later development of respiratory allergies and asthma. The role of food allergy in otitis media is controversial and probably very rare. Similarly, asthmatic reactions to food additives can occur but are uncommon. Food-induced asthma is more common in young pediatric patients, especially those with atopic dermatitis, than in older children and adults. Respiratory symptoms, especially asthma, induced by food allergens are considered risk factors for fatal and near-fatal anaphylactic reactions.

Studies have demonstrated that foods can elicit airway hyperreactivity and asthmatic responses, so evaluation for food allergy should be considered among patients with recalcitrant or otherwise unexplained acute, severe asthma exacerbations; asthma triggered following ingestion of particular foods; and asthma and other manifestations of food allergy (e.g., anaphylaxis, moderate to severe atopic dermatitis). Practice parameters for the diagnosis and treatment of asthma have been published and highlight the potential role of food allergy in asthma in some patients.[65]

HELPFUL WEBSITES

The Food Allergy and Anaphylaxis Network website (www.foodallergy.org)
The International Food Information Council website (www.ific.org)

REFERENCES

1. Sampson HA: Food allergy. Part 1: Immunopathogenesis and clinical disorders, J Allergy Clin Immnunol 103:717-728, 1999.
2. Woods RK, Weiner J, Abramson M, et al: Patient perceptions of food-induced asthma, N Z J Med 26:504-512, 1996.
3. Bock SA: Prospective appraisal of complaints of adverse reactions to foods in children during the first 3 years of life, Pediatrics 79:683-688, 1987.
4. Niestijl Jansen JJ, Kardinaal AFM, Huijbers G, et al: Prevalence of food allergy and intolerance in the adult Dutch population, J Allergy Clin Immunol 93:446-456, 1994.
5. Onorato J, Merland N, Terral C, et al: Placebo-controlled double-blind food challenges in asthma, J Allergy Clin Immunol 78:1139-1146, 1986.
6. Nekam KL: Nutritional triggers in asthma, Acta Microbiol Immunol Hung 45:113-117, 1998.
7. Kanny G, Moneret-Vautrin D-A, Flabbee J, et al: Population study of food allergy in France, J Allergy Clin Immunol 108:133-140, 2001.
8. Woods RK et al: Reported food intolerance and respiratory symptoms in young adults, Eur Respir J 11:151-155, 1998.
9. Tariq SM, Matthews SM, Hakin EA, et al: Egg allergy in infancy predicts respiratory allergic disease by 4 years of age, Pediatr Allergy Immunol 11:162-167, 2000.
10. Rhodes HL, Sporik R, Thomas P, et al: Early life risk factors for adult asthma: a birth cohort study of subjects at risk, J Allergy Clin Immunol 108:720-725, 2001.
11. Sicherer SH, Furlong TJ, Munoz-Furlong A, et al: A voluntary registry for peanut and tree nut allergy: characteristics of the first 5149 registrants, J Allergy Clin Immunol 108:128-32, 2001.
12. Sicherer SH: Is food allergy causing your patient's asthma symptoms? J Respir Dis 21:127-136, 2000.
13. Platts-Mills TAE: The role of immunoglobulin E in allergy and asthma, Am J Respir Crit Care Med 164:S1-S5, 2001.
14. Bock SA, Atkins FM: Patterns of food hypersensitivity during sixteen years of double-blind placebo-controlled oral food challenges, J Pediatr 117:561-567, 1990.
15. Burks AW, James JM, Hiegel A, et al: Atopic dermatitis and food hypersensitivity reactions, J Pediatr 132:132-136, 1998.
16. Sampson HA, McCaskill CM: Food hypersensitivity and atopic dermatitis: evaluation of 113 patients, J Pediatr 107:669-675, 1985.
17. James JM: Anaphylactic reactions to foods, Immunol Allergy Clin North Am 21:653-667, 2001.
18. Sampson HA, Mendelson L, Rosen JP: Fatal and near-fatal food anaphylaxis reactions in children, N Engl J Med 327:380-384, 1992.
19. Yuninger JY, Sweeney KG, Sturner WQ, et al: Fatal food-induced anaphylaxis, J Am Med Assoc 260:1450-1452, 1988.
20. Abramson M, Kutin J, Rosier M, et al: Morbidity, medication and trigger factors in a community sample of adults with asthma, Med J Aust 162:78-81, 1995.
21. Weber RW: Food additives and allergy, Ann Allergy 70:183-190, 1993.
22. Woods RK, Weiner JM, Thien F, et al: The effects of monosodium glutamate in adults with asthma who perceive themselves to be monosodium glutamate-intolerant, J Allergy Clin Immunol 101:762-771, 1998.
23. Yang WH, Drouin MA, Herbert M, et al: The monosodium glutamate symptom complex: assessment in a double-blind, placebo-controlled, randomized study, J Allergy Clin Immunol 99:757-762, 1997.

24. Daroca P, Crespo JF, Reano M, et al: Asthma and rhinitis induced by exposure to raw green beans and chards, *Ann Allergy Asthma Immunol* 85:215-218, 2000.

25. Crespo JF, Pascual C, Dominguez C, et al: Allergic reactions associated with airborne fish particles in IgE-mediated fish hypersensitive patients, *Allergy* 50:257-261, 1995.

26. Sicherer DH, Furlong TJ, DeSimone J, et al: Self-reported peanut allergic reactions on commercial airlines, *J Allergy Clin Immunol* 103:186-189, 1999.

27. Baur X, Posch A: Characterized allergens causing bakers' asthma, *Allergy* 53:562-566, 1998.

28. Crespo JF, Rodriguez J, Vives R, et al: Occupational IgE-mediated allergy after exposure to lupine seed flour, *J Allergy Clin Immunol* 108:295-297, 2001.

29. James JM, Bernhisel-Broadbent J, Sampson HA: Respiratory reactions provoked by double-blind food challenges in children, *Am J Respir Crit Care Med* 149:59-64, 1994.

30. Pinnock CB, Graham NM, Mylvaganam A, et al: Relationship between milk intake and mucus production in adult volunteers challenged with rhinovirus-2, *Am Rev Respir Dis* 141:352-356, 1990.

31. Woods RK, Weiner JM, Abramson M, et al: Do dairy products induce bronchoconstriction in adults with asthma? *J Allergy Clin Immunol* 101:45-50, 1998.

32. Raphael G, Raphael M, Kaliner M: Gustatory rhinitis: a syndrome of food-induced rhinorrhea, *J Allergy Clin Immunol* 83:110-115, 1989.

33. Nsouli TM, Nsouli SM, Linde RE, et al: Role of food allergy in serous otitis media, *Ann Allergy* 73:215-219, 1994.

34. Bernstein JM: The role of IgE-mediated hypersensitivity in the development of otitis media with effusion: a review, *Otolaryngol Head Neck Surg* 109:611-620, 1993.

35. Juntti H, Tikkanen S, Kokkonen J, et al: Cow's milk allergy is associated with recurrent otitis media during childhood, *Acta Otolaryngol* 119: 867-873, 1999.

36. Heiner DC, Sears JW: Chronic respiratory disease associated with multiple circulation precipitins to cow's milk, *Am J Dis Child* 100:500-502, 1960.

37. Lee SK, Kniker WT, Cook CD, et al: Cow's milk-induced pulmonary disease in children, *Adv Pediatr* 25:39-57, 1978.

38. Novembre E, de Martino M, Vierucci A: Foods and respiratory allergy, *J Allergy Clin Immunol* 81:1059-1065, 1988.

39. Oehling A, Baena Cagnani CE: Food allergy and child asthma, *Allergol et Immunopathol* 8:7-14, 1980.

40. Businco L, Falconieri P, Giampietro P, et al: Food allergy and asthma, *Pediatr Pulmonary (Suppl)* 11:59-60, 1995.

41. Yazicioglu M, Baspinar I, Ones U, et al: Egg and milk allergy in asthmatic children: assessment by immulite allergy panel, skin prick tests and double-blind placebo-controlled food challenges, *Allergol et Immunopathol* 27:287-293, 1999.

42. Hill DJ, Firer MA, Shelton MJ, et al: Manifestations of milk allergy in infancy: clinical and immunological findings, *J Pediatr* 109:270-276, 1986.

43. Bock SA: Respiratory reactions induced by food challenges in children with pulmonary disease, *Pediatr Allergy Immunol* 3:188-194, 1992.

44. James JM, Eigenmann PA, Eggleston PA, et al: Airway reactivity changes in asthmatic patients undergoing blinded food challenges, *Am J Respir Crit Care Med* 153:597-603, 1996.

45. Zwetchkenbawn JF, Skufca R, Nelson HS: An examination of food hypersensitivity as a cause of increased bronchial responsiveness to inhaled methacholine, *J Allergy Clin Immunol* 88:360-364, 1991.

46. Sicherer DH, Burks AW, Sampson HA: Clinical features of acute allergic reactions to peanut and tree nuts in children, *Immunol Allergy Clin North Am* 102:6, 1998.

47. Cianferoni A, Novembre E, Mugnaini L, et al: Clinical features of acute anaphylaxis in patients admitted to a university hospital: an 11-year retrospective review (1985-1996), *Ann Allergy Asthma Immunol* 87:27-32, 2001.

48. James JM, Burks AW: Foods, *Immunol Clin N Am* 15:477-488, 1995.

49. Roesler TA, Barry PC, Bock SA: Factitious food allergy and failure to thrive, *Arch Pediatr Adolesc Med* 148:1150-1155, 1994.

50. Sampson HA: Food allergy: diagnosis and management, *J Allergy Clin Immunol* 103:981-989, 1999.

51. Bock SA, Buckley J, Holst A, et al: Proper use of skin tests with food extracts in diagnosis of food hypersensitivity, *Clin Allergy* 8:559-564, 1978.

52. Price GW, Hogan AD, Farris AH, et al: Sensitization (IgE antibody) to food allergens in wheezing infants and children, *J Allergy Clin Immunol* 96:266-270, 1995.

53. Sampson HA, Ho D: Relationship between food-specific IgE concentrations and the risk of positive food challenges in children and adolescents, *J Allergy Clin Immunol* 100:444-451, 1997.

54. Sampson HA: Utility of food specific IgE concentrations in predicting symptomatic food allergy, *J Allergy Clin Immunol* 107:891-896, 2001.

55. Wraith DG, Merret J, Roth A, et al: Recognition of food-allergic patients and their allergens by the RAST technique and clinical investigation, *Clin Allergy* 9:25-36, 1979.

56. James JM, Sampson HA: An overview of food hypersensitivity, *Pediatr Allergy Immunol* 3:67-78, 1992.

57. Condemi JJ: Unproved diagnostic and therapeutic techniques. In Metcalfe DD, Sampson HA, Simon RA, eds: *Food allergy: adverse reactions to foods and food additives*, ed 2, London, 1997, Blackwell Scientific Publications.

58. James JM: Unproven diagnostic and therapeutic techniques, *Curr Allergy Asthma Rep* 2:87-91, 2002.

59. Bock SA, Sampson HA, Atkins FM, et al: Double-blind placebo-controlled food challenge (DBPCFC) as an office procedure: a manual, *J Allergy Clin Immunol* 82:986-997, 1988.

60. David TJ, Waddington E, Stanton RHJ: Nutritional hazards of elimination diets in children with atopic dermatitis, *Arch Dis Child* 59:323-325, 1984.

61. McGowan M, Gibney MJ: Calcium intakes in individuals on diets for the management of cow's milk allergy: a case control study, *Eur J Clin Nutr* 47:609-616, 1993.

62. Davidovits M, Levy Y, Avramovitz T, et al: Calcium-deficiency rickets in a four-year-old boy with milk allergy, *J Pediatr* 122:249-251, 1993.

63. Gern J, Yang E, Evrard HM, et al: Allergic reactions to milk-contaminated "nondairy" products, *N Engl J Med* 324:976-979, 1991.

64. Barnes-Koerner C, Sampson HA: Diets and nutrition. In Metcalfe DD, Sampson HA, Simon RA, eds: *Food allergy: adverse reactions to foods and food additives*, ed 2, London, 1997, Blackwell Scientific Publications.

65. Spector SL, Nicklas RA: Practice parameters for the diagnosis and treatment of asthma, *J Allergy Clin Immunol* 96:707-870, 1995.

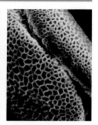

CHAPTER 51

Atopic Dermatitis and Food Hypersensitivity

STACIE M. JONES ■ WESLEY BURKS

Atopic dermatitis (AD) is a complex, chronic disorder that has been referred to as "the itch that rashes." The origin of AD is multifactorial, including many commonly encountered triggers. In 1892 Besnier[1] used the term *neurodermatitis* to describe a chronic, pruritic skin condition seen in patients with a nervous disorder. This familial disorder was termed *prurigo Besnier* because of its intensely pruritic quality. In the early 1900s, Coca and Cooke[2] noted the occurrence of a similar disorder with other diseases such as asthma and hay fever and used the term *atopy* to refer to the allergic constellation of these diseases. The term *atopic dermatitis* was then coined by Wise and Sulzberger[3] in 1933 to comprehensively describe this inheritable skin disorder. Since its earliest description, AD has had one primary feature recognized by clinicians and patients alike: intense pruritus triggered by a variety of stimuli. In this chapter, we explore how the ingestion of specific foods can trigger the condition of AD.

A strong correlation exists with AD and other atopic conditions such as asthma and allergic rhinitis. Approximately 50% of patients with AD will develop disease in the first year of life, and as many as 50% to 80% of children with AD will develop allergic respiratory disease later in life. In addition many clinicians note the peculiar tendency of AD and asthma to alternate in their courses in some patients. Because of these early historical observations, investigators have explored the role of various allergens as triggers for the pathogenesis of AD (Table 51-1).

Food allergy has been strongly correlated with the development and persistence of AD, especially during infancy and early childhood. The skin is the site that is most often involved in food hypersensitivity reactions. For most skin manifestations of food hypersensitivity, pruritus is a hallmark of the disease.

PATHOPHYSIOLOGY

In the early twentieth century, Schloss,[4] Talbot,[5] and Blackfan[6] published case reports of patients who had improvement in their AD after avoiding specific foods in their diet. Subsequent conflicting reports spurred controversy related to the role of specific food allergens in the pathogenesis of AD.[7] This controversy has continued into the twenty-first century, although there now is significant laboratory and clinical evidence that would suggest the debate is no longer valid. Recent studies have demonstrated that allergen-induced, IgE-mediated mast cell activation has as its end product hypersensitivity reactions characterized by tissue (i.e., skin) infiltration of monocytes and lymphocytes.[8,9] The pattern of cytokine expression found in lymphocytes infiltrating acute AD lesions are predominantly those of the T helper cell type 2 (Th2) (interleukin [IL]-4, IL-5, and IL-13).[10,11] In addition, these cytokines promote influx of activated eosinophils and release of eosinophil products.[10-13] IgE-bearing Langerhans cells that are up-regulated by these cytokines are highly efficient at presenting allergens to T cells, activating a combined Th1/Th2 profile in chronic lesions. Thus it appears that IgE antibody and the Th2 cytokine milieu combine to play a major role in the pathogenesis of these lesions.

Several recent articles have speculated on the role of food-specific T cells in the pathophysiology of AD.[14-16] In some patients who may have a delayed response to foods, these authors and others hypothesize that the reactions may occur via high-affinity IgE receptors expressed on Langerhans and dendritic cells leading to allergen-specific T cell responses capable of promoting IgE production and delayed-type hypersensitivity reactions.

LABORATORY INVESTIGATION

Several studies support a role for food-specific IgE antibody in the pathogenesis of AD. Patients have been shown to have elevated concentrations of total IgE and food-specific IgE antibodies.[17,18] More than 50 years ago, Walzer[19] and Wilson and Walzer[20] demonstrated that the ingestion of foods would allow food antigens to penetrate the gastrointestinal barrier and then be transported in the circulation to IgE-bearing mast cells in the skin. More recent investigations have shown that in children with food-specific IgE antibodies undergoing oral food challenges, positive challenges were accompanied by increases in plasma histamine concentration,[21] elaboration of eosinophil products,[22] and activation of plasma eosinophils[23] (Table 51-2).

Children with AD who were chronically ingesting foods to which they are allergic have been found to have increased "spontaneous" basophil histamine release (SBHR) from peripheral blood basophils *in vitro* compared with children without food allergy or normal subjects.[24] After placement on the appropriate elimination diet, food-allergic children experienced significant clearing of their skin and a significant fall in their SBHR.[24] Other studies have shown that peripheral

Allergic Triggers of Atopic Dermatitis

Food allergens (most common)
Milk
Eggs
Peanuts
Soy
Wheat
Shellfish
Fish

Aeroallergens
Pollen
Mold
Dust mite
Animal dander
Cockroach

Microorganisms
Bacteria
  Staphylococcus aureus
  Streptococcus species
Fungi/yeasts
  Pityrosporum ovale/orbiculare
  Trichophytan species
  Other yeast species (e.g., *Candida, Malazassia*)

blood mononuclear cells from food-allergic patients with high SBHR elaborate specific cytokines termed histamine-releasing factors (HRFs) that activate basophils from food-sensitive, but not food-insensitive, patients. Furthermore, passive sensitization experiments *in vitro* with basophils from nonatopic donors and IgE from patients allergic to specific foods showed that basophils could be rendered sensitive to HRFs.[24]

Food allergen–specific T cells have been cloned from normal skin and active skin lesions in patients with AD.[25,26] There has been some disagreement in the literature about the validity of *in vitro* lymphocyte-proliferation response to specific foods in this disorder. There appears to be an increase in antigen-specific lymphocyte proliferation, but there is considerable overlap in individual responses. Cutaneous lymphocyte-associated antigen (CLA) is a homing molecule that interacts with E-selectin and directs T cells to the skin. A study compared patients with milk-induced AD with control subjects with milk-induced gastrointestinal reactions without AD and with nonatopic control subjects.[25] Casein-reactive T cells from

Laboratory Investigation of Atopic Dermatitis and Food Hypersensitivity

Positive food challenges produce increases in
  Plasma histamine concentrations
  Activation of plasma eosinophils and eosinophil products
Patients ingesting foods to which they are allergic have
  Increased spontaneous basophil histamine release
  Histamine-releasing factors that activate basophils from food-sensitive patients
Patients with milk allergy have
  Higher expression of milk-specific activated cutaneous lymphocyte antigen

children with milk-induced AD had a significantly higher expression of CLA than *Candida albicans*–reactive T cells from the same patients and either casein or *C. albicans*–reactive T cells from the control groups.[25]

Multiple clinical studies have addressed the role of food allergy in AD. Investigators have shown that elimination of the relevant food allergen can lead to improvement in skin symptoms and that repeat challenge can lead to recurrence of symptoms. Additionally, the disease can be delayed by prophylactically eliminating highly allergenic foods (e.g., milk, eggs) from the diets of genetically at-risk infants and possibly breast-feeding mothers.[27]

A number of studies have addressed the therapeutic effect of dietary elimination in the treatment of AD. Atherton et al[28] reported that two thirds of children with AD between the ages of 2 and 8 years showed marked improvement during a double-blind crossover trial of milk and egg exclusion. However, there were problems in this study, including high dropout and exclusion rates as well as confounding variables such as environmental factors and other triggers of AD. Another trial by Neild et al[29] was able to demonstrate improvement in some patients during the milk and egg exclusion phase, but no significant difference was seen in 40 patients completing the crossover trial. Another study by Juto et al[30] reported that approximately one third of AD patients had resolution of their rash and that one half improved on a highly restricted diet. The cumulative results of these studies support the role for food allergy in the exacerbation of AD. Certainly, most of the trials failed to control confounding factors such as other trigger factors, as well as the placebo effect or observer bias.

In one of the original prospective follow-up studies, Sampson and Scanlon[31] studied 34 patients with AD, of whom 17 had food allergy diagnosed by double-blind, placebo-controlled food challenges (DBPCFCs). These patients were placed on an appropriate allergen elimination and experienced significant improvement in their clinical symptoms. At 1- to 2-year and 3- to 4-year follow-ups, the subjects were compared with control subjects who did not have food allergy and to children with food allergy who were not compliant with their diet. Food-allergic patients with appropriate dietary restriction demonstrated highly significant improvement in their AD compared with the control groups, and their time frame for outgrowing their food sensitivity was reduced.

Lever et al[32] performed a randomized controlled trial of egg elimination in young children with AD and a positive radioallergosorbent test (RAST) to eggs who presented to their dermatology clinic. At the end of this study, egg allergy was confirmed by oral challenge, and 55 children who were allergic to egg were ultimately identified. There was a significant decrease in the skin area affected, as well as symptom scores in the children avoiding eggs compared with the control subjects (percent involvement, 21.9% to 18.9%; symptom score, 36.7 to 33.5).

Oral food challenges have been used to demonstrate that food allergens can induce symptoms of rash and pruritus in children with food allergy–related AD. Sampson and Scanlon,[31] Sampson and McCaskill,[33] Sampson and Metcalfe,[34] and Eigenmann et al[35] published a number of articles using DBPCFCs to identify causal food proteins that are involved as trigger factors of AD. In studies during the past 20 years, they have conducted more than 2000 oral food challenges in more than 700 patients with greater than 40% of the challenges resulting in reactions. In their studies, as well as others to follow, they show that cutaneous reactions occurred in 75% of the positive challenges, generally consisting of pruritic, morbiliform, or macular eruptions in the predilection sites for AD. Isolated skin symptoms were seen in only 30% of the reactions; gastrointestinal (50%) and respiratory (45%) reactions also occurred. Almost all reactions occurred within the first hour of beginning the oral challenges. Clinical reactions to egg, milk, wheat, and soy accounted for almost 75% of the reactions. Some patients had repeated reactions during a series of daily challenges and had increasingly severe AD, further showing that ingestion of the causal food protein can trigger itching and scratching with recrudescence of typical lesions of AD.

Subsequent studies confirmed that a limited number of foods cause clinical symptoms in younger patients with AD.[36,37] Milk, eggs, and peanuts generally cause more than 75% of the IgE-mediated reactions. If soy, wheat, fish, and tree nuts are added to this list of foods, more than 98% of the foods that cause clinical symptoms would be identified.

Additional studies have been done to show that patients with AD could have their disease ameliorated through elimination of causal food proteins and that reintroduction of these proteins would elicit symptoms. Dietary intervention has been attempted during pregnancy, lactation, and early feeding in "at-risk" infants. In two series, infants from atopic families whose mothers excluded eggs, milk, and fish from their diets during lactation (prophylaxis group) had significantly less AD and food allergy compared at 18 months with those infants whose mothers' diets were unrestricted.[38,39] Follow-up at 4 years showed that the prophylaxis group had less AD, but there was no difference in food allergy or respiratory allergy.[39] In a comprehensive, prospective, randomized allergy prevention trial, Zeiger,[40] Zeiger and Heller,[41] and Zeiger et al[42,43] compared the benefits of maternal and infant food allergen avoidance on the prevention of allergic disease in infants at high risk for allergic disease. Breast-feeding was encouraged in both prophylaxis and control groups. In the prophylaxis group, eggs, cow's milk, and peanuts were restricted from the diets of lactating mothers; a casein hydrolysate formula was used for supplementation or weaning, and solid food introduction was delayed. The control infants received cow's milk formula for supplementation and the American Academy of Pediatrics' recommendations for infant feeding were followed (peanuts, nuts, and fish are not recommended in the first 3 years). The results show that the prevalence of AD in food allergy in the prophylaxis group was reduced significantly in the first 2 years compared with the control group; however, the period prevalence of AD was no longer significant beyond 2 years. These studies also failed to show that treatment of at-risk infants could modify allergic disease after 2 years of age. A recent meta-analysis concluded that exclusive breast-feeding during the first 3 months of life is associated with lower incidence rates of AD during childhood in children with a family history of atopy.[44] The authors concluded that breast-feeding should be strongly recommended to mothers of infants with a family history of atopy as a possible means of preventing AD. Recent studies have speculated on the possibility of delayed reactions to food playing a part in exacerbations of AD in certain patients.[14-16,45,46] These investigators and others have concluded

that a positive atopy patch test (APT; discussed later) with T cell infiltration of the skin correlates with clinical late-phase reactions and is associated with T cell–mediated allergen-specific immune responses.[14]

EPIDEMIOLOGY OF FOOD ALLERGY IN ATOPIC DERMATITIS

The prevalence of food allergy in patients with AD varies with the age of the patient and severity of AD. Burks et al[36,37] diagnosed food allergy in approximately 35% of 165 patients with AD referred to both university allergy and university dermatology clinics. Because many of the patients were referred to an allergist, it was possible that there was an ascertainment bias favoring food allergy in those patients with AD. Eigenmann et al[35] undertook a study to address this potential bias by studying 63 unselected children with moderate to severe AD who were referred to a university dermatologist. After an evaluation including oral food challenges, 37% of these patients were diagnosed with food allergy. In another study by Guillet and Guillet[47] that evaluated more than 250 children with AD, they noted that increased severity of AD in the younger patients was directly correlated with the presence of food allergy. Additional studies in adults with severe AD are relatively limited and have not shown a significant role for food allergy[48] or success in reducing symptoms during trials of elimination diets.[49]

DIAGNOSIS

General Approach

The diagnosis of food allergy in AD is complicated by several factors related to the disease: (1) the immediate response to ingestion of causal foods is apparently down-regulated with repetitive ingestion, making obvious "cause-and-effect" relations by history difficult to establish; (2) other environmental trigger factors (other allergens, irritants, infection) may play a role in the waxing and waning of the disease, obscuring the effect of dietary changes; and (3) patients have the ability to generate IgE to multiple allergens, many not associated with clinical symptoms, making diagnosis based solely on laboratory testing impossible (Table 51-3).

A complete medical history must include any pertinent details concerning the dietary history (e.g., timing of the reaction after ingestion, specific foods involved, recurrence of symptoms) and any acute reactions (e.g., hives, asthma, exacerbation of AD, etc.) following particular food ingestions (Figure 51-1). For breast-fed infants, a maternal dietary

---

TABLE 51-3 Factors Related to Atopic Dermatitis that Complicate the Diagnosis of Food Allergy

- Immediate response to ingestion of causal foods is apparently down-regulated with repetitive ingestion, making obvious "cause-and-effect" relations by history difficult to establish.
- Other environmental trigger factors (other allergens, irritants, infection) may play a role in the waxing and waning of the disease, obscuring the effect of dietary changes.
- Patients have the ability to generate IgE to multiple allergens, making diagnosis based solely on laboratory testing impossible.

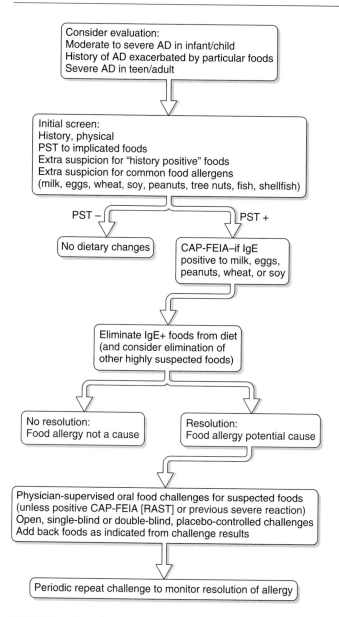

FIGURE 51-1 General approach to evaluation of food allergy in atopic dermatitis *(AD)*. *PST,* Prick skin test. (From Sicherer SH, Sampson HA: *J Allergy Clin Immunol* 104:S114-S122, 1999.)

TABLE 51-4 Foods Responsible for the Majority of Food-Allergic Reactions

Infants	Children	Older Children/Adults
Cow's milk	Cow's milk	Peanuts
Eggs	Eggs	Tree nuts
Peanuts	Peanuts	Fish
Soy	Soy	Shellfish
	Wheat	
	Tree nuts (walnut, cashew, etc.)	
	Fish	
	Shellfish	

From Sicherer SH, Sampson HA: *J Allergy Clin Immunol* 104:S114-S122, 1999.

wheat, fish, and tree nuts (walnut, cashew, pecan) by using PSTs or RAST[35,37] with additional testing for other suspected foods obtained by the history or given by the parents. If PSTs reveal specific IgE to certain foods, then determining the quantity of food-specific IgE antibodies (e.g., CAP-FEIA Pharmacia) to the positive allergens would indicate whether food challenges are necessary. After the laboratory studies are performed, the best initial treatment would be elimination of that suspected food from the diet, followed by a food challenge if indicated. No further testing or food challenges may be necessary in cases of severe, acute reactions or if dramatic improvement in skin disease occurs. Because symptoms are chronic in AD and often a large number of foods are implicated, it is often necessary to perform diagnostic oral food challenges.

IN VIVO AND IN VITRO LABORATORY TESTING

Currently several methods are available for detecting food-specific IgE. PSTs are often performed by using a device such as a bifurcated needle or lance to puncture the skin through a glycerinated extract of food with appropriate positive (histamine) and negative (saline-glycerin) controls. A positive response is a wheal of 3 mm or larger 15 minutes after placement of the skin test. PSTs are most informative when negative because the negative predictive value (NPV) of the tests is very high (> 95%).[55,56] Conversely, the positive predictive value (PPV) is generally 30% to 50%[55,56] and must be correlated with the clinical history and food challenges. In interpreting these studies, the positive PST result in isolation cannot be considered proof of a clinically relevant food reaction. On the other hand, a negative food-specific test virtually rules out IgE-mediated food allergy. Intradermal allergy skin tests with food extracts should not be performed because of an unacceptably high false-positive rate and a much higher risk for adverse reactions.[56] In the case of fruits and vegetables, it may be necessary to use fresh fruits and vegetables in a prick-by-prick method because the fresh products are more reliable than the commercially available skin test extracts (because of the lability of the allergens).

Although slightly less sensitive than skin prick tests, *in vitro* tests for specific IgE antibodies (RASTs) are practical in the screening of food allergy in most office settings. Like skin

history is also helpful because of the passage of food proteins in breast milk. As indicated by the patient's history and the most common foods triggering the disease, selected foods are evaluated by tests for specific IgE (e.g., prick skin test [PST], RAST). A small number of foods account for more than 90% of reactions[33,37,50] (Table 51-4). In children, the most common foods causing reactions are eggs, milk, peanuts, soy, wheat, tree nuts, and fish. In children with AD and food allergy, two thirds are reactive to eggs.[51] In adults, peanuts, tree nuts, fish, and shellfish are most frequently implicated in significant food-allergic reactions, but as previously mentioned, food allergy as a cause for AD in adults is not frequently seen. Food additives have been documented to cause flaring of AD but with a much lower prevalence.[52-54]

The best general approach is to screen children with moderate to severe AD for sensitivity to eggs, milk, peanuts, soy,

tests, a negative result is very reliable in ruling out an IgE-mediated reaction to a particular food, but a positive result has low specificity. In two studies by Sampson and Ho[57] and Sampson,[58] the investigators compared the role of DBPCFCs with the serum concentration levels of food-specific IgE antibody obtained by using the Pharmacia CAP system (FEIA; kU/L) in several hundred patients (Table 51-5). For certain allergens (eggs, milk, peanuts, and fish), CAP-FEIA levels exist that correlate very highly with clinical reactivity (see Table 51-5). Those patients with concentrations of food-specific IgE above these defined values would likely react on ingestion of the food and therefore would not likely need further evaluation. Unless indicated by previous history, an oral challenge may be needed to confirm reactivity for children with levels falling below the 90% or 95% PPV. Patients with specific IgE levels that are more than 95% NPV would not need further evaluation unless indicated in their clinical history.

The APT (patients had foods placed in solution and then on uninvolved skin for 48 to 72 hours before reading) has been advocated in recent articles[14-16,45] as an additional means of diagnosing food allergy in patients with AD. Some authors use the APT in diagnosing only patients with possible delayed food reactions, whereas others use the test after either allergy PSTs or RAST studies.

Other tests have been studied, including measurements of IgG$_4$ antibody, provocation-neutralization, cytotoxicity, applied kinesiology, and others that have not been shown to be useful for the diagnosis of food allergy in this disease.[59]

Patients with AD will often have positive skin tests and/or RASTs to several members of a botanical family (e.g., wheat and grass) or animal species (e.g., egg and chicken), more likely indicating immunologic cross-reactivity but not symptomatic intrabotanical or intraspecies cross-reactivity. In an initial study, legume cross-reactivity was evaluated in 69 children with AD by use of PST, RAST, and immunoblot analyses.[60,61] Immunologic reactivity was demonstrated in most patients; however, only 2 patients were symptomatic to more than one legume when challenged. Both of the patients had a history of severe allergic reaction to peanut and mild reactions to soy challenge. Similar studies with cereal grains have shown significant IgE cross-reactivity but very little (about 20%) clinical cross-reactivity.[62] More than 50% of children allergic to eggs have IgE antibodies to chicken meat, but few (about

5%) have clinical reactivity. Additionally, approximately 50% of children who are allergic to milk have a positive PST or RAST to beef but only 10% of these exhibit clinical symptoms. There appears to be more cross-reactivity among the food families from shellfish, fish, and tree nuts once an allergy to one type of these foods is identified. However, the practice of avoiding all foods within a botanical family when one member is suspected of provoking allergic symptoms generally appears to be unwarranted (except for tree nuts, fish, and shellfish).

ORAL FOOD CHALLENGES

Oral food challenges are invaluable in the appropriate diagnosis and management of patients with AD and possible food allergy. Oral challenges are also necessary to evaluate the resolution (or development of tolerance) of the specific food allergy. However, oral challenges are contraindicated when there is a clear, recent history of food-induced airway reactivity or anaphylaxis. Additionally, patients should not be instructed to perform home food challenges because of the potential risk of severe allergic reactions.[63] DBPCFCs are considered the gold standard for diagnosing food allergy.[50,55,64] Certainly in evaluating any scientific literature, DBFCFCs should be part of any major contribution to this literature. If allergic reactions to only a few foods are suspected, single-blind or open challenges may be useful to screen for reactivity. One caveat in this situation is that these challenges are subject to observer and patient bias and may overestimate the reactivity. In blinded food challenges, the patient must have the food antigen blinded in a material to mask the taste and smell of the food (grape or apple juice). On completing the blinded portion, patients must take the food openly to confirm the blinded portion of the challenge.

MANAGEMENT

For the best clinical results, the elimination of the offending food, when properly diagnosed, should be added to medical management of AD. The elimination of food proteins can often be a difficult task. Incomplete elimination of the offending food can lead to confusion and inconclusive results during an open trial of dietary elimination. For example, in a

TABLE 51-5 Performance Characteristics of 90% Specificity Diagnostic Decision Points Generated in the Prospective Study in Diagnosing Food Allergy in 100 Consecutive Children and Adolescents Referred for Evaluation of Food Hypersensitivity

Allergen	Decision Point (kU/L)	Sensitivity (%)	Specificity (%)	Efficiency (%)	PPV (%)	NPV (%)
Eggs	7	61	95	68	98	38
Milk	15	57	94	69	95	53
Peanuts	14	57	100	84	100	36
Fish	3	63	91	87	56	93
Soybean	30	44	94	81	73	82
Wheat	26	61	92	84	74	87

From Sampson HA: *J Allergy Clin Immunol* 107:891-896, 2001.
PPV, Positive predictive value; *NPV*, negative predictive value.
Given are PPV and NPV of food-specific IgE concentrations for predicting reactions on oral challenge by using the Pharmacia CAP-RAST System FEIA.
As seen in Table 51-4, the PPVs for eggs, milk, and peanuts on the basis of the 90% specificity values are excellent (i.e., 98% to 100%) but are less predictive for fish, wheat, and soy (i.e., 56%, 73%, and 74%, respectively).

milk-free diet, patients must be instructed not only to avoid all milk products but also to read all food labels to identify "hidden" sources of cow's milk protein. The terms on labels may include words such as *casein, whey, lactalbumin, caramel color,* and *nougat,* which indicate the presence of cow's milk. Recent studies[65] indicate that it is difficult even for patients with nutritional counseling to always understand the food label. Patients and parents must be aware that the food protein, as opposed to sugar or fat, is the primary reason for the hypersensitivity reaction and is the substance that needs to be avoided in the diet. For example, lactose-free milk contains cow's milk protein, and many egg substitutes contain chicken egg proteins. Conversely, peanut oil and soy oil generally do contain allergenic food protein unless the processing method is one in which the protein is not completely eliminated (as with cold pressed or "extruded" oil).[66]

Accidental ingestion of known allergenic foods, despite good nutritional counseling, is relatively common. The Food Allergy and Anaphylaxis Network, Fairfax, VA (800-929-4040, www.foodallergy.org) is a lay organization that provides valuable educational materials to assist families, physicians, and schools in the difficult task of eliminating allergenic foods and in the appropriate treatment of accidental food ingestions. An emergency plan must be in place to treat severe reactions (respiratory reactions, anaphylaxis) caused by accidental ingestion of these foods. Patients with previously severe, acute reactions, those with underlying asthma, and patients allergic to peanuts, tree nuts, fish, and shellfish may be more at risk for acute, severe reactions. Injectable epinephrine (an appropriate dose) and oral antihistamines should be readily available to treat these patients at all times. Equally important, when multiple foods are eliminated from the diet, it is prudent to enlist the help of a dietitian in formulating a nutritionally balanced diet.[67]

NATURAL HISTORY

Most children outgrow their allergies to milk, eggs, wheat, and soy[68] (Table 51-6). Patients allergic to peanuts, tree nuts, fish, and shellfish are much less likely to lose their clinical reactivity.[69] It does appear, however, that approximately 20% of patients who have a reaction to peanuts early in life may outgrow their sensitivity. Approximately one third of children with AD and food allergy lost or outgrew their clinical reactivity over 1 to 3 years with strict adherence to dietary elimination, which was believed to have aided in a more timely recovery.[31] Clinical reactivity is lost over time more quickly than the loss of

TABLE 51-6 Natural History of Food Hypersensitivity

Food allergy often outgrown by school age
Milk
Eggs
Soy
Wheat

Food allergy often *not* outgrown by school age
Peanuts
Tree nuts
Fish
Shellfish

BOX 51-1	**KEY CONCEPTS**
	Food Allergy Pearls

- About one third of children with moderate to severe atopic dermatitis (AD) are affected by food hypersensitivity.
- The younger the child and the more severe the eczema, the more likely the child is affected by food hypersensitivity.
- Egg allergy is the most common food hypersensitivity in children with AD; egg, milk, and peanut allergy account for about 80% of food allergy diagnosed by food challenge in children with AD.
- Appropriate diagnosis of food allergy and elimination of the responsible food allergen lead to significant clearing of the eczematous lesions in the majority of children with AD and food allergy.
- Infants with AD and egg allergy are at high risk for developing respiratory allergy and asthma.

food-specific IgE measured by PST or RAST testing. Certainly children with food allergy need to be followed at regular intervals with appropriate oral challenges to determine when they outgrow their food sensitivity.

CONCLUSIONS

The triggers associated with disease pathogenesis and clinical symptoms for patients with AD are vast (Box 51-1). The role of allergens, particularly food allergens, early in life is clearly very important. A careful history and appropriate diagnostic testing coupled with a comprehensive treatment program can be disease modifying and life altering for patients with AD.

HELPFUL WEBSITE

The Food Allergy and Anaphylaxis Network website (www.foodallergy.org)

REFERENCES

1. Besnier E: Premiere note et observations preliminaires pour sevir d'introduction a l'etude des prurigos diathesiques, *Ann de Dermatol* 23:634, 1892.
2. Coca AF, Cooke RA: On the classification of the phenomena of hypersensitiveness, *J Immunol* 8:163-182, 1923.
3. Wise F, Sulzberger MB: Eczematous eruptions. In: *Year Book of Dermatology and Syphilogy,* Chicago, 1933, Year Book Medical.
4. Schloss OM: Allergy to common foods, *Trans Am Pediatr Soc* 27:62-68, 1915.
5. Talbot FB: Eczema in childhood, *Med Clin North Am* 985-996, 1918.
6. Blackfan KD: A consideration of certain aspects of protein hypersensitiveness in children, *Am J Med Sci* 160:341-350, 1920.
7. Hanifin JM: Critical evaluation of food and mite allergy in the management of atopic dermatitis, *J Dermatol* 24:495-503, 1997.
8. Solley GO, Gleich GJ, Jordon RE, et al: The late phase of the immediate wheal and flare skin reaction. Its dependence upon IgE antibodies, *J Clin Invest* 58:408-420, 1976.
9. Lemanske R, Kaliner M: Late-phase allergic reactions. In Middleton E, Reed C, Ellis E, et al, eds: *Allergy: principles and practice,* ed 3, St Louis, 1988, Mosby.
10. Hamid Q, Boguniewicz M, Leung DY: Differential *in situ* cytokine gene expression in acute versus chronic atopic dermatitis, *J Clin Invest* 94:870-876, 1994.

11. Hamid Q, Naseer T, Minshall EM, et al: *In vivo* expression of IL-12 and IL-13 in atopic dermatitis, *J Allergy Clin Immunol* 98:225-231, 1996.

12. Tsicopoulos A, Hamid Q, Varney V, et al: Preferential messenger RNA expression of Th1-type cells (IFN-gamma+, IL- 2+) in classical delayed-type (tuberculin) hypersensitivity reactions in human skin, *J Immunol* 148:2058-2061, 1992.

13. Leiferman KM, Ackerman SJ, Sampson HA, et al: Dermal deposition of eosinophil-granule major basic protein in atopic dermatitis: comparison with onchocerciasis, *N Engl J Med* 313:282-285, 1985.

14. Niggemann B, Reibel S, Wahn U: The atopy patch test (APT): a useful tool for the diagnosis of food allergy in children with atopic dermatitis, *Allergy* 55:281-285, 2000.

15. Niggemann B, Reibel S, Roehr CC, et al: Predictors of positive food challenge outcome in non-IgE-mediated reactions to food in children with atopic dermatitis, *J Allergy Clin Immunol* 108:1053-1058, 2001.

16. Kekki OM, Turjanmaa K, Isolauri E: Differences in skin-prick and patch-test reactivity are related to the heterogeneity of atopic eczema in infants, *Allergy* 52:755-759, 1997.

17. Johnson EE, Irons JS, Patterson R, et al: Serum IgE concentration in atopic dermatitis. Relationship to severity of disease and presence of atopic respiratory disease, *J Allergy Clin Immunol* 54:94-99, 1974.

18. Hoffman DR: Food allergy in children: RAST studies with milk and egg. In Evans RI, ed: *Advances in diagnosis of allergy: RAST*, New York, 1975, Stratton.

19. Walzer M: Studies in absorption of undigested proteins in human beings: I. A simple direct method of studying the absorption of undigested protein, *J Immunol* 14:143-174, 1927.

20. Wilson SJ, Walzer M: Absorption of undigested proteins in human beings, IV: absorption of unaltered egg protein in infants, *Am J Dis Child* 50:49-54, 1935.

21. Sampson HA, Jolie PL: Increased plasma histamine concentrations after food challenges in children with atopic dermatitis, *N Engl J Med* 311: 372-376, 1984.

22. Suomalainen H, Soppi E, Isolauri E: Evidence for eosinophil activation in cow's milk allergy, *Pediatr Allergy Immunol* 5:27-31, 1994.

23. Magnarin M, Knowles A, Ventura A, et al: A role for eosinophils in the pathogenesis of skin lesions in patients with food-sensitive atopic dermatitis, *J Allergy Clin Immunol* 96:200-208, 1995.

24. Sampson HA, Broadbent KR, Bernhisel-Broadbent J: Spontaneous release of histamine from basophils and histamine-releasing factor in patients with atopic dermatitis and food hypersensitivity, *N Engl J Med* 321:228-232, 1989.

25. Abernathy-Carver KJ, Sampson HA, Picker LJ, et al: Milk-induced eczema is associated with the expansion of T cells expressing cutaneous lymphocyte antigen, *J Clin Invest* 95:913-918, 1995.

26. Van Reijsen FC, Bruijnzeel-Koomen CA, Kalthoff FS, et al: Skin-derived aeroallergen-specific T-cell clones of Th2 phenotype in patients with atopic dermatitis, *J Allergy Clin Immunol* 90:184-193, 1992.

27. Zeiger RS: Dietary aspects of food allergy prevention in infants and children, *J Pediatr Gastroenterol Nutr* 30:S77-S86, 2000.

28. Atherton DJ, Sewell M, Soothill JF, et al: A double-blind controlled crossover trial of an antigen-avoidance diet in atopic eczema, *Lancet* 1:401-403, 1978.

29. Neild VS, Marsden RA, Bailes JA, et al: Egg and milk exclusion diets in atopic eczema, *Br J Dermatol* 114:117-123, 1986.

30. Juto P, Engberg S, Winberg J: Treatment of infantile atopic dermatitis with a strict elimination diet, *Clin Allergy* 8:493-500, 1978.

31. Sampson HA, Scanlon SM: Natural history of food hypersensitivity in children with atopic dermatitis, *J Pediatr* 115:23-27, 1989.

32. Lever R, MacDonald C, Waugh P, et al: Randomised controlled trial of advice on an egg exclusion diet in young children with atopic eczema and sensitivity to eggs, *Pediatr Allergy Immunol* 9:13-19, 1998.

33. Sampson HA, McCaskill CC: Food hypersensitivity and atopic dermatitis: evaluation of 113 patients, *J Pediatr* 107:669-675, 1985.

34. Sampson HA, Metcalfe DD: Food allergies, *JAMA* 268:2840-2844, 1992.

35. Eigenmann PA, Sicherer SH, Borkowski TA, et al: Prevalence of IgE-mediated food allergy among children with atopic dermatitis, *Pediatrics* 101:E8, 1998.

36. Burks AW, Mallory SB, Williams LW, et al: Atopic dermatitis: clinical relevance of food hypersensitivity reactions, *J Pediatr* 113:447-451, 1988.

37. Burks AW, James JM, Hiegel A, et al: Atopic dermatitis and food hypersensitivity reactions, *J Pediatr* 132:132-136, 1998.

38. Hattevig G, Kjellman B, Sigurs N, et al: Effect of maternal avoidance of eggs, cow's milk and fish during lactation upon allergic manifestations in infants, *Clin Exp Allergy* 19:27-32, 1989.

39. Sigurs N, Hattevig G, Kjellman B: Maternal avoidance of eggs, cow's milk, and fish during lactation: effect on allergic manifestations, skin-prick tests, and specific IgE antibodies in children at age 4 years, *Pediatrics* 89:735-739, 1992.

40. Zeiger RS: Prevention of food allergy in infancy, *Ann Allergy* 65:430-442, 1990.

41. Zeiger RS, Heller S: The development and prediction of atopy in high-risk children: follow-up at age seven years in a prospective randomized study of combined maternal and infant food allergen avoidance, *J Allergy Clin Immunol* 95:1179-1190, 1995.

42. Zeiger RS, Heller S, Mellon MH, et al: Effect of combined maternal and infant food-allergen avoidance on development of atopy in early infancy: a randomized study, *J Allergy Clin Immunol* 84:72-89, 1989.

43. Zeiger R, Heller S, Mellon M, et al: Genetic and environmental factors affecting the development of atopy through age 4 in children of atopic patents: a prospective randomized Study of food allergen avoidance, *Pediatr Allergy Immunol* 3:110-127, 1992.

44. Gdalevich M, Mimouni D, David M, et al: Breast-feeding and the onset of atopic dermatitis in childhood: a systematic review and meta-analysis of prospective studies, *J Am Acad Dermatol* 45:520-527, 2001.

45. Turjanmaa K: "Atopy patch tests" in the diagnosis of delayed food hypersensitivity, *Allerg Immunol (Paris)* 34:95-97, 2002.

46. Roehr CC, Reibel S, Ziegert M, et al: Atopy patch tests, together with determination of specific IgE levels, reduce the need for oral food challenges in children with atopic dermatitis, *J Allergy Clin Immunol* 107:548-553, 2001.

47. Guillet G, Guillet MH: Natural history of sensitizations in atopic dermatitis: a 3-year follow- up in 250 children: food allergy and high risk of respiratory symptoms, *Arch Dermatol* 128:187-192, 1992.

48. Maat-Bleeker F, Bruijnzeel-Koomen C: Food allergy in adults with atopic dermatitis, *Monogr Allergy* 32:157-163, 1996.

49. Munkvad M, Danielsen L, Hoj L, et al: Antigen-free diet in adult patients with atopic dermatitis: a double- blind controlled study, *Acta Derm Venereol* 64:524-528, 1984.

50. Bock SA, Atkins FM: Patterns of food hypersensitivity during sixteen years of double-blind, placebo-controlled food challenges, *J Pediatr* 117:561-567, 1990.

51. Sampson HA: Food sensitivity and the pathogenesis of atopic dermatitis, *J R Soc Med* 90:2-8, 1997.

52. Young E, Patel S, Stoneham M, et al: The prevalence of reaction to food additives in a survey population, *J R Coll Physicians Lond* 21:241-247, 1987.

53. Fuglsang G, Madsen G, Halken S, et al: Adverse reactions to food additives in children with atopic symptoms, *Allergy* 49:31-37, 1994.

54. Schwartz HJ: Food allergy: Adverse reactions to foods and food additives. In Metcalfe DD, Sampson HA, Simon RA, eds: *Asthma and food additives*, ed 2, 1997, Blackwell Science.

55. Sampson HA, Albergo R: Comparison of results of skin tests, RAST, and double-blind, placebo-controlled food challenges in children with atopic dermatitis, *J Allergy Clin Immunol* 74:26-33, 1984.

56. Bock SA, Buckley J, Holst A, et al: Proper use of skin tests with food extracts in diagnosis of hypersensitivity to food in children, *Clin Allergy* 7:375-383, 1977.

57. Sampson HA, Ho DG: Relationship between food-specific IgE concentrations and the risk of positive food challenges in children and adolescents, *J Allergy Clin Immunol* 100:444-451, 1997.

58. Sampson HA: Utility of food-specific IgE concentrations in predicting symptomatic food allergy, *J Allergy Clin Immunol* 107:891-896, 2001.

59. Terr A.I., Salvaggio JE: Controversial concepts in allergy and clinical immunology. In Bierman CW, Pearlman DS, Shapiro GG, et al, eds: *Allergy, asthma and immunology from infancy to adulthood*, ed 3, Philadelphia, 1996, WB Saunders.

60. Bernhisel-Broadbent J, Sampson HA: Cross-allergenicity in the legume botanical family in children with food hypersensitivity, *J Allergy Clin Immunol* 83:435-440, 1989.

61. Bernhisel-Broadbent J, Taylor S, Sampson HA: Cross-allergenicity in the legume botanical family in children with food hypersensitivity. II. Laboratory correlates, *J Allergy Clin Immunol* 84:701-709, 1989.

62. Jones SM, Magnolfi CF, Cooke SK, et al: Immunologic cross-reactivity among cereal grains and grasses in children with food hypersensitivity, *J Allergy Clin Immunol* 96:341-351, 1995.

63. David TJ: Hazards of challenge tests in atopic dermatitis, *Allergy* 44: 101-107, 1989.

64. Bock SA, Sampson HA, Atkins FM, et al: Double-blind, placebo-controlled food challenge (DBPCFC) as an office procedure: a manual, *J Allergy Clin Immunol* 82:986-997, 1988.

65. Joshi, J, Mofidi S, Sicherer SH: Interpretation of food labels by parents of food allergic children (abstract), *J Allergy Clin Immunol* 109:S91, 2002.

66. Hourihane JO, Bedwani SJ, Dean TP, et al: Randomised, double blind, crossover challenge study of allergenicity of peanut oils in subjects allergic to peanuts, *Br Med J* 314:1084-1088, 1997.

67. Salman S, Christie L, Burks W, et al: Dietary intakes of children with food allergies: comparison of the food guide pyramid and the recommended dietary allowances, *J Allergy Clin Immunol* 109:S214, 2002.

68. Bock SA: The natural history of food sensitivity, *J Allergy Clin Immunol* 69:173-177, 1982.

69. Skolnick HS, Conover-Walker MK, Koerner CB, et al: The natural history of peanut allergy, *J Allergy Clin Immunol* 107:367-374, 2001.

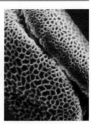

CHAPTER 52

Management of Food Allergy

SHIDEH MOFIDI ■ HUGH A. SAMPSON

The management of food allergy consists primarily of educating patients and their families on how to avoid specific food allergens. In addition, the child (if appropriate) and all caregivers must be taught to recognize early symptoms of an allergic reaction and to initiate treatment. Diagnosis and management of food hypersensitivities require a team approach involving the physician, registered dietitian, and nurse in addition to other allied health members such as the pharmacist and speech, occupational, and feeding therapists. Accurate identification of the allergenic foods is the first critical step of management of food allergies, as discussed in Chapter 45. The removal of the identified allergens from the diet either for a prolonged period or as a diagnostic intervention is the next step. Education about allergen avoidance and hidden sources of the suspect foods is essential. Finally, providing an adequate diet appropriate for growth and development of the child despite the removal of particular foods from the diet is essential in the management of children with food allergies. As discussed here, some medications may alter the course of hypersensitivity responses, but new immunomodulatory approaches hold promise for "treating" IgE-mediated food hypersensitivity.

If a child is allergic to a single food, the nutritional adequacy of the diet may not be compromised. However, if several major foods such as milk, egg, soy, and wheat are restricted from the diet, the impact on the quality of the diet is significant. Children with multiple food allergies are at risk for growth and nutritional deficiencies.

GROWTH AND NUTRITIONAL NEEDS OF INFANTS AND CHILDREN WITH FOOD HYPERSENSITIVITY

Assessment of Growth

Assessment of growth and nutrition is fundamental to the care of any infant or child. The same principles of assessing growth that are used for healthy children should be used for children with food allergies. Growth is assessed primarily by comparing values for weight, length, weight-to-length ratios, and head circumference against National Center for Health Statistics growth standards for boys and girls.[1] However, it is important to realize that these measurements alone have shortcomings.[2-5] Growth velocity is a more sensitive index than weight or length obtained at a specific time point. Growth velocity is a measure of changes in the parameters over time and should be used when assessing the nutritional status of infants and children. Height velocity and weight-to-length ratios are excellent measures of stature. Recumbent length should be used in infants younger than 2 years, having the infant lie supine on a flat surface and using a length board fitted against the soles of the feet and the crown of the head. A stadiometer or a height board should be used for children older than 2 years who can follow directions. Body mass index is useful after 2 years of age. Failure to achieve normal growth rates or growth velocity suggests the need to recheck measurements primarily and, if obtained correctly, to assess nutritional intake.

Food/Symptom Diaries and Food Labels

Assessing nutritional needs of infants and children can be accomplished by checking 24-hour recalls or 3-day diet records. A 24-hour recall can be easily used in the first 4 to 6 months of life because of the simple nature of the infant's intake. It is usually simple to recall the number of feedings either by breast-feeding or bottle-feeding and the amount consumed each time. Estimating the amount of breast milk may be difficult unless expressed milk is used. A 3-day diet record is beneficial for a child 6 months and older because day-to-day intake is more varied.

Food/symptom diaries are also an important component of the diagnostic process. Besides providing information that can be used to assess the adequacy of the diet, they serve as another means to check on foods consumed and the timing of the symptoms. Details such as the time of the meal or snack, the brand name if commercially prepared, specific ingredients if homemade, the amount consumed, and any accompanying symptoms should be recorded. Provision of the actual labels from the foods consumed enhances the evaluation provided by the dietitian.

Reviewing the food diaries can be a starting point for the dietitian to identify a particular food that is common to different products and is repeatedly causing similar symptoms. It also can reveal hidden sources of the food allergen or unknown sources of contamination. On occasion, particular foods that a family believes they are avoiding are in fact present in the diet and have actually been tolerated. This form of documentation essentially narrows the list of possible suspect foods for the child or can identify the presence of certain allergenic foods in the diet. It is highly unlikely that the child is allergic to everything he or she eats. In fact, it is much more likely that the child is receiving a particular food allergen in different forms and in different foods, prompting an expanding list of foods to avoid. Virtually any food protein can cause an allergic reaction; however, most children are sensitive to less than three foods. In children, egg, milk, peanuts, soy, wheat, tree nuts, and fish are responsible for 90% of the adverse food reactions.[6,7]

The list of foods and the timing of the meals consumed by the child are also helpful in assessing other factors that may be affecting the child's eating behavior and appetite, which can help facilitate directive counseling. Using alternative foods similar to what is recorded in the diet diary can also significantly enhance compliance with the restricted diet.

Nutritional Needs

Assessment of the quality of the diet and also degree of compliance is necessary to prevent future problems in growth and development. Particular attention should be made to calories, protein, and fat intake in addition to particular vitamins, minerals, and trace elements for children with food allergies. Another issue of concern is the distribution of carbohydrates, protein, and fats in the diet, which are altered and need to be addressed. Modifications in food choices should be made to ensure sufficient macronutrients, micronutrients, and energy intake.

Calories and Protein

Provision of adequate nutrients for appropriate growth and development of infants and children with food allergies is central in planning the diet. Nutrient requirements for infants and children with food allergies are similar to the requirements for healthy children based upon age and can be obtained from the Recommended Dietary Allowances (RDAs)

and, since 1998, the Dietary Reference Intakes (DRIs).[8,9] These published guidelines are updated periodically based on the current scientific research by The Food and Nutrition Board of the National Academy of Sciences. The DRI project has been divided into seven nutrient groups, and so far DRIs have been established for the first three groups: vitamins, minerals, and certain trace elements. Currently, the panel is working on establishing guidelines for macronutrients, including protein. Recommended intakes of protein and energy for normal healthy individuals based on the 1989 RDAs are provided in Table 52-1.

Provision of adequate essential amino acids by assuring sufficient intake of complete proteins and/or complementary proteins is critical for the diet of a child with multiple food allergies. Several factors affect nitrogen requirements, including the form and quantity in which nitrogen is consumed. Jones et al[10] reported increased nitrogen losses in healthy individuals receiving L-amino acids as their source of protein equivalent in comparison to individuals receiving intact whole protein. Hence, intake of adequate protein to cover nitrogen losses caused by poor utilization of amino acid–based formulas and protein hydrolysates, in addition to sufficient energy intake, should be recommended for children with food allergies.

Use of protein hydrolysates and/or amino acid–based elemental formulas may be necessary if sufficient intake of good-quality protein is compromised. For a child with moderate to severe atopic dermatitis, increased needs for calories and protein should be considered based on the degree of skin involvement.

Fats

It is important to note that providing adequate fats is critical to the diet of an allergic individual and obviously most crucial to the diet of infants and children. This is not only to provide adequate calories but also to meet essential fatty acid (EFA)

TABLE 52-1 Recommended Intakes of High-Quality Reference Protein and Calories for Normal Healthy Individuals Based on 1989 Recommended Dietary Allowances

Age (yr)	Weight (kg)	Protein (g/kg/day)	Energy (kcal/kg/day)
Infants			
0 to 0.5	6	2.2	108
0.5 to 1	9	1.6	98
Children			
1 to 3	13	1.2	102
4 to 6	20	1.1	90
7 to 10	28	1.0	70
Males			
11 to 14	45	1.0	55
15 to 18	66	0.9	45
19+	72 to 79	0.8	40
Females			
11 to 14	46	1.0	47
15 to 18	55	0.8	40
19+	58-65	0.8	38
Pregnancy		Add 10 g/day	Add 300 kcal/day
Lactation, first 6 mo		Add 15 g/day	Add 500 kcal/day
Lactation, second 6 mo		Add 12 g/day	Add 500 kcal/day

Modified from the Food and Nutrition Board, National Research Council: *Recommended dietary allowances*, ed 10, Washington, DC, 1989, National Academy Press.

requirements of the child. The fatty acids essential for humans are linoleic (C18:2n-6) and alpha-linolenic (C18:3n-3) acids. Linoleic acid and its derivative, arachidonic acid (C20:4n-6), function as precursors for eicosanoids, which include prostaglandins and leukotrienes involved in cell signaling mechanisms. Alpha-linolenic acid and its derivatives, eicosapentaenoic acid (C20:5n-3) and docosahexaenoic acid (C22:6n-3), function as important components of the brain and the retina of the eye. The optimum requirements for EFA of the n-3 and n-6 families for infants are still not known, although normal growth of infants depends on an adequate supply of EFAs. The Committee on Nutrition of the American Academy of Pediatrics (AAP) recommends that 2.7% (range, 1% to 4.5%) of energy intake be linoleic acid and that 1% of energy intake be linolenic acid.[11] This should ensure an adequate supply of EFA for tissue proliferation, membrane integrity, and eicosanoid formation. Kaila et al[12] studied the fatty acid content of alternative formulas used during infancy for children with cow's milk allergy. They analyzed two soy-based formulas, two casein hydrolysates, three whey hydrolysates, and two amino acid–based formulas with human milk as the control by gas chromatography. The quantity of fatty acids in the formulas analyzed was within the same range as breast milk and in the recommended range for linoleic acid intake. However, the linoleic–to–alpha-linolenic acid ratio, which is a prerequisite for the balanced synthesis of n-6 and n-3 very long-chain polyunsaturated fatty acids, was 1.5 to 2.5 times higher than the recommended amount in three of the studied formulas. The fatty acid composition of these formulas met the nutritional recommendations for healthy infants, but in children with food allergies, the effects of such elevations on inflammatory reactions are unknown and need further exploration.

Vegetable oils (except for coconut oil) are predominantly unsaturated with high quantities of linoleic acid and small amounts of linolenic acid. Major sources of linolenic acid include fish, fish oils, and oil extracted from seeds of *Oenothera biennis* (evening primrose). Fatty acids in the diet should be varied so that an equivalent blend of saturated, monounsaturated, and polyunsaturated fatty acids is provided. Typically, animal proteins provide adequate amounts of saturated fatty acids. Use of vegetable oils such as safflower, canola, corn, soybean, and olive oil is recommended to supply monounsaturated and polyunsaturated fatty acids and the necessary EFAs for the allergic individual.[13]

Carbohydrates

Carbohydrates are the primary source of energy for the body and provide between 40% and 60% of the caloric requirement. Grains, fruits, and vegetables are all good sources of carbohydrates. Complex carbohydrates should be emphasized in the diet not only for their nutrient contribution but also to provide fiber to the diet.

Vitamins, Minerals, and Trace Elements

The adequacy of vitamins, minerals, and trace elements is dependent on the variety of the foods in the diet. When one food or a food group is eliminated in the diet, alternative sources of nutrients that are lost through the elimination diet need to be identified. These diet limitations may be either from elimination diets instituted to determine if a suspect food is allergenic or by personal preference. Either way, the risk of nutritional deficiencies should be considered. The RDAs and DRIs for vitamins, minerals, and trace elements can be used as guidelines for children with food allergies. However, specific nutrient needs of children with food allergies are not known. Recently, Salman et al[14] reviewed the nutritional intake of a group of children (1 to 9 years of age) with known food allergies. Several nutrients, including calcium, iron, vitamin D, vitamin E, and zinc, were noted to be problem nutrients and were provided at less than 67% of the RDAs.

Table 52-2 can be helpful in determining which vitamins and minerals will be affected by the child's food restrictions. For example, if the allergy is to a food group that is a major contributor to the diet such as in cow's milk allergy, all dairy products should be avoided. Consequently, calcium, phosphorus, riboflavin, pantothenic acid, vitamin B_{12}, vitamin A, and vitamin D will need to be supplied from other sources. It is rather difficult to obtain adequate calcium from nondairy foods. There are, however, alternate drinks (soy and rice) and juices that are enriched with calcium. Milk-free calcium supplements can also be considered for use with milk-allergic children. Use of calcium-fortified juices that come in juice box form is discouraged because contamination with milk protein has been noted in several different products that come in juice box form (H.A. Sampson, personal communication). Juices that are from bottles or cans and/or in frozen form are not contaminated with milk protein. Intake of other foods in the diet needs to be evaluated to determine if an adequate amount of, for example, vitamin A is provided and, if necessary, to stress intake of foods high in vitamin A. Appendices I and II provide tables of food sources for vitamins, minerals, and trace elements that can help in the selection of particular foods based on their nutrient contribution to ensure an adequate diet for the allergic child.

Use of Supplemental Modules in Food Allergy

Several categories of supplements should be considered to enhance the intake of particular nutrients in children with food allergies. Complete formulas, vitamins, and mineral

---

TABLE 52-2 Vitamins and Minerals Provided by Different Food Allergens

Allergen	Vitamin and Minerals
Milk	Vitamin A, vitamin D, riboflavin, pantothenic acid, vitamin B_{12}, calcium, and phosphorus
Eggs	Vitamin B_{12}, riboflavin, pantothenic acid, biotin, and selenium
Soy	Thiamin, riboflavin, pyridoxine, folate, calcium, phosphorus, magnesium, iron, and zinc
Wheat	Thiamin, riboflavin, niacin, iron, and folate if fortified
Peanuts	Vitamin E, niacin, magnesium, manganese, and chromium

preparations and even fortified foods can help meet some of the nutrient requirements for the allergic child.

Complete Formulas

Several studies have looked at the use of protein hydrolysates or elemental formulas in infants and children with food allergies. Use of protein hydrosylates has been used with varying degrees of success in children with cow's milk allergy.[15-23] Amino acid–based formulas have been reported to effectively alleviate residual symptoms that did not completely resolve with protein hydrolysates.[17,24-26] Recently, two studies specifically addressed growth of children with multiple food allergies.[25,27] Isolauri et al[27] focused on growth in children with cow's milk allergy. In a group of 100 infants (> 12 months old) with cow's milk allergy and their age-matched healthy controls, length and weight for length index were noted to be decreased. The age at the onset of symptoms and the elimination diet were found to be major contributors to growth problems. Niggeman et al[25] looked at the efficacy of amino acid–based

formula versus extensively hydrolyzed cow's milk formula in children with cow's milk allergy and found improved growth specifically in length, despite similar intakes of calories. Use of any of these formulas, depending on the child's reactions, is highly recommended, especially if sufficient high-quality protein cannot be obtained from the foods allowed in the diet of the child with multiple food hypersensitivities.

Table 52-3 provides a comparison of the currently available protein hydrolysates (Nutramigen and Alimentum) and elemental formulas (Neocate, Neocate One+, and EleCare) that can be used for children with multiple food allergies. Nutramigen, Alimentum, and Neocate are available in 20 calories per ounce as the standard dilution with capability of concentrating. Neocate One+ and EleCare are available as 30 calories per ounce. Nutrient sources and selected nutrition information for each of the formulas per 100 g and per 100 calories are also provided to help with the selection of the most appropriate formula for the child. One hundred fifty milliliters of Nutramigen, Alimentum, or Neocate at 20 calories per ounce is

TABLE 52-3 Comparison of Protein Hydrolysates and Elemental Amino Acid Formulas

	Nutramigen*	Alimentum†	Neocate‡	Neocate One+‡	EleCare†
Preparation availability	Powder and RTF	Powder and RTF	Powder	Powder	Powder
Caloric density					
Standard solution (kcal/oz)	20	20	20	30	30
Can be prepared to other dilutions	Yes	Yes	Yes	Yes	Yes
Nutrition information	100 g powder/ 100 kcal RTF (150 ml)	100 g powder/ 100 kcal RTF (150 ml)	100 g powder/ 100 kcal (150 ml) mixed as 20 kcal/oz dilution	100 g/100 kcal (100 ml) mixed as 30 kcal/oz dilution	100 g/100 kcal (100 ml) mixed as 30 kcal/oz dilution
Calories	492/100	509/100	420/100	400/100	475/100
Protein (g)	14.2/2.8	14/2.75	13/3.1	10/2.5	14.3/3.01
Fat (g)	25/5	28.2/5.54	19/4.5	14/3.5	22.6/4.76
Carbohydrate (g)	55/11	51.9/10.2	49/11.7	58.4/14.6	51/10.7
Vitamin B_{12} (μg)	1.48/0.3	2.29/0.45	0.7/0.17	0.28/0.07	2.0/0.42
Calcium (mg)	460/94	534/105	522/124	248/62	515/108
Phosphorus (mg)	310/63	381/75	392/93.1	248/62	385/81
Iron (mg)	8.9/1.8	9.2/1.8	7.8/1.85	3.1/0.77	8.4/1.77
Zinc (mg)	4.9/1	3.81/0.75	7/1.66	3.1/0.77	5.3/1.12
Energy distribution (percent of total calories)					
Percent protein	11	11	12	10	15
Percent fat	45	48	47	32	42
Percent carbohydrate	44	41	41	58	43
Nutrient sources					
Protein source	Casein hydrolysate	Casein hydrolysate	Free L-amino acids	Free L-amino acids	Free L-amino acids
Carbohydrate source	Glucose polymers, modified corn starch	Sucrose, maltodextrin (powder), tapioca starch (RTF)	Corn syrup solids	Corn syrup solids	Corn syrup solids
Fat source	Corn oil	MCT oil, safflower oil, and soy oil	MCT oil and safflower oil	MCT oil, canola oil, and safflower oil	Safflower oil, MCT oil, and soy oil
Osmolality					
mOsm/kg water	320	320	360	610	596

RTF, Ready to feed; *MCT*, medium chain triglycerides.
*Mead Johnson Nutritionals, Evansville, Ind.
†Ross Products Division, Columbus, Ohio.
‡Scientific Hospital Supplies, Gaithersburg, Md.

calorically equivalent to 100 ml of Neocate One+ and EleCare at 30 calories per ounce. Review of the provision of the other nutrients is important to ensure an adequate intake of not only calories but also protein, calcium, zinc, vitamin B_{12}, and others based on the specific diet limitations of the child. For children who have trouble consuming sufficient quantities of formula to meet their growth needs, advancement to a more concentrated dilution of the formula may be appropriate. Care should be taken in advancing a child slowly from 20 to, for example, 30 calories per ounce by transitioning in several steps to avoid intolerance problems with the adjustment.

Continued use of these commercially prepared formulas as a supplement is sometimes recommended for children with multiple food allergies because providing sufficient nutrients may not be possible, because of limitations placed on the type of foods allowed or the quantity required to get adequate amounts of the necessary nutrients. It is common to see infants doing well on breast milk or commercially prepared complete formulas during the first year of life and then fail to thrive after the use of formulas or breast milk is discontinued. Use of formula as a supplement to table foods is even more critical for children who not only are avoiding the major sources of dietary protein for their age (milk, egg, and soy) but also are restricting meats either as a prophylactic measure or because of child or parental preference. If meats are allowed in the diet, sufficient quantities should be consumed to provide protein and other nutrients that are nutritionally required. Reviewing the intake of infant foods/table foods with the family before considering discontinuation of formula is strongly recommended. Encouraging the family to work on getting more meats in the diet and reviewing the child's intake at 3-month intervals may simply provide a safety net for the child until sufficient amounts of all the nutrients can be provided from the allowed list of foods. As the intake of meats or other foods increases, the quantity of formula can be reduced, signifying the decreased dependence on the nutrient contribution from the formula. This slow transition can also prevent situations in which failure to thrive is encountered after switching from a combination of formula/breast milk/infant foods to only table foods.

Vitamin and Mineral Supplements

A multivitamin and mineral supplement can also offer a safety net in relation to providing adequate vitamins and minerals. Unfortunately, most supplements that are marketed as milk free are potentially contaminated with milk proteins (e.g., lactose filler) and create problems for the milk-allergic child. Care should be taken in choosing a supplement that meets the child's needs. The manufacturer should be contacted to assess the possibility of contaminating food allergens. Concerns regarding cross-contamination are further discussed later.

Fortified Foods

Use of fortified baby cereals is another way to supplement the diets of children with multiple food allergies. For example, Beechnut Rice or Oat Cereal is fortified with vitamins and minerals to provide 25% calcium, 45% iron, 25% zinc, and 25% vitamin B_{12} of daily values in addition to several other vitamins in a 1/4-cup serving (15 g). The addition of even one serving of this cereal to the restricted diet of the food-allergic child can help provide several of the needed nutrients and serve as a supplement.

TABLE 52-4 Checklist to Determine Adequacy of Intake

- Is the child growing appropriately? Is the child continuing on his or her own growth curve?
- Is the quantity of breast milk or formula sufficient to promote growth?
- Are there additional foods in the diet that are not appropriate for age or based on the child's allergies?
- Is the quantity of other liquids in the diet such as juice, rice milk, or herbal/colic remedies appropriate for age?
- Is the quality of protein and fat in the diet appropriate?
- Are there sufficient vitamins, minerals, and trace elements in the diet based on the child's food allergies?
- Are supplements used appropriately to provide the missing nutrients?

Adequacy of Intake and Use of Alternate Milk Sources in Food Allergies

A frequent review of a child's growth chart, with emphasis on growth velocity, is the easiest way to monitor growth of infants and children with food allergies. Reviewing the quantity of breast milk, formula, or other liquids and foods provided is an important anticipatory step to prevent future problems. Alternate milk products are frequently used as alternatives to breast milk or commercially prepared infant formulas. Vitamins and minerals should be added to these products to prevent nutrient deficiencies. Some milk substitutes are not appropriate for feeding milk-allergic infants. For example, goat's milk is an alternate milk product that is commonly recommended for infants with cow's milk allergy. In a study of children with confirmed cow's milk allergy, 24 of 26 reacted to goat's milk in a double-blind, placebo-controlled food challenge (DBPCFC).[28] Rice milk is another alternate milk that is recommended for infants and children with cow's milk allergy. Enriched rice milk is a good source of calcium and vitamin D; however, it lacks sufficient protein, fat, and other nutrients that are necessary for growth of infants and children (Table 52-4).

ELIMINATION DIETS

Elimination diets should be undertaken with caution, especially if a number of foods or food groups are restricted. Several reports have documented misuse of elimination diets resulting in inadequate caloric intake and failure to thrive in different patient populations.[29-34] Accurate identification of the offending allergens is critical not only to get resolution of symptoms by eliminating the food, but also to avoid unnecessary restriction of foods from the diet. Verification of the foods avoided via food challenges is also important to determine whether it is necessary to continue to avoid the food and if not, to add the particular food safely back into the diet.[35,36]

When elimination diets are used in the diagnostic process, it should be for a specified trial period. The symptoms attributed to the food should resolve and then reappear when the food is reintroduced. The duration of the diet can be from 1 week for acute symptoms such as hives to as long as 8 weeks for chronic symptoms such as vomiting and diarrhea, depending on the suspected disorder. In some gastrointestinal food allergies, an elemental diet using amino acid–based formulas may be required before significant resolution of gut pathology is observed by endoscopy and biopsy.[37] In food protein–induced enterocolitis syndrome (FPIES) (see Chapter 48), which is a symptom complex of profuse vomiting and diarrhea, symptoms completely resolve when the responsible food protein is removed from the diet.[38] Most often cow's milk or soy is responsible for the symptoms observed in FPIES, although other food proteins such as egg, wheat, rice, oat, chicken, and fish have also been noted to induce enterocolitis symptoms.[38-40]

When more than one particular food allergen is suspected, a limited "eat only" (oligoantigenic) diet is prescribed. The foods allowed are those that cannot be related to exacerbation of symptoms or were negative on testing. An example of an oligoantigenic diet is one in which rice and rice products; corn and corn products; cooked fruits and vegetables such as apples, pears, grapes, peaches, carrots, broccoli, spinach, squash, and sweet potato; and chicken and turkey may be allowed. Individualization is absolutely critical in this type of an elimination diet, not only for selection of allowed foods but also for the likelihood of compliance. If the symptoms attributed to the food persist, a thorough review of the diet is necessary to ensure that no other potential food allergens have been inadvertently added to the diet. For example, popcorn would be allowed in the oligoantigenic diet as listed; however, if the individual is consuming packaged popcorn, most products either contain butter or are contaminated with milk protein from the packaging lines. Homemade popcorn should be the only form allowed in such a diet. If a source of contamination cannot be found, reassessment of the allowed foods may be necessary to determine if a causal food is still in the diet.

Other forms of elimination diets include elimination of a particular food or food groups, such as milk and milk products, and an elemental diet consisting of an amino acid–based elemental formula with the addition of a single food such as rice or corn. Occasionally, if protein hydrolysates are tolerated, they can be continued in the elimination diet. If the anticipated resolution of symptoms is not achieved, changing to an elemental formula would be indicated. Food selected for the diet should only include those of which the patient has no history of experiencing reactions and can be provided in different forms. For example, white rice, brown rice, rice bread, rice cakes, rice cereals, rice pasta, rice puffs, and rice milk can be used in a rice-only diet. For a corn-only diet, corn on the cob; canned, fresh, or frozen corn; corn cereals; corn chips; corn pasta; popcorn; and polenta can be used. It is important to provide different textures so that the child's oral skills and needs are satisfied but also to be able to continue the transitioning with textures as appropriate for the child's age and feeding skills. The type of elimination diet will depend on the clinical history and results of tests for IgE antibody.[41,42] Elemental diets are frequently required in gastrointestinal disorders associated with multiple food allergies such as allergic eosinophilic esophagitis (AEE) or gastroenteritis (AEG).[41,43,44]

Independent of the underlying condition responsible for allergic symptoms, procuring the assistance of a dietitian for a child with multiple food allergies is essential for formulating an adequate diet to promote appropriate growth and development despite the elimination of a food. If the diet is modified for a short period of time to determine the impact on the child by eliminating several foods, a complete nutritional evaluation may not be necessary. However, if the elimination diet is long term (exceeding 2 weeks), a full nutritional assessment is crucial so that sufficient nutrients are provided to promote appropriate growth and to ensure proper institution of alternate food sources in the diet.

Allergen-Free Diets and Label Reading

Dietary elimination of any of the major allergens such as egg, milk, wheat, soy, or peanut is not a simple procedure. Simply telling a patient to "avoid milk" is like telling a diabetic patient to "take insulin." Particular allergens may be hidden in unsuspected foods, such as milk or egg proteins in bread products, milk or soy proteins in canned tuna fish, peanut flour in cakes, sauces, or chili, and peanut butter as the "glue" that holds together egg rolls.[45] A number of complicating factors exist when attempting to use lists of approved products because they may become outdated very quickly. The use of kosher symbols also may inadvertently mislead patients into thinking a product is always "milk free." Some kosher products may contain small amounts of milk protein because of inadequately cleaned equipment or differences in rabbinical laws. If any lists of allowed foods are generated for any of the allergens, frequent calls should be made to the food manufacturer to ensure the continued appropriateness of the particular product. Food Allergy Appendix D is a listing of common foods containing various food allergens.

Adherence and compliance to an elimination diet are greatly affected by the number of foods eliminated. If the child's allergy is to a nonessential food such as banana, having to avoid it is an inconvenience but very possible. However, if the child is allergic to a dietary staple such as egg, eliminating it from the diet is very difficult. Education regarding elimination of egg protein in the diet will include not only avoidance of egg-based foods (mayonnaise, ice cream, quiche) but also learning to identify words used on food labels that may indicate the presence of egg protein or a "hidden ingredient" in the food. On looking at a food labels, parents should be able to recognize terms that can be easily identified to be an egg byproduct (egg white), terms that are not so obvious (ovomucoid, globulin), or terms that may or may not be egg based (lecithin, natural flavor).[46,47] Food Allergy Appendix E contains terms used on labels that indicate the presence of food allergens for milk, egg, wheat, soy, and peanuts. These are available as "How to Read a Label" cards from the Food Allergy and Anaphylaxis Network (FAAN) (1-800-929-4040 or www.foodallergy.org) to help parents with this somewhat tricky task. Teaching parents how to replace the egg in the diet and to provide an alternative source of nutrients lost through the elimination of egg is essential. It is also important to prepare egg-free baked goods that have appropriate texture and taste. The Food Allergy & Anaphylaxis Network's Cookbook and several other resources are available with recipes that do not use milk, egg, soy, wheat, peanut, and tree nuts. Most of the egg substitutes available in the market are made with egg whites, which would still pose a problem to the egg-allergic child. There are ways to replace an egg, such as baking powder, oil and water, or apricot puree, to resemble the function or the color of an egg in a baked product.[48] A potato-based egg substitute is also available that can be used in place of eggs in baked goods.

Sometimes the removal of a particular food protein requires that a large number of products be removed from the diet. For example, if the child is wheat allergic, virtually all commercial breads, cereals, baked goods, and pastas need to be eliminated from the diet. Wheat is not only a main ingredient for a large number of products, but it is one of the common starches used in many processed foods. In this situation, educating the parents to experiment with the use of other grain flours such as rice, oat, potato, and barley to prepare baked goods such as breads, muffins, pancakes, cakes, and cookies may provide several alternative foods for the child. Use of alternate grain crackers, rice cakes, and pastas (rice, corn, potato, and quinoa) can help provide some normalcy to the diet of the allergic child. Needless to say, palatability of these products will determine the degree of compliance to the restricted diet. Using some of these commercial products and preparing some products at home will provide variety and other necessary nutrients (calories, carbohydrates, protein, fats, vitamins, and minerals) in appropriate proportions for the child's diet.

Table 52-5 is a sample menu that eliminates all major food allergens. Quantities of foods in this sample menu must be individualized to meet the child's nutritional needs. Contacting the manufacturer to ensure the purity of the foods, depending on the child's allergies, is critical.

Cross-Contamination

Another major source of hidden allergens is cross-contamination. Contact of one food with another even in trace amounts can pose a problem for a highly allergic child. Cross-contaminations can be caused by processing errors, where an ingredient is added to a batch of food by mistake, or by processing on shared lines, where the equipment is not adequately cleaned. It also can occur when purchasing food items from bulk bins or at a deli counter, where, for example, the same slicer is used for cutting both meats and cheese, or from accidents in food preparation at home, where the same knife is used for peanut butter and then simply wiped clean and used for jelly to make a sandwich. In the food industry, the use of leftover products, or "rework," to the next batch of products is a common practice. For example, the addition of a small amount of cookie dough, which has had the nuts filtered out, to a new batch of chocolate chip cookies will add nut residues and possibly enough protein to elicit an allergic reaction in a nut-allergic child. Some manufacturers are adding warning labels to their packaging such as "may contain. . ." to alert consumers to potential cross-contamination.

In January 2001, the U. S. Food and Drug Administration reported an investigation of food companies in which 25% of the products contained undeclared allergenic ingredients, often from cross-contamination.[49] A review of 221 telephone calls regarding allergic reactions made to FAAN over a 24-month period demonstrated that 70 (32%) of the calls concerned reactions after the ingestion of a purchased products and the remainder concerned label changes or errors.[50] Milk and peanut were implicated in 84% and 60% of cases, respectively. The majority of the problems reported were caused by cross-contamination by unlabeled allergen (28%), a visible ingredient that was not on the label (26%), and change in product ingredients (22%). The other calls, ranging from 1% to 7%, included incorrect contents in the package, an outer package label that differed from individual package labels, ambiguous wording, a "pareve" label with milk labeled as an ingredient, an English label placed over a foreign product label, and different package sizes of the same product containing different ingredients.

Using kosher products may seem to be a viable option for individuals who are milk allergic because kosher dietary laws prohibit use of milk or milk products in combination with meat. Therefore a product labeled with a "D" for dairy should not contain any meat and a product labeled "pareve" (neutral) should contain neither milk nor meat products. Under most major kosher supervision agencies, any product containing material derived from milk as an ingredient that is intentionally put into a product would be marked with a "D" next to the

---

TABLE 52-5 Sample Menu Eliminating All Major Food Allergens*

Breakfast	Calcium-fortified orange juice or enriched rice milk
	Cooked plain oatmeal with sugar and cinnamon
	Fruit salad made with apples, grapes, pears, and orange sections
Lunch	Hamburger with ground beef, lettuce, tomato, and milk-free/soy-free bun
	French fries with catsup or baked potato with milk-free/soy-free margarine
	Green salad made with lettuce, cucumber, tomato, and carrot curls
	Homemade vinegar and oil dressing
	Enriched rice milk
	Banana or apple
Dinner	Baked chicken
	White or brown rice
	Mixed vegetables made with carrots, broccoli, cauliflower, and zucchini
	Milk-free/soy-free margarine
	Canned peaches
	Enriched rice milk
Snacks	Milk-free/peanut-free rice cakes
	Milk-free/wheat-free corn or rice puffs
	Fresh fruit (apple, banana, grapes)
	Carrot and celery sticks
	Applesauce

*Contacting the manufacturer to ensure the safety of the food for the individual child is necessary. Amounts of food in this sample menu must be individualized to meet the child's nutrient needs.

kosher symbol. However, some agencies allow products, which contain no intentionally added milk products, to be marked with a "DE" if they are packaged on shared dairy equipment. Under Jewish law, a food product may contain a very small amount of milk and still be considered "pareve." Even though food manufacturers adhere to "good manufacturing practice" guidelines, there are reports of adverse reactions after ingestion of products either specifically intended to be "nondairy" or not appropriately labeled to have milk as an ingredient.[51-54] Products such as hot dogs, "pareve" labeled soy and other dairy-free desserts, lemon sorbet, dairy-free cookies and muffins, and dairy-free ice cream sandwiches have been implicated in a number of studies.[51-54]

FOOD CHALLENGES

As discussed in Chapter 45, oral food challenges are used to identify, confirm, or rule out a suspected allergy to foods. They also can be used to determine if a patient has lost his or her clinical reactivity to a food. When several foods are in question as possible causal foods and the elimination of those foods from the diet resulted in the resolution of symptoms, an oral food challenge to each food is warranted. However, if a number of foods were eliminated based on positive IgE tests (skin and blood tests) that previously were tolerated without any problems, adding those foods back to the diet generally does not warrant a physician-supervised food challenge. Food challenges in a patient with a recent history of severe anaphylaxis is contraindicated. However, a physician-supervised challenge to determine resolution of the allergy may be performed in some settings.[36]

The selection of the food for the challenge is determined by the history and/or results of food-specific IgE tests. Foods that are identified by positive IgE tests with no obvious history of significant reactivity or that are unlikely to provoke a reaction may be screened with open food challenges.[35,36] Caution should be exercised for suspected non–IgE-mediated conditions such as AEE or AEG, for which IgE tests are usually negative.[42] Physician-supervised challenges based on the history and prior reactions to the food in question may be warranted to determine if clinical tolerance has developed. If no history of acute reactions exists in addition to no evidence of IgE antibodies, the foods may be added to the diet one at a time every 5 to 7 days.[41] Biopsy after elimination, which allows for normalization of gut pathology and then after reintroduction, which could result in an inflammatory response, can help identify responsible food triggers. Longer time periods and multiple doses may be required to elicit reaction in some of these gastrointestinal disorders.

Suspected food allergens should be eliminated for at least 7 to 14 days before the food challenge for IgE-mediated disorders and up to 12 weeks for some gastrointestinal disorders. The patient should also be off antihistamines long enough to promote a normal histamine response.[36]

For IgE-mediated reactions, 8 to 10 g of the dry food or double for wet foods (meat and fish) is mixed in the vehicle of choice. For non–IgE-mediated reactions such as in FPIES, 0.15 to 0.3 g of protein/kg of weight of the individual and no more than 8 to 10 g of the dry food is given in the vehicle of choice.[38] A repeat of the morning challenge or an open challenge is often performed to provide more reassurance of resolution of the allergies. In non–IgE-mediated hypersensitivities, such as AEG or AEE, feeding of the food in an open form over several days may be necessary to elicit a reaction.

Food challenges are performed in a fasting state, with sequentially increasing doses of the food given over a 90-minute period for IgE-mediated reactions, but the dose and the timing between doses are frequently individualized based on the patient's history of reaction. The patient is evaluated for the development of symptoms throughout the challenge. Emergency medications should be available on site before the start of the food challenge. Food challenges must be conducted under the supervision of trained medical personnel in a facility equipped to treat anaphylactic reactions.[35,36]

Food challenges can be open (patient and clinician are aware of the challenge content), single blind (patient is unaware but clinician is aware of the challenge content), or double blind, placebo controlled (neither patient nor clinician is aware of the challenge content).[35,36] In an office setting, performing a DBPCFC may not be practical, whereas a single-blind food challenge (SBFC) would provide similar information to the physician in less time. In that situation, the challenge substance is given in the proposed vehicle followed by an open challenge.

Double-Blind, Placebo-Controlled Food Challenge

A DBPCFC is considered the gold standard for the diagnosis of food allergy. It is useful in a clinic setting because it removes bias in the diagnosis of allergy to a particular food; however, it is very labor intensive. Masking oral food challenges can be challenging. Although capsules can be used in adults, many challenges require more creative ideas, especially when trying to persuade children to cooperate with the food challenge. Table 52-6 outlines foods and vehicles used in the administration of these challenges. Care should be taken to use challenge substances that are "clean" and free of contamination. In addition, the individual must not be allergic to the placebo selected. Flours of wheat, rye, oat, rice, barley, corn, potato, and soy can be added to almost any food vehicle. Dried milk and egg powders are also available and can be added to the vehicle of choice if appropriate. Meats and fish can be masked in another tolerated meat, although masking the aroma of fish is more difficult. Fortunately, most fish-allergic patients tolerate canned tuna fish, so this can be used as a vehicle to mask fish challenges. Vehicles are selected to mask the taste, odor, texture, and color of the challenge food. The selection of the vehicle is limited only by what the child likes or is willing to eat or drink. Formulas and applesauce function as very good vehicles that can be used for infants and toddlers. Other vehicles used for masking purposes are fruit juices, oatmeal, puddings, potato pancakes, mashed potato, ground meat patties, and fruit shakes. The placebo should have properties similar to the test food, and the challenges should have a similar look, smell, and texture. For older children, a similar "mouth feel" and taste are also helpful to prevent bias.

The order in which the challenges are administered is randomized, and neither the patient nor the clinician administering the challenge knows which is the test food and which is placebo. Usually, one food is tested per day with either the placebo or the test food in the morning followed by the other challenge in the afternoon. A negative challenge should be followed by an open feeding of the food to rule out a false-negative challenge.

TABLE 52-6 Foods and Vehicles Used in the Administration of Challenges

Food	Challenge Substance	Placebo Suggestions	Vehicles
Eggs	Pasteurized dehydrated egg whites	Corn starch, oat flour, white rice flour	Mashed potato, oatmeal, applesauce, milk-free chocolate pudding
Milk	Nonfat dry milk powder or Lactaid milk	Corn starch, white flour, white rice flour	Rice or soy milk, infant formulas, applesauce, milk-free chocolate pudding
Wheat	Arrowhead Mills white or whole wheat flour	White rice flour, oat flour, barley flour	Applesauce, oatmeal, milk-free chocolate pudding
Soy	Arrowhead Mills soy flour, Ener-G Foods Soy Quik, Isomil formula	White rice flour, corn flour, oat flour, safe formula	Applesauce, oatmeal, milk-free chocolate pudding, safe formula
Peanuts	Peanut flour, peanut butter, crushed peanut (mortar and pestle)	Grain flour, safe tree nut flour or butter	Oatmeal, tomato-based meatballs, home-made chocolate
Tree nuts	Crushed suspected nut from the shell	Safe crushed nut from the shell, peanut butter	Peanut butter, milk-free chocolate pudding
Fish	Suspected fish	Safe fish or canned tuna	Safe fish patties, canned tuna
Shellfish	Suspected shellfish	Safe shellfish, canned tuna	Safe fish patties, canned tuna
Corn	Arrowhead Mills corn flour, corn grits	Rice flour, oat flour	Applesauce, oatmeal, milk-free chocolate pudding
Meats	Suspected meat	Safe meat	Meat patties

Single-Blind Food Challenge

The food being challenged is disguised to the patient but not to the clinician conducting the challenge. Because this process eliminates subject bias, it is most reliable to document the absence of symptoms. Vehicles used to mask the food in an SBFC are similar to those used in a DBPCFC. When more than one food is to be tested, an equal number of placebo and test food challenges are not always given.

Open Food Challenge

Open challenges may be done to confirm lack of reactivity to a food or may follow double-blind or single-blind challenges. Normal portions of the food are cooked in such a way that the food is usually consumed and given to the patient. In some cases, the normal portion of the food may be mixed in a vehicle that the child likes in order to facilitate the intake of the challenge for younger children. For example, mixing 4 to 6 ounces of soy milk in the child's current formula may enhance acceptance of the new taste so that you can proceed with the challenge in a timely fashion. The advantage of an open challenge is that it is quick, easy, and a good screening tool; however, it is prone to bias by both the clinician and the patient. If an open challenge is suspected to be falsely positive, a follow-up DBPCFC is warranted.[35,36]

FEEDING THE FOOD-ALLERGIC INFANT

The AAP recommends breast-feeding as the optimal source of nutrition for infants through the first year of life or longer.[55] Several studies have looked at the presence of certain food allergens in breast milk sufficient to induce reactions in infants.[56-58] These studies showed that milk and peanut protein were secreted in the breast milk of lactating women after maternal ingestion of these foods. Hence, the AAP, the European Society for Paediatric Allergology and Clinical Immunology, and the European Society for Paediatric Gastroenterology, Hepatology, and Nutrition all recommend complete exclusion of the causal protein from the maternal diet.[59,60] The AAP specifically suggests restricting milk, egg, fish, peanuts, and tree nuts in the maternal diet if symptoms of food allergy are noted in the infant.[59]

As a consequence of these recommendations, lactating mothers on such diets may also be at nutritional risk. The adequacy of the diets of the breast-feeding mothers who are avoiding a number of food allergens has not specifically been studied. The nutrients that are provided in peanuts, tree nuts, and fish can certainly be replaced by modifications of food choices for the mother. Such a task is not so simple in relation to milk and eggs because both are ubiquitous in our food supply and limit food choices greatly. The restricted diet is not limited to the avoidance of the above-mentioned allergens but also includes additional foods that may be perceived as a problem food for either the mother or the child, which will further limit food choices. This is another situation in which the number of foods on the avoidance list can expand markedly while the number of allowed foods decreases dramatically. Alternate sources of the nutrients provided by milk and egg should be instituted in the diet, and adequate intake of protein, calories, and calcium must be specifically emphasized for the mother. This may become an overwhelming and frustrating task for the mother to monitor her own diet along with the anxiety that comes with having an atopic infant. Eliciting the assistance of a dietitian to help with food choices and to assist in providing adequate nutrition for the mother and the infant is recommended.

Protein hydrolysates or amino acid–based formulas may be used to supplement "at risk" infants or when weaning to ensure adequate nutrition for the infant. Isolauri et al[61] studied 100 infants with atopic dermatitis who were exclusively breastfed. Some improvement was achieved by instituting a maternal elimination diet, although the infant's atopic symptoms resolved completely after the cessation of breast-feeding and institution of an amino acid–based formula. In addition, growth and nutritional parameters of the infants were noted to improve. The single most important factor contributing to the growth and nutrition of atopic infants was found to be the length of time between the onset of symptoms and cessation of breast-feeding.[61]

Because infants with food allergies have a limited number and type of foods allowed, introduction to a bottle, even in exclusively breast-fed babies, should be considered. This facilitates introduction of other formulas as needed. Providing one bottle a day of expressed breast milk for exclusively breast-fed babies helps not only with allowing some flexibility in the mother's schedule but also with maintaining the skills needed for the infant to suck from a bottle if needed based on the outcome of the allergic evaluation.

Solids

The introduction of solids (Beikost) during the first 4 months of life has been associated with a higher risk of atopic dermatitis.[62] Several studies recommend avoidance of solids for the first 6 months of life with delayed introduction of the allergenic foods.[63-66] The Committee on Nutrition of the AAP also recommends delayed introduction of solids until 6 months of age.[59] In a healthy infant, the timing of introducing solid feedings depends on neurologic and gastrointestinal maturation of the infant.[67] The infant should be able to sit and to coordinate chewing and swallowing nonliquid foods. The oral-motor skills needed to transfer food from the front of the tongue to the back of the mouth are also necessary. The ability to digest and absorb proteins, fats, and carbohydrates should be sufficiently mature by 4 to 6 months of age. Usually it is at that time that cereals, pureed fruits, vegetables, and eventually meats are introduced. Obviously a great variation exists among infants in achieving these goals. Infants generally indicate their readiness by opening their mouths and leaning forward in the sitting position. Similarly, infants indicate satiety or lack of interest or readiness by turning away. The decision to introduce solid foods should be individualized and based on the infant's developmental ability. Infants may aspirate food if they do not have the necessary oral-motor skills. Hence, types of foods and textures need to commensurate with age or developmental level of the child.

For children with a positive history of food allergies, a modified schedule of food introduction can be used (Table 52-7). As discussed previously, breast-feeding and/or supplemental feeding of a hydrolyzed formula can be suggested for the first 6 months of life. Solids are delayed until 6 months of age or when the child shows readiness. Single-ingredient foods should be introduced first, with 5 to 7 days between each new food to permit identification of any problems. Selection of foods is also individualized based on the child's history or family history. Infant cereals (rice or oat) are a good first choice because the texture can be manipulated to the tolerance of the infant. Additionally, cereals can play an important role in replenishing the infant's iron stores. Orange vegetables (squash, sweet potato, and carrots) followed by fruits (apple, pear, banana, plum, peach, and apricot) can be introduced next. Green vegetables (spinach, peas, and green beans) may be added, followed by grains (rice or oat, corn, white potato, barley, and wheat) and then meats (lamb, pork, turkey, chicken, and beef). The AAP recommends delaying the introduction of milk or soy to after 1 year of age, eggs to after 2 years of age, and peanuts, tree nuts, fish, and shellfish to after

---

TABLE 52-7 Sample Feeding Schedule for a Child with a Positive History of Food Allergies

- Breast-feeding with or without formula-feeding with a hydrolyzed formula
- At 6 months: rice cereal or other single-grain source (Beechnut)
- At 7 months: orange vegetables (squash, sweet potato, and carrots for 5 to 7 days each)
- At 8 to 10 months: fruits (apple, pear, banana, plum, peach, and apricot for 5 to 7 days each)
- At 8 to 10 months: green vegetables (spinach, broccoli, peas, and green beans for 5 to 7 days each)
- At 10 to 11 months: grains (oats, corn, white potato, barley, and wheat for 5 to 7 days each)
- At 12 months: meats (lamb, pork, turkey, chicken, and beef for 5 to 7 days each)
- Continue to introduce new foods (other fruits and vegetables) one at a time and watch for signs of an allergic reaction
- Delaying the introduction of the eight major allergens may prevent, decrease the severity of, or delay the onset of food allergies by allowing the immune system to mature before it is exposed to highly allergenic foods.
    After 1 year of age, introduce milk and soy
    After 2 years of age, introduce egg
    Between 3 and 4 years of age, introduce peanuts, tree nuts, fish, and shellfish

---

3 years of age.[59] It is important to educate the families in reading labels of baby foods to ensure complete avoidance of the major allergens. For example, a jar of "Green Beans and Potatoes" baby food mix contains "water, green beans, potatoes, brown rice, flour, nonfat dry milk, unsalted butter, and onions" (Tender Harvest Green Beans and Potatoes; Gerber Products Company). This product is certainly inappropriate for a child with cow's milk allergy. It is important to stress to families to read all labels every time and to either mix single-ingredient baby foods together for the desired combination or to prepare the desired mixture from scratch at home.

For a child who is on a few foods during infancy, either because of allergic symptoms noted from specific foods or as a prophylactic measure, advancing textures to the appropriate developmental stage is critical to prevent feeding problems. Advancing from pureed sweet potato, for example, to mashed, then diced, then well cooked chunks, and finally to French fried sweet potatoes allows the child to experiment and master different textures and finger-feeding to achieve appropriate feeding skills.

PSYCHOLOGIC CONCERNS

As with any chronic illness, dealing with food allergies is a disruption of normal daily life. The families with food-allergic children must live with constant uncertainties and fear. Their normal daily activities are potentially affected by issues such as label reading, concerns for cross-contamination, and various exposures that may occur in school or even in social settings.

The course of the disease is variable, with some children tolerating small quantities or allergen in some foods and others not tolerating the same foods. There could be several members of the family who have allergies to different foods, requiring the preparation of different meals for each individual. There are time-consuming care demands, not only involving the calling of companies to check on particular products and in special cleaning of utensils and equipment required and the preparation of all foods but also extra precautions in dealing with everyday activities such as shopping, going out to dinner, going away on a trip, summer camp, play dates, etc. An exceptional level of anxiety is generated for both the child and the family every time they present for a food challenge and/or for their annual clinic visits. Some parents have expressed disappointment when the levels of food-specific IgE remain elevated, indicating that a challenge is not warranted, or when their child fails a food challenge. Both of these situations generate a feeling of dissatisfaction, often with the child feeling that they let down his or her parents. Also, the children were hoping to have outgrown their allergies so that they can be like their other friends, eating whatever they want.

As with any chronic illness, the whole family dynamics are disrupted. It affects not only the allergic child but also the unaffected siblings. Most important, food develops a subjective role. After hours of calling the companies to check on the ingredients and issues of cross-contamination, a particular item is prepared with the hope that it will please the child's palate. In one quick turn, the child may not feel like eating that particular food that day; not like the texture, not like it aesthetically, or not like the taste. After all of the time and preparation, not only are the parents disappointed that what they thought would be a success was not, but they then must find something else to feed their child.

The psychologic burden of peanut allergy has specifically been studied by Primeau et al.[68] Disruption in daily activities and family relations was identified as factors affecting children and adults with peanut allergy. Sicherer et al[69] specifically looked at the impact of food allergy on quality of life of food-allergic children. The Children's Health Questionnaire (CHQ-PF50),[70] which is a general tool that focuses on physical and psychologic functioning, was utilized to determine the impact of food allergy on parental perceptions of physical and psychologic functioning. A random sample of 400 members of FAAN with children aged 5 to 18 received the questionnaire. The questionnaires were completed by 253 parents with 68% allergic to one or two foods, and the remainder to more than two foods. Childhood food allergy was noted to have a significant impact on general health perceptions, emotional impact on the parent, and limitation of family activities, with the number of foods avoided as a major contributor.

Effective education is necessary to support development of appropriate self-management skills not only for the parents and caretakers, but also for the allergic child and his or her siblings. Empowering children encourages them to take control of their lives and further enhances compliance.

MANAGEMENT

A number of medications such as H_1 and H_2 antihistamines, ketotifin, corticosteroids and leukotriene inhibitors have been utilized in an attempt to modify symptoms of food-allergic disorders. Antihistamines may partially mask symptoms of oral allergy syndrome[71] and IgE-mediated skin symptoms, but overall they have minimal efficacy in blocking systemic reactions. Oral corticosteroids are generally effective in alleviating chronic IgE-mediated disorders, (e.g., atopic dermatitis or asthma) and non–IgE-mediated gastrointestinal disorders, such as AEE or AEG and dietary-induced enteropathy, but the side effects of prolonged steroid use are generally unacceptable.

Some anecdotal studies have suggested that oral cromolyn sodium is effective in treating IgE-mediated food allergies and AEG, but appropriately controlled studies are lacking or fail to show efficacy.[72]

A number of anecdotal reports have appeared in the literature supporting a therapeutic role for immunotherapy in food hypersensitivity. Nelson utilized "standard" immunotherapy in six peanut-allergic patients and found that two of the six patients could tolerate larger quantities of peanuts for a prolonged period following rush therapy, but the adverse reaction rate was unacceptable for standard clinical practice.[73] Consequently, alternative strategies to treat food-allergic patients are being explored.

A recent study evaluated the use of anti-IgE antibody in the treatment of patients with peanut allergy. Using "humanized" monoclonal antibodies (TNX-901; Tanox, Inc., Houston, TX) specific for the $C_\epsilon 3$ domain of IgE (portion of the IgE Fc region that binds to the Fc_ϵ receptor), investigators found that anti-IgE therapy leads to a dose-dependent increase in the amount of peanut protein that peanut-allergic patients tolerated during DBPCFCs.[74] A less traditional approach, Chinese herbal medication, may also provide an effective form of therapy for food-allergic patients. It was shown to prevent anaphylactic symptoms in a murine model of peanut anaphylaxis.[75]

The most urgent form of therapy required for the treatment of food allergy involves early management of food-induced anaphylactic reactions. The treatment of food-induced anaphylaxis is similar to the treatment of anaphylaxis provoked by other causes, as reviewed in Chapter 60. A review of fatal anaphylactic reactions suggests that the longer the initial therapy is delayed, the greater the incidence of complications and deaths.[76-78] Certain factors place some individuals at increased risk for more severe anaphylactic reactions: (1) history of a previous anaphylactic reaction; (2) history of asthma, especially if poorly controlled; (3) allergy to peanuts, nuts, fish, and shellfish; (4) teenage patients; and (5) patients on beta blockers or angiotensin-converting enzyme inhibitors. Education is imperative to ensure the patient and his or her family understand how to avoid all forms of the food allergen and the potential severity of a reaction if the food is inadvertently ingested. Accidental food ingestion is likely despite avoidance measures, so immediate treatment should be available for such emergencies. Treatment protocols should be prescribed by the patient's physician, and caretakers and/or school staff should have written instructions by the physician and signed by the parents. A sample plan can be downloaded from the FAAN's website (www.foodallergy.org). "Epinephrine is the first drug that should be used in the emergency management of a child having a potentially life-threatening allergic reaction. There are no contraindications to the use of epinephrine for a life-threatening allergic reaction."[79] Children at risk for anaphylaxis should carry medical information concerning their condition, such as a Medic Alert bracelet, emergency medications (EpiPen and liquid diphenhydramine), and their treatment plan, with them at all times.

FUTURE IMMUNOMODULATORY APPROACHES

Several novel immunotherapeutic strategies are being examined as treatment modalities for food allergy: (1) humanized anti-IgE monoclonal antibody therapy, (2) "engineered" (mutated) allergen protein immunotherapy, (3) antigen-immunostimulatory sequence-modulated immunotherapy, (4) peptide immunotherapy, (5) plasmid-DNA immunotherapy, and (6) cytokine-modulated immunotherapy.[80]

Because IgE-mediated allergic diseases are the result of an overproduction of T helper cell type 2 (Th2) cytokines by allergen-specific CD4+ T cells, a number of immunomodulatory strategies have been investigated in murine models of peanut-induced anaphylaxis. In one approach, the major allergenic proteins of peanut (Ara h 1, Ara h 2, and Ara h 3) have been identified, sequenced, and cloned. The DNA that codes for these proteins has been "engineered" to eliminate IgE binding sites on the recombinant protein so it can be injected into an allergic patient without provoking an allergic reaction and to retain T cell activation sites so it can induce "desensitization." When these engineered proteins were injected into peanut-allergic mice, they reversed their allergic sensitivity and prevented anaphylaxis when the mice were fed peanut.[81]

Oligonucleotide immunostimulatory sequences (ISS-ODNs) containing unmethylated palindromic CpG motifs have been shown to possess immunomodulatory properties that decrease airway hyperreactivity, lung eosinophilia, and allergen-specific IgE production when administered during allergen sensitization.[82,83] These nucleotide sequences activate antigen-presenting cells (primarily monocytes) to secrete interferon (IFN)-α/β, interleukin (IL)-6, IL-12, and IL-18 and natural killer cells to secrete IFN-γ, both of which promote Th1 responses. In preliminary studies, our group has demonstrated that the use of ISS-ODNs as adjuvants with native proteins also may be an effective form of immunotherapy to prevent IgE-mediated peanut allergy.

Another approach being investigated is the use of overlapping peptides. Vaccines comprised of small peptides (10 to 20 amino acids in length) that represent the entire length of a specific food protein are generated. These peptides are too small to cross-link IgE molecules on mast cells; they cannot activate an immediate reaction but do provide antigen-presenting cells with all of the possible T cell binding ("activation") sites necessary to promote "desensitization." Preliminary studies in our anaphylactic mouse model with peptides (20 amino acids in length) demonstrated that peanut-allergic mice could be "desensitized" with this approach. Oldfield et al[84] used a similar approach in cat-allergic patients and demonstrated that repeated injections of peptides generated from Fel d 1, the major cat allergen, lead to suppression of both the early- and late-phase reactions, thus providing a potentially effective form of immunotherapy. A number of exciting new immunotherapeutic strategies are being evaluated by a number of investigators. With the increasing interest in this area, effective forms of therapy for IgE-mediated food allergies should be available in the next several years.

CONCLUSIONS

Currently, the treatment of food allergy is directed at complete avoidance of the offending food allergens, and its success is dependent on the correct identification of the allergens and complete exclusion of the allergens from the diet. Independent of the condition triggering the symptoms of hypersensitivity, whether it is an IgE- or non–IgE-mediated hypersensitivity, the suspect foods that are repeatedly causing symptoms have to be eliminated from the diet. Resolution of symptoms

---

BOX 52-1   **KEY CONCEPTS**
Key Points in the Management of Food Allergy

- Dietary elimination of any of the major allergens, such as egg, milk, wheat, soy, or peanut, requires education and close attention to food labels and food composition.
- Instructing the patient and family to read all food labels to avoid hidden sources of the suspected food and to avoid potential sources of contamination is critical.
- Monitoring growth is a simple way to gauge adequacy of intake.
- Use of complete formulas may be recommended to prevent possible growth and nutritional problems. Continued use of the complete formulas is also recommended until there are sufficient quantities of the compromised nutrients based on the foods avoided.
- Delayed introduction of solids until 6 months of age is recommended by the American Academy of Pediatrics. Delayed introduction of the major allergens such as milk or soy to after 1 year of age, eggs to after 2 years of age, and peanuts, tree nuts, fish, and shellfish to after 3 years of age is also recommended in a child with a positive family history of food allergies.
- One new food should be introduced to the diet every 5 to 7 days, whether it is introduction of a new food to an infant or reintroduction of foods after an elimination diet. Types of foods and textures will need to be commensurate with age or developmental level and the child's history.
- Effective education is necessary to support the development of a child/family that is not only nutritionally sufficient but allows them to master the necessary skills needed to cope with and minimize the level of uncertainty in their lives. Education empowers children and allows them to achieve some degree of control of their lives.
- New immunomodulatory therapies, such as anti-IgE antibodies and "engineered" recombinant proteins, are being evaluated and show promise for more effective, "proactive" therapy of IgE-mediated food allergies.

---

should be noted on elimination of the offending allergens. Verification of the foods avoided via food challenges is also important to determine whether it is necessary to continue to avoid the food and, if not, to add the particular food safely back to the diet. Eliciting the assistance of a dietitian for a child with multiple food allergies is essential to formulating an adequate diet to promote appropriate growth and development despite the elimination of a food. A number of new immunomodulatory therapies are under intense study and may provide more proactive therapy for patients with IgE-mediated food allergy in the next few years (Box 52-1).

HELPFUL WEBSITES

The Allergic Reaction Central website (www.allergic-reactions.com)
The American Dietetic Association website (www.eatright.org)

The Food Allergy Initiative website (www.foodallergyinitiative.org)
The Food Allergy News for Kids website (www.fankids.org)
The International Food Information Council website (www.ific.org)
The MedicAlert website (www.medicalert.org)
The National Coalition for Food Safe Schools website (www.foodsafeschools.org)
The Food Allergy and Anaphylaxis Network (FAAN) website (www.foodallergy.org)

REFERENCES

1. Kuczmarski RJ, Ogden CL, Guo SS, et al: 2000 CDC growth charts for the United States: methods and development. National Center for Health Statistics, *Vital Health Stat* 11(246), 2002. URL: www.cdc.gov/growthcharts.
2. Queen PM, Wilson SE: Growth and nutrient requirements of infants. In Grand RJ, Sutphen JL, Dietz WH, eds: *Pediatric nutrition: theory & practice*, Boston, 1987, Butterworths.
3. Queen PM, Henry RR: Growth and nutrient requirements of children. In Grand RJ, Sutphen JL, Dietz WH, eds: *Pediatric nutrition: theory & practice*, Boston, 1987, Butterworths.
4. Leleiko NS, Stawski C, Benkov K, et al: The nutritional assessment of the pediatric patient. In Grand RJ, Sutphen JL, Dietz WH, eds: *Pediatric nutrition: theory & practice*, Boston, 1987, Butterworths.
5. Bessler S: Nutritional assessment. In Samour PQ, Helm KK, Lang CE, eds: *Handbook of pediatric nutrition*, ed 2, Gaithersburg, Md, 1999, Aspen.
6. Sampson HA, McCaskill CM. Food hypersensitivity and atopic dermatitis: evaluation of 113 patients, *J Pediatr* 107:669-675, 1985.
7. Bock SA, Atkins FM: Patterns of food hypersensitivity during sixteen years of double-blind placebo-controlled oral food challenges, *J Pediatr* 117:561-567, 1990.
8. Food and Nutrition Board, National Research Council: *Recommended dietary allowances*, ed 10, Washington, DC, 1989, National Academy Press.
9. Food and Nutrition Board, Institute of Medicine: *Dietary reference intakes: applications in dietary assessment: a report of the Subcommittee on Interpretation and Uses of Dietary Reference Intakes and the Standing Committee on the Scientific Evaluation of Dietary Reference Intakes*, Washington, DC, 2000, National Academy Press.
10. Jones BJM, Lees R, Andrews J, et al: Comparison of an elemental and polymeric enteral diet in patients with normal gastrointestinal function, *Gut* 24:78-84, 1983.
11. Jones PJH, Kubow S: Lipids, sterols, and their metabolites. In Shils ME, Olson JA, Shike M, et al, eds: *Modern nutrition in health and disease*, ed 9, Baltimore, 1999, Williams & Wilkins.
12. Kaila M, Salo MK, Isolauri E: Fatty acids in substitute formulas for cow's milk allergy, *Allergy* 54:74-77, 1999.
13. Goodnight SH Jr, Harris WS, Connor WE, et al: Polyunsaturated fatty acids, hyperlipidemia, and thrombosis, *Arteriosclerosis* 2:87-113, 1982.
14. Salman S, Christie L, Burks AW, et al: Dietary intakes of children with food allergies: comparison of the food guide pyramid and the Recommended Dietary Allowances, *J Allergy Clin Immunol* 109:S214, 2002.
15. Merritt RJ, Carter M, Haight M, et al: Whey protein hydrolysate formula for infants with gastrointestinal intolerance to cow milk and soy protein in infant formulas, *J Pediatr Gastroenterol Nutr* 11:78-82, 1990.
16. Sampson HA, Bernhisel-Broadbent J, Yang E, et al: Safety of casein hydrolysate formula in children with cow milk allergy, *J Pediatr* 118:71-74, 1991.
17. Isolauri E, Sutas Y, Makinen-Kiljunen S, et al: Efficacy and safety of hydrolyzed cow milk and amino acid-derived formulas in infants with cow milk allergy, *J Pediatr* 127:550-557, 1995.
18. de Boissieu D, Matarazzo P, Dupont C: Allergy to extensively hydrolyzed cow milk proteins in infants: identification and treatment with an amino acid-based formula, *J Pediatr* 131:744-747, 1997.
19. Vanderhoof JA, Murray ND, Kaufman SS, et al: Intolerance to protein hydrolysate infant formulas: an under recognized cause of gastrointestinal symptoms in infants, *J Pediatr* 131:741-744, 1997.
20. Oldæus G, Anjou K, Moran JR, et al: Extensively and partially hydrolyzed infant formulas for allergy prophylaxis, *Arch Dis Child* 77:4-10, 1997.
21. Chandra RK: Five-year follow-up of high-risk infants with family history of allergy who were exclusively breast-fed or fed partial whey hydrolysate, soy, and conventional cow's milk formulas, *J Pediatr Gastroenterol Nutr* 24:380-388, 1997.
22. Halken S, Hansen KS, Jacobsen HP, et al: Comparison of a partially hydrolyzed infant formula with two extensively hydrolyzed formulas for allergy prevention: a prospective, randomized study, *Pediatr Allergy Immunol* 11:149-161, 2000.
23. Giampietro PG, Kjellman N-IM, Oldæus G, et al: Hypoallergenicity of an extensively hydrolyzed whey formula, *Pediatr Allergy Immunol* 12:83-86, 2001.
24. Sampson HA, James JM, Bernhisel-Broadbent J: Safety of an amino acid-derived infant formula in children allergic to cow milk, *Pediatrics* 40:463-465, 1992.
25. Niggeman B, Christaine B, Dupont C, et al: Prospective, controlled, multi-center study on the effect of an amino acid based formula in infants with cow's milk allergy/intolerance and atopic dermatitis, *Pediatr Allergy Immunol* 12:78-82, 2001.
26. Sicherer SH, Noone SA, Koerner CB, et al: Hypoallergenicity and efficacy of an amino acid-based formula in children with cow's milk and multiple food hypersensitivities, *J Pediatr* 138:688-693, 2001.
27. Isolauri E, Sutas Y, Salo MK, et al: Elimination diet in cow's milk allergy: risk for impaired growth in young children, *J Pediatr* 132:1004-1009, 1998.
28. Bellioni-Businco B, Paganelli R, Lucenti P, et al: Allergenicity of goat's milk in children with cow's milk allergy, *J Allergy Clin Immunol* 103:1191-1194, 1999.
29. Bierman CW, Shapiro GG, Christie DL, et al: Allergy grand round: eczema, rickets, and food allergy, *J Allergy Clin Immunol* 61:119-127, 1978.
30. Lloyd-Still JD: Chronic diarrhea of childhood and the misuse of elimination diets, *J Pediatr* 95:10-13, 1979.
31. David TJ, Waddington E, Stanton RHJ: Nutritional hazards of elimination diets in children with atopic dermatitis, *Arch Dis Child* 59:323-325, 1984.
32. Podleski WK: Elimination diet therapy in allergic children: a word of caution, *Am J Dis Child* 139:330, 1985:
33. Arvola T, Holmberg-Marttila D: Benefits and risks of elimination diets, *Ann Med* 31:293-298, 1999.
34. Liu T, Howard RM, Mancini AJ, et al: Kwashiorkor in the United States: fad diets, perceived and true milk allergy, and nutritional ignorance, *Arch Dermatol* 137:630-636, 2001.
35. Bock SA, Sampson HA, Atkins FM, et al: Double-blind, placebo-controlled food challenge (DBPCFC) as an office procedure: a manual, *J Allergy Clin Immunol* 82:986-997, 1988.
36. Sicherer SH: Food allergy: when and how to perform oral food challenges, *Pediatr Allergy Immunol* 10:226-234, 1999.
37. Kelly KJ: Eosinophillic gastroenteritis, *J Pediatr Gastroenterol Nutr* 30:S28-S35, 2000.
38. Powell GK: Food protein-induced enterocolitis of infancy: differential diagnosis and management, *Comp Ther* 12:28-37, 1986.
39. Sicherer SH, Eigenmann PA, Sampson HA: Clinical features of food protein-induced enterocolitis syndrome, *J Pediatr* 133:214-219, 1988.
40. Nowak-Wegrzyn AH, Sampson HA, Wood RA, et al: Food protein-induced enterocolitis syndrome (FPIES) caused by oat, *J Allergy Clin Immunol* 107:S195, 2001.
41. Sampson HA, Sicherer SH, Birnbaum AH: American Gastroenterological Association (AGA) technical review on the evaluation of food allergy in gastrointestinal disorders, *Gastroenterology* 120:1026-1040, 2001.
42. Spergel JM, Beausoleil JL, Mascarenhas M, et al: The use of skin prick rests and patch tests to identify causative foods in eosinophilic esophagitis, *J Allergy Clin Immunol* 109:363-368, 2002.
43. Kelly KJ, Lazenby AJ, Rowe PC, et al: Eosinophilic esophagitis attributed to gastroesophageal reflux: improvement with an amino acid based formula, *Gastroenterology* 109:1503-1512, 1995.
44. Justinich C, Katz A, Gurbindo C, et al: Elemental diet improves steroid-dependent eosinophilic gastroenteritis and reverses growth failure, *J Pediatr Gastroenterol Nutr* 23:81-85, 1996.
45. Steinman HA: "Hidden" allergens in food, *J Allergy Clin Immunol* 98:241-250, 1996.
46. Koerner CB, Sampson HA: Diets and nutrition. In Metcalfe DD, Sampson HA, Simon RA, eds: *Adverse reactions to foods and food additives*, Oxford, 1996, Blackwell Scientific.
47. Koerner CB, Hays TL: Nutrition basics in food allergy, *Immunol Allergy Clin North Am* 19:583-603, 1999.
48. Food Allergy & Anaphylaxis Network: *How to read a label for an egg-free diet*, Fairfax, Va, 2000, The Network.

49. U.S. Food and Drug Administration, Center for Food Safety and Applied Nutrition, Office of Scientific Analysis and Support: *Food allergen partnership. January 2001.* Available at: http//:www.cfsan.fda.gov/~dms/alrgpart.html. Accessed May 11, 2002.

50. Altschul AS, Scherrer DL, Munoz-Furlong A, et al: Manufacturing and labeling issues for commercial products: relevance to food allergy, *J Allergy Clin Immunol* 108:468, 2001.

51. Gern JE, Yang E, Evrard HM, et al: Allergic reactions to milk-contaminated "non-dairy" products, *N Engl J Med* 324:976-979, 1991.

52. Jones RT, Squillace DL, Yunginger JW: Anaphylaxis in a milk-allergic child after ingestion of milk-contaminated kosher-pareve-labeled "dairy-free" dessert, *Ann Allergy* 68:223-227, 1992.

53. Laoprasert N, Wallen ND, Jones RT, et al: Anaphylaxis in a milk-allergic child following ingestion of lemon sorbet containing trace quantities of milk, *J Food Prot* 61:1522-1524, 1998.

54. Mofidi S, Bardina L, Chatchatee P, et al: Reactions to food products labeled dairy-free: quantity of milk contaminant, *J Allergy Clin Immunol,* 105:S138, 2000.

55. Gartner LM, Black LS, Eaton AP, et al, for the American Academy of Pediatrics Committee on Nutrition: Breastfeeding and the use of human milk, *Pediatrics* 100:1035-1039, 1997.

56. Jarvinen KM, Makinen-Kiljunen S, Suomalainen H: Cow's milk challenge through human milk evokes immune responses in infants with cow's milk allergy, *J Pediatr* 135:506-512, 1999.

57. Jarvinen KM, Suomalainen H: Development of cow's milk allergy in breast-fed infants, *Clin Exp Allergy* 31:978-987, 2001.

58. Vadas P, Wai Y, Burks AW, et al: Detection of peanut allergens in breast milk of lactating women, *JAMA* 285:1746-1748, 2001.

59. Baker SS, Cochran WJ, Greer FR, et al, for the American Academy of Pediatrics Committee on Nutrition: Hypoallergenic infant formulas, *Pediatrics* 106:346-349, 2000.

60. Host A, Koletzko B, Dreborg S, et al: Dietary products used in infants for treatment and prevention of food allergy. Joint statement of the European Society for Paediatric Allergology and Clinical Immunology (ESPACI), Committee on Hypoallergenic Formulas and the European Society for Paediatric Gastroenterology, Hepatology and Nutrition (ESPGHAN) Committee on Nutrition, *Arch Dis Child* 81:80-84, 1999.

61. Isolaurie E, Tahvanainen A, Peltola T, et al: Breast-feeding of allergic infants, *J Pediatr* 134:27-32, 1999.

62. Fergusson DM, Horwood LJ, Shannon FT: Early solid feeding and recurrent childhood eczema: a 10-year longitudinal study, *Pediatrics* 86:541-546, 1990.

63. Gern JE, Lemanske RF Jr: Pediatric allergy: can it be prevented? *Immunol Allergy Clin North Am* 19:233-252, 1999.

64. Zeiger RS, Heller S, Mellon MH, et al: Effect of combined maternal and infant food-allergen avoidance on development of atopy in early infancy: a randomized study, *J Allergy Clin Immunol* 84:72-89, 1989.

65. Zeiger RS: Secondary prevention of allergic disease: an adjunct to primary prevention, *Pediatr Allergy Immunol* 6:127-138, 1995.

66. Zeiger RS: Prevention of food allergy in infants and children, *Immunol Allergy Clin North Am* 19:619-646, 1999.

67. Akers SM, Groh-Wargo SL: Normal nutrition during infancy. In Samour PQ, Helm KK, Lang CE, eds: *Handbook of pediatric nutrition,* ed 2, Gaithersburg, Md, 1999, Aspen.

68. Primeau MN, Kagan R, Joseph L, et al: The psychological burden of peanut allergy as perceived by adults with peanut allergy and the parents of peanut-allergic children, *Clin Exp Allergy* 30:1135-1143, 2000.

69. Sicherer SH, Noone SA, Munoz-Furlong A: The impact of food allergy on quality of life, *Ann Allergy Asthma Immunol* 87:461-464, 2001.

70. Landgraf J, Abetz L, Ware JE: *The child health questionnaire (CHQ): a user's manual,* Boston, 1996, The Health Institute.

71. Bindslev-Jensen C, Vibits A, Stahl Skov P, et al: Oral allergy syndrome: the effect of astemizole, *Allergy* 46:610-613, 1991.

72. Burks AW, Sampson HA: Double-blind placebo-controlled trial of oral cromolyn in children with atopic dermatitis and documented food hypersensitivity, *J Allergy Clin Immunol* 81:417-423, 1988.

73. Nelson HS, Lahr J, Rule R, et al: Treatment of anaphylactic sensitivity to peanuts by immunotherapy with injections of aqueous peanut extract, *J Allergy Clin Immunol* 99:744-751, 1997.

74. Leung DYM, Sampson HA, Yunginger JW, et al: Effect of anti-IgE therapy (TNX-901) on hypersensitivity threshold by oral food challenge in patients with severe peanut allergy, *N Engl J Med* 2003; in press.

75. Li XM, Zhang TF, Huang CK, et al: Food Allergy Herbal Formula-1 (FAHF-1) blocks peanut-induced anaphylaxis in a murine model, *J Allergy Clin Immunol* 108:639-646, 2001.

76. Yunginger JW, Sweeney KG, Sturner WQ, et al: Fatal food-induced anaphylaxis, *JAMA* 260:1450-1452, 1988.

77. Sampson HA, Mendelson LM, Rosen JP: Fatal and near-fatal anaphylactic reactions to food in children and adolescents, *N Engl J Med* 327:380-384, 1992.

78. Bock SA, Munoz-Furlong A, Sampson HA: Fatalities caused by anaphylactic reactions to foods, *J Allergy Clin Immunol* 107:191-193, 2001.

79. AAAAI Board of Directors. Anaphylaxis in schools and other child-care settings, *J Allergy Clin Immunol* 102:173-176, 1998.

80. Sampson HA: Immunological approaches to the treatment of food allergy, *Pediatr Allergy Immunol* 12:91-96, 2001.

81. Li XM, Serebrisky D, Lee SY, et al: A murine model of peanut anaphylaxis: T- and B-cell responses to a major peanut allergen mimic human responses, *J Allergy Clin Immunol* 106:150-158, 2000.

82. Broide D, Schwarze J, Tighe H, et al: Immunostimulatory DNA sequences inhibit IL-5, eosinophilic inflammation, and airway hyperresponsiveness in mice, *J Immunol* 161:7054-7062, 1998.

83. Kline JN, Krieg AM, Waldschmidt TJ, et al: CpG oligodeoxynucleotides do not require Th1 cytokines to prevent eosinophilic airway inflammation in a murine model of asthma, *J Allergy Clin Immunol* 104:1258-1264, 1999.

84. Oldfield WL, Kay AB, Larche M: Allergen-derived T cell peptide-induced late asthmatic reactions precede the induction of antigen-specific hyporesponsiveness in atopic allergic asthmatic subjects, *J Immunol* 167:1734-1739, 2001.

Allergic Skin and Eye Diseases

DONALD Y.M. LEUNG

CHAPTER **53**

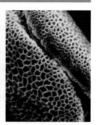

Atopic Dermatitis

DONALD Y.M. LEUNG

Atopic dermatitis (AD) is a highly pruritic chronic inflammatory skin disease that commonly presents during early childhood.[1] It is frequently associated with a personal or family history of respiratory allergy and can have profound effects on patients' lives, career choices, and social interactions.[2] Recent interest in AD has been sparked by reports of its increasing prevalence.[3] Management approaches in AD have evolved from our understanding of the mechanisms underlying this skin disease.

EPIDEMIOLOGY

AD is a common skin disease with a lifetime prevalence in children of 10% to 20% in the United States, Northern and Western Europe, Japan, and other westernized countries.[4] A recent study in Portland found that 17% of school-aged children had AD.[5] This represents the culmination of a twofold to threefold increase in the prevalence of AD since the 1970s. Interestingly, the prevalence of AD is much lower in agricultural countries such as China, Eastern Europe, rural Africa, and Central Asia.

Wide variations in prevalence have been observed among similar ethnic groups of common genetic background, suggesting that environmental factors are critical in determining disease expression.[6] Some of the potential risk factors that have received attention as being associated with the rise in atopic disease include small family size, increased income and education both in whites and blacks, migration from rural to urban environments, and increased use of antibiotics, that is, the so-called "Western Lifestyle." These observations are supported by recent studies demonstrating that allergic responses are driven by T helper cell type 2 (Th2) immune responses, whereas infections are induced by Th1 immune responses.[7] Th1 responses antagonize the development of Th2 cells. Therefore a decreased number of infections or the lack of Th1 polarizing signals (such as endotoxin) during early childhood could predispose to enhanced Th2 allergic responses (see Chapters 1 and 2).

DIAGNOSIS AND DIFFERENTIAL DIAGNOSIS

Clinical features of AD are listed in Table 53-1.[8] Of the major features, pruritus and chronic or relapsing eczematous dermatitis with typical distribution are essential for diagnosis. Intense pruritus and cutaneous reactivity are cardinal features of AD. Pruritus may be intermittent throughout the day but is usually worse at night. Its consequences are scratching, prurigo papules, lichenification, and eczematous skin lesions. Patients with AD also have a reduced threshold for pruritus. As a result, allergens, reduced humidity, excessive sweating, and low concentrations of irritants (e.g., wool, acrylic, soaps, and detergents) can exacerbate pruritus and scratching.

During infancy AD is generally more acute with excoriation, vesicles over erythematous skin, and serous exudate, and the rash primarily involves the face, scalp, and the extensor surfaces of the extremities (Figure 53-1); the diaper area is usually spared. In older children and in those who have long-standing skin disease, the patient develops chronic AD with lichenification (Figure 53-2) and localization of the rash to the flexural folds of the extremities. AD often subsides as the patient grows older, leaving an adult with skin that is prone to itching and inflammation when exposed to exogenous irritants. At all stages of AD, patients usually have dry lackluster skin. Chronic hand eczema, the most common form of occupational skin disease, may be the primary manifestation of many adults with AD. Other features, including exogenous allergy or elevated IgE, are variable although commonly seen in AD.

Table 53-2 lists a number of inflammatory skin diseases, immunodeficiencies, skin malignancies, genetic disorders, infectious diseases, and infestations that share symptoms and signs with AD. These should be considered and ruled out

TABLE 53-1 Clinical Features of Atopic Dermatitis*

Essential features
- Pruritus
- Facial and extensor eczema in infants and children
- Flexural eczema in adults
- Chronic or relapsing dermatitis

Frequently associated features
- Personal or family history of atopic disease
- Xerosis
- Cutaneous infections
- Nonspecific dermatitis of the hands or feet
- Elevated serum IgE levels
- Positive immediate-type allergy skin tests
- Early age of onset

Other features
- Ichthyosis, palmar hyperlinearity, keratosis pilaris
- Pityriasis alba
- Nipple eczema
- White dermatographism and delayed blanch response
- Anterior subcapsular cataracts, keratoconus
- Dennie-Morgan infraorbital folds, orbital darkening
- Facial erythema or pallor
- Perifollicular accentuation

*Other skin conditions that may mimic atopic dermatitis should be excluded (see Table 53-2).

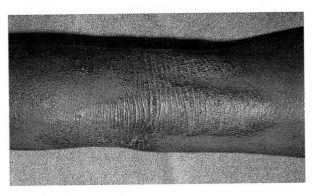

FIGURE 53-2 Adolescent with lichenification of the popliteal fossa from chronic atopic dermatitis. (From Weston WL, Morelli JG, Lane A, eds: *Color textbook of pediatric dermatology*, ed 3, St Louis, 2002, Mosby.)

Adolescents who present with an eczematous dermatitis with no history of childhood eczema, respiratory allergy, or atopic family history may have allergic contact dermatitis (see Chapter 55). A contact allergen should be considered in any patient whose AD does not respond to appropriate therapy. Of note, topical glucocorticoid contact allergy has been reported increasingly in patients with chronic dermatitis on topical corticosteroid therapy. Eczematous dermatitis has also been

before a diagnosis of AD is made. Infants presenting in the first year of life with failure to thrive, diarrhea, a generalized scaling erythematous rash, and recurrent cutaneous and/or systemic infections should be evaluated for severe combined immunodeficiency syndrome (see Chapter 9). Wiskott-Aldrich syndrome is an X-linked recessive disorder characterized by thrombocytopenia, variable abnormalities in humoral and cellular immunity, and recurrent severe bacterial infections. It is associated with cutaneous findings almost indistinguishable from AD. The hyperimmunoglobulin-E syndrome is characterized by elevated serum IgE levels, defective T and B cell function, recurrent deep-seated bacterial infections including cutaneous abscesses caused by *Staphylococcus aureus* and/or pruritic skin disease caused by *S. aureus* pustulosis, or recalcitrant dermatophytosis.

TABLE 53-2 Differential Diagnosis of Atopic Dermatitis

Congenital disorders
- Netherton's syndrome
- Familial keratosis pilaris

Chronic dermatoses
- Seborrheic dermatitis
- Contact dermatitis (allergic or irritant)
- Nummular eczema
- Psoriasis
- Ichthyoses

Infections and infestations
- Scabies
- Human immunodeficiency virus–associated dermatitis
- Dermatophytosis

Malignancies
- Cutaneous T cell lymphoma (mycosis fungoides/Sézary syndrome)
- Letterer-Siwe disease

Autoimmune disorders
- Dermatitis herpetiformis
- Pemphigus foliaceus
- Graft-versus-host disease
- Dermatomyositis

Immunodeficiencies
- Wiskott-Aldrich syndrome
- Severe combined immunodeficiency syndrome
- Hyper-IgE syndrome

Metabolic disorders
- Zinc deficiency
- Pyridoxine (vitamin B_6) and niacin
- Multiple carboxylase deficiency
- Phenylketonuria

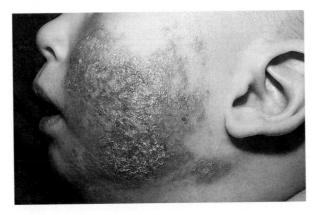

FIGURE 53-1 Infant with acute atopic dermatitis. Note the oozing and crusting skin lesions. (From Weston WL, Morelli JG, Lane A, eds: *Color textbook of pediatric dermatology*, ed 3, St Louis, 2002, Mosby.)

reported with human immunodeficiency virus as well as with a variety of infestations such as scabies. Other conditions that can be confused with AD include psoriasis, ichthyosis, and seborrheic dermatitis.

PATHOGENESIS

Interactions between susceptibility genes, the host's environment, pharmacologic abnormalities, and immunologic factors contribute to the pathogenesis of AD. The belief that AD has an immunologic basis is supported by the observation that primary T cell immunodeficiency disorders are frequently associated with elevated serum IgE levels and eczematoid skin lesions. Clearing of the skin rash occurs following correction of the immunologic defect by successful bone marrow transplantation.[9]

Systemic Immune Response

Most patients with AD have peripheral blood eosinophilia and increased serum IgE levels.[10] Nearly 80% of children with AD develop allergic rhinitis or asthma. Because serum IgE level is strongly associated with the prevalence of asthma, it suggests that allergen sensitization through the skin predisposes the patient to respiratory disease because of its effects on the systemic allergic response.[11] Indeed, when mice are sensitized epicutaneously with protein antigen, it induces allergic dermatitis, elevated serum IgE, airway eosinophilia, and hyperresponsiveness to methacholine. This suggests that epicutaneous exposure to allergen in AD enhances the development of allergic asthma.[12]

An increased frequency of skin homing T cells producing interleukin (IL)-4, IL-5, and IL-13 but little interferon (IFN)-γ has been found in the peripheral blood of patients with AD.[13] These immunologic alterations are important because IL-4 and IL-13 are the only cytokines that induce germline transcription at the Cε exon, thereby promoting isotype switching to IgE. IL-4 and IL-13 also induce the expression of vascular adhesion molecules such as vascular cell adhesion molecule-1 involved in eosinophil infiltration and down-regulate Th1-type cytokine activity. IL-5 plays a key role in the development, activation, and cell survival of eosinophils. In contrast, IFN-γ inhibits IgE synthesis as well as the proliferation of Th2 cells and expression of the IL-4 receptor on T cells. The decreased IFN-γ produced by T cells from AD patients may be the result of reduced production of IL-18.[14] Cytotoxic T cells have also been found to be depleted in AD.[15]

A number of determinants support Th2 cell development in AD. These include the cytokine milieu in which T cell development is taking placing, pharmacologic factors, the costimulatory signals used during T cell activation, and the antigen-presenting cell (APC).[11] In this regard, IL-4 promotes Th2 cell development, whereas IL-12, produced by macrophages, dendritic cells, or eosinophils, induces Th1 cells. Mononuclear cells from patients with AD have increased cyclic adenosine monophosphate (cAMP)–phosphodiesterase (PDE) enzyme activity.[16] This cellular abnormality contributes to the increased IgE synthesis by B cells and IL-4 production by T cells in AD as IgE and IL-4 production is decreased *in vitro* by PDE inhibitors.

Activation of resting T cells following engagement of T cell receptors with the MHC plus peptide complex on APC requires co-stimulatory signals, for example, interactions between CD80 or CD86 on APCs and CD28 on T cells. The expression of the co-stimulatory molecule, CD86, on B cells of AD patients is significantly higher than in normal patients or patients with psoriasis.[17] Importantly, total serum IgE from AD patients and normal subjects correlated significantly with CD86 expression on B cells. Anti-human CD86 but not CD80 mAb significantly decreased IgE production by peripheral blood mononuclear cells stimulated with IL-4 and anti-CD40 mAb. These data support the concept that CD86 expression in AD promotes IgE synthesis. IL-4 and IL-13 have also been found to induce CD86 expression on B cells, thereby providing an amplification loop for IgE synthesis in AD.

Skin Immunopathology

Pathology

Clinically *unaffected* skin of AD patients exhibits mild epidermal hyperplasia and a sparse perivascular T cell infiltrate.[18] Acute eczematous skin lesions are characterized by marked intercellular edema (spongiosis) of the epidermis. Dendritic APCs such as Langerhans cells (LC), and macrophages in lesional and, to a lesser extent, in nonlesional skin of AD patients have surface-bound IgE molecules. In the dermis of the acute lesion there is a marked perivenular T cell infiltrate with occasional monocyte-macrophages. The critical role of T cells in AD is suggested by the obligate role of T cells in mouse models of AD.[19] The lymphocytic infiltrate consists predominantly of activated memory T cells bearing CD3, CD4, and CD45 RO, suggesting a previous encounter with antigen). Eosinophils, basophils, and neutrophils are rarely present in acute AD; mast cells are found in normal numbers but in various stages of degranulation.

Chronic lichenified lesions are characterized by a hyperplastic epidermis with elongation of the rete ridges, prominent hyperkeratosis, and minimal spongiosis. There is an increased number of IgE-bearing LCs in the epidermis, and macrophages dominate the dermal mononuclear cell infiltrate. The number of mast cells are increased in number but are generally fully granulated. Increased numbers of eosinophils are observed in chronic AD skin lesions. Eosinophils secrete cytokines and mediators that augment allergic inflammation and induce tissue injury in AD through the production of reactive oxygen intermediates and release of toxic granule proteins.

Cytokine Expression

Th2- and Th1-type cytokines contribute to the pathogenesis of skin inflammation in AD. As compared with the skin of normal controls, unaffected skin of AD patients have an increased number of cells expressing IL-4 and IL-13, but not IL-5, IL-12, or IFN-γ, mRNA.[18,20] Acute and chronic skin lesions, when compared to normal skin or uninvolved skin of AD patients, have significantly greater numbers of cells that are positive for IL-4, IL-5, and IL-13 mRNA. However, acute AD does not contain significant numbers of IFN-γ or IL-12 mRNA-expressing cells.

Chronic AD skin lesions have significantly fewer IL-4 and IL-13 mRNA-expressing cells, but greater numbers of IL-5, granulocyte-macrophage colony-stimulating factor (GM-CSF), IL-12, and IFN-γ mRNA-expressing cells than acute

AD. IL-5 and GM-CSF probably contribute to the increased numbers of eosinophils and macrophages. The increased expression of IL-12 in chronic AD skin lesions is of interest in that cytokine plays a key role in IFN-γ induction. Its expression in eosinophils and/or macrophages may initiate the switch to Th1 or Th0 cell development in chronic AD.

Activated T cells infiltrating the skin of AD patients have also been found to induce keratinocyte apoptosis, which contributes to the spongiotic process found in AD skin lesions.[21] This process is mediated by IFN-γ, which up-regulates *Fas* on keratinocytes. The lethal hit is delivered to keratinocytes by *Fas*-ligand expressed on the surface of T cells that invade the epidermis and soluble *Fas*-ligand released from T cells.

Antigen-Presenting Cells

AD skin contains an increased number of IgE-bearing LCs, which appear to play an important role in cutaneous allergen presentation to Th2 cells.[22] In this regard, IgE-bearing LCs from AD skin lesions but not LCs that lack surface IgE are capable of presenting house dust mite allergen to T cells. These results suggest that cell-bound IgE on LCs facilitate capture and internalization of allergens into LCs before their processing and antigen presentation to T cells. IgE-bearing LCs that have captured allergen are likely to activate memory Th2 cells in atopic skin but may also migrate to the lymph nodes to stimulate naive T cells there to expand the pool of systemic Th2 cells.

Binding of IgE to LCs occurs primarily via high-affinity IgE receptors. The clinical importance of these IgE receptors on LCs is supported by the observation that the presence of FcεRI-expressing LCs bearing IgE molecules is required to provoke eczematous skin lesions by application of aeroallergens on uninvolved skin of AD patients. In contrast to mast cells and basophils where the FcεRI is a tetrameric structure constitutively expressed at high levels, this receptor on LCs lacks the classic β chain and its expression varies depending on the donor. Normal individuals and patients with respiratory allergy have low-level surface expression of FcεRI on their LCs, whereas FcεRI is expressed at high levels in the inflammatory environment of AD. High-level FcεRI expression enhances not only binding and uptake of allergens but the activation of LCs upon receptor ligation.

LCs in the lesional skin of AD predominantly express CD86 as compared to CD80.[23,24] Furthermore, antibodies to B7.2 completely inhibited T cell proliferation stimulated with *Dermatophagoides pteronyssinus* (house dust mite antigen) in the presence of LCs. These data suggest that CD86 expression on LCs plays an important role as co-stimulatory molecules for T cell activation and may account for the increased Th2 responses that occur after repeated antigen presentation by LCs.

Inflammatory Cell Infiltration

IL-16, a chemoattractant for CD4+ T cells, is increased in acute AD skin lesions.[25,26] The C-C chemokines, RANTES, monocyte chemotactic protein-4, and eotaxin have also been found to be increased in AD skin lesions and likely contribute to the chemotaxis of eosinophils and Th2 lymphocytes into the skin.[27-29] Recent studies suggest a role for cutaneous T cell-attracting chemokine (CTACK/CCL27) in the preferential attraction of CLA+ T cells to the skin.[30] The chemokine receptor CCR3, which is found on eosinophils and Th2 lymphocytes and can mediate the action of eotaxin, RANTES, and MCP-4,

has been reported to be increased in nonlesional and lesional skin of patients with AD.[28] Selective recruitment of CCR4 expressing Th2 cells into AD skin may also be mediated by the monocyte-derived chemokine and thymus- and activation-regulated chemokines, which are increased in AD.[31-33]

Chronic Skin Inflammation

Chronic AD is linked to the prolonged survival of eosinophils and monocyte-macrophages in atopic skin. IL-5 expression during chronic AD likely plays a role in prolonging eosinophil survival and enhancement of their function. In chronic AD the increased GM-CSF expression plays an important role in maintaining the survival and function of monocytes, LCs, and eosinophils.[34] Epidermal keratinocytes from AD patients have significantly higher levels of RANTES expression following stimulation with tumor necrosis factor (TNF)-α and IFN-γ than keratinocytes from psoriasis patients.[35] This may serve as one mechanism by which the TNF-α and IFN-γ production during chronic AD enhances the chronicity and severity of eczema. Mechanical trauma can also induce the release of TNF-α and many other proinflammatory cytokines from epidermal keratinocytes. Thus, chronic scratching plays a role in the perpetuation and elicitation of skin inflammation in AD.

GENETICS

AD is familially transmitted with a strong maternal influence. There has been considerable interest in the potential role of chromosome 5q31-33 as it contains a clustered family of cytokine genes, that is, IL-3, IL-4, IL-5, IL-13, and GM-CSF, which are expressed by Th2 cells.[36] A case-control comparison has suggested a genotypic association between the T allele of the -590C/T polymorphism of the IL-4 gene promoter region with AD. Because the T allele is associated with increased IL-4 gene promoter activity compared with the C allele, this suggests that genetic differences in transcriptional activity of the IL-4 gene influence AD predisposition. In addition, an association of AD with a gain-of-function mutation in the alpha subunit of the IL-4 receptor has been reported. These data support the concept that IL-4 gene expression plays a critical role in the expression of AD. A functional mutation in the promoter region of the C-C chemokine RANTES and an IL-13 coding region variant may also be involved in the pathogenesis of AD. These candidate gene approaches have, therefore, identified genes that suggest that AD has a common genetic basis with other atopic diseases.

A significant association between a specific polymorphism in the mast cell chymase gene and AD has been identified that has no association with asthma or allergic rhinitis.[37] This finding suggests that a genetic variant of mast cell chymase, which is a serine protease secreted by skin mast cells, may have organ-specific effects and contribute to the genetic susceptibility for AD. AD has also been associated with a low-producer transforming growth factor beta cytokine genotype.[38] Because transforming growth factor beta is an important regulatory gene that down-regulates T cell activation, a low production genotype may contribute to increased skin inflammation.

Two genome-wide linkage studies have identified susceptibility loci for AD. A study by Lee et al[39] suggested linkage for AD on chromosome 3q21, a region that encodes the costimulatory molecules CD80 and CD86. In contrast, Cookson et al[40] reported linkage of AD to chromosome 1q21 and 17q25, identifying loci that closely coincide with regions linked to psoriasis. This suggests that AD is influenced by genes that modulate skin responses independent of allergic mechanisms.

IMMUNOLOGIC TRIGGERS

Foods

Well-controlled studies have demonstrated that food allergens induce skin rashes in children with AD.[41] Based on double-blind, placebo-controlled food challenges approximately 40% of infants and young children with moderate to severe AD have food allergy. Food allergies in AD patients induce eczematous dermatitis and contribute to severity of skin disease in some patients,[42] whereas in others urticarial reactions, contact urticaria, or other noncutaneous symptom complexes are elicited. Removal of food allergens from the patient's diet can lead to significant clinical improvement but requires a great deal of education because most of the common allergens (e.g., egg, milk, wheat, soy, and peanut) contaminate many foods and are therefore difficult to avoid.[43]

Infants and young children with food allergy generally have positive immediate skin tests or serum IgE directed to various foods. Positive food challenges are accompanied by significant increases in plasma histamine levels and eosinophil activation. Importantly, food allergen-specific T cells have been cloned from the skin lesions of patients with AD, providing direct evidence that foods can contribute to skin inflammation.[44] In mouse models of AD, oral sensitization with foods results in the elicitation of eczematous skin lesions on repeat oral food challenges.[45] In patients, however, immediate skin tests for specific allergens do not always indicate clinical sensitivity. Therefore clinically relevant food allergy must be verified by controlled food challenges or carefully investigating the effects of a food elimination diet, which is being done in the absence of other exacerbating factors.

Aeroallergens

A number of well-controlled studies have demonstrated that pruritus and eczematoid skin lesions develop after intranasal or bronchial inhalation challenge with aeroallergens, but not placebo in AD patients sensitized to inhalant allergens.[46] Epicutaneous application of aeroallergens by patch test techniques on uninvolved atopic skin elicits eczematoid reactions in 30% to 50% of patients with AD.[47] Positive reactions have been observed to dust mite, weeds, animal dander, and molds. In contrast, patients with respiratory allergy and healthy volunteers rarely have positive allergen patch tests.

Several studies have examined whether avoidance of aeroallergens results in clinical improvement of AD. Most of these reports have involved uncontrolled trials in which patients were placed in mite-free environments, for example, hospital rooms in which acaricides or impermeable mattress covers were used. Such methods have invariably led to improvement in AD. One double-blind, placebo-controlled study using a combination of effective mite-reduction measures, as compared to no treatment, in the home has reported that a reduction in house dust mites is associated with significantly greater improvement in AD.[48-50]

Laboratory data supporting a role for inhalants include the finding of IgE antibody to specific inhalant allergens in most patients with AD. Indeed, a recent study found that 95% of sera from AD patients had IgE to house dust mites as compared to 42% of asthmatic subjects.[51] The degree of sensitization to aeroallergens is directly associated with the severity of AD.[52] The isolation from AD skin lesions and allergen patch test sites of T cells that selectively respond to *D. pteronyssinus* (Der p1) and other aeroallergens provides further evidence that the immune response in AD skin can be elicited by aeroallergens.[47]

Staphylococcus Aureus

Patients with AD have an increased tendency to develop bacterial (Figure 53-3), viral (Figure 53-4) and fungal skin infections. *S. aureus* is found in over 90% of AD skin lesions. The density of *S. aureus* on inflamed AD lesions without clinical superinfection can reach up to 10^7 colony-forming units per cm² on lesional skin. The importance of *S. aureus* is supported by the observation that even AD patients without overt infection show a greater reduction in severity of skin disease when treated with a combination of antistaphylococcal antibiotics and topical corticosteroids as compared to topical corticosteroids alone.[53]

One strategy by which *S. aureus* exacerbates or maintains skin inflammation in AD is by secreting a group of toxins known to act as superantigens, which stimulate marked activation of T cells and macrophages. The skin lesions of over half of AD patients have *S. aureus* that secrete superantigens such as enterotoxins A, B, and toxic shock syndrome toxin-1.[54,55] An analysis of the peripheral blood skin homing CLA+ T cells from these patients as well as T cells in their skin lesions reveals that they have undergone a beta region of the T cell receptor variable chain expansion consistent with superantigenic stimulation.[56,57] Most AD patients make specific IgE antibodies directed against the staphylococcal superantigens found on their skin.[54,55] Basophils from patients with IgE antibodies directed to superantigens release histamine on exposure to the relevant superantigen, but not in response to superantigens to which they have no specific IgE.[54] This raises the interesting possibility that superantigens induce specific

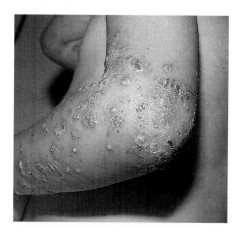

FIGURE 53-3 Patient with atopic dermatitis who is secondarily infected with *Staphylococcus aureus*. Note multiple pustules and areas of crusting. (From Weston WL, Morelli JG, Lane A, eds: *Color textbook of pediatric dermatology*, ed 3, St Louis, 2002, Mosby.)

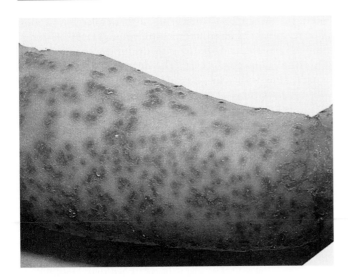

FIGURE 53-4 Eczema herpeticum, the primary skin manifestation of herpes simplex in atopic dermatitis. (From Fireman P, Slavin R, eds: *Atlas of allergies,* ed 2, London, 1996, Mosby-Wolfe.)

IgE in AD patients and mast cell degranulation *in vivo* when the superantigens penetrate their disrupted epidermal barrier. This promotes the itch-scratch cycle critical to the evolution of skin rashes in AD.

A correlation has also been found between the presence of IgE anti-superantigens and severity of AD.[55] Utilizing a humanized murine model of skin inflammation, the combination of *S. aureus* superantigen plus allergen has been shown to have an additive effect in inducing skin inflammation.[58] Superantigens can also augment allergen-specific IgE synthesis and induce corticosteroid resistance, suggesting that several mechanisms exist by which superantigens could aggravate the severity of AD.[59,60] Fulfilling Koch's postulates, application of the superantigen staphylococcal enterotoxin B (SEB) to the skin can induce skin changes of erythema and induration accompanied by the infiltration of T cells that are selectively expanded in response to SEB.[61,62] Furthermore, in a prospective study of patients recovering from toxic shock syndrome, it was found that 14 of 68 patients developed chronic eczematoid dermatitis whereas no patients recovering from gram-negative sepsis developed eczema.[63] These investigators concluded that superantigens may induce an atopic process in the skin. It is therefore of interest that superantigens have been demonstrated to induce T cell expression of the skin homing receptor via stimulation of IL-12 production.[64]

Increased binding of *S. aureus* to AD skin is likely related to underlying atopic skin, inflammation. This concept is supported by several lines of investigation. First, it has been found that treatment with topical corticosteroids or tacrolimus will reduce *S. aureus* counts on atopic skin, although they have no antibiotic actions.[65,66] Second, acute inflammatory lesions have more *S. aureus* than chronic AD skin lesions or normal-looking atopic skin. Scratching likely enhances *S. aureus* binding by disturbing the skin barrier and exposing extracellular matrix molecules known to act as adhesins for *S. aureus,* for example, fibronectin and collagens. Finally, in studies of *S. aureus* binding to skin lesions of mice undergoing Th1 versus Th2 inflammatory responses, bacterial binding was significantly greater at skin sites with Th2-mediated inflammation.[67]

Importantly, this increased bacterial binding did not occur in IL-4 gene knockout mice, indicating that IL-4 plays a crucial role in the enhancement of *S. aureus* binding to skin. IL-4 appears to enhance *S. aureus* binding to the skin by inducing the synthesis of fibronectin, an important *S. aureus* adhesin. Interestingly studies of human AD have found a role for fibrinogen in the binding of *S. aureus* to atopic skin.[68] Because acute exudative lesions likely have increased plasma-derived fibrinogen, this may provide a mechanism for further binding of *S. aureus* to acute AD lesions.

The highly increased binding of *S. aureus* to AD skin is not enough to account for the highly increased numbers of *S. aureus* found on AD as compared to normal skin. Once bound to AD skin, *S. aureus* must therefore rapidly proliferate as the result of impaired local immune responses. Two major classes of antimicrobial peptides are known in mammalian skin: β-*defensins* and *cathelicidins.* They have been shown to have antimicrobial activities against bacterial, fungal, and viral pathogens. The mechanism of action for these cationic antimicrobial peptides involves disruption of the microbial membrane or the penetration of the microbial membranes to interfere with intracellular functions. Recently we have found that AD is markedly deficient in the production of β-defensins and cathelicidins.[69]

Autoallergens

In the 1920s several investigators reported that human skin dander could trigger immediate hypersensitivity reactions in the skin of patients with severe AD, suggesting that they made IgE against autoantigens in the skin.[70] The potential molecular basis for these observations was recently demonstrated by Valenta et al[71] who reported that the majority of sera from patients with severe AD contain IgE antibodies directed against human proteins. One of these IgE-reactive autoantigens has been cloned from a human epithelial cDNA expression library and designated *Hom s 1*, which is a 55kDa cytoplasmic protein in skin keratinocytes.[72] Such antibodies were not detected in patients with chronic urticaria, systemic lupus erythematosus, and graft-versus-host disease or in health controls. Although the autoallergens characterized to date have mainly been intracellular proteins, they have been detected in IgE immune complexes of AD sera, suggesting that release of these autoallergens from damaged tissues could trigger responses mediated by IgE or T cells. This concept is supported by the recent observation that IgE autoallergen titers decreased with resolution of AD.[73] These data suggest that, whereas IgE immune responses are initiated by environmental allergens, allergic inflammation can be maintained by human endogenous antigens, particularly in severe AD.

MANAGEMENT

Successful management of AD requires a multipronged approach involving skin hydration, pharmacologic therapy, and the identification and elimination of flare factors such as irritants, allergens, infectious agents, and emotional stressors (Figure 53-5).[74] Treatment plans should be individualized to address each patient's skin disease reaction pattern and trigger factors that are unique to the patient. In patients refractory to conventional forms of therapy, alternative antiinflammatory and immunomodulatory agents may be necessary.

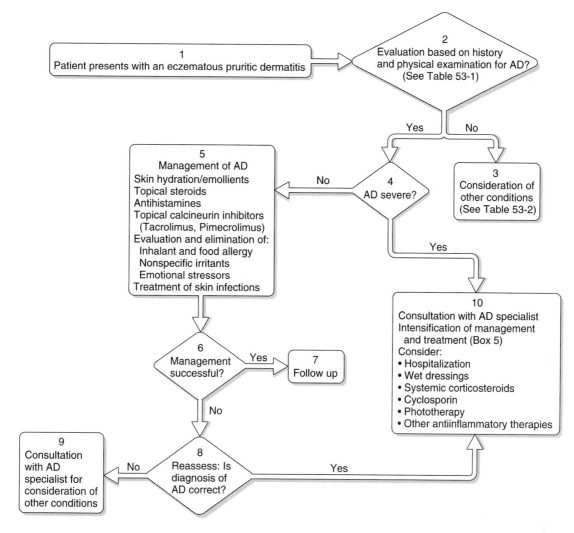

FIGURE 53-5 Clinical algorithm for diagnosis and management of atopic dermatitis.

Cutaneous Hydration

Patients with AD have a marked decrease in skin barrier function associated with reduced ceramide levels and enhanced transepidermal water loss.[75] This leads to dry skin (xerosis) contributing to disease morbidity by the development of microfissures and cracks, which serve as portals of entry for skin pathogens, irritants, and allergens. Lukewarm soaking baths for at least 20 minutes, followed by the application of an occlusive emollient to retain moisture can give patients excellent symptomatic relief. Use of an effective emollient combined with hydration therapy will help to restore and preserve the stratum corneum barrier.

Hydration, by baths or wet dressings, promotes transepidermal penetration of topical glucocorticoids. Dressings may also serve as an effective barrier against persistent scratching, allowing more rapid healing of excoriated lesions. Wet dressings are recommended for use on severely affected or chronically involved areas of dermatitis refractory to skin care. Overuse of wet dressings may result in maceration of the skin and may be complicated by secondary infection. Wet dressings

or baths also have the potential to promote drying and fissuring of the skin if not followed by topical emollient use. Thus, wet dressing therapy is reserved for poorly controlled AD and should be closely monitored by a physician.

Topical Glucocorticoids

Glucocorticoids have been the cornerstone of anti-inflammatory treatment for over 50 years. Because of potential side effects, most physicians use topical glucocorticoids for control of acute exacerbation of AD. However, recent studies suggest that once control of AD is achieved with a daily regimen of topical glucocorticoid, long-term control can be maintained with twice-weekly applications of topical fluticasone to areas that have healed but are prone to developing eczema.[76]

Patients should be carefully instructed in the use of topical glucocorticoids to avoid potential side effects. The potent fluorinated glucocorticoids should be avoided on the face, the genitalia, and the intertriginous areas. Patients should be instructed to apply topical glucocorticoids to their skin lesions and to use emollients over uninvolved skin. Failure of a patient to respond to topical glucocorticoids is sometimes because of an inadequate supply. It is important to remember that it takes approximately 30 g of cream or ointment to cover the entire skin surface of an adult once. To treat the entire body twice daily for 2 weeks requires approximately 840 g (2 lb) of topical glucocorticoids.

There are seven classes of topical glucocorticoids, ranked according to their potency based on vasoconstrictor assays. Because of their potential side effects the ultrahigh-potency glucocorticoids should be used only for very short periods of time and in areas that are lichenified, but not on the face or intertriginous areas. The goal is to use emollients to enhance skin hydration and lower-potency glucocorticoids for maintenance therapy.

Side effects from topical glucocorticoids are directly related to the potency ranking of the compound and the length of use, so it is incumbent on the clinician to balance the need for a more potent steroid with the potential for side effects. In addition, ointments have a greater potential to occlude the epidermis, resulting in enhanced systemic absorption compared to creams. Side effects from topical glucocorticoids can be divided into local side effects and systemic side effects resulting from suppression of the hypothalamic-pituitary-adrenal axis. Local side effects include the development of striae and skin atrophy; systemic side effects are related to the potency of the topical glucocorticoid, the site of application, the occlusiveness of the preparation, the percentage of the body surface area covered, and the length of use. The potential for potent topical glucocorticoid to cause adrenal suppression is greatest in infants and young children.

Topical Calcineurin Inhibitors

Tacrolimus

Topically applied FK-506 or tacrolimus, a calcineurin inhibitor that acts by binding to FK binding protein, has been successfully used in the treatment of AD.[77] Tacrolimus inhibits the activation of a number of key cells involved in AD, including T cells, LCs, mast cells, and keratinocytes.[78] AD patients receiving this form of therapy can have markedly diminished pruritus within 3 days of initiating therapy. Skin biopsy results after treatment demonstrates markedly diminished T cell and eosinophilic infiltrates as well as decreased FcεRI expression on both LCs and inflammatory dendritic epidermal cells. Multicenter, blinded, vehicle-controlled Phase 3 trials with tacrolimus ointment, 0.03% and 0.1%, in both adults and children with AD have shown tacrolimus to be both safe and effective.[79-81] Local burning sensation has been the only common adverse event. In adults but not children a dose-response effect was seen between 0.03% and 0.1% tacrolimus, particularly for patients with severe skin disease. Long-term open-label studies with tacrolimus ointment applied on up to 100% body surface area have been performed in adults and children with demonstrated sustained efficacy and no significant side effects, for example, no increased skin infections have been observed.[82] In addition, unlike topical corticosteroids, tacrolimus ointment does not cause cutaneous atrophy and has been used safely for facial and eyelid eczema. Tacrolimus ointment (Protopic) 0.03% has been approved by the Food and Drug Administration (FDA) for short-term and intermittent long-term use in moderate-severe AD for children 2 to 15 years of age and in formulations of 0.03% as well as 0.1% for adults.

Pimecrolimus

Ascomycin compounds, that act by binding to macrophilin 12 to interfere with calcineurin action, have been developed in topical and oral forms that appear to have preferential drug distribution to the skin. Like tacrolimus, they inhibit Th1 and Th2 cytokine production, reduce antigen-presenting capacity of dendritic cells, and have also been shown to inhibit mediator release from mast cells and basophils.[83] Multicenter, blinded, vehicle-controlled Phase 3 trials with pimecrolimus ointment, 1%, in both adults and children with AD have shown pimecrolimus to be both safe and effective,[84,85] with little systemic absorption.[86] Pimecrolimus cream ointment (Elidel) 1% has been approved by the FDA for short-term and intermittent long-term use in mild-moderate AD for patients 2 years of age and over. Because of its lack of skin toxicity including absence of skin atrophy, several studies have explored its use as a prophylactic anti-inflammatory agent used to prevent relapses of AD. These studies have demonstrated that treatment with Elidel at the earliest signs of AD significantly reduces the incidence of flares and decreases the use of corticosteroids.[87]

Identification and Elimination of Triggering Factors

Patients with AD are more susceptible to irritants than are normal individuals. Thus it is important to identify and eliminate aggravating factors that trigger the itch-scratch cycle. These include soaps or detergents, chemicals, smoke, abrasive clothing, and extremes of temperature and humidity. Alcohol and astringents found in toiletries are drying. When soaps are used, they should have minimal defatting activity and a neutral pH. Using a liquid rather than powder detergent and adding a second rinse cycle will facilitate removal of the detergent.

Recommendations regarding environmental living conditions should include temperature and humidity control to avoid problems related to heat, humidity, and perspiration. Every attempt should be made to allow children to be as normally active as possible. Certain sports such as swimming may be better tolerated than other sports involving intense perspiration, physical contact, or heavy clothing and equipment, but chlorine should be rinsed off immediately after swimming and the skin lubricated. Although ultraviolet light may be beneficial to some patients with AD, sunscreens should be used to avoid sunburn.

Specific Allergens

Potential allergens can be identified by taking a careful history and carrying out selective skin prick tests. Negative skin tests or serum tests for allergen-specific IgE have a high predictive value for ruling out suspected allergens. Positive skin or *in vitro* tests, particularly to foods, often do not correlate with clinical symptoms and should be confirmed with controlled food challenges and elimination diets. Avoidance of foods implicated in controlled challenges has been shown to result in clinical improvement.[41,42] Infants who do not improve on formulas containing hydrolyzed proteins should be fed more elemental formulas.[88] Extensive elimination diets, which in some cases can be nutritionally deficient, are rarely if ever required because even with multiple positive skin tests, the majority of patients will react to three or fewer foods on controlled challenge. Most food-allergic children, however, outgrow their food hypersensitivity in the first few years of life so food allergy is not a common trigger factor in older patients with AD. In patients allergic to dust mites, prolonged avoidance of dust mites has been found to result in improvement of AD. Avoidance measures include using dust mite–proof casings on pillows, mattresses, and box springs; washing bedding in hot water weekly; removing bedroom carpeting; and decreasing indoor humidity levels with air conditioning. Because there are many triggers contributing to the flares of AD, attention should be focused on identifying and controlling the flare factors that are important to the individual patient.

Emotional Stressors

AD patients often respond to frustration, embarrassment, or other stressful events with increased pruritus and scratching. In some instances, scratching is simply habitual and less commonly associated with significant secondary gain. Stress can also lead to immunologic changes in patients with AD.[89,90] Psychologic evaluation or counseling should be considered in patients who have difficulty with emotional triggers or psychologic problems contributing to difficulty in managing their disease. Relaxation, behavioral modification, or biofeedback may be helpful in patients who scratch habitually.

Infectious Agents

Antistaphylococcal antibiotics are very helpful in the treatment of patients who are heavily colonized or infected with *S. aureus*.[91] Erythromycin and the newer macrolide antibiotics (azithromycin and clarithromycin) are usually beneficial for patients who are not colonized with a resistant *S. aureus* strain. However, for macrolide-resistant *S. aureus,* a penicillinase-resistant penicillin (dicloxacillin, oxacillin, or cloxacillin) may be preferred. First-generation cephalosporins also offer effective coverage for both staphylococci and streptococci. Topical mupirocin or fusidic acid offers some utility in the treatment of localized impetiginized lesions; however, in patients with extensive superinfection, a course of systemic antibiotics is most practical.

AD can be complicated by recurrent viral skin infections that may reflect local defects in T cell function. The most serious viral infection is Herpes simplex, which can affect patients of all ages, resulting in Kaposi's varicelliform eruption or eczema herpeticum. After an incubation period of 5 to 12 days, multiple, itchy, vesiculopustular lesions erupt in a disseminated pattern; vesicular lesions are umbilicated, tend to crop, and often become hemorrhagic and crusted. These lesions may coalesce to large, denuded, and bleeding areas that can extend over the entire body. Herpes simplex can provoke recurrent dermatitis and may be misdiagnosed as *S. aureus* infection. The presence of punched-out erosions, vesicles, and/or infected skin lesions that fail to respond to oral antibiotics should initiate a search for herpes simplex. This can be

diagnosed by a Giemsa-stained Tzanck smear of cells scraped from the vesicle base or by viral culture. For suspected infection caused by herpes simplex, topical glucocorticoids are best discontinued, at least temporarily. Antiviral treatment for cutaneous herpes simplex infections is of critical importance in the patient with widespread AD because life-threatening dissemination has been reported.

In patients with AD, smallpox vaccination or even exposure to vaccinated individuals may cause a severe widespread skin rash called *eczema vaccinatum* similar in appearance to eczema herpeticum.[92] An increased risk of fatalities resulting from eczema vaccinatum has been reported in AD. Even if not fatal, eczema vaccinatum is often associated with severe scarring and lifelong complications following recovery from this illness. As the medical community prepares for potential bioterrorism attacks with smallpox, it is important to weigh the risks versus the benefits of smallpox vaccination in patients with AD.

Patients with AD have an increased prevalence of *Trichophyton rubrum* infections compared to non-atopic controls. There has been particular interest in the role of *Malassezia furfur* (*Pityrosporum ovale*) in AD. *M. furfur* is a lipophilic yeast commonly present in the seborrheic areas of the skin. IgE antibodies against *M. furfur* are commonly found in AD patients and most frequently in patients with head and neck dermatitis.[93] In contrast, IgE sensitization to *M. furfur* is rarely observed in normal controls or asthma patients. Positive allergen patch test reactions to this yeast have also been demonstrated. The potential importance of *M. furfur* as well as other dermatophyte infections is further supported by the reduction of AD skin severity in such patients following treatment with antifungal agents.

Control of Pruritus

The treatment of pruritus in AD should be directed primarily at the underlying causes. Reduction of skin inflammation and dryness with topical glucocorticoids and skin hydration, respectively, will often symptomatically reduce pruritus. Inhaled and ingested allergens should be eliminated if documented to cause skin rash in controlled challenges. Systemic antihistamines act primarily by blocking the H_1 receptors in the dermis and thereby ameliorate histamine-induced pruritus. However, histamine is only one of many mediators that can induce pruritus of the skin, so certain patients may derive minimal benefit from antihistaminic therapy. Some antihistamines are also mild anxiolytic agents and may offer symptomatic relief through their tranquilizing and sedative effects. Studies of newer nonsedating antihistamines have shown variable results in the effectiveness of controlling pruritus in AD patients although they may be useful in the subset of AD patients with concomitant urticaria.[94]

Because pruritus is usually worse at night, the sedating antihistamines, for example, hydroxyzine or diphenhydramine, may offer an advantage with their soporific side effects when used at bedtime. Doxepin hydrochloride has both tricyclic antidepressant and H_1- and H_2-histamine receptor blocking effects. Thus, it may be useful in treating children and adolescents who do not respond to H_1 sedating antihistamines. If nocturnal pruritus remains severe, short-term use of a sedative to allow adequate rest may be appropriate. Treatment of

AD with topical antihistamines is generally not recommended because of potential cutaneous sensitization. However, short-term (1 week) application of topical 5% doxepin cream has been reported to reduce pruritus without sensitization. It is noteworthy that sedation is a side effect of widespread application of doxepin cream.

Tar Preparations

Coal tar preparations may have antipruritic and antiinflammatory effects on the skin. The antiinflammatory properties of tars, however, are not well characterized and are usually not as pronounced as those of topical glucocorticoids. Tar shampoos can be beneficial for scalp dermatitis and are often helpful in reducing the concentration and frequency of topical glucocorticoid applications. Tar preparations should not be used on acutely inflamed skin because this often results in skin irritation. Side effects associated with tars include folliculitis and photosensitivity. There is a theoretic risk of tar being a carcinogen based on observational studies of workers using tar components in their occupations.

Phototherapy

Natural sunlight is frequently beneficial to patients with AD; however, if the sunlight occurs in the setting of high heat or humidity, thereby triggering sweating and pruritus, it may be deleterious to patients. Broad-band ultraviolet B, broad-band ultraviolet A, narrow-band ultraviolet B (311 nm), UVA-1 (340 to 400 nm), and combined UVAB phototherapy can be useful adjuncts in the treatment of AD.[95] Photochemotherapy with PUVA may be indicated in patients with severe, widespread AD even though studies comparing it with other modes of phototherapy are limited. Short-term adverse effects with phototherapy may include erythema, skin pain, pruritus, and pigmentation; long-term adverse effects include premature skin aging and cutaneous malignancies.

Systemic Therapy

Systemic Glucocorticoids

The use of systemic glucocorticoids, such as oral prednisone, is rarely indicated in the treatment of chronic AD. The dramatic clinical improvement that may occur with systemic glucocorticoids is frequently associated with a severe rebound flare of AD following the discontinuation of systemic glucocorticoids. Short courses of oral glucocorticoids may be appropriate for an acute exacerbation of AD while other treatment measures are being instituted. If a short course of oral glucocorticoids is given, it is important to taper the dosage and begin intensified skin care, particularly with topical glucocorticoids and frequent bathing followed by application of emollients, in order to prevent rebound flaring of AD.

Allergen Immunotherapy

Unlike allergic rhinitis and extrinsic asthma, immunotherapy with aeroallergens has not been proven to be efficacious in the treatment of AD. There are anecdotal reports of both disease exacerbation and improvement. Well-controlled studies are still required to determine the role for immunotherapy with this disease, and this form of treatment for AD should be reserved for individuals who have a clear, demonstrable history of aeroallergen-induced AD, for example, seasonal exacerbations to pollen.

Interferon-γ

IFN-γ is known to suppress IgE responses and down-regulate Th2 cell proliferation and function. Several studies of patients with AD, including a multicenter, double-blinded, placebo-controlled trial, have demonstrated that treatment with recombinant IFN-γ results in clinical improvement.[96] Reduction in clinical severity of AD was correlated with the ability of IFN-γ to decrease total circulating eosinophil counts. Influenza-like symptoms are commonly observed side effects seen early in the treatment course.

Cyclosporine

Cyclosporine is a potent immunosuppressive drug that acts primarily on T cells by suppressing cytokine transcription. The drug binds to an intracellular protein, cyclophilin, and this complex in turn inhibits calcineurin, a molecule required for initiation of cytokine gene transcription. Multiple studies have demonstrated that patients with severe AD, refractory to conventional treatment, can benefit from short-term cyclosporine treatment with reduced skin disease and improved quality of life.[97] However, discontinuation of treatment generally results in rapid relapse of skin disease. Elevated serum creatinine or more significant renal impairment and hypertension are specific side effects that are of concern when cyclosporine is used.

Antimetabolites

Mycophenolate mofetil (MMF), a purine biosynthesis inhibitor used as an immunosuppressant in organ transplantation, has been used for treatment of refractory inflammatory skin disorders.[98] Short-term oral MMF as monotherapy has been reported in open-label studies to result in clearing of skin lesions in adults with AD resistant to other treatment, including topical and oral steroids and PUVA. The drug has generally been well tolerated with the exception of one patient developing herpes retinitis that may have been secondary to this immunosuppressive agent. Dose-related bone marrow suppression has also been observed. Of note, not all patients benefit from treatment so the medication should be discontinued if patients do not respond within 4 to 8 weeks. Dose finding and well-controlled studies are needed for this drug.

Methotrexate is an antimetabolite with potent inhibitory effects on inflammatory cytokine synthesis and cell chemotaxis. It has been used for AD patients with recalcitrant disease even though controlled trials are lacking. Dosing is more frequent than the weekly dosing used for psoriasis. Azathioprine is a purine analogue with antiinflammatory and antiproliferative effects; it has been used for severe AD, although no controlled trials have been reported. Myelosuppression is a significant adverse effect, and thiopurinemethyl transferase levels may predict individuals at risk.

Other Therapies

Leukocytes from patients with AD have increased cAMP-PDE enzyme activity. Monocytes from AD patients produce elevated levels of prostaglandin E$_2$ and IL-10, which both inhibit IFN-γ production by T cells. Clinical studies using topical application of high-potency PDE inhibitors have demonstrated clinical benefit in AD.[16]

<table>
<tr><td>

BOX 53-1

KEY CONCEPTS

Atopic Dermatitis

- Atopic dermatitis (AD) affects 10% to 20% of children.
- AD is a genetically transmitted chronic inflammatory allergic skin disease.
- Skin-homing T cells express T helper cell type 2 (Th2) cytokines that induce IgE and eosinophilia.
- Antigen-presenting cells in the skin (e.g., Langerhans cells) express surface-bound IgE molecules.
- Transition from acute to chronic AD is associated with a switch from predominantly Th2 cytokines to a combination of Th1 and Th2 cytokine gene expression.
- Immunologic triggers include foods, aeroallergens, microbial agents, and autoallergens.

</td></tr>
</table>

By virtue of its immunomodulatory and antiinflammatory actions, intravenous immunoglobulin has been used effectively in the treatment of a number of immune-mediated diseases (see Chapter 17). High-dose intravenous immunoglobulin has been reported to reduce skin inflammation in patients with refractory AD.[99] The benefits of intravenous immunoglobulin therapy in AD, however, can be rather short-lived, that is, the effects are gone within 3 weeks. Therefore it is important to intensify local skin care in combination with such alternative therapies.

Several studies have suggested that patients with AD benefit from treatment with traditional Chinese herbal therapy.[100] The beneficial response of Chinese herbal therapy, however, is often temporary, and its effects may wear off despite continued treatment. The possibility of hepatic toxicity, cardiac side effects, or idiosyncratic reactions remains a concern. The specific ingredients of the herbs also remain to be elucidated and some preparations have been found to be contaminated with corticosteroids. AD is an illness associated with a multitude of immunoregulatory abnormalities and future directions in therapy are likely to focus on a number of different immunologic targets in this illness.

BOX 53-2

THERAPEUTIC PRINCIPLES
Atopic Dermatitis

Skin hydration and emollients are needed to repair skin barrier function.

Topical antiinflammatory agents (corticosteroids, pimecrolimus, tacrolimus) are the cornerstones of therapy for acute flares and prevention of relapses.

Avoidance of food and inhalant allergens may prevent flares.

Antimicrobial therapy is often useful in poorly controlled patients.

Sedating antihistamines may promote sleeping at night.

Nonsedating antihistamines may be useful for patients with concomitant urticaria or coexisting respiratory allergy.

Considerations for refractory patients include phototherapy, systemic glucocorticoids, cyclosporin, interferon-γ, mycophenolate, and methotrexate.

CONCLUSIONS

AD is a common genetically transmitted inflammatory skin disease frequently found in association with respiratory allergy (Box 53-1). The keys to management are skin hydration; use of effective topical antiinflammatory agents such as corticosteroids, tacrolimus, or pimecrolimus; and avoidance of allergenic triggers and skin irritants (Box 53-2). With a better understanding of the immunoregulatory abnormalities underlying AD, new paradigms are emerging to more effectively treat acute flares of AD and to prevent relapses of this skin condition.

HELPFUL WEBSITES

The American Academy of Dermatology website (www.aad.org/)

The American Academy of Family Physicians website (www.aafp.org/afp/990915ap/1191.html)

The National Eczema Association for Science and Education website (www.nationaleczema.org/)

The American Academy of Allergy, Asthma, and Immunology website (www.aaaai.org/)

REFERENCES

1. Bieber T, Leung DYM, eds: *Atopic dermatitis*, New York, 2002, Marcel Dekker.
2. Finlay AY: Quality of life in atopic dermatitis, *J Am Acad Dermatol* 45:S64-S66, 2001.
3. Schultz-Larsen F, Hanifin JM: Epidemiology of atopic dermatitis, *Immunol Allergy Clin North Am* 22:1-24, 2002.
4. Williams H, Robertson C, Stewart A, et al: Worldwide variations in the prevalence of symptoms of atopic eczema in the International Study of Asthma and Allergies in Childhood, *J Allergy Clin Immunol* 103:125-138, 1999.
5. Laughter D, Istvan JA, Tofte SJ, et al: The prevalence of atopic dermatitis in Oregon schoolchildren, *J Am Acad Dermatol* 43:649-655, 2000.
6. von Mutius E: The environmental predictors of allergic disease, *J Allergy Clin Immunol* 105:9-19, 2000.
7. Romagnani S: The role of lymphocytes in allergic disease, *J Allergy Clin Immunol* 105:399-408, 2000.
8. Williams HC: Diagnostic criteria for atopic dermatitis: where do we go from here? *Arch Dermatol* 135:583-586, 1999.
9. Saurat JH: Eczema in primary immune-deficiencies: clues to the pathogenesis of atopic dermatitis with special reference to the Wiskott-Aldrich syndrome, *Acta Dermatol Venereol Suppl (Stockh)* 114:125-128, 1985.
10. Leung DY: Atopic dermatitis: new insights and opportunities for therapeutic intervention, *J Allergy Clin Immunol* 105:860-876, 2000.
11. Beck LA, Leung DY: Allergen sensitization through the skin induces systemic allergic responses, *J Allergy Clin Immunol* 106:S258-S263, 2000.
12. Spergel JM, Mizoguchi E, Brewer JP, et al: Epicutaneous sensitization with protein antigen induces localized allergic dermatitis and hyperresponsiveness to methacholine after single exposure to aerosolized antigen in mice, *J Clin Invest* 101:1614-1622, 1998.
13. Akdis M, Simon HU, Weigl L, et al: Skin homing (cutaneous lymphocyte-associated antigen-positive) CD8+ T cells respond to superantigen and contribute to eosinophilia and IgE production in atopic dermatitis, *J Immunol* 163:466-475, 1999.
14. Higashi N, Gesser B, Kawana S, et al: Expression of IL-18 mRNA and secretion of IL-18 are reduced in monocytes from patients with atopic dermatitis, *J Allergy Clin Immunol* 108:607-614, 2001.
15. Ambach A, Bonnekoh B, Gollnick H: Perforin hyperreleasability and depletion in cytotoxic T cells from patients with exacerbated atopic dermatitis and asymptomatic rhinoconjunctivitis allergica, *J Allergy Clin Immunol* 107:878-886, 2001.
16. Hanifin JM, Chan SC, Cheng JB, et al: Type 4 phosphodiesterase inhibitors have clinical and *in vitro* anti-inflammatory effects in atopic dermatitis, *J Invest Dermatol* 107:51-56, 1996.
17. Jirapongsananuruk O, Hofer MF, Trumble AE, et al: Enhanced expression of B7.2 (CD86) in patients with atopic dermatitis: a potential role in the modulation of IgE synthesis, *J Immunol* 160:4622-4627, 1998.

18. Hamid Q, Boguniewicz M, Leung DY: Differential *in situ* cytokine gene expression in acute versus chronic atopic dermatitis, *J Clin Invest* 94:870-876, 1994.

19. Woodward AL, Spergel JM, Alenius H, et al: An obligate role for T-cell receptor alpha beta+ T cells but not T-cell receptor gamma delta+ T cells, B cells, or CD40/CD40L interactions in a mouse model of atopic dermatitis, *J Allergy Clin Immunol* 107:359-366, 2001.

20. Hamid Q, Naseer T, Minshall EM, et al: *In vivo* expression of IL-12 and IL-13 in atopic dermatitis, *J Allergy Clin Immunol* 98:225-231, 1996.

21. Trautmann A, Akdis M, Schmid-Grendelmeier P, et al: Targeting keratinocyte apoptosis in the treatment of atopic dermatitis and allergic contact dermatitis, *J Allergy Clin Immunol* 108:839-846, 2001.

22. von Bubnoff D, Geiger E, Bieber T: Antigen-presenting cells in allergy, *J Allergy Clin Immunol* 108:329-339, 2001.

23. Ohki O, Yokozeki H, Katayama I, et al: Functional CD86 (B7-2/B70) is predominantly expressed on Langerhans cells in atopic dermatitis, *Br J Dermatol* 136:838-845, 1997.

24. Schuller E, Teichmann B, Haberstok J, et al: *In situ* expression of the co-stimulatory molecules CD80 and CD86 on Langerhans cells and inflammatory dendritic epidermal cells (IDEC) in atopic dermatitis, *Arch Dermatol Res* 293:448-454, 2001.

25. Laberge S, Ghaffar O, Boguniewicz M, et al: Association of increased CD4+ T-cell infiltration with increased IL-16 gene expression in atopic dermatitis, *J Allergy Clin Immunol* 102:645-650, 1998.

26. Reich K, Hugo S, Middel P, et al: Evidence for a role of Langerhans cell-derived IL-16 in atopic dermatitis, *J Allergy Clin Immunol* 109:681-687, 2002.

27. Taha RA, Minshall EM, Leung DY, et al: Evidence for increased expression of eotaxin and monocyte chemotactic protein-4 in atopic dermatitis, *J Allergy Clin Immunol* 105:1002-1007, 2000.

28. Yawalkar N, Uguccioni M, Scharer J, et al: Enhanced expression of eotaxin and CCR3 in atopic dermatitis, *J Invest Dermatol* 113:43-48, 1999.

29. Morita E, Kameyoshi Y, Hiragun T, et al: The C-C chemokines, RANTES and eotaxin, in atopic dermatitis, *Allergy* 56:194-195, 2001.

30. Morales J, Homey B, Vicari AP, et al: CTACK, a skin-associated chemokine that preferentially attracts skin-homing memory T cells, *Proc Natl Acad Sci U S A* 96:14470-14475, 1999.

31. Galli G, Chantry D, Annunziato F, et al: Macrophage-derived chemokine production by activated human T cells *in vitro* and *in vivo*: preferential association with the production of type 2 cytokines, *Eur J Immunol* 30:204-210, 2000.

32. Kakinuma T, Nakamura K, Wakugawa M, et al: Thymus and activation-regulated chemokine in atopic dermatitis: serum thymus and activation-regulated chemokine level is closely related with disease activity, *J Allergy Clin Immunol* 107:535-541, 2001.

33. Nakatani T, Kaburagi Y, Shimada Y, et al: CCR4 memory CD4+ T lymphocytes are increased in peripheral blood and lesional skin from patients with atopic dermatitis, *J Allergy Clin Immunol* 107:353-358, 2001.

34. Bratton DL, Hamid Q, Boguniewicz M, et al: Granulocyte macrophage colony-stimulating factor contributes to enhanced monocyte survival in chronic atopic dermatitis, *J Clin Invest* 95:211-218, 1995.

35. Giustizieri ML, Mascia F, Frezzolini A, et al: Keratinocytes from patients with atopic dermatitis and psoriasis show a distinct chemokine production profile in response to T cell-derived cytokines, *J Allergy Clin Immunol* 107:871-877, 2001.

36. Forrest S, Dunn K, Elliott K, et al: Identifying genes predisposing to atopic eczema, *J Allergy Clin Immunol* 104:1066-1070, 1999.

37. Mao XQ, Shirakawa T, Yoshikawa T, et al: Association between genetic variants of mast-cell chymase and eczema, *Lancet* 348:581-583, 1996.

38. Arkwright PD, Chase JM, Babbage S, et al: Atopic dermatitis is associated with a low-producer transforming growth factor β₁ cytokine genotype, *J Allergy Clin Immunol* 108:281-284, 2001.

39. Lee YA, Wahn U, Kehrt R, et al: A major susceptibility locus for atopic dermatitis maps to chromosome 3q21, *Nat Genet* 26:470-473, 2000.

40. Cookson WO, Ubhi B, Lawrence R, et al: Genetic linkage of childhood atopic dermatitis to psoriasis susceptibility loci, *Nat Genet* 27:372-373, 2001.

41. Sampson HA: Food allergy. Part 1. Immunopathogenesis and clinical disorders, *J Allergy Clin Immunol* 103:717-728, 1999.

42. Guillet G, Guillet MH: Natural history of sensitizations in atopic dermatitis. A 3-year follow-up in 250 children: food allergy and high risk of respiratory symptoms, *Arch Dermatol* 128:187-192, 1992.

43. Lever R, MacDonald C, Waugh P, et al: Randomised controlled trial of advice on an egg exclusion diet in young children with atopic eczema and sensitivity to eggs, *Pediatr Allergy Immunol* 9:13-19, 1998.

44. van Reijsen FC, Felius A, Wauters EA, et al: T-cell reactivity for a peanut-derived epitope in the skin of a young infant with atopic dermatitis, *J Allergy Clin Immunol* 101:207-209, 1998.

45. Li XM, Kleiner G, Huang CK, et al: Murine model of atopic dermatitis associated with food hypersensitivity, *J Allergy Clin Immunol* 107:693-702, 2001.

46. Tupker RA, De Monchy JG, Coenraads PJ, et al: Induction of atopic dermatitis by inhalation of house dust mite, *J Allergy Clin Immunol* 97:1064-1070, 1996.

47. Wheatley LM, Platts-Mills TAE: Role of inhalant allergens in atopic dermatitis. In Leung DYM, Greaves MW, eds: *Allergic skin disease: a multidisciplinary approach*, New York, 2000, Marcel Dekker.

48. Tan BB, Weald D, Strickland I, et al: Double-blind controlled trial of effect of house dust-mite allergen avoidance on atopic dermatitis, *Lancet* 347:15-18, 1996.

49. Gutgesell C, Heise S, Seubert S, et al: Double-blind placebo-controlled house dust mite control measures in adult patients with atopic dermatitis, *Br J Dermatol* 145:70-74, 2001.

50. Holm L, Bengtsson A, van Hage-Hamsten M, et al: Effectiveness of occlusive bedding in the treatment of atopic dermatitis—a placebo-controlled trial of 12 months' duration, *Allergy* 56:152-158, 2001.

51. Scalabrin DM, Bavbek S, Perzanowski MS, et al: Use of specific IgE in assessing the relevance of fungal and dust mite allergens to atopic dermatitis: a comparison with asthmatic and nonasthmatic control subjects, *J Allergy Clin Immunol* 104:1273-1279, 1999.

52. Schafer T, Heinrich J, Wjst M, et al: Association between severity of atopic eczema and degree of sensitization to aeroallergens in schoolchildren, *J Allergy Clin Immunol* 104:1280-1284, 1999.

53. Leyden JJ, Kligman AM: The case for steroid-antibiotic combinations, *Br J Dermatol* 96:179-187, 1977.

54. Leung DY, Harbeck R, Bina P, et al: Presence of IgE antibodies to staphylococcal exotoxins on the skin of patients with atopic dermatitis: evidence for a new group of allergens, *J Clin Invest* 92:1374-1380, 1993.

55. Breuer K, Wittmann M, Bosche B, et al: Severe atopic dermatitis is associated with sensitization to staphylococcal enterotoxin B (SEB), *Allergy* 55:551-555, 2000.

56. Bunikowski R, Mielke ME, Skarabis H, et al: Evidence for a disease-promoting effect of *Staphylococcus aureus*-derived exotoxins in atopic dermatitis, *J Allergy Clin Immunol* 105:814-819, 2000.

57. Strickland I, Hauk PJ, Trumble AE: Evidence for superantigen involvement in skin homing of T cells in atopic dermatitis, *J Invest Dermatol* 112:249-253, 1999.

58. Herz U, Schnoy N, Borelli S, et al: A human-SCID mouse model for allergic immune response bacterial superantigen enhances skin inflammation and suppresses IgE production, *J Invest Dermatol* 110:224-231, 1998.

59. Hofer MF, Harbeck RJ, Schlievert PM, et al: Staphylococcal toxins augment specific IgE responses by atopic patients exposed to allergen, *J Invest Dermatol* 112:171-176, 1999.

60. Hauk PJ, Hamid QA, Chrousos GP, et al: Induction of corticosteroid insensitivity in human PBMCs by microbial superantigens, *J Allergy Clin Immunol* 105:782-787, 2000.

61. Strange P, Skov L, Lisby S, et al: Staphylococcal enterotoxin B applied on intact normal and intact atopic skin induces dermatitis, *Arch Dermatol* 132:27-33, 1996.

62. Skov L, Olsen JV, Giorno R, et al: Application of Staphylococcal enterotoxin B on normal and atopic skin induces up-regulation of T cells by a superantigen-mediated mechanism, *J Allergy Clin Immunol* 105:820-826, 2000.

63. Michie CA, Davis T: Atopic dermatitis and staphylococcal superantigens, *Lancet* 347:324, 1996.

64. Leung DY, Gately M, Trumble A, et al: Bacterial superantigens induce T cell expression of the skin-selective homing receptor, the cutaneous lymphocyte-associated antigen, via stimulation of interleukin 12 production, *J Exp Med* 181:747-753, 1995.

65. Nilsson EJ, Henning CG, Magnusson J: Topical corticosteroids and *Staphylococcus aureus* in atopic dermatitis, *J Am Acad Dermatol* 27:29-34, 1992.

66. Remitz A, Kyllonen H, Granlund H, et al: Tacrolimus ointment reduces staphylococcal colonization of atopic dermatitis lesions, *J Allergy Clin Immunol* 107:196-197, 2001.

67. Cho SH, Strickland I, Tomkinson A, et al: Preferential binding of *Staphylococcus aureus* to skin sites of Th2-mediated inflammation in a murine model, *J Invest Dermatol* 116:658-663, 2001.

68. Cho SH, Strickland I, Boguniewicz M, et al: Fibronectin and fibrinogen contribute to the enhanced binding of *Staphylococcus aureus* to atopic skin, *J Allergy Clin Immunol* 108:269-274, 2001.

69. Ong PY, Ohtake T, Brandt C, et al: Decreased anti-microbial peptides contribute to increased infections in atopic dermatitis, *N Engl J Med* 347:1151-1160, 2002.

70. Keller P: Beitrag zu den beziehungen von asthma und ekzem, *Arch Derm Syph Berl* 148:82, 1924.

71. Valenta R, Seiberler S, Natter S, et al: Autoallergy: a pathogenetic factor in atopic dermatitis? *J Allergy Clin Immunol* 105:432-437, 2000.

72. Valenta R, Natter S, Seiberler S, et al: Molecular characterization of an autoallergen, Hom s 1, identified by serum IgE from atopic dermatitis patients, *J Invest Dermatol* 111:1178-1183, 1998.

73. Kinaciyan T, Natter S, Kraft D, et al: IgE autoantibodies monitored in a patient with atopic dermatitis under cyclosporin A treatment reflect tissue damage, *J Allergy Clin Immunol* 109:717-719, 2002.

74. Hoare C, Li Wan Po A, Williams H: Systematic review of treatments for atopic eczema, *Health Technol Assess* 4:1-191, 2000.

75. Imokawa G: Lipid abnormalities in atopic dermatitis, *J Am Acad Dermatol* 45:S29-S32, 2001.

76. Van Der Meer JB, Glazenburg EJ, Mulder PG, et al: The management of moderate to severe atopic dermatitis in adults with topical fluticasone propionate. The Netherlands Adult Atopic Dermatitis Study Group, *Br J Dermatol* 140:1114-1121, 1999.

77. Reitamo S: Tacrolimus: a new topical immunomodulatory therapy for atopic dermatitis, *J Allergy Clin Immunol* 107:445-448, 2001.

78. Wollenberg A, Sharma S, von Bubnoff D, et al: Topical tacrolimus (FK506) leads to profound phenotypic and functional alterations of epidermal antigen-presenting dendritic cells in atopic dermatitis, *J Allergy Clin Immunol* 107:519-525, 2001.

79. Reitamo S, Van Leent EJ, Ho V, et al: Efficacy and safety of tacrolimus ointment compared with that of hydrocortisone acetate ointment in children with atopic dermatitis, *J Allergy Clin Immunol* 109:539-546, 2002.

80. Reitamo S, Rustin M, Ruzicka T, et al: Efficacy and safety of tacrolimus ointment compared with that of hydrocortisone butyrate ointment in adult patients with atopic dermatitis, *J Allergy Clin Immunol* 109: 547-555, 2002.

81. Paller A, Eichenfield LF, Leung DY, et al: A 12-week study of tacrolimus ointment for the treatment of atopic dermatitis in pediatric patients, *J Am Acad Dermatol* 44:S47-S57, 2001.

82. Kang S, Lucky AW, Pariser D, et al: Long-term safety and efficacy of tacrolimus ointment for the treatment of atopic dermatitis in children, *J Am Acad Dermatol* 44:S58-S64, 2001.

83. Zuberbier T, Chong SU, Grunow K, et al: The ascomycin macrolactam pimecrolimus (Elidel, SDZ ASM 981) is a potent inhibitor of mediator release from human dermal mast cells and peripheral blood basophils, *J Allergy Clin Immunol* 108:275-280, 2001.

84. Luger T, Van Leent EJ, Graeber M, et al: SDZ ASM 981: an emerging safe and effective treatment for atopic dermatitis, *Br J Dermatol* 144:788-794, 2001.

85. Eichenfield LF, Lucky AW, Boguniewicz M, et al: Safety and efficacy of pimecrolimus (ASM 981) cream 1% in the treatment of mild and moderate atopic dermatitis in children and adolescents, *J Am Acad Dermatol* 46:495-504, 2002.

86. Van Leent EJ, Ebelin ME, Burtin P, et al: Low systemic exposure after repeated topical application of Pimecrolimus (Elidel, SD Z ASM 981) in patients with atopic dermatitis, *Dermatology* 204:63-68, 2002.

87. Kapp A, Papp K, Bingham A, et al: Long-term management of atopic dermatitis in infants with topical pimecrolimus, a non-steroid anti-inflammatory drug, *J Allergy Clin Immunol* 110:277-284, 2002.

88. Woodmansee DP, Christiansen SC: Improvement in atopic dermatitis in infants with the introduction of an elemental formula, *J Allergy Clin Immunol* 108:309, 2001.

89. Schmid-Ott G, Jaeger B, Meyer S, et al: Different expression of cytokine and membrane molecules by circulating lymphocytes on acute mental stress in patients with atopic dermatitis in comparison with healthy controls, *J Allergy Clin Immunol* 108:455-462, 2001.

90. Schmid-Ott G, Jaeger B, Adamek C, et al: Levels of circulating CD8(+) T lymphocytes, natural killer cells, and eosinophils increase upon acute psychosocial stress in patients with atopic dermatitis, *J Allergy Clin Immunol* 107:171-177, 2001.

91. Boguniewicz M, Sampson H, Leung SB, et al: Effects of cefuroxime axetil on *Staphylococcus aureus* colonization and superantigen production in atopic dermatitis, *J Allergy Clin Immunol* 108:651-652, 2001.

92. Fritz SB, Singer AM, Revan VB, et al: Bioterrorism: relevance to allergy and immunology in clinical practice, *J Allergy Clin Immunol* 109: 214-228, 2002.

93. Zargari A, Eshaghi H, Back O, et al: Serum IgE reactivity to *Malassezia furfur* extract and recombinant *M. furfur* allergens in patients with atopic dermatitis, *Acta Derm Venereol* 81:418-422, 2001.

94. Simons FE: Prevention of acute urticaria in young children with atopic dermatitis, *J Allergy Clin Immunol* 107:703-706, 2001.

95. Tzaneva S, Seeber A, Schwaiger M, et al: High-dose versus medium-dose UVA1 phototherapy for patients with severe generalized atopic dermatitis, *J Am Acad Dermatol* 45:503-507, 2001.

96. Hanifin JM, Schneider LC, Leung DY, et al: Recombinant interferon gamma therapy for atopic dermatitis, *J Am Acad Dermatol* 28:189-197, 1993.

97. Granlund H, Erkko P, Remitz A, et al: Comparison of cyclosporin and UVAB phototherapy for intermittent one-year treatment of atopic dermatitis, *Acta Derm Venereol* 81:22-27, 2001.

98. Grundmann-Kollmann M, Podda M, Ochsendorf F, et al: Mycophenolate mofetil is effective in the treatment of atopic dermatitis, *Arch Dermatol* 137:870-873, 2001.

99. Jolles S: A review of high-dose intravenous immunoglobulin treatment for atopic dermatitis, *Clin Exp Dermatol* 27:3-7, 2002.

100. Koo J, Arain S: Traditional Chinese medicine for the treatment of dermatologic disorders, *Arch Dermatol* 134:1388-1393, 1998.

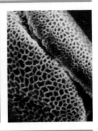

CHAPTER 54

Urticaria and Angioedema

BRUCE L. ZURAW

Urticaria (hives) typically present as a pruritic generalized eruption with erythematous circumscribed borders and pale, slightly elevated centers (Figure 54-1, *A*). Angioedema is characterized by an asymmetric non-dependent swelling that is generally not pruritic (see Figure 54-1, *B*). The pathophysiology of urticaria and angioedema is similar, resulting from leakage of plasma into the superficial skin in urticaria and into the deeper skin layers in angioedema. Recognition of urticaria and angioedema is generally obvious, and often made by the patient or the patient's family.

Based on their distinctive appearance and course, urticaria and angioedema are generally easily diagnosed. In contrast, these disorders are often frustratingly difficult to treat and their cause is elusive. Affected patients may manifest symptoms that range from transient and mildly annoying hives to severe and potentially fatal angioedema. Quality of life has been reported to be moderately to severely impaired in patients with chronic urticaria.[1] An efficient and cost-effective approach to the management of urticaria and angioedema depends on a careful assessment of the characteristics and likely cause of the swelling. This chapter provides a framework to differentiate the various types of urticaria and angioedema, then outlines a directed evaluation and treatment plan based on the etiology (Box 54-1).

EPIDEMIOLOGY/ETIOLOGY

Epidemiology

Urticaria and angioedema are commonly encountered in the general population.[2] It is generally assumed that urticaria and angioedema occur more frequently in adults than in children, although accurate figures are not available and the majority of the published information is based on observations made in adult patients.[3]

Urticaria and/or angioedema is conventionally classified as either *acute* or *chronic,* defined as the continuous or frequent occurrence of lesions for longer than 6 weeks. Although it is arbitrary, this distinction is important because it has significant implications regarding the cause, course, and treatment of the swelling. The majority of patients with urticaria or angioedema experience acute swelling, and this is thought to be particularly true in children. Urticaria is more common than angioedema, although they frequently present concurrently. Approximately 50% of affected patients have both urticaria and angioedema, 40% urticaria alone, and 10% only angioedema.[4]

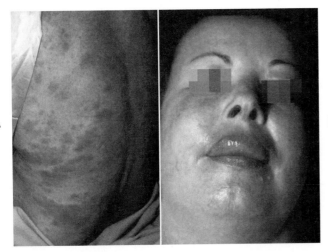

FIGURE 54-1 Typical examples of swelling. **A,** Diffuse urticaria with areas of confluence. **B,** Angioedema of the upper lip and left eye.

BOX 54-1	**KEY CONCEPTS** *Urticaria and Angioedema*

- The distinction between acute and chronic urticaria/angioedema has important diagnostic and therapeutic implications.
- The most common type of swelling in children is acute urticaria/angioedema.
- Cause of acute urticaria can usually be determined and is most likely to involve IgE-mediated reactions, viral infections, or bites and stings.
- Cause of chronic urticaria/angioedema is typically idiopathic; however, physical stimuli often contribute to the symptoms.
- Chronic urticaria/angioedema must be distinguished from urticarial vasculitis.
- Recurrent angioedema without urticaria suggests the possibility of hereditary angioedema.
- Most cases of chronic urticaria/angioedema resolve within 3 to 4 years.

Surveys in the United States and Denmark have indicated that 15% to 23% of the populace experience urticaria at least once during their lifetime.[2,5] Among children, the prevalence of urticaria/angioedema has been estimated to be about 6% to 7%. Whereas atopic individuals are at increased risk for acute urticaria/angioedema as well as some forms of physical urticaria, most patients with chronic urticaria/angioedema are surprisingly not atopic.

Etiology

The vast majority of urticaria/angioedema cases are caused by mast cell degranulation. The immediate consequence of mast cell degranulation is a wheal and flare response that is indistinguishable from an urticarial lesion. Although mast cell degranulation is accompanied by the release of a variety of preformed and newly formed mediators, histamine has long been known to be the primary mediator of the immediate wheal (which is largely abrogated by pretreatment with antihistamines). A delayed inflammatory response resulting from mast cell degranulation termed the *late-phase cutaneous response* consists of variable amounts of erythema and induration that begin in 1 to 2 hours, peak at 6 to 12 hours, and persist for up to 24 hours after degranulation.[6] The late-phase cutaneous response is mediated by a variety of mast cell mediators (including cytokines, chemokines, and leukotrienes) that recruit inflammatory cells into the site of degranulation. Taken together, these observations have been interpreted to suggest that mast cell degranulation is a final common pathway linking most of the diverse types of urticaria/angioedema.

The classic model of mast cell degranulation is through binding of allergen to specific immunoglobulin E (IgE) with resulting cross-linking of high-affinity FcεR displayed on the cell surface. IgE-mediated mast cell degranulation in response to allergen exposure is probably responsible for the majority of acute urticaria or angioedema in children. The most common sources of allergen that trigger IgE-mediated urticaria or angioedema are drugs and foods. Interestingly, *in vitro* stimulation of peripheral blood mononuclear cells obtained from children with milk-induced urticaria using milk protein results in specific activation of lymphocytes expressing the skin homing receptor cutaneous lymphocyte antigen (CLA).[7] Furthermore, the lesional skin of acute urticaria patients demonstrates increased expression of tumor necrosis factor alpha as well as E-selectin (the CLA counterligand).[8,9]

A significant proportion of acute urticaria/angioedema cases as well as the vast majority of cases of *chronic* urticaria or angioedema cannot be linked to IgE-mediated allergy. In these cases, nonimmunologic mechanisms or immune processes not involving IgE may also feed into the final common pathway of mast cell stimulation, histamine release, and resultant urticaria/angioedema. A variety of non-IgE stimuli can lead to mast cell degranulation and manifestation of acute or chronic urticaria/angioedema, including direct mast cell degranulators, viral infections, anaphylatoxins, various peptides/proteins, and several types of physical stimuli.

Understanding the cause of chronic idiopathic urticaria remains a particular challenge, as one rarely finds a direct relationship between the disease and exposure to an external agent or infection. The skin of patients with chronic urticaria demonstrates a non-necrotizing mononuclear cell infiltrate around small venules.[10] Immunohistochemical and *in situ*

hybridization studies showed increased numbers of basophils, eosinophils, and T helper cells (interleukin [IL]-4, IL-5, interferon gamma mRNA+ T cells) in chronic urticaria skin compared to normal. The cause of these inflammatory changes remains uncertain; however, recent studies have suggested an autoimmune link. Approximately 40% of patients with chronic urticaria have been found to possess circulating autoantibodies that contribute to mast cell degranulation,[11] with specificity for IgE or the high-affinity FcεR.[12-16] An increased prevalence of thyroid antimicrosomal and antithyroglobulin antibodies has also been found in urticaria/angioedema patients, and about half of these have goiters or abnormal thyroid function.[17] Conversely, an increased cumulative prevalence of urticaria/angioedema has been found in thyroid disease patients with antimicrosomal and antithyroglobulin antibodies (primarily Hashimoto's thyroiditis) but not in patients with other types of thyroid disease.[18] Supporting an autoimmune pathogenesis, patients with chronic idiopathic urticaria have also been shown to have an increased frequency of HLA DRB1*04 (DR4) and DQB1*0302 (DQ8) compared to normal controls.[19] Finally, several biologically active proteins that are generated during inflammation are able to induce mast cell degranulation, including the anaphylatoxin C5a, neuropeptides, and eosinophilic major basic protein.[20-22]

Rare cases of severe urticaria/angioedema associated with marked weight gain, pronounced leukocytosis, and striking eosinophilia have been described and the syndrome has become known as the *Gleich syndrome.*[23] These patients have been found to have increased serum levels of IL-5 and other cytokines during attacks.[24] Gleich syndrome patients are also notable for their good response to treatment with corticosteroids, and they also differ from cases of hypereosinophilic syndrome by the absence of cardiac involvement. Other cases of urticaria/angioedema have been reported in association with parathyroid disease, polycythemia vera, hemolytic uremic syndrome, and pregnancy.

A separate group of familial swelling disorders needs to be distinguished. Genetic causes of swelling are transmitted as autosomal dominant traits and include hereditary angioedema (HAE); Muckle-Wells syndrome (urticaria, deafness, and amyloidosis); vibratory angioedema; familial cold autoinflammatory syndrome (formally called *familial cold urticaria);* familial localized heat urticaria of delayed type; erythropoietic protoporphyria with solar urticaria; C3 inactivator deficiency with urticaria; and serum carboxypeptidase N deficiency with angioedema. With the exception of HAE (which has a prevalence reported to be as high as 1 per 10,000),[25] all are very rare.

HAE presents as recurrent angioedema in the absence of urticaria and is caused by a functional deficiency of the plasma protein C1 inhibitor (C1 INH), which is the primary inactivator of the contact system proteases plasma kallikrein and Hageman factor (coagulation factor XIIa) as well as the complement proteases C1r and C1s.[26] Two major types of HAE have been described. The classic type (or Type I), found in 85% of the patients with HAE, is characterized by low C1 INH antigenic functional levels; the other 15% of the patients have variant HAE (or type II) and have C1 INH levels that are normal or elevated immunologically, but their C1 INH shows little or no activity in functional tests. C1 INH deficiency may also be acquired; however, this occurs primarily in older adults and has not been reported in children. Acquired C1

INH deficiency may be caused by an autoantibody directed against C1 INH or an underlying disease, particularly lymphoreticular malignancies. HAE is caused by mutations in the C1 INH gene, and over 100 different mutations of the C1 INH gene have been reported in HAE patients.[27-30] Interestingly, the location of the C1 INH mutation determines whether the HAE is Type I or Type II. A novel familial estrogen-dependent form of recurrent angioedema has also been described. This syndrome closely resembles HAE but only affects females and is characterized by normal C1 INH function.[31,32] Familial cold autoinflammatory syndrome and Muckle-Wells syndrome have recently been shown to be associated with mutations in a newly described gene that encodes cryopyrin.[33]

DIFFERENTIAL DIAGNOSIS

Recognition of urticaria and angioedema is generally obvious on examination, and the single most important step in the differential diagnosis is to visualize the lesions during swelling. If there is uncertainty about the diagnosis of urticaria, the fact that the individual skin lesions seldom last for more than a few hours (up to 24 hours) distinguishes it from almost all other skin diseases. In addition, urticarial lesions blanch with pressure and new hives frequently develop as the older ones fade. If the lesions do not itch, the diagnosis should be reconsidered. Unlike edema, angioedema is not dependent and is typically not symmetrical. Figure 54-2 presents an algorithm for the approach to the differential diagnosis.

Acute Urticaria/Angioedema

A cause of acute urticaria/angioedema can frequently be determined. Most cases in children will be secondary to IgE-mediated reactions or viral infections. Drugs that frequently cause urticaria or angioedema on an IgE-mediated basis include penicillin and other antibiotics. In addition to the IgE-mediated mechanism, drugs may also cause urticaria/angioedema by a serum sickness reaction. The onset of serum sickness reactions is delayed about 7 to 21 days, and the cutaneous manifestations commonly are accompanied by fever, arthralgias, and lymphadenopathy. The most common foods associated with IgE-mediated urticaria or angioedema depend, in large part, on the age of the patient. In younger children, egg, milk, soy, peanut, and wheat are the most common allergens, whereas fish, seafood, nuts, and peanuts are common offenders in older children. Urticaria and angioedema are the most common manifestations of anaphylactic reactions to insect stings and bites. Although the association usually is obvious in patients attacked by *Hymenoptera* or imported fire ants, Triatoma (kissing bug) reactions may present a diagnostic problem because these insects generally inflict essentially painless bites during the night.[34] Very different is the papular urticaria produced by insects such as bedbugs, fleas, or mites. These are observed most often on the legs of children, are less evanescent than most hives, and are caused by immunologic reactions to the saliva of the insect.

Ingestion or injection of direct mast cell degranulation substances such as strawberries, narcotic drugs, polymyxin antibiotics, D-tubocurarine, dextran volume expanders, or thiamine can cause hives. In pediatric practice many cases of acute transient urticaria appear to be associated with the common viral illnesses of childhood, but evidence for a leukocytoclastic vasculitis generally is lacking and its mechanism is unclear in most instances. Infections (particularly herpes and *Mycoplasma pneumoniae*) and less frequently drugs can cause erythema multiforme.[35] In its milder form, this non–IgE-mediated disease may be misdiagnosed as urticaria; however, erythema multiforme may be distinguished by the lack of prominent pruritus and the persistence of the lesions, which may be ringed (target lesions) or bullous. Urticaria may also occur following contact with an offending agent. These lesions are often produced by agents that actually penetrate the skin,

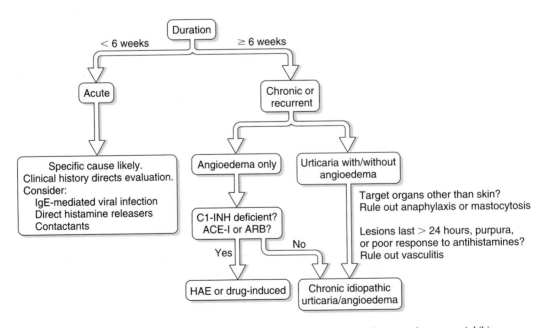

FIGURE 54-2 Diagnostic algorithm for urticaria/angioedema. *ACE-I*, Angiotensin-converting enzyme inhibitor; *ARB*, angiotensin II receptor blocker; *HAE*, hereditary angioedema.

such as nettles, Portuguese man-of-war, other forms of sea life, moth and butterfly scales, tarantula hairs, and caterpillar foot processes. Other substances, however, can produce urticaria on contact with intact skin. Examples include latex, drugs, foods, chemicals used on the job, benzoic acid, sorbic acid, and numerous other agents that can produce either non-immunologically or immunologically mediated reactions.[36]

Chronic Urticaria/Angioedema

The underlying cause of mast cell degranulation in the majority of patients with chronic urticaria/angioedema cannot be determined, and these patients are said to have chronic idiopathic urticaria/angioedema. This is a diagnosis of exclusion, based on history, examination, and carefully selected testing. Contrary to earlier claims, food allergy almost never can be implicated as the cause of chronic urticaria/angioedema. Moreover, claims that food additives are a common cause of chronic urticaria/angioedema are controversial and not supported by more recent studies.[37] A variety of parasitic infestations have been associated with urticaria/angioedema, the prevalence of such obviously varying with geographic locale. Substantial eosinophilia, elevated IgE level, abdominal symptoms, or foreign travel might suggest this diagnosis. In the past chronic focal infections in the teeth, gums, paranasal sinuses, tonsils, gall bladder, or genitourinary tract were thought to be a common cause of urticaria/angioedema just as they were thought to cause a variety of other diseases. However, in a study of 106 chronic urticaria/angioedema patients by Rorsman,[38] only 4 of 63 improved after a focal infection was treated. Most recently, *Helicobacter pylori* infection has been suggested as a link to chronic urticaria; however, further studies are needed to establish whether there is a direct relationship.[39]

The physical urticarias are intriguing conditions in which mast cell degranulation is precipitated by discrete physical stimuli. Physical urticaria is typically encountered in the setting of chronic idiopathic urticaria/angioedema. The percentage of children with chronic urticaria who have a physical component ranges from 1% to 10% for the more common types (dermographism, cholinergic, and cold-induced).[3] Documentation of physical urticaria is important for therapeutic purposes and because it largely precludes the need to consider other diagnoses. Table 54-1 describes several of the more common physical urticarias. A variety of provoking stimuli have been described, including mechanical (pressure or stroking), thermal (heat or cold), solar, and aquagenic. In its mildest form dermographism may occur in up to 2% to 5% of the general population; however, symptomatic dermographism (Figure 54-3) can account for the majority of hives in some patients with chronic urticaria.[2] Delayed pressure urticaria is more angioedematous than urticarial and causes significant morbidity.[1] Primary acquired cold urticaria is often seen in children. The physician should be aware that patients with acquired cold urticaria have drowned when exposed to cold water, presumably because of massive swelling with subsequent hypotension. It is therefore essential that patients with this condition be warned to avoid cold water and never to swim alone. Cholinergic urticaria (Figure 54-4) is relatively common in children, may be confused with exercise-induced anaphylaxis, and can be associated with angioedema, wheezing, or even syncope.[40] Persistent cholinergic erythema, a variant of cholinergic urticaria, can be mistaken for a drug eruption or cutaneous mastocytosis.[41] It is important to note that many patients have been described who have combinations of physical urticarias, such as cold and cholinergic urticaria, cold and localized heat urticaria, or dermographism with cold urticaria. Although the sera of patients with several types of physical urticaria (dermographism, cold urticaria, and solar urticaria) sometimes contain IgE that can passively transfer the activity, the antigen specificity of the IgE is unknown.

Mast cell degranulation and whealing may also occur because of a primary disorder of the mast cells. Mastocytosis is a disease of mast cell proliferation which has recently be recognized to result in many cases from somatic mutations in *c*-kit, a tyrosine kinase membrane receptor for stem cell factor that regulates mast cell proliferation.[42] The most common forms of mastocytosis in children are solitary mastocytomas or diffuse maculopapular urticaria pigmentosa. Although urtication of affected skin following stroking (Darier's sign) is a cardinal sign of mastocytosis, diffuse urticaria is not encountered in mastocytosis. Furthermore, the dermographism in urticaria pigmentosa is not linear but is associated with the pigmented papules and macules caused by mast cell infiltration.

Anaphylaxis that is not caused by any external allergen has been termed *idiopathic anaphylaxis,* and this syndrome often includes a prominent component of urticaria and/or angioedema.[43] Some idiopathic anaphylaxis patients have systemic symptoms such as diarrhea, wheezing, hypotension, and generalized flushing, whereas others may have only recurrent life-threatening angioedema.[44] Idiopathic anaphylaxis that presents with purely cutaneous symptoms can be indistinguishable from severe recurrent angioedema. The angioedema of idiopathic anaphylaxis can also resemble HAE; however, a positive family history as well as complement abnormalities will clearly identify HAE.

Although not common in children, urticarial vasculitis must be distinguished from chronic idiopathic urticaria/angioedema. When flagrant, urticarial vasculitis can be easily distinguished by the presence of palpable purpura and bruising or discoloration that persists after the hive disappears. Persistence of individual urticarial lesions for more than 24 hours together with a poor response to antihistamine therapy suggest the possibility of urticarial vasculitis even in the absence of palpable purpura and bruising or discoloration. As discussed previously, most patients with chronic urticaria/angioedema have a mononuclear cell infiltrate around lesional venules. Urticarial vasculitis typically shows variable degrees of polymorphonuclear neutrophil infiltration, leukocytoclasis with nuclear dust, endothelial cell proliferation, fibrinoid deposits, and/or erythrocyte extravasation. Immunofluorescent staining often shows deposition of immunoglobulin and complement.

Urticarial vasculitis spans a wide range of problems, from the relatively benign normocomplementemic cutaneous hypersensitivity vasculitis to the hypocomplementemic urticarial vasculitis syndrome.[45] In children, most cases of cutaneous vasculitis represent Henoch-Schönlein purpura or hypersensitivity vasculitis.[46] Adults, by contrast, are much more likely than children to manifest urticarial vasculitis as part of an underlying connective tissue disease such as systemic lupus erythematosus, Sjögren's syndrome, essential mixed cryoglobulinemia, or polymyositis. The hypocomplementemic urticarial vasculitis syndrome is rarely seen in children.[47] This severe

TABLE 54-1 Major Physical Urticaria Syndromes

Type	Provoking Stimuli	Diagnostic Test	Comment
Mechanically provoked			
Dermographism (urticaria factitia)	Rubbing or scratching of skin causes linear wheals.	Stroking the skin (especially the back) elicits linear wheal.	Primary (idiopathic or allergic) or secondary (urticaria pigmentosa or transient following virus or drug reaction)
Delayed dermographism	Same	Same	Rare
Delayed-pressure urticaria	At least 2 hr after pressure is applied to the skin, deep, painful swelling develops, especially involving the palms, soles, and buttocks.	Attach two sandbags or jugs of fluid (5-15 lbs) to either end of a strap and apply over the shoulder or thigh for 10-15 min. A positive test exhibits linear wheals or swelling after several hours.	Can be disabling and may be associated constitutional symptoms such as malaise, fever, arthralgia, headache, and leukocytosis
Immediate-pressure urticaria	Hives develop within 1-2 min of pressure.	Several minutes of pressure elicit hives.	Rare; seen in conjunction with hypereosinophilic syndrome
Thermally provoked			
Acquired cold urticaria	Change in skin temperature rapidly provokes urticaria.	Place ice cube on extremity for 3-5 min, then observe for pruritic welt and surrounding erythema as the skin rewarms over subsequent 5-15 min.	Relatively common, may occur transiently with exposure to drugs or with infections; other rare cases may be associated with cryoproteins or may be transferable by serum
Familial cold autoinflammatory syndrome	Intermittent episodes of rash, arthralgia, fever, and conjunctivitis occur after generalized exposure to cold.	Symptoms occur 2-4 hr after exposure to cold blowing air.	Autosomal-dominant inflammatory disorder previously called familial cold "urticaria"; results from mutation of cryopyrin gene
Cholinergic urticaria	Heat, exertion, or emotional upsets cause small punctate wheals with prominent erythematous flare.	Methacholine cutaneous challenge is sometimes helpful; better to reproduce the lesions by exercising in a warm environment or while wearing a wet suit or plastic occlusive suit.	Differs from exercise-induced anaphylaxis in that it features smaller wheals and is induced by heat as well as by exercise but does not cause patients to collapse
Localized heat urticaria	Urtication occurs at sites of contact with a warm stimulus.	Hold a test tube containing warm water against the skin for 5 min.	Rare
Miscellaneous provoked			
Solar urticaria	Urticaria develops in areas of skin exposed to sunlight.	Controlled exposure to light; can be divided depending on the wavelength of light eliciting the lesions.	Types include genetic abnormality in protoporphyrin IX metabolism as well as types that can be passively transferred by IgE in serum
Aquagenic urticaria	Tiny perifollicular urticarial lesions develop after contact with water of any temperature.	Apply towel soaked in 37° C water to the skin for 30 min.	Rare

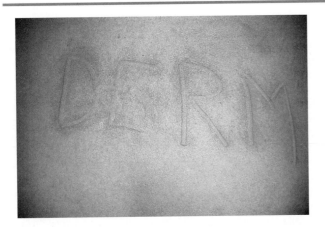

FIGURE 54-3 Dermatographism. (From Weston WL, Morelli JG, Lane A, eds: *Color textbook of pediatric dermatology*, ed 3, St Louis, 2002, Mosby.)

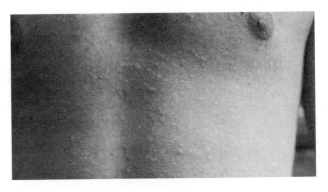

FIGURE 54-4 Cholingergic urticaria. (From Fireman P, Slavin R, eds: *Atlas of allergies*, ed 2, London, 1996, Mosby-Wolfe.)

form of urticarial vasculitis is characterized by ocular inflammation, glomerulonephritis, and obstructive pulmonary diseases in addition to recurrent urticaria vasculitis and angioedema. It may also be accompanied by a 7s C1q precipitin.[48]

Angioedema

Like urticaria, angioedema is also usually an obvious diagnosis. Angioedematous swellings are associated with little or no itching, probably because of fewer sensory nerve endings in the deep dermis and subcutaneous tissue where the swelling is located. In contrast to most other forms of edema, angioedema does not characteristically occur in dependent areas, and is often asymmetric and transient (although often recurrent). Angioedema is usually associated with urticaria; recurrent angioedema without urticaria should suggest a possible diagnosis of HAE. This is particularly important to recognize and treat because of its potential morbidity and mortality. Angioedema may also occur during the treatment of hypertension with angiotensin-converting enzyme (ACE) inhibitors or less commonly with angiotensin II receptor blockers.[49] There are also several forms of facial edema that can be confused with angioedema, including the granulomatous cheilitis accompanying Crohn's disease and the Melkersson-Rosenthal syndrome (a rare syndrome of recurrent orofacial swelling, relapsing facial paralysis, and fissured tongue).

EVALUATION AND MANAGEMENT

History

A discerning history is the most important diagnostic procedure in the evaluation of urticaria/angioedema, and dictates which if any of the large number of etiologic possibilities should be pursued. One first should determine whether the urticaria or angioedema is acute or chronic, the duration of the individual lesions, and the presence of pruritus. Obtaining clues about pathogenesis can be aided by the types of questions used to assess patients with other types of potentially allergic disease. *When* do hives and angioedema occur (time of year, month, week, and day)? *Where* do lesions occur (effect of travel, onset in specific locales)? *What* has the patient suspected? Specific inquiry then should be made about the agents that have most frequently been implicated in causing urticaria or angioedema, such as drugs (including over-the-counter products), foreign sera, foods, food additives, psychologic factors, inhalants, bites and stings, direct contact of skin with various agents, connective tissue diseases, and exposure to physical agents.

The history should elicit information about factors that may influence the severity of urticaria/angioedema. In many or most patients with urticaria, the disease is aggravated by vasodilating stimuli, such as heat, exercise, emotional stress, alcoholic drinks, fever, and hyperthyroidism. Premenstrual exacerbations also are common. Aspirin causes exacerbations of chronic urticaria or angioedema in up to 30% of patients, but hives generally continue even when aspirin is assiduously avoided. Other cyclooxygenase (COX)-1 inhibiting nonsteroidal antiinflammatory drugs (NSAIDs) have a similar effect, and urticaria/angioedema has also been reported in patients taking COX-2 inhibitors.[50] A retrospective random review of 1007 charts of atopic children revealed a surprisingly high rate of NSAID-induced facial angioedema.

Although the overall rate of NSAID-induced facial angioedema was 4%, the rate among the 493 children less than 6 years old was 2%.[51] Angioedema occurring during the treatment of hypertension by ACE inhibitors may be related to the kininase activity of this enzyme.

Patients with HAE manifest a unique set of symptoms that must be assessed when evaluating a patient with recurrent angioedema.[52] The duration of swelling in HAE is longer than idiopathic angioedema, typically lasting 72 or more hours. The swelling in HAE attacks generally increases over 12 to 24 hours and slowly subsides over the subsequent 48 to 72 hours. Although the precipitating stimulus is usually obscure, many attacks appear to be triggered by minor trauma or stress. Attacks may be preceded by a nonpruritic erythematous rash that may have a serpentine shape. HAE often shows a striking periodicity with attacks of angioedema followed by several weeks or more during which the patient does not swell. Daily episodes of angioedema suggest a diagnosis other than HAE. The swelling may affect the extremities, face, gastrointestinal tract, or upper airway. Recurrent school absences because of abdominal pain may be a presenting symptom of HAE because of angioedema of the abdominal wall. It is not unusual to obtain a history of a normal exploratory laparotomy for presumed appendicitis. A positive family history of angioedema can often be elicited; however, up to 20% of HAE patients have *de novo* mutations.[53] HAE typically presents around puberty, although symptoms may begin in younger children and then worsen at puberty. It is often very helpful to ask whether the patient has ever been treated for the angioedema with antihistamines, corticosteroids, or epinephrine as these medications do not have any significant benefit for the angioedema in HAE.

Physical Examination

A complete physical examination is important, especially in cases of chronic urticaria and angioedema, to rule out an underlying condition such as a connective tissue, viral, or endocrine disease. Urticarial lesions typically are generalized and may involve any part of the body, and individual lesions often coalesce into large lesions. Angioedema typically involves loose connective tissue such as the face or mucous membranes involving the lips or tongue. Occasionally, the appearance of the lesions gives a clue as to the type of urticaria being encountered: linear wheals suggest dermographism; small wheals surrounded by large areas of erythema suggest cholinergic urticaria; wheals limited to exposed areas suggest solar or cold urticaria; and wheals mainly on the lower extremities suggest papular urticaria or urticarial vasculitis.

Diagnostic Procedures

The laboratory evaluation of patients with urticaria or angioedema must be tailored to the clinical situation. If the history or physical examination provide any clues to the cause of the urticaria/angioedema, the evaluation should be pursued using the appropriate tests. Acute urticaria, in general, does not require specific laboratory evaluation except to document the suspected cause (e.g., skin testing to confirm IgE-mediated food allergy). Table 54-2 summarizes the limited laboratory evaluation that should be performed in patients with chronic urticaria/angioedema to exclude important underlying disease. Because the cause of chronic urticaria or angioedema is

TABLE 54-2 Suggested Testing for Chronic Urticaria/Angioedema of Unknown Etiology

Basic Tests	Discretionary Tests Based on
Complete blood count with differential	If vasculitis is suspected:
Erythrocyte sedimentation rate	Antinuclear antibody
Urinalysis	Skin biopsy
Liver function tests	CH_{50}
Thyroid function and autoantibodies	If liver function tests abnormal:
Anti-FcεR autoantibody (if available)	Serology for viral hepatitis

not related to extrinsic allergen exposure in the vast majority of cases, routine skin testing is not cost effective and typically only increases the frustration of both the patient and physician when no culprit is identified. Patients with a suggestive history of physical urticaria may be challenged to confirm the diagnosis (see Table 54-1). Patients with recurrent angioedema without urticaria should be evaluated for HAE (Table 54-3).

TREATMENT

Reassurance is an important aspect of therapy for urticaria/angioedema. Skin lesions are often more frightening in appearance than the generally favorable prognosis warrants. Acute urticaria/angioedema lasts less than 6 weeks as long as contact with the provoking agent is recognized and avoided; 50% of patients with chronic idiopathic urticaria/angioedema experience remission within 3 to 5 years.[4] Patients and their families should be told (1) that there will be a spontaneous remission after weeks, months, or years; (2) that urticaria/angioedema *per se* does not lead to any irreversible damage to one's health; and (3) that the disease usually can be controlled by one or more of a variety of medications while awaiting a spontaneous remission. Patients should be made aware of the need for an emergency room visit if laryngeal edema occurs. If the patient has experienced laryngeal edema, many physicians would prescribe and instruct the patient in the use of self-injectable epinephrine. However, one should

avoid generating undue anxiety about laryngeal edema because the only known fatalities from this cause have been in patients with HAE, angiotensin-converting enzyme inhibitor–associated angioedema, or anaphylactic reactions.

Guidelines for treating patients with urticaria/angioedema are summarized in Box 54-2. Obviously the preferred treatment is avoidance of causative agents when these can be identified and when avoidance is feasible. This generally is the case when allergy to drugs, foods, inhalants, insects, or contactants is involved. An explanation of the disease process and its triggers should also be helpful for patients with physical urticaria such as dermographism, cholinergic urticaria, and delayed-pressure urticaria. Common sense avoidance measures should be reviewed with patients afflicted with cold or solar urticaria, and the former should be forewarned about the dangers of swimming in cool water and of swimming alone. Sunscreens can help protect against light of 285- to 320-nm wavelength. Treatment of any discovered underlying disease is imperative, and genetic counseling should be provided to families with hereditary forms of these conditions. In addition, patients should avoid, to the extent feasible, the previously mentioned potentiating factors such as alcoholic drinks, heat, exertion, and aspirin.

Antihistamines are the mainstay of treatment for acute or chronic urticaria/angioedema (Figure 54-5). Used at a sufficient dose, they alleviate pruritus and suppress hive formation. Corticosteroids should not be used except in extraordinary circumstances such as hypocomplementemic urticarial vasculitis or delayed-pressure urticaria. Most first-generation H_1 antihistamines have some degrees of effectiveness in mild urticaria, but among the commonly employed drugs of this type, hydroxyzine and doxepin have greater potency. Side effects, especially drowsiness, are substantial problems, however, and have limited the usefulness of these drugs, particularly in children.[54] Second-generation H_1 antagonists cross the blood-brain barrier poorly, producing much less drowsiness, and have thus become the preferred drugs for many physicians in the treatment of urticaria/angioedema.

TABLE 54-3 Complement Evaluation of Patients with Recurrent Angioedema

Assay	Idiopathic Angioedema	Type I HAE	Type II HAE	Acquired C1 INH Deficiency	Vasculitis
C4	nl	Low	Low	Low	Low or nl
C4d/C4 ratio	nl	High	High	High	High or nl
C1 INH level	nl	Low	nl	Low	nl
C1 INH function	nl	Low	Low	Low	nl
C1q	nl	nl	nl	Low	Low or nl
C3	nl	nl	nl	nl	Low or nl

HAE, Hereditary angioedema; *INH*, inhibitor; *nl*, normal.

BOX 54-2

THERAPEUTIC PRINCIPLES
Treatment of Urticaria/Angioedema

Avoidance of known provoking stimuli can greatly improve treatment outcomes.

H_1 antihistamines are the mainstay of treatment, and second-generation H_1 antihistamines are preferred because they have fewer side effects.

Difficult cases may require treatment with various combinations of second-generation H_1 antihistamines, first-generation H_1 antihistamines, H_2 antihistamines, and leukotriene receptor antagonists.

Delayed-pressure urticaria does not generally respond well to antihistamines.

Corticosteroids should be avoided whenever possible and in particular for the treatment of chronic urticaria/angioedema without delayed-pressure urticaria.

The angioedema of hereditary angioedema does not respond to antihistamines, corticosteroids, or epinephrine; oropharyngeal attacks of hereditary angioedema must be treated as a medical emergency.

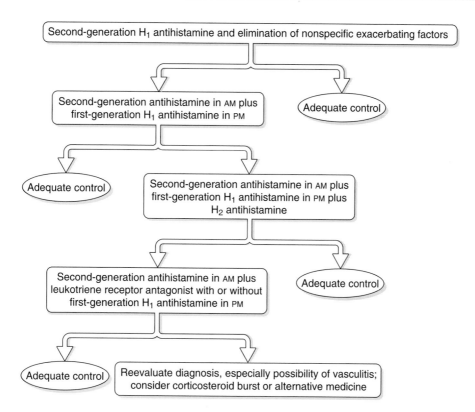

FIGURE 54-5 Therapeutic algorithm for chronic urticaria/angioedema.

The most commonly used second-generation H_1 antihistamines in the United States are cetirizine, desloratadine, and fexofenadine. Each of these has been shown to be well tolerated and effective for the treatment of urticaria/angioedema. The recommended doses of cetirizine are 10 mg/day in children 6 or older and 5 mg in children 2 to 5 years old.[55] Cetirizine syrup (0.25 mg/kg twice daily) was reported to be well tolerated and able to suppress the development of hives in 1- to 2-year-old children with atopic dermatitis who were at high risk of developing urticaria.[56] Desloratadine is used at a dose of 5 mg/day to treat urticaria in children aged 12 or older,[57] whereas loratadine (which is metabolized to desloratadine) has been safely used at 5 mg/day in children as young as 2 years.[58] The recommended dosage of fexofenadine for the treatment of urticaria is 60 mg twice daily in children 12 years or older and 30 mg twice daily in children 6 to 11 years.[59,60]

If a second-generation H_1 antihistamine by itself does not provide adequate relief, one should try using a combination of different medications. A sedating H_1 antihistamine given at bedtime can be used in conjunction with a second-generation H_1 antihistamine in the morning. Because the cutaneous vasculature expresses H_2 as well as the more abundant H_1 receptors, the addition of an H_2 antihistamine (e.g., cimetidine or ranitidine) may provide significant benefit for patients who are refractory to H_1 antihistamines alone. Leukotriene receptor antagonists have shown some promise in the treatment of urticaria/angioedema,[61] and can be added to an antihistamine regimen. The addition of ephedrine or terbutaline is another option but is generally not effective and is often associated with significant side effects.

Almost all patients will respond to antihistamine therapy. Lack of response should raise the question of an underlying urticarial vasculitis. It should be emphasized, however, that the physician must document the continuing hives by direct observation. Furthermore, it is often helpful to counsel the patient and patient's family that the goal of therapy is not to totally suppress the swelling, but rather to minimize the urticaria/angioedema to the point that it is tolerable. In those patients who require additional therapy, a variety of drugs have been reported to be helpful, although most of the reports are anecdotal. Recent reports, however, suggest that cyclosporine may be safely used to treat resistant chronic urticaria.[62,63] Corticosteroids are clearly effective in controlling urticaria/angioedema as well as urticarial vasculitis; however, the potential side effects from chronic use of corticosteroids mandates that they be used at the lowest possible dose that controls the swelling for the shortest period of time that is reasonable. Urticarial vasculitis has been reported to respond favorably to hydroxychloroquine, which has a superior safety profile compared to that of corticosteroids.[64]

The pharmacologic treatment of cold urticaria and delayed-pressure urticaria merits specific comment. Cyproheptadine is thought to be particularly effective for the treatment of cold urticaria,[65] although its side effects may include substantial weight gain because of stimulated appetite. Because the less sedating antihistamines are sufficiently effective to treat all but the most severe cases of cold urticaria, it is still wise to try one of these antihistamines first. Delayed pressure urticaria is a particularly difficult problem as it typically does not respond well to any antihistamine. Although some patients appear to be helped by cetirizine,[66] most patients with delayed pressure urticaria require systemic corticosteroids, which should be used at the lowest possible dosage.

As might be expected from its differing pathogenesis, the angioedema seen in HAE does not respond to the drugs employed in treating other forms of urticaria/angioedema. Treatment of HAE is best considered in three settings: long-term prophylaxis, short-term prophylaxis, and treatment of acute attacks. Long-term prophylaxis is meant to decrease the frequency and/or severity of swelling. Many children with HAE do not require long-term prophylactic therapy; however, patients with frequent severe attacks or with a history of serious attacks involving the upper airway should be treated prophylactically. The best tolerated and most effective long-term prophylactic drugs are the synthetic anabolic androgens; the antifibrinolytic drug epsilon aminocaproic acid is a second choice. The anabolic androgens stanozolol 2 mg/day or danazol 200 mg/day will generally give reasonable control of the angioedema, although they often provide sufficient control at lower doses. Side effects of these medications are dose-dependent and of concern, particularly in girls and pre-pubertal boys.[67] Oxandralone (2.5 to 7.5 mg/day) is another anabolic androgen that has been used to treat acquired immunodeficiency wasting syndrome in children and has recently begun to be used to treat HAE patients. Compared with stanozolol or danazol, oxandralone is equally effective but may have fewer side effects. All the anabolic androgens increase C1 INH and C4 levels; however, symptomatic benefit is achieved at doses less than those required to significantly change the complement levels. Therefore it is important to base the dosage on the clinical effect and not the laboratory values. Short-term prophylaxis for HAE is indicated before expected trauma, such as surgery or dental procedures. High-dose anabolic androgen therapy (stanozolol 2 mg three times daily) begun 7 to 10 days before the procedure gives excellent protection. Alternatively, the patient can be infused with two units of fresh frozen plasma before the procedure.

The management of acute attacks is primarily concerned with symptomatic control of the swelling as there is no medication for control of the angioedema currently available in the United States. Abdominal attacks require aggressive intravenous replacement of the fluid loss that occurs because of third spacing, as well as control of pain and nausea with parenteral narcotic and antiemetic drugs. Oropharyngeal attacks may lead to death secondary to asphyxiation, and therefore require hospitalization for careful monitoring of airway patency. If the airway is threatened, the patient should be intubated by an experienced physician, with the capability for emergency tracheostomy immediately available. Once intubated, an HAE patient should not be extubated until the swelling has resolved. Acute angioedema of the extremities does not typically require treatment.

Replacement therapy with purified C1 INH is available in Europe and elsewhere but not in the United States. C1 INH replacement therapy works extremely well to treat acute episodes of angioedema as well as for short-term prophylaxis.[68,69] It is hoped that this medicine will become available in the United States in the near future.

CONCLUSIONS

Urticaria and angioedema are common clinical problems whose manifestations range from trivial and intermittent to life threatening. To minimize spending time and money unnecessarily on complicated workups while simultaneously not overlooking important diagnoses, the clinician must be able to characterize urticaria/angioedema by chronicity, type, and, increasingly, by pathogenesis. With careful detective work, the cause of acute urticaria/angioedema can often be determined and appropriate interventions can be instituted that should lead to prompt resolution of the problem. A discrete cause of chronic urticaria, by contrast, is rarely established, forcing the clinician into the role of suppressing symptoms but not curing the problem. Although frequently frustrating for both the patient and the physician, the treatment of chronic urticaria can almost always achieve adequate results until the swelling disorder spontaneously remits.

HELPFUL WEBSITES

The American Contact Dermatitis Society website (www.contactderm.org/)
The American Academy of Dermatology website (www.aad.org/)
The American Academy of Allergy, Asthma, and Immunology website (www.aaaai.org)
The Hereditary Angioedema (HAE) Association website (www.hereditaryangioedema.com)

REFERENCES

1. Poon E, Seed PT, Greaves MW, et al: The extent and nature of disability in different urticarial conditions, *Br J Dermatol* 140:667-671, 1999.
2. Mathews KP: Urticaria and angioedema, *J Allergy Clin Immunol* 72:1-14, 1983.
3. Greaves MW: Chronic urticaria in childhood, *Allergy* 55:309-320, 2000.
4. Champion RH, Roberts S, Carpenter RG, et al: Urticaria and angioedema: a review of 554 patients, *Br J Dermatol* 81:588-597, 1969.
5. Swinny B: The atopic factor in urticaria, *South Med J* 34:855-858, 1941.
6. Atkins PC, Zweiman B: The IgE-mediated late-phase skin response: unraveling the enigma, *J Allergy Clin Immunol* 79:12-15, 1987.
7. Beyer K, Castro R, Feidel C, et al: Milk-induced urticaria is associated with the expansion of T cells expressing cutaneous lymphocyte antigen, *J Allergy Clin Immunol* 109:688-693, 2002.
8. Haas N, Schadendorf D, Henz BM: Differential endothelial adhesion molecule expression in early and late whealing reactions, *Intl Arch Allergy Immunol* 115:210-214, 1998.
9. Hermes B, Prochazka AK, Haas N, et al: Upregulation of TNF-alpha and IL-3 expression in lesional and uninvolved skin in different types of urticaria, *J Allergy Clin Immunol* 103:307-314, 1999.
10. Natbony SF, Phillips ME, Elias JM, et al: Histologic studies of chronic idiopathic urticaria, *J Allergy Clin Immunol* 71:177-183, 1983.
11. Kikuchi Y, Kaplan AP: Mechanisms of autoimmune activation of basophils in chronic urticaria, *J Allergy Clin Immunol* 107:1056-1062, 2001.
12. Gruber BL, Baeza ML, Marchese MJ, et al: Prevalence and functional role of anti-IgE autoantibodies in urticarial syndromes, *J Invest Dermatol* 90:213-217, 1988.
13. Grattan C, Francis DM, Hide M, et al: Detection of circulating histamine-releasing autoantibodies with functional properties of anti-IgE in chronic urticaria, *Clin Exp Allergy* 21:695-704, 1991.
14. Hide M, Francis DM, Grattan CE, et al: Autoantibodies against the high-affinity IgE receptor as a cause of histamine release in chronic urticaria, *N Engl J Med* 328:1599-1604, 1993.
15. Tong LJ, Balakrishnan G, Kochan JP, et al: Assessment of autoimmunity in patients with chronic urticaria, *J Allergy Clin Immunol* 99:461-465, 1997.
16. Fiebiger E, Maurer D, Holub H, et al: Serum IgG autoantibodies directed against the alpha chain of Fc epsilon RI: a selective marker and pathogenetic factor for a distinct subset of chronic urticaria patients? *J Clin Invest* 96:2606-2612, 1995.
17. Leznoff A, Sussman GL: Syndrome of idiopathic chronic urticaria and angioedema with thyroid autoimmunity: a study of 90 patients, *J Allergy Clin Immunol* 84:66-71, 1989.
18. Lanigan SW, Short P, Moult P: The association of chronic urticaria and thyroid autoimmunity, *Clin Exp Dermatol* 12:335-338, 1987.

19. O'Donnell BF, O'Neill CM, Francis DM, et al: Human leucocyte antigen class II associations in chronic idiopathic urticaria, *Br J Dermatol* 140:853-858, 1999.
20. Zheutlin LM, Ackerman SJ, Gleich GJ, et al: Stimulation of basophil and rat mast cell histamine release by eosinophil granule-derived cationic proteins, *J Immunol* 133:2180-2185, 1984.
21. Goetzl EJ, Chernov T, Reynold F, et al: Neuropeptide regulation of the expression of immediate hypersensitivity, *J Immunol* 135:802-805, 1985.
22. Kikuchi Y, Kaplan AP: A role for C5a in augmenting IgG-dependent histamine release from basophils in chronic urticaria, *J Allergy Clin Immunol* 109:114-118, 2002.
23. Gleich GJ, Schroeter AL, Marcoux JP, et al: Episodic angioedema associated with eosinophilia, *N Engl J Med* 310:1621-1626, 1984.
24. Butterfield JH, Leiferman KM, Abrams J, et al: Elevated serum levels of interleukin-5 in patients with the syndrome of episodic angioedema and eosinophilia, *Blood* 79:688-692, 1992.
25. Nzeako UC, Frigas E, Tremaine WJ: Hereditary angioedema: a broad review for clinicians, *Arch Intern Med* 161:2417-2429, 2001.
26. Davis AE III: C1 inhibitor and hereditary angioneurotic edema, *Ann Rev Immunol* 6:595-628, 1988.
27. Donaldson VH, Bissler JJ: C1 inhibitors and their genes: an update, *J Lab Clin Med* 119:330-333, 1992.
28. Bissler JJ, Aulak KS, Donaldson VH, et al: Molecular defects in hereditary angioneurotic edema, *Proc Assoc Am Physicians* 109:164-173, 1997.
29. Verpy E, Biasotto M, Brai M, et al: Exhaustive mutation scanning by fluorescence-assisted mismatch analysis discloses new genotype-phenotype correlations in angioedema [see comments], *Am J Hum Genet* 59:308-319, 1996.
30. Zuraw BL, Herschbach J: Detection of C1 inhibitor mutations in patients with hereditary angioedema, *J Allergy Clin Immunol* 105:541-546, 2000.
31. Binkley KE, Davis A III: Clinical, biochemical, and genetic characterization of a novel estrogen-dependent inherited form of angioedema, *J Allergy Clin Immunol* 106:546-550, 2000.
32. Bork K, Barnstedt SE, Koch P, et al: Hereditary angioedema with normal C1-inhibitor activity in women, *Lancet* 356:213-217, 2000.
33. Hoffman HM, Mueller JL, Broide DH, et al: Mutation of a new gene encoding a putative pyrin-like protein causes familial cold autoinflammatory syndrome and Muckle-Wells syndrome, *Nat Genet* 29:301-305, 2001.
34. Rohr AS, Marshall NA, Saxon A: Successful immunotherapy for Triatoma protracta-induced anaphylaxis, *J Allergy Clin Immunol* 73:369-375, 1984.
35. Leaute-Labreze C, Lamireau T, Chawki D, et al: Diagnosis, classification, and management of erythema multiforme and Stevens-Johnson syndrome, *Arch Dis Child* 83:347-352, 2000.
36. Burdick AE, Mathias C: The contact urticaria syndrome, *Derm Clin* 3:71-84, 1985.
37. Simon RA: Additive-induced urticaria: experience with monosodium glutamate (MSG), *J Nutr* 130:1063S-1066S, 2000.
38. Rorsman H: Basophilic leukopenia in different forms of urticaria, *Acta Allergol* 17:168-184, 1962.
39. Greaves MW: Pathophysiology of chronic urticaria, *Int Arch Allergy Immunol* 127:3-9, 2002.
40. Lawrence CM, Jorizzo JL, Kobza-Black A, et al: Cholinergic urticaria with associated angio-oedema, *Br J Dermatol* 105:543-550, 1981.
41. Black AK: Unusual urticarias, *J Dermatol* 28:632-634, 2001.
42. Metcalfe DD, Akin C: Mastocytosis: molecular mechanisms and clinical disease heterogeneity, *Leuk Res* 25:577-582, 2001.
43. Hogan MB, Kelly MA, Wilson NW: Idiopathic anaphylaxis in children, *Ann Allergy Asthma Immunol* 81:140-142, 1998.
44. Ditto AM, Krasnick J, Greenberger PA, et al: Pediatric idiopathic anaphylaxis: experience with 22 patients, *J Allergy Clin Immunol* 100:320-326, 1997.
45. Wisnieski JJ: Urticarial vasculitis, *Curr Opin Rheumatol* 12:24-31, 2000.
46. Blanco R, Martinez-Taboada VM, Rodriguez-Valverde V, et al: Cutaneous vasculitis in children and adults: associated diseases and etiologic factors in 303 patients, *Medicine (Baltimore)* 77:403-418, 1998.
47. Cadnapaphornchai MA, Saulsbury FT, Norwood VF: Hypocomplementemic urticarial vasculitis: report of a pediatric case, *Pediatr Nephrol* 14:328-331, 2000.
48. Zeiss CR, Burch FX, Marder RJ, et al: A hypocomplementemic vasculitic urticarial syndrome, *Am J Med* 68:867-875, 1980.
49. Warner KK, Visconti JA, Tschampel MM: Angiotensin II receptor blockers in patients with ACE inhibitor-induced angioedema, *Ann Pharmacother* 34:526-528, 2000.
50. Kelkar PS, Butterfield JH, Teaford HG: Urticaria and angioedema from cyclooxygenase-2 inhibitors, *J Rheumatol* 28:2553-2554, 2001.
51. Capriles-Behrens E, Caplin J, Sanchez-Borges M: NSAID facial angioedema in a selected pediatric atopic population, *J Invest Allergol Clin Immunol* 10:277-279, 2000.
52. Frank MM, Gelfand JA, Atkinson JP: Hereditary angioedema: the clinical syndrome and its management, *Ann Intern Med* 84:586-593, 1976.
53. Pappalardo E, Cicardi M, Duponchel C, et al: Frequent de novo mutations and exon deletions in the C1 inhibitor gene of patients with angioedema, *J Allergy Clin Immunol* 106:1147-1154, 2000.
54. Qidwai JC, Watson GS, Weiler JM: Sedation, cognition, and antihistamines, *Curr Allergy Asthma Rep* 2:216-222, 2002.
55. La Rosa M, Leonardi S, Marchese G, et al: Double-blind multicenter study on the efficacy and tolerability of cetirizine compared with oxatomide in chronic idiopathic urticaria in preschool children, *Ann Allergy Asthma Immunol* 87:48-53, 2001.
56. Simons FE: Prevention of acute urticaria in young children with atopic dermatitis, *J Allergy Clin Immunol* 107:703-706, 2001.
57. Ring J, Hein R, Gauger A, et al: Once-daily desloratadine improves the signs and symptoms of chronic idiopathic urticaria: a randomized, double-blind, placebo-controlled study, *Int J Dermatol* 40:72-76, 2001.
58. Salmun LM, Herron JM, Banfield C, et al: The pharmacokinetics, electrocardiographic effects, and tolerability of loratadine syrup in children aged 2 to 5 years, *Clin Ther* 22:613-621, 2000.
59. Nelson HS, Reynolds R, Mason J: Fexofenadine HCl is safe and effective for treatment of chronic idiopathic urticaria, *Ann Allergy Asthma Immunol* 84:517-522, 2000.
60. Thompson AK, Finn AF, Schoenwetter WF: Effect of 60 mg twice-daily fexofenadine HCl on quality of life, work and classroom productivity, and regular activity in patients with chronic idiopathic urticaria, *J Am Acad Dermatol* 43:24-30, 2000.
61. Aprile A, Lucarelli S, Vagnucci B, et al: The use of antileukotrienes in paediatrics, *Eur Rev Med Pharmacol Sci* 5:53-57, 2001.
62. Loria MP, Dambra PP, D'Oronzio L, et al: Cyclosporin A in patients affected by chronic idiopathic urticaria: a therapeutic alternative, *Immunopharmacol Immunotoxicol* 23:205-213, 2001.
63. Grattan CE, O'Donnell BF, Francis DM, et al: Randomized double-blind study of cyclosporin in chronic 'idiopathic' urticaria, *Br J Dermatol* 143:365-372, 2000.
64. Lopez LR, Davis KC, Kohler PF, et al: The hypocomplementemic urticarial-vasculitis syndrome: therapeutic response to hydroxychloroquine, *J Allergy Clin Immunol* 73:600-603, 1984.
65. Wanderer AA: Essential acquired cold urticaria, *J Allergy Clin Immunol* 85:531-532, 1990.
66. Kontou-Fili K, Maniatakou G, Paleologos G, et al: Cetirizine inhibits delayed pressure urticaria. Part 2: skin biopsy findings, *Ann Allergy* 65:520-522, 1990.
67. Cicardi M, Castelli R, Zingale LC, et al: Side effects of long-term prophylaxis with attenuated androgens in hereditary angioedema: comparison of treated and untreated patients, *J Allergy Clin Immunol* 99:194-196, 1997.
68. Waytes AT, Rosen FS, Frank MM: Treatment of hereditary angioedema with a vapor-heated C1 inhibitor concentrate, *N Engl J Med* 334:1630-1634, 1996.
69. Bork K, Barnstedt SE: Treatment of 193 episodes of laryngeal edema with C1 inhibitor concentrate in patients with hereditary angioedema, *Arch Intern Med* 161:714-718, 2001.

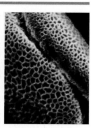

CHAPTER 55

Contact Dermatitis

MARK BOGUNIEWICZ ▪ VINCENT S. BELTRANI

Contact dermatitis includes a spectrum of inflammatory skin reactions induced by exposure to external agents. It is a common skin problem that affects patients of all ages, including infants and children. Clinically, contact dermatitis most commonly manifests as a dermatitis or eczema, but it can present as urticaria, phototoxic or photoallergic reactions, hypopigmentation or hyperpigmentation, and even acne. The more

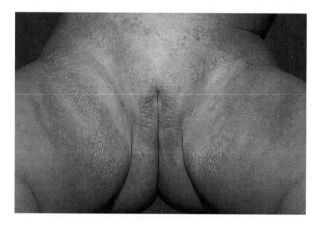

FIGURE 55-1 Irritant diaper dermatitis. (From Weston WL, Morelli JG, Lane A, eds: *Color textbook of pediatric dermatology*, ed 3, St Louis, 2002, Mosby.)

common irritant contact reaction results from tissue damage caused by contact with irritants, whereas contact with allergens causes allergic contact dermatitis. The former is seen commonly in young children as diaper dermatitis (Figure 55-1), whereas nickel (Figure 55-2) and poison ivy (Figure 55-3) are often causes of allergic contact dermatitis in the pediatric population.[1]

An estimated 85,000 chemicals exist in the world, and the majority of these agents, when applied to the skin, induce an irritant contact dermatitis. Approximately 2800 substances have been identified as contact allergens.[2] Identifying the responsible agent is essential for the appropriate management of patients with contact dermatitis. The diagnosis is usually inferred by the clinical presentation, which must then be supported by a history of exposure to the offending agent. It is only when the implicated agent is identified and strictly avoided that resolution occurs. When avoidance is not achieved, the condition may become chronic and disabling and significantly affect the quality of life of children and their families.

EPIDEMIOLOGY

The prevalence of contact allergy to common allergens in the general population is largely unknown because almost all patch test studies have been performed in selected groups

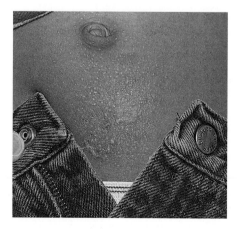

FIGURE 55-2 Allergic contact dermatitis in a young child to nickel. (From Weston WL, Morelli JG, Lane A, eds: *Color textbook of pediatric dermatology*, ed 3, St Louis, 2002, Mosby.)

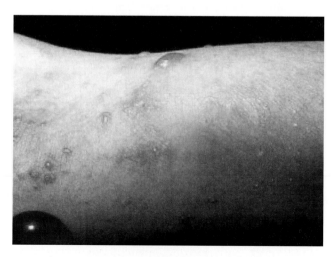

FIGURE 55-3 Poison ivy dermatitis with characteristic linear vesicles.

rather than in the general population. A recent study in a Danish population aged 15 to 41 years showed prevalence increasing from 15.9% to 18.6% between 1990 and 1998.[3] However, the number of subjects studied was relatively small for an epidemiologic survey. Subsequently, Schafer et al[4] conducted a population-based nested case-controlled study of 1141 adults in Germany with patch testing to 25 standard allergens. Forty percent of subjects exhibited at least one positive reaction, most frequently to fragrance mix (15.9%), nickel (13.1%), thimerosal (4.7%), and balsam of Peru (3.8%). Women were more sensitized more frequently than were men (50.2% versus 29.9%). A frequency estimate for overall contact sensitization for the general adult population based on these findings is 28%.

Prevalence of diaper dermatitis, an irritant contact dermatitis, in infants has been estimated to be 7% to 35% with a peak incidence between ages 9 and 12 months.[5] However, a more recent large-scale study in Great Britain demonstrated an incidence of 25% in the first 4 weeks of life alone.[6] Other forms of contact dermatitis in children were believed to be uncommon, but several studies suggest an increasing prevalence, possibly because of an increase in the practice of ear piercing, which may cause nickel sensitization.[7] A cross-sectional study of 1501 children aged 12 to 16 years using questionnaires ($N = 1438$), examination ($N = 1340$), and patch testing ($N = 1146$) found that the point prevalence of contact allergy was 15.2% (girls versus boys, 19.4% versus 10.3%; $P < 0.001$), and present or past allergic contact dermatitis was found in 7.2% (girls versus boys, 11.3% versus 2.5%).[8] Contact allergy to nickel (8.6%) and fragrance mix (1.8%) was most common. In other studies looking specifically at pediatric populations, up to 52% showed positive reactions on patch testing.[9-20]

In a study designed to look specifically at infants and young children, Bruckner et al[21] found that 24.5% of asymptomatic children aged 6 months to 5 years were sensitized to one or more contact allergens. Approximately one half of the sensitized children were younger than 18 months. Nickel (12.9%) and thimerosal (9.4%) were the most prevalent allergens, with the distribution between males and females equal. With respect to race, in a large study of more than 9000 individuals, DeLeo et al[22] found no difference in the overall response rate to allergens on patch testing between white and black patients, although reactivity to specific allergens differed, likely reflecting differences in exposures rather than a genetic basis.

PATHOGENESIS

Irritant Contact Dermatitis

Irritant contact dermatitis is a polymorphous syndrome resulting from contact with agents that abrade, irritate, or traumatize the skin. Irritation is usually a cytotoxic event produced by a wide variety of chemicals, detergents, solvents, alcohol, creams, lotions, ointments, and powders and by environmental factors such as wetting, drying, perspiration, and temperature extremes. A major finding after exposure to skin irritants is perturbation of the skin barrier with an associated increase in transepidermal water loss. The mechanism associated with this barrier perturbation may include disorganization of the lipid bilayers in the epidermis.[23] In addition, these changes can stimulate an array of cytokine production in the epidermis, including interleukin (IL)-1α and -β, tumor necrosis factor (TNF)-α, and granulocyte-monocyte colony-stimulating factor (GM-CSF).[24]

Although allergens are not implicated in irritant contact dermatitis, the skin-associated immune system is clearly involved, and historically few differences were noted when irritant and allergic contact dermatitis were compared immunohistopathologically.[25] An important difference between the two forms of contact dermatitis is that the irritant form does not require prior sensitization and immunologic memory is not involved in the clinical manifestation. The cellular infiltrate includes CD4+ T cells with a T helper cell type 1 (Th1)–type profile.[26] A number of studies have identified the epidermal keratinocyte as a key effector cell in the initiation and propagation of contact irritancy. Keratinocytes, which make up the majority of cells in the epidermis, can release both preformed and newly synthesized cytokines, as well as upregulate major histocompatibility complex (MHC) class II molecules and induce adhesion molecules in response to irritants.[27] These mediators can cause direct tissue damage, activating the underlying mast cells, which in turn release their proinflammatory mediators. This is recognized by the increase in dermal mast cell density, and their mediators are thought to be largely responsible for the vasodilation that occurs in the early stages of acute irritant dermatitis. Other mast cell pleiotropic proinflammatory cytokines are thought to stimulate leukocyte recruitment and activation in the acute inflammatory responses. The "final" cellular damage results from inflammatory mediators released by activated, nonsensitized T cells. The interactions between epidermal keratinocytes, mast cells and the inflammatory mediators they release, endothelial cells, and infiltrating leukocytes in irritant contact dermatitis are certainly complex, and the precise mechanisms remain to be elucidated. The inflammatory response is dose and time dependent. Any impairment to the epidermal barrier layer (e.g., fissuring, overhydration) renders the skin more susceptible to an irritant effect. The clinical presentation of irritant contact dermatitis is usually restricted to the skin site directly in contact with the offending agents, with little or no extension beyond the site of contact. The evolution and resolution of irritant contact dermatitis are less predictable than those of allergic contact dermatitis.

Allergic Contact Dermatitis

Allergic contact dermatitis is recognized as the prototypic cutaneous cell–mediated hypersensitivity reaction in which a distinct type of dendritic cell, the epidermal Langerhans cells, plays a pivotal role.[28] The offending agent, acting as an antigen, initiates the immunologic reaction at the site of contact with the skin. Most environmental allergens are haptens (>500 daltons) that bind to carrier proteins to form complete antigens before they can cause sensitization. The importance of the carrier is suggested by the observation that potent contact sensitizers, when complexed to nonimmunogenic carriers, induce tolerance rather than sensitization. MHC class II molecules on the surface of antigen-presenting Langerhans cells act as carriers for contact allergens. The antigen must be in solution (usually sweat) to reach the antigen-presenting cells (APCs) in the epidermis. The thickness and integrity of the skin influence the allergic response. Thus thinner sites such as the eyelids, earlobes, and genital skin are most vulnerable, whereas the thicker palms and soles are more resistant.

Exposure patterns determine the clinical appearance and course of the dermatitis. Exposure to the antigen may be episodic, such as poison ivy, or protracted, such as nickel in snaps or jewelry.

The immune response of allergic contact dermatitis requires completion of both an afferent and an efferent limb. The afferent limb consists of the hapten gaining entrance to the epidermis, activating keratinocytes to release inflammatory cytokines and chemokines including TNF-α, GM-CSF, IL-1β, IL-10, and macrophage inflammatory protein (MIP)-2. The latter in turn activate Langerhans cells, other dendritic cells, and endothelial cells, leading to an accumulation of even more dendritic cells at the site of antigen contact. In addition, the release of IL-1α by epidermal Langerhans cells promotes their egress from the epidermis. After the uptake of antigen, Langerhans cells process it while migrating to regional lymph nodes, where they present it to naive T cells. An important property of Langerhans cells and dendritic cells is their ability to present exogenous antigens on both MHC class I and class II molecules. This cross-priming leads to the activation of both CD4+ and CD8+ hapten-specific T cells.[29] Although classic delayed-type hypersensitivity reactions are mediated primarily by CD4+ cells, contact dermatitis to haptens is mediated primarily by CD8+ cells with a Th1-type cytokine profile.[30,31] Other cytokines released during the sensitization process have been implicated in directing the type of immune response mounted by T cells. It has been shown that IL-10 converts Langerhans cells and dendritic cells from potent inducers of a primary immune response to hapten-specific tolerizing cells as discussed later. A significant decrease in mRNA signals for IL-1α, IL-1β, and TNF-α confirms the immunomodulatory role of this cytokine in contact hypersensitivity reactions. On the other hand, IL-12, which is released by Langerhans cells and dendritic cells, is known to be a strong inducer of the Th1 response.

On subsequent contact of the skin with a hapten, that is, during the elicitation phase of allergic contact dermatitis, other APCs, including macrophages, dermal dendritic cells, or even less professional APCs such as MHC class II–expressing endothelial cells, may stimulate antigen-specific memory T cells and contribute to the initiation of the local inflammatory response (the dermatitis reaction). The sensitized T cells home in on the hapten-provoked skin site, releasing their inflammatory mediators, which results in epidermal spongiosis ("eczema"). Secondary or subsequent hapten exposure shortens the period of latency from contact to appearance of the rash (anamnesis).

Of interest, recent evidence suggests that a significant number of nickel-specific T cells isolated from allergic subjects can be directly activated by the metal in the absence of professional APCs.[32] T-T nickel presentation was MHC class II restricted, independent of CD28 triggering, and was followed by CD25, CD80, CD86 up-regulation, cytokine release, and cell proliferation. The results demonstrate that the epitopes recognized by APC-independent T cell clones do not require processing. Thus in T-T presentation the epitopes were generated by a direct interaction of the hapten with MHC class II molecules expressed on T cells. Nevertheless, not all of the processing-independent clones belonged to the APC-independent subtype, suggesting that independence from APC processing was necessary but not sufficient for T-T presentation. It is likely that fewer epitopes are generated by

T cells on interaction with nickel, whereas professional APCs may display a broader spectrum of nickel epitopes. These data suggest that in the efferent phase of allergic contact dermatitis, T lymphocytes can simultaneously act as effector cells and APCs. In particular, the subset of APC-independent lymphocytes may play a role in the initiation and rapid amplification of the cutaneous allergic reaction, representing a subset of nickel-reactive T cells not requiring professional APCs for complete functional activation.

Keratinocyte Apoptosis and Eczema

Spongiosis is a well-established histologic hallmark of the epidermis in eczema. It is characterized by the diminution and rounding of keratinocytes (condensation), widening of intercellular spaces, and stretching of remaining intercellular contacts, resulting in a spongelike appearance of the epidermis that progresses sometimes to the formation of small intraepidermal vesicles. The function and integrity of the epidermis are dependent on specific cell surface adhesion molecules. Trautmann et al[33] made the important observation that activated T cells infiltrating the skin in eczematous dermatoses induced keratinocyte apoptosis, resulting in spongiosis. In the current study, they investigated the effects of immunomodulatory agents on an *in vitro* model of eczematous dermatitis using keratinocyte/T cell co-cultures. In addition, these authors performed *in vivo* studies in allergic contact dermatitis, demonstrating resolution of epidermal spongiosis and cellular infiltrate in skin successfully treated with both topical corticosteroids and tacrolimus 0.1% ointment.[34]

T Cell Recruitment in Allergic Contact Dermatitis

The recruitment of T cells into the skin is regulated by the expression of the specific skin homing receptor, cutaneous lymphocyte–associated antigen (CLA), which mediates rolling of T cells over activated endothelial cells expressing E-selectin.[35] In addition, chemokine receptors have been proposed as important regulators of the tissue targeting of T cells. In this respect, CLA+ T cells co-express the chemokine receptor CCR4, the ligand for thymus and activation-regulated chemokine TARC (CCL17) and macrophage-derived chemokine (CCL22). CCR4 triggered by TARC exposed on the endothelial cell surface during inflammatory skin disorders is thought to augment integrin-dependent firm adhesion of T cells to endothelial intercellular adhesion molecule (ICAM)-1.[36] T cell migration into peripheral tissues mostly depends on their chemokine receptor profiles. Th1-type cells express high levels of CCR5 and CXCR3, interacting with MIP-1β (CCL4) and interferon gamma (IFN-γ)–inducible protein 10 (CXCL10), respectively, whereas Th2-type cells express primarily CCR3, CCR4, and CCR8 and interact with eotaxin (CCL11), TARC and MDC, and I-309 (CCL1).[37]

Epidermal keratinocytes have been shown to be an important source of inflammatory mediators for the initiation and amplification of skin immune responses. Treatment with IFN-γ or IFN-γ plus TNF-α induces keratinocytes to express ICAM-1 and MHC class II molecules and to release a number of chemokines and cytokines, including IL-1, TNF-α, and GM-CSF.[38] IL-17, a cytokine produced by both skin-infiltrating Th1-type and Th2-type T cells, modulates many of the effects induced by IFN-γ. Of note, IL-4, a Th2 cytokine, acts synergistically with the Th1 cytokine IFN-γ to enhance keratinocyte ICAM-1 expression and release of the CXCR3 agonistic chemokines, IP-10, monokines induced by IFN-γ (Mig; CXCL9), and IFN-inducible T cell α-chemoattractant (I-TAC; CXCL11), thus augmenting both recruitment and retention of Th1-type cells in lesional skin.[39]

Effector T Cells in Allergic Contact Dermatitis

Both CD4 and CD8 T cells participate in allergic contact dermatitis, with CD8 T cells predominating in effector mechanisms of tissue damage.[40] Budinger et al[41] demonstrated that nickel-responsive peripheral T cells from patients with nickel-induced contact dermatitis showed a significant overexpression of T cell receptor (TCR)–Vβ17, and the frequency of TCR-Vβ17+ T cells correlated significantly with the *in vitro* reactivity of peripheral blood mononuclear cells to nickel. In addition, the cutaneous infiltrate of nickel-induced patch test reactions consisted primarily of Vβ17+ T cells, suggesting that T cells with a restricted TCR-Vβ repertoire predominate in nickel-induced contact dermatitis and may be crucial in the effector phase of nickel hypersensitivity. Of note, these nickel-specific T cells produced IL-5 but not IFN-γ, consistent with a Th2-type cytokine profile. Other studies have shown nickel-specific T cells with a Th1-type profile[42]; in addition, nickel-specific CD4+ Th1-type cells have been shown to be cytotoxic (along with CD8+ T cells) against keratinocytes, whereas Th2-type nickel-reactive T cells were not.[43]

Regulatory T Cells in Allergic Contact Dermatitis

Cavani et al[44] described nickel-specific CD4+ T cells from nickel-allergic subjects that secrete predominantly IL-10, which blocks the maturation of dendritic cells including IL-12 release, thus impairing their capacity to activate specific T effector lymphocytes. Thus regulatory T cells may limit excessive tissue damage and participate in the resolution of allergic contact dermatitis.

DIFFERENTIAL DIAGNOSIS

A number of both eczematous and noneczematous dermatoses should be considered in the evaluation of a child with suspected contact dermatitis (Table 55-1). Seborrheic and atopic dermatitis occur commonly, whereas psoriasis and zinc deficiency are less common. Contact dermatitis may be superimposed on atopic dermatitis and should be suspected when eczema appears to flare with treatment of the underlying dermatitis. At times, contact dermatitis may be superimposed on atopic dermatitis and should be suspected when eczema appears to flare with treatment of the underlying dermatitis.

EVALUATION AND MANAGEMENT

Spectrum of Contact Dermatitis

A broad spectrum of adverse cutaneous reactions can result from the interaction of an external agent with the skin, whether the reaction is mediated by an irritant or allergen. Contact dermatitis can be described as acute, subacute, or chronic. Acute dermatitis can present with erythematous

TABLE 55-1 Differential Diagnosis of Contact Dermatitis

Other eczematous dermatoses
  Seborrheic dermatitis
  Atopic dermatitis
  Nummular eczema
  Neurodermatitis (lichen simplex chronicus)
  Acrodermatitis enteropathica
  Psoriasis
Noneczematous dermatoses
  Dermatophytosis
  Bullous impetigo
  Vesicular viral eruptions
  Urticarial vasculitis
  Mycosis fungoides
  Erythroderma related to adverse drug reaction, Sézary syndrome, psoriasis (generalized contact dermatitis)

papules, vesicles, and even bullae. Chronic dermatitis is characterized by pruritus, erythema, scaling, fissuring, excoriations, and lichenification. Less common clinical presentations of contact dermatitis that may be overlooked include urticaria, acneiform, and pigmentary changes. A broader spectrum of irritant contact dermatitis, including *acute, acute delayed, cumulative, traumatic,* and *subjective,* has been described.[45]

DIAGNOSIS OF CONTACT DERMATITIS

History

A careful history should elicit that the site of the skin problem was in contact with the offending agent within 36 hours before the initial appearance of the rash. Unfortunately, although history can strongly suggest the cause of contact dermatitis, relying solely on the history other than with obvious nickel reactions and a few other allergens may confirm sensitization in only 10% to 20% of patients with allergic contact dermatitis. The evolution of the skin reaction is influenced by many factors, including the patient's skin age, color, ambient conditions, and the relationship to home, school, work, and/or recreational exposures. Contact urticaria is often associated with respiratory symptoms such as itchy eyes, sneezing, and/or wheezing. Frequency of hand washing and the cleansers used should be noted. Frequent causes of irritant contact dermatitis include water, soaps/detergents, and the juices of food products. The patient's medical history may be a contributing factor. The impaired epidermal barrier layer of all atopics, with or without active dermatitis, subjects them to a greater risk for both allergic sensitization and irritation. Because the majority of contact reactions present as eczematous eruptions, it is essential to note clinical evolution from acute vesiculation to chronic lichenification. The history should also review response to all prior treatment.

Physical Examination

The physical examination precludes that the physician can recognize specific skin changes. The objective findings include the appropriate identification of all the primary and secondary skin lesions, such as macules, papules, and so on, each of which may be secondarily affected by color, crusts, excoriations, and other factors.

Exposed areas, especially the hands and face, are the sites most frequently involved in contact dermatitis. Hand dermatitis deserves special consideration not only because it is extremely common but also because the differential diagnosis can be challenging. Because the palmar skin is much thicker than the dorsum of the hands, allergic contact dermatitis rarely involves the palms, occurring most often on the thinner skin between the fingers and the dorsum of the hands.

Although contact dermatitis is considered to be the most common cause of eyelid dermatitis, it is believed that 25% of patients with atopic dermatitis may have a chronic eyelid dermatitis. In evaluating patients with eyelid dermatitis, one must note if other areas of the body are involved. Chronic eyelid dermatitis is more often due to cosmetics applied to other areas of the body (e.g., nails, scalp) than to cosmetics that are directly applied to the eye area. Because of increased exposure, extreme sensitivity, susceptibility to irritants and allergens (including aeroallergens), and easy accessibility to rubbing, the eyelids are easily inflamed. The history should also take note of the use of eyelash curlers (especially in nickel-sensitive patients) and facial tissues (which may contain fragrances, formaldehyde, or benzalkonium chloride). Shampoos, conditioners, hair sprays, gels, and mousses may cause eyelid dermatitis without causing scalp or forehead lesions. Paraphenylenediamine (PPD) and ammonium persulfate can cause urticaria and/or eyelid edema.

Similar to eyelid dermatitis, facial dermatitis may occur secondary to allergens transferred to the face from other regions of the body. Most commercially available cosmetics are virtually free of sensitizing components, but allergic contact dermatitis in response to moisturizers, sunscreens, foundations, and powders does occur and usually produces a symmetric dermatitis. Rubber-sensitive individuals may react to rubber sponges, masks, balloons, children's toys, and other products that are in contact with the face. A spouse's fragrance and cosmetics may produce a unilateral facial eruption.

The scalp skin is relatively resistant to allergens in shampoos and hair dyes, and the dermatitis may be manifest on the face or eyelids. Severe burns of the scalp and hair can be caused by the misuse of hair straighteners and relaxers. The manufacturers of hair dyes recommend that the client be patch tested with the product before each application.

The thin intertriginous skin of the neck is vulnerable to irritant reactions from "perms," hair dyes, shampoos, and conditioners. "Berloque" dermatitis from certain perfumes or nail polish presents as localized areas of eczema. Nickel-sensitive individuals may react from wearing a necklace or from zippers.

Allergic contact dermatitis can be caused by deodorants but not antiperspirants. These agents cause a dermatitis involving the entire axillary vault, whereas textile allergic contact dermatitis spares the apex of the vault. Irritant contact dermatitis can occur from shaving and depilating agents.

Allergic contact dermatitis must be considered in all patients with persistent stasis dermatitis caused by the increased use of medications on the impaired skin. Local absorption of the topical medication has also been noted to produce an "autosensitization," resulting in a generalized "id" reaction. Shaving agents, moisturizers, and rubber in the elastic of socks can cause allergic reactions.

Medication, douches, spermicides, sprays, and cleaners can cause contact dermatitis in the genital area. Fragrances found in liners, toilet paper, soap, and bubble baths can cause a reaction in sensitized patients. Contraceptive devices can affect rubber (especially latex)-sensitive individuals. Ammonia and/or the acidity of urine may cause an irritant dermatitis, especially in incontinent patients. The ingestion of spices, antibiotics, or laxatives may cause anal itching.

PATCH TESTING

The patch test remains the gold standard for confirming allergic contact dermatitis. The paradox of patch testing lies in its deceptive simplicity. Although the application of antigens for patch testing is rather simple, antigen selection and patch test interpretation require an experienced clinician (Box 55-1).

Selection of Appropriate Subjects to Test

The higher the index of suspicion, the more frequent the diagnosis of allergic contact dermatitis. Indeed, the observation that the greatest abuse of patch testing is its lack of use holds true even for the pediatric population. There are no well-documented reports of how often patch testing is performed in the pediatric population. The personal experience of one of the authors (V.S.B.) and personal contact with personnel at several large patch test clinics in New York City revealed that fewer than 1% of patients tested during the past 5 years were children. It is important for the clinician to remember that the majority of patients will be allergic to a single allergen or a single group of allergens and that there is a risk of false-positive patch test results. Some patients will benefit more from direct therapeutic intervention (i.e., allergen avoidance) than from patch testing. Ideally, one needs to know the value of all the clinical data before patch testing in predicting a clinically relevant response to any of the allergens tested. Patch testing should be considered for any patient with a chronic, pruritic, or recurrently eczematous or lichenified dermatitis. Virtually any eczematous lesion could be caused or aggravated by a contactant (Box 55-2).

Immunocompromised patients, including those on oral

BOX 55-1 **KEY CONCEPTS**
Evaluation and Management of Contact Dermatitis

- Irritant contact dermatitis is much more common than allergic contact dermatitis.
- Response to a contactant is influenced by factors related to the agent, the host, the exposure, and the environment.
- The higher the index of suspicion for allergic contact dermatitis, the more frequent the correct diagnosis.
- The greatest abuse of patch testing is lack of use.
- Patch testing is indicated for any persistent eczematous eruption on the dorsum of the hands but rarely for palmar rashes.
- Patients with a suggestive history or physical findings but negative results on Thin-layer Rapid-Use Epicutaneous Test should be considered for further evaluation in a patch testing clinic.

BOX
55-2

KEY CONCEPTS

Approach to Patch Testing in Allergic Contact Dermatitis

- Understand the underlying pathophysiology.
- Select the proper patient to test.
- Never test with an unknown substance.
- Apply the patches properly, and instruct the patient or family in proper care.
- Interpret the patch test results correctly.
- Determine the relevance of the results.
- Counsel the patient and/or family.

steroids or those on chemotherapy, are not appropriate candidates for patch testing. Ideally, the dermatitis should be quiescent. The skin site where the patch tests are to be applied should have had no potent steroid applied for 5 to 7 days before testing. Patients should avoid sun or ultraviolet light exposure for 96 hours. Systemic antihistamines have no effect on patch test results. Of note, human immunodeficiency virus–positive patients can react to contact allergens if they are sensitive to them.

Patch Testing Procedure

It has been suggested that the concentration of allergens used for children should be less than those for adults, but we now know that children tolerate adult concentrations well.[46] Standardized criteria for patch testing have been set by the Task Force on Contact Dermatitis of the American Academy of Dermatology. All results are dependent on the recommended protocol for application, removal, and interpretation of results. Patch testing is typically done on the upper back between the spine and scapulae. Patients are instructed to keep the back dry during the procedure, avoiding showers and excessive perspiration. In infants and small children, patch tests can be covered with fabric adhesive tape or a stockinette vest.

In the United States, one approved product is available for patch testing, the Thin-layer Rapid-Use Epicutaneous (T.R.U.E.) Test (manufactured by Mekos Laboratories AS, Herredsvejen, Denmark, and distributed by Cardinal Health [800-TRUE-TEST]). This constitutes a standard battery of 23 allergens and a negative control (Table 55-2). The allergens are in a vehicle attached to an adhesive backing. Comparative results of the T.R.U.E. Test and Finn Chamber method have shown a 64% to 98% concordance in results, depending on the allergen. However, a more recent study suggested that false-negative results may occur with the T.R.U.E. Test, particularly with fragrance mix and rubber additives (thiuram and carba mix).[47] A number of other standardized allergens are available from Canada (Trolab, Pharmascience Inc, Montreal [514-340-1114]; Chemotechnique, Toronto [416-242-6167]) and Europe and can be tested individually with the Finn Chamber attached to the back with Scanpor tape. Clinicians need to be aware of the limitations of each system of patch testing for individual allergens.[48] Caution should be exercised when testing for nonstandardized antigens to avoid adverse effects and false-positive responses. Ideally, at least two control subjects should be tested with any non-standardized allergen. Patch testing should never be performed with an unknown substance.

Patch testing should be scheduled for an initial reading 48

TABLE 55-2 Thin-layer Rapid Use Epicutaneous Test Antigens

Antigen	Common Exposures
Nickel sulfate	Snaps, jewelry
Wool alcohols (lanolin)	Cosmetics, soaps, topical medications, moisturizers
Neomycin sulfate	Topical antibiotics
Potassium dichromate	Chrome-tanned leather, cement
Caine mix	Topical anesthetics
Fragrance mix	Fragrances, scented household products
Colophony	Cosmetics, adhesives, household products
Paraben mix	Preservative in topical formulations, cosmetics
Balsam of Peru	Foods, cosmetics, fragrances, topical medications
Ethylenediamine dihydrochloride	Topical medications, eyedrops
Cobalt dichloride	Metal-plated objects, paints
p-tert-Butylphenol formaldehyde resin	Fabrics, waterproof glues
Epoxy resin	Two-part adhesives
Carba mix	Rubber products, shampoos, disinfectants
Black rubber mix	All black rubber products, some hair dyes
CL+ ME− Isothiazolinone	Cosmetics, skin care products, topical medications
Quaternium-15	Preservative in cosmetics and skin care products
Mercaptobenzothiazole	Rubber products, adhesives
p-Phenylenediamine	Permanent or semipermanent hair dyes, cosmetics, printing ink
Formaldehyde	Fabric finishes, cosmetics
Mercapto mix	Rubber products, glues for leather and plastics
Thimerosal	Preservative in contact lens solutions, cosmetics, injectable drugs
Thiuram mix	Rubber products, adhesives

TABLE 55-3 Patch Test Interpretation

Grade	Patch Test Grading	Clinical Interpretation of Grading
0	No reaction	No evidence for contact allergy
+/−	Mild erythema only	Doubtful for contact allergy
1+	50% of patch test site erythematous with edema	Possible (versus false-positive) contact allergy
2+	50% of patch test site with erythematous papules	Probable contact allergy
3+	50% of patch test site with vesicles or bullae	Definite contact allergy

hours after application, when the patches are removed, with the final definitive reading usually at 72 to 96 hours. Patch test results should be evaluated 30 minutes after removal of the tape and patch test materials. Allowance for the irritative effect from the adhesive material must be considered. The American Contact Dermatitis Society has established a grading system that is almost universally recognized (Table 55-3). Alternative grading with the T.R.U.E. Test is shown in Figure 55-4. Relevance of positive reactions to the clinical presentation needs to be carefully evaluated. Conversely, patients with negative results may need to be referred for more complete testing to a Patch Test clinic.

Additional tests used less frequently in the diagnosis of contact dermatitis include skin biopsy to differentiate from other diseases (listed in Table 55-1). Prick or intradermal testing may be helpful, especially in the evaluation of contact urticaria. Contact urticaria can also be evaluated with an "open" patch test as an alternative to the prick or intradermal test. Potassium hydroxide preparation for fungal hyphae or cultures may be needed to identify fungal disease. The Repeat Open Application Test, or exaggerated use test, which involves application of the allergen to the antecubital fossa twice daily for 1 week, is applicable for "leave-on" but not "wash-off" products.

ALLERGENS OF PARTICULAR IMPORTANCE IN CHILDREN

Nickel

Nickel is often reported as the most common allergen in children (see Figure 55-2). It is more common in girls than boys, and ear piercing is the most important predisposing factor.[7] In females, nickel sensitivity may increase the risk of developing hand eczema.[49] Of note, the nickel in stainless steel is not normally biologically available. The presence of releasable nickel from the surface of any object can be detected using the dimethylglyoxime spot test; a pink color indicates the presence of releasable nickel. Dietary avoidance of nickel is not usually

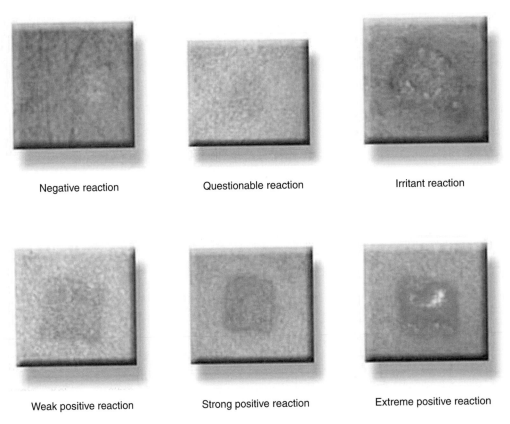

Negative reaction

Questionable reaction

Irritant reaction

Weak positive reaction

Strong positive reaction

Extreme positive reaction

FIGURE 55-4 Patch test grading.

advocated. Reactions to cobalt generally occur in association with nickel, whereas isolated cobalt sensitivity is rare.

Chromate

Chromate is found in leather, especially shoes, where chromium salts are used in the tanning process. Metallic chromium is not an allergen. Chromate sensitivity can be associated with hand or foot dermatitis, which can persist even after chromate avoidance.

Thimerosal

Thimerosal is a preservative that is widely used in vaccines. Although many children react to it on patch testing, these are rarely of clinical significance and individuals reacting to thimerosal typically have no reactions when given vaccines containing this preservative.[50] Data from the North American Contact Dermatitis Group reported thimerosal as the fifth most common allergen, inducing allergic reactions in 11% of patch-tested patients. However, in only 17% of patients with sensitivity to thimerosal was the patch test result considered clinically relevant to their dermatitis, ranking thimerosal last in relevance among the 50 allergens tested.[51] Thimerosal was named the Contact (Non)allergen of the Year 2002 and will be removed from the recommended screening tray in 2003.

Aluminum

Aluminum may cause cutaneous granulomas in response to vaccines containing aluminum hydroxide. These tend to resolve spontaneously, although children subsequently have positive patch tests to metallic aluminum or their salts.[52] The aluminum sensitivity appears to be lost with time as it occurs rarely in adults.

Rubber Chemicals

Rubber chemicals including thiuram mix, mercaptobenzothiazole, and mercapto mix are used in the manufacturing of rubber products including dipped (e.g., balloons, gloves) and molded (e.g., pacifiers, handle bars) products.

SPECIAL CONSIDERATIONS

Diaper Dermatitis

Diaper dermatitis represents the most common dermatologic disorder of infancy[53] (see Figure 55-1). It results from contact with irritants in the diaper environment, including feces and urine with associated friction, occlusion, and maceration. There has also been an association with bottle-feeding, maturity of the infant, and intestinal carriage of *Candida albicans.* Treatment usually involves increasing the frequency of diaper changes using superabsorbent disposable diapers and applying topical agents such as low-potency corticosteroids and barrier ointments or creams. When secondary *C. albicans* infection is present, a topical antifungal agent is beneficial.

There has been a definite decrease in the incidence of diaper dermatitis because of the improvement of diaper materials. In this respect, the introduction of disposable diapers, especially those with superabsorbent gel capable of absorbing water 50 times its own weight, has contributed to the positive trends.[54]

Foot Dermatitis

In their evaluation of contact dermatitis in children, Romaguera and Vilaplana[9] found that foot eczema was the most frequent localization. Irritant dermatitis of the feet may occur in children because of excessive perspiration or the use of synthetic footwear. Children can also develop allergic sensitization to rubber accelerators, dichromates, or cements used in manufacturing shoes. Topical medications can also cause allergic contact dermatitis of feet in children. The dorsal aspect of the foot is more commonly involved in allergic contact dermatitis, whereas irritant dermatitis can involve either the dorsum or sole. The majority of patients with contact dermatitis of the feet also have hyperhidrosis. Sweaty sock dermatitis needs to be distinguished from contact dermatitis, atopic dermatitis, and tinea pedis. Patients should be encouraged to wear cotton socks and to change them frequently, along with breathable footwear. Occasionally, a dusting powder (Zea-SORB) may be needed.

Perioral Dermatitis and Cheilitis

Children who lick or chew their lips, suck their thumb, or drool excessively may develop perioral dermatitis or cheilitis. Juices of foods and even chewing gum ingredients may contribute to skin irritation of these areas. Cinnamon flavorings and peppermint are the most common causes of allergic cheilitis from toothpastes.[55] In addition, some patients can develop an idiosyncratic response to various exogenous factors, especially potent topical corticosteroids on the face.

Plant Dermatitis (Phytodermatoses)

A number of plants can cause irritant reactions through mechanical or chemical injury. Most mechanical injury from plants is trivial, although inoculation of cactus hairs can give rise to pruritus. Implanted cacti spines can be removed by applying sticky tape to the skin and gently peeling it off. "Itching powder" from rose hip hairs has caused maculopapular and sometimes pustular eruptions at sites of contact. Chemical irritants caused by oxalate crystals results from contact with mustard, horseradish, and capsaicinoids in chili peppers. Contact with stinging nettles injects a mixture of inflammatory mediators, including histamine causing a hive, and an unidentified neurotoxin that causes localized numbness and tingling.

Plants of the *Toxicodendron* group, including poison ivy and poison oak, are the most common causes of allergic plant dermatitis in children in the United States. Even newborns can be sensitized to the oleoresin (urushiol). Because this is a potent antigen, the clinical reaction typically results in vesicles and bullae, often with a characteristic linear pattern (see Figure 55-3). Of note, the fluid content of vesicles is not antigenic. On the other hand, the oleoresin can be transferred by handling exposed animals, clothing, or sports equipment, for example, although soap and water inactivate the antigen. Urishiol is also found in cashew nut trees, Japanese lacquer, Ginkgo biloba, and mango skin, and the ingestion of cashews or contact with mango skin can cause a similar rash. Rhus patch testing is not recommended because it has a significant sensitizing capacity.

Of note, *Ambrosia* species, which include ragweed, can cause allergic plant dermatitis when pollinating in both atopic and nonatopic individuals. Repeated contact with ornamental cut flowers, including *Alstromeria* (the lily and tulip family of plants), can result in an allergic contact dermatitis that presents with a fissured dermatitis of the fingertips. Finally, plants that contain furocoumarins (psoralens), including parsley, parsnips, and wild carrots, can cause phytotoxic reactions. These reactions occur when the skin, contaminated with psoralens, is exposed to ultraviolet A light. They occur typically during the summer months, when psoralens are most abundant in wild garden plants and children are playing outdoors.

Topical Medications

Frequent self-treatment or treatment by the parent for various minor skin conditions results in sensitization and contact reactions. The topical application of anesthetics, antihistamines, antibiotics, and even antiinflammatory drugs along with preservatives or fragrances may be implicated. Neomycin is a frequent and potent sensitizer in children, as is diphenhydramine in topical form. Contact allergy to topical corticosteroids can be difficult to recognize and diagnose.[56] It should be suspected in any patient whose skin condition worsens with the application of a corticosteroid. There have been a number of reports of contact allergy to budesonide nasal spray with stomatitis with budesonide for oral inhalation.[57] Patch testing to corticosteroids is not standardized, is complicated by the concurrent antiinflammatory actions of the medication, and should be performed by clinicians familiar with this problem. Corticosteroids representative of different groupings typically used in patch testing include tixocortol, triamcinolone, dexamethasone, and budesonide. Sensitized patients must be instructed to avoid the systemic use of those drugs.

Contact Dermatitis of the Mucous Membranes

Although oral and mucus membrane contact reactions are rare, contact sensitivity has been described as a factor in recurrent oral ulcerations. Objectively, changes may be barely visible or may vary from a mild erythema to a fiery red color, with or without edema. Dental and mouth care products contain abrasives and sensitizing chemicals. Cinnamon flavorings and peppermint are probably the most common cause of allergic stomatitis from dentifrices and chewing gum. The metals used in dentistry that have been responsible for contact dermatitis include mercury, chromate, nickel, gold, cobalt, beryllium, and palladium. Of these metals, mercury has most often been implicated as a producer of allergic reactions.

Contact Dermatitis to Cosmetics

Cosmetics and personal hygiene products are ubiquitous in today's society. Exposure to a legion of potential allergens occurs regularly with the use of such products. It is not unusual for these products to manifest as contact allergy in sites distant from the sites on which the agent is applied. This phenomenon is termed *ectopic contact dermatitis* and requires diligent evaluation to elucidate the cause of the eruption. Fragrances are one of the most common causes of allergic contact dermatitis in the United States. They can be in cosmetics and personal hygiene products either overtly to add an appealing scent or to mask unpleasant odors. The term *unscented* can erroneously suggest that a product does not contain fragrance when in fact a masking fragrance can be present. *Fragrance-free* products are typically free of classic fragrance ingredients and generally acceptable for the allergic patient. The fragrance mix that is popularly used for testing contains eight different fragrances and will detect approximately 85% of fragrance-allergic individuals. Diagnosing fragrance allergy is essential for appropriate avoidance. However, because current labeling laws do not require manufacturers to label the specific fragrance present in a product, consumers are left eliminating far more materials from their activities of daily living than may be necessary.

Preservatives are present in most aqueous based cosmetics and personal hygiene products to prevent rancidity. These preservatives are grouped into two broad categories: formaldehyde releasers and nonformaldehyde releasers. Individuals who are allergic to formaldehyde cannot use any of the formaldehyde releasers. Common sensitizers that are formaldehyde releasers include quaternium-15, whereas thimerosal, benzalkonium chloride, and parabens are nonformaldehyde releasers. Excipients, including propylene glycol, ethylenediamine, and lanolin, are inert substances that make up the base of a product and serve to solubilize, sequester, thicken, foam, or lubricate the active component in a product. They can cause allergic contact dermatitis or, in higher concentrations, can act as irritants.

Hair products are second only to skin care products as the most common cause of cosmetic allergy. In addition to routine hair care products, intermittent cosmetic hair products such as permanent or semi-permanent hair dye and permanent wave solutions are commonly used. Adolescents working in hair salons may be exposed to PPD, the most common allergen affecting hairdressers. Glycerol thioglycolate is the active ingredient in permanent wave solutions. Nail cosmetics and glues have become increasingly popular and fashionable. There are several varieties of sculpting nails and the currently marketed products contain various methacrylate ester monomers, dimethacrylates, and trimethacrylates as well as cyanoacrylate-based glues. Clinical allergy to acrylics in nails can present locally at the distal digit or ectopically on the eyelids and face. Patch testing to a variety of acrylates and nail polish resin may be necessary to delineate the causative agent. Sunscreens are frequently present in cosmetics such as moisturizers, lip preparations, and foundations. As a group they are the most common cause of photoallergic contact dermatitis. *Chemical-free* sun blocks use physical blocking agents instead of photoactive chemicals and include titanium dioxide and zinc oxide, which are rarely sensitizers.

Systemic Allergic Contact Dermatitis

Patients allergic to ethylenediamine may react systemically with exposure to systemic aminophylline and antihistamines of the piperazine or ethanolamine family. Patients sensitized to topical diphenhydramine or neomycin can develop a systemic reaction from the systemic administration of these drugs. Reactions have been noted in patients sensitized to topical corticosteroids with the administration of corticosteroids systemically or intraarticularly. Nickel-sensitive patients may develop systemic reactions from the ingestion of nickel in tap water or foods cooked in nickel utensils and from eating canned foods.

Contact urticaria is discussed in Chapter 54.

TREATMENT

The mainstay of treatment for contact dermatitis is complete avoidance of contact with the offending agent. Thus identification of the putative agent remains the key to resolving the problem. All other measures are palliative and temporary. Whereas mechanical barriers against contacts, such as protective gloves, clothing, and barrier creams, are helpful in some cases, results are often disappointing. Once the offending agent is identified, patients and/or families must be educated and ideally provided with a list of potential sources of exposure and, wherever possible, given substitute, nonrelated agents (usually listed in textbooks, such as Fisher's *Contact Dermatitis*[58] or Marks & DeLeo's *Contact and Occupational Dermatitis*[59]). After removal of the offending agent, topical therapy may be used. Cool compresses are usually soothing and mildly antipruritic. The addition of aluminum subacetate, calamine, or colloidal oatmeal is of questionable value. In chronic eruptions, emollients, lubricants, and moisturizers may be used, but they should be nonsensitizing and fragrance free. Soaps and nonalkaline cleansers should be avoided. Rarely, antibiotics may be needed for secondary infection.

Topical antiinflammatory agents, primarily corticosteroids, are most effective when treating localized dermatitis. Patients with sensitivity to preservatives can use preservative-free corticosteroids such as Synalar Ointment, Aristocort Ointment, or Diprosone Ointment. Low-potency corticosteroids are recommended for the thinner skin, and high-potency corticosteroids are indicated for thickened, lichenified lesions. Ointments are generally more potent and more occlusive and contain less sensitizing preservatives than creams and lotions. Of note, high-potency corticosteroids should not be used for diaper dermatitis, yet a recent survey revealed that a combination antifungal-corticosteroid product containing betamethasone dipropionate was used in 6% of encounters.[60] Oral, intramuscular, or parenteral corticosteroids should be reserved for severe widespread acute eczema, which may be seen with poison ivy. Because the course of allergic contact dermatitis, after removal of the offending agent, varies from 14 to 28 days, systemic antiinflammatory drugs may need to be administered at appropriate doses (prednisone 0.5 to 1.0 mg/kg/day) for an extended period.

Topical calcineurin inhibitors, approved for use in children with atopic dermatitis 2 years of age and older (see Chapter 53), have been used in both animal models and patients with allergic contact dermatitis.[61,62] These immunomodulatory agents do not induce skin atrophy and may be especially valuable in treating facial or eyelid dermatitis. Burning or stinging has been the primary adverse reaction seen with these novel agents, although less so in pediatric patients.

Antihistamines may offer some benefit in contact urticaria. They are less effective for pruritus associated with eczematous reactions, although sedating antihistamines may offer some relief. Patient care must be individualized. Patient education regarding the nature of the dermatitis, triggering agents, irritant factors plus instruction for avoidance, and appropriate substitutes will not only aid in clearing the dermatitis but also prevent or minimize recurrences. At the present, hyposensitization of patients with allergic contact dermatitis is not a viable therapy.[63]

CONCLUSIONS

Contact dermatitis includes irritant and allergic forms and can affect patients of any age. It can affect the quality of life of children and their families. Patch testing remains the gold standard for diagnosis of allergic contact dermatitis, and negative results in the face of a convincing clinical presentation should prompt consideration for further evaluation by a specialist in contact dermatitis. New insights into the immune mechanisms involved may lead to better treatment strategies, including induction of tolerance, especially with difficult-to-avoid allergens.

HELPFUL WEBSITES

Thin-layer Rapid-Use Epicutaneous (T.R.U.E.) Test website (www.truetest.com)
The American Academy of Dermatology website (www.aad.org)

REFERENCES

1. Mortz CG, Andersen KE: Allergic contact dermatitis in children and adolescents, *Contact Dermatitis* 41:121-130, 1999.
2. Beltrani VS, Beltrani VP: Contact dermatitis, *Ann Allergy Asthma Immunol* 78:160-173; quiz 174-176, 1997.
3. Nielsen NH, Linneberg A, Menne T, et al: Allergic contact sensitization in an adult Danish population: two cross-sectional surveys eight years apart (the Copenhagen Allergy Study), *Acta Derm Venereol* 81:31-34, 2001.
4. Schafer T, Bohler E, Ruhdorfer S, et al: Epidemiology of contact allergy in adults, *Allergy* 56:1192-1196, 2001.
5. Jordon WE, Lawson KD, Berg RW, et al: Diaper dermatitis: frequency and severity among a general infant population, *Pediatr Dermatol* 3:198-207, 1986.
6. Philipp R, Hughes A, Golding J: Getting to the bottom of nappy rash. ALSPAC Survey Team. Avon Longitudinal Study of Pregnancy and Childhood, *Br J Gen Pract* 47:493-497, 1997.
7. Larsson Stymme B, Widstromm L: Ear piercing—a cause of nickel allergy in schoolgirls? *Contact Dermatitis* 13:289-293, 1985.
8. Mortz CG, Lauritsen JM, Bindslev-Jensen C, et al: Prevalence of atopic dermatitis, asthma, allergic rhinitis, and hand and contact dermatitis in adolescents. The Odense Adolescence Cohort Study on Atopic Diseases and Dermatitis, *Br J Dermatol* 144:523-532, 2001.
9. Romaguera C, Vilaplana J: Contact dermatitis in children: 6 years experience (1992-1997), *Contact Dermatitis* 39:277-280, 1998.
10. Manzini BM, Ferdani G, Simonetti V, et al: Contact sensitization in children, *Pediatr Dermatol* 15:12-17, 1998.
11. Shah M, Lewis FM, Gawkrodger DJ: Patch testing in children and adolescents: five years' experience and follow-up, *J Am Acad Dermatol* 37:964-968, 1997.
12. Stables GI, Forsyth A, Lever RS: Patch testing in children, *Contact Dermatitis* 34:341-344, 1996.
13. Wilkowska A, Grubska-Suchanek E, Karwacka I, et al: Contact allergy in children, *Cutis* 58:176-180, 1996.
14. Rudzki E, Rebandel P: Contact dermatitis in children, *Contact Dermatitis* 34:66-67, 1996.
15. Katsarou A, Koufou V, Armenaka M, et al: Patch tests in children: a review of 14 years experience, *Contact Dermatitis* 34:70-71, 1996.
16. Wantke F, Hemmer W, Jarisch R, et al: Patch test reactions in children, adults and the elderly: a comparative study in patients with suspected allergic contact dermatitis, *Contact Dermatitis* 34:316-319, 1996.
17. Sevila A, Romaguera C, Vilaplana J, et al: Contact dermatitis in children, *Contact Dermatitis* 30:292-294, 1994.
18. Goncalo S, Goncalo M, Azenha A, et al: Allergic contact dermatitis in children: a multicenter study of the Portuguese Contact Dermatitis Group (GPEDC), *Contact Dermatitis* 26:112-115, 1992.

19. Rademaker M, Forsyth A: Contact dermatitis in children, *Contact Dermatitis* 20:104-107, 1989.

20. Balato N, Lembo G, Patruno C, et al: Patch testing in children, *Contact Dermatitis* 20:305-307, 1989.

21. Bruckner AL, Weston WL, Morelli JG: Does sensitization to contact allergens begin in infancy? *Pediatrics* 105:e3, 2000.

22. DeLeo VA, Taylor SC, Belsito DV, et al: The effect of race and ethnicity on patch test results, *J Am Acad Dermatol* 46:S107-S112, 2002.

23. Fartasch M, Schnetz E, Diepgen TL: Characterization of detergent-induced barrier alterations—effect of barrier cream on irritation, *J Invest Dermatol Symp Proc* 3:121-127, 1998.

24. Wood LC, Jackson SM, Elias PM, et al: Cutaneous barrier perturbation stimulates cytokine production in the epidermis of mice, *J Clin Invest* 90:482-487, 1992.

25. Brasch J, Burgard J, Sterry W: Common pathogenetic pathways in allergic and irritant contact dermatitis, *J Invest Dermatol* 98:166-170, 1992.

26. Hoefakker S, Caubo M, van 't Erve EH, et al: *In vivo* cytokine profiles in allergic and irritant contact dermatitis, *Contact Dermatitis* 33:258-266, 1995.

27. Lisby S, Baadsgaard O: Mechanisms of irritant contact dermatitis. In Rycroft RJG, Menne T, Frosch PJ, et al, eds: *Textbook of contact dertmatitis*, London, 2001, Springer-Verlag.

28. Novak N, Bieber T: The skin as a target for allergic diseases, *Allergy* 55:103-107, 2000.

29. Krasteva M, Kehren J, Horand F, et al: Dual role of dendritic cells in the induction and down-regulation of antigen-specific cutaneous inflammation, *J Immunol* 160:1181-1190, 1998.

30. Grabbe S, Schwarz T: Immunoregulatory mechanisms involved in elicitation of allergic contact hypersensitivity, *Immunol Today* 19:37-44, 1998.

31. Xu H, DiIulio NA, Fairchild RL: T cell populations primed by hapten sensitization in contact sensitivity are distinguished by polarized patterns of cytokine production: interferon gamma-producing (Tc1) effector CD8+ T cells and interleukin (Il) 4/Il-10-producing (Th2) negative regulatory CD4+ T cells, *J Exp Med* 183:1001-1012, 1996.

32. Nasorri F, Sebastiani S, Mariani V, et al: Activation of nickel-specific CD4+ T lymphocytes in the absence of professional antigen-presenting cells, *J Invest Dermatol* 118:172-179, 2002.

33. Trautmann A, Akdis M, Kleemann D, et al: T cell-mediated Fas-induced keratinocyte apoptosis plays a key pathogenetic role in eczematous dermatitis, *J Clin Invest* 106:25-35, 2000.

34. Trautmann A, Akdis M, Schmid-Grendelmeier P, et al: Targeting keratinocyte apoptosis in the treatment of atopic dermatitis and allergic contact dermatitis, *J Allergy Clin Immunol* 108:839-846, 2001.

35. Robert C, Kupper TS: Inflammatory skin diseases, T cells, and immune surveillance, *N Engl J Med* 341:1817-1828, 1999.

36. Campbell JJ, Haraldsen G, Pan J, et al: The chemokine receptor CCR4 in vascular recognition by cutaneous but not intestinal memory T cells, *Nature* 400:776-780, 1999.

37. Sallusto F, Mackay CR, Lanzavecchia A: The role of chemokine receptors in primary, effector, and memory immune responses, *Annu Rev Immunol* 18:593-620, 2000.

38. Albanesi C, Scarponi C, Cavani A, et al: Interleukin-17 is produced by both Th1 and Th2 lymphocytes, and modulates interferon-gamma- and interleukin-4-induced activation of human keratinocytes, *J Invest Dermatol* 115:81-87, 2000.

39. Cavani A, Albanesi C, Traidl C, et al: Effector and regulatory T cells in allergic contact dermatitis, *Trends Immunol* 22:118-120, 2001.

40. Martin S, Lappin MB, Kohler J, et al: Peptide immunization indicates that CD8+ T cells are the dominant effector cells in trinitrophenyl-specific contact hypersensitivity, *J Invest Dermatol* 115:260-266, 2000.

41. Budinger L, Neuser N, Totzke U, et al: Preferential usage of TCR-Vbeta17 by peripheral and cutaneous T cells in nickel-induced contact dermatitis, *J Immunol* 167:6038-6044, 2001.

42. Kapsenberg ML, Wierenga EA, Stiekema FE, et al: Th1 lymphokine production profiles of nickel-specific CD4+ T-lymphocyte clones from nickel contact allergic and non-allergic individuals, *J Invest Dermatol* 98:59-63, 1992.

43. Cavani A, Mei D, Guerra E, et al: Patients with allergic contact dermatitis to nickel and nonallergic individuals display different nickel-specific T cell responses. Evidence for the presence of effector CD8+ and regulatory CD4+ T cells, *J Invest Dermatol* 111:621-628, 1998.

44. Cavani A, Nasorri F, Prezzi C, et al: Human CD4+ T lymphocytes with remarkable regulatory functions on dendritic cells and nickel-specific Th1 immune responses, *J Invest Dermatol* 114:295-302, 2000.

45. Iliev D, Elsner P: Clinical irritant contact dermatitis syndromes, *Immunol Allergy Clin North Am* 17:365-375, 1997.

46. Weston WL, Weston JA, Kinoshita J, et al: Prevalence of positive epicutaneous tests among infants, children, and adolescents, *Pediatrics* 78: 1070-1074, 1986.

47. Sherertz EF, Fransway AF, Belsito DV, et al: Patch testing discordance alert: false-negative findings with rubber additives and fragrances, *J Am Acad Dermatol* 45:313-314, 2001.

48. Suneja T, Belsito DV: Comparative study of Finn Chambers and T.R.U.E. test methodologies in detecting the relevant allergens inducing contact dermatitis, *J Am Acad Dermatol* 45:836-839, 2001.

49. Christensen OB, Moller H: Nickel allergy and hand eczema, *Contact Dermatitis* 1:129-135, 1975.

50. Wantke F, Demmer CM, Gotz M, et al: Contact dermatitis from thimerosal: 2 years' experience with ethylmercuric chloride in patch testing thimerosal-sensitive patients, *Contact Dermatitis* 30:115-117, 1994.

51. Marks JG Jr, Belsito DV, DeLeo VA, et al: North American Contact Dermatitis Group patch-test results, 1996-1998, *Arch Dermatol* 136:272-273, 2000.

52. Kaaber K, Nielsen AO, Veien NK: Vaccination granulomas and aluminum allergy: course and prognostic factors, *Contact Dermatitis* 26:304-306, 1992.

53. Ward DB, Fleischer AB Jr, Feldman SR, et al: Characterization of diaper dermatitis in the United States, *Arch Pediatr Adolesc Med* 154:943-946, 2000.

54. Bonifazi E: Napkin dermatitis—causative factors. In Harper J, Oranje A, Prose N, eds: *Textbook of pediatric dermatology*, London, 2000, Blackwell Scientific Publications.

55. Sainio EL, Kanerva L: Contact allergens in toothpastes and a review of their hypersensitivity, *Contact Dermatitis* 33:100-105, 1995.

56. Matura M, Goossens A: Contact allergy to corticosteroids, *Allergy* 55: 698-704, 2000.

57. Gonzalo Garijo MA, Bobadilla Gonzalez P: Cutaneous-mucosal allergic contact reaction due to topical corticosteroids, *Allergy* 50:833-836, 1995.

58. Fisher AA, ed: *Contact dermatitis*, Philadelphia, 1986, Lea & Febiger.

59. Marks JG Jr, DeLeo VA: *Contact and occupational dermatology*, St Louis, 1992, Mosby.

60. Ward DB, Fleischer AB Jr, Feldman SR, et al: Characterization of diaper dermatitis in the United States, *Arch Pediatr Adolesc Med* 154:943-946, 2000.

61. Queille-Roussel C, Graeber M, Thurston M, et al: SDZ ASM 981 is the first non-steroid that suppresses established nickel contact dermatitis elicited by allergen challenge, *Contact Dermatitis* 42:349-350, 2000.

62. Gupta AK, Adamiak A, Chow M: Tacrolimus: a review of its use for the management of dermatoses, *J Eur Acad Dermatol Venereol* 16:100-114, 2002.

63. Marks JG Jr, Trautlein JJ, Epstein WL, et al: Oral hyposensitization to poison ivy and poison oak, *Arch Dermatol* 123:476-478, 1987.

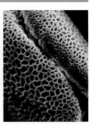

CHAPTER 56

Allergic and Immunologic Eye Disease

LEONARD BIELORY ■ TODD M. WILSON ■ RUDOLPH S. WAGNER

Allergic disease affects as many as 25% of the pediatric population. The direct costs attributable to upper airway allergies are estimated to be 5.9 billion, and children 12 years and younger account for 38% (2.3 billion) of this total.[1] Allergic eye involvement is very common. In one study of 5000 allergic children, 32% had ocular disease as the single manifestation of their allergies.[2] Although frequent, ocular allergy is certainly not the sole culprit of pediatric "red eye," which is why the clinician must be able to accurately distinguish an allergic response from nonallergic insults on the eye. This chapter provides an overview of pediatric allergic eye disease as well as a clinical approach to proper diagnosis and treatment.

EYE ANATOMY, HISTOLOGY, AND IMMUNE FUNCTION

The eye is a common target of inflammation by both local and systemic hypersensitivity reactions. Because of the eye's considerable vascularization and sensitivity of these vessels, particularly in the conjunctiva, ocular inflammation can be quite pronounced. Besides scaring the parents of affected children, ocular inflammation can pose a formidable diagnostic challenge to clinicians so a solid understanding of the eye's anatomy, histology, and immune function is essential.

The eye is basically constructed of four layers that are predominantly involved in immunologic reactions (Figure 56-1):

1. the anterior portion, consisting of the eyelids, conjunctiva, and tear fluid layer, providing the eye's primary barrier against environmental aeroallergens, chemicals, and infectious agents;
2. the collagenous sclera, involved in rheumatic (connective tissue) disorders;
3. the highly vascular uvea, involved in systemic inflammatory reactions associated with circulating immune complexes and cell-mediated hypersensitivity reactions; and
4. the retina, an extension of the central nervous system.

The eye is immunologically distinctive because it lacks formed lymph nodes in the orbit, lacrimal gland, eyelids, and conjunctiva. Interestingly, the spleen appears to function as the primary lymphoid organ for intraocular reactions.[3] Immunologic hypersensitivity reactions involving the eye incorporate the spectrum of the classic Gell and Coombs classification and include mast cells, cytotoxic antibodies, circulating immune complexes, and cell-mediated receptors[4,5] (Table 56-1).

Eyelids

Designed to protect, moisten, and cleanse the ocular surface, the eyelids are the first line of defense for the eye. The palpebral skin is extremely thin compared with the dermal thickness elsewhere on the human body (0.55 mm compared with the thickness of the integument of the face, measuring about 2 mm), which explains the common extensive involvement of this portion of the eye in minor inflammatory insults.

Conjunctiva

The conjunctiva consists of a thin mucous membrane that extends from the limbus of the eye to the lid margin of the eyelid. It is the most immunologically active tissue of the external eye and undergoes lymphoid hyperplasia in response to vari-

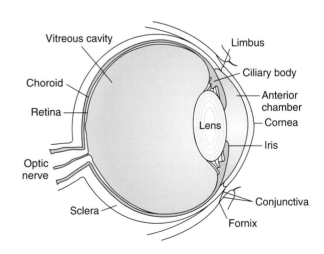

FIGURE 56-1 Cross-section of the eye. Sagittal cross-sectional view of the human eye revealing the parts commonly involved in immunologic reactions: eyelids (blepharitis and dermatitis); conjunctiva (conjunctivitis); cornea (keratitis); sclera (episcleritis and scleritis); optic nerve (neuritis); iris (iritis); vitreous (vitreitis); choroids (choroiditis); and retina (retinitis). The last four parts involve the inner portion of the eye (the uveal tract) and are classified as forms of uveitis.

TABLE 56-1 Categories of Pediatric Ocular Inflammation

Category	Recognition Component	Soluble Mediators	Time Course	Cellular Response	Clinical Example
IgE/mast cell	IgE	Leukotrienes Arachidonates Histamine	Seconds Minutes	Eosinophils Neutrophils Basophils	Allergic conjunctivitis Anaphylaxis Vernal keratoconjunctivitis
Cytotoxic antibody	IgG IgM	Complement	Hours Days	Neutrophils Macrophages	Mooren's ulcer Pemphigus Pemphigoid
Immune complex	IgG IgM	Complement	Hours Days	Neutrophils Eosinophils Lymphocytes	Serum sickness uveitis Corneal immune rings Lens-induced uveitis Behçet's syndrome Kawasaki's disease Vasculitis
Delayed hypersensitivity	Lymphocytes Monocytes	Lymphokines Monokines	Days Weeks	Lymphocytes Monocytes Eosinophils Basophils	Corneal allograft rejection Sympathetic ophthalmia Sarcoid-induced uveitis

ous stimulants.[6] Anatomically, the conjunctiva is divided into three parts: the bulbar conjunctiva covers the anterior portion of the sclera; the palpebral conjunctiva lines the inner surface of the eyelids; and the space bounded by the bulbar and palpebral conjunctiva is the fornix, or the conjunctival sac. In addition, the conjunctiva is composed of two histologically distinctive layers: the epithelium and substantia propria. The epithelial layer is composed of two to five cells of stratified columnar cells, whereas the lamina propria is composed of loose connective tissue.

Inflammatory cells such as mast cells, eosinophils, and basophils normally do not reside in the ocular epithelium; instead these cells are found in the substantia propria. Mast cells at a concentration of up to $6000/mm^3$ are present in this layer whereas the other inflammatory cells migrate into the tissue in response to various stimuli. The predominant form ($> 95\%$) of mast cells is the connective tissue type (MC_{TC}) that contains both chymase and tryptase.[7-9] However, in chronic forms of allergic conjunctivitis there is an increase in mucosal-type mast cells (MC_T), which produce tryptase only, followed by migration of these cells to the epithelial layer.[8] Epithelial cells have also been found to have an extensive proinflammatory capability in the production of various cytokines such as tumor necrosis factor alpha (TNF-α), interleukin (IL)-6, and IL-10 as well as various adhesion molecules such as intracellular adhesion molecules-1 (ICAM-1).

Various mononuclear cells including Langerhans cells, CD3+ lymphocytes, and CD4+/CD8+ lymphocytes are also an active component of the anterior surface immune response that is primarily found in the epithelial layer. Langerhans' cells, which serve as antigen-presenting cells in the skin, have a similar role in the eye.[9] The primary lymphoid organ for intraocular reactions is the spleen. Lymphatics from the lateral conjunctiva drain to the preauricular nodes (e.g., parotid node) just anterior to the tragus of the ear. The nasal conjunctival lymphatics drain to the submandibular nodes. It is generally believed that activated conjunctival lymphocytes travel first to these regional lymph nodes, then to the spleen, and ultimately back to the conjunctiva.

Tear Film

Tear secretion begins at approximately 2 to 4 weeks after birth. The conjunctival surface is bathed with a thin layer of tear film, which is composed of an outer lipid layer, a middle aqueous layer, and an inner mucoprotein layer. Goblet cells that produce mucin are distributed along the conjunctival surface. Mucin is important in decreasing the surface tension of the tear film, thus maintaining a moist hydrophobic corneal surface. This mixture decreases the evaporation rate of the aqueous portion. The aqueous portion of the tear film contains a variety of solutes, including electrolytes, carbohydrates, ureas, amino acids, lipids, enzymes, tear-specific prealbumin, and immunologically active proteins, including immunoglobulin A (IgA), IgG, IgM, IgE, tryptase, histamine, lysozyme, lactoferrin, ceruloplasmin, and vitronectin.

Uveal Tract

The uveal tract comprises the iris, ciliary body, and choroids, each of which possesses a rich vascular architecture and pigment. The pigment acts as a filtering system, and the ciliary body is involved in the production of aqueous humor. As is the case with other structures that produce filtrates (including the renal glomerulus [urine] and the choroid plexus [cerebrospinal fluid]), it is a common site for the deposition of immune complexes. In addition, disturbances in aqueous humor production or outflow obstructions may cause increased intraocular pressure (IOP; i.e., glaucoma). There are congenital forms of glaucoma that are not specifically associated with immunologic disorders but must be considered in the differential diagnosis of pediatric conjunctivitis.

DIFFERENTIAL DIAGNOSIS

The differential diagnosis of pediatric red eye can be broadly divided into four categories: allergic, infectious, immunologic, and nonspecific (Figure 56-2). Each category possesses distinct signs and symptoms. These indicators are

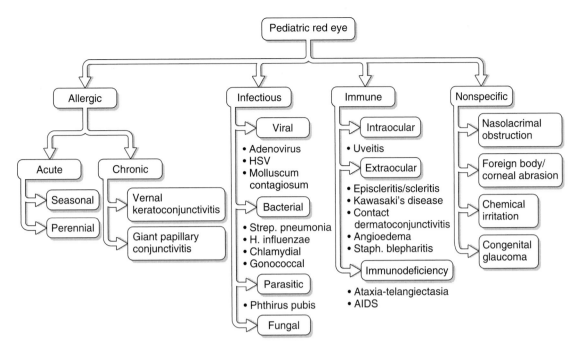

FIGURE 56-2 The differential diagnosis of pediatric "red eye" includes infectious agents (e.g., chlamydial disease, adenovirus), allergic conditions (e.g., SAC, PAC, GPC, VKC), immunologic disorders (e.g, Kawasaki's disease, uveitis, ataxia-telangiectasia), and nonspecific causes (e.g., foreign body, chemical irritation, nasolacrimal obstruction).

summarized in the supplied table and can be used as a guide to delineate pediatric "red eye" (Table 56-2).

HISTORY

A detailed and accurate history is the most important element in distinguishing allergic from nonallergic causes of pediatric conjunctivitis. Generally, this information is obtained from the parents or guardian, yet an astute clinician must not overlook input from the verbal child. Not only may the child's information prove clinically insightful, but this interaction helps establish good rapport with the child, which will be beneficial during the eye examination.

When evaluating a newborn, a full prenatal history must be obtained. This includes any developmental delays and maternal infections such as herpes simplex virus, chlamydia, or human immunodeficiency virus (HIV). Was the pregnancy preterm or postterm, a C-section or a vaginal delivery? Were there any complications? Ocular trauma from forceps or vacuum delivery has been known to occur. In addition, ocular medications such as silver nitrate and erythromycin given at childbirth may cause chemical irritation.

In the older child, a detailed history may reveal recent exposure to individuals with conjunctivitis or upper respiratory tract infection either within the family or school; such a history may help confirm an adenovirus in an endemic area. Family history is particularly important when inherited disorders are suspected. Accidental trauma resulting in corneal abrasions or ocular foreign bodies may also occur. This is especially true in the curious and mobile toddler. Yet, when these "accidents" occur frequently, child abuse must be considered; in these circumstances, a thorough social history is merited.

In teenagers, a sexual history may suggest a chlamydial or a neisserial infection. Frequently, the patient will not mention the use of over-the-counter topical medications such as vasoconstrictors or artificial tears, cosmetics, or contact lens wear. Direct questioning will often reveal the use of these products or other topical and systemic medications, all capable of producing inflammation (conjunctivitis medicamentosa or toxic keratopathy). As with all allergies, environmental factors and time of onset must be addressed, including seasonal variation and exposure to smoking, cleaning supplies, pets, air conditioning, carpets, and other sources of irritants.

Many of the symptoms of allergic conjunctivitis are nonspecific, such as tearing, irritation, stinging, burning, and photophobia. Symptoms tend to improve with cool, rainy weather and are exacerbated by warm, dry weather. The true hallmark of allergic conjunctivitis is itching. This pruritus can be mild or prominent and may last from hours to days. A stringy or ropy discharge is also characteristic of allergy. The discharge may range from serous to purulent. A purulent discharge accompanied by morning crusting and difficulty opening the lids is more characteristic of bacterial causes, especially gram-negative organisms such as *Neisseria* and *Haemophilus* (Figures 56-3 and 56-4). Most environmental allergens affect both eyes at once, although a unilateral reaction may result if the one eye is inoculated with animal hair or dander. Ocular pain is not typically associated with allergic conjunctivitis and suggests an extraocular process such as a corneal abrasion, scleritis or foreign body, or an intraocular process such as uveitis.

EYE EXAMINATION

Once a complete history is obtained, a thorough eye examination is necessary to confirm the diagnosis. Although a seemingly daunting task in a child, one does not need to be a pediatric ophthalmologist to perform a routine examination. Simple observation alone can be quite revealing. The eye

TABLE 56-2 Differential Diagnosis of Pediatric Conjunctivitis

	Predominant Cell Type	Chemosis	Lymph Node	Cobblestoning	Discharge	Lid Involvement	Pruritis	Gritty Sensation	Pain	Seasonal Variation
Allergic										
AC	Mast cell	+	-	-	Clear mucoid	-	+	+/-	-	+
VKC	Lymph EOS	+/-	-	++	Stringy mucoid	+	++	+/-	+/- if cornea is involved	+
GPC	Lymph EOS	+/-	-	++	Clear white	-	++	+	-	+/-
Infectious										
Bacterial	PMN	+/-	+	-	++ Mucopurulent	-	-	+	+/-	+/-
Viral	PMN Monolymph	+/-	++	+/-	Clear mucoid	-	-	+	+/-	+/-
Chlamydial	Monolymph	+/-	+/-	+	++ Mucopurulent	-	-	+	+/-	+/-
Immunologic										
Kawasaki's disease	PMN, lymph	+/-	++	-	Serous mucoid	-	+/-	+/-	+/-	-
Uveitis	Lymph	-	-	-	-	-	-	-	++	-
Sarcoidosis	Lymph	-	-	-	-	Grey, flat papules	-	-	+/-	-
JRA	Lymph	-	-	-	-	-	-	-	++	-
Episcleritis	Lymph	-	-	-	-	-	+	-	+/-	-
Contact dermato-conjunctivitis	Lymph	+/-	-	-	+/-	++	+	-	+/- if cornea is involved	-
Angioedema	Mast cell	++	-	-	-	+++	+/-	-	-	-
Ataxia-telangiectasia	-	-	-	-	-	-	-	-	-	-
Staphylococcal blepharitis	Monolymph	+/-	-	-	++ Mucopurulent	++	+	++	+/- if cornea is involved	-
Nonspecific										
Congenital entropion/ epiblepharon	-	-	-	-	Serous watery	++	-	+	+++	-
Congenital glaucoma	-	-	-	-	Serous	+/-	-	+/-	+++	-
Corneal abrasion	-	-	-	-	Serous watery	+	-	+/-	+++	-
Chemical	-	-	-	-	Serous mucoid	++	-	+/-	+++	-
Nasolacrimal obstruction	PMN if secondary infection	-	-	-	Mucopurulent	+	-	+/-	+/-	-

AC, Allergic conjunctivitis; *EOS*, eosinophil; *VKC*, vernal keratoconjunctivitis; *GPC*, giant papillary conjunctivitis; *PMN*, polymorphonuclear; *JRA*, juvenile rheumatoid arthritis.

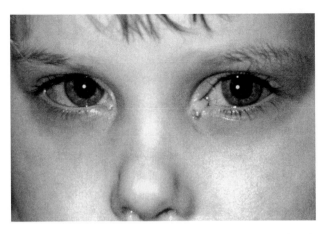

FIGURE 56-3 Bilateral conjunctival vascular injection and purulent discharge in a child with *Haemophilus influenzae* bacterial conjunctivitis.

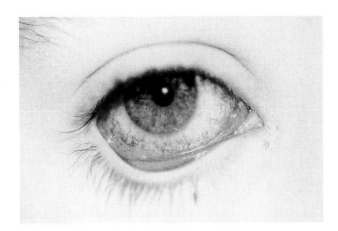

FIGURE 56-4 Mild inferior bulbar conjunctival vascular injection in viral conjunctivitis.

should be carefully examined for evidence of eyelid involvement such as blepharitis, dermatitis, swelling, discoloration, ptosis, or blepharospasm (Table 56-3). Conjunctival involvement may present with chemosis, hyperemia, cicatrization, or papillae formation on the palpebral and bulbar membranes. The presence of increased or abnormal secretions should also be noted. A funduscopic examination should be performed to detect such conditions as uveitis (often associated with autoimmune disorders) and cataracts (associated with atopic disorders and chronic steroid use).

Begin the examination with simple inspection of the face and area surrounding the eye. Allergic "clues" may be present. A horizontal skin crease on the nose (nasal salute) suggests a history of allergic rhinitis. Allergic shiners, which are ecchymotic-looking areas beneath the eyes thought to result from impaired venous return from the skin and subcutaneous tissues, have also been described in the allergic patient (Figure 56-5). Angioedema is the swelling of the dermis of which the conjunctiva is one of the most commonly involved sites in a variety of systemic hypersensitivity reactions. Patients typically exhibit periorbital edema, which is more prominent around the lower lids secondary to gravity. Nonallergic indicators may also be present. Eyelid or nasal vesicular eruptions are often seen in ophthalmic zoster. Scratches and scars on the face or eyelid suggest ocular injury. In addition, palpation of the sinuses and the preauricular and cervical chain lymph nodes are of diagnostic importance.

Next, the conjunctiva should be thoroughly inspected. Examination of the bulbar conjunctiva is performed by looking directly at the eye and asking the patient to look up and then down while gently retracting the opposite lid. Examine the palpebral (tarsal) conjunctiva by grasping the upper lid at its base with a cotton swab on the superior portion of the lid while gently pulling the lid out and up as the patient looks down. To return the lid to its normal position, have the patient look up. The lower tarsal conjunctiva is examined by everting the lower eyelid while placing a finger near the lid margins and drawing downward. A "milky" appearance of the conjunctiva is characteristic of allergy and is the result of the obscuring of blood vessels by conjunctival edema (Figure 56-6). In contrast, a velvety, beefy-red conjunctiva with purulent discharge suggests a viral or bacterial etiology.

Conjunctival inflammation can further be delineated by the presence of follicles or papillae. Follicles appear as grayish, clear, or yellow bumps varying in diameter from a pinpoint to 2 mm, with conjunctival vessels on their surfaces; they are generally distinguishable from papillae, which contain a centrally located tuft of vessels. Although a fine papillary reaction is nonspecific, giant papillae (greater than 1 mm) on the upper tarsal conjunctiva indicate an allergic source. Papillae are generally not seen in active viral or bacterial conjunctivitis. However, the presence of follicles, a lymphocytic response in the conjunctiva, is a specific finding that occurs primarily in viral and chlamydial infections.

The cornea is best examined with a slit lamp biomicroscope, although many important clinical features can be seen with the naked eye or with the use of an ophthalmoscope. The cornea should be perfectly smooth and transparent. Dusting of the cornea may indicate punctate epithelial keratitis. A localized corneal defect may suggest erosion or a larger ulcer that could be related to major basic protein deposition. Surface lesions can best be demonstrated by applying fluorescein dye to the eye, preferably following the instillation of a topical anesthetic drop (Figure 56-7). The end of the fluorescein strip is touched to the marginal tear meniscus. When the patient blinks the dye is dispersed throughout the ocular surface and stains wherever an epithelial defect exists as in a corneal or conjunctival abrasion. A light utilizing a cobalt filter will best demonstrate the abnormal accumulations of the dye. Most modern ophthalmoscopes are equipped with a cobalt blue filter, and many penlights have an attachable adapter. A Woods lamp, used by dermatologists to demonstrate tinea infections, will also cause the dye to fluoresce. Mucus adhering to the corneal or conjunctival surface is considered pathologic.

The limbus is the zone immediately surrounding the cornea that becomes intensely inflamed with a deep pink coloration in cases of anterior uveitis or iritis, the so-called ciliary flush. Discrete swellings with small white dots are indicative of degenerating cellular debris, which is commonly seen in vernal conjunctivitis. The anterior chamber is examined for clearness or cloudiness of the aqueous humor and for the presence of blood, either diffuse or settled out (i.e., hyphema) or the settling out of pus (i.e., hypopyon). A shallow anterior chamber suggests narrow-angle glaucoma and is a

TABLE 56-3 Ocular Clinical Signs

Disorder	Description
Blepharitis	Inflammation of the eyelids; sometimes associated with the loss of eyelashes (madarosis).
Chalazion	A chronic, granulomatous inflammation of the meibomian gland.
Chemosis	Edema of the conjunctiva due to transudate leaking through fenestrated conjunctival capillaries.
Epiphora	Excessive tearing; may be due to increased tear production or, more commonly, congenital obstruction of the nasolacrimal drainage system. This may occur in as many as 20% of infants, but resolves spontaneously in most cases before 1 year of age.[86] Children with chronic sinusitis and/or rhinitis may have intermittent nasolacrimal duct obstruction since the distal nasolacrimal duct drains below the inferior meatus. Congenital glaucoma may also present with epiphora but has other characteristic findings (e.g., corneal enlargement, photophobia, and eventually corneal edema presenting as a corneal haze) usually within the first year of life.*
Hordeolum	Synonymous with a sty.
Keratitis	Inflammation and infection of the corneal surface, stroma, and endothelium, with numerous causes.
Leukocoria	A white pupil; seen in patients with Chédiak-Higashi syndrome (a neutrophil defect), retinoblastoma, cataracts, and retrolental fibroplasia.
Papillae	Large, hard, polygonal, flat-topped excrescences of the conjunctiva seen in many inflammatory and allergic ocular conditions.
Phlyctenule	The formation of a small, gray, circumscribed lesion at the corneal limbus that has been associated with staphylococcal sensitivity, tuberculosis, and malnutrition.
Proptosis	Forward protrusion of the eye or eyes.
Ptosis	Drooping of the eyelid, which may have neurogenic, muscular, or congenital causes. Conditions specific to the eyelid that may cause a ptotic lid include chalazia, tumors, and preseptal cellulitis.
Scleritis	Inflammation of the tunic that surrounds the ocular globe. Episcleritis presents as a red, somewhat painful eye in which the inflammatory reaction is located below the conjunctiva and only over the globe of the eye. The presence of scleritis should prompt a search for other systemic immune-mediated disorders.
Trichiasis	In-turned eyelashes; usually results from the softening of the tarsal plate within the eyelid.
Trantas' dots	Pale, grayish-red, uneven nodules with a gelatinous composition seen at the limbal conjunctiva in vernal conjunctivitis.

*Data from Seidman DJ, Nelson LB, Calhoun JH, et al: *Pediatrics* 77:399-404, 1986.

contraindication for the use of mydriatic agents. An estimate of the anterior chamber depth can be made by illuminating it from the side with a penlight; if the iris creates a shadow on the far side from the light, then there is a high index of suspicion for increased IOP (i.e., glaucoma).

ALLERGIC DISORDERS

Conjunctivitis caused by IgE-mast cell-mediated reactions is the most common hypersensitivity response of the eye.[10] An estimated 50 million mast cells reside at the interface of the conjunctiva.[11] Direct exposure of the ocular mucosal surface to the environment stimulates these mast cells, clinically producing allergic conjunctivitis. In addition, the conjunctivas are infiltrated with inflammatory cells such as neutrophils, eosinophils, lymphocytes, and macrophages. Interestingly, acute forms of allergic conjunctivitis lack an eosinophilic predominance as seen in asthma. However, eosinophils and other immunologic active cells are prevalent in the more chronic forms.

Seasonal Allergic Conjunctivitis

Seasonal allergic conjunctivitis (SAC) is the most common allergic conjunctivitis, representing over half of all cases. As its name implies, its symptoms are seasonal and related to specific aeroallergens. Symptoms predominate in the spring and

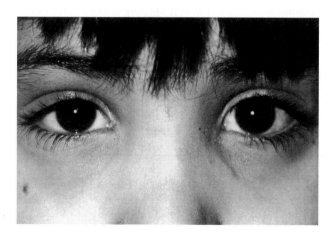

FIGURE 56-5 Bilateral "allergic shiners" of the lower eyelids in a child with chronic allergies.

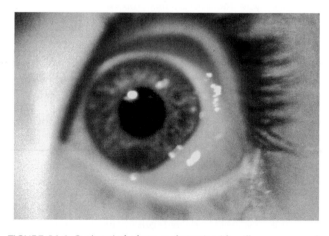

FIGURE 56-6 Conjunctival edema or chemosis with milky appearance obscuring conjunctival vessels in an acute allergic reaction.

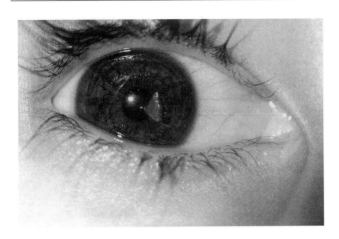

FIGURE 56-7 Triangular corneal abrasion highlighted with fluorescein dye.

in some areas during the fall (Indian summer). Grass pollen is thought to produce the most ocular symptoms. Commonly associated with nasal or pharyngeal symptoms, patients report itchy eyes and/or a burning sensation with watery discharge. A white exudate may be present that turns stringy in the chronic form of the condition. The conjunctiva will appear milky or pale pink and is accompanied by vascular congestion. This congestion may progress to conjunctival swelling (chemosis). Symptoms are usually bilateral but not always symmetric in degree of involvement. SAC rarely results in permanent visual impairment but can interfere greatly with daily activities.

Perennial Allergic Conjunctivitis

Perennial allergic conjunctivitis (PAC) is actually considered a variant of SAC that persists throughout the year. Dust mites, animal dander, and feathers are the most common allergens. Symptoms are analogous to SAC and 79% of PAC patients will have seasonal exacerbations. In addition, both PAC and SAC are similar in distribution of age, sex, and associated symptoms of asthma or eczema. The prevalence of PAC has been reported to be lower than that of SAC (3.5:10,000) although subjectively more severe,[12] but with the increasing prevalence of the allergies as reported in the International Survey for Asthma and Allergic Conditions study, this may be clearly underrepresented.

Vernal Keratoconjunctivitis

Vernal keratoconjunctivitis (VKC) is a severe bilateral, recurrent, chronic ocular inflammatory process of the upper tarsal conjunctival surface. It has a marked seasonal incidence, and its frequent onset in the spring has led to use of the term *vernal catarrh*. It occurs most frequently in children and young adults who have a history of seasonal allergy, asthma, and eczema. The age of onset for VKC is usually before puberty, with boys being affected twice as often as girls. After puberty it becomes equally distributed among the sexes and "burns out" by the third decade of life (about 4 to 10 years after onset). VKC may threaten sight if the cornea is involved and is more common in persons of Asian or African origin.

Symptoms include intense pruritus exacerbated by time and exposure to wind, dust, bright light, hot weather, or physical exertion associated with sweating. Associated symptoms involving the cornea include photophobia, foreign body sensation, and lacrimation. Signs include conjunctival hyperemia with papillary hypertrophy ("cobblestoning") reaching 7 to 8 mm in diameter in the upper tarsal plate; a thin, copious, milk-white, fibrinous secretion composed of eosinophils, epithelial cells, and Charcot-Leyden granules; limbal or conjunctival "yellowish-white points" (Horner's points and Trantas' dots) lasting 2 to 7 days; an extra lower eyelid crease (Dennie's line); corneal ulcers infiltrated with Charcot-Leyden crystals; or pseudomembrane formation of the upper lid when everted and exposed to heat (Maxwell-Lyon's sign; Figure 56-8). Although vernal conjunctivitis is a bilateral disease, it may affect one eye more than the other.

VKC is characterized by conjunctival infiltration with eosinophils, degranulated mast cells, basophils, plasma cells, lymphocytes, and macrophages. Degranulated eosinophils and their toxic enzymes (e.g., major basic proteins) have been found in the conjunctiva and in the periphery of corneal ulcers, a fact that may suggest their etiopathogenic role in many of the problems associated with vernal conjunctivitis.[13,14] MC_T cells are increased in the conjunctiva of these patients.[15] Tears from vernal conjunctivitis patients have been found to contain higher levels of leukotrienes and histamine (16 ng/ml) when compared to controls (5 ng/ml).[16] Tears from vernal conjunctivitis patients also contain major basic protein, Charcot-Leyden crystals, basophils, IgE and IgG specific for aeroallergens (e.g., ragweed pollen), and eosinophils (in 90% of cases).[17] The tear-specific IgE does not correlate with the positive immediate skin tests the vernal conjunctivitis patient may have, thus reflecting that it represents more than a chronic allergic response.

Giant Papillary Conjunctivitis

Giant papillary conjunctivitis (GPC) is associated with the infiltrations of basophils, eosinophils, plasma cells, and lymphocytes and is suggestive of process mediated by mixed mast cells and lymphocytes. GPC has been directly linked to the continued use of contact lenses. There is an increase in symptoms during spring pollen season. Symptoms include itching; signs include a white or clear exudate upon awakening that chronically becomes thick and stringy. The patient may develop Trantas' dots, limbal infiltration, and bulbar conjunctival

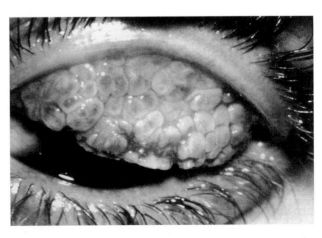

FIGURE 56-8 Conjunctival hyperemia with papillary hypertrophy (cobblestoning) on an everted palpebral conjunctiva of the upper eyelid in a patient with vernal conjunctivitis.

hyperemia and edema. Upper tarsal papillary hypertrophy ("cobblestoning") has been described in 5% to 10% of soft and 3% to 4% of hard contact lens wearers. The contact lens polymer, preservative (thimerosal), and proteinaceous deposits on the surface of the lens have been implicated as causing GPC, but this remains controversial. Analysis of the glycoprotein deposits on disposable soft contact lenses have revealed that the higher the water content, the higher the protein integration into the lens. The deposits have been analyzed and contain lysozyme, tear-specific prealbumin, and the heavy chain components of IgG.[18]

IMMUNOLOGIC DISORDERS

Kawasaki's Disease

Kawasaki's disease, also known as *mucocutaneous lymph node syndrome,* is an acute exanthematous illness that almost exclusively affects children. Fifty percent of cases occur predominantly in males below the age of 2, with an increased prevalence in individuals of Japanese ancestry. Five of the following six criteria must be present for diagnosis: (1) fever, (2) bilateral conjunctival injection, (3) changes in upper respiratory tract mucous membrane, (4) changes in skin and nails, (5) maculopapular cutaneous eruptions, and (6) cervical lymphadenopathy. The cutaneous eruption characteristically involves the extremities and desquamates in the later stages. The disease may occur in cyclic epidemics, and the current theory is that an infectious agent (a *Rickettsia*-like organism has been demonstrated by electron microscopy) causes a hypersensitivity response. Although most cases of Kawasaki's disease are benign and self-limited, 2% of Japanese Kawasaki's disease cases (nearly all male) experience sudden cardiac death.[19] This is because of acute thrombosis of aneurysmally dilated coronary arteries secondary to direct vasculitic involvement.

The most typical ocular finding is bilateral nonexudative conjunctival vasodilatation, typically involving the bulbar conjunctiva. Anterior uveitis is seen in 66% of patients, and is usually mild, bilateral and symmetric[20]; superficial punctate keratitis is seen in 12% of patients. Vitreous opacifications and papilledema have been reported. Choroiditis has been reported and pathologically demonstrated in a case of infantile periarteritis nodosa, which may be indistinguishable from Kawasaki's disease. On magnetic resonance imaging of the brain, deep white matter lesions, typically of the vasculopathic lesions of systemic vasculitis as opposed to the periventricular lesions more characteristic of multiple sclerosis, have been seen.

Uveitis

Uveitis may be anatomically classified as anterior, intermediate, posterior, and diffuse. Patients typically complain of diminished or hazy vision accompanied by black floating spots. Severe pain, photophobia, and blurred vision occur in cases of acute iritis or iridocyclitis. The major signs in anterior uveitis are pupillary miosis and ciliary/perilimbal flush, which is a peculiar injection seen adjacent to the limbus that can be easily confused with conjunctivitis. Vitreal cells and cellular aggregates are characteristic of intermediate uveitis and can be seen with the direct ophthalmoscope. Cells, flare, keratic precipitates on the corneal endothelium, and exudates with membranes covering the ciliary body can be visualized with the slit lamp and indirect ophthalmoscopy.

Anterior uveitis may be confused with conjunctivitis because its primary manifestations are a red eye and tearing; ocular pain and photophobia are also present. Anterior uveitis may be an isolated phenomenon that presents to an ophthalmologist or is associated with a systemic autoimmune disorder that presents to a general practitioner. It is found in approximately 50% of the cases of human leukocyte group A (HLA) spondyloarthropathy (e.g., ankylosing spondylitis, Reiter's syndrome), as well as in inflammatory bowel disease (e.g., Crohn's disease). Anterior uveitis is linked to the HLA-B27 genotype and systemic immunologic disorders, such as ankylosing spondylitis (sacroileitis) and Reiter's syndrome; infections, such as Klebsiella bowel infections (resulting from molecular mimicry), brucellosis, syphilis, and tuberculosis; as well as HLA-B5, -Bw22, -A29, and -D5 genotypes. The inflammatory response in the anterior chamber of the eye results in an increased concentration of proteins (flare [i.e., Tyndall effect]), a constricted pupil (miosis) with an afferent pupillary defect (a poor response to illumination), or cells in the aqueous humor. White blood cells can form a hypopyon or stick to the endothelial surface of the cornea, forming keratic precipitates. The sequelae of anterior uveitis may be acute, which may result in synechia (adhesions of the posterior iris to the anterior capsule of the lens), angle-closure glaucoma (blockage of the drainage of the aqueous humor), and cataract formation.

Posterior uveitis commonly presents with inflammatory cells in the vitreous, retinal vasculitis, and macular edema, which threatens vision. Posterior uveitis caused by toxoplasmosis occurs as the result of congenital transmission. Serologic assays for toxoplasmosis (enzyme-linked immunosorbent assay or immunofluorescent antibody) assist in the diagnosis.[21]

Panuveitis is involvement of all three portions of the uveal track, including the anterior, intermediate (pards plana), and posterior sections. In an Israeli study it was clearly linked (over 95% of cases) to a systemic autoimmune disorder, such as Behçet's disease.[22]

Sarcoidosis

Although rare, sarcoidosis does occur in children and 50% to 80% will have eye involvement. Sarcoidosis is associated with any type of anterior, intermediate, posterior, or diffuse nongranulomatous uveitis. Classically, noncaseating granulomas appear as "mutton fat precipitates," obstructive glaucoma, Koeppe nodules at the pupillary margin, or sheathing of vessels ("candle wax drippings"). The ocular inflammatory response may occur independent of any evidence of systemic involvement. Diagnostic tests include biopsy of the conjunctival or lacrimal granulomas, serum angiotensin-converting enzyme and lysozyme, chest radiograph for hilar adenopathy, and gallium scan. Biopsy of the lacrimal gland, the conjunctiva, or the periocular skin is useful only when direct visualization reveals a nodule. Other granulomatous processes involving the eye include toxocariasis, tuberculosis, and histoplasmosis, which may occur months to years after the primary infection.

Juvenile Rheumatoid Arthritis

Juvenile rheumatoid arthritis (JRA) accounts for 70% of chronic arthritis in children. Three subtypes of JRA exist: (1) systemic JRA, which occurs in 10% to 20% of affected children and is usually characterized by a febrile onset, lymphadenopathy, and evanescent rash; (2) polyarticular JRA, which occurs in 30% to 40% of affected children and is characterized by involvement of multiple (> 4) joints with few systemic manifestations; and (3) pauciarticular JRA, which occurs in 40% to 50% of affected children and is characterized by no more than four joints involved, usually larger joints and a positive antinuclear antibody (~75%). Anterior uveitis can develop in all types, although it is seen most often in pauciarticular JRA (~25%). JRA is associated with chronic bilateral iridocyclitis and Russell bodies (large crystalline deposits of immunoglobulin in the iris). The exact mechanism of ocular destruction is thought to be autoimmune based, although the specificity is much debated. S-antigen, histone 3, and type II collagen have all been proposed targets of humoral autoimmunity. Ocular manifestations do not parallel the patient's arthritis; instead, onset generally occurs within 7 years after joint inflammation, so frequent screening and early detection is crucial to decrease vision loss.

Blepharitis

Blepharitis is defined as an inflammation of the eyelids, sometimes associated with the loss of eyelashes (madarosis). It is one of the most common causes of pediatric red eye and is often misdiagnosed as an ocular allergy. In children, the two most common forms of blepharitis include staphylococcal blepharitis and meibomian gland obstruction.

As its name implies, staphylococcal blepharitis is characterized by colonization of the lid margin with *Staphylococcus aureus*. Antigenic products, such as staphylococcal superantigens, and not the colonization itself are being discussed as having a primary role in the induction of chronic eyelid eczema. Supporting the role of a noninfectious etiology are the relatively normal tear concentrations of antiinfection proteins (lysozyme, lactoferrin), including IgA and IgG antibodies.[23] Patients typically complain of persistent burning, itching, tearing, and a feeling of "dryness." These symptoms tend to be more severe in the morning and an exudative crust may be present, which causes the child's eye to become "glued shut." The signs of staphylococcal blepharitis include dilated blood vessels, erythema, scales, collarettes of exudative material around the eyelash bases, and foamy exudates in the tear film. Conjunctival injection and even a form of chronic papillary conjunctivitis may occur. In addition, corneal immune deposits may cause severe photophobia. Treatment is directed towards eyelid hygiene with detergents (baby shampoo) and steroid ointments applied to the lid margin. Within several weeks to months, the patient usually improves and becomes asymptomatic.

Meibomian gland obstruction may result in an acute infection (internal hordeolum or stye) but more commonly it produces a chalazion. A chalazion is a localized granulomatous inflammation caused by an accumulation of lipids and waxes within the meibomian gland. Clinically this results in edema, erythema, and burning of the eyelid, which over time may evolve into a firm, painless nodule. Bilateral eye involvement and conjunctivitis may also be present, which further contribute to its allergic mimicry; once again, eyelid hygiene is the mainstay of therapy.

Phthirus pubis, the pubic or crab louse, has a predilection for eyelash infestation[24] and may also cause blepharitis. Often, the lice may be visualized with direct inspection. Involvement

of the eyelashes in prepubertal children should raise the suspicion of sexual abuse.

Episcleritis

Inflammation of the scleral surface is termed *episcleritis.* It occurs mainly in adolescents and young adults, presenting as a localized injection of the conjunctiva around the lateral rectus muscle insertion (Figure 56-9). Typically, the inflammation is bilateral and accompanied by ocular pain. The presence of pain and absence of pruritis distinguishes episcleritis from allergic conjunctivitis. Episcleritis is self-limited and usually not associated with systemic disease.

Contact Dermatoconjunctivitis

Contact dermatitis involving the eyelids frequently causes the patient to seek medical attention for a cutaneous reaction that elsewhere on the skin would be of less concern. The eyelid skin, being soft, pliable, and thin, increases the eyelid susceptibility to contact dermatitis. The eyelid skin is capable of developing significant swelling and redness with minor degrees of inflammation; cosmetics are a major offender. Ironically, contact dermatitis of the lids and periorbital area more often is caused by cosmetics applied to the hair, face, or fingernails than by cosmetics applied to the eye area. In addition, preservatives such as thimerosal, which are found in contact lens cleaning solutions, have been shown by patch tests to be among the culprits. Because of the high incidence of irritant false-positive reactions, patch testing is generally used as a confirmatory tool, not as the first line of investigation. As yet no diagnostic test exists for irritant contact dermatitis.

Angioedema

Angioedema is the swelling of the dermis of which the conjunctiva is one of the most commonly involved sites in a variety of systemic hypersensitivity reactions. A documented local IgE–mast cell sensitization has been reported to papain enzyme in contact lens cleaning solution in which serum specific IgE to papain and chymopapain were detected.[25] The anatomy of the eyelid consists of loose epidermal tissue that provides an extensive reservoir for edema to even minor allergic

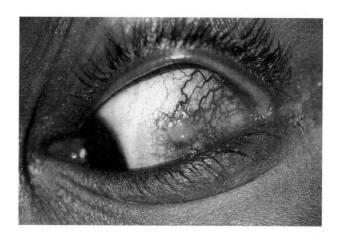

FIGURE 56-9 Localized bulbar conjunctival vascular injection in a patient with nodular episcleritis.

reactions but should also include the differential diagnosis of periorbital cellulitis, which may be life threatening.

Ataxia-Telangiectasia

Louis-Bar's Syndrome

Ataxia-telangiectasia presents with large tortuous vessels on the bulbar conjunctiva, most prominent in the exposed canthal regions[26] (Figure 56-10). This finding typically becomes evident between 1 and 6 years of age and may become more prominent with time. There are no other signs or symptoms of conjunctivitis. These children eventually develop ataxia and some recurrent sinopulmonary infection. Hypogammaglobulinemia and absent or deficient IgA have been reported in this condition.[27]

Acquired Immunodeficiency Syndrome

Children stricken with acquired immunodeficiency syndrome (AIDS) rarely have eye involvement. Cytomegalovirus retinitis is the most frequently encountered disorder, affecting approximately 7% of children with AIDS, and can lead to permanent vision loss if untreated. It is characterized by regions of intraretinal hemorrhage and white areas of edematous retina. HIV cotton-wool spot retinitis, herpes zoster retinitis, and toxoplasmosis retinitis have also been documented in children.

TREATMENT

Once an allergic etiology is identified, treatment is approached in a stepwise fashion. Treatment may be divided into primary, secondary, and tertiary interventions (Table 56-4).

Primary Intervention

Environmental Control

Avoidance of allergens remains the first option in the management of any ocular disorder.[28]

Cold Compresses

Cold compresses provide considerable symptomatic relief, especially from ocular pruritus. In general, all ocular

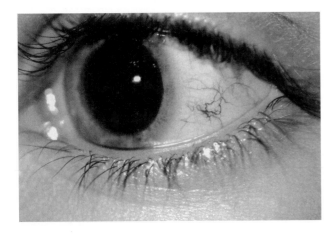

FIGURE 56-10 Tortuous conjunctival vessels on the bulbar conjunctiva in a patient with ataxia-telangiectasia.

medications provide additional subjective relief when refrigerated and immediately applied in a cold state.

Lubrication

Tear substitutes consist of saline combined with a wetting and viscosity agent, such as methylcellulose or polyvinyl alcohol. Artificial tears can be applied topically 2 to 4 times daily, as necessary. This primarily assists in the direct removal and dilution of allergens that may come in contact with the ocular surface. Ocular lubricants also vary by class, osmolarity, and electrolyte composition; no product has yet emerged as a clear favorite. Parents should be given the name of one or two brands from each class of lubricant to try until a suitable product or combination of products is found.

Secondary Intervention

Decongestants

Topical decongestants act primarily as vasoconstrictors that are highly effective in reducing erythema and are widely used in combination with topical antihistamines.[29] The decongestants are applied topically 2 to 4 times daily as necessary. They have no effect in diminishing the allergic inflammatory response. Vasocon-A is the only antihistamine/decongestant proven effective to treat the signs and symptoms (itch and redness) of allergic conjunctivitis. The usual dose is 1 to 2 drops per eye every 2 hours, up to four times daily. The primary contraindication is for narrow-angle glaucoma. Excessive use of these agents has been associated with a rebound phenomenon (a form of conjunctivitis medicamentosa).

Antihistamines

In the conjunctiva, histamine receptor 1 (H_1) stimulation principally mediates the symptom of pruritus whereas the H_2 receptor appears to be clinically involved in vasodilation.[30-33] Although topical antihistamines can be used alone to treat allergic conjunctivitis, they have been shown to have a synergistic effect when used in combination with a vasoconstrictor or when the agents themselves have been shown to have effects on other mediators of allergic inflammation. Dosing is 1 to 4 times daily and is safe for children 3 years and older.

Information on oral antihistamine use in the treatment of allergic conjunctivitis is commonly buried within studies on allergic rhinitis instead of *rhinoconjunctivitis*. Oral antihistamines, especially the older generation (e.g., chlorpheniramine), appear to have an effect on excessive tearing (lacrimation and epiphora).[34] Another assessment tool has been ocular challenge testing, which has shown that oral antihistamines, such as terfenadine or loratadine, can increase the tolerance to a dose of specific allergen treatment in children and adults severalfold.[35,36] Oral antihistamines can offer relief from the symptoms of ocular allergy but have a delayed onset of action. Newer, second-generation H_1 receptor (nonsedating) antagonists are less likely to cause unwanted sedative or anticholinergic (dry eye) effects than was the case with earlier compounds.[37]

In general, the older topical antihistamines are known to be irritating to the eye, especially with prolonged use. This is associated with the risk of developing sensitivity reactions that can further aggravate ocular allergies. One must keep in mind that ciliary muscle paralysis, mydriasis, and photophobia may result with the older topical antihistamines that are nonselective and block muscarinic receptors in addition to H_1

TABLE 56-4 Overview for the Treatment of Pediatric Ocular Allergic Disorders in a Stepwise Format

Therapeutic Intervention	Clinical Rationale	Pharmaceutic Agents	Comments
Primary			
Avoidance	Effective, simple in theory, typically difficult in practice		>30% symptom improvement
Cold compresses	Decrease nerve c-fiber stimulation, reduce superficial vasodilation		Effective for mild-moderate symptoms
Preservative-free tears	Lavage, dilutional effect	Artificial tears	Extremely soothing, recommend refrigeration to improve symptomatic relief, inexpensive OTC, safe for all ages, comfortable, use as needed
Secondary			
Topical antihistamine and decongestants	Antihistamine relieves pruritus, vasoconstrictor relieves injection	Antazoline naphazoline, Pheniramine naphazoline	No prescription required, quick onset, more effective than systemic antihistamines, limited duration of action, frequent dosing required
Topical antihistamine and mast cell stabilizer (plus other mechanisms)	Single agent with multiple actions, has immediate and prophylactic activity, eliminates need for 2-drug therapy, comfort enhances patient compliance	Olopatadine (Patanol), ketotifen (Zaditor), azelastine (Optivar)	Twice daily dosing, dual acting agents, antihistamine, mast cell stabilizer, inhibitor of inflammatory mediators, more effective at relieving symptoms than other classes of agents, longer duration of action, safe and effective for 3 years and older
Topical mast cell stabilizers	Safe and effective for allergic diseases, especially those associated with corneal changes	Cromolyn (Crolom), lodoxamide (Alomide), nedocromil (Alocril), pemirolast (Alamast)	Cromolyn relieves mild-to-moderate symptoms of vernal keratoconjunctivitis, vernal conjunctivitis, vernal keratitis; Lodoxamide is highly potent
Topical antihistamines	Relieves signs and symptoms of pruritus and erythema	Levocabastine (Livostin), emedastine (Emadine)	Dosing 1-4 times daily, safe and effective for 3 years and older
Topical NSAIDs	Relieves pruritus	Ketorolac (Acular)	Stinging and/or burning on instillation experienced by up to 40% of patients
Tertiary			
Topical corticosteroids	Relieves all facets of the inflammatory response including erythema, edema, and pruritus	Loteprednol (Lotemax, Alrex), rimexolone (Vexol), fluorometholone (FML)	Appropriate for short-term use only, contraindicated in patients with viral infections
Immunotherapy	Identify and modulate allergen sensitivity		Adjunctive, although may be considered in secondary treatment in conjunction with allergic rhinitis
Ancillary			
Oral antihistamines	Mildly effective for pruritus	Loratadine, fexofenadine, cetirizine	May cause dry eyes, worsening allergy symptoms, may not effectively resolve the ocular signs and symptoms of allergy

NSAID, Nonsteroidal antiinflammatory drug; *OTC,* over the counter.

receptors. Interestingly, this effect is more pronounced in patients with lighter irides and has not been reported with the newer topical agents. Also related to muscarinic receptor blockade is the risk for angle-closure glaucoma.

Mast Cell Stabilizers

Cromolyn. Cromolyn 4% (Crolom) is the prototypic mast cell stabilizer. The efficacy of the medication appears to be dependent on the concentration of the solution used (i.e.,

a 1% solution with no effect, a 2% solution with a possible effect, and a 4% solution with a probable effect).[38-49] After many years of clinical use the possible mechanisms for cromolyn are still unclear. At first it was thought that the material had an effect on phosphodiesterase or cyclic adenosine monophosphate, and most recently it appears that cromolyn may inhibit B lymphocytes switching from μ (IgM) to ε (IgE) heavy chains, which is a novel potential mechanism for the prevention of disorders mediated by mast cells.[39,40] Sodium cromolyn was originally approved for more severe forms of conjunctivitis (GPC, VKC) but many physicians have used it for the treatment of allergic conjunctivitis with an excellent safety record, although the original studies reflecting its clinical efficacy were marginal for allergic conjunctivitis when compared to placebo[41,42] and in some animal models.[43] Cromolyn sodium 4% ophthalmic solution is applied 4 to 6 times daily with the dosage being decreased incrementally to twice daily as symptoms permit. It is approved for children 3 years and older. The major adverse effect is burning and stinging, which has been reported in 13% to 77% of patients treated.

Lodoxamide. Lodoxamide 0.1% (Alomide) is a mast cell stabilizer that is approximately 2500 times more potent than cromolyn in the prevention of histamine release in several animal models.[44] Lodoxamide is effective in reducing tryptase and histamine levels and the recruitment of inflammatory cells in the tear fluid after allergen challenge[45,46] as well as tear eosinophil cationic protein[47] and leukotrienes (BLT and CysLT$_1$) when compared to cromolyn. In early clinical trials lodoxamide (0.1%) was shown to deliver greater and earlier relief in patients with more chronic forms, such as VKC, including upper tarsal papillae, limbal signs (papillae, hyperemia, and Trantas' dots), and conjunctival discharge, and to improve epithelial defects seen in the chronic forms of conjunctivitis (VKC, GPC) more than cromolyn.[48] Overall, lodoxamide appears to be significantly more effective than placebo[49] and as effective as levocabastine.[50] However, its clinical efficacy vis-à-vis cromolyn remains unclear. In a study of allergic conjunctivitis it was only perceived by the patient to be clinically better than that perceived by the physician. In patients with allergic conjunctivitis, it is approved for the treatment of vernal conjunctivitis at a concentration of 0.1% four times daily. Lodoxamide may be used continuously for 3 months in children aged older than 2 years.

Pemirolast. Pemirolast potassium 0.1% (Alamast) is a novel mast cell stabilizer for the prevention and relief of ocular manifestations of allergic conjunctivitis. It was originally marketed as a tablet formulation in 1991 for the treatment of bronchial asthma and allergic rhinitis and was subsequently developed and registered in Japan as an ophthalmic formulation for the treatment of allergic and vernal conjunctivitis.[51] It has been studied in children as young as 2 years of age, with no reports of serious adverse events. In the rat model the ocular instillation of pemirolast appears to have a potency more than 100 times that of sodium cromolyn, although in some *in vitro* models was found to be equivalent to cromolyn.[52] The usual regimen is 1 to 2 drops four times a day for each eye.

Multiple-Action Agents

Olopatadine. Olopatadine 0.01%, another new agent, possesses antihistaminic activity and minimal mast cell stabilizing effects.[53-55] Olopatadine was approximately ten times more potent as an inhibitor of cytokine secretion (50% inhibitory concentration 1.7 to 5.5 nmol/L) than predicted from binding data whereas antazofine and pheniramine were far less potent (20 to 140 times) in functional assays, including TNF-α mediator release from human conjunctival mast cells.[54-57] It has been shown to be significantly more effective than placebo in relieving itching and redness for up to 8 hours.[55] In a study comparing to another multiple-action

agent, ketotifen, olopatadine fared only slightly better over 2 weeks.[56]

Ketotifen. Ketotifen 0.025% (Zaditor) is a benzocycloheptathiophene that has been shown to display several antimediator properties, including strong H$_1$ receptor antagonism and inhibition of leukotriene formation.[57,58] Ketotifen has been used as an orally active prophylactic agent for the management of bronchial asthma and allergic disorders. Ketotifen has also been shown to have pronounced antihistaminic and antianaphylactic properties that result in moderate to marked symptom improvement in the majority of patients with atopic dermatitis, seasonal or perennial rhinitis, allergic conjunctivitis, chronic or acute urticaria, and food allergy.[59] It has been reported in several studies to have a mild stinging affect on the conjunctival surface. Ketotifen is distinguished from the cromones (sodium cromolyn and nedocromil) by a conjoint antihistamine effect.

Azelastine. Azelastine 0.05% (Optivar) is a second-generation H$_1$ receptor antagonist that was first shown to be clinically effective in relieving the symptoms of allergic rhinitis following oral or intranasal administration.[60,61] In a pediatric SAC study comparing the effects of azelastine with levocabastine eye drops, the response rate of the azelastine eye drop group (74%) was significantly higher than that of the placebo group (39%) and comparable to that of the levocabastine group.[62] Apart from the ability to inhibit histamine release from mast cells and to prevent the activation of inflammatory cells, it is likely that the antiallergic potency of azelastine is partially the result of down-regulation of ICAM-1 expression during the early- and late-phase components of ocular allergic response that probably leads to a reduction of inflammatory cell adhesion to epithelial cells, confirming the prophylactic properties of azelastine.[63] It is safe to use in children 3 years and older.

Nedocromil. Nedocromil 2% (Alocril) is a pyranoquinoline dicarboxylic acid that has potent inhibitory activities on various allergic inflammatory cells, such as mast cells and eosinophils. Nedocromil appears to be able to stabilize mast cells and inhibit histamine release more than cromolyn.[64] Nedocromil has been shown to improve clinical symptoms in the control of ocular pruritus and irritation when compared against placebo in the treatment of SAC.[65-72] Its safety profile is similar to that of sodium cromolyn but is more potent and can be given just twice daily. The results of several placebo-controlled studies have shown that nedocromil is effective in alleviating the signs and symptoms of SAC and provided relief in approximately 80% of patients.[66] In a comparative study, nedocromil sodium eye drops (2%) were more efficacious than sodium cromolyn for hyperaemia, keratitis, papillae, and pannus and took less time to have an effect for itching, grittiness, hyperemia, and keratitis.[67]

Nonsteroidal Antiinflammatory Drugs

Topically applied inhibitors of the cyclooxygenase system (1% suprofen)[68] have been used in the treatment of VKC.[69,70] Ocufen (diclofenac) is one of three topical nonsteroidal antiinflammatory drugs (NSAIDs) approved for the treatment of intraocular inflammatory disorders. Another topically applied NSAID (0.03% flurbiprofen) has been examined in the treatment of allergic conjunctivitis and was found to decrease conjunctival, ciliary, and episcleral hyperemia and ocular pruritus when compared with the control (vehicle-treated eyes). Pruritus is associated with prostaglandin release, as it has been shown that prostaglandins can lower the threshold of human skin to histamine-induced pruritus (itching) that may also be the primary benefit of these medications in the eye.

Ketorolac Tromethamine. Ketorolac tromethamine (Acular, Allergan) was approved in November 1992 for the treatment of allergic conjunctivitis. Ketorolac, a pyrazolon, is an NSAID, with its primary mechanism of action on the arachidonic acid cascade by binding cyclooxygenase to block the production of prostaglandins but does not inhibit lipoxygenase or the formation of leukotrienes. Clinical studies have shown that prostanoids are associated with ocular itching and conjunctival hyperemia and thus inhibitors of this cascade such as topical ketorolac can interfere with ocular itch and hyperemia produced by antigen-induced and SAC.[71-73] NSAIDs (e.g., ketorolac) do not mask ocular infections, affect wound healing, increase IOP, or contribute to cataract formation, unlike topical corticosteroids. Although only ketorolac tromethamine is currently approved by the Food and Drug Administration (FDA) for use in acute SAC, a recent study compared diclofenac sodium with ketorolac tromethamine, with the results for both agents being similar.[71] Treatment group differences were observed for the pain/soreness score with an advantage observed for the diclofenac sodium group over ketorolac tromethamine (20.7% versus 3.2%).

NSAIDs of the indole (indomethacin, sulindac, tolmetin), pyrazolon (phenylbutazone, oxyphenabutazone, apazone), propionic acid (ibuprofen, flurbiprofen, ketaprofen, naproxen), and fenamate derivatives have been developed for topical treatment of inflammatory conditions of the eye but have been associated with a low-to-moderate incidence of burning and stinging.

Tertiary Intervention

Topical Corticosteroids

When topically administered medications such as antihistamines, vasoconstrictors, cromolyn sodium, and other multiple-action agents are ineffective, milder topical steroids are a consideration. Topical corticosteroids are highly effective in the treatment of acute and chronic forms of allergic conjunctivitis and are even required for control of some of the more severe variants of conjunctivitis including vernal conjunctivitis and GPC. However, the local administrations of these medications are not without possible localized ocular complications including increased IOP (e.g., in glaucoma), viral infections, and cataract formation. Topically or systemically administered steroids will produce a transient rise in IOP in susceptible individuals; this trait is thought to be genetically influenced.[72-75] Unlike efficacy, which varies among the steroid esters, IOP effects are consistent among the different esters of the same corticosteroid base.

Loteprednol. Loteprednol 0.2% (Alrex) is an ophthalmic suspension approved for the treatment of ocular allergy. Its more potent partner, loteprednol 0.5% (Lotemax), is approved to treat more advanced ocular and postoperative inflammatory conditions. Alrex is the first topical corticosteroid to be FDA approved for the treatment of ocular allergy. One of its unique features is its claim to be a site-specific steroid (i.e., the active drug resides at the target tissue long enough to render a therapeutic effect but rarely long enough to cause secondary effects such as increased IOP and posterior subcapsular cataract development). The 0.5% loteprednol formulation has been shown to be effective in reducing the signs and symptoms of GPC, acute anterior uveitis, and inflammation following cataract extraction with intraocular lens implantation.[72] It has also been shown to be effective as prophylactic treatment for the ocular signs and symptoms of SAC. In using this intervention beginning before the onset of the allergy season and continuing for 6 weeks, the majority of patients (94%) never develop any symptoms and none of them had an IOP increase of at least 10 mm Hg.[73] In another placebo-controlled study of loteprednol (0.2%) versus placebo, a reduction in severity was seen in both loteprednol and placebo groups for bulbar conjunctival injection and itching over the first 2 weeks. However, clinical resolution (the proportion of patients with the sign or symptom no longer present) at visit 4 (day 14) strongly favored loteprednol-treated patients over placebo-treated patients.[74] In a study of patients with GPC associated with contact lens use, the proportion of patients treated with loteprednol (78%) demonstrated an improvement in papillae.[75] Although in this study 7% of patients taking loteprednol had an IOP increase of at least 10 mm Hg on at least one visit during the study, after discontinuation of loteprednol, IOP returned to normal levels.

It is recommended that only patients with more chronic forms of allergic conjunctivitis use topical steroids in a routine manner. Ophthalmologic consultation should be obtained for any patient using ocular steroids for more than 2 weeks to assess cataract formation or increased IOP. Consultation is also merited for any persistent ocular complaint or if the use of strong topical steroids or systemic steroids is being considered.

Immunotherapy

The efficacy of allergen immunotherapy is well established, although it appears that allergic rhinitis may respond better to treatment than allergic conjunctivitis.[76] The very first report of the use of immunotherapy in 1911 measured the patient's resistance during experiments of pollen extracts to excite a conjunctival reaction.[77] However, one must consider that at present, studies have focused primarily on nasal symptoms and rarely use ocular provocation as a primary end point. In one pediatric study specifically evaluating the alterations made by bronchial and ocular challenge tests in patients being desensitized to a specific mold allergen, cladosporium, the results revealed that fewer medications were used and higher doses of topically applied allergen were required to induce allergic symptoms of redness, pruritus, and swelling.[78] Similarly, allergic patients who had asthma and rhinoconjunctivitis when exposed to animal dander (Fel d-I allergen), immunotherapy clearly improved the overall symptoms of rhinoconjunctivitis, decreased the use of allergy medications, and required a tenfold increase in the dose of allergen to induce a positive OCT reaction after 1 year of immunotherapy with the specific cat allergen.[79] Symptom assessment postchallenge for ragweed-sensitive patients treated for at least 2 years with specific ragweed immunotherapy revealed that nasal symptoms responded more than ocular symptoms when compared with controls.[80] The effect of immunotherapy specific for Japanese cedar (*Cryptomeria japonica*) pollinosis had reduced the daily total symptom medication score not only in cedar but also in the cross-allergenic Japanese cypress (*Chamaecyparis obtusa*) pollination season but not significantly.[81] Thus immunotherapy plays more of an important role in the "long-term" control of rhinoconjunctivitis.

New Directions and Future Developments

Novel treatments of ocular allergy include medications that are commonly used in organ transplantation such as cyclosporine and tacrolimus. Cyclosporine is a fungal antimetabolite that has known antiinflammatory properties. It acts on IL-l, which has an immunomodulatory effect on the activation of T lymphocytes. Recent studies and reports on the use of topical cyclosporine in cases of VKC have demonstrated marked and lasting improvement in symptoms.[82] Tacrolimus is a macrolide antibiotic that acts primarily on T lymphocytes by inhibiting the production of lymphokines, particularly IL-2. It has been effective in the treatment of immune-mediated ocular diseases such as corneal graft rejection, keratitis, scleritis, ocular pemphigoid, and uveitis. The drug is approximately 100 times as potent as cyclosporine. Both tacrolimus and cyclosporine have been shown *in vitro* to inhibit histamine release.[83]

Alternative delivery systems for the topical agents are also under investigation. A liposomal drug delivery system is currently being developed that provides increased therapeutic activity with decreased toxicity. Liposome-encased compounds have been shown to have a greater penetrating effect into the cornea, aqueous humor, vitreous humor, and conjunctiva. Immunization approaches using "naked plasmid" DNA (pDNA) are being pursued as well. This approach induces an altered antiallergic immune state in which there is a preference for the T helper cell type 1 response, producing

primarily IgG2a whereas allergens would normally induce IgG1 and IgE responses.[84,85] Additional areas of future research include cytokine antagonists and anti-IgE therapy.[86]

CONCLUSIONS

Ocular allergies in children encompass a spectrum of clinical disorders. A basic understanding of the eye's immune response coupled with a stepwise diagnostic approach facilitates proper diagnosis and treatment (Boxes 56-1 and 56-2). As we develop a greater understanding of the biomolecular mechanisms of these disease states, treatment will progress from symptomatic relief to more directed therapeutic interventions.

REFERENCES

1. Ray NF, Baraniuk JN, Thamer M, et al: Direct expenditures for the treatment of allergic rhinoconjunctivitis in 1996, including the contributions of related airway illnesses, *J Allergy Clin Immunol* 103:401-407, 1999.
2. Marrache F, Brunet D, Frandeboeuf J, et al: The role of ocular manifestations in childhood allergy syndromes, *Rev Fr Allergrol Immunol Clin* 18:151-155, 1978.
3. Bielory L: Allergic disorders of the eye. In Rich R, ed: *Principles and practices of clinical immunology*, St Louis, 1996, Mosby.
4. Freidlaender MH: Immunologic aspects of disease of the eye. Chapter 10 in primer on allergic and immunologic diseases, *JAMA* 258:2916-2919, 1987.
5. Bielory L: Allergic and immunological disorders of the eye. Part I: Immunology of the eye, *J Allergy Clin Immunol* 106:805-816, 2000.
6. Isaacson P, Wright DH: Extranodal malignant lymphoma arising from mucosa-associated lymphoid tissue, *Cancer* 53:2515-2524, 1984.
7. Irani AA, Butrus SI, Tabbara KF, et al: Human conjunctival mast cells: distribution of MC$_T$ and MC$_{TC}$ in vernal conjunctivitis and giant papillary conjunctivitis, *J Allergy Clin Immunol* 86:34-40, 1990.
8. Irani AA: Ocular mast cells and mediators. In Bielory L, ed: *Ocular allergy, immunology and Allergy Clinics of North America*, Philadelphia, 1997, WB Saunders.
9. Gillette TE, Chandler JW, Geiner JV: Langerhans' cells of the ocular surface, *Ophthalmology* 89:700-711, 1982.
10. Friedlaender MH: Current concepts in ocular allergy, *Ann Allergy* 67:5-13, 1991.
11. Allansmith MR: Immunology of the external ocular tissues, *J Am Optom Assoc* 61:16-22, 1990.
12. Dart JK, Buckley RJ, Monnickendan M, et al: Perennial allergic conjunctivitis: definition, clinical characteristics and prevalence: a comparison with seasonal allergic conjunctivitis, *Trans Ophthalmol Soc UK* 105:513-520, 1986.

13. Trocme SD, Gleich GJ, Zeiske JD: Eosinophil granule major basic protein inhibits corneal epithelial wound healing *in vitro* (abstract), *Invest Ophthalmol Vis Sci* 32:1161, 1991.

14. Trocme SD, Kephart GM, Allansmith, MR, et al: Conjunctival deposition of eosinophil granule major basic protein in vernal keratoconjunctivitis and contact lens associated giant papillary conjunctivitis, *Am J Ophthalmol* 108:57-63, 1989.

15. Irani AM, Butrus SI, Tabbara KF, et al: Human conjunctival mast cells: distribution of MC_T and MC_{TC} in vernal conjunctivitis and giant papillary conjunctivitis, *J Allergy Clin Immunol* 86:34-40, 1990.

16. Abelson MB, Baird RS, Allansmith MR: Tear histamine levels in vernal conjunctivitis and other ocular inflammations, *Ophthalmology* 87:812-814, 1980.

17. Udell IJ, Gleich GJ, Allansmith MR, et al: Eosinophilic major basic protein and Charcot-Leyden crystal protein in human tears, *Am J Ophthalmol* 92:824-828, 1981.

18. Tripathi PC, Tripathi RC: Analysis of glycoprotein deposits on disposable contact lenses, *Invest Ophthalmol Vis Sci* 33:121-125, 1992.

19. Dreborg S, Agrell B, Foucard T, et al: A double-blind, multicenter immunotherapy trial in children, using a purified and standardized *Cladosporium herbarum* preparation. I. Clinical results, *Allergy* 41:131-140, 1986.

20. Bligard CA: Kawasaki disease and its diagnosis, *Pediatr Dermatol* 4:75-84, 1987.

21. Rosenbaum JT: An algorithm for the systemic evaluation of patients with uveitis: guidelines for the consultant, *Semin Arthritis Rheum* 19:248-257, 1990.

22. Weiner A, Ben Ezra D: Clinical patterns and associated conditions in chronic uveitis, *Am J Ophthalmol* 112:151-158, 1991.

23. Dougherty JM, McCulley JP: Tear measurements in chronic blepharitis, *Ann Ophthalmol* 17:53-57, 1985.

24. Hogan DJ, Schachner L, Tanglertsampan C: Diagnosis and treatment of childhood scabies and pediculosis, *Pediatr Clin North Am* 36:941-957, 1991.

25. Berstein DI, Gallagher JS, Grad M, et al: Local ocular anaphylaxis to papain enzyme contained in a contact lens cleaning solution, *J Allergy Clin Immunol* 74:258-260, 1984.

26. Boder E, Sedgwick R: Ataxia-telangiectasia: a familial syndrome of progressive cerebellar ataxia, oculocutaneous telangiectasia and frequent pulmonary infection, *Pediatrics* 21:526-554, 1958.

27. Harley RD, Baird HW, Craven EM: Ataxia-telangiectasia: report of seven cases, *Arch Ophthalmol* 77:582-592, 1967.

28. Ciprandi G, Buscaglia S, Cerqueti PM, et al: Drug treatment of allergic conjunctivitis: a review of the evidence, *Drugs* 43:154-176, 1992.

29. Abelson MB, Paradis A, George MA, et al: Effects of Vasocon-A in the allergen challenge model of acute allergic conjunctivitis, *Arch Ophthalmol* 108:520-524, 1990.

30. Abelson ME, Udell IJ: H_2-receptors in the human ocular surface, *Arch Ophthalmol* 99:302-304, 1981.

31. Jaanus SD: Oral and topical antihistamines: pharmacologic properties and therapeutic potential in ocular allergic disease, *J Am Optom Assoc* 69:77-87, 1998.

32. Sharif NA, Wiernas TK, Griffin EW, et al: Pharmacology of [3H] pyrilamine binding and of the histamine induced inositol phosphates generation, intracellular Ca^{2+}-mobilization and cytokine release from human corneal epithelial cells, *Br J Pharmacol* 125:1336-1344, 1998.

33. Yanni JM, Sharif NA, Gamache DA, et al: A current appreciation of sites for pharmacological intervention in allergic conjunctivitis: effects of new topical ocular drugs, *Acta Ophthalmol Scand Suppl* 228:33-37, 1999.

34. Bielory L: The role of antihistamines in ocular allergy, *Am J Med* 113:34S-37S, 2002.

35. Kjellman NI, Andersson B: Terfenadine reduces skin and conjunctival reactivity in grass pollen allergic children, *Clin Allergy* 16:441-449, 1986.

36. Ciprandi G, Euscaglia S, Pesce GP, et al: Protective effect of loratadine on specific conjunctival provocation test, *Int Arch Allergy Appl Immunol* 96:344-347, 1991.

37. Hingorani M, Lightman S: Therapeutic options in ocular allergic disease, *Drugs* 50:208-221, 1995.

38. Azevedo M, Castel-Branco MG, Oliveira JF, et al: Double-blind comparison of levocabastine eye drops with sodium cromoglycate and placebo in the treatment of seasonal allergic conjunctivitis, *Clin Exp Allergy* 21:689-694, 1991.

39. Kimata H, Yoshida A, Ishioka C, et al: Disodium cromoglycate (DSCG) selectively inhibits IgE production and enhances IgG4 production by human B cell *in vitro*, *Clin Exp Immunol* 84:395-399, 1991.

40. Loh RK, Jabara HH, Geha RS: Disodium cromoglycate inhibits S mu--> S epsilon deletional switch recombination and IgE synthesis in human B cells, *J Exp Med* 180:663-671, 1994.

41. Friday GA, Biglan AW, Hiles DA, et al: Treatment of ragweed allergic conjunctivitis with cromolyn sodium 4% ophthalmic solution, *Am J Ophthalmol* 95:169-174, 1983.

42. Sorkin EM, Ward A: Ocular sodium cromoglycate: an overview of its therapeutic efficacy in allergic eye disease, *Drugs* 31:131-148, 1986.

43. Kamei C, Izushi K, Tasaka K: Inhibitory effect of levocabastine on experimental allergic conjunctivitis in guinea pigs, *J Pharmacobiodyn* 14:467-473, 1991.

44. Johnson HG, White GJ: Development of new antiallergic drugs (cromolyn sodium, lodoxamide tromethamine): What is the role of cholinergic stimulation in the biphasic dose response? *Monogr Allergy* 14:299-306, 1979.

45. Leonardi AA, Smith LM, Fregona IA, et al: Tear histamine and histaminase during the early (EPR) and late (LPR) phases of the allergic reaction and the effects of lodoxamide, *Eur J Ophthalmol* 6:106-112, 1996.

46. Bonini S, Schiavone M, Bonini S, et al: Efficacy of lodoxamide eye drops on mast cells and eosinophils after allergen challenge in allergic conjunctivitis, *Ophthalmology* 104:849-853, 1997.

47. Leonardia A, Borghesan F, Avarello A, et al: Effect of lodoxamide and disodium cromoglycate on tear eosinophil cationic protein in vernal keratoconjunctivitis, *Br J Ophthalmol* 81:23-26, 1997.

48. Santos CI, Huang AJ, Abelson MB, et al: Efficacy of lodoxarnide 0.1% ophthalmic solution in resolving corneal epitheliopathy associated with vernal keratoconjunctivitis, *Am J Ophthalmol* 117:488-497, 1994.

49. Cerqueti PM, Ricca V, Tosca MA, et al: Lodoxamide treatment of allergic conjunctivitis, *Int Arch Allergy Immunol* 105:185-189, 1994.

50. Richard C, Trinquand C, Bloch-Michel E: Comparison of topical 0.05% levocabastine and 0.1% lodoxamide in patients with allergic conjunctivitis. Study Group, *Eur J Ophthalmol* 8:207-216, 1998.

51. Nakagawa Y, IIkuhara Y, Higasida M, et al: Suppression of conjunctival provocation by 0.1 % pemirolast potassium ophthalmic solution in VKC, *Areruga* 43:1405-1408, 1994.

52. Yanni JM, Miller ST; Gamache DA, et al: Comparative effects of topical ocular antiallergy drugs on human conjunctival mast cells, *Ann Allergy Asthma Immunol* 79:541-545, 1997.

53. Sharif NA. Xu SX. Miller ST, et al: Characterization of the ocular antiallergic and antihistaminic effects of olopatadine (AL-4943A), a novel drug for treating ocular allergic diseases, *J Pharmacol Exp Ther* 278:1252-1261, 1996.

54. Yanni JM, Stephens DJ, Miller ST, et al: The in vitro and in vivo ocular pharmacology of olopatadine (AL-4943A), an effective anti-allergic/antihistaminic agent, *J Ocul Pharmacol Ther* 12:389-400, 1996.

55. Abelson MB, Spitalny L: Combined analysis of two studies using the conjunctival allergen challenge model to evaluate olopatadine hydrochloride, a new ophthalmic antiallergic agent with dual activity, *Am J Ophthalmol* 125:797-804, 1998.

56. Aguilar A: Comparative study of clinical efficacy and tolerance in seasonal allergic conjunctivitis management with 0.1% olopatadine hydrochloride versus 0.05% kerotifen fumarate, *Acta Ophthalmol Scand* 78:52-55, 2000.

57. Tomioka H, Yoshida S, Tanaka M, et al: Inhibition of chemical mediator release from human leukocytes by a new antiasthma drug, HC 20-511 (ketotifen), *Monogr Allergy* 14:313-317, 1979.

58. Nishimura N, Ito K, Tomioka H, et al: Inhibition of chemical mediator release from human leukocytes and lung *in vitro* by a novel antiallergic agent, KB-2413, *Immunopharmacol Immunotoxicol* 9:511-521, 1987.

59. Grant SM, Goa KL, Fitton A, et al: Ketotifen: a review of its pharmacodynamic and pharmacokinetic properties, and therapeutic use in asthma and allergic disorders, *Drugs* 40:412-448, 1990.

60. McTavish D, Sorkin EM: Azelastine: a review of its pharmacodynamic and pharmacokinetic properties, and therapeutic potential, *Drugs* 38:778-800, 1989.

61. McNeelyW, Wiseman LR: Intranasal azelastine: a review of its efficacy in the management of allergic rhinitis, *Drugs* 56:91-114, 1998.

62. Sabbah A, Marzetto M: Azelastine eye drops in the treatment of seasonal allergic conjunctivitis or rhinoconjunctivitis in young children, *Curr Med Res Opin* 14:161-170, 1998.

63. Ciprandi G, Buscaglia S, Pesce G, et al: Allergic subjects express intercellular adhesion molecule-1 (ICAM-1 or CD54) on epithelial cells of conjunctiva after allergen challenge, *J Allergy Clin Immunol* 91:783-792, 1993.

64. Gonzalez JP, Brogden RN: Nedocromil sodium: a preliminary review of its pharmacodynamic and pharmacokinetic properties, and therapeutic efficacy in the treatment of reversible obstructive airways disease, *Drugs* 34:560-577, 1987.

65. Leino M, Carlson C, Latvala AL, et al: Double-blind group comparative study of 2% nedocromil sodium eye drops with placebo eye drops in the treatment of seasonal allergic conjunctivitis, *Ann Allergy* 64:398-402, 1990.

66. Verin P: Treating severe eye allergy, *Clin Exp Allergy* 28:44-48, 1998.

67. Verin PH, Dicker ID, Mortemousque B: Nedocromil sodium eye drops are more effective than sodium cromoglycate eye drops for the long-term management of vernal keratoconjunctivitis, *Clin Exp Allergy* 29:529-536, 1999.

68. Wood TS, Stewart RH, Bowman RW, et al: Suprofen treatment of contact lens associated giant papillary conjunctivitis, *Ophthalmology* 95:822-826, 1988.

69. Abelson MB, Butrus SI, Weston JH: Aspirin therapy in vernal conjunctivitis, *Am J Ophthalmol* 95:502-505, 1983.

70. Meyer E, Kraus E, Zonis S: Efficacy of antiprostaglandin therapy in vernal conjunctivitis, *Br J Ophthalmol* 71:497-499, 1987.

71. Tauber J, Raizman MB, Ostrov CS, et al: A multicenter comparison of the ocular efficacy and safety of diclofenac 0.1 % solution with that of ketorolac 0.5% solution in patients with acute seasonal allergic conjunctivitis, *J Ocul Pharmacol Ther* 14:137-145, 1998.

72. Howes JF: Loteprednol etabonate: a review of ophthalmic clinical studies, *Pharmazie* 55:178-183, 2000.

73. Dell SJ, Shulman DG, Lowry GM, et al: A controlled evaluation of the efficacy and safety of loteprednol etabonate in the prophylactic treatment of seasonal allergic conjunctivitis. Loteprednol Allergic Conjunctivitis Study Group, *Am J Ophthalmol* 123:791-797, 1997.

74. Dell SJ, Lowry GM, Northcutt JA, et al: A randomized, double-masked, placebo-controlled parallel study of 2% loteprednol etabonate in patients with seasonal allergic conjunctivitis, *J Allergy Clin Immunol* 102:251-255, 1998.

75. Friedlaender MH, Howes J: A double-masked, placebo-controlled evaluation of the efficacy and safety of loteprednol etabonate in the treatment of giant papillary conjunctivitis. The Loteprednol Etabonate Giant Papillary Conjunctivitis Study Group I, *Am J Ophthalmol* 123:455-464, 1997.

76. Bielory L, Mongia A: Current immunotherapy treatment of ocular allergy, *Curr Opin Allergy Immunol* 2:447-452, 2002.

77. Noon L, Cantab B: Prophylactic inoculation against hay fever, *Lancet* 1572-1573, 1911.

78. Dreborg S, Agrell B, Foucard T, et al: A double-blind, multicenter immunotherapy trial in children, using a purified and standardized Cladosporium herbarum preparation. I. Clinical results, *Allergy* 41:131-140, 1986.

79. Alvarez-Cuesta E, Cuesta-Herranz J, Puyana-Ruiz J, et al: Monoclonal antibody standardized cat extract immunotherapy: risk-benefit effects from a double-blind placebo study, *J Allergy Clin Immunol* 93:556-566, 1994.

80. Donovan JP, Buckeridge DL, Briscoe MP, et al: Efficacy of immunotherapy to ragweed antigen tested by controlled antigen exposure, *Ann Allergy Asthma Immunol* 77:74-80, 1996.

81. Ito Y, Takahashi Y, Fujita T, et al: Clinical effects of immunotherapy on Japanese cedar pollinosis in the season of cedar and cypress pollination, *Auris Nasus Larynx* 24:163-170, 1997.

82. Mendicute], Aranzasti C, Eder F, et al: Topical cyclosporine A 2% in the treatment of vernal keratoconjunctivitis, *Eye* 11:75-78, 1997.

83. Sperr WR, Agis H, Semper H, et al: Inhibition of allergen induced histamine release from human basophils by cyclosporine A and FK-506, *Int Arch Allergy Immunol* 114:68-73, 1997.

84. Spiegelberg HL, Orozco EM, Roman M, et al: DNA immunization: a novel approach to allergen-specific immunotherapy, *Allergy* 52:964-970, 1997.

85. Beck L, Spiegelberg HL: The polyclonal and antigen-specific IgE and IgG subclass response of mice injected with ovalbumin in alum or complete Freund's adjuvant, *Cell Immunol* 123:1-8, 1989.

86. Bielory L: Allergic and immunologic disorders of the eye. Part II: Ocular allergy, *J Allergy Clin Immunol* 106:1019-1032, 2000.

DRUG ALLERGY AND ANAPHYLAXIS

DONALD Y.M. LEUNG

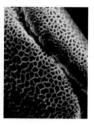

CHAPTER 57

Drug Allergy

ROLAND SOLENSKY ■ LOUIS M. MENDELSON

The clinician is frequently confronted with patients who have histories of various medication allergies. In the pediatric population, antibiotics are by far the most commonly implicated medications in allergic reactions. This chapter will concentrate on the clinical management of pediatric patients who present with a history of drug allergy, and basic science will only be included as it relates to diagnosis and treatment. Because of space limitations, the entire wide spectrum of all drug hypersensitivity disorders is unable to be addressed (Table 57-1). Instead, our discussion will focus on the most clinically relevant reactions—to antibiotics, aspirin (ASA) and other nonsteroidal antiinflammatory drugs (NSAIDs), and local anesthetics.

ETIOLOGY/EPIDEMIOLOGY

Patients and physicians commonly refer to all adverse drug reactions (ADRs) as being "allergic," but the term drug allergy, or drug hypersensitivity, should be applied only to those reactions that are known (or presumed) to be mediated by an immunologic mechanism. ADRs are broadly divided into predictable and unpredictable reactions (Table 57-2). The majority of ADRs are predictable in nature, and examples of these reactions include medication side effects (such as β-agonist–associated tremor) and drug-drug interactions (such as cardiac arrhythmia from the combination of terfenadine and erythromycin). Allergic reactions are a type of unpredictable reaction and they are thought to account for less than 10% of all ADRs.[1]

The overall incidence of allergic drug reactions is difficult to estimate accurately due to the wide spectrum of disorders they encompass and a lack of accurate diagnostic tests. There are limited epidemiological data for specific types of hypersensitivity disorders in pediatric patients. For example, the incidence of anaphylaxis in children and adolescents who received intramuscular injections of penicillin G was 1.23[2] and 2.17[3] per 10,000 injections. In a large pediatric practice, 7.3%

of children developed cutaneous eruptions due to oral antibiotics (although no testing or challenges were performed to confirm an allergy).[4]

While true drug allergy is relatively uncommon, many more children are labeled as being "allergic" to various medications, particularly antibiotics, and end up carrying the label into adulthood. These patients are frequently treated with alternate medications that may be more toxic, less effective, or more expensive. Hence, an important and often underappreciated aspect of drug allergy is the morbidity, mortality and economic cost associated with the unnecessary withholding of indicated therapy.

Risk factors for the development of drug allergy are poorly understood and most of the limited data come from studies on penicillin allergy in adult subjects. The presence of atopy is not a risk factor for drug allergy,[5] although patients with asthma may be more prone to having severe reactions (as is the case with food allergies[6]). The parental route of administration and repeated courses of the same or cross-reacting antibiotic appear to favor the development of immediate-type drug allergy.[7] Genetic susceptibility has been described for several types of drug allergy.[8,9] Patients with "multiple drug allergy syndrome" may have an inherent predilection to develop hypersensitivity reactions to more than one non−cross-reacting medication,[10,11] but the existence of this condition is controversial.[12]

There is no single classification scheme that is able to account for all allergic drug reactions. The widely used Gell and Coombs classification scheme of type I to type IV hypersensitivity reactions can be applied to some drug-induced allergic reactions (Table 57-3). Certain reactions cannot be categorized into any classification scheme despite the fact that we have insight into their underlying mechanism. In other instances, reactions cannot be classified because the mechanism responsible for their elicitation is not understood.

Most medications, due to their relatively small size, are unable to elicit an immune response independently. Drugs must

TABLE 57-1 Partial List of Pediatric Drug Hypersensitivity Disorders

Multisystem
Anaphylaxis
Serum-sickness and serum sickness–like reactions
Drug fever
Hypersensitivity syndrome
Vasculitis
Lupus erythematosus–like syndrome
Generalized lymphadenopathy

Skin
Urticaria/angioedema
Stevens-Johnson syndrome
Toxic epidermal necrolysis
Fixed drug eruption
Maculopapular or morbilliform rashes
Contact dermatitis
Photosensitivity
Erythema nodosum

Bone marrow
Hemolytic anemia
Thrombocytopenia
Neutropenia
Aplastic anemia
Eosinophilia

Lung
Bronchospasm
Pneumonitis
Pulmonary edema
Pulmonary infiltrates with eosinophilia

Kidney
Interstitial nephritis
Nephrotic syndrome

Liver
Hepatitis
Cholestasis

Heart
Myocarditis

TABLE 57-3 Gell and Coombs Classification Scheme for Allergic Reactions

Type	Mechanism	Example
Type I	IgE antibodies leading to mast cell/basophil degranulation	Penicillin—anaphylaxis
Type II	IgG/IgM-mediated cytotoxic reaction against cell surface	Quinidine—hemolytic anemia
Type III	Immune complex deposition reaction	Cephalexin—serum sickness
Type IV	Delayed T cell–mediated reaction	Neomycin—contact dermatitis

undergo spontaneous degradation) to reactive intermediates in order to bind to proteins. Frequently, the identity of the intermediates is not known, making it impossible to develop accurate diagnostic tests for drug allergy.

DIAGNOSTIC TESTS

This section will familiarize the reader with the available diagnostic tests for antibiotic allergy. A full discussion of how to apply these tests in clinical situations follows in the Evaluation and Management section. ASA/NSAIDs and local anesthetics, which are diagnosed by provocative challenges rather than testing, are discussed only in the section on Evaluation and Management.

Penicillins

The immunochemistry of penicillin, as it relates to IgE-mediated reactions, was elucidated in the 1960s,[13-15] allowing for the development of validated diagnostic skin test reagents. Under physiologic conditions, 95% of penicillin spontaneously degrades to penicilloyl—also called the major antigenic determinant (Figure 57-1). The remaining portion of penicillin degrades mainly to penicilloate and penilloate, which, along with penicillin, are called the minor antigenic determinants (see Figure 57-1). Penicilloyl is commercially available for skin testing as Pre-Pen (Hollister-Stier), as is aqueous penicillin G. Penicilloate and penilloate, which are often produced in a mixture (minor determinant mixture [MDM]), are not commercially available in the United States. Nevertheless, many allergists have access to MDM,[16] presumably from local medical centers.

Penicillin skin testing is particularly useful because of its high negative predictive value. In large series that used both major and minor determinants, only 1% to 3% of skin test-negative patients experienced mild, self-limited reactions.[5,17,18] Penicillin-induced anaphylaxis has never been reported in a skin test-negative individual challenged with the medication.[19] Skin testing with Pre-Pen and penicillin G alone (without MDM) fails to detect about 10% to 20% of truly allergic patients.[5,17] Since about 10% of patients who report a penicillin allergy are truly allergic, omitting MDM from skin testing misses about 1% to 2% (10% to 20% of 10%) of "all comers" who are labeled penicillin allergic.

first covalently bind to larger carrier molecules such as tissue or serum proteins to act as complete multivalent antigens. This process is called haptenation and the drugs act as haptens. The elicited immune response may be humoral (with the production of specific antibodies), cellular (with the generation of specific T cells), or both. Most drugs are not reactive in their native state and must be enzymatically metabolized (or

TABLE 57-2 Classification of Adverse Drug Reactions

Predictable reactions occur in otherwise normal patients, are generally dose-dependent, and are related to the known pharmacologic actions of the drug. Unpredictable reactions occur only in susceptible individuals, are dose-independent, and are not related to the pharmacologic actions of the drug.

Reactions	Example
Predictable	
Overdosage	Acetaminophen—hepatic necrosis
Side effect	Albuterol—tremor
Secondary effect	Clindamycin—*Clostridium difficile* pseudomembranous colitis
Drug-drug interaction	Terfenadine/erythromycin—torsade de pointes arrhythmia
Unpredictable	
Intolerance	Aspirin—tinnitus (at usual dose)
Idiosyncratic	Chloroquine—hemolytic anemia in G6PD-deficient patient
Allergic	Penicillin—anaphylaxis
Pseudoallergic	Radiocontrast material—anaphylactoid reaction

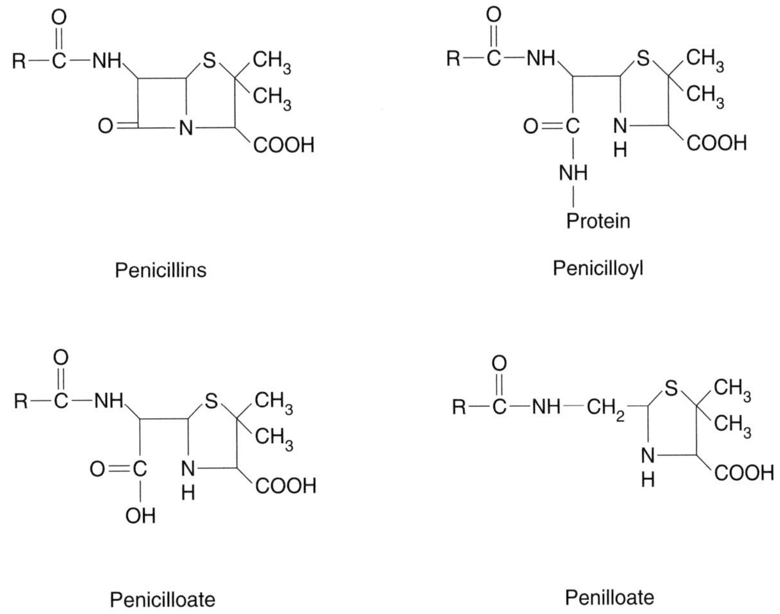

FIGURE 57-1 Structures of major and minor penicillin antigenic determinants. The R-group side chain determines the specific penicillin.

In the last decade a subset of patients who are able to tolerate penicillin but develop allergic reactions to particular semi-synthetic penicillins has been recognized. These individuals do not mount an immune response to the core beta-lactam portion of the molecule, but rather form IgE antibodies directed against particular R group side chains (see Figure 57-1).[20] Skin testing with major and minor penicillin determinants is negative, whereas nonirritating concentrations of the culprit semisynthetic penicillin produce a positive response. For amoxicillin and ampicillin, concentrations up to 25 mg/ml have been reported to be nonirritating for intradermal testing.[20,21] While the predictive value of such testing is not well established, a positive response is suggestive of an immediate-type allergy. Hence, for patients who reacted to a semi-synthetic penicillin, skin testing should be performed with the specific antibiotic in addition to the major and minor deter-minants. Table 57-4 summarizes the commonly used penicillin skin test reagents.

Immediate-type penicillin skin testing should be performed only by experienced personnel in a setting prepared to treat possible allergic reactions. Epicutaneous testing should precede intradermal tests, and appropriate positive (histamine) and negative (normal saline) controls should be used. When carried out in this manner, penicillin skin testing is safe.[5,17,18] A positive response to both prick and intradermal testing is defined by the diameter of the wheal, which should be 3 mm or greater than that of the negative control.[22]

There are no validated tests for penicillin-induced delayed maculopapular eruptions. Delayed intradermal skin tests and patch tests have been found to be positive in some patients by European investigators,[23,24] but these findings have not been reproduced in the United States[25] (and authors' unpublished observations in 50 patients).

Non-penicillin Antibiotics

Unfortunately, for antibiotics other than penicillin, we lack insight into the relevant allergenic determinants that are produced by metabolism or degradation. As a result, there is no available validated skin testing for these antibiotics. Skin testing with the native antibiotic can be helpful, since a positive response using a concentration that is known to be nonirritating strongly suggests the presence of drug-specific IgE antibodies.[22] A negative response, however, does not rule out an allergy. To determine a nonirritating concentration for a given antibiotic, one can refer to previous reports or skin test several nonallergic volunteers. A helpful reference is a recent report of nonirritating concentrations of 17 commonly used antibiotics, as determined in 25 healthy subjects (Table 57-5).[26] The skin testing procedure, precautions, and interpretation for non-penicillins are identical to those outlined for penicillin earlier.

TABLE 57-4 Commonly Used Penicillin Skin Testing Reagents

Reagent	Concentration	Comment
Penicilloyl-polylysine	6×10^{-5} M	Commercially available as Pre-Pen
Penicillin G	10,000 units/ml	Commercially available
Penicilloate/penilloate	0.01 M	Not commercially available in United States, requires synthesis
Ampicillin (intravenous)	1-25 mg/ml	Commercially available
Amoxicillin (intravenous)	1-25 mg/ml	Not commercially available in the United States, requires synthesis

TABLE 57-5 Nonirritating Concentrations of Commonly Used Antibiotics*

Antibiotic	Full-Strength Concentration (mg/ml)	Nonirritating Concentration (Dilution from Full Strength)
Cefotaxime	100	Tenfold
Cefuroxime	100	Tenfold
Cefazolin	330	Tenfold
Ceftazidime	100	Tenfold
Ceftriaxone	100	Tenfold
Tobramycin	40	Tenfold
Ticarcillin	200	Tenfold
Clindamycin	150	Tenfold
Trimethoprim-sulfa	80 (sulfa component)	100-fold
Gentamycin	40	100-fold
Aztreonam	50	1000-fold
Levofloxacin	25	1000-fold
Erythromycin	50	1000-fold
Nafcillin	250	10,000-fold
Vancomycin	50	10,000-fold
Azithromycin	100	10,000-fold
Ciprofloxacin	10	10,000,000-fold

Data from Empedrad RB, Earl HS, Gruchalla RS: *J Allergy Clin Immunol* 105:S272, 2000.

*Skin testing was performed intradermally with intravenous formulations of the antibiotics.

EVALUATION AND MANAGEMENT

Penicillins

Patient history is known to be an unreliable predictor of allergy,[27] and thus one cannot rely on it to rule out the presence of penicillin allergy. The ideal time to perform skin testing for evaluation of penicillin allergy in children is when they are well and not in immediate need of the antibiotic.[22] Testing in acute situations when children are sick is generally difficult if not impossible to accomplish. Up to 10% of patients are labeled penicillin allergic, but about 90% of them lack penicillin-specific IgE and could receive β-lactams safely.[28] These children are commonly denied access not only to penicillins but also other β-lactams, which leaves the clinician with few acceptable antibiotic choices. Usually, once a label of penicillin allergy is made, it is carried indefinitely into adulthood. Patients with a history of penicillin allergy are frequently treated with broad-spectrum antibiotics,[29,30] the use of which contributes to the development of multiple-drug–resistant bacteria.[31,32] It is known that more judicious use of broad-spectrum antibiotics can help reduce the spread of antibiotic resistance.[32,33] One way to achieve this goal is to identify, via "elective" skin testing, the numerous children and adolescents who are mistakenly labeled as "penicillin allergic."

If penicillin skin testing is positive, penicillins should be avoided and alternate antibiotics should be used (Figure 57-2). If the patient develops an absolute need for penicillin, rapid desensitization can be performed (see section on treat-

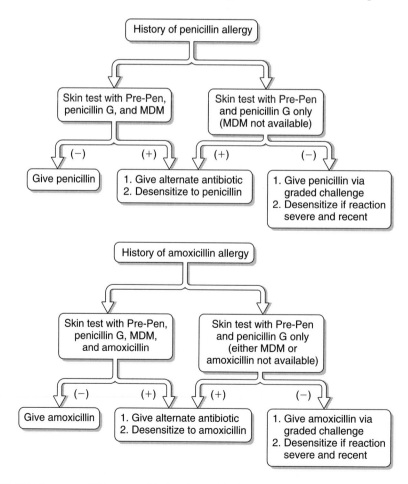

FIGURE 57-2 Structures of β-lactam antibiotics, all of which share a common four-member β-lactam ring.

ment options). In the vast majority of children with a history of penicillin allergy, skin testing is negative.[28] Despite the test's excellent negative predictive value, patients, their parents, and referring physicians are frequently reluctant to "trust" the results, and consequently β-lactam antibiotics are not prescribed.[34,35] To unequivocally prove the medication's safety and to alleviate patients' and physicians' concerns, an oral challenge with the identical antibiotic that caused the previous reaction should be performed.

In the past, there was a theoretical concern that patients may become resensitized (or redevelop their allergy) by a course of penicillin, placing them at risk of an immediate reaction during subsequent exposure. However, evidence does not suggest that children are at increased risk of becoming resensitized. Mendelson et al[28] reported that among 240 history-positive/skin test-negative children and adolescents, only 1% converted to a positive skin test following a course of penicillin. These findings have been confirmed in an additional 1500 pediatric patients by the authors (unpublished observations).

In patients whose histories are clearly consistent with a serum sickness–like reaction or desquamative-type reactions (such as Stevens-Johnson syndrome or toxic epidermal necrolysis), skin testing should not be performed and penicillin should be avoided indefinitely.

Cephalosporins

Patients with a History of Penicillin Allergy

Penicillins and cephalosporins share a common β-lactam ring (Figure 57-3) and early *in vitro* studies indicated extensive immunologic cross-reactivity between these compounds.[36,37] While the exact clinical cross-reactivity is not known, it appears to be quite low. Because most "penicillin-allergic" patients identified by history lack penicillin-specific IgE antibodies, the most informative clinical studies are those in which patients with positive penicillin skin tests are challenged with cephalosporins (Table 57-6). In addition to the very low rate of cross-reactivity, it is interesting to point out that nearly all of the positive challenges occurred with cephalosporins that share a similar R group side chain with benzylpenicillin. Hence, it is possible that the observed cross-reactivity was the result of side chain–specific determinants rather than the core β-lactam portion of the molecules. There are recent reports of patients with selective allergic cross-reactivity between a particular penicillin and cephalosporin that share identical R groups (Table 57-7).[21,38]

Figure 57-4 outlines the clinical approach to children with a history of penicillin allergy who require treatment with cephalosporins. As mentioned previously, the most practical time to perform skin testing is when children are well. Patients who have negative penicillin skin tests are not at increased risk of having an allergic reaction to cephalosporins and therefore can receive them safely. If skin testing is positive, the clinician has one of three options—an alternate non–cross-reacting antibiotic, graded challenge, or desensitization (see Figure 57-4). Under most circumstances, these authors would recommend a graded challenge (see section on treatment options) with a particular cephalosporin that would subsequently be useful and available to treat sinopulmonary infections.

Patients with a History of Cephalosporin Allergy

The clinical situation of patients who have reacted to a cephalosporin and require treatment with penicillin is straightforward and based on penicillin skin test results (Figure 57-5). Patients who test negative may safely receive penicillins, whereas those who are positive should receive an alternate antibiotic or undergo desensitization (if there is an absolute need for penicillin).

The evaluation of patients with a history of cephalosporin allergy who require the same or another cephalosporin is more difficult due to a lack of standardized validated skin testing reagents (see Figure 57-5). Skin testing with nonirritating concentrations of native cephalosporins can be of some value, especially if it is positive, but its negative predictive value is uncertain. Additionally, there are no definitive data on the extent of cross-reactivity among different cephalosporins, and hence, the safety of administering a given cephalosporin to a patient who has previously experienced an allergic reaction to another cephalosporin. The general belief is that the allergic

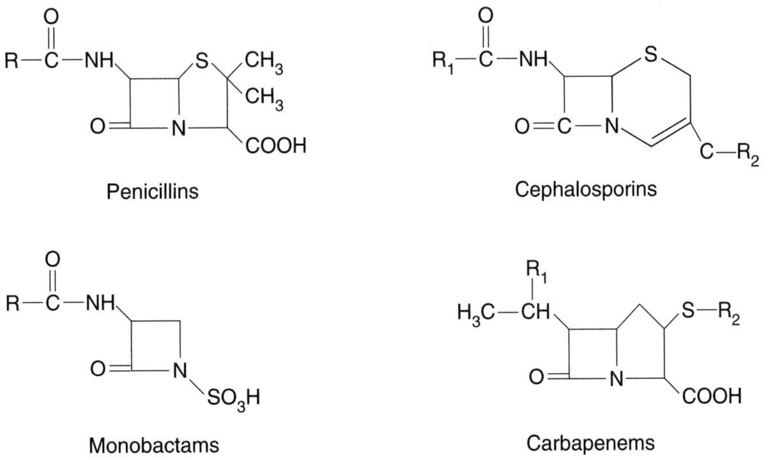

FIGURE 57-3 Management of pediatric patients with a history of penicillin or amoxicillin allergy. Ideally, skin testing is performed on an elective basis, not in situations of acute need.

TABLE 57-6 Summary of Published Reports in which Cephalosporins Were Administered to Patients with Positive Penicillin Skin Tests[a]

Reference (No.)	No. of Patients	No. of Reactions (%)	Comment
Girard[45]	23	2 (8.7)	Both reactions to cephaloridine[b]
Assem, Vickers[46]	3	3 (100)	All reactions to cephaloridine[b]
Warrington et al[c]	3	0	
Solley, Gleich, VanDellen[d]	27	0	
Saxon et al[e]	62	1 (1.6)	Specific cephalosporin not reported
Blanca et al[f]	17	2 (11.8)	Both reactions to cefamandole†
Shepherd, Burton[g]	9	0	
Audicana et al[h]	12	0	
Novalbos et al[i]	23	0	
TOTAL	179	8 (4.5)	

[a]All patients had positive skin test responses to Pre-Pen, Penicillin G, and/or minor determinant mixture. Patients negative to the major and minor penicillin determinants but positive to amoxicillin or ampicillin are not included.

[b]These cephalosporins have R group side chains similar to benzylpenicillin.

[c]From Warrington RJ, Simons FER, Ho HW, et al: *Can Med Assoc J* 118:787-791, 1978.

[d]From Solley GO, Gleich GJ, VanDellen RG: *J Allergy Clin Immunol* 69:238-244, 1982.

[e]From Saxon A, Beall GN, Rohr AS, et al: *Ann Intern Med* 107:204-215, 1987.

[f]From Blanca M, Fernandez J, Miranda A, et al: *J Allergy Clin Immunol* 83:381-385, 1989.

[g]From Shepherd GM, Burton DA: *J Allergy Clin Immunol* 91:262, 1993.

[h]From Audicana M, Bernaola G, Urrutia I, et al: *Allergy* 49:108-113, 1994.

[i]From Novalbos A, Sastre J, Cuesta J, et al: *Clin Exp Allergy* 31:438-443, 2001.

TABLE 57-7 Beta-lactam Antibiotics with Identical R Group Side Chains*

	amoxicillin	ampicillin	aztreonam	benzylpenicillin	cefaclor	cefadroxil	cefamandole	cefazolin	cefepime	cefixime	cefmenoxime	cefonicid	cefotaxime	cefotetan	cefoxitin	cefpodoxime	ceftazidime	ceftizoxime	ceftriaxone	cefuroxime	cephalexin	cephaloridine	cephalothin	cephradine	imipenem	loracarbef	meropenem
amoxicillin	X					1																					
ampicillin		X			1																1			1		1	
aztreonam			X														1										
benzylpenicillin				X																							
cefaclor		1			X																			1		2	
cefadroxil	1					X																					
cefamandole							X					1															
cefazolin								X																			
cefepime									X								1										
cefixime										X																	
cefmenoxime											X		1					1									
cefonicid							1					X															
cefotaxime											1		X			1		1									
cefotetan														X													
cefoxitin															X							1	1				
cefpodoxime													1			X											
ceftazidime			1						1								X										
ceftizoxime											1		1					X									
ceftriaxone																			X	1							
cefuroxime																			1	X							
cephalexin		1																			X					1	
cephaloridine															1							X	1				
cephalothin															1							1	X				
cephradine		1			1																			X			
imipenem																									X		
loracarbef		1			2																1					X	
meropenem																											X

Modified from Poley GE, Slater JE: Drug and vaccine allergy, *Immunol Allergy Clin North Am* 19:409-422, 1999.

*1 or 2 indicates number of shared side chains.

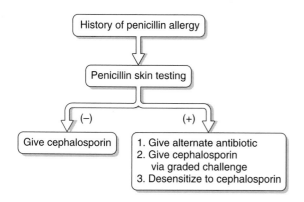

FIGURE 57-4 Administration of cephalosporins to pediatric patients with a history of penicillin allergy. (From Bernstein IL, Gruchalla RS, Lee RE, et al: *Ann Allergy Asthma Immunol* 83:665-700, 1999.)

response to cephalosporins is directed at the R group side chains, rather than the β-lactam portion of the molecule and that patients who have reacted to one cephalosporin can tolerate other cephalosporins with dissimilar side chains.[22] A recent report in which 30 cephalosporin-allergic adult patients underwent skin testing with several different cephalosporins

placed some doubt on this theory.[39] About half of the subjects had positive skin responses only to the cephalosporin that caused their reactions, whereas the other half reacted to various cephalosporins—including ones with different R groups. The results suggest that some cephalosporin-allergic patients form cross-reacting IgE antibodies, but none of the patients were challenged to confirm this suspicion.

Other β-Lactam Antibiotics

Monobactams

Monobactams differ from other β-lactams by their monocyclic ring structure (see Figure 57-3), and aztreonam is the prototype drug in this class. *In vitro* studies showed no immunologic cross-reactivity between aztreonam and either penicillin or cephalosporins, with the exception of ceftazidime—which shares an R group side chain identical with aztreonam (see Table 57-7).[40,41] Lack of clinical cross-reactivity has been confirmed in numerous penicillin skin test–positive subjects who were challenged and tolerated aztreonam.[42,43] Therefore patients who are allergic to penicillins or cephalosporins (except for ceftazidime) can safely receive aztreonam. Conversely, patients who have reacted to aztreonam can safely receive penicillins and cephalosporins (except for ceftazidime).

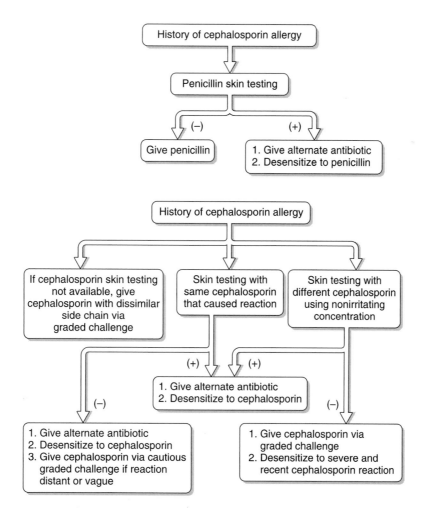

FIGURE 57-5 Management of pediatric patients with a history of cephalosporin allergy. (From Bernstein IL, Gruchalla RS, Lee RE, et al: *Ann Allergy Asthma Immunol* 83:665-700, 1999).

Carbapenems

Based on skin test results, imipenem (see Figure 57-3) appears to have extensive cross-reactivity with penicillin. Of 20 adult patients with positive penicillin skin tests, half also had positive responses to imipenem, but none of the subjects was challenged with imipenem.[44] Interestingly, this rate of skin test cross-reactivity is similar to that observed with first-generation cephalosporins in penicillin-allergic patients.[45,46] While there are no published reports of imipenem challenges in penicillin skin test–positive patients, McConnell et al[47] reviewed records of 63 inpatients with reported penicillin allergy (by history) who received imipenem and found that only 4 (6%) experienced mild cutaneous reactions. Pending further data, carbapenems should be administered cautiously (via desensitization or graded challenge) to patients who have positive penicillin skin tests, whereas penicillin skin test–negative individuals can safely receive carbapenems.

Non−β-Lactam Antibiotics

The lack of reliable diagnostic tests for non−β-lactam antibiotics makes evaluation of children who have reacted to one of these medications more challenging. As discussed earlier, some information can be gleaned from skin testing with nonirritating concentrations of the native antibiotics, but an immediate-type allergy cannot be ruled out. Consequently, unlike penicillin allergy, it is not practical to evaluate these patients on an elective basis. Unless the previous reaction was clearly predictable in nature, such as emesis from erythromycin, the medication should simply be avoided in the future. Evaluation with skin testing should be performed only if readministration of the culprit antibiotic is being considered. If skin testing with a nonirritating concentration of the antibiotic is positive, the medication should be avoided. If such a patient develops an absolute need for the drug, acute desensitization should be performed. If skin testing is negative, either desensitization or a graded challenge can be performed—depending on the "strength" of the history of the previous reaction. The total dose of the antibiotic used in skin testing can be used as a starting point for desensitization or graded challenge (see section on treatment options). Patients who previously experienced Stevens-Johnson syndrome, toxic epidermal necrolysis, or serum sickness should not be given the same antibiotic.

Aside from the β-lactams, the two most commonly used antibiotics in children are macrolides and sulfonamides; a brief discussion of these antibiotics follows.

Sulfonamides

The majority of adverse reactions to sulfonamide antibiotics are non−IgE-mediated delayed cutaneous reactions.[48] They vary from benign, self-limited maculopapular/morbilliform eruptions to severe, potentially life-threatening reactions such as Stevens-Johnson syndrome and toxic epidermal necrolysis. Metabolism of sulfonamides produces a number of reactive intermediates that appear to play a pivotal role in various allergic reactions.[48] Despite this knowledge, there are no *in vitro* or *in vivo* tests that can predict a patient's risk of developing an adverse reaction to sulfonamides. A provocative challenge with a sulfonamide remains the only way to determine whether a patient is truly allergic, but this should be reserved for cases in which alternate antibiotics cannot be substituted and if the previous reaction was not severe. Because of the propensity of sulfonamides to cause severe desquamative-type reactions, most children who have reacted to a member of the family should simply avoid all sulfa antibiotics. The use of non-arylamine–containing sulfa drugs such as diuretics, oral hypoglycemics, celecoxib, and rofecoxib is not contraindicated.[48]

Patients with human immunodeficiency virus (HIV) are at particularly high risk of developing various cutaneous reactions from sulfonamides.[48] Unfortunately, these patients are also likely to require treatment with trimethoprim-sulfamethoxazole (TMP-SMX), since it is the antibiotic of choice for both prophylaxis and acute treatment of *Pneumocystis carinii* pneumonia. Various TMP-SMX "desensitization" protocols ranging in length from a few hours to several weeks have been reported in adult and pediatric patients with HIV.[49,50] "Desensitization" is probably a misnomer for these procedures. They are most likely types of graded challenges during which mild reactions are often "treated through.[48]"

Macrolides

Hypersensitivity reactions to macrolides appear to be uncommon. While there are no published studies addressing the degree of allergic cross-reactivity among the different macrolides, our clinical experience is that it is very low. This observation may partly be due to the structural difference between azithromycin (which is an azalide) and erythromycin or clarithromycin. In children who have reacted to a given macrolide antibiotic, it is reasonable to evaluate the safety of another macrolide. This can be done via skin testing (using a nonirritating concentration of the native antibiotic) followed by a graded challenge, assuming testing is negative. If testing is positive and there is an absolute need to treat the patient with a macrolide, rapid desensitization can be performed.[51]

Local Anesthetics

True hypersensitivity reactions to local anesthetics in children are extremely uncommon and usually consist of a delayed contact dermatitis; anaphylaxis from local anesthetics occurs very rarely, if ever.[52] Most adverse reactions are vasovagal, anxiety or toxic reactions, or predictable side effects of epinephrine. Unfortunately, patients who experience any adverse reaction are frequently labeled as being "allergic" and told to avoid all "caines" in the future. Evaluation of children with a supposed allergy to local anesthetics serves to alleviate dentists' or physicians' concerns and may prevent these patients from being subjected to the increased risk of general anesthesia. Figure 57-6 summarizes the approach to children with previous reactions to local anesthetics. Data from patch testing suggest there is cross-reactivity among the benzoate esters but not among the amides (Table 57-8).[52] While these findings may have no significance on immediate-type reactions, it is generally recommended that if a patient previously reacted to an ester, an amide should be used in evaluation for readministration. If the identity of the previous local anesthetic is not known or if it was an amide, another amide can be used. Additionally, during skin testing and challenge, one should attempt to employ the same agent that will subsequently be used by the dentist or physician.

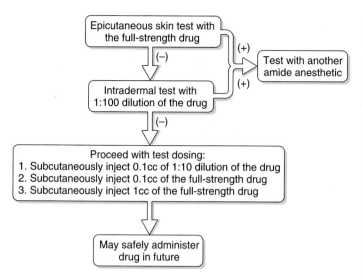

FIGURE 57-6 Management of pediatric patients with previous reactions to local anesthetics. Intervals between steps are 15 minutes. Generally, an amide is used because the benzoate esters cross-react immunologically whereas the amides do not, and frequently patients do not know which drug they reacted to previously. (Data from Patterson R, DeSwarte RD, Greenberger PA, et al: *Allergy Proc* 15:239-264, 1994.)

Acetylsalicylic Acid and Other Nonsteroidal Antiinflammatory Drugs

ASA and other NSAIDs have been associated with five types of allergic and pseudo-allergic reactions (Table 57-9).[53] Reactions that are caused by modifying effects on arachidonic acid metabolism—namely respiratory reactions and urticarial reactions (in patients with underlying chronic urticaria) show cross-reactivity with other NSAIDs, as one would expect. Asthmatics with proven ASA sensitivity, however, can safely receive tartrazine, azo and non-azo dyes, sulfites, monosodium glutamate, and usual doses of acetaminophen (although a minority of patients experiences mild reactions above 1000 mg).[53,54] Recently, drugs that selectively block the cyclooxygenase-2 (COX-2) enzyme, such as rofecoxib, have also been found to be safe in ASA-sensitive asthmatics.[55] Unlike respiratory reactions, acute urticarial or anaphylactic reactions in otherwise normal individuals are medication specific. Hence it is reasonable to perform graded challenges in these individuals with another NSAID to identify an agent that can be safely used in the future. Not uncommonly, patients with acute urticarial reactions are mistakenly told to avoid all NSAIDs indefinitely.

With the exception of respiratory reactions in asthmatics, there are no data on the incidences of these reactions in

TABLE 57-8 Benzoate Esters and Amides Constituting the Two Major Classes of Local Anesthetics*

Generic Name	Available Forms	Examples of Trade Names
Benzoate esters		
Benzocaine	Topical	Orajel, Hurricane, Lanacaine, many others
Butamben picrate	Topical	Butesin
Chloroprocaine	Injectable	Nesacaine
Cocaine	Topical	Cocaine
Procaine	Injectable	Novocain
Proparacaine	Ophthalmic	Alcaine, Opthcaine, Opthetic
Tetracaine	Injectable, topical, ophthalmic	Pontocaine
Amides		
Bupivacaine	Injectable	Marcaine, Sensorcaine
Dibucaine	Topical	Nupercaine
Etidocaine	Injectable	Duranest, Durnest MPF
Lidocaine	Injectable, topical	Xylocaine, Dilocaine, Nervocaine, many others
Mepivacaine	Injectable	Carbocaine, Polocaine, Isocaine
Prilocaine	Injectable	Citanest
Ropivacaine	Injectable	Naropin
Combination		
Lidocaine/Prilocaine	Topical	EMLA

*Patch testing data indicate there is cross-reactivity among the esters but not the amides.

TABLE 57-9 Major Types of Hypersensitivity Reactions to ASA and Other NSAIDs

Reaction Type	Underlying Disease	Cross-Reactions	COX-1 Inhibition	Other Immunologic Mechanisms
Cross-reacting respiratory	Asthma, rhinitis, polyposis	ASA/NSAIDs	Yes	None
Cross-reacting urticaria	Chronic urticaria	ASA/NSAIDs	Yes	None
Urticaria/anaphylaxis	None	None	No	IgE-mediated (presumed)
Aseptic meningitis (only NSAIDs)	None	None	No	Delayed hypersensitivity (presumed)
Hypersensitivity pneumonitis (only NSAIDs)	None	None	No	Delayed hypersensitivity (presumed)

Modified from Stevenson DD: *Immunol Allergy Clin North Am* 18:773-798, 1998.
ASA, Acetylsalicylic acid; *NSAIDs*, nonsteroidal antiinflammatory drugs; *COX*, cyclooxygenase; *IgE*, immunoglobulin E.

children; however, clinical experience suggests that it is low. This observation may be partly the result of the infrequent use of ASA caused by concerns of Reye's syndrome in children. The incidence of ASA sensitivity in children with asthma has been investigated in five prospective studies in which blinded oral challenges were performed.[56-60] The rate of positive challenges varied from 0% (mean age of patients 9.6 years) to 28% (mean age 13.6 years). Overall, these data indicate that ASA sensitivity in asthmatic children under the age of 10 is rare, but thereafter it begins to approach the reported incidence in adults.

TREATMENT OPTIONS

Desensitization

Acute desensitization to a drug should be considered in children who have an IgE-mediated allergy to a medication and no acceptable alternate treatment is available. The aim of desensitization is to convert a child who is highly allergic to a drug to a state in which they can tolerate treatment with the medication. Although most published desensitization protocols involve penicillin, the principle has been applied successfully to other antibiotics, including cephalosporins, sulfonamides, vancomycin, macrolides, quinolones, aminoglycosides, pentamidine, and antituberculin agents.[61] Rapid desensitization is thought to somehow render mast cells unresponsive to the drug used in the procedure, but the exact immunologic mechanism is unknown. Desensitization can be performed either by the oral or intravenous route. Tables 57-10 to 57-12 list representative protocols for penicillin desensitization, and these can be modified and used for other antibiotics as well.

Several principles of management have been derived from studies on penicillin desensitization[62-65] and presumably they hold true for other drugs also. First, the amount of drug the patient tolerated during skin testing determines a safe initial dose for desensitization, which generally translates to 1/10,000 or less of the full therapeutic dose. Second, doubling the dose

TABLE 57-10 Penicillin Oral Desensitization Protocol

Step*	Penicillin (mg/ml)	Amount (ml)	Dose Given (mg)	Cumulative Dose (mg)
1	0.5	0.1	0.05	0.05
2	0.5	0.2	0.1	0.15
3	0.5	0.4	0.2	0.35
4	0.5	0.8	0.4	0.75
5	0.5	1.6	0.8	1.55
6	0.5	3.2	1.6	3.15
7	0.5	6.4	3.2	6.35
8	5	1.2	6	12.35
9	5	2.4	12	24.35
10	5	5	25	49.35
11	50	1	50	100
12	50	2	100	200
13	50	4	200	400
14	50	8	400	800

Observe patient for 30 minutes, then give full therapeutic dose by the desired route.

Modified from Sullivan TJ: Drug allergy. In Middleton E, Reed CE, Ellis EF, et al, eds. *Allergy: principles and practice*, ed 4, St Louis, 1993, Mosby.
*Interval between doses is 15 minutes.

TABLE 57-11 Penicillin Intravenous Desensitization Protocol with Drug Added by Piggyback Infusion

Step*	Penicillin (mg/ml)	Amount (ml)	Dose Given (mg)	Cumulative Dose (mg)
1	0.1	0.1	0.01	0.01
2	0.1	0.2	0.02	0.03
3	0.1	0.4	0.04	0.07
4	0.1	0.8	0.08	0.15
5	0.1	1.6	0.16	0.31
6	1	0.32	0.32	0.63
7	1	0.64	0.64	1.27
8	1	1.2	1.2	2.47
9	10	0.24	2.4	4.87
10	10	0.48	4.8	10
11	10	1	10	20
12	10	2	20	40
13	100	0.4	40	80
14	100	0.8	80	160
15	100	1.6	160	320
16	1000	0.32	320	640
17	1000	0.64	640	1280

Observe patient for 30 minutes, then give full therapeutic dose by the desired route.

Modified from Sullivan TJ: Drug allergy. In Middleton E, Reed CE, Ellis EF, et al, eds: *Allergy: principles and practice*, ed 4, St Louis, 1993, Mosby.
*Interval between doses is 15 minutes.

every 15 minutes until the recommended dose is reached is effective in nearly all instances. Mild reactions occur in about a third of patients, but no fatal or life-threatening reactions have been reported. Third, desensitization does not prevent

TABLE 57-12 Penicillin Intravenous Desensitization Protocol Using a Continuous Infusion Pump

Step*	Penicillin (mg/ml)	Amount (ml)	Dose Given (mg)	Cumulative Dose (mg)
1	0.001	4	0.001	0.001
2	0.001	8	0.002	0.003
3	0.001	16	0.004	0.007
4	0.001	32	0.008	0.015
5	0.001	60	0.015	0.03
6	0.001	120	0.03	0.06
7	0.001	240	0.06	0.12
8	0.1	5	0.125	0.245
9	0.1	10	0.25	0.495
10	0.1	20	0.5	1
11	0.1	40	1	2
12	0.1	80	2	4
13	0.1	160	4	8
14	10	3	7.5	15
15	10	6	15	30
16	10	12	30	60
17	10	25	62.5	123
18	10	50	125	250
19	10	100	250	500
20	10	200	500	1000

Observe patient for 30 minutes, then give full therapeutic dose by the desired route.

*Interval between doses is 15 minutes.

non-IgE reactions such as serum sickness, hemolytic anemia, or interstitial nephritis from occurring. Fourth, for the patient to remain desensitized, it is necessary to administer it on a twice-daily basis. If penicillin is discontinued for more than 48 hours, the patient is again at risk of developing anaphylaxis and desensitization needs to be repeated.

Rapid desensitization should be performed only by a physician experienced in the procedure, in a hospital setting, with intravenous access and necessary medications and equipment to treat anaphylaxis. The hospital pharmacy staff should be consulted prior to the procedure to assist with preparation of the required drug dilutions. Generally oral desensitization is preferred, but taste may be an issue in younger children or some medications may not be available in an oral form, in which case the intravenous route can be used. Patients should not be pretreated with corticosteroids or antihistamines because they may mask early signs of an allergic reaction. If mild reactions do occur, they should be treated and the dose not be advanced until they have resolved.

Graded Challenge

Graded challenge, also known as test dosing, refers to a cautious administration of a medication to a patient who is unlikely to be truly allergic to it. Unlike desensitization, test dosing does not modify the immune system to accept a medication to which an allergy exists. Graded challenges are most commonly undertaken with medications for which testing cannot adequately rule out an allergy, such as cephalosporins, other non-penicillin antibiotics, or penicillin skin testing when MDM is not available. Children who previously experienced severe reactions or who are suspected to be allergic to a medication should undergo desensitization rather than graded challenge.

Most graded challenges can be safely carried in an office without intravenous access but with preparedness to treat potential allergic reactions including anaphylaxis. The pace of the challenge and degree of caution exercised depend on the likelihood that the patient may be allergic and the physician's experience and comfort level with the procedure. Generally, the starting dose is 1/10 to 1/100 of the full dose and approximately fivefold increasing doses are administered every 30 minutes until the full therapeutic dose is reached. At the first sign of any allergic reaction, the procedure should be abandoned and the patient should be treated appropriately. If at a later point the patient requires the medication, it should be administered only via formal desensitization.

CONCLUSIONS

Children commonly experience adverse reactions to medications, many of which are falsely labeled as being allergic and subsequently avoided due to a fear of causing a severe life-threatening reaction (Box 57-1). If a child has reacted to several different medications, such as antibiotics, physicians are often at their "wit's end" about how to approach future inevitable treatment courses. Likewise, parents of patients are apprehensive and concerned that their child may "die" because of a lack of safe medications. Using the tools (Box 57-2) discussed in this chapter, physicians can play an important role in helping to sort out which medications a child can safely receive, and in many cases prevent them from needlessly being labeled as allergic for the rest of their lives.

BOX 57-1 **KEY CONCEPTS**
Drug Allergy

- Children are commonly labeled as being allergic to various medications and a thorough allergy evaluation can help determine which patients are truly at risk of a severe reaction.
- The majority of children labeled as allergic to medications, particularly antibiotics, can take them without fear of a severe reaction.
- The ideal time to evaluate drug allergy in children is when they are well and not in acute need of treatment.

BOX 57-2 **THERAPEUTIC PRINCIPLES**

1. Penicillin allergy
   a. About 10% of children are labeled as being "penicillin allergic."
   b. The vast majority of children with the label of penicillin allergy can safely take all β-lactam antibiotics without fear of an allergic reaction.
   c. The only accurate way to determine whether a child has an IgE-mediated allergy to penicillin is by skin testing with the appropriate penicillin reagents.
   d. To unequivocally prove the safety of penicillin to the patient, parents, and the referring physician, an oral challenge should be undertaken.
   e. The ideal time to evaluate penicillin allergy in children is when they are well and not in immediate need of antibiotic treatment.
   f. Physicians should make an effort to evaluate penicillin allergy in children and not allow them to unnecessarily carry the label into adulthood.

2. Allergy to non-penicillin antibiotics
   a. There are no validated skin testing reagents to accurately rule out an IgE-mediated allergy.
   b. Skin testing with nonirritating concentrations of antibiotics can assist the clinician in evaluating a possible allergy.
   c. Graded challenge or desensitization can be used in situations where need for an antibiotic arises.

3. Allergy to local anesthetics
   a. True immediate-type allergic reactions to local anesthetics are very rare.
   b. Skin testing followed by graded challenge rules out an allergy to local anesthetics in virtually all children.

4. Acetylsalicylic acid/nonsteroidal antiinflammatory drug (NSAID) allergy
   a. Reactions to NSAIDs appear to be less frequent in children than they are in adults.
   b. Reactions in patients with underlying asthma or chronic urticaria are cross-reactive among all NSAIDs.
   c. Reactions in patients without underlying asthma or chronic urticaria, including anaphylaxis/angioedema/urticaria, are medication specific.

REFERENCES

1. DeSchazo RD: Allergic reactions to drugs and biologic agents, *JAMA* 278:1895-1906, 1997.
2. International Rheumatic Fever Study Group: Allergic reactions to long-term benzathine penicillin prophylaxis for rheumatic fever, *Lancet* 337:1308-1310, 1991.
3. Napoli DC, Neeno TA: Anaphylaxis to benzathine penicillin G, *Pediatr Asthma Allergy Immunol* 14:329-332, 2000.
4. Ibia EO, Schwartz RH, Wiederman BL: Antibiotic rashes in children: a survey in a private practice setting, *Arch Dermatol* 136:849-854, 2000.
5. Gadde J, Spence M, Wheeler B, et al: Clinical experience with penicillin skin testing in a large inner-city STD Clinic, *JAMA* 270:2456-2463, 1993.
6. Bock SA, Munoz-Furlong A, Sampson HA, et al: Fatalities due to anaphylactic reactions to foods, *J Allergy Clin Immunol* 107:191-193, 2001.
7. Adkinson NF: Risk factors for drug allergy, *J Allergy Clin Immunol* 74:567-572, 1984.
8. Roujeau JC, Huynh TN, Bracq C, et al: Genetic susceptibility to toxic epidermal necrolysis, *Arch Dermatol* 123:1171-1173, 1987.
9. Wooley PH, Griffin J, Panayi GS, et al: HLA-DR antigens and toxic reactions to sodium aurothiomalate and D-penicillamine in patients with rheumatoid arthritis, *N Engl J Med* 303:300-302, 1980.
10. Kamada MM, Twarog F, Leung DYM: Multiple antibiotic sensitivity in a pediatric population, *Allergy Proc* 12:347-350, 1991.
11. Moseley EK, Sullivan TJ: Allergic reactions to antimicrobial drugs in patients with a history of prior drug allergy (abstract), *J Allergy Clin Immunol* 87:226, 1991.
12. Khoury L, Warrington R: The multiple drug allergy syndrome: A matched-control retrospective study in patients allergic to penicillin, *J Allergy Clin Immunol* 98:462-464, 1996.
13. Parker CW, deWeck AL, Kern M, et al: The preparation and some properties of penicillenic acid derivatives relevant to penicillin hypersensitivity, *J Exp Med* 115:803-819, 1962.
14. Levine BB, Ovary Z: Studies on the mechanism of the formation of the penicillin antigen. III. The N-(D-alpha-benzyl-penicilloyl) group as an antigenic determinant responsible for hypersensitivity to penicillin G, *J Exp Med* 114:875-904, 1961.
15. Levine BB, Redmond AP: Minor haptenic determinant-specific reagins of penicillin hypersensitivity in man, *Int Arch Allergy Appl Immunol* 35:445-455, 1969.
16. Wickern GM, Nish WA, Bitner AS, et al: Allergy to beta-lactams: a survey of current practices, *J Allergy Clin Immunol* 94:725-731, 1994.
17. Sogn DD, Evans R, Shepherd GM, et al: Results of the National Institute of Allergy and Infectious Diseases collaborative clinical trial to test the predictive value of skin testing with major and minor penicillin derivatives in hospitalized adults, *Arch Intern Med* 152:1025-1032, 1992.
18. Sullivan TJ, Wedner HJ, Shatz GS, et al: Skin testing to detect penicillin allergy, *J Allergy Clin Immunol* 68:171-180, 1981.
19. DeSwarte RD, Patterson R: Drug allergy. In Patterson R, Grammer LC, Greenberger PA, eds: *Allergic diseases: diagnosis and management*, ed 5, Philadelphia, 1997, Lippincott-Raven.
20. Blanca M, Vega JM, Garcia J, et al: Allergy to penicillin with good tolerance to other penicillins: study of the incidence in subjects allergic to betalactams, *Clin Exp Allergy* 20:475-481, 1990.
21. Sastre J, Quijano LD, Novalbos A, et al: Clinical cross-reactivity between amoxicillin and cephadroxil in patients allergic to amoxicillin and with good tolerance of penicillin, *Allergy* 51:383-386, 1996.
22. Bernstein IL, Gruchalla RS, Lee RE, et al: Disease management of drug hypersensitivity: a practice parameter, *Ann Allergy Asthma Immunol* 83:665-700, 1999.
23. Romano A, Quaratino D, Papa G, et al: Aminopenicillin allergy, *Arch Dis Child* 76:513-517, 1997.
24. Romano A, Quaratino D, DiFonso M, et al: A diagnostic protocol for evaluating nonimmediate reactions to aminopenicillins, *J Allergy Clin Immunol* 103:1186-1190, 1999.
25. Primeau MN, Hamilton RG, Whitmore E, et al: Negative patch tests and skin tests in patients with delayed cutaneous to penicillins (abstract), *J Allergy Clin Immunol* 109:S267, 2002.
26. Empedrad RB, Earl HS, Gruchalla RS: Determination of nonirritating concentrations of commonly used antimicrobial drugs (abstract), *J Allergy Clin Immunol* 105:S272, 2000.
27. Solensky R, Earl HS, Gruchalla RS: Penicillin allergy: prevalence of vague history in skin test-positive patients, *Ann Allergy Asthma Immunol* 85:195-199, 2000.
28. Mendelson LM, Ressler C, Rosen JP, et al: Routine elective penicillin allergy skin testing in children and adolescents: study of sensitization, *J Allergy Clin Immunol* 73:76-81, 1984.
29. Solensky R, Earl HS, Gruchalla RS: Clinical approach to penicillin allergic patients: a survey, *Ann Allergy Asthma Immunol* 84:329-333, 2000.
30. Lee CE, Zembower TR, Fotis MA, et al: The incidence of antimicrobial allergies in hospitalized patients: implications regarding prescribing patterns and emerging bacterial resistance, *Arch Intern Med* 160:2819-2822, 2000.
31. Murray BE: Vancomycin-resistant enterococcal infections, *N Engl J Med* 342:710-721, 2000.
32. Rao GG: Risk factors for the spread of antibiotic-resistant bacteria, *Drugs* 55:323-330, 1998.
33. Hospital Infection Control Practices Advisory Committee (HICPAC): Recommendations for preventing the spread of vancomycin resistance, *MMWR* 44(RR-12):1-13, 1995.
34. Warrington RJ, Tsai EL: The value of routine penicillin skin testing in an outpatient population, *J Allergy Clin Immunol* 109:S268, 2002.
35. Lacuesta GA, Moote DW, Payton K, et al: Follow-up of patients with negative skin tests to penicillin (abstract), *J Allergy Clin Immunol* 109:S143, 2002.
36. Abraham GN, Petz LD, Fudenberg HH: Immunohaematological cross-allergenicity between penicillin and cephalothin in humans, *Clin Exp Immunol* 3:343-357, 1968.
37. Batchelor FR, Dewdney JM, Weston RD, et al: The immunogenicity of cephalosporin derivatives and their cross-reaction with penicillin, *Immunol* 10:21-33, 1966.
38. Miranda A, Blanca M, Vega JM, et al: Cross-reactivity between a penicillin and a cephalosporin with the same side chain, *J Allergy Clin Immunol* 98:671-677, 1996.
39. Romano A, Mayorga C, Torres MJ, et al: Immediate allergic reactions to cephalosporins: cross reactivity and selective responses, *J Allergy Clin Immunol* 106:1177-1183, 2000.
40. Adkinson NF, Swabb EA, Sugerman AA: Immunology of the monobactam aztreonam, *Antimicrob Agents Chemother* 25:93-97, 1984.
41. Saxon A, Swabb EA, Adkinson NF: Investigation into the immunologic cross-reactivity of aztreonam with other beta-lactam antibiotics, *Am J Med* 78:19-26, 1985.
42. Adkinson NF: Immunogenicity and cross-allergenicity of aztreonam, *Am J Med* 88:S3-S14, 1990.
43. Vega JM, Blanca M, Garcia JJ, et al: Tolerance to aztreonam in patients allergic to betalactam antibiotics, *Allergy* 46:196-202, 1991.
44. Saxon A, Adelman DC, Patel A, et al: Imipenem cross-reactivity with penicillin in humans, *J Allergy Clin Immunol* 82:213-217, 1988.
45. Girard JP: Common antigenic determinants of penicillin G, ampicillin and the cephlosporins demonstrated in men, *Int Arch Allergy* 33:428-438, 1968.
46. Assem ESK, Vickers MR: Tests for penicilin allergy in man II. The immunological cross-reaction between penicillins and cephalosporins, *Immunology* 27:255-269, 1974.
47. McConnell SA, Penzak SR, Warmack TS, et al: Incidence of imipenem hypersensitivity reactions in febrile neutropenic marrow transplant patients with a history of penicillin allergy, *Clin Infect Dis* 31:1512-1514, 2000.
48. Cribb AE, Lee BL, Trepanier LA, et al: Adverse reactions to sulphonamide and sulphonamide-trimethoprim antimicrobials: clinical syndromes and pathogenesis, *Adverse Drug React Toxicol Rev* 15:9-50, 1996.
49. Demoly P, Messaad D, Sahla H, et al: Six-hour trimethoprim-sulfamethoxazole-graded challenge in HIV-infected patients, *J Allergy Clin Immunol* 102:1033-1036, 1998.
50. Yango MC, Kim K, Evans R: Oral desensitization to trimethoprim-sulfamethoxazole in pediatric patients, *Immunol Allergy Practice* 56:17-24, 1992.
51. Laurie S, Khan D: Successful clarithromycin desensitization in a macrolide-sensitive patient (abstract), *Ann Allergy Asthma Immunol* 84:116, 2000.
52. Soto-Aguilar MC, deSchazo RD, Dawson ES: Approach to the patient with suspected local anesthetic sensitivity, *Immunol Allergy Clin North Am* 18:851-865, 1998.
53. Stevenson DD: Adverse reactions to nonsteroidal anti-inflammatory drugs, *Immunol Allergy Clin North Am* 18:773-798, 1998.
54. Settipane RA, Shrank PJ, Simon RA, et al: Prevalence of cross-sensitivity with acetaminophen in aspirin-sensitive asthmatic subjects, *J Allergy Clin Immunol* 96:480-485, 1995.

55. Stevenson DD, Simon RA: Lack of cross-reactivity between rofecoxib and aspirin in aspirin-sensitive patients with asthma, *J Allergy Clin Immunol* 108:47-51, 2001.

56. Fisher TJ, Guilfoile TD, Kesarwala HH, et al: Adverse pulmonary responses to aspirin and acetaminophen in chronic childhood asthma, *Pediatrics* 71:313-318, 1983.

57. Vedanthan PK, Menon MM, Bell TD, et al: Aspirin and tartrazine oral challenge: incidence of adverse response in chronic childhood asthma, *J Allergy Clin Immunol* 60:8-13, 1977.

58. Rachelefsky GS, Coulson A, Siegel SC, et al: Aspirin intolerance in chronic childhood asthma: detected by oral challenge, *Pediatrics* 56:443-448, 1975.

59. Schuhl JF, Pereyra JG: Oral acetylsalicylic acid (aspirin) challenge in asthmatic children, *Clin Allergy* 9:83-88, 1979.

60. Towns SJ, Mellis CM: Role of acetyl salicylic acid and sodium metabisulfite in chronic childhood asthma, *Pediatrics* 73:631-637, 1984.

61. Solensky R, Mendelson LM: Systemic reactions to antibiotics, *Immunol Allergy Clin North Am* 21:679-697, 2001.

62. Borish L, Tamir R, Rosenwasser LJ: Intravenous desensitization to beta-lactam antibiotics, *J Allergy Clin Immunol* 80:314-319, 1987.

63. Sullivan TJ, Yecies LD, Shatz GS, et al: Desensitization of patients allergic to penicillin using orally administered beta-lactam antibiotics, *J Allergy Clin Immunol* 69:275-282, 1982.

64. Stark BJ, Earl HS, Gross GN, et al: Acute and chronic desensitization of penicillin-allergic patients using oral penicillin, *J Allergy Clin Immunol* 79:523-532, 1987.

65. Wendel GD, Stark BJ, Jamison RB, et al: Penicillin allergy and desensitization in serious infections during pregnancy, *N Engl J Med* 312:1229-1232, 1985.

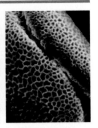

CHAPTER 58

Latex Allergy

GORDON L. SUSSMAN ■ STEPHEN D. BETSCHEL ■ DONALD H. BEEZHOLD

It has been more than 20 years since natural rubber latex (NRL) has been recognized as a cause of type I allergy.[1] Latex gloves are the major source of NRL allergens. Since the implementation of universal precautions to help contain the spread of the human immunodeficiency virus, the use of latex examination gloves has increased dramatically, from 2 billion gloves used annually in 1985 to 22 billion in 1999.[2] An increased number of allergic reactions to latex has paralleled this increase in latex use and has become a significant problem in the healthcare environment.[3] This chapter presents an overview of latex allergy and reviews the determinants of the relevant allergens and the clinical presentations of latex hypersensitivity. An outline of the investigation and treatment principles are also provided.

ETIOLOGY

The cytosol from the lactiferous layer of the cultivated rubber tree, *Hevea brasiliensis*, is the predominant source of commercially produced latex.[4] Latex is processed to produce the multitude of natural rubber products that are ubiquitous in today's environment. The majority of extracted rubber is coagulated dry rubber and used for the manufacture of goods such as tires for vehicles, rubber seals, and other molded rubber products, which are a rare source of latex allergens.[5] A minority of harvested rubber is used for the manufacture of dipped products, which are produced from ammoniated and noncoagulated rubber. Dipped products, which include condoms, medical examination gloves, catheters, and balloons, are the primary reservoir of latex allergens.

The principal structural component of latex is *cis*-1,4-polyisoprene, which is found as a spherical rubber particle derived from the enzymatic conversion of sucrose. *cis*-1,4-Polyisoprene is coated with lipid, phospholipid, and protein. Proteins, which constitute 1% to 2% of NRL, are the major allergens and are closely associated with the rubber particles in the serum or are organized into organelles called lutoids. Some of these are pathogenesis-related (PR) proteins that are functionally responsible for the plant's protection against infection and infestation. These include proteins with lysozyme and chitinase activity; hevein, a fungitoxic protein; and hevamine.

The proteins causing latex allergy are present in both raw latex and processed rubber products.[6,7] They correspond to proteins originating from the rubber plant itself and are not introduced into the manufacturing process. However, during the manufacture of dipped rubber products, several low-molecular-weight antioxidants (phenylenediamine), accelerators (thiurams, carbamates, thiazoles), and preservatives are added. The clinical manifestation of reactions to these additives is primarily an allergic contact dermatitis. The latex-derived proteins present in the dipped products can leach out of the rubber with skin moisture and be absorbed into the skin or associated with cornstarch powder inside the gloves.[8-13] The latex allergens can be easily aerosolized when the gloves are donned as a consequence of their adherence to the cornstarch powder, resulting in the sensitization of persons who inhale the allergens or an exacerbation of allergic symptoms in patients who are already sensitized.[7]

Numerous investigators have contributed to the characterization of allergens contained in latex. Table 58-1 lists the currently identified latex allergens.[14-36] Specific latex proteins have been shown to be important in sensitization of specific high-risk groups for latex allergy. Hev b 5, Hev b 6, and Hev b 7 are allergens recognized by IgE and responsible for sensitization in the majority of health care workers (93%)[37] and latex-allergic children.[38] Children with spina bifida represent a distinct group of latex-allergic patients with a unique IgE binding pattern compared with those of other populations of latex-allergic individuals.

Hev b 1 and Hev b 3 share 47% structural homology and are major allergens in children with congenital abnormalities, including those with spina bifida, with greater than 80% having IgE that binds to these allergens.[39-41] Hev b 7 has recently been shown to be an important allergen not only for latex-allergic patients (45%) but also among latex-allergic children with spina bifida (39.5%).[42] However, as with health care workers, children with spina bifida tend to be sensitized to multiple Hevea determinants and monosensitization is uncommon.

Clinical and immunochemical cross-reactivity between latex and foods is well recognized and has been termed the *latex-fruit syndrome*.[43-45] Several latex allergens cross-react with pollen proteins or foods including banana, avocado, kiwi, chestnut, potato, and papaya.[44,46] Brehler et al[47] investigated 136 patients with latex allergy using a radioallergosorbent test (RAST) for 12 foods commonly involved in latex-food reactions and found that 69% of patients were positive to at least one food, with 49% positive to multiple foods. We found that

TABLE 58-1 Allergenic Proteins Derived from Natural Rubber Latex

Biosynthesis and coagulations

Hev b 1	Rubber elongation factor[14-16]
Hev b 3	Small rubber particle protein[17,18]
Hev b 7	Patatin[19-21]

Pathogenesis-related proteins

Hev b 2	Beta-1,3-glucanase[22,23]
Hev b 6.01	Prohevein[19]
Hev b 6.02	Hevein[24-27]
Hev b 6.03	C-terminal fragment[24]
Hev b 11	Chitinase[28]
Hevamine	Lysozyme[19]

Structural proteins and housekeeping enzymes

Hev b 4	Microhelix protein complex[23]
Hev b 5	Proline-rich acidic latex protein[29,30]
Hev b 8	Profilin[31-33]
Hev b 9	Enolase[34,35]
Hev b 10	Manganese superoxide dismutase[34,36]

among 47 latex-allergic adults, 100 of 376 food skin tests were positive, with up to 50% associated with clinical reactions to specific foods and some of these reactions resulting in serious anaphylactic events.[48] In patients with fruit allergy but without latex allergy risk factors, 86% of the 57 patients had IgE antibody detected using RAST, but 11% demonstrated clinical reactions to latex.[49]

A recent publication suggested that there might be clinical value in differentiating individuals with isolated food, pollen, or latex sensitization.[50] Levy et al[50] investigated adults with latex allergy and pollinosis ($N = 24$) and without pollinosis ($N = 20$), plus a group with pollinosis but without latex allergy ($N = 25$), for allergies to 12 foods commonly associated with latex and pollen allergy. In patients with latex allergy alone, reactions were documented to banana ($N = 4$), avocado ($N = 4$), kiwi ($N = 2$), melon ($N = 1$), and peach ($N = 1$). Those with pollinosis were more likely to react to Rosaceae foods and celery. In the groups with pollen allergy, positive skin test responses to the foods were found in 45%, but for isolated latex allergy, only 24% of responses were positive. Reactions to banana, avocado, and kiwi accounted for nearly 50% of reactions in those with latex allergy.

The molecular mimicry that is responsible for cross-reactive symptoms has been the focus of much research. A number of plant proteins can be classified as belonging to distinct PR-protein groups that share structural and functional homology. The principal PR-proteins in latex that give rise to cross-reactivity with foods are the beta-1,3-glucanases, basic class I chitinases, and chitinases similar to potato wound–inducible proteins, which are classified as PR-type proteins PR-2, PR-3, and PR-4, respectively.[51]

The PR-2 type proteins are phylogenetically conserved, homologous proteins that are recognized by IgE from food-allergic patients with hypersensitivity to banana, potato, and tomato.[52] The amount of beta-1,3-glucanase expression has been shown to increase in banana fruit during ripening, suggesting that there are varying amounts of allergens within the same species of fruit.[53]

The PR-3 type proteins are abundantly found in seed-producing plants. Chitinases function as part of the plant's defense mechanism against pathogens. These proteins contain an N-terminal hevein domain of approximately 40 amino acid residues with putative chitin-binding properties. Latex prohevein (Hev b 6.01) belongs to the group of chitin-binding proteins with a hevein domain. Hevein (Hev b 6.02), a 43–amino acid polypeptide cleavage product derived from prohevein, is found in latex that shares sequence similarities with PR-3 and PR-4 proteins. This cleavage product contributes to the increased prevalence of fruit allergies in individuals allergic to latex. Relevant allergens of chestnut and avocado have been identified by N-terminal amino acid sequencing as class I chitinases containing hevein domains.[54] Two major IgE-binding proteins from banana have been identified as class I chitinases with a hevein-like domain further explaining the cross-reactivity between Hevea latex and fruits.[55] Furthermore, an inducible 18.7-kD protein that is produced in wounded turnip plants was shown to be recognized by IgE from individuals with NRL allergy.[56] The peptide sequence of this protein shares 70% protein homology with Hev b 6.01. It also shares greater than 70% homology with wound-induced proteins from tomato and potato. In summary, the data indicate that Hev b 6.01 is responsible for much of the cross-reactivity of latex with other plants.

EPIDEMIOLOGY

General Population

The ability of latex to provide an effective physical barrier because of its strength, elasticity, and tactile properties has made it an effective product for many applications in the health care industry. Studies of the prevalence of latex allergy vary greatly. This variation is probably because of different levels of exposure and methods used for estimating latex sensitization or allergy. Recent reports in the scientific literature suggest that latex sensitization in the general population is between 1% and 6.5% depending on the method of detection.[57-59] Using skin prick testing Novembre et al,[60] evaluated 453 consecutive children seen at a university allergy clinic and found that 3% had a positive skin test to latex. A study from Finland reported latex sensitivity was less than 1% in the general population using skin prick testing. However, using serologic testing, Ownby et al[61] reported latex-specific IgE antibodies to be present in 6.5% of 1000 blood donors. Similar findings were documented by other investigators who used *in vitro* serologic methods to estimate latex sensitivity.[62,63] Such dramatic differences in the prevalence likely reflect the poor specificity of the *in vitro* tests used with respect to the extensive cross-reactivity with foods and inhalant allergens. Clearly, we know that 6% of the general population is not clinically allergic to latex.

High-Risk Groups

Distinct groups are at risk for latex allergy with respect to amount of latex exposure. The populations most at risk are atopic individuals, health care workers, and children with spina bifida or other congenital anomalies. In the health care industry, workers at risk of developing latex allergy because of ongoing latex exposure include, but are not limited to, physicians, nurses, aides, dentists, dental hygienists, operating room employees, laboratory technicians, and housekeeping personnel. Studies of health care workers found the prevalence of latex allergy to be between 5% and 15%.[64-67] Furthermore, among sensitized workers, there is variability in the manifestations of clinical symptoms or signs of latex allergy. One study of latex-exposed hospital workers found that 54% of those sensitized had latex-induced asthma, with an overall prevalence of latex asthma of 2.5%.[68]

Several reasons have been suggested to account for the high prevalence of latex allergy in health care workers.[69] Major factors responsible for the development of latex allergy have included the increased use of latex gloves since the introduction of universal precautions and the requirement that employers provide gloves for their employees. Also, some manufacturers may have produced more allergenic gloves because of changes in materials, processing, or manufacturing procedures to meet this increased demand for latex gloves.[70] Because of the increased reports of latex allergy over the past decade, physicians are also recognizing the signs and symptoms of latex allergy and may be better at diagnosis.

Frequent surgical intervention in children has been shown to increase the risk of latex allergy.[71-73] This includes children with cerebral palsy,[74-76] esophageal atresia,[77] gastroschisis, and omphalocele.[78] The prevalence of latex allergy in patients with spina bifida has been reported to be as high as 60%.[79] Patients with multiple surgeries are also included in this group, especially if these surgeries are performed at an early age.[80] This exceptionally high prevalence may also be secondary to the frequent exposure to latex as part of these patient's daily management such as intermittent bladder catheterizations, manual bowel disimpaction, routine examinations, and diagnostic testing.

Although health care workers and individuals without spina bifida who have had multiple surgeries show a high incidence of latex allergy, their risk is still much lower than the risk for children with spina bifida (up to 15% versus up to 60%, respectively). This difference has led some investigators to suggest that patients with spina bifida may have a genetic predisposition to develop latex allergy with an early shift to preferentially produce latex-specific IgE antibody because of early exposure.[81]

The most important factor in latex sensitization has been shown by several investigators to be the total amount of exposure to latex. In a cross-sectional study of dental students in Ontario, Tarlo et al[82] found no evidence of latex allergy among 20 first- and second-year students. However, among third-year students the prevalence had increased to 6% and further to 10% among fourth-year students. In another study involving 1351 health care workers, employees who worked in hospital departments with increased use of surgical gloves had a higher prevalence of skin test reactivity to latex.[83] Furthermore, among patients with spina bifida, it has been shown that not only does the number of surgical procedures correlate positively with the development of latex allergy[84,85] but also latex avoidance in a group of spina bifida patients younger than 2 years decreased the seroconversion rate from 43% to 0%.[86]

CLINICAL MANIFESTATIONS

Local Reactions

Irritant Contact Dermatitis

The most common reaction to latex products is the development of nonallergic, irritated, dry areas on the skin in those who wear latex gloves. These clinical reactions are not immune mediated and are the result of repeated hand washing, the use of soaps, and the cornstarch powder that is added to

the latex gloves during their manufacture. Irritant contact hand dermatitis may lead to breaches in the skin barrier that can result in antigen penetration, predisposing to sensitization and leading to an IgE response in some individuals.[86]

Allergic Contact Dermatitis

Allergic dermatitis is a cell-mediated delayed hypersensitivity type IV immunologic response that occurs 24 to 48 hours after contact with the offending cause. The reaction is frequently a result of the low-molecular-weight antioxidants and accelerators added to the latex during the manufacturing process. Thiuram compounds found in rubber are the most common cause of contact dermatitis.[3] Carbamates and mercaptobenzothiazole are other common sensitizers in NRL products. The diagnosis of an allergic contact dermatitis is suspected on the basis of clinical history and the morphology and distribution of the skin lesions. A specific diagnosis is confirmed by patch testing with the suspected chemical additives.

Contact Urticaria

Contact urticaria is a common manifestation and is often the presenting symptom of type I latex allergy. In health care workers with latex sensitivity, up to 80% reported contact urticaria.[87,88] The symptoms of contact urticaria include redness, itching, and wheal-and-flare at the site of glove exposure. These reactions are often but not always IgE mediated and caused by the NRL proteins.

Rhinitis and Asthma

The ability of latex allergens to be adsorbed to glove powder and aerosolized and dispersed when the gloves are donned and discarded can lead to direct immunologic stimulation of the airways.[89-92] These inhaled particles directly contribute to latex-induced occupational asthma,[93] which is often irreversible unless identified early.[94]

Systemic Reactions

Allergenic proteins derived from the natural rubber sensitize patients and subsequently can cause a wide spectrum of allergic clinical responses. The mechanism is a type I, IgE-mediated hypersensitivity that occurs in predisposed patients resulting in mast cell degranulation and the release of potent mediators of anaphylaxis.[95-97] These chemical mediators include histamine, tryptase, leukotrienes, prostaglandins, kinins, platelet activating factor, and chemokines that result in vasodilation, increased vascular permeability, and bronchoconstriction and manifest as urticaria, angioedema, wheezing, and hypotension.

Reactions characterized by cutaneous exposure to latex allergens are generally less severe than those caused by mucosal or inhalant exposure, which may manifest as rhinoconjunctivitis, asthma,[98] anaphylaxis,[99,100] and even death.[101] Serious anaphylactic reactions to latex have occurred in many different settings and have generally involved mucosal exposures during vaginal deliveries,[102] vaginal examinations,[99,103] medical procedures such as barium enemas,[101] rectal manometry,[104] dental procedures,[105] and, intraabdominal and genitourinary surgery.[6,78,106] However, severe anaphylactic reactions have also been reported from percutaneous and inhalant exposures.[3]

DIAGNOSIS

History

The diagnosis of latex allergy relies mainly on a thorough patient history. However, even a complete history cannot identify all patients at risk.[107] Figure 58-1 outlines a decision tree to aid in the steps that should be taken in making a diagnosis of latex allergy. All patients should be asked about latex, drug, and food allergies. A more detailed history should be taken from those identified as having a possible latex sensitivity. These patients should be referred for further evaluation of these historical details and allergy confirmation. When assessing for a possible latex allergy, three principal areas must be addressed: (1) the presence of compatible clinical symptoms including urticaria, pruritis, angioedema, conjunctivitis, rhinitis, asthma, or anaphylaxis during exposure to NRL gloves, balloons, or other latex-containing devices; reactions occurring during surgical or dental procedures and rectal or pelvic examination are also important; (2) the presence of any of the accepted risk factors including spina bifida and congenital urologic problems; occupational (health care, industrial); multiple dental or medical surgical procedures; asthma, eczema, or rhinitis; food rashes; and allergic reactions to fruits or vegetables; and (3) a prior history of unexplained anaphylaxis or unexplained intraoperative reactions. Table 58-2 outlines a simplified questionnaire to help address these points.

Allergy Testing

Individuals identified with a possible history of latex allergy should be referred for further assessment. In addition, those

TABLE 58-2 Simplified Questionnaire for the Identification of Latex Allergy
Medical history
Presence of atopy including hay fever, food allergy (especially reactions to banana, avocado, potato, and tomato), eczema, and asthma
Surgical history
Multiple surgeries
Intraoperative events consistent with anaphylaxis (episodes of urticaria or angioedema, respiratory distress, difficulty with ventilation), hypotension, reactions during dental procedures and radiologic procedures (barium enema)
Occupational history
History of latex exposure; type of latex device, nature, and duration of exposure
Work-related symptoms of possible latex allergy
Cutaneous symptoms including hand dermatitis, eczema, and urticaria
Upper respiratory symptoms including nasal rhinorrhea, pruritis, and sneezing
Lower respiratory symptoms including cough, wheeze, and shortness of breath
Other symptoms, including itchy hands, localized angioedema, possible systemic anaphylactic symptoms with use of household latex cleaning gloves, balloons, condoms, and diaphragms

individuals who have no known clinical symptoms related to latex sensitivity but belong to those high-risk groups mentioned earlier should also have further evaluation. After an anaphylactic reaction, skin tests may be rendered negative. It is reasonable to perform skin testing after an anaphylactic

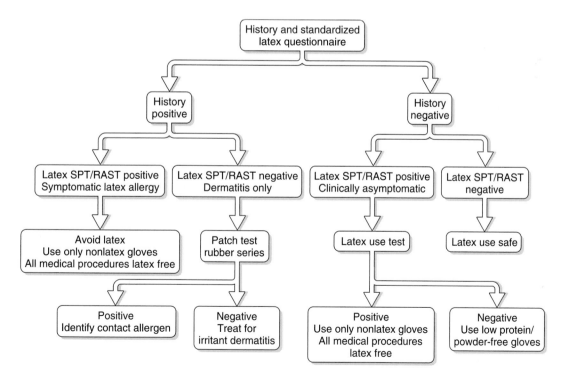

FIGURE 58-1 Investigational decision tree for the diagnosis of latex allergy. Patients are divided into those with positive or negative histories and those with positive or negative results from skin testing, and a management outcome for these patients is given. Patients with negative histories do not receive skin testing unless they are categorized as high risk. *RAST,* Radioallergosorbent testing; *SPT,* skin prick testing. (From Sussman G, Beezhold D: *Ann Intern Med* 122:43-46, 1995.)

episode with the recognition that if the reaction is negative the patient should be brought back and tested 4 to 6 weeks after the systemic reaction. In the interim, until confirmatory testing can be done, latex exposure should be completely avoided in these patients. After diagnosis, the hospitalized latex-allergic patient should have proper documentation and identification of latex allergy on an armband and in the medical chart. Latex allergy signs should be posted on the bed and at the entrance to the patient's room. Nonhospitalized patients should wear a medic alert bracelet and be fully educated regarding possible hidden exposures to latex.

Skin Prick Testing

Presently, skin prick testing is the diagnostic test of choice. Skin testing extracts to determine latex protein allergy have included nonammoniated latex, high- or low-ammoniated latex, Hevea leaf extracts, and NRL glove solutions. Lack of standardization of skin testing reagents has complicated testing because not all countries have access to commercially prepared extracts. Presently there is no skin test reagent available in the United States. This has resulted in the use of glove extracts being prepared by soaking premeasured amounts of glove material in diluent solutions for varying lengths of time.[57] This must be done with extreme caution because gloves contain variable allergen levels. One study demonstrated a 3000-fold difference among gloves from different manufacturers.[108] Today, because of improved manufacturing procedures, the concentration of allergens in NRL gloves is significantly reduced, making it more difficult to prepare a reliable skin test extract.

Commercial extracts are currently used in some countries.[109] One particular extract (Greer Laboratories) studied in the United States was shown to have a sensitivity of 99% and a specificity of 96%.[110] However, this reagent is not presently licensed for use by the Food and Drug Administration (FDA) in the United States, although it is nearing licensure.

Given the variability of allergen composition and lack of uniformly standardized reagents, skin testing should be done only by qualified specialists with full resuscitation equipment and medications available in the event of possible allergic reactions to the testing material.

Measurement of Latex-Specific IgE Antibodies

The use of *in vitro* serologic testing such as the RAST is very sensitive for specific populations, such as the spina bifida population, who have very high titers of latex-specific IgE. However, these assays are not very useful as a screening tool. A recent study compared three of the currently available quantitative modifications of the RAST for latex-specific IgE: CAP RAST (Pharmacia Biotech), microplate AlaSTAT (Diagnostic Products Corp.), and HY-TEC-EIA (HYTEC).[110] Intraassay agreement was 96%. CAP and AlaSTAT produced about 25% false-negative results. HY-TEC produced 27% false-positive results. Although these tests provide a useful means to confirm latex allergy, they are not completely reliable and caution should be used when patients have convincing clinical stories with discordant serologic testing. The patients who fall into this category may be challenged with a provocation test.

Provocation Tests

These tests are done when there is discrepancy between the patient's history and other forms of testing. They are contraindicated when there is a history of anaphylaxis. Individuals are tested by wearing a piece of a latex glove on a wet finger, and if there is no response then the entire glove is donned on a wet hand. A nonlatex glove is worn on the opposite hand as a negative control. The presence of pruritis, erythema, and rash within 15 to 30 minutes is considered positive. This type of testing has limitations that include lack of blinding, variable antigen concentrations in the gloves, and risk of systemic reaction. Furthermore, it is very difficult to evaluate false-negative provocation tests.

Modifications have been made to the provocation test to help circumvent some of these limitations; this has included the use of goggles and a face mask fitted with a filter to prevent respiratory symptoms. The hands are washed, the skin is pricked in three places on the wet volar surface of the hand, and gloves are placed on both hands with a liner used on the control side. Circular pressure is applied 50 times over these sites, and the patient is observed for up to 30 minutes.[111] A second stage can also be added if there is a negative result. The patient blows up the NRL glove and expels it gently on his or her face. A 20% drop in peak expiratory flow rates would constitute a positive test.[110] It is difficult to blind the patients during these challenges and to quantify the latex allergenic exposure. A more elaborate method uses a hooded exposure chamber and an air pump to introduce respirable latex particles in a graded and quantitative manner with appropriate masking. This procedure requires specialized equipment and laboratory space and is costly and labor intensive. However, this last method may be useful when the history and other testing are discordant and can quantify the severity of clinical latex sensitivity in research centers.[112]

MANAGEMENT

Avoidance

The cornerstone in managing latex allergy, and presently the only means to prevent allergic reactions, is avoidance of latex-containing products. Avoidance can be directed at those individuals who are at high risk for developing latex allergy but have not yet developed allergic symptoms, such as patients with spina bifida, health care workers, and children requiring multiple surgical interventions. In contrast, more focused avoidance efforts can be directed at asymptomatic patients who are detected to be sensitized to latex and known symptomatic patients. These patients should strive for a latex-safe environment, and they should wear a latex allergy identification bracelet. They should be educated regarding the possible cross-reactivity of the foods that share common antigens with latex (see earlier), especially if these foods are consumed for the first time.

A "latex-safe environment" is defined as an area where every effort is made to remove, reduce, contain, or separate by distance from allergic patients latex particulates or latex-containing products. Latex allergy should be clearly designated with appropriate warning signs on the patient's charts, room, and bed. Latex-containing products include but are not limited to gloves, catheters, drains, intravenous equipment, surgical tapes, adhesives, electrocardiogram pads, bandages, tourniquets, blood pressure cuffs, ventilation and airway equipment, syringe stoppers, and medication containers with stoppers. In the United States, the FDA has stipulated that all medical products and packaging containing latex be specifically labeled.[113]

All hospital workers who are in direct contact with latex-allergic patients should wear only nonlatex gloves. Powder-free, low-protein gloves can be worn by workers who do not have to care directly for latex-allergic patients but are caring for other patients in the vicinity of a patient with latex allergy. Powdered gloves have been incriminated because of their ability to disseminate latex allergens via aerosolization. Because of potential protein transfer, personnel not in contact with latex-allergic patients but handling equipment that may eventually come in contact with latex-allergic patients should wear nonlatex gloves.[114] For example, Swartz et al[115] reported on latex-allergic patients reacting to food prepared by fast-food workers donning latex gloves. Previously, caution was used when using gloves labeled "hypoallergenic" because these gloves were not necessarily latex free. They were designated as hypoallergenic because of the reduction in additives used in the manufacturing of the gloves that contribute to contact dermatitis, not the IgE-mediated reactions. The FDA has subsequently banned the term *hypoallergenic* with respect to latex gloves.

Prevention in the Workplace

The National Institute for Occupational Safety and Health and the Occupational Safety and Health Administration of the U.S. Department of Labor have developed recommendations for both employers and workers to help minimize exposure to latex and reduce the development of latex allergy.[116] Some of the specific recommendations include using nonlatex for activities not likely to involve contact with infectious agents; using powder-free, low-protein latex gloves when handing infectious agents; and using appropriate work practices to reduce likely exposure to latex.

Medical Prophylaxis

The effectiveness of premedication of patients with latex allergy before undergoing surgery has not been established to be an effective strategy and is presently not recommended. Two case reports differ as to whether treatment with glucocorticosteroids and antihistamines prevents or modifies the severity of allergic reactions.[117,118] By extrapolating from the experience of pretreating patients with allergy to radiocontrast dye,[119-121] a number of empiric regimens have been suggested but none have been compared in controlled trials.[122-124] Premedication cannot replace vigilant antigen avoidance even though it theoretically could reduce the severity of a potential reaction. Pharmacologic pretreatment is also controversial because it may mask the early signs of an anaphylactic reaction, which could delay early intervention.

FUTURE INTERVENTIONS

Other means by which to control latex allergy must continue to be considered because avoidance is not always reliable and the role of premedication is unproved. Latex allergy is an IgE-mediated disease and in theory could be treatable with immunotherapy. One of the major obstacles of this approach is identifying the relevant allergens to use for this purpose. A case report demonstrated that oral latex desensitization was possible in six health care workers who had severe latex allergy using noncompounded ammoniated latex.[125] After the hyposensitization protocol, the latex skin test size was reduced significantly in each of these reported patients and all were able to return to work without significant symptoms despite continued latex exposure.

Another case report documented the treatment of a latex-allergic patient using increasing weekly doses of a latex vaccine (ALK-Abello).[126] The vaccine was administered subcutaneously in incrementally increasing dosages until a systemic reaction occurred. At this point the dose was reduced slightly and maintained using weekly injections. Clinical symptoms improved, skin test reactivity decreased to latex-specific allergens, and the patient returned to work in an environment with significant levels of latex exposure. These few case reports do not support the use of routine latex immunotherapy currently; however, they may hold promise for the future.

A number of the latex allergens have been cloned and produced using recombinant technology. This should allow for more controlled diagnostic testing once all of the relevant allergens have been identified and cloned. By combining recombinant allergen technology with epitope-specific immunotherapy and possibly DNA vaccine immunotherapy, it may not be long before specific immunotherapy will extend to the treatment of latex allergy.

CONCLUSIONS

Latex allergy is a serious medical problem with enormous economic ramifications. The relevant issues related to latex allergy are summarized in Box 58-1. Significant strides have been made to characterize the antigens responsible for the development of latex allergy and to broaden understanding of the cross-reactivity of antigens that exist in our environment. Because of this diversity, the diagnosis can be elusive as a result of the variable clinical manifestations of latex allergy. One's threshold to refer a patient suspected of having a latex allergy should be low because there is no gold standard for making the diagnosis. A specialist qualified to discern the nuances of the appropriate investigations and treat the complications of the latex allergy testing should be involved in the patient's care. Once the diagnosis has been made, the mainstay of treatment is avoidance of latex allergens and patient education. Premedication and immunotherapy at this point are still investigational but may yield promising treatment options in the future. Box 58-2 provides an outline of the key therapeutic principles that should be considered when managing a patient with latex allergy.

HELPFUL WEBSITE

The National Latex Allergy Network website (http://latex-allergy.org/)

BOX 58-1	KEY CONCEPTS

Latex Allergy

- Natural rubber latex (NRL) is an important cause of type 1 (IgE-mediated) allergy, resulting in a broad spectrum of clinical manifestations that can range from local reactions to severe life-threatening systemic reactions.
- NRL contains several proteins that have been implicated in the pathogenesis of latex allergy. Many of these proteins cross-react with antigens from foods including, but not limited to, banana, avocado, and kiwi.
- Early identification of latex sensitization is essential to avoid future allergic reactions by unknown exposure. Diagnosis is confirmed by presence of latex-specific IgE antibody using skin prick testing or radioallergosorbent test.
- Avoidance of NRL allergens and clinically cross-reactive foods remains the cornerstone of treatment. This is especially important during medical, dental, and surgical procedures.
- Immunotherapy shows promise for the future management of latex-sensitized patients, but at this point it is still experimental.

BOX 58-2	THERAPEUTIC PRINCIPLES

AVOIDANCE

High-risk, nonsensitized individuals should
Prevent sensitization by using only low-protein, powder-free gloves.

Avoid all contact with latex from birth if spina bifida is a health-related factor.

Latex-sensitized individuals should
Strive for a "latex-safe environment" by removing, reducing, containing, or separating by distance latex particulates or latex-containing products by using latex-free gloves and avoiding products containing latex allergens.

Be educated about possible cross-reactivity with foods sharing common latex epitopes.

Wear latex allergy identification bracelets.

Caring for latex-sensitized individuals
Health care workers should use only nonlatex gloves while working with latex-allergic patients.

Patients with latex allergy should be clearly identified while in the hospital.

MEDICAL PROPHYLAXIS

Pretreatment of patients before surgical intervention with corticosteroids and antihistamines has not been shown to be effective.

IMMUNOTHERAPY

Although immunotherapy shows promise for future therapeutic intervention in latex-allergic patients, it is currently too early in development to be recommended.

REFERENCES

1. Nutter AF: Contact urticaria to rubber, *Br J Dermatol* 101:597-598, 1979.
2. Surgeon's and patient examination gloves: reclassification and medical glove guidance manual availability; proposed rule and notice, *Fed Reg* 64:146, July 30, 1999.
3. Sussman GL, Tarlo S, Dolovich J: The spectrum of IgE-mediated responses to latex, *JAMA* 265:2844-2847, 1991.
4. Archer BL, Barnard D, Cockbain EG, et al: Structure, composition and biochemistry of Hevea latex. In Bateman L, ed: *The chemistry and physics of rubber-like substances,* New York, 1963, John Wiley & Sons.
5. Ohm RF: *The Vanderbilt rubber handbook,* ed 13, Norwalk, Conn, 1990, RT Vanderbilt.
6. Slater JE: Rubber anaphylaxis, *N Engl J Med* 320:1126-1131, 1989.
7. Bubak ME, Reed CE, Fransway AF, et al: Allergic reactions to latex among health-care workers, *Mayo Clin Proc* 67:1075-1079, 1992.
8. Yunginger JW, Jones RT, Fransway AF, et al: Extractable latex allergens and proteins in disposable medical gloves and other rubber products, *J Allergy Clin Immunol* 93:836-841, 1994.
9. Jaeger D, Kleinhans D, Czuppon AB, et al: Latex-specific proteins causing immediate-type cutaneous, nasal, bronchial, and systemic reactions, *J Allergy Clin Immunol* 89:759-764, 1992.
10. Beezhold D, Beck WC: Surgical glove powders bind latex antigens, *Arch Surg* 127:1354-1359, 1992.
11. Seaton A, Cherrie B, Tunrbull J: Rubber glove asthma, *Br Med J* 296:531-535, 1988.
12. Baur X, Jager D: Airborne antigens from latex gloves, *Lancet* 335:912-917, 1990.
13. Tomazic VJ, Shampaine EL, Lamanna A, et al: Cornstarch powder on latex products is an allergen carrier, *J Allergy Clin Immunol* 93:751-758, 1994.
14. Czuppon AB, Chen Z, Rennert S, et al: The rubber elongation factor of rubber trees *(Hevea brasiliensis)* is the major allergen in latex, *J Allergy Clin Immunol* 92:690-695, 1993.
15. Goyvaerts E, Dennis M, Light D: Cloning and sequencing of the cDNA encoding tree rubber elongation factor of *Hevea brasiliensis, Plant Physiol* 97:317-321, 1991.
16. Attanyaka DP, Kekwick RG, Franklin FC: Molecular cloning and nucleotide sequencing of the rubber elongation factor gene from *Hevea brasiliensis, Plant Mol Biol* 16:1079-1081, 1991.
17. Wagner B, Krebitz M, Buck D, et al: Cloning, expression, and characterization of recombinant Hev b 3, a *Hevea brasiliensis* protein associated with latex allergy in patients with spina bifida, *J Allergy Clin Immunol* 104:1084-1092, 1999.
18. Yeang HY, Ward MA, Zamri AS, et al: Amino acid sequence similarity of Hev b 3 to two previously reported 27- and 23-kDa latex proteins allergenic to spina bifida patients, *Allergy* 53:513-519, 1998.
19. Beezhold DH, Sussman GL, Kostyal DA, et al: Identification of a 46-kD latex protein allergen in health care workers, *Clin Exp Immunol* 98:408-413, 1994.
20. Kostyal DA, Hickey VL, Noti JD, et al: Cloning and characterization of a latex allergen (Hev b 7): homology to patatin, a plant PLA2, *Clin Exp Immunol* 112:355-362, 1998.
21. Sowka S, Wagner S, Krebitz M, et al: cDNA cloning of the 43-kDa latex allergen Hev b 7 with sequence similarity to patatins and its expression in the yeast *Pichia pastoris, Eur J Biochem* 255:213-219, 1998.
22. Chye ML, Cheung KY: Beta-1,3-glucanase is highly-expressed in laticifers of *Hevea brasiliensis, Plant Mol Biol* 29:397-402, 1995.
23. Sunderasan E, Hamzah S, Hamid S, et al: Latex B-serum b-1,3-glucanase (Hev b II) and a component of the microhelix (Hev b IV) are major latex allergens, *J Nat Rubb Res* 10:82-99, 1995.
24. Beezhold DH, Kostyal DA, Sussman GL: IgE epitope analysis of the hevein preprotein: a major latex allergen, *Clin Exp Immunol* 108:114-121, 1997.
25. Lee H., Broekaert WF, Railhel NV: Co- and post-translational processing of the hevein preproprotein of latex of the rubber tree *(Hevea brasiliensis), J Biol Chem* 266:15944-15948, 1991.
26. Chen Z, Posch A, Lohaus C, et al: Isolation and identification of hevein as a major IgE-binding polypeptide in Hevea latex, *J Allergy Clin Immunol* 99:402-409, 1997.
27. Alenius H, Kalkkinen N, Reunala T, et al: The main IgE-binding epitope of a major latex allergen, prohevein, is present in its N-terminal 43-amino acid fragment, hevein, *J Immunol* 156:1618-1622, 1996.
28. O'Riordain G, Radaver C, Hoffmann-Sommergruber K, et al: Cloning and molecular characterization of the *Hevea brasiliensis* allergen Hev b 11, a class 1 chitinase, *Clin Exp Allergy* 32:455-462, 2002.

29. Slater JE, Vedvick T, Arthur-Smith A, et al: Identification, cloning and sequence of a major allergen (Hev b 5) from natural rubber latex *(Hevea brasiliensis), J Biol Chem* 271:25394-25399, 1996.

30. Akasawa A, Hsieh LS, Martin BM, et al: A novel acidic allergen, Hev b 5, in latex: purification, cloning, and characterization, *J Biol Chem* 271:25389-25393, 1996.

31. Neito A, Mazon A, Estornell F, et al: Profilin, a relevant allergen in lates allergy, *J Allergy Clin Immunol* 101:5207-5211, 1998.

32. Fuchs T, Spitzauer S, Vente C, et al: Natural latex, grass pollen, and weed pollen share IgE epitopes, *J Allergy Clin Immunol* 100:356-364, 1997.

33. Vallier P, Balland S, Harf R, et al: Identification of profilin as an IgE-binding component in latex from *Hevea brasiliensis:* clinical implications, *Clin Exp Allergy* 25:332-339, 1995.

34. Posch A, Chen Z, Wheeler C, et al: Characterization and identification of latex allergens by two-dimensional electrophoresis and protein microsequencing, *J Allergy Clin Immunol* 99:385-395, 1997.

35. Posch A, Chen Z, Dunn MJ, et al: Latex allergen database, *Electrophoresis* 18:2803-2810, 1997.

36. Kurup VP, Alenius H, Kelly KJ, et al: A two-dimensional electrophoretic analysis of latex peptides reacting with IgE and IgG antibodies from patients with latex allergy, *Int Arch Allergy Immunol* 109:58-67, 1996.

37. Yip L, Hickey V, Wagner B, et al: Skin prick test reactivity to recombinant latex allergens, *Int Arch Allergy Immunol* 121:292-299, 2000.

38. Slater JE, Vedvick T, Arthur-Smith A, et al: Identification, cloning, and sequence of a major allergen (Hev b 5) from natural rubber latex *(Hevea brasiliensis), J Biol Chem* 271:25394-25399, 1996.

39. Yeang HY, Cheong KF, Sunderasan E, et al: The 14.6 kd rubber elongation factor (Hev b 1) and 24 kd (Hev b 3) rubber particle proteins are recognized by IgE from patients with spina bifida and latex allergy, *J Allergy Clin Immunol* 98:628-632, 1996.

40. Wagner B, Krebitz M, Buck D et al: Cloning, expression, and characterization of recombinant Hev b 3, a *Hevea brasiliensis* protein associated with latex allergy in patients with spina bifida, *J Allergy Clin Immunol* 104:1084-1092, 1999.

41. Chen Z, Posch A, Lohaus C, et al: Isolation and identification of hevein as a major IgE-binding polypeptide in Hevea latex, *J Allergy Clin Immunol* 99:402-409, 1997.

42. Wagner B, Buck D, Hafner C, et al: Hev b 7 is a Hevea brasiliensis protein associated with latex allergy in children with spina bifida, *J Allergy Clin Immunol* 108:621-627, 2001.

43. Llatser R, Zambrano C, Guillaumet B: Anaphylaxis to natural rubber latex in a girl with food allergy, *Pediatrics* 94:736-737, 1994.

44. Blanco C, Carrillo T, Castillo R, et al: Latex allergy: clinical features and cross-reactivity with fruits, *Ann Allergy* 73:309-314, 1994.

45. M'Raihi L, Charpin D, Pons A, et al: Cross-reactivity between latex and banana, *J Allergy Clin Immunol* 87:129-130, 1991.

46. Nel A, Gujuluva C: Latex antigens: identification and use in clinical and experimental studies, including cross-reactivity with food and pollen allergens, *Ann Allergy Asthma Immunol* 81:388-401, 1998.

47. Brehler R, Theissen U, Mohr C, et al: "Latex-fruit syndrome": frequency of cross-reacting IgE antibodies, *Allergy* 52:404-410, 1997.

48. Beezhold DH, Sussman GL, Liss GM, et al: Latex allergy can induce clinical reactions to specific foods, *Clin Exp Allergy* 26:416-422, 1996.

49. Garcia JC, Moyano JC, Alverez M, et al: Latex allergy in fruit allergic patients, *Allergy* 53:532-536, 1998.

50. Levy DA, Mounedji N, Noirot C, et al: Allergic sensitization and clinical reactions to latex, food and pollen in adult patients, *Clin Exp Allergy* 30:270-275, 2000.

51. Van Loon LC, Van Strien EA: The families of pathogenesis-related proteins, their activities, and comparative analysis of PR-1 type proteins. *Physiol Mol Plant Pathol* 55:85-97, 1999.

52. Yagami T, Sato M, Nakamura A, et al: Plant defense-related enzymes as latex antigens, *J Allergy Clin Immunol* 101:379-385, 1998.

53. Clendennen SK, May GD: Differential gene expression in ripening banana fruit, *Plant Physiol* 115:463-469, 1997.

54. Diaz-Perales A, Collada C, Blanco C, et al: Class I chitinases with hevein-like domains, but not class II enzymes, are relevant chestnut and avocado allergens, *J Allergy Clin Immunol* 102:127-133, 1998.

55. Sanchez-Monge R, Blanco C, Díaz-Perales A, et al: Isolation and characterization of major banana allergens: identification as fruit class I chitinases, *Clin Exp Allergy* 29:673-680, 1999.

56. Hänninen AR, Mikkola JH, Kalkkinen N, et al: Increased allergen production in turnip (Brassica rapa) by treatments activating defense mechanisms, *J Allergy Clin Immunol* 104:194-201, 1999.

57. Turjanmaa K: Incidence of immediate allergy to latex gloves in hospital personnel, *Contact Dermatitis* 17:270-275, 1987.

58. Turjanmaa K, Makinen-Kiljunen S, Reunala T, et al: Natural rubber latex allergy: the European experience, *Immunol Allergy Clin North Am* 15:71-88, 2000.

59. Sussman GL: Latex allergy: an overview, *Can J Allergy Clin Immunol* 5:317-322, 2000.

60. Novembre E, Bernardini R, Brizzi I, et al: The prevalence of latex allergy in children seen in a university hospital allergy clinic, *Allergy* 52:101-105, 1997.

61. Ownby DR, Ownby HE, McCullough JA, et al: The prevalence of anti-latex IgE antibodies in 100 volunteer blood donors, *J Allergy Clin Immunol* 97:1188-1193, 1996.

62. Merrett TG, Merrett J, Kekwick R: The prevalence of immunoglobulin E antibodies to the proteins of rubber (Hevea brasiliensis) latex and grass *(Phleum pratense)* pollen in sera of British blood donors, *Clin Exp Allergy* 29:1572-1578, 1999.

63. Porri, P, Lemiere C, Bernbaum J, et al: Prevalence of latex sensitization in subjects attending health screening: implications for a perioperative screening, *Clin Exp Allergy* 27:413-417, 1997.

64. Lagier F, Vervloet D, Lhermet I, et al: Prevalence of latex allergy in operating room nurses, *J Allergy Clin Immunol* 90:319-322, 1992.

65. Kaczmarek RG, Silverman BG, Gross TP, et al: Prevalence of latex-specific IgE antibodies in hospital personnel, *Ann Allergy Asthma Immunol* 76:51-56, 1996.

66. Yassin MS, Lierl MB, Fischer TJ, et al: Latex allergy in hospital employees, *Ann Allergy* 72:245-249, 1994.

67. Liss GM, Sussman GL, Deal K, et al: Latex allergy: epidemiological study of 1351 hospital workers, *Occup Environ Med* 54:335-342, 1997.

68. Vandenplas O, Delwiche J-P, Evrard G, et al: Prevalence of occupational asthma due to latex among hospital personnel, *Am J Respir Crit Care Med* 151:54-60, 1995.

69. Truscott W: The industry perspective on latex, *Immunol Allergy Clin North Am* 15:89-122, 1995.

70. Hunt LW, Fransway AF, Reed CE, et al: An epidemic of occupational allergy to latex involving health care workers, *J Occup Environ Med* 37:1204-1209, 1995.

71. Porri F, Pradal M, Rud C, et al: Is systematic preoperative screening for muscle relaxant and latex allergy advisable? *Allergy* 50:374-377, 1995.

72. Means LJ, Rescorla FJ: Latex anaphylaxis: report of occurrence in two pediatric surgical patients and review of the literature, *J Pediatr Surg* 30:748-750, 1995.

73. Burrow GH, Vincent KA, Krajbich KI, et al: Latex allergy in non-spina bifida patients: unfamiliar intra-operative anaphylaxis, *Aust N Z J Surg* 68:183-187, 1998.

74. Slater JE: Latex allergy, *Ann Allergy* 70:1-6, 1993.

75. Hodgson CA, Andersen BD: Latex allergy: an unfamiliar cause of intra-operative cardiovascular collapse, *Anaesthesia* 49:507-509, 1994.

76. Dormans JP, Templeton JJ, Edmonds C, et al: Intraoperative anaphylaxis due to exposure to latex (natural rubber) in children, *J Bone Joint Surg* 76:1688-1691, 1994.

77. Kam PCA, Lee MSM, Thompson JF: Latex allergy: an emerging clinical and occupational health problem, *Anaesthesia* 52:570-572, 1997.

78. Gerber AC, Jörg W, Zbinden S, et al: Severe intraoperative anaphylaxis to surgical gloves: latex allergy, an unfamiliar condition, *Anesthesiology* 71:800-804, 1989.

79. Yassin MS, Sanyurah S, Lierl MB, et al: Evaluation of latex allergy in patients with meningomyelocele, *J Allergy Clin Immunol* 89:224-228, 1992.

80. Kwittken PL, Sweinberg SK, Campbell DE, et al: Latex hypersensitivity in children: clinical presentation and detection of latex-specific immunoglobulin E, *Pediatrics* 95:693-697, 1995.

81. Konz KR, Chia JK, Kurup VP, et al: Comparison of latex hypersensitivity among patients with neurologic defects, *J Allergy Clin Immunol* 95:950-954, 1995.

82. Tarlo SM, Sussman GL, Holness DL: Latex sensitivity in dental students and staff: a cross-sectional study, *J Allergy Clin Immunol* 99:396-401, 1997.

83. Liss GM, Sussman GL: Latex sensitization: occupational versus general population prevalence rates, *Am J Ind Med* 35:196-200, 1999.

84. De Swert LF, Van Laer KM, Verpoorten CM, et al: Determination of independent risk factors and comparative analysis of diagnostic methods for immediate type latex allergy in spina bifida patients, *Clin Exp Allergy* 27:1067-1076, 1997.

85. Kelly KJ, Pearson ML, Kurup VP, et al: A cluster of anaphylactic reactions in children with spina bifida during general anesthesia: epidemiologic features, risk factors, and latex hypersensitivity, *J Allergy Clin Immunol* 94:53-61, 1994.

86. Cremer R, Hoppe A, Kleine-Diepenbruck U, et al: Longitudinal study on latex sensitization in children with spina bifida, *Pediatr Allergy Immunol* 9:40-43, 1998.

87. Hunt LW, Fransway AF, Reed CE, et al: An epidemic of occupational allergy to latex involving health care workers, *J Occup Environ Med* 37:1204-1208, 1995.

88. Charous BL, Hamilton RG, Yunginger JW: Occupational latex exposure: characteristics of contact and systemic reactions in 47 workers, *J Allergy Clin Immunol* 94:12-16, 1994.

89. Charous BL: The puzzle of latex allergy: some answers, still more questions, *Ann Allergy* 73:277-281, 1994.

90. Lagier F, Badier M, Charpin D, et al: Latex as aeroallergen, *Lancet* 336:516-517, 1990.

91. Jaeger D, Kleinhans D, Czuppon AB, et al: Latex-specific proteins causing immediate-type cutaneous, nasal, bronchial, and systemic reactions, *J Allergy Clin Immunol* 89:759-768, 1992.

92. Tomazic VJ, Shampaine EL, Lamanna A, et al: Cornstarch powder on latex products is an allergen carrier, *J Allergy Clin Immunol* 93:751-758, 1994.

93. Swanson MC, Bubak ME, Hunt LW, et al: Quantification of occupational latex aeroallergens in a medical center, *J Allergy Clin Immunol* 94:445-451, 1994.

94. Vandenplas O, Charous B, Tarlo S: Latex allergy. In Bernstein I, Chan-Yeung M, Malo J-L, et al, eds: *Asthma in the workplace*, ed 2, New York, 1999, Marcel Dekker.

95. Moudgil GC: Anaesthesia and allergic drug reactions, *Can Anaesth Soc J* 33:400-403, 1986.

96. Serafin WE, Austen KF: Mediators of immediate hypersensitivity reactions, *N Engl J Med* 317:30-34, 1987.

97. Bochner BS, Lichtenstein LM: Anaphylaxis, *N Engl J Med* 324:1785-1789, 1991.

98. Seaton A, Cherrie B, Turnbull J: Rubber glove asthma, *Br Med J* 296:531-535, 1988.

99. Axelsson IGK, Johansson SGO, Wrangsjo K: IgE-mediated anaphylactoid reactions to rubber, *Allergy* 42:46-53, 1987.

100. Axelsson IGK, Eriksson M, Wrangsjö K: Anaphylaxis and angioedema due to rubber allergy in children, *Acta Paediatr Scand* 77:314-319, 1988.

101. Ownby DR, Tomlanovich M, Sammons N, et al: Anaphylaxis associated with latex allergy during barium enema examination, *AJR Am J Roentgenol* 156:903-908, 1991.

102. Laurent J, Malet R, Smiejan JM, et al: Latex hypersensitivity after natural delivery, *J Allergy Clin Immunol* 89:779-784, 1992.

103. Mansell P, Reckless JP, Lovell CR: Severe anaphylactic reaction to latex rubber surgical gloves, *Br Dent J* 178:86-87, 1995.

104. Sondheimer JM, Pearlman DS, Baily WC: Systemic anaphylaxis during rectal manometry with a latex balloon, *Am J Gastroenterol* 84:975-978, 1989.

105. Grattan CEH, Kennedy CTC: Angioedema during dental treatment, *Contact Dermatitis* 13:333-336, 1985.

106. Schwartz HJ: Latex a potential hidden "food" allergen in fast food restaurants, *J Allergy Clin Immunol* 95:139-144, 1990.

107. Sussman G, Beezhold D: Allergy to latex rubber, *Ann Intern Med* 122:43-46, 1995.

108. Jones RT, Scheppmann DL, Heilman DK, et al: Prospective study of extractable latex allergen contents of disposable gloves, *Ann Allergy* 73:321-325, 1994.

109. Blanco C, Carrillo T, Ortega N, et al: Comparison of skin-prick test and specific serum IgE determination for the diagnosis of latex allergy, *Clin Exp Allergy* 28:971-976, 1998.

110. Hamilton RG, Adkinson NF Jr: Multi-Center Latex Skin Testing Study Task Force. Diagnosis of natural rubber latex allergy: multicenter latex skin testing efficacy study, *J Allergy Clin Immunol* 102:482-490, 1998.

111. Hamilton RG, Adkinson NF Jr: Validation of the latex glove provocation procedure in latex-allergic subjects, *Ann Allergy Asthma Immunol* 79:266-272, 1997.

112. Kurtz KM, Hamilton RG, Adkinson NF Jr: Role and application of provocation in the diagnosis of occupational latex allergy, *Ann Allergy Asthma Immunol* 83:634-639, 1999.

113. Food and Drug Administration: Natural rubber-containing medical devices: user labeling, *Fed Reg* 62:51021, 1997.

114. Beezhold DH, Reschke JE, Allen JH, et al: Latex protein: a hidden "food" allergen? *Allergy Asthma Proc* 21:301-306, 2000.

115. Schwartz J, Braude BM, Gilmour RF, et al: Intraoperative anaphylaxis to latex, *Can J Anesth* 37:589-592, 1990.

116. NIOSH Alert: *Preventing allergic reactions to natural rubber latex in the workplace*, Cincinnati, Ohio, 1997, Department of Health and Human Services. Pub No. 97-135.

117. Sockin SM, Young MC: Preoperative prophylaxis of latex anaphylaxis, *J Allergy Clin Immunol* 87:269-274, 1991.

118. Kwittken PL, Becker J, Oyefara B, et al: Latex hypersensitivity reactions despite prophylaxis, *Allergy Proc* 13:123-127, 1992.

119. Bielory L, Kaliner MA: Anaphylactoid reactions to radiocontrast materials, *Int Anesthesiol Clin* 23:97-100, 1985.

120. Greenberger PA, Patterson R, Tapio CM: Prophylaxis against repeated radiocontrast media reactions in 857 cases: adverse experience with cimeditine and safety of beta-adrenergic antagonists, *Arch Intern Med* 145:2197-2200, 1985.

121. Lasser EC, Berry CC, Talner EB, et al: Pretreatment with corticosteroids to alleviate reactions to intravenous contrast material, *N Engl J Med* 317:845-849, 1987.

122. Moneret-Vautrin DA, Laxenaire MC, Bavoux F: Allergic shock to latex and ethylene oxide during surgery for spina bifida, *Anesthesiology* 73:556-559, 1990.

123. Pasquariello CA, Lowe DA, Schwartz RE: Intraoperative anaphylaxis to latex, *Pediatrics* 91:983-987, 1993.

124. Tosi LL, Slater JE, Shaer C, et al: Latex allergy in spina bifida patients: prevalence and surgical implications, *J Pediatr Orthop* 13:709, 1993.

125. Toci GR, Shah SR, Beezhold DH, et al: Oral latex desensitization in healthcare providers. *Can J Allergy Clin Immunol* 7:83-91, 2002.

126. Pereira C, Rico P, Lourenco M, et al: Specific immunotherapy for occupational latex allergy, *Allergy* 54:291-293, 1999.

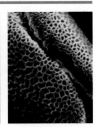

CHAPTER 59

Insect Sting Anaphylaxis

ROBERT E. REISMAN

Stinging insect allergy is a relatively common medical problem, estimated to affect at least 0.3% to 3% of the population and responsible for at least 40 deaths per year in the United States[1] and considerable anxiety in lifestyle modification. During the past 25 years, the pathogenesis, diagnosis, and treatment of allergic reactions caused by insect stings have been clarified, and reliable guidelines have been established for the assessment of this allergic disease. The availability of purified insect venoms and the clinical application of measurements of venom-specific IgE (skin test, radioallergosorbent test [RAST], and serum venom–specific IgG) provided the appropriate tools to understand and modulate this disease process. Criteria have been established for the use of venom as a diagnostic skin test reagent, correlating with the presence of potential clinical insect sting allergy. Insect venom immunotherapy (VIT) is remarkably effective in individuals at potential risk of insect sting anaphylaxis, inducing a permanent "cure" in many individuals.

There remain pertinent unresolved issues, including the identification of individuals who may be at risk for initial insect sting anaphylaxis, further insight into factors that affect the natural history of venom allergy, and objective criteria with which to define the adequate duration of VIT. More recent observations that require resolution are the rare occurrence of sting reactions in people with negative venom skin tests[2,3] and elevation of baseline serum tryptase levels in some people who have more severe allergic reactions.[4]

This chapter reviews the general concepts relating to insect sting allergy and, in particular, addresses those aspects that are more relevant to children.

EPIDEMIOLOGY/ETIOLOGY

Development of Insect Sting Allergy

At present, no predictive criteria identify individuals at risk of acquiring an insect sting allergy. The majority of people who have had insect sting anaphylaxis have tolerated prior stings without reaction. In general, no time relationship exists between the last uneventful sting and the subsequent sting that leads to an allergic reaction.[5] A further confusing observation is the occurrence of initial insect sting anaphylaxis after the first known insect sting, primarily in children, raising the issue of the cause of sensitization or the pathogenesis of this initial reaction.[6] As insect stings always cause pain, in contrast to insect bites, the history in this regard seems reliable.

In the past, there has been a common misconception that large local reactions after insect stings, particularly those that were increasing in size with each sting, might precede an anaphylactic reaction. These large local reactions are defined as reactions extending from the sting site, often peaking in 24 to 48 hours and lasting up to 1 week. For example, the swelling from a sting on the finger may extend to the wrist or elbow. Clinical observations in recent years indicate that these large local reactions tend to be repetitive with a very low incidence, perhaps less than 5%, of subsequent systemic allergic reactions.[7]

Venoms are potent sensitizing substances. For example, individuals who collect snake venoms often develop inhalant-type allergy to venom. The occurrence of many simultaneous stings, such as 100 to 200 stings, can sensitize individuals for subsequent single-sting anaphylaxis. This potential problem is now recognized more often because of the increasing spread of the "killer bees," which may inflict several hundred stings at one time.[8]

Demographic Studies

Demographic studies suggest that the incidence of insect sting allergy in the general population ranges between 0.4% to 3%. Approximately 33% to 40% of individuals who have insect sting anaphylaxis are atopic. There is a 2:1 male/female ratio that is probably a reflection of exposure rather than any specific sex predilection. The majority of reactions that do occur are in younger individuals, although the fatality rate is greater in adults.[9-12] It is estimated that 40 to 50 deaths per year occur in the United States as the result of insect sting anaphylaxis. Most individuals had no warning or indication of their allergies and had tolerated prior stings with no difficulty.

The Insects

Insects that sting are members of the order Hymenoptera of the class Insecta. There are two major subgroups: vespids, which include the yellow jacket, hornet, and wasp; and aphids, which include the honeybee and bumblebee. In most parts of the United States, yellow jackets are the principal cause of allergic reactions. These insects nest in the ground or in the walls of homes and are frequently disturbed by lawn mowing, gardening, or other outdoor activities. Yellow jackets feed on substances containing sugar and are commonly attracted to food and garbage. Hornets nest in shrubs and trees and are disturbed by activities such as trimming hedges. Wasps are more prevalent early in the summer season. In some areas of the country, such as Texas, they are the most frequent cause of sting reactions. Honeybees and bumblebees are docile and sting only when provoked. People have received multiple stings from honeybees when their hives, which contain thousands of insects, were threatened.

The stinging apparatus originates in the abdomen of the female insect. It consists of a sac containing venom attached to a barbed stinger. The honeybee's stinger has multiple barbs, which usually cause the stinging apparatus to detach from the insect, leading to its death. In contrast, the stingers of vespids have few barbs and these insects can inflict multiple stings.

Africanized honeybees, or the "killer bees," have received much publicity.[8] They entered this country in south Texas and are now present in Arizona and California. They were introduced into Brazil from Africa in 1956 for the purpose of more productive pollination and have gradually spread north. The venom components of the Africanized honeybees and the domesticated European honeybees that are found throughout the United States are similar. The venom of the Africanized honeybee is no more allergic or toxic than that of the European honeybee. However, African honeybees are much more aggressive. Massive stinging incidents have occurred, leading to death from venom toxicity. Africanized honeybees are expected to continue to move northward, although they do not survive well in colder climates.

The fire ant, *Solenopsis invicta,* is a nonwinged Hymenopteran. This insect is found in the southeastern and south central United States, especially along the Gulf Coast. They have now spread to California. The fire ant attaches itself to a person by biting with its jaws. It then pivots around its head and stings at multiple sites in a circular pattern. The stinger is located on the abdomen. Within 24 hours a sterile pustule develops, which is diagnostic of the fire ant's sting. Allergic reactions to fire ant stings are becoming increasingly common in the southern United States.[13,14]

Unlike insect stings, insect bites rarely cause anaphylaxis. Biting insects such as mosquitoes deposit salivary gland secretions that have no relation to venom allergens. Anaphylaxis has been described after the bites of deer flies, bed bugs, and black flies. Large local reactions, however, are much more common, and recent studies suggest that the reactions to mosquito bites may be associated with IgE and perhaps IgG antibodies.

These large local reactions from mosquito bites are more common in young children. Over time and with repeated exposure, the reactions become less intense and are less frequent problems in adolescents and adults. Elevated titers of salivary gland–specific IgE and IgG correlate with the intensity of the local reactions and appear to be the responsible immunologic mediators of the reactions.[15,16]

DIFFERENTIAL DIAGNOSIS: REACTION TO INSECT STINGS

Normal Reaction

The usual or normal reaction to an insect sting consists of localized pain, swelling, and erythema at the site of the sting. This reaction usually subsides within several hours. Little treatment is needed other than analgesics and cold compresses.

Large Local Reactions

More extensive local reactions are common. Swelling extends from a sting site over a large area, often peaking at 48 hours and lasting as long as 7 days. Fatigue and nausea may develop. The cause of these large local reactions has not been established, although they may be mediated by IgE antibodies. After a large local reaction occurs, most people, including children, have positive skin tests to venom, suggesting the possibility of an allergic pathogenesis.[7,17] Medical treatment usually consists of aspirin or antihistamines. If the swelling is extensive and disabling, systemic steroids such as prednisone 40 mg/day taken orally for 2 or 3 days is beneficial.

On occasion, large local reactions are confused with cellulitis. However, cellulitis rarely develops after an insect sting; I have never seen that occur. A common therapeutic error, particularly in emergency department settings, is to treat with antibiotics. In addition, tetanus prophylaxis is unnecessary.

In people who have had large local reactions from stings, the risk for subsequent re-sting anaphylaxis is very low. In our study of a large series of people, the risk of anaphylaxis was about 5%.[7] In one study of children, the risk of anaphylaxis was only 2%.[17] In this latter study, most children had positive skin tests, which became less reactive over time.

People who have had large local reactions do not require venom skin tests and they generally are not candidates for VIT. Also, in our study the occurrence of subsequent large local reactions was not affected by VIT.[7] However, one recent case report indicated that VIT could have been helpful in reducing the large local reaction in a patient who was repeatedly exposed to insect stings.[18]

Toxic Reactions

Toxic reactions to constituents of venom may occur after many simultaneous stings (50 to 100). The reaction has the same clinical characteristics as anaphylaxis. Exposure to large amounts of insect venom frequently stimulates production of IgE antibodies. People may have positive venom skin tests after toxic reactions. If they do, they are at potential risk for allergic reactions to subsequent single stings.

Unusual Reactions

There have been rare reports of vasculitis, nephrosis, neuritis, encephalitis, and serum sickness occurring in a temporal relationship to insect stings.[19] Sometimes anaphylaxis has preceded these reactions. The symptoms usually start several days to several weeks after the sting and may last for a long period.

Serum sickness, characterized by urticaria, joint pain, and fever, may occur approximately 7 to 10 days after an insect sting.[20] An immune pathogenesis is suggested by consistent findings of venom-specific IgE and, on occasion, venom-specific IgG. People who have had venom-induced serum sickness may be at risk for acute anaphylaxis after subsequent insect stings and may therefore be candidates for VIT, which provides protection from subsequent sting reactions.

Anaphylaxis

Other than a prior reaction, no clinical criteria or predictors identify people at potential risk for anaphylaxis from insect stings. The clinical features of anaphylaxis from an insect sting are the same as those from anaphylaxis from any other cause. The most common symptoms are dermal: generalized urticaria, flushing, and angioedema. Life-threatening symptoms include edema of the upper airways, circulatory collapse with shock and hypotension, and bronchospasm. The symptoms usually start within 10 to 15 minutes after a sting; on occasion reactions have occurred as long as 72 hours later. Compared with adults, children have a higher incidence of dermal (hives, angioedema) reactions only and a lower incidence of more severe anaphylactic symptoms.[21]

Severe anaphylaxis, however, may occur at any age, but most deaths from anaphylaxis have occurred in adults. In our study[22] of 158 patients with severe anaphylaxis, there was a fairly uniform age distribution. Of the reactions, 21% occurred in children younger than 10 years old, and an additional 19% occurred in people between the ages of 11 and 20. There were 45 patients who had the most severe reactions as defined by loss of consciousness. This reaction was more common in adults; 24% of those were younger than 20.

EVALUATION AND MANAGEMENT

Natural History of Insect Sting Anaphylaxis

To assess appropriate intervention, it is necessary to understand the natural history of any disease process. This is particularly true of insect sting allergy. Extracts prepared by crushing or grinding whole insect bodies were used for more than 40 years for diagnosis and treatment. It was generally accepted that these extracts were therapeutically potent and provided protection against further sting reactions. It is now clear that these whole body extracts are impotent, lack sufficient venom contact, are unreliable for diagnosis, and are ineffective for treatment. The only explanation for the mistaken confidence in these extracts was the failure to understand the natural history of insect sting allergy. Individuals may spontaneously lose their clinical sensitivity.

Observations of individuals who have had allergic reactions from insect stings and who did not receive VIT have provided insight into the natural history of this allergy and suggest that insect sting allergy is a self-limiting process for many people. In the initial study[23] that documented the efficacy of VIT, 40% of people treated with either placebo or whole body extracts failed to react to subsequent stings. These observations were extended in a study of a large number of people who had insect sting reactions and were observed without treatment.[5] Overall, the incidence of field re-sting reactions was higher in adults than in children but averaged about 60%. There was no relationship between the time interval between the sting reaction and subsequent re-sting. The severity of the anaphylactic symptoms was an important criterion. The individuals with more severe reactions had a higher incidence of re-sting reactions. Finally, when a re-sting reaction did occur, the symptoms were generally similar to those that had occurred previously.

Studies of reactions to intentional insect sting challenges in people who have had prior reactions and had positive skin tests have showed similar results. Reaction rates to these intentional re-stings have varied from 25% to 60%.[24-26] Unfortunately, no immunologic criteria, such as skin test reactivity or titers of serum venom–specific IgE or IgG, distinguish or identify sting challenge reactors from nonreactors.

Children who have dermal reactions (urticaria, angioedema) only, without other allergic symptoms, are a very specific subgroup. These children have a very low re-sting reaction rate, and when reaction does occur, it tends to be of similar intensity.[27] In the Johns Hopkins University study, 84 re-stings occurred in 36 children receiving VIT with a very low systemic allergic re-sting rate (1.2%). There were 196 re-stings in 86 children who did not receive VIT with 18 reactions, a reaction rate of 18.6% per patient and 9.2% per re-sting. Of the reactions that did occur, 16 were milder and 2 were the same in severity. None were more severe. In the large study of field re-stings,[5] 64 children had dermal symptoms only with the initial reaction; 30% had re-sting reactions, of which two were of moderate intensity and one was of severe intensity. Thus three children had more severe symptoms with a re-sting. Overall these data suggest that children who have dermal reactions only have a very benign prognosis and generally do not retain their allergic sensitivity.

Diagnosis and Detection of Venom-Specific IgE

Venom Skin Tests

The diagnosis of potential venom allergy is dependent on the history of insect sting anaphylaxis and the presence of venom-specific IgE, usually detected by the immediate skin test reaction. Both of these components are necessary to document the diagnosis of insect sting allergy and the possibility of administering VIT.

A positive venom skin test without a history of an allergic reaction does not indicate a risk for venom anaphylaxis. The majority of people who have had large local insect sting reactions do have positive venom skin tests but, as noted earlier, have a small risk of anaphylaxis. Some individuals who have a "normal" insect sting will have a transient positive skin test.

Five commercial venoms (honeybee, yellow jacket, Polistes wasp, yellow hornet, and white-faced hornet) are available for testing and treatment. People suspected of having insect sting allergy are usually tested with all five venoms. Intradermal skin tests are performed starting with venom doses usually around 0.001 μg/ml and testing up to a concentration of 1 μg/ml.[28] Greater venom concentrations may cause irritative reactions that are not immunologically specific.

Skin tests with extracts prepared from whole bodies of fire ants appear to be reliable in identifying allergic individuals with few false-positive reactions in nonallergic controls.[13,14] Fire ant venom, which is not commercially available at present, has been collected and compared with fire ant whole body extract. The results of skin tests and in vitro tests show that venom is a better diagnostic antigen. However, whole body extracts can be prepared that apparently contain sufficient allergen and are reliable for skin test diagnosis. These results suggest that the allergens responsible for reactions can be preserved in the preparation of these whole body extracts, but future availability of fire ant venom may provide a more potent, reliable material.

In Vitro Measurement of Venom-Specific IgE

Venom-specific IgE can also be measured in the serum by in vitro tests (RASTs). In general, the skin test is a more sensitive test for the detection of venom-specific IgE than the in vitro test. In addition, the sensitivity of the RAST may vary from laboratory to laboratory. The skin test remains a preferred test for the diagnosis of venom allergy. When skin tests cannot be performed or reliably interpreted, such as in people with dermatographism, or when they give equivocal results in the presence of a highly suspect history, measurement of serum venom–specific IgE may be helpful.

Chipps et al[29] reported 44 children (mean age, 9.6 years) who had had allergic reactions to an insect sting and positive venom skin tests. Venom-specific IgE was detected in 77% of the children. In our studies[22] of people with serious anaphylaxis, 144 of 149 people had positive venom skin tests. Five people had negative skin tests up to a venom testing concentration of 0.1 μg/ml; three of these people had positive RASTs and one had a borderline RAST. The one person with negative skin tests (0.1 μg/ml) and a negative RAST was tested 10 years after the sting reaction.

Recently, people have been described who had a history of venom anaphylaxis, had negative venom skin tests, and reacted again to a subsequent intentional sting challenge.[2] This observation has raised the issue of the accuracy or reliability of the venom skin test. These individuals represent a very small percentage of people who have had allergic reactions to insect stings.

Although the issue of the approach to the negative skin test reactor who has had moderate to severe sting anaphylaxis is still under review, the current recommendation is to perform a RAST. If the RAST is positive, VIT would be indicated. If the RAST is negative, skin tests should be repeated in 3 to 6 months. People with a history of a moderately severe reaction should be advised about the potential sensitivity and to carry emergency medication.[2,3]

Baseline serum tryptase levels have been found to be elevated in some people who had insect sting anaphylaxis, particularly in people who have had more severe symptoms. This has led to a search for mast cell disease in these people. It is postulated that with an increased number of mast cells, venom may release mediators on either an immunologic or a nonimmunologic basis and lead to more severe symptoms. These people may require more intensive VIT, as discussed later.[4]

THERAPY

Acute Reaction

The medical treatment for acute anaphylaxis is the same as that for anaphylaxis from any cause and is detailed in Chapter 60. Epinephrine is the drug of choice and should be administered as soon as possible, even if symptoms are mild. The use of other medications depends on the symptom complex and includes antihistamines, steroids, oxygen, and vasopressors. Specific attention should be directed at the airway patency because upper airway swelling has been a major cause of death.

If the insect stinger remains in the skin, which most frequently occurs after a honeybee sting, it should be gently flicked off. Care should be take to avoid squeezing the sac, which could deposit more venom. Because the venom is deposited very quickly after the sting, this procedure may not be very helpful unless it is done immediately after the sting.

Prophylaxis

Individuals at risk of an allergic reaction are advised to use precautions to avoid subsequent stings. When outside, especially when involved in activities that might increase insect exposure such as gardening, these individuals should wear slacks, long-sleeve shirts, and shoes. Cosmetics, perfumes, and hair sprays, which attract insects, should be avoided. Light-colored clothing is less likely to attract insects. Particular care should be taken outside around food and garbage, which especially attracts yellow jackets. Individuals at risk are advised to carry epinephrine, available in preloaded syringes for self-administration. As mentioned earlier, epinephrine should be administered at the earliest sign of an acute allergic reaction from an insect sting. Studies comparing individuals who have had fatal allergic reactions with individuals who have had serious nonfatal reactions suggest that the use of epinephrine may be the decisive factor in determining the outcome.[30]

An obvious problem is how long people should keep epinephrine available; at this time, no clear-cut answer to that question is available. This recommendation for availability of epinephrine is not a benign recommendation. Patients and families are often concerned about having it available in all situations, including school, work, and home, and, as indicated in a recent study, must be continually reeducated regarding its use.[31] Currently, conversion to a negative skin test is often used as a criterion to indicate loss of clinical sensitivity and to advise patients and families that continued availability of epinephrine is no longer necessary.

Venom Immunotherapy

Insect venom extracts for diagnosis and therapy have been available for approximately 25 years. Although some questions remain, the concepts of the treatment have been fairly well established. This therapy is remarkably effective, preventing subsequent allergic reactions in more than 98% of treated patients and, in many instances, providing a permanent "cure." Major remaining issues relate to the refining of the selection process for people requiring VIT and refining criteria for duration of treatment.

TREATMENT: VENOM IMMUNOTHERAPY

Patient Selection

Potential candidates for VIT are people who have had an allergic reaction from an insect sting and have a positive venom skin test or elevated levels of serum venom–specific IgE (Table 59-1). As noted, studies of the natural history of insect sting allergy have shown that only approximately 60% or less of these individuals will have a subsequent reaction when re-stung.[5] The incidence of these sting reactions is influenced by age and the nature of the anaphylactic symptoms. Adults are more likely to have re-sting reactions than children, and the more severe the symptoms, the more likely it is that the reaction will recur. These observations influence the decision regarding patient selection for immunotherapy. Children with dermal (hives, angioedema) reactions only have a very benign prognosis, do not require immunotherapy,[27] and can be managed with availability of epinephrine. Individuals of any age who have had severe allergic reactions should be advised to receive VIT; this is particularly true of people who have had loss of consciousness. Current recommendations are to administer VIT to adults who have had mild to moderate allergic sting reactions. This decision may

TABLE 59-1 Indications for Venom Immunotherapy in Patients with Positive Venom Skin Tests or Elevated Titers of Venom-Specific IgE (RAST)*

Insect Sting Reaction	Venom Immunotherapy
"Normal" transient pain swelling	No
Extensive local swelling	No†
Anaphylaxis	
Severe	Yes
Moderate	Yes
Mild, dermal only	
Children	No
Adults	Yes‡
Serum sickness	Yes
Toxic	Yes

Modified from Reisman RE: Allergy to stinging insects. In Grammer LC, Greenberger PA, eds: *Patterson's allergic diseases*, ed 6, Philadelphia, 2002, Lippincott Williams & Wilkins.

*Venom immunotherapy is not indicated for individuals with negative venom skin tests and negative radioallergosorbent tests (RASTs).

†Venom immunotherapy might be effective and a trial might be advisable if sting risk is high (see text).

‡Patients in this group might be managed without venom (see text).

require evaluation of other risk factors such as co-existing medical problems, concomitant medication use, patient lifestyle, and risk of sting exposure. People who have had serum sickness–like reactions are also candidates for VIT. If these individuals are reexposed to venom, they are at potential risk for acute anaphylaxis.

A diagnostic sting challenge has been suggested as a criterion for initiating VIT. This approach has been suggested because of the repeated observations that only 60% or less of individuals thought to be at risk for a sting reaction because of a history of a prior reaction and the presence of a positive skin test do react when re-stung. The problems with the sting challenge relate to its safety, reliability, and practicality. Observations of both field stings and intentional sting challenges have shown similar results. Approximately 20% of people who initially tolerate a re-sting with no difficulty react after another subsequent sting.[5,32] More important, this diagnostic sting challenge raises serious medical and ethical issues. Life-threatening reactions have occurred after intentional sting challenges in patients who did not receive VIT. It is my opinion that patients who have a high risk of serious anaphylaxis, such as adults who have had prior severe reactions, should not be intentionally rechallenged and should be given immunotherapy on the basis of their history and skin test reactivity, recognizing that some of these patients may not need therapy. Furthermore, in the United States it is highly impractical to have sufficient referral centers for diagnostic challenge studies.

Hauk et al[33] conducted sting challenges in 113 children with histories of sting anaphylaxis; children who had had life-threatening anaphylaxis were omitted. Two challenges were performed at 2- to 6-week intervals. The authors concluded that the dual-sting challenge was the best predictor of reactions to subsequent stings and need for VIT. They also stated that these challenge procedures were not recommended for adults because of increased risk.

Venom Selection

The commercial venom product brochure recommends treatment with all venoms to which there are positive skin tests. As a result, many people are treated with multiple venoms, despite the history of a single-sting reaction. The basic issue is really whether multiple skin test reactions represent specific venom allergy or cross-reactivity among different venoms. Extensive studies of venom cross-reactivity can be summarized as follows.[34-37]

- Extensive cross-reactivity exists between the two major North American hornet venoms, yellow hornet and bald-faced hornet.
- Extensive cross-reactivity exists between yellow jacket and hornet venoms.
- Limited cross-reactivity exists between yellow jacket and Polistes venoms.
- A more complex relationship exists between honeybee and vespid venoms. There may be no cross-reaction, extensive cross-reaction, or reaction to a major allergen in one venom cross-reacting with a minor allergen in the other venom.

The practical application of these data suggest that almost all people who have had allergic reactions to yellow jacket or hornet stings should be expected to have positive skin test reactions to both of these venoms. In this situation, VIT with one venom, more commonly yellow jacket, provides adequate protection.[38] Approximately 50% of people who have had yellow jacket or hornet sting reactions also have positive skin test reactions to Polistes venom. Polistes VIT is not necessary. The converse is also true, with half of the people who have had Polistes sting reactions having positive skin tests to yellow jacket or hornet venom and requiring treatment with Polistes venom only.

People who have had positive skin tests to both yellow jacket and honeybee venoms are more difficult to treat with single venoms, unless the history of the offending insect is clear.

The implications of these observations for therapy are clear. If the offending insect can be identified accurately or if there is a significant difference in the degree of skin test reactivity, knowledge of these cross-reactions should lead to single-venom therapy whenever possible, despite the presence of multiple positive skin test reactions. This is particularly true in children in whom the administration of a single venom is much better tolerated than the administration of three or four venoms.

Bumblebees, which are solitary bees, are rare causes of insect sting reactions. Recently, however, exposure to bumblebees has become a potential occupational hazard because of their use in greenhouses for pollination. Bumblebee venom is not commercially available at the present for diagnosis and treatment. People who have had allergic reactions to bumblebee stings should be tested with honeybee venom but may not react because of sensitivity to an allergen specific to the bumblebee venom.[39] If skin test reactions to honeybee venom are positive, it can be used for immunotherapy.

Immunotherapy with whole body fire ant extract appears to be quite effective. Because this extract is a good diagnostic agent, this therapeutic response could be anticipated. One study that compared the results of fire ant re-stings in whole body extract–treated patients and untreated patients confirmed the effectiveness of treatment.[40] In the treatment group, there were 47 re-stings with one systemic reaction in contrast to the 11 untreated control patients, in whom 11 restings in 6 patients all resulted in systemic reactions.

Allergic reactions to fire ant stings are more common in children and have been reported in children as young as 15 to 39 months old.[41] No data are available for children who have had cutaneous allergic reactions only and on whether they could be managed with emergency medication, analogous to children who react to the winged Hymenoptera.

Dosing Schedule

VIT is administered in a manner similar to other forms of immunotherapy (Tables 59-2 and 59-3). Treatment is initiated in small doses, usually from 0.01 to 0.1 μg, and incremental doses are given until the maintenance dose is reached, traditionally 100 μg. The selection of a starting dose is really based on the intensity of the skin test reaction rather than on the nature of the allergic symptoms. A number of dosing regimens have been suggested. A commonly used schedule suggests the use of two or three injections during weekly buildup phases with doses doubled or tripled at 30-minute intervals. Maintenance doses can then be reached in 4 to 6 weeks. Rush desensitization therapy has also been given with multiple doses administered, often in a hospital setting, over a period of 2 or 3 days to 1 week. The more rapid schedules appear to be accompanied by a more rapid increase in venom-specific IgG. A slower schedule used for other types of allergen immunotherapy is the weekly administration of a single-venom dose. Reported immunotherapy reaction rates with both rapid and slower schedules vary but are not significantly different. The critical issue is to reach the top maintenance dose.

Once the top maintenance dose is reached, it can be administered every 4 weeks during the first year. The maintenance interval can then be extended to 6 weeks after the first year and to 8 weeks after the second year. This has been done with no loss of clinical effectiveness or increase in reaction rate. More recent studies indicate that the interval can be extended to 3 months with no difficulty.[42] The top maintenance dose for a single venom is 100 μg; 50 μg has been given as the

TABLE 59-2 General Venom Immunotherapy Dosing Guidelines

Initial dose	Dose of 0.01 to 0.1 μg, depending on degree of skin test reaction
Incremental doses	Schedules vary from "rush" therapy, administering multiple venom injections over several days, to traditional once-weekly injections (see Table 59-3).
Maintenance dose	Doses of 50 to 100 μg of single venoms, 300 μg of mixed vespid venom
Maintenance interval	4 wk 1st yr 6 wk 2nd yr 8 wk 3rd yr
Duration of therapy	Stop if skin test becomes negative or if the finite time, 3 to 5 yr, has been reached (see text).

From Reisman RE: Allergy to stinging insects. In Grammer LC, Greenberger PA, eds: *Patterson's allergic diseases*, ed 6, Philadelphia, 2002, Lippincott Williams & Wilkins.

TABLE 59-3 Representative Examples of Venom Immunotherapy Dosing Schedules[a]

	Traditional	Modified Rush	Rush
Day			
1	0.1	0.1	0.1†
		0.3	0.3
		0.6	0.6
			1.0
			3.0
			5.0
			10.0
2			20.0
			35.0
			50.0‡
			75.0
3			100.0
Week			
1	0.3	1.0	
		3.0	
2		5.0	100
		10.0	Repeat every 4 wk
3	3.0	20.0	
4	5.0	35.0	
5	10.0	50.0‡	
6	20.0	65.0	
7	35.0	80.0	
8	50.0‡	100.0	
9	65.0		
10	80.0	100.0	
11	100.0	Repeat every 4 wk	
12			
13	100.0		
	Repeat every 4 wk		

From Reisman RE: Allergy to stinging insects. In Grammer LC, Greenberger PA, eds: *Patterson's allergic diseases*, ed 6, Philadelphia, 2002, Lippincott Williams & Wilkins.

*Starting dose may vary depending on patient's skin test sensitivity. Subsequent doses modified by local or systemic reactions. Doses expressed in micrograms.

†Sequential venom doses administered on same day at 20- to 30-minute intervals.

‡Fifty micrograms may be used as top dose.

top dose with good results.[38] A mixed vespid venom preparation that contains the two hornet venoms and yellow jacket venom is available for therapy. The top dose of this preparation is 300 μg.

Venom Immunotherapy Reactions

VIT may cause reactions similar to those induced by other types of allergenic extracts. These reactions may pose a more difficult clinical problem because to ensure protection, it is necessary to administer maximum venom doses. Reduction of doses, as done with other forms of allergenic extracts, may not be clinically effective. Fortunately, reactions to VIT are uncommon, and the majority of people are able to reach maintenance doses.

Large Local Reactions

Venoms are intrinsically irritating and cause pain at the injection site. Local swelling may occur and can cause considerable morbidity. Several approaches are available to minimize these reactions. The venom dose can be split into two injections, thus limiting the amount of venom delivered at one site. The addition of a small amount of epinephrine with the venom may minimize the immediate local swelling. If the swelling is extensive and particularly delayed in onset, the addition of a small amount of steroid with the venom usually effectively inhibits this large local reaction. Administration of an antihistamine 30 to 60 minutes before the venom injection may also be beneficial.

Systemic Reactions

Systemic reactions to VIT are quite rare and much less common than those induced by pollen immunotherapy. After a reaction, the next dose is usually reduced approximately 25%, and subsequent doses are slowly increased. If people are receiving multiple venoms, it might be advisable to administer single venoms on separate days.

Generalized Fatigue

Another reaction occasionally noted after injections of other allergenic extracts such as mold and dust, but more frequently venom, is the occurrence of generalized fatigue and aching, sometimes associated with a large local swelling. Successful treatment of this reaction is usually accomplished with the administration of aspirin approximately 30 minutes before the injection and every 4 hours thereafter for 1 to 2 days if needed. If symptoms are severe, steroids such as prednisone administered daily for several days can be helpful.

Other Reactions

There have been no identified adverse reactions caused by long-term VIT. Injections appear to be safe during pregnancy with no effect on the pregnancy or the fetus.

Monitoring of Venom Immunotherapy

VIT is associated with initially increasing titers of serum venom–specific IgG, occasionally increasing and subsequently decreasing titers of serum venom–specific IgE, and highly successful clinical response. A minority of people will develop negative venom skin tests while receiving VIT. As described later, this is one criterion for stopping treatment. Repeat venom skin tests approximately every 2 years are recommended. In a study of 62 children,[43] 28 developed a negative venom skin test to one or more venoms after 3 years of VIT. However, only two children converted to negative tests with all treatment venoms.

Stimulation of venom-specific IgG has been associated with clinical immunity to insect stings. For individual patients, however, there is no absolute titer that is directly related to successful treatment. In my opinion, the overall success rate of VIT and review of relative data do not support the routine measurement of venom-specific IgG.[44,45]

Results

VIT is highly effective in preventing subsequent anaphylaxis in people at risk. Repeat anaphylaxis occurs in only about 2% to 5% of people treated after re-stings.[46] In my experience with children and adults,[38] 258 re-stings in 108 people led to three systemic reactions (2.7% per patient, 1.2% per re-sting). Graft et al[46] reported that during a 3- to 6-year period, 200 restings in 49 VIT-treated children resulted in only four mild systemic reactions (98% efficacy). A recent study of children

receiving bee VIT reported five reactors in 55 children after field re-stings.[48]

VIT treatment significantly improves quality-of-life issues for patients and family compared with recommended treatment with epinephrine availability only.[49]

Treatment Failures

VIT is very effective, protecting approximately 98% of treated people. If a re-sting reaction does occur, it is initially advisable to determine whether the appropriate venom has been administered. Culprit insect identification is important and repeat testing may be necessary to verify specific venom sensitivity. If the specific treatment is correct, then the venom dose should be increased by 50% to 100%. For example, if the maintenance dose is 100 μg, it should be increased to 150 or 200 μg. Increasing the venom dose has been shown to be highly effective, preventing subsequent re-sting reactions.[50]

Duration of Therapy

The question of duration of treatment or when it is safe to discontinue VIT has been a persistent issue (Table 59-4). Several criteria have been suggested as reliable guidelines: these include conversion to a negative venom skin test, a fall in serum venom–specific IgE to undetectable levels, and a finite period of treatment (3 to 5 years), regardless of the persistence of skin test reactivity or serum antibody.

A position statement from the Insect Committee of the American Academy of Allergy, Asthma and Immunology has addressed this issue,[51] and these conclusions are supported by recently published studies.[52-54] These data strongly suggest that conversion to a negative venom skin test is an absolute criterion for stopping VIT.[53-55] However, there have been several anecdotal reports of people who continue to have allergic reactions to insect stings, apparently despite the presence of a negative venom skin test, which suggests the need for continuous monitoring of this guideline.

It appears that 3 to 5 years of VIT is adequate for the large majority of people who have had mild to moderate anaphylactic reactions, despite the persistence of a positive skin test.[51-55] The re-sting reaction rate after cessation of VIT is low, generally in the range of 5% to 10%. People who have had severe anaphylactic symptoms such as hypotension, laryngeal edema, or loss of consciousness have a higher risk of repeated severe systemic reactions if therapy is discontinued. For this

---

TABLE 59-4   Venom Immunotherapy: When to Stop

Suggested criteria for stopping venom immunotherapy
   Conversion to a negative venom skin test
   Persistence of positive venom skin test: 3 to 5 years of therapy
Factors that may influence decision to stop therapy
   Severe anaphylactic symptoms, such as loss of consciousness, caused by insect sting
   Systemic reactions to venom immunotherapy
   Unchanged venom skin test sensitivity during venom immunotherapy
   Honeybee venom allergy (compared with vespid venom allergy)
   Presence of significant medical problems, such as cardiovascular disease
   Access to emergency medical care

reason, I currently recommend that individuals who have had severe symptoms and retain positive venom skin tests receive VIT indefinitely, which, at this point, can be administered every 8 to 12 weeks. Other suggested risk factors that have been associated with the occurrence of re-sting reactions after cessation of VIT include systemic reactions to VIT, persistence of significant skin test reactivity, and honeybee venom allergy compared with vespid venom allergy. These decisions regarding the cessation of therapy also should include consideration of other medical problems, concomitant medication, patient lifestyle, and patient preference.

CONCLUSIONS

Insect sting anaphylaxis is a relatively common problem, estimated to affect at least 0.3% to 3% of the population and responsible for at least 40 deaths per year in the United States (see Boxes 59-1 and 59-2). The allergic reactions are mediated

---

BOX 59-1	**KEY CONCEPTS**
	Differential Diagnoses: Reaction to Insect Stings

- Insect stings always cause pain at the sting site associated with some swelling and erythema.
- Large local reactions from insect stings tend to recur after subsequent re-stings, with little risk of developing anaphylaxis.
- Many simultaneous stings (50 to 100) may sensitize a person for risk of subsequent single sting–induced anaphylaxis.
- Unusual reactions, usually involving neurologic or vascular pathology, have occurred in a temporal relationship to insect stings.
- No absolute criteria predict the occurrence of initial venom-induced anaphylaxis. Serious anaphylactic reactions may occur at any age; fatalities are more common in adults.

BOX 59-2	**KEY CONCEPTS**
	Evaluation and Management

- Approximately 60% or less of people who have had an anaphylactic reaction from an insect sting and have positive venom skin tests will have another reaction to a subsequent re-sting.
- The risk of a re-sting reaction is related to age and severity of the initial reaction. Re-sting reactions are more likely to occur in adults than in children and in people who have had more severe reactions.
- The venom skin test is the preferred diagnostic test to detect potential insect sting allergy. The radioallergosorbent test, for measurement of serum venom–specific IgE, is indicated when the skin test cannot be done or the reaction is equivocal.
- People at risk for insect sting anaphylaxis should (1) be educated regarding measures to avoid stings, (2) carry emergency medication, particularly epinephrine, and (3) be advised to receive venom immunotherapy.

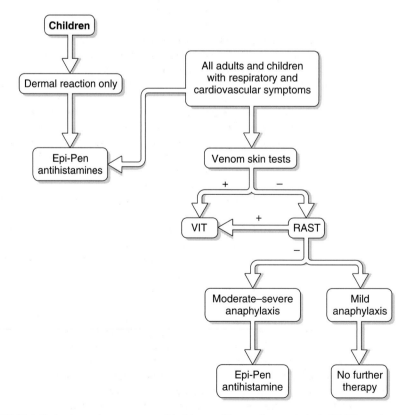

FIGURE 59-1 Evaluation and management of the history of insect sting anaphylaxis. *VIT,* Venom immunotherapy; *RAST,* radioallergosorbent test.

by IgE antibodies directed at constituents in insect venoms. In addition, increasing numbers of reactions occur from fire ant stings and nonwinged Hymenopterans present in the southeastern United States and slowly extending westward. Anaphylactic symptoms are typical of those occurring from any cause. The majority of reactions in children are mild and frequently only dermal (hives, angioedema). The more severe reactions such as shock and loss of consciousness can occur at any age but are relatively more common in adults. After sting anaphylaxis, about 50% of unselected people will continue to have allergic reactions to subsequent stings. The natural history of the disease process is influenced by the severity of the anaphylactic symptoms. Children with dermal reactions have only a benign course and are unlikely to have recurrent reactions. (Figure 59-1 illustrates a clinical algorithm of evaluation and management of insect sting anaphylaxis.) People with more severe reactions are more likely to have repeat anaphylaxis. People with a history of insect sting anaphylaxis and positive venom skin tests should have epinephrine available and are candidates for subsequent VIT, which provides almost 100% protection against subsequent resting reactions. Recommendations for the duration of VIT are still evolving. VIT therapy can be stopped if skin test reactions become negative; for most people, 3 to 5 years of therapy appears adequate despite the persistence of these positive tests. People who have had life-threatening reactions such as loss of consciousness and retain positive venom skin tests should receive VIT indefinitely.

REFERENCES

1. Barnard JH: Studies of 400 Hymenoptera sting deaths in the United States, *J Allergy Clin Immunol* 52:259-264, 1973.
2. Golden DB, Kagey-Sobotka A, Norman PS, et al: Insect sting allergy with negative venom skin test responses, *J Allergy Clin Immunol* 107:897-901, 2001.
3. Reisman RE: Insect sting allergy: the dilemma of the negative skin test reactor, *J Allergy Clin Immunol* 107:781-782, 2001.
4. Ludolph-Hauser D, Rueff F, Fries C, et al: Constitutively raised serum concentrations of mast-cell tryptase and severe anaphylactic reactions to Hymenoptera stings, *Lancet* 357:361-362, 2001.
5. Reisman RE: Natural history of insect sting allergy: relationship of severity of symptoms of initial sting anaphylaxis to re-sting reactions, *J Allergy Clin Immunol* 90:335-339, 1992.
6. Reisman RE, Osur SL: Allergic reactions following first insect sting exposure, *Ann Allergy* 59:429-432, 1987.
7. Mauriello PM, Barde SH, Georgitis JW, et al: Natural history of large local reactions from stinging insects, *J Allergy Clin Immunol* 74:494-498, 1984.
8. McKenna WR: Killer bees: what the allergist should know, *Pediatr Asthma Allergy Immunol* 4:275-285, 1992.
9. Chaffee FH: The prevalence of bee sting allergy in an allergic population, *Acta Allergol* 25:292-293, 1970.
10. Settipane GA, Boyd GK: Prevalence of bee sting allergy in 4,992 Boy Scouts, *Acta Allergol* 25:286-291, 1970.
11. Golden DB: Epidemiology of allergy to insect venoms and stings, *Allergy Proc* 10:103-107, 1989.
12. Lockey RF, Turkeltaub PC, Baird-Warren IA, et al: The Hymenoptera venom study, I, 1979-1982: demographics and history-sting data, *J Allergy Clin Immunol* 82:370-381, 1988.
13. Kemp SF, deShazo RD, Moffitt JE, et al: Expanding habitat of the imported fire ant (Solenopsis invicta): a public health concern, *J Allergy Clin Immunol* 105:683-691, 2000.
14. Stafford CT: Hypersensitivity to fire ant venom, *Ann Allergy Asthma Immunol* 77:87-95, 1996.
15. Peng Z, Ho MK, Ye C, et al: Evidence of natural desensitization to mosquito salivary allergens—mosquito saliva—specific IgE and IgG levels in 424 infants, children and adolescents (abstract), *J Allergy Clin Immunol* 109:S271, 2002.
16. Peng Z, Simons FE: A prospective study of naturally acquired sensitization and subsequent desensitization to mosquito bites and concurrent antibody responses, *J Allergy Clin Immunol* 101:284-286, 1998.
17. Graft DF, Schuberth KC, Kagey-Sobotka A, et al: A prospective study of the natural history of large local reactions after Hymenoptera stings in children, *J Pediatr* 104:664-668, 1984.
18. Hamilton RG, Golden DB, Kagey-Sobotka A, et al: Case report of venom immunotherapy for a patient with large local reactions, *Ann Allergy Asthma Immunol* 87:134-137, 2001.
19. Light WC, Reisman RE, Shimizu M, et al: Unusual reactions following insect stings. Clinical features and immunologic analysis, *J Allergy Clin Immunol* 59:391-397, 1977.
20. Reisman RE, Livingston A: Late-onset allergic reactions, including serum sickness, after insect stings, *J Allergy Clin Immunol* 84:331-337, 1989.
21. Golden DBK, Lichtenstein LM: Insect sting allergy. In Kaplan AP, ed: *Allergy*, New York, 1985, Churchill Livingstone.
22. Lantner R, Reisman RE: Clinical and immunologic features and subsequent course of patients with severe insect-sting anaphylaxis, *J Allergy Clin Immunol* 84:900-906, 1989.
23. Hunt KJ, Valentine MD, Sobotka AK, et al: A controlled trial of immunotherapy in insect hypersensitivity, *N Engl J Med* 299:157-161, 1978.
24. Blaauw PJ, Smithuis LO: The evaluation of the common diagnostic methods of hypersensitivity for bee and yellow jacket venom by means of an in-hospital insect sting, *J Allergy Clin Immunol* 75:556-562, 1985.
25. Parker JL, Santrach PJ, Dahlberg MJ, et al: Evaluation of Hymenoptera-sting sensitivity with deliberate sting challenges: inadequacy of present diagnostic methods, *J Allergy Clin Immunol* 69:200-207, 1982.
26. van der Linden PW, Hack CE, Struyvenberg A, et al: Insect-sting challenge in 324 subjects with a previous anaphylactic reaction: current criteria for insect-venom hypersensitivity do not predict the occurrence and the severity of anaphylaxis, *J Allergy Clin Immunol* 94:151-159, 1994.
27. Valentine MD, Schuberth KC, Kagey-Sobotka A, et al: The value of immunotherapy with venom in children with allergy to insect stings, *N Engl J Med* 323:1601-1603, 1990.
28. Hunt KJ, Valentine MD, Sobotka AK, et al: Diagnosis of allergy to stinging insects by skin testing with Hymenoptera venoms, *Ann Intern Med* 85:56-59, 1976.
29. Chipps BE, Valentine MD, Kagey-Sobotka A, et al: Diagnosis and treatment of anaphylactic reactions to Hymenoptera stings in children, *J Pediatr* 97:177-184, 1980.
30. Barnard JH: Nonfatal results in third-degree anaphylaxis from Hymenoptera stings, *J Allergy* 45:92-96, 1970.
31. Goldberg A, Confino-Cohen R: Insect sting-inflicted systemic reactions: attitudes of patients with insect venom allergy regarding after-sting behavior and proper administration of epinephrine, *J Allergy Clin Immunol* 106:1184-1189, 2000.
32. Franken HH, Dubois AE, Minkema HJ, et al: Lack of reproducibility of a single negative sting challenge response in the assessment of anaphylactic risk in patients with suspected yellow jacket hypersensitivity, *J Allergy Clin Immunol* 93:431-436, 1994.
33. Hauk P, Friedl K, Kaufmehl K, et al: Subsequent insect stings in children with hypersensitivity to Hymenoptera, *J Pediatr* 126:185-190, 1995.
34. Mueller U, Reisman R, Wypych J, et al: Comparison of vespid venoms collected by electrostimulation and by venom sac extraction, *J Allergy Clin Immunol* 68:254-261, 1981.
35. Reisman RE, Mueller U, Wypych J, et al: Comparison of the allergenicity and antigenicity of yellow jacket and hornet venoms, *J Allergy Clin Immunol* 69:268-274, 1982.
36. Reisman RE, Wypych JI, Mueller UR, et al: Comparison of the allergenicity and antigenicity of Polistes venom and other vespid venoms, *J Allergy Clin Immunol* 70:281-287, 1982.
37. Reisman RE, Muller UR, Wypych JI, et al: Studies of coexisting honeybee and vespid-venom sensitivity, *J Allergy Clin Immunol* 73:246-252, 1984.
38. Reisman RE, Livingston A: Venom immunotherapy: 10 years of experience with administration of single venoms and 50 micrograms maintenance doses, *J Allergy Clin Immunol* 89:1189-1195, 1992.
39. Hoffman DR, El-Choufani SE, Smith MM, et al: Occupational allergy to bumblebees: allergens of Bombus terrestris, *J Allergy Clin Immunol* 108:855-860, 2001.
40. Freeman TM, Hylander R, Ortiz A, et al: Imported fire ant immunotherapy: effectiveness of whole body extracts, *J Allergy Clin Immunol* 90:210-215, 1992.
41. Bahna SL, Strimas JH, Reed MA, et al: Imported fire ant allergy in young children: skin reactivity and serum IgE antibodies to venom and whole body extract, *J Allergy Clin Immunol* 82:419-424, 1988.
42. Goldberg A, Confino-Cohen R: Maintenance venom immunotherapy administered at 3-month intervals is both safe and efficacious, *J Allergy Clin Immunol* 107:902-906, 2001.

43. Graft DF, Schuberth KC, Kagey-Sobotka A, et al: The development of negative skin tests in children treated with venom immunotherapy, *J Allergy Clin Immunol* 73:61-68, 1984.

44. Golden DB, Lawrence ID, Hamilton RH, et al: Clinical correlation of the venom-specific IgG antibody level during maintenance venom immunotherapy, *J Allergy Clin Immunol* 90:386-393, 1992.

45. Reisman RE: Should routine measurements of serum venom-specific IgG be a standard of practice in patients receiving venom immunotherapy? *J Allergy Clin Immunol* 90:282-284, 1992.

46. Mueller UR: *Insect sting allergy,* New York, 1990, Gustav Fischer Verlag.

47. Graft DF, Schuberth KC, Kagey-Sobotka A, et al: Assessment of prolonged venom immunotherapy in children, *J Allergy Clin Immunol* 80:162-169, 1987.

48. Gold SG: A six year review of bee venom immunotherapy in children (abstract), *J Allergy Clin Immunol* 109:S202, 2002.

49. Elberink HO, Munchy JD, Guyatt A, et al: Insect venom allergy and the burden of the treatment (BoT): Epipen vs venom immunotherapy (VIT) (abstract), *J Allergy Clin Immunol* 109:S80, 2002.

50. Rueff F, Wenderoth A, Przybilla B: Patients still reacting to a sting challenge while receiving conventional Hymenoptera venom immunotherapy are protected by increased venom doses, *J Allergy Clin Immunol* 108:1027-1032, 2001.

51. American Academy of Allergy, Asthma and Immunology Position Statement. The discontinuation of Hymenoptera venom immunotherapy. Report from the Committee on Insects, *J Allergy Clin Immunol* 101:573-575, 1998.

52. Golden DB, Kwiterovich KA, Kagey-Sobotka A, et al: Discontinuing venom immunotherapy: extended observations, *J Allergy Clin Immunol* 101:298-305, 1998.

53. Lerch E, Müller UR: Long-term protection after stopping venom immunotherapy: results of re-stings in 200 patients, *J Allergy Clin Immunol* 101:606-612, 1998.

54. van Halteren HK, van der Linden PW, Burgers JA, et al: Discontinuation of yellow jacket venom immunotherapy: follow-up of 75 patients by means of deliberate sting challenge, *J Allergy Clin Immunol* 100:767-770, 1997.

55. Reisman RE: Duration of venom immunotherapy: relationship to the severity of symptoms of initial insect sting anaphylaxis, *J Allergy Clin Immunol* 92:831-836, 1993.

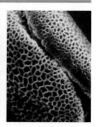

CHAPTER 60

General Treatment of Anaphylaxis

MICHAEL C. YOUNG

Anaphylaxis is the most catastrophic consequence of all allergic disorders, a medical emergency requiring prompt recognition of symptoms and immediate treatment. Anaphylaxis is a potentially fatal multisystem syndrome resulting from the massive release of inflammatory mediators from mast cells and basophils. Typically, the symptoms can be cutaneous, respiratory, gastrointestinal, and/or cardiovascular.[1-5] Anaphylactic reactions can be mild, involving only urticaria, or they can be life-threatening with upper airway angioedema or hypotension and cardiovascular shock.[3,6] These symptoms often have an explosive onset, occurring within seconds to minutes of exposure to the triggering agent, but can also be delayed for several hours after the initial exposure. The acute anaphylactic event can be followed by a late-phase or biphasic reaction occurring 3 to 8 hours after the initial reaction. Biphasic anaphylaxis occurs in 5% to 20% of anaphylactic reactions.[7-13] Protracted anaphylaxis lasting 3 to 21 days has been reported.[7,10,11] Over 50% of fatal anaphylaxis occurs within the first hour.[5] Common triggers for anaphylaxis in children are food, drugs, Hymenoptera stings, drugs, and latex.[10,14,15] Exercise, allergen immunotherapy injections, and vaccinations can also be causes of anaphylaxis in children.[15] In large series of patients with anaphylaxis, no etiology could be found in 20% to 37%; these patients were classified as having idiopathic anaphylaxis.[16-19] Idiopathic anaphylaxis has been reported in children but is rare.[20,21] Anaphylactoid (non–IgE-mediated) reactions may occur on the first exposure, whereas IgE-mediated and immunologically mediated anaphylactic reactions require sensitization from a previous exposure unless there is cross-reactivity.[3,4] For the purposes of this discussion of treatment, no distinction is made between anaphylactic and anaphylactoid reactions because the symptoms are clinically indistinguishable. Table 60-1 lists the causes of anaphylactic and anaphylactoid reactions reported in children.

EPIDEMIOLOGY

The true incidence of anaphylaxis is unknown because it is not a reportable condition.[3,22,23] Estimates of the risk of anaphylaxis per person in the United States range from less than 1% to 3%.[5,18] Neugut and colleagues performed a meta-analysis on studies of food, drug, stinging insect, and latex anaphylaxis in the medical literature and calculated estimates of the prevalence of anaphylaxis for the general population of the United States.[24] They concluded that between 3.3 and 4.3

million Americans are at risk for anaphylaxis, which is approximately 1.24% to 16.76% of the U.S. population.[24] Fatal anaphylaxis is rare. It is estimated that there are 500 fatalities from penicillin anaphylaxis per year and 40 fatalities from Hymenoptera stings per year.[25] Food anaphylaxis accounts for approximately 125 to 150 fatalities per year.[26,27] More than 90% of fatal food anaphylaxis is caused by peanut and tree nut hypersensitivity.[28] Allergen immunotherapy injections can result in anaphylactic reactions. Estimates of fatal anaphylaxis from immunotherapy are approximately one in 2 million injections.[29] Latex anaphylaxis is estimated to cause approximately 3 fatalities per year.[24]

Anaphylaxis occurs in all age groups but is more common in adults, which may partially be a function of increased time for exposure and sensitization. The incidence of anaphylaxis in children is unknown. In the several large series of anaphylaxis published, the age ranges and mean ages are given but not the age distributions. In Yocum's 5-year retrospective epidemiologic study of anaphylaxis in 1255 Olmsted County, Minnesota residents, the 133 patients presenting with anaphylaxis had a mean age of 29 years with a range of 6 months to 89 years.[18] In Kemp's review of 266 cases of anaphylaxis,[17] the age range of patients was 12 to 75 years with a mean age of 38 years. Yocum and Khan[16] reviewed 179 patients with anaphylaxis with a mean age of 36 years; no age range was given. Brown and colleagues[19] reviewed 142 patients presenting to an emergency department in Australia from 1998 to 1999 with a mean age of 35.3 years and an age range from 14 to 88 years. Cianferoni and colleagues[30] did a retrospective chart review of all admissions to a university hospital in Florence, Italy and found 107 patients presenting with 113 episodes of anaphylaxis, with a mean age of 42 years ± 18 years. Alonso and colleagues reviewed 81 patients with idiopathic anaphylaxis in Spain with a mean age of 30 ± 17.3 years with an age range of 5 to 73 years.[31] Alves and Shieikh[32] reviewed 2320 emergency admissions over a 4-year period to the National Health Service in the United Kingdom and found that 385 patients (17%) were children under the age of 16 years. There are seven published series of anaphylaxis in children. In the largest study, Lee and Greenes[13] reported 106 patients with a median age of 8 years ranging from 6 months to 21 years. Stratifying their patients by age, they found 3.7% less than age 1 year, 30% from age 1 to 5 years, 35% from 6 to 11 years, and 31.5% from 12 to 21 years.[13] Dibs and Baker found in their series of 50 children a median age of 7 years; 42% were between ages 1

TABLE 60-1 Common Causes of Anaphylaxis in Children*

Food: peanuts, tree nuts (walnut, hazelnut, cashew, pistachio, Brazil nut), milk, eggs, fish, shellfish (shrimp, crab, lobster, clam, scallop, oyster), seeds (sesame, cottonseed, pine nuts, psyllium), fruits (apples, banana, kiwi, peaches, oranges, melon), grains (wheat)

Drugs: penicillins, cephalosporins, sulfonamides, nonsteroidal antiinflammatory agents, opiates, muscle relaxants, vancomycin, dextran, thiamine, vitamin B_{12}, insulin, thiopental, local anesthetics

Hymenoptera venom: honeybee, yellow jacket, wasp, hornet, fire ant

Latex

Allergen immunotherapy

Exercise: food-specific exercise, postprandial (non–food-specific) exercise

Vaccinations: tetanus, measles, mumps, influenza

Miscellaneous: radiocontrast media, gammaglobulin, cold temperature, chemotherapeutic agents (asparaginase, cyclosporine, methotrexate, vincristine, 5-fluorouracil), blood products, inhalants (dust and storage mites, grass pollen)

Idiopathic

*In order of frequency.

to 5 years, 25% from age 6 to 11 years, and 33% from age 12 to 19 years.[14] Ditto and colleagues reported 22 children diagnosed with idiopathic anaphylaxis, with an age range at presentation from 3 years to 17 years; 14% were between the of 1 and 5 years, 41% between 6 and 11 years, and 45% from age 12 to 17 years.[20] Novembre and colleagues reviewed anaphylaxis in 76 children with an age range of 1 month to 16 years with a mean age of 6.1 ± 4.6 years.[15] Sampson and colleagues reported 13 children with fatal and near-fatal food anaphylaxis ranging in age from 2 to 16 years; 12 of the 13 patients were age 8 years and older.[10] Hogan and colleagues reviewed 8 children with idiopathic anaphylaxis with an age range at presentation of 11 months to 19 years. Six (75%) of the children were age 9 years and older.[21] Macdougall and associates reviewed severe and fatal food anaphylaxis under age 16 years in the United Kingdom and Ireland with retrospective data from 1990 to 1998 and prospective data from 1998 to 2000.[33] Eight fatalities from food anaphylaxis occurred in patients between the ages of 3 months and 15 years; an average age of 10.4 years was identified.[33] From the prospective data, 55 children with severe nonfatal reactions were identified but the age distribution of these patients was not given. Combining data from these studies, the average age of anaphylaxis in children can be estimated to be approximately 9 years.

CLINICAL MANIFESTATIONS

The signs and symptoms of anaphylaxis are highly variable, involve multiple organ systems, and can range from mild cutaneous symptoms to a fatal reaction. The successful treatment of anaphylaxis is dependent upon the prompt, early recognition of these signs and symptoms.

The symptoms of anaphylaxis in children and adults are similar. Dermatologic symptoms are the most common manifestations of an anaphylactic reaction, occurring in 90% of patients reported in all series of anaphylaxis published including all pediatrics series.[14-21,30,31] Ninety-two percent of the 106 children in the series reported by Lee and Greenes presented

with dermatologic symptoms, including urticaria, angioedema, flushing, and warmth.[13] In the pediatric anaphylaxis series of Dibs and Baker, the dermatologic symptoms were urticaria (31%), erythema (11%), angioedema of the face or lips (11%), extremity edema (2%), pruritis (4%), and "other rashes" (2%).[14] In the series of pediatric idiopathic anaphylaxis of Ditto et al, urticaria and/or angioedema occurred in all 22 patients.[20] When the only symptom that occurs with an allergic reaction is urticaria, the diagnosis of anaphylaxis can sometimes be difficult for the patient or family to ascertain. The urticaria associated with anaphylaxis is an explosive, rapidly evolving eruption occurring over seconds to minutes as opposed to an isolated cutaneous allergic reaction that is stable and nonprogressive. The severity of an allergic reaction is often heralded by the rapidity of onset of symptoms, with pruritis, flushing, urticaria, and angioedema.[5,34] However, despite the fact that urticaria and angioedema are the most common symptoms of anaphylaxis, the absence of dermatologic symptoms does not rule out the diagnosis of anaphylaxis.[26,35] Hypotension and cardiovascular shock can occur in isolation without any associated symptoms, including dermatologic symptoms.[35] A rapidly developing anaphylactic reaction may present with shock, only to be followed by cutaneous symptoms.[5] Urticaria, facial and upper-airway angioedema, and bronchospasm are commonly associated with food ingestion whereas hypotension and cardiovascular shock are more often associated with injected allergens such as insect stings and intravenous medications.[6] It is interesting that in Sampson's study of fatal and near-fatal food anaphylaxis, only one of the six patients with a fatal reaction had dermatologic symptoms, whereas dermatologic symptoms occurred in all seven patients who survived their anaphylaxis.[10]

Lieberman[35] reviewed the frequency of presenting symptoms from four series of anaphylaxis and found them to be very similar: urticaria and angioedema (87%), flush (50%), dyspnea/wheeze (46%), gastrointestinal symptoms (30%), hypotension/syncope/dizziness (30%), and rhinitis (18%). The review of 266 patients with anaphylaxis by Kemp and colleagues[17] showed urticaria and angioedema in 90%; flushing (28%); generalized pruritis (4%); dyspnea and wheezing (60%); upper-airway symptoms such as swelling of the tongue and throat, dysphagia, choking, and dysphonia (24%); hypotension (49%); and nausea, vomiting, diarrhea, and abdominal pain (46%). Neurologic symptoms such as headache (5%), blurred vision (2%), and seizures (2%) also occurred.[17] Some patients have described a sense of impending doom,[6,13,36] which in a young nonverbal child might be manifested as severe fright and irritability. In the 106 children with anaphylaxis reported by Lee and Greenes,[13] the most common presenting symptoms were dermatologic (92%), followed by upper respiratory, such as stridor, drooling, and oropharyngeal swelling (78%); lower respiratory, such as chest tightness and wheezing (58%); gastrointestinal (GI) (37%); cardiovascular, including weak pulses, arrhythmias, and hypotension (30%); neurologic (27%); and 13% had diaphoresis, tingling, or a sense of impending doom. Of the initial presenting symptoms of 50 children with anaphylaxis reported by Dibs and Baker,[14] dermatologic symptoms were the most common (60%), followed by respiratory symptoms (25%), which included wheezing, upper airway obstructive symptoms, hoarseness, stridor, and dysphagia. Neurologic symptoms such as irritability, lethargy, tremor, syncope, and seizures (5%); GI symptoms (4%); and cardiovascular symptoms consisting of hypotension and cardiac arrhythmias (2%) were less common on initial presentation.[14] When the entire episode of anaphylaxis was assessed, 93% of the children had dermatologic and respiratory symptoms, 26% had cardiovascular symptoms, and 26% had neurologic symptoms whereas GI symptoms occurred in 13%.[14] In the series of 76 children with anaphylaxis by Novembre et al,[15] the frequencies for dermatologic symptoms were 78%, respiratory symptoms 79%, cardiovascular symptoms 25%, and GI symptoms 24%. Dermatologic and respiratory symptoms had an earlier onset than cardiovascular and GI symptoms.[15] In the series of 22 children with idiopathic anaphylaxis by Ditto et al,[20] every child had urticaria and/or angioedema, 41% had respiratory symptoms with bronchospasm, 18% had hypotension and dizziness, and 4% had GI symptoms. In Hogan's series of 8 children with idiopathic anaphylaxis,[21] all 8 (100%) had dermatologic symptoms, 6 (75%) had respiratory symptoms, and 6 (75%) had GI symptoms. Hypotension and loss of consciousness occurred in 5 children (63%).[21]

Fortunately, fatal anaphylaxis in children remains uncommon. In the largest series of pediatric anaphylaxis of 106 patients by Lee and Greenes,[13] there were two fatalities (2%), both patients with food allergies. In the other four series of pediatric anaphylaxis totaling 156 patients, there were no fatalities.[14,15,20,21] The most common etiology in the two largest series of pediatric anaphylaxis is food allergy. Forty-seven percent of the 106 patients in the Lee and Greenes study[13] and 57% of the 76 children in the Novembre et al study[15] had food allergy as the trigger for their anaphylaxis. In the Dibs and Baker study of 50 children with anaphylaxis,[14] food allergy was the etiology in 25%, whereas latex was the leading cause in 27% of cases. The difference between the first two studies and the Dibs and Baker study[14] is that the latter study included hospitalized patients who developed anaphylaxis as inpatients, whereas the Lee and Greenes study[13] was an emergency department population with all outpatients and the Novembre et al study[15] examined outpatients referred to an allergy and immunology clinic of which only four patients had their anaphylactic episodes in a hospital. Alves and Sheikh[32] found that emergency admissions for food-related anaphylaxis were highest for infants less than age 1 year (62%) and declined with increasing age to 48% for age 1 to 5 years, 32% for age 6 to 10 years, 26% for age 11 to 15 years, and 4% for adults greater than age 55 years. In contrast, admissions for drug anaphylaxis increased with increasing age while insect venom anaphylaxis admissions were stable in all age groups except for the infancy group, which had no admissions.[32] Fatal anaphylaxis from Hymenoptera stings is more common in the adult age group, where there is a higher incidence of underlying cardiovascular disease.[37]

A history of asthma seems to be a risk factor for fatal anaphylaxis. In Sampson's et al study of fatal and near-fatal food anaphylaxis in children,[10] all 13 patients had asthma. In all 6 patients who died, their fatal symptoms involved bronchospasm and respiratory distress despite the fact that their asthma was well controlled. Similarly, in Yunginger's report of fatal food anaphylaxis of 7 patients ages 11 to 40 years,[38] 5 of the 7 fatalities had a history of asthma. Settipane[39] reviewed 9 patients with fatal and near-fatal anaphylaxis to peanuts and found 7 of the 9 had a previous history of asthma. In Macdougall's study,[33] the severity of anaphylaxis was strongly

correlated with a history of asthma: fatal (100% with asthma), near-fatal (83%), and severe (57%) versus non-severe (37%). Settipane[39] also reports data showing that Hymenoptera sting anaphylaxis in asthma patients is twice as likely to have a bronchospastic or respiratory component than in nonasthmatic patients. Unstable asthma is one of the risk factors associated with systemic reactions and fatal anaphylaxis to allergen immunotherapy.[40,41] The mechanism of the more severe anaphylactic reactions suffered by asthma patients may be its greater reactivity to the mediators released during anaphylaxis such as histamine, leukotrienes, and prostaglandins.[39] Pumphrey and Nicholls[42] reviewed 48 cases of fatal food anaphylaxis and found 46 (96%) were taking inhaled asthma medication with 20 (42%) dying of bronchospasm and 14 (29%) dying of a combination of asthma and upper-airway obstruction. Bock and colleagues[28] reviewed 32 cases of fatal food anaphylaxis and found that in the fatalities where data were available, 96% had asthma. The acute onset of severe bronchospasm in a previously well-controlled asthmatic should always raise the suspicion of anaphpylaxis.[43]

In Sampson's series[10] and Bock's series[28] of patients with fatal food-induced anaphylaxis, failure to administer epinephrine or lack of available epinephrine was the problem in 100% and 90% of fatalities, respectively. In Yunginger's series of 7 cases of fatal food anaphylaxis,[38] 57% had no epinephrine administered, and one patient received a late, suboptimal dose.

Fatalities occurred away from home in 83% of Sampson's patients,[10] 84% of Bock's patients,[28] and 86% of Yunginger's patients,[38] most likely because it is more difficult to respond to a medical emergency in a public place than in the home. Failure to administer epinephrine promptly and early in the course of anaphylaxis is the most important risk factor for a fatal reaction.

TREATMENT

Anaphylaxis is a life-threatening medical emergency requiring prompt recognition of symptoms and immediate institution of treatment. The treatment must consist of the simultaneous administration of epinephrine and adjunctive pharmacologic agents as well as the institution of basic measures of cardiopulmonary resuscitation to support the airway and maintain adequate oxygenation and circulation. Given the labile nature of acute anaphylaxis, meticulous monitoring of vital signs, airway patency, cardiac output, and tissue perfusion are essential. Anticipation of all possible life-threatening consequences of anaphylaxis including upper-airway obstruction, bronchospasm, and cardiovascular collapse as well as the preparedness to act quickly to reverse them is the key to successful management. All patients presenting with anaphylaxis should be placed on supplemental 100% oxygen and large-bore intravenous lines should be inserted so that hypovolemic shock can be quickly treated.[34] Equipment and personnel should be available for intubation and mechanical ventilation as well as for performing an emergency surgical airway for laryngeal obstruction. Endotracheal intubation is preferably performed early, before the loss of significant landmarks from angioedema and obstruction. The protocol for the treatment of acute anaphylaxis is summarized in Box 60-1. Table 60-2 lists recommended equipment that should be available for the office treatment of acute anaphylaxis. The individual pharmacologic agents are reviewed below.

THERAPEUTIC PRINCIPLES
Management of Acute Anaphylaxis

IMMEDIATE

Rapid assessment of airway, breathing, circulation, dermatologic examination, and mental status

Epinephrine 0.01 mg/kg (1:1000) IM, repeat every 20 minutes as needed

Oxygen 100%, secure and maintain airway

Start large-bore intravenous line for venous access and fluids

Intravenous fluids, 10-20 ml/kg, repeat as necessary

Frequent vital signs, cardiac monitor, pulse oximetry

Rapid history for acute triggering event, known allergy and anaphylaxis history, current medications, history of asthma symptoms, concomitant medical conditions

SUBACUTE

H_1 antagonist, diphenhydramine 1-2 mg/kg PO, IM, IV

Corticosteroids, administered PO (prednisone 1 mg/kg) or IV methylprednisolone 1-2 mg/kg or nebulized albuterol 1.25-2.5 mg every 20 minutes or continuously

SECONDARY

H_2 antagonist, ranitidine 1.5 mg/kg administered PO or IV

Glucagon 0.1 mg/kg IV if refractory to initial treatment above, and/or if patient is receiving β-blockers

Observe at least 4 hours for biphasic anaphylaxis

DISPOSITION

If still symptomatic, admit for further treatment.

If unstable vital signs, angioedema of upper airway, or refractory bronchospasm, admit patient to intensive care unit.

If symptoms have resolved without biphasic response, discharge patient on 72 hours of antihistamine, prednisone, and, if bronchospasm occurred with episode, albuterol metered-dose inhaler.

Discuss allergen trigger and avoidance and Epi-Pen instructions and prescription.

Follow up with allergist.

TABLE 60-2 Office Equipment for the Management of Acute Anaphylaxis

Stethoscope
Sphygmomanometer
Tourniquets
Syringes
Epinephrine 1:1000 (aqueous)
Oxygen tank with mask, nasal prongs
Intravenous fluids, 2 L
Intravenous setup, large-bore catheters
Oral airway, Ambu bag
Diphenhydramine, injectable
Albuterol nebulizer solution
Compressor nebulizer
Methylprednisolone/hydrocortisone, injectable
Ranitidine, injectable
Glucagon, injectable
Laryngoscope
Endotracheal tube

---

tropic and chronotropic effects on cardiac muscle, cause bronchodilation, and increase the production of intracellular cyclic AMP, thereby inhibiting mast cell mediator release.[49,51-53] The vasoconstrictor properties of epinephrine can prevent or decrease systemic absorption of antigen such as that from an insect sting or injected medication, if the epinephrine is injected directly into the site of the sting or injection.[5]

Despite the universal acceptance of epinephrine as the drug of choice in the treatment of anaphylaxis and cardiopulmonary resuscitation, the recommended route of administration as well as the dosages for adults and children vary considerably in the literature.[52,53,56-60] Because of the unpredictable onset and explosive nature of acute anaphylaxis, as well as a usually prompt response to treatment, clinical therapeutic trials are difficult to perform.[57] Therefore, treatment recommendations have traditionally been based on clinical experience, anecdotal reports, and knowledge of pathophysiology and pharmacology, as well as animal studies.[57-59]

The Practice Parameters for the Diagnosis and Management of Anaphylaxis was prepared jointly by the Joint Task Force on Practice Parameters of the American College of Allergy, Asthma, and Immunology, American Academy of Allergy, Asthma, and Immunology, and the Joint Council of Allergy, Asthma, and Immunology and published in 1998.[45] Specific recommendations are stated for the use of epinephrine. The dosage of epinephrine recommended for the treatment of acute anaphylaxis in adults is 0.2 ml (0.2 mg) to 0.5 ml (0.5 mg) of a 1:1000 (1 mg/ml) weight per volume (w/v) dilution, every 10 to 15 minutes up to a maximum of 1 ml (1 mg) per dose.[45] In children, the recommended dose is 0.01 ml (0.01 mg)/kg body weight up to a maximum of 0.5 ml (0.5 mg) per dose of 1:1000 (1 mg/ml) w/v dilution, repeated every 15 minutes for two doses and then every 4 hours as needed.[45,61] This concurs with Fisher's recommendation[57] but is slightly different from the 0.3 to 0.5 mg of 1:1000 w/v epinephrine recommended by other authors.[3,53,62,63] Interestingly, the British National Formulary recommends 0.5 to 1 mg of 1:1000 w/v epinephrine, whereas the Swedish recommend a 0.5- to 0.8-mg dose.[52] The Project Team of the Resuscitation Council (UK) recommends dosing of epinephrine based not on body weight but on age: age less than 2 years, 62.5 µg; age

Epinephrine

Epinephrine is universally recommended as the drug of choice in the treatment of acute anaphylaxis.[3-5,34,44-48] Epinephrine is a potent catecholamine with both α-adrenergic and β-adrenergic properties.[49-51] The actions of epinephrine reverse all the pathophysiologic features of anaphylaxis.[52] Hypotension, peripheral vasodilation, increased vasopermeability, urticaria, and angioedema are all reversed by the α-adrenergic stimulation from epinephrine.[49,53] The success of cardiopulmonary resuscitation is often dependent upon restoration of aortic diastolic pressure.[54] Increased aortic pressure enhances myocardial perfusion and cerebral perfusion is improved by increased carotid arterial pressure, both of which are results of arterial vasoconstriction and selective redistribution of cardiac output from the α-adrenergic effects of epinephrine.[55] The β agonist properties of epinephrine have positive ino-

2 to 5 years, 125 µg; age 6 to 11 years, 250 µg; and age greater than 11 years, up to 500 µg with a repeat dose after 5 minutes if necessary.[47] The most current recommendation for epinephrine dosage, published in 2002 by Sampson,[43] is 0.01 ml/kg every 10 to 20 minutes up to a maximum of 0.3 to 0.5 ml of 1:1000 w/v dilution. The differences in efficacy between these dosage variations have not been defined by clinical trials but presumably are clinically minor.

There are few data on the amount of epinephrine needed to reverse an anaphylactic reaction. Korenblat and colleagues[64] reviewed 105 anaphylactic reactions in 88 patients, age range 4 to 76 years, mean age 31 ± 16 years, in a retrospective study. Thirty-eight patients (35%) required more than one injection of epinephrine to reverse symptoms of anaphylaxis.[64] Of the 13 children (less than age 11 years) in the study, 6 (46%) required multiple injections of epinephrine.[64] The number of epinephrine doses required to reverse anaphylaxis correlated with the severity of the reaction but even some mild cases of anaphylaxis required more than one dose of epinephrine.[64]

In animal studies high-dose epinephrine in the range of 0.1 mg/kg to 0.2 mg/kg improved myocardial and cerebral perfusion as well as survival outcomes.[55] A nonblinded study of high-dose epinephrine (0.2 mg/kg) in 20 children with cardiac arrest showed improved survival and neurologic outcome compared with a historical cohort control group.[65] Unfortunately, subsequent adult and pediatric studies failed to show any advantage of high-dose epinephrine over standard-dose epinephrine.[55] Furthermore, high doses and overdoses of epinephrine can be associated with tachycardia, hypertension, arrhythmia, and increasing myocardial oxygen consumption, resulting in myocardial ischemia and necrosis.[50,53,59,66]

Epinephrine is available for out-of-hospital use by parents and patients in a user-friendly preloaded autoinjector, Epi-Pen and Epi-Pen Jr (Dey Laboratories, Napa, California). It is a single-use device. Epi-Pen dispenses one 0.3-mg dose of 1:1000 w/v aqueous epinephrine solution, and Epi-Pen Jr dispenses one 0.15-mg dose.[67] The Epi-Pen and Epi-Pen Jr autoinjectors are administered intramuscularly into the vastus lateralis muscle of the thigh.[67] The Epi-Pen dose is appropriate for a 30-kg person, and the Epi-Pen Jr dose is appropriate for a 15-kg child. Given the choice of only two fixed-dose autoinjector formulations of epinephrine for the entire range of all body weights and ages, the potential is great for overdosing and underdosing. Simons and colleagues reviewed epinephrine prescriptions dispensed in the province of Manitoba, Canada over a 4-year period and found the age range for Epi-Pen prescriptions ranged from age 1 year, 8 months to 16 years, 11 months and the age range for Epi-Pen Jr prescriptions was age 2 months to 16 years.[68] The mean age of transition from Epi-Pen Jr to Epi-Pen was 6 years, 6 months ± 2 years, an age where less than 3% of children have reached a weight of 30 kg.[68] Simons and others[68] calculate the possibility that potential overdosing can occur with 6.7% of epinephrine prescriptions and underdosing can potentially affect 0.6% of epinephrine prescriptions. The prescribing physician is faced with the dilemma of which dose of Epi-Pen to use for the "in-between" body weights and body weights below 15 kg and whether to err on the side of giving an overdose or underdose.[69] The Epi-Pen Jr package insert gives the prescribing physician latitude and flexibility in dosing based upon "careful assessment of the individual patient and . . . the life-threatening nature of their reactions."[67] If the prescribing

physician considers doses less than 0.15 mg, "other formulations of injectable epinephrine should be considered."[67] Because of the difficulties of administering small, precisely measured doses of epinephrine from a syringe in a difficult situation "when hands are shaking and a needle is exposed,"[69] Simons and colleagues[68] sought to address this dilemma in two studies. In the first study, 18 parents of children at risk for anaphylaxis were evaluated in their ability to accurately draw up 0.09 ml of epinephrine in a timed test, and their performance was compared to 18 resident physicians, 18 general duty nurses, and 18 emergency department nurses acting as controls.[70] Most parents were unable to draw up the epinephrine dose rapidly or accurately; a number of parents were unable to open the ampule, get air out of a syringe, and locate the injection site.[70] There was a fortyfold range in the epinephrine concentration drawn up by the parent group compared to the control group of health professionals.[70] Simons et al[70] concluded that prescribing the Epi-Pen Jr for infants who weigh less than 10 kg, despite potentially delivering an overdose, appears preferable to the ampule/syringe/needle technique, which might lead to a late dose, overdose, underdose, or no dose at all. In the second study, the rate and extent of epinephrine absorption in children between 15 and 30 kg was measured following administration of Epi-Pen and Epi-Pen Jr.[71] Ten children participated, with a mean age of 5.4 ± 0.4 years and a mean weight of 18.0 ± 0.6 kg. Five children receiving Epi-Pen Jr at a dose of 0.008 to 0.009 mg/kg reached a plasma epinephrine concentration of 2037 ± 541 pg/ml.[71] The five children who received Epi-Pen at a dose of 0.01 to 0.014 mg/kg had a plasma epinephrine concentration of 2289 ± 405 pg/ml.[71] Peak epinephrine plasma concentrations were reached in 16 ± 3 minutes with Epi-Pen Jr and 15 ± 3 minutes with Epi-Pen.[71] Systolic blood pressure was higher 30 minutes after Epi-Pen administration than after Epi-Pen Jr.[71] All 10 children experienced some transient adverse effect after either Epi-Pen or Epi-Pen Jr such as pallor (100%), tremor (80%), anxiety (70%), cardiac symptoms such as palpitations, "pounding or racing heart" (50%), headache (20%), and nausea (20%).[71] Simons et al[71] concluded that the benefits of prompt epinephrine administration outweigh the risks of transient adverse pharmacologic reactions. For the child between 15 kg and 30 kg, the clinical decision to prescribe Epi-Pen Jr or Epi-Pen must be based on the actual weight and how close it is to 15 or 30 kg, the severity of prior anaphylactic reactions, a concomitant history of asthma, and ease of access to emergency medical services.[71] It seems reasonable to recommend the development of additional epinephrine autoinjectors available in several smaller sizes, such as 0.05 mg and 0.1 mg, to allow for more precise milligram-per-kilogram dosing for the very young child.[69-71]

In addition to the controversies concerning the dosing of epinephrine, there have been controversies in the literature regarding the route of administration of epinephrine: subcutaneous, intramuscular, inhaled, and intravenous. For example, subcutaneous epinephrine has been recommended for mild anaphylaxis, whereas the intramuscular route is recommended for more severe reactions.[34,53,63] Simons and colleagues[72] have also made significant contributions toward settling these issues. A prospective, randomized, blinded, parallel-group study of 17 children with anaphylaxis to food, Hymenoptera venom, and other agents was performed in which a dose of 0.01 mg/kg epinephrine up to a maximum of

0.3 ml was injected subcutaneously or intramuscularly by Epi-Pen. Plasma epinephrine concentrations, heart rate, blood pressure, and adverse effects were compared between the two treatment groups. In the 9 children receiving subcutaneous epinephrine, the maximum plasma epinephrine concentration was 1802 ± 214 pg/ml, reached at a mean time of 34 ± 14 minutes with only 2 children reaching maximum plasma concentration by 5 minutes.[72] In contrast, in the 8 children receiving intramuscular epinephrine by Epi-Pen, the mean maximum plasma epinephrine concentration was 2136 ± 351 pg/ml, reached at a mean time of 8 ± 2 minutes, with 6 children reaching maximum plasma levels by 5 minutes.[72] There were no serious adverse effects observed for any child in the study; transient minor effects were noted: tremor (94%), pallor (82%), headache (24%), tingling of extremities (18%), and nausea (6%).[72] Because of the delayed absorption of subcutaneously administered epinephrine in children, the authors concluded that the preferred route of administration of epinephrine in children is intramuscular.[72] Simons and colleagues[73] extended these observations to adults in a randomized, blinded, parallel-group, controlled study of 13 adult males with a mean age of 26 ± 2 years and mean weight of 85 ± 5 kg. Epinephrine 0.3 mg was injected intramuscularly by ampule or Epi-Pen into either the thigh or deltoid muscle. Subcutaneous epinephrine 0.3 mg by ampule was injected into the arm. Intramuscular epinephrine injected into the thigh gave ninefold to fourteenfold higher peak plasma epinephrine concentrations compared to intramuscular epinephrine injected into the deltoid muscle or subcutaneous epinephrine injected into the arm.[73] The authors hypothesize that the greater absorption of epinephrine from the thigh compared to the arm is because of the greater vascularity of the vastus lateralis muscle compared to the deltoid muscle.[73]

The convincing evidence of these two studies by Simons and colleagues[73] indicates that epinephrine should be administered intramuscularly into the thigh in the treatment of acute anaphylaxis. The most current recommendations reflect this new data.[43,74] There is a concern that in some patients, particularly women, the 14.29 mm length (1/2 inch) of the Epi-Pen needle may result in a subcutaneous injection instead of an intramuscular injection because of the presence of the fat pad thickness over the vastus lateralis muscle.[75,76]

Inhalation of epinephrine from a metered-dose inhaler has been recommended as a safe, non-invasive alternative to epinephrine by injection.[77,78] Fifteen to 30 puffs of epinephrine from a metered-dose inhaler yield plasma concentrations equivalent to 0.3 mg injected subcutaneously.[77] Administration of a sympathomimetic amine, oxymetazoline hydrochloride by nonprescription nasal spray, was reported to successfully reverse an anaphylactic reaction to ketoprofen involving upper-airway angioedema in a 39-year-old woman with a history of aspirin and NSAID allergy.[79] The rationale for using these alternate routes of administration is ease of use and better acceptance by patients, widespread nonprescription availability, and directed concentration of the medication to a common site of anaphylaxis—the upper airway.[80] Simons et al[80] sought to measure plasma epinephrine levels following inhalation of epinephrine by prospectively studying 19 children ages 6 to 14 years, all with a history of anaphylaxis and of whom 15 (79%) also had concomitant asthma. Each child was instructed to take the number of inhalations of epinephrine calculated to increase plasma epinephrine concentrations,

ranging from 10 to 20 puffs. Only 4 (21%) of the children were able to take the required number of puffs.[80] There was a wide range in plasma epinephrine concentrations as well as a wide range in the time to achieve peak concentrations of 32.7 ± 62 minutes.[80] Fourteen (79%) of the children complained that the inhalations tasted bad and many complained of the difficulty of taking so many inhalations.[80] Given these problems, epinephrine by inhalation is an unreliable method to treat acute anaphylaxis in children and certainly no substitute for the recommended route of intramuscular injection.[80]

When the patient with anaphylaxis presents with hypotension, cardiovascular shock, or cardiopulmonary arrest, epinephrine is administered intravenously.* Because intravenous epinephrine increases the risk of supraventricular and ventricular tachyarrhythmias, hypertension, and myocardial ischemia and necrosis, slow administration and dilution of the epinephrine to a 1:100,000 w/v dilution are recommended.[34,45,50,53,59] Although there has been some controversy in the literature regarding the dosage of intravenous epinephrine for anaphylactic shock,[59,60] the current consensus is 0.01 mg/kg (0.1 mg/kg of 1:10,000 dilution or 0.01 mg/kg of 1:100,000 dilution).[34,50] Continuous intravenous epinephrine infusion at a rate of 0.1 to 0.2 μg/kg/min can be titrated by increasing in increments of 0.1 μg/kg/min to a maximum of 1.5 μg/kg/min to maintain blood pressure and vital signs. Low-dose infusions have more β-adrenergic effect, whereas higher-dose infusions have more α-adrenergic effect with vasoconstriction.[51] Because hypoxemia and acidosis can affect the responsiveness of tissues to epinephrine, these conditions must be corrected before epinephrine is administered.[54] Patients receiving intravenous epinephrine need to have it administered through a secure intravenous line and never mixed with bicarbonate as alkaline pH conditions will inactivate epinephrine.[50] Patients need to be under continuous telemetry with monitoring of cardiovascular parameters and oxygenation.[50] If intravascular access cannot be established, epinephrine can be absorbed endotracheally at a dose of 0.1 mg/kg (1:1000 dilution) despite unpredictable absorption and plasma concentrations from the upper airway.[50]

Fluid Replacement

Loss of up to 50% of intravascular volume from third spacing of fluid because of increased vasopermeability from anaphylaxis can result in profound hypotension unresponsive to epinephrine. Twenty-five percent of fatal anaphylaxis is caused by circulatory failure with hypotension.[59] Correction of hypovolemic shock with rapid fluid replacement together with epinephrine administration is a major goal of treatment.[66] Hypotensive patients should be placed in the Trendelenburg position.[81] Volume expansion can be achieved with a large-bore intravenous line and a bolus of crystalloid (lactated Ringer's solution or normal saline solution) or colloid (5% albumin or hydroxyethyl starch) at a rate of 10 to 20 ml/kg in the first 5 minutes and repeated as necessary.[52,81,82] Children can receive up to 30 ml/kg of fluid volume in the first hour.[82] There are differences of opinion as to whether to administer crystalloid or colloid, but the material used is less important than the rate of administration of volume.[59,66,83] Large volumes may be required. Central venous pressure,

*References 5, 34, 43, 45, 48, 52-54, 57, 59.

heart rate, and hematocrit should be monitored to prevent fluid overload.[66]

Antihistamines

Antihistamines are not appropriate monotherapy for the treatment of acute anaphylaxis. Slow-acting antihistamines, even at maximal doses, cannot overcome the massive, explosive mediator release seen in acute anaphylaxis, and the high concentration of histamine-occupying receptors will simply overwhelm any competitive receptor antagonist.[5,52] Antihistamines do not prevent mediator release and they do not have any effect on other mediators released in anaphylaxis such as leukotrienes, prostaglandins, platelet-activating factor, and others.[5,52] H_1 receptor antagonists will mitigate the dermal symptoms of pruritis, urticaria, and angioedema and may prevent relapse of symptoms. Antihistamines are unlikely to be harmful and may be beneficial so it is reasonable that after the patient has been treated with epinephrine and fluids, and has stable cardiorespiratory status, antihistamines can be added to the regimen. Diphenhydramine, the most commonly used H_1 antagonist, can be given orally, intramuscularly, or intravenously at a dose of 1 to 2 mg/kg up to maximum adult dose of 50 mg every 6 hours.[34,45] Other rapidly absorbed H_1 antagonists may be substituted: hydroxyzine 12.5 to 25 mg or chlorpheniramine 10 to 20 mg intramuscularly or intravenously.[34,47,83] Intravenous infusions of antihistamines should be administered slowly, as too rapid a rate of infusion can cause hypotension.[47,83] Antihistamine therapy can be continued for 48 hours to saturate H_1 receptors and prevent relapse of symptoms.

The combination therapy of H_1 and H_2 antagonists is recommended by many authorities in the treatment of acute anaphylaxis.[34,45,52,66,81,85] H_2 receptors mediate the effect of histamine on the atria and ventricles, whereas H_1 receptors mediate the effect of histamine on coronary arteries.[84] There are case reports of H_2 antagonists used successfully in persistent hypotension and refractory anaphylactic shock.[5,52,66] Late-phase cutaneous responses can be blocked by combination H_1 and H_2 therapy.[7] H_2 antagonists may work synergistically with H_1 antagonists.[81] Lieberman concluded from a review of the literature that the combination of H_1 and H_2 antagonists is more effective than the use of H_1 antagonists alone in the prevention of anaphylaxis caused by a variety of agents, including plasma expanders and anesthetic agents such as muscle relaxants, radiocontrast material, and chymopapain.[85] Despite the lack of controlled studies, based on this information, H_2 antagonists such as ranitidine (1.5 mg/kg up to 50 mg intramuscularly or intravenously) are recommended in combination with H_1 antagonists in treatment of acute anaphylaxis to minimize the deleterious cardiac effects of histamine and to reverse epinephrine-resistant shock.[45,59,66,85]

Corticosteroids

The use of corticosteroids, like the use of antihistamines, is considered ancillary to the use of epinephrine, fluids, and oxygen in the acute treatment of anaphylaxis. The onset of action of corticosteroids is even more delayed than that of antihistamines, a minimum of 1 to 2 hours and usually 4 to 6 hours for initial effects to be clinically evident. Corticosteroids are therefore of limited benefit for acute anaphylaxis. Given this time course of action, corticosteroids should be administered after the initial stabilization of the patient. As with antihistamines, there are no controlled studies on the use of corticosteroids in the management of acute anaphylaxis. The use of corticosteroids is based upon knowledge of its pharmacologic properties, including inhibiting of mediator synthesis and release, increasing tissue responsiveness to beta-adrenergic agents, decreasing IgE receptor expression, and decreasing neutrophil and platelet aggregation.[59,66] Its use in the management of anaphylaxis is based upon its utility and effectiveness in the treatment of acute asthma, especially in the abrogation of the late-phase asthmatic response. Although it is not clear that the pathophysiology of the biphasic response of anaphylaxis is the same as that of the late asthmatic response, both involve an IgE-mediated reaction[8] and the generation of leukotrienes and chemotactic mediators, the time course of which is characteristically several hours following the initial response. Late-phase reactions occurring in IgE-mediated reactions of the nose, lung, and skin are abrogated by systemic corticosteroids.[7] Based on these theoretic benefits, many authorities recommend the administration of systemic corticosteroids as part of the treatment of acute anaphylaxis to prevent or attenuate the biphasic response and for patients with bronchospasm as part of their presentation.* In addition, patients who have received corticosteroids within the previous several months may have HPA axis suppression and should be covered with stress doses of hydrocortisone during treatment of their anaphylaxis.[26,85] There is no established preparation or dose. Hydrocortisone 4 to 8 mg/kg or methylprednisolone 1 to 2 mg/kg intravenously every 6 hours may be given.[26,59,82,85] Unfortunately, in three studies of biphasic anaphylaxis, including one in children, there was no benefit of corticosteroid treatment in preventing the biphasic response.[7,8,13] Therefore, even with the early administration of corticosteroids, all patients with an anaphylactic reaction, regardless of their early responses to treatment, must be observed for at least 4 to 6 hours in a hospital facility in the event a biphasic response occurs. Severe anaphylactic reactions require at least a 24-hour hospitalization; Lee and Greenes[13] found that 2% of their pediatric patients with anaphylaxis benefited from such a 24-hour observation period. It is common practice to discharge patients with a minimum 72-hour coverage with both antihistamines and oral steroids.[43]

Bronchodilators

For the asthmatic undergoing anaphylaxis, epinephrine should be given first, and if bronchospasm persists, then inhaled albuterol should be administered. Nebulized albuterol 1.25 to 2.5 mg every 20 minutes or by continuous nebulization should be administered for bronchospasm refractory to epinephrine.[5,34,43] As in the treatment of acute asthma, nebulized ipratropium bromide can be added for synergistic effect with albuterol at a dose of 0.5 mg.[34] Given the association of asthma and anaphylaxis, it is important for the patient at risk for anaphylaxis, especially food-induced anaphylaxis, to maintain good control of asthma with a maintenance regimen and appropriate action plan. Supplemental oxygen and close monitoring of oxygenation are vital to the treatment of anaphylaxis with bronchospasm. Aminophylline by intravenous infusion may be considered for bronchospasm resistant to

*References 2, 3, 5, 26, 47, 59, 85.

epinephrine, nebulized bronchodilators, and steroids in the patient on a beta blocker. Aminophylline functions independent of the β receptor by increasing intracellular cAMP, which may potentiate the effect of epinephrine on inhibiting mediator release.[59] Aminophylline is a bronchodilator and stimulates respiratory muscles and diaphragmatic contractility.[59,66] However, because of its possible cardiac toxicity and potential to cause arrhythmias, especially with concomitant β-adrenergic agents, aminophylline should be avoided in anaphylactic shock.[59,66]

Glucagon

Glucagon has positive chronotropic and inotropic effects on the heart and reverses bronchospasm by directly increasing intracellular cAMP independent of the β-adrenergic receptor.[5,52,66] This mechanism of action enables glucagon to be particularly useful in treating anaphylaxis in a beta-blocked patient in whom the beta agonist effects of epinephrine would be attenuated.[86] Although not widely used in pediatrics, beta blockers are used in some children for migraine prophylaxis. Beta-blocker therapy is associated with an increase in the severity and possibly an increased incidence of anaphylaxis.[86-88] In a beta-blocked patient with acute anaphylaxis, glucagon 0.025 to 0.1 mg/kg up to 1 mg can be administered intravenously every 20 minutes if initial treatment with epinephrine fails to reverse the initial symptoms.[5] Glucagon can also be considered for treatment of anaphylaxis refractory to standard initial treatment with epinephrine, fluids, H_1 and H_2 antagonists, and corticosteroids.[34,85]

Other Pharmacologic Agents

For treatment of hypotension refractory to epinephrine, fluid replacement, combination H_1 and H_2 antagonists, and glucagon, vasopressor agents are indicated. As long as central venous pressure (CVP) is less than 12 mm Hg, high-volume fluid replacement can be continued.[34] Dopamine is the vasopressor of choice in anaphylactic shock and should be started at 5 μg/kg/min titrated to systolic blood pressure, especially if the CVP is greater than 12 mm Hg.[5,34] At this stage of clinical severity, the patient should be under the care of a critical care specialist.

DISPOSITION AND FOLLOW-UP

Patients who have successfully responded to the initial treatment of acute anaphylaxis need to be observed for at least 4 hours in the emergency department for biphasic anaphylaxis, as 90% of biphasic reactions occur within 4 hours of the initial reaction.[43,59] Patients who have moderate to severe anaphylaxis with hypotension, bronchospasm, and/or laryngeal edema need a minimum observation period of 8 to 24 hours following stabilization of vital signs and normalization of clinical status.[47,52,81] Measurement of elevated serum β-tryptase is diagnostic of anaphylaxis and can help to distinguish it from other disorders, particularly if the clinical presentation involves hypotension without other manifestations of anaphylaxis.[90] However, normal tryptase levels do not rule out the diagnosis of anaphylaxis, especially if the reaction is very mild or the patient has food-induced anaphylaxis that has not been associated with elevation of serum β-tryptase

levels.[10,26] Serum β-tryptase peaks 1 to 2 hours after the onset of symptoms, and remains elevated for 4 to 6 hours after, and can be detected even after 12 hours.[45] Tryptase is a relatively stable compound and can be ordered retrospectively on stored serum 1 to 2 days old to document the diagnosis of anaphylaxis.[45]

Discharge medications should consist of at least 72 hours of maintenance antihistamine therapy with diphenhydramine or hydroxyzine or low and nonsedating antihistamines such as cetirizine (5 mg/day for weight less than 30 kg, 10 mg/day for 30 kg and greater), loratidine (5 mg/day for age less than 6 years, 10 mg/day for age 6 years and greater), or fexofenadine (30 mg twice daily for age less than 12 years, 60 mg twice daily for age 12 and greater).[43] In addition, treatment with 72 hours of oral prednisone 1 mg/kg/day is recommended for coverage of potential biphasic responses[43] and longer treatment with a tapering schedule may be necessary for the patient with bronchospasm, angioedema, hypotension, and biphasic or protracted anaphylaxis. Oral ranitidine may be useful as an adjunct to H_1 antagonists and prednisone as well as protecting against the GI side effects of oral corticosteroids. Patients with bronchospasm and anaphylaxis without a prior history of asthma need to be discharged with an albuterol metered-dose inhaler with instructions on its use in the event of recurrent bronchospasm.[34] All patients need to be discharged with an epinephrine autoinjector (Epi-Pen or Epi-Pen Jr) with instructions on its technique of administration and use. Ideally, a minimum of three should be dispensed, two available to the patient or parent for use in an acute episode and one for the home or school. There should be a thorough discussion of avoidance strategies against the trigger factor, and if the trigger is unknown, referral to an allergist for a complete diagnostic evaluation should be arranged.

TREATMENT OF IDIOPATHIC ANAPHYLAXIS

When no clear trigger or allergen is identified as the cause of the anaphylaxis, the diagnosis of idiopathic anaphylaxis is made. The management of acute episodes of idiopathic anaphylaxis is identical to the treatment of acute anaphylaxis. Unlike antigen-induced anaphylaxis, recurrent episodes of idiopathic anaphylaxis can be prevented by the use of maintenance oral corticosteroids.[20,21,89] Patients with idiopathic anaphylaxis who have more than six episodes per year are treated with oral prednisone 1 to 2 mg/kg/day for 1 week or until symptoms are controlled and then tapered slowly by 5 to 10 mg/mo to alternate-day prednisone 1 to 2 mg/kg.[20] As the frequency of anaphylactic episodes decreases, the alternate-day dosage is further tapered on a weekly basis, titrating against symptoms to the lowest dose that maintains control. In addition, the prophylactic regimen consists of maintenance antihistamines such as hydroxyzine 2 mg/kg/day in combination with oral albuterol 0.1 to 0.2 mg/kg three times daily.[20] In the largest series of pediatric anaphylaxis, of 22 patients, 2 (9%) were steroid-dependent and 7 (32%) were in complete remission on follow-up.[20] Ketotifen was added to the regimen of three steroid-dependent patients and one child was able to taper off prednisone completely.[20] For four children with throat angioedema, inhaled beclomethasone dipropionate was added to the regimen with successful results.[20]

FUTURE THERAPIES FOR ANAPHYLAXIS

A promising future therapy for the prevention of anaphylaxis in general may be the administration of humanized anti-IgE antibodies. This treatment has already been studied in asthma and is currently undergoing trials for the prevention of peanut anaphylaxis. Another potential area of interest may be the use of leukotriene modifiers in the treatment of acute anaphylaxis, particularly with respect to its effect on biphasic and protracted anaphylaxis.

There is considerable ongoing research in the modification of specific inhalant and food allergens with molecular biologic techniques. The success of these allergen-specific therapies should have a positive impact on the future incidence of anaphylaxis.

EDUCATION AND PREVENTION OF ANAPHYLAXIS

Education and prevention are the hallmarks of good allergy care and this is especially true for anaphylaxis, the most deadly of all allergic diseases. By identifying the offending triggers and formulating a comprehensive avoidance strategy and action plan, morbidity and mortality of subsequent episodes of anaphylaxis can hopefully be decreased. This process can begin with a referral to an allergy specialist for a thorough allergy history, appropriate diagnostic testing, and recommendations for avoidance. Skin testing and serum IgE-specific (RAST and immunoCAP) testing are available for foods, inhalants, insect venoms, drugs (penicillin), vaccines (measles-mumps-rubella, influenza), and latex. For specific allergic disorders, specific therapies are available such as insect venom immunotherapy; acute and long-term drug desensitization to penicillin, aspirin, and insulin; and pretreatment of radiocontrast media reactions with antihistamines and corticosteroids. These specific allergic disorders and their evaluation and management are reviewed elsewhere in this book. For the patient with a history of asthma, the asthma regimen needs to be optimized as well to minimize possible complications from asthma during any subsequent episodes of anaphylaxis. Concomitant medication use such as beta blockers, ACE inhibitors, and MAO inhibitors that may exacerbate anaphylaxis or its treatment should be discontinued. The treatment plan centers on teaching the patient and family the signs and symptoms of anaphylaxis because early recognition of anaphylaxis and early administration of epinephrine correlate with good outcome.[10] An algorithm for the evaluation and management of the child with anaphylaxis is presented in Figure 60-1.

Educating the patient and family on using the Epi-Pen with the proper technique is of great importance. There are a number of studies documenting problems with patient education, compliance, poor technique, and even more disconcerting problems of physicians underprescribing epinephrine, failing to provide teaching on the use of Epi-Pen, prescribing errors in dose, and lacking knowledge among physicians in the actual use of the device.[69] In Huang's study of 98 patients,[91] 16% did not know the circumstances for use of the Epi-Pen, 92% did not have the use of the device demonstrated to them by the physician in their doctor's office, and 60% did not know how to administer the device. Sicherer and colleagues[92] studied 101 families of food-allergic children and found that 68% were unable to demonstrate the correct use of Epi-Pen; only 71% had their Epi-Pen in their possession, of whom 45% had expired Epi-Pen; and 23% did not have Epi-Pen in their school. In the same study, surprisingly only 21% of attending pediatricians and 36% of residents correctly demonstrated the device.[92] Blyth and Sundrum[93] had similar findings in a study of 25 children and their families. Seventy-six percent were unable to demonstrate the correct technique of administration, 12% had the incorrect dose of Epi-Pen, and 48% had no follow-up arrangements in place. Gold and Sainsbury[94] studied 68 children and their families and found that 76% were unable to recall the steps required to use the Epi-Pen, only 40% had the Epi-Pen and an action plan in place at school, and the Epi-Pen was used in only 29% of recurrent anaphylactic reactions. Oral antihistamines were used to treat symptoms 76% of the time, and when Epi-Pen was used, it was often after a trial of antihistamines first.[94] An even more disturbing study by Grouhi and colleagues[95] surveyed 122 physicians composed of emergency physicians, family practitioners, and pediatricians and found that 81% had no placebo Epi-Pen trainer to educate their patients, 75% were unable themselves to demonstrate the device (with the major mistake being forgetting to hold the device in site for 10 seconds), and 76% did not know the two available doses. These studies highlight the importance of educating both patients and their families as well as physicians. Patients need to practice using the Epi-Pen with a trainer device or with expired devices. They also need to note the expiration dates of their devices and obtain replacement Epi-Pen in a timely fashion. Simons and colleagues[96] did address the issue of expired Epi-Pen and found that the epinephrine content of expired devices correlated inversely with the number of months past the expiration date. They recommend using an expired device if no other epinephrine source is available, provided no discoloration or precipitate is observed, as the potential benefit of a suboptimal dose is greater than no epinephrine dose at all.[96]

Studies of fatal food-induced anaphylaxis show that most fatalities occur outside the home, with children dying usually in the school setting and adults dying in eating establishments.[10,28,38,97] Guidelines for management of anaphylaxis in schools have been published, emphasizing the identification of the child with life-threatening allergies, having a written individual health care action plan for that child, education of school staff in avoidance strategies, and training nonmedical staff in the use of Epi-Pen, which must be "easily accessible" in the classroom or, if the child is old enough to self-administer, in the child's possession.[98] The restaurant and food industries also need to be made more aware of the growing population of food-allergic consumers and be educated on the need for informative, unambiguous, and user-friendly labeling; address the issues of cross-contamination in food preparation, processing, and packaging; and train restaurant staff to be more knowledgeable about allergies and to listen to their customers' needs and requests. Patients and families need to be knowledgeable about their local emergency services network and who the first responder to an emergency call will be and whether they will be equipped and trained to administer epinephrine. Wearing a MedicAlert bracelet can be another way to optimize on-site care, particularly if there is no adult accessible to convey medical information regarding the child. Educating the public and increasing awareness of food allergies and other potentially lethal allergies are important in promoting understanding to patients and families as well as

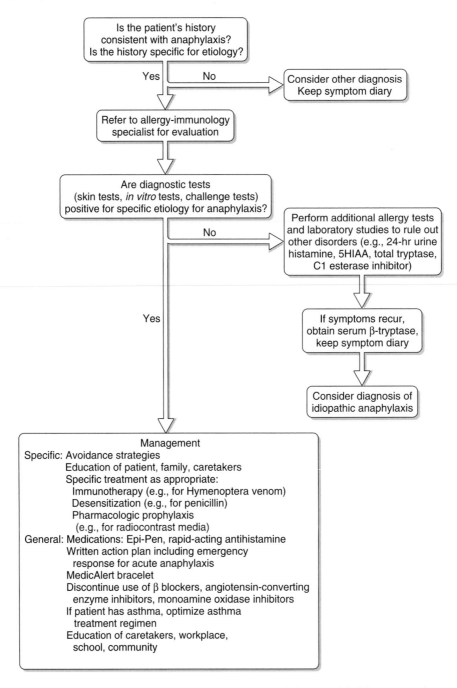

FIGURE 60-1 Algorithm for the evaluation and management of anaphylaxis. (Modified from Joint Task Force on Practice Parameters: *J Allergy Clin Immunol* 101:S466-S468, 1988.)

improving the general climate for safety and health. The Food Allergy and Anaphylaxis Network has been one of the most valuable resources for patients, families, health care professionals, and the general public in disseminating practical advice and up-to-date scientific information, promoting research, and being active in the food industry and legislative issues as well. They can be contacted at 800-929-4040 or www. foodallergy.org.

CONCLUSIONS

Box 60-2 summarizes the key concepts of the treatment and management of anaphylaxis. Anaphylaxis is a life-threatening,

potentially fatal disorder that in children is often caused by food hypersensitivity but may also be caused by allergy to insect venom, medication, and latex. The most common food allergies resulting in fatal anaphylaxis are peanut and tree nut hypersensitivities. The medication of choice for acute anaphylaxis is intramuscular epinephrine. Patients who are at risk for anaphylaxis must be provided with epinephrine autoinjectors (Epi-Pen or Epi-Pen Jr) for self-administration. Failure to administer epinephrine early and a history of asthma are risk factors for fatal anaphylaxis. The patient undergoing an acute anaphylactic reaction must be quickly assessed for the ABCs of cardiopulmonary resuscitation: airway, breathing, and circulation. After epinephrine is given, oxygen, fluid

- Anaphylaxis is a life-threatening multi-system reaction in children most often triggered by food, but also by medications, stinging insect venom, and latex.
- Peanut and tree nuts are the most common causes of fatal anaphylaxis in children.
- Cutaneous symptoms are the most commonly occurring symptoms in acute anaphylaxis but the absence of cutaneous symptoms does not preclude the diagnosis of anaphylaxis.
- Of fatal anaphylaxis, 50% occurs within the first hour. The most important risk factor for a fatal outcome is the delay of administration of epinephrine.
- The treatment of acute anaphylaxis is intramuscular epinephrine. H_1, H_2 antagonists, systemic corticosteroids, and bronchodilators are secondary medications to be given *after* epinephrine has been administered.
- Of patients with anaphylaxis, 5% to 20% have biphasic anaphylaxis, a late-phase of anaphylactic symptoms usually occurring 4 to 6 hours after the acute reaction. Pretreatment with corticosteroids and antihistamines is often ineffective in preventing biphasic anaphylaxis.
- Patients experiencing acute anaphylaxis need to be observed in a medical facility for a minimum of 4 hours after initial treatment, to monitor for signs and symptoms of biphasic anaphylaxis.
- Patients with anaphylaxis need a thorough, comprehensive allergy-immunology evaluation to diagnose the specific etiology. The physician and family need to implement a written action plan detailing the early recognition of signs and symptoms of anaphylaxis, and the use of an epinephrine auto-injector for self-administration EpiPen, for pre-hospital treatment.
- Because fatal anaphylaxis occurs despite timely and appropriate treatment, successful avoidance strategies and education remain the mainstay of management.

replacement, and airway support are critical components of therapy. H_1 and H_1 antagonists and corticosteroids are administered as second-line therapies to ameliorate symptoms and attenuate the biphasic response, which can occur in 5% to 20% of acute anaphylactic reactions. Unfortunately, patients can have fatal outcomes even with maximal therapy. Therefore prevention and education are of paramount importance in the management of the child at risk for anaphylaxis. Identification of the triggers with an allergy evaluation is important so that the family can then formulate avoidance strategies, particularly with regard to learning all the various forms the allergen can take, such as food proteins being "hidden" in other foods and cross-reacting substances, and learning to read labels. It is essential for the patient and family to recognize the signs and symptoms of anaphylaxis and to have a detailed written action plan so that appropriate intervention can occur in a timely manner. Learning the proper use of the Epi-Pen device and using it at the right time is the cornerstone of pre-hospital treatment. Education of the public, particularly with regard to the school setting, will promote a safer environment and conditions more conducive to a rapid, timely response to a medical emergency. It is hoped that new directions in therapy will eventually provide definitive treatment for anaphylaxis of all etiologies.

REFERENCES

1. Austen KF: Systemic anaphylaxis in the human being, *N Engl J Med* 291:661-664, 1974.
2. Sheffer AL: Anaphylaxis, *J Allergy Clin Immunol* 75:227-234, 1985.
3. Bochner BS, Lichtenstein LM: Anaphylaxis, *N Engl J Med* 324:1785-1790, 1991.
4. Yunginger JW: Anaphylaxis, *Ann Allergy* 69:87-96, 1992.
5. Kemp SF: Current concepts in pathophysiology, diagnosis, and management of anaphylaxis, *Immunol Allergy Clin North Am* 21:611-634, 2001.
6. Ewan PW: Anaphylaxis, *Br Med J* 316:1442-1445, 1998.
7. Stark BJ, Sullivan TJ: Biphasic and protracted anaphylaxis, *J Allergy Clin Immunol* 78:76-83, 1986.
8. Popa VT, Lerner SA: Biphasic systemic anaphylactic reaction: three illustrative cases, *Ann Allergy* 53: 151-155, 1984.
9. Douglas DM, Sukenick E, Andrade WP, et al: Biphasic systemic anaphylaxis: an inpatient and outpatient study, *J Allergy Clin Immunol* 93: 977-985, 1994.
10. Sampson HA, Mendelson L, Rosen JP: Fatal and near-fatal anaphylactic reactions to food in children and adolescents, *N Engl J Med* 327:380-384, 1992.
11. Brady WJ, Luber S, Carter CT, et al: Multiphasic anaphylaxis: an uncommon event in the emergency department, *Acad Emerg Med* 4:193-197, 1996.
12. Brazil E, MacNamara AF: "Not so immediate" hypersensitivity—the danger of biphasic anaphylactic reactions, *J Accid Emerg Med* 15:252-253, 1998.
13. Lee JM, Greenes DS: Biphasic anaphylactic reactions in pediatrics, *Pediatrics* 106:762-766, 2000.
14. Dibs SD, Baker MD: Anaphylaxis in children: a 5-year experience, *Pediatrics* 99:e7, 1999.
15. Novembre E, Cianferoni A, Bernardini R, et al: Anaphylaxis in children: clinical and allergologic features, *Pediatrics* 101:e8, 1998.
16. Yocum MW, Khan DA: Assessment of patients who have experienced anaphylaxis: a 3- year survey, *Mayo Clinic Proc* 69:16-23, 1994.
17. Kemp SF, Lockey RF, Wolf BL, et al: Anaphylaxis: a review of 266 cases, *Arch Int Med* 155:1749-1754, 1995.
18. Yocum MW, Butterfield JH, Klein JS, et al: Epidemiology of anaphylaxis in Olmsted county: a population-based study, *J Allergy Clin Immunol* 104:452-456, 1999.
19. Brown AF, McKinnon D, Chu K: Emergency department anaphylaxis: a review of 142 patients in a single year, *J Allergy Clin Immunol* 108: 861-868, 2001.
20. Ditto AM, Krasnick J, Greenberger PA, et al: Pediatric idiopathic anaphylaxis: experience with 22 patients, *J Allergy Clin Immunol* 100:320-326, 1997.
21. Hogan, MB, Kelly MA, Wilson NW: Idiopathic anaphylaxis in children, *Ann Allergy Asthma Immunol* 81:140-142, 1998.
22. Winbury SL, Lieberman P: Anaphylaxis, *Immunol Allergy Clin North Am* 15:447-475, 1995.
23. Ewan PW: Anaphylaxis, *Br Med J* 316:1442-1445, 1998.
24. Neugut AI, Ghatak AT, Miller RL: Anaphylaxis in the United States, *Arch Intern Med* 161:15-21, 2001.
25. Herrera AM, deShazo RD: Current concepts in anaphylaxis, *Immunol Allergy Clin North Am* 12: 517-534, 1992.
26. Sampson HA: Fatal food-induced anaphylaxis, *Allergy* 53:125-130, 1998.
27. Burks W, Bannon GA, Sicherer S, et al: Peanut-induced anaphylactic reactions, *Int Arch Allergy Immunol* 119:165-172, 1999.
28. Bock SA, Munoz-Furlong A, Sampson HA: Fatalities due to anaphylactic reactions to food, *J Allergy Clin Immunol* 107:191-193, 2001.
29. Crockett RE, Lockey RF: Vaccine hypersensitivity, *Immunol Allergy Clin North Am* 21:707-743, 2001.
30. Cianferoni A, Novembre E, Mugnaini L, et al: Clinical features of acute anaphylaxis in patients admitted to a university hospital: an 11-year retrospective review (1985-1996), *Ann Allergy Asthma Immunol* 87:27-32, 2001.
31. Alonso, MA, Dominguez JS, Sanchez-Hernandez JJ, et al: Idiopathic anaphylaxis: a descriptive study of 81 patients in Spain, *Ann Allergy Asthma Immunol* 88:313-318, 2002.
32. Alves B, Sheikh A: Age specific aetiology of anaphylaxis, *Arch Dis Child* 85:349, 2001.

33. Macdougall CF, Cant AJ, Colver AF: How dangerous is food allergy in childhood? The incidence of severe and fatal allergic reactions across the UK and Ireland, *Arch Dis Child* 86:236-239, 2002.

34. Muelleman RL, Tran TP: Allergy, Hypersensitivity and Anaphylaxis. In Marx JA, Hockberger RS, Walls RM, eds: *Rosen's emergency medicine*, ed 5, St Louis, 2002, Mosby.

35. Lieberman P: Unique clinical presentations of anaphylaxis, *Immunol Allergy Clin North Am* 21:813-825, 2001.

36. Weiler JM: Anaphylaxis in the general population: a frequent and occasionally fatal disorder that is underrecognized, *J Allergy Clin Immunol* 104:271-273, 1999.

37. Reisman RE: Hymenoptera, *Immunol Allergy Clin North Am* 15:567-574, 1995.

38. Yunginger JW, Sweeney KG, Sturner WQ, et al: Fatal food-induced anaphylaxis, *JAMA* 260:1450-1452, 1988.

39. Settipane GA: Anaphylactic deaths in asthmatic patients, *Allergy Proc* 10:271-274, 1989.

40. Lockey RS, Benedict LM, Turkeltaub P, et al: Fatalities from immunotherapy and skin testing, *J Allergy Clin Immunol* 79:660-666, 1987.

41. Reid MJ, Lockey RS, Turkeltaub P et al: Surveys of fatalities from skin testing and immunotherapy, *J Allergy Clin Immunol* 192:6-15, 1993.

42. Pumphrey RSD, Nicholls JM: Epinephrine-resistant food anaphylaxis, *Lancet* 355:1099, 2000.

43. Sampson HA: Peanut allergy, *N Engl J Med* 346:1294-1299, 2002.

44. AAAI Board of Directors: The use of epinephrine in the treatment of anaphylaxis, *J Allergy Clin Immunol* 94:666-668, 1994.

45. Nicklas RA, Bernstein IL, Li JT, et al: The diagnosis and management of anaphylaxis, *J Allergy Clin Immunol* 101:S465-S528, 1998.

46. Fisher M: Treatment of acute anaphylaxis, *Br Med J* 311:731-733, 1995.

47. Project Team of the Resuscitation Council (UK): Emergency medical treatment of anaphylactic reactions, *J Accid Emerg Med* 16:243-247, 1999.

48. Cummins RO, Hazinski MR, Baskett PJF, et al: Guidelines 2000 for cardiopulmonary resuscitation and emergency cardiovascular care, Part 8. Advanced challenges in resuscitation, *Circulation* 102:I-241–I-243, 2000.

49. Hoffman BB: Catecholamines, sympathomimetic drugs, and adrenergic receptor anatagonists. In Hardman JG, Limbird LE, Gilman AG, eds: *Goodman & Gilman's the pharmacologic basis of therapeutics*, ed 10, New York, 2001, McGraw-Hill.

50. Cummins RO, Hazinski MR, Baskett PJF, et al: Guidelines 2000 for cardiopulmonary resuscitation and emergency cardiovascular care, Part 10. Pediatric advanced life support, *Circulation* 102:I-291–I-342, 2000.

51. Zaritsky A, Chernow B: Use of catecholamines in pediatrics, *J Pediatr* 105:341-350, 1984.

52. Brown AFT: Anaphylactic shock: mechanisms and treatment, *J Accid Emerg Med* 12:89-100, 1995.

53. Barach EM, Nowak RM, Lee TG, et al: Epinephrine for treatment of anaphylactic shock, *JAMA* 251:2118-2122, 1984.

54. American College of Cardiology, American Heart Association Task Force: Pediatric advanced life support, *JAMA* 268:2262-2275, 1992.

55. Niemann JT: Cardiopulmonary resuscitation, *N Engl J Med* 327:1075-1080, 1992.

56. Longmore JM: The use of adrenaline in anaphylaxis, *Br Med J* 298:1496, 1989.

57. Fisher M: Treating anaphylaxis with sympathomimetic drugs, *Br Med J* 305:1107-1108, 1992.

58. Stoloff R, Adams SL, Orfan N, et al: Emergency medical recognition and management of idiopathic anaphylaxis, *J Emerg Med* 10:693-698, 1992.

59. Brown AFT: Therapeutic controversies in the management of acute anaphylaxis, *J Accid Emerg Med* 15:89-95, 1998.

60. Brown AFT: Intramuscular or intravenous adrenaline in acute, severe anaphylaxis? *J Accid Emerg Med* 17:152, 2000.

61. Taketomo CK, Hodding JH, Kraus DM: Epinephrine, Pediatric Dosage Handbook, ed 7, Hudson (Cleveland), 2000, Lexi-Comp.

62. Sim TC: Anaphylaxis, how to manage and prevent this medical emergency, *Postgrad Med* 92:277-296, 1992.

63. Freeman TM: Anaphylaxis, diagnosis and treatment, *Primary Care* 25:809-817, 1998.

64. Korenblat P, Lundie MJ, Dankner RE, et al: A retrospective study of epinephrine administration for anaphylaxis: how many doses are needed? *Allergy Asthma Proc* 20:383-386, 1999.

65. Goetting MG, Paradis NA: High-dose epinephrine improves outcome from pediatric cardiac arrest, *Ann Emerg Med* 20:22-26, 1991.

66. Perkin RM, Anas NG: Mechanisms and management of anaphylactic shock not responding to traditional therapy, *Ann Allergy* 54:202-208, 1985.

67. EpiPen and EpiPen Jr. In Physician's Desk Reference, ed 56, Montvale, NJ, 2002, Medical Economics.

68. Simons FER, Peterson S, Black CD: Epinephrine dispensing for the out-of-hospital treatment of anaphylaxis in infants and children: A population-based study, *Ann Allergy Asthma Immunol* 86:622-626, 2001.

69. Sicherer SH: Self-injectable epinephrine: no size fits all! *Ann Allergy* 86:597-598, 2001.

70. Simons FER, Chan ES, Gu X, et al: Epinephrine for the out-of-hospital (first-aid) treatment of anaphylaxis in infants: Is the ampule/syringe/needle method practical? *J Allergy Clin Immunol* 108:1040-1044, 2001.

71. Simons FER, Gu X, Silver NA, et al: EpiPen Jr versus EpiPen in young children weighing 15 to 30 kg at risk for anaphylaxis, *J Allergy Clin Immunol* 109:171-175, 2002.

72. Simons FER, Roberts JR, Gu X, et al: Epinephrine absorption in children with a history of anaphylaxis, *J Allergy Clin Immunol* 101:33-37, 1998.

73. Simons FER, Gu X, Simons, KJ: Epinephrine absorption in adults: intramuscular versus subcutaneous injection, *J Allergy Clin Immunol* 108:871-873, 2001.

74. Hughes G, Fitzharris P: Managing acute anaphylaxis, *Br Med J* 319:1-2, 1999.

75. Chowdhury BA, Meyer RJ: Intramuscular versus subcutaneous injection of epinephrine in the treatment of anaphylaxis (letter), *J Allergy Clin Immunol* 109:720, 2002.

76. Simons FER, Gu X, Simons KJ: Intramuscular versus subcutaneous injection of epinephrine in the treatment of anaphylaxis (reply), *J Allergy Clin Immunol* 109:720-721, 2002.

77. Warren JB, Doble N, Dalton N, et al: Systemic absorption of inhaled epinephrine, *Clin Pharm Ther* 40:673-678, 1986.

78. Warren JB: Anaphylaxis, *N Engl J Med* 325:1658, 1991.

79. Kim KT, Kwong FK, Klaustermeyer WB: Use of non-prescription decongestant to abort anaphylaxis (letter), *N Engl J Med* 341:439,1993.

80. Simons FER, Gu X, Johnston LM, et al: Can epinephrine inhalations be substituted for epinephrine injection in children at risk for systemic anaphylaxis? *Pediatrics* 106:1040-1044, 2000.

81. Kulick RM, Ruddy RM: Allergic emergencies. In Fleisher G, Ludwig S, eds: *Textbook of pediatric emergency medicine*, ed 4, Philadelphia, 2000, Lippincott Williams & Wilkins.

82. Saryan JA, O'Loughlin JM: Anaphylaxis in children, *Pediatr Ann* 21:590-598, 1992.

83. Lieberman P: Anaphylaxis: guidelines for prevention and management, *J Respir Dis* 16:456-462, 1995.

84. Lieberman P: The use of antihistamines in the prevention and treatment of anaphylaxis and anaphylactoid reactions, *J Allergy Clin Immunol* 86:684-686, 1990.

85. Lieberman P: Anaphylaxis and anaphylactoid reactions. In Middleton E, Reed CE, Ellis EF, et al, eds: *Allergy: principles and practice*, ed 5, St Louis, 1998, Mosby.

86. Zaloga GP, Delacey W, Holmboe E, et al: Glucagon reversal of hypotension in a case of anaphylactoid shock, *Ann Intern Med* 105:65-66, 1986.

87. Toogood JH: Beta-blocker therapy and the risk of anaphylaxis, *Can Med Assoc J* 136:929-933, 1987.

88. Toogood JH: Risk of anaphylaxis in patients receiving beta-blocker drugs, *J Allergy Clin Immunol* 81:1-5,1988.

89. Patterson R, Stoloff RS, Greenberger PA, et al: Algorithms for the diagnosis and management of idiopathic anaphylaxis, *Ann Allergy* 71:40-44, 1993.

90. Schwartz LB, Metcalfe DD, Miller JS, et al: Tryptase levels as an indicator of mast-cell activation in systemic anaphylaxis and mastocytosis, *N Engl J Med* 316:1622-1626, 1987.

91. Huang S: A survey of Epi-PEN use in patients with a history of anaphylaxis, *J Allergy Clin Immunol* 102:525-526, 1998.

92. Sicherer S, Forman JA, Noone SA: Use assessment of self-administered epinephrine among food-allergic children and pediatricians, *Pediatrics* 105:359-362, 2000.

93. Blyth TP, Sundrum R: Adrenaline autoinjectors and schoolchildren: a community based study, *Arch Dis Child* 86:26-27, 2002.

94. Gold MS, Sainsbury R: First aid anaphylaxis management in children who were prescribed an epinephrine autoinjector device (EpiPen), *J Allergy Clin Immunol* 106:171-176, 2000.

95. Grouhi M, Alshehri M, Hummel D, et al: Anaphylaxis and epinephrine autoinjector training: who will teach the teachers?, *J Allergy Clin Immunol* 103:190-193, 1999.

96. Simons FER, Gu X, Simons KJ: Outdated EpiPen and EpiPen Jr autoinjectors: past their prime? *J Allergy Clin Immunol* 105:1025-1030, 2000.

97. Pumphrey RSH: Lessons for management of anaphylaxis from a study of fatal reactions, *Clin Exp Allergy* 30:1144-1150, 2000.

98. AAAAI Board of Directors: Anaphylaxis in schools and other childcare settings, *J Allergy Clin Immunol* 102:173-176, 1998.

AUTOANTIBODIES IN PEDIATRIC RHEUMATOLOGIC DISEASES

AUTOANTIBODIES ASSOCIATED WITH SYSTEMIC LUPUS ERYTHEMATOSUS

ANTINUCLEAR ANTIBODY (ANA)

Positive in 98% of patients with systemic lupus erythematosus (SLE)

Positive in 13.3% of normal population at titer of 1:160

May also be positive in scleroderma, Sjögren's syndrome, rheumatoid arthritis, polyarteritis nodosa, dermatomyositis, polymyositis

Pattern of staining is helpful in determining particular type of antinuclear antibody (see below)

Homogeneous staining

Anti–double-stranded (ds) DNA

50% of patients with SLE, suggests more serious disease

Titer correlates with disease activity

Anti-histone

Associated with drug-induced lupus

Speckled pattern

Anti-Smith (anti-Sm)

25% of patients with SLE

Most specific antibody test for SLE

Antiribonucleoprotein (anti-RNP, anti–U1-RNP)

25% of patients with SLE

Also associated with mixed connective tissue disease (MCTD)

Anti-Ro/SSA

30% of patients with SLE

Also associated with Sjögren's syndrome, neonatal lupus, photosensitivity

Anti-La/SSB

15% of patients with SLE

Occurs in association with SSA

Antiphospholipid, Anticardiolipin, Lupus Anticoagulant, Anti-β_2 glycoprotein I (β_2-GPI)

33% of patients with SLE

One third of patients with anti-phospholipid antibodies have thrombotic/embolic events

AUTOANTIBODIES IN JUVENILE RHEUMATOID ARTHRITIS

ANA positivity in patients with pauciarticular juvenile rheumatoid arthritis (JRA) is associated with increased risk of uveitis

Rheumatoid factor positivity in polyarticular JRA is associated with more chronic disease course

AUTOANTIBODIES IN SCLERODERMA

Anti-centromere and anti–Scl-70 and others are associated with scleroderma

AUTOANTIBODIES ASSOCIATED WITH SYSTEMIC VASCULITIDES

ANTINEUTROPHIL CYTOPLASMIC ANTIBODY (ANCA)

Cytoplasmic ANCA (c-ANCA) is highly specific for Wegener's granulomatosis

Perinuclear ANCA (p-ANCA) is associated with microscopic polyangiitis, Churg-Strauss syndrome, IBD-associated vasculitis, and other vasculitides

ANTIGLOMERULAR BASEMENT MEMBRANE (GBM)

Associated with Goodpasture's syndrome

AUTOANTIBODIES ASSOCIATED WITH OTHER AUTOIMMUNE DISEASES

Addison's disease: antiadrenal antibodies

Celiac disease and dermatitis herpetiformis: antigliadin, antiendomysial, antireticulin, and anti-tissue transglutaminase antibodies

Chronic active hepatitis: anti-smooth muscle antibodies

Diabetes mellitus type I: anti-islet cell antibodies

Myasthenia gravis: anti-acetylcholine receptor antibodies

Pemphigoid: anti BP230 and BP180 (bullous pemphigoid)

Pemphigus: antidesmoglein and antiplakoglobulin

Pernicious anemia: anti-intrinsic factor antibodies

Primary biliary cirrhosis: antimitochondrial antibodies

Thyroid disease: antithyroid peroxidase, antithyroglobulin, and antithyrotropin receptor antibodies

TABLE 1 Relative Size of Lymphocyte Subpopulations in Blood*

Lymphocyte Subpopulations	Neonatal (N = 20)	1 wk–2 mo (N = 13)	2-5 mo (N = 46)	5-9 mo (N = 105)	9-15 mo (N = 70)	15-24 mo (N = 33)	2-5 yr (N = 33)	5-10 yr (N = 35)	10-16 yr (N = 23)	Adults (N = 51)
CD19+ B lymphocytes	12% (5-22)	15% (4-26)	24% (14-39)	21% (13-35)	25% (15-39)	28% (17-41)	24% (14-44)	18% (10-31)	16% (8-24)	12% (6-19)
CD3+ T lymphocytes	62% (28-76)	72% (60-85)	63% (48-75)	66% (50-77)	65% (54-76)	64% (39-73)	64% (43-76)	69% (55-78)	67% (52-78)	72% (55-83)
CD3+/CD4+ T lymphocytes	41% (17-52)	55% (41-68)	45% (33-58)	45% (33-58)	44% (31-54)	41% (25-50)	37% (23-48)	35% (27-53)	39% (25-48)	44% (28-57)
CD3+/CD8+ T lymphocytes	24% (10-41)	16% (9-23)	17% (11-25)	18% (13-26)	18% (12-28)	20% (11-32)	24% (14-33)	28% (19-34)	23% (9-35)	24% (10-39)
CD4/CD8 ratio per CD3+	1.8 (1.0-2.6)	3.8 (1.3-6.3)	2.7 (1.7-3.9)	2.5 (1.6-3.8)	2.4 (1.3-3.9)	1.9 (0.9-3.7)	1.6 (0.9-2.9)	1.2 (0.9-2.6)	1.7 (0.9-3.4)	1.9 (1.0-3.6)
CD3+/HLA-DR+ T lymphocytes	2% (1-6)	5% (1-38)	3% (1-9)	3% (1-7)	4% (2-8)	6% (3-12)	6% (3-13)	7% (3-14)	4% (1-8)	5% (2-12)
CD3−/CD16-56+ NK cells	20% (6-58)	8% (3-23)	6% (2-14)	5% (2-13)	7% (3-17)	8% (3-16)	10% (4-23)	12% (4-26)	15% (6-27)	13% (7-31)

From Comans-Bitter WM, de Groot R, van den Beemd R, et al: *J Pediatr* 130:388-393, 1997.

*The relative frequencies are expressed within the lymphocyte population: median and percentiles (5th to 95th percentiles).

TABLE 2 Absolute Size of Lymphocyte Subpopulations in Blood*

Lymphocyte Subpopulations	Neonatal (N = 20)	1 wk–2 mo (N = 13)	2-5 mo (N = 46)	5-9 mo (N = 105)	9-15 mo (N = 70)	15-24 mo (N = 33)	2-5 yr (N = 33)	5-10 yr (N = 35)	10-16 yr (N = 23)	Adults (N = 51)
Lymphocytes	4.8 (0.7-7.3)	6.7 (3.5-13.1)	5.9 (3.7-9.6)	6.0 (3.8-9.9)	5.5 (2.6-10.4)	5.6 (2.7-11.9)	3.3 (1.7-6.9)	2.8 (1.1-5.9)	2.2 (1.0-5.3)	1.8 (1.0-2.8)
CD19+ B lymphocytes	0.6 (0.04-1.1)	1.0 (0.6-1.9)	1.3 (0.6-3.0)	1.3 (0.7-2.5)	1.4 (0.6-2.7)	1.3 (0.6-3.1)	0.8 (0.2-2.1)	0.5 (0.2-1.6)	0.3 (0.2-0.6)	0.2 (0.1-0.5)
CD3+ T lymphocytes	2.8 (0.6-5.0)	4.6 (2.3-7.0)	3.6 (2.3-6.5)	3.8 (2.4-6.9)	3.4 (1.6-6.7)	3.5 (1.4-8.0)	2.3 (0.9-4.5)	1.9 (0.7-4.2)	1.5 (0.8-3.5)	1.2 (0.7-2.1)
CD3+/CD4+ T lymphocytes	1.9 (0.4-3.5)	3.5 (1.7-5.3)	2.5 (1.5-5.0)	2.8 (1.4-5.1)	2.3 (1.0-4.6)	2.2 (0.9-5.5)	1.3 (0.5-2.4)	1.0 (0.3-2.0)	0.8 (0.4-2.1)	0.7 (0.3-1.4)
CD3+/CD8+ T lymphocytes	1.1 (0.2-1.9)	1.0 (0.4-1.7)	1.0 (0.5-1.6)	1.1 (0.6-2.2)	1.1 (0.4-2.1)	1.2 (0.4-2.3)	0.8 (0.3-1.6)	0.8 (0.3-1.8)	0.4 (0.2-1.2)	0.4 (0.2-0.9)
CD3+/HLA-DR+ T lymphocytes	0.09 (0.03-0.4)	0.3 (0.03-3.4)	0.2 (0.07-0.5)	0.2 (0.07-0.5)	0.2 (0.1-0.6)	0.2 (0.1-0.7)	0.2 (0.08-0.4)	0.2 (0.05-0.7)	0.06 (0.02-0.2)	0.09 (0.03-0.2)
CD3−/CD16-56+ NK cells	1.0 (0.1-1.9)	0.5 (0.2-1.4)	0.3 (0.1-1.3)	0.3 (0.1-1.0)	0.4 (0.2-1.2)	0.4 (0.1-1.4)	0.4 (0.1-1.0)	0.3 (0.09-0.9)	0.3 (0.07-1.2)	0.3 (0.09-0.6)

From Comans-Bitter WM, de Groot R, van den Beemd R, et al: *J Pediatr* 130:388-393, 1997.

*Absolute counts (× 10⁹/L): median and percentiles (5th to 95th percentiles).

TABLE 3 Reference Ranges for Serum Immunoglobulins and Specific Antibody Levels*

Age	IgG (mg/dl)	IgA (mg/dl)	IgM (mg/dl)	
0-1 mo	700-1300	0-11	5-30	
1-4 mo	280-750	6-50	15-70	
4-7 mo	200-1200	8-90	10-90	
7-13 mo	300-1500	16-100	25-115	
13 mo–3 yr	400-1300	20-230	30-120	
3-6 yr	600-1500	50-150	22-100	
6 yr–adult	639-1344	70-312	56-352	

Age	IgG1 (mg/dl)	IgG2 (mg/dl)	IgG3 (g/dl)	IgG4 (mg/dl)
Cord	435-1084	143-453	27-146	1-47
0-3 mo	218-496	40-167	4-23	1-120
3-6 mo	143-394	23-147	4-100	1-120
6-9 mo	190-388	37-60	12-62	1-120
9 mo–2 yr	286-680	30-327	13-82	1-120
2-4 yr	381-884	70-443	17-90	1-120
4-6 yr	292-816	83-513	8-111	2-112
6-8 yr	422-802	113-480	15-133	1-138
8-10 yr	456-938	163-513	26-113	1-95
10-12 yr	456-952	147-493	12-179	1-153
12-14 yr	347-993	140-440	23-117	1-143
Adult	422-1292	117-747	41-129	10-67

	Tetanus Toxoid (IU/ml)	PRP (HIB) (ng/ml)	Pneumococcus (ng/ml)	
Protective level	0.15	1000	1000	
Adequate response	Fourfold rise	Fourfold rise	Fourfold rise	

Age	Isohemagglutinin Titer†	Anti-A	Anti-B	
0-6 mo		Unpredictable	Unpredictable	
6 mo–2 yr		≥ 1:4-8	≥ 1:4-8	
2-10 yr		1:4-256	1:16-256	
10 yr–adult		≥ 1:4-8	≥ 1:4-8	

*These are normal ranges from the laboratories of Children's Hospital, Boston, Mass. (except isohemagglutinins). Normal ranges are method-dependent and should be validated for each laboratory. These reference ranges are intended for educational purposes only.
†From Fong SW, Qaqundah BY, Taylor WF: *Transfusion* 14:551-559, 1974.
PRP, Polyribosylribitolphosphate; *HIB*, *Haemophilus influenzae* type B.
Disclaimer: The ordering and interpretation of laboratory testing in pediatric rheumatic disease must occur in the context of the patient's history and physical examination and under the guidance of an experienced pediatric rheumatologist.[1,2]

REFERENCES

1. D'Cruz D: Testing for autoimmunity in humans, *Toxicol Lett* 127:93-100, 2002.

2. Wallace DJ, Hahn BH, eds: *Dubois' lupus erythematosus,* ed 6, Baltimore, 2001, Lippincott Williams & Wilkins.

Appendix II
Food Allergy

A   FUNCTIONS AND FOOD SOURCES OF VITAMINS

VITAMIN NAME	CHIEF FUNCTIONS IN THE BODY	SIGNIFICANT SOURCES
Vitamin A	Visual adaptation to light and dark, growth of skin and mucous membrane	Retinol (animal foods): Liver, egg yolk, fortified milk, cheese, cream, butter, fortified margarine Carotene (plant foods): Spinach, other dark leafy green vegetables, broccoli, deep orange fruits (apricots, cantaloupe), vegetables (squash, carrots, sweet potato, pumpkin)
Vitamin D	Absorption of calcium and phosphorus, calcification of bones	Self-synthesis from sunlight; fortified milk, fortified margarine, eggs, liver, fish oils
Vitamin E	Antioxidant, stabilization of cell membranes, protection of polyunsaturated fatty acids and vitamin A	Polyunsaturated plant oils, green leafy vegetables, wheat germ, whole-grain products, nuts, seeds
Vitamin K	Normal blood clotting	Bacterial synthesis in the digestive tract; green leafy vegetables, milk and dairy products, meats, eggs, cereals
Thiamine (B_1)	Coenzyme in carbohydrate metabolism; normal function of the heart, nerves, and muscle	Pork, beef, liver, whole or enriched grains, legumes, nuts
Riboflavin (B_2)	Coenzyme in protein and energy metabolism	Milk, yogurt, cottage cheese, meat, leafy green vegetables, whole or enriched grains and cereals
Niacin (B_3)	Coenzyme in energy production, health of skin, normal activity of stomach, intestines, and nervous system	Meat, peanuts, legumes, and whole or enriched grains
Pyridoxine (B_6)	Coenzyme in amino acid metabolism, helps convert tryptophan to niacin, heme formation	Grains, seeds, liver, meats, milk, eggs, vegetables
Cyanocobalamin (B_{12})	Coenzyme in synthesis of heme in hemoglobin, normal blood cell formation	Animal products (meat, fish, poultry, shellfish, milk, cheese, eggs)
Folic acid	Part of DNA, growth and development of red blood cells	Liver, leafy green vegetables, legumes, seeds, yeast
Pantothenic acid	Part of coenzyme A (used in energy metabolism); formation of fat, cholesterol, and heme; activation of amino acids	Meats, cereals, legumes, milk, fruits, vegetables

A   FUNCTIONS AND FOOD SOURCES OF VITAMINS—cont'd

VITAMIN NAME	CHIEF FUNCTIONS IN THE BODY	SIGNIFICANT SOURCES
Biotin	Part of coenzyme A (used in energy metabolism); involved in lipid synthesis, amino acid metabolism, glycogen synthesis	Liver, egg yolk, soy flour, cereals, tomatoes, yeast
Vitamin C	Collagen synthesis (strengthens blood vessel walls, forms scar tissue and matrix for bone growth), antioxidant, thyroxine synthesis, strengthens resistance to infection, helps with absorption of iron	Citrus fruits, tomatoes, cabbage, dark leafy green vegetables, broccoli, chard, turnip greens, potatoes, peppers, cantaloupe, strawberries, melons, papayas, mangos

B   FUNCTIONS AND FOOD SOURCES OF MINERALS AND TRACE ELEMENTS

MINERAL NAME	CHIEF FUNCTIONS IN THE BODY	SIGNIFICANT SOURCES
Calcium	Bone and teeth formation; involved in normal muscle contraction and relaxation, nerve functioning, blood clotting, blood pressure	Milk and milk products, small fish (with bones), greens, legumes, calcium-fortified tofu, calcium-fortified juices, calcium-fortified rice, soy, and potato milks
Chloride	Part of hydrochloric acid found in the stomach, necessary for proper digestion	Salt, soy sauce, moderate quantities in whole unprocessed foods, large amounts in processed foods
Chromium	Cofactor for insulin	Molasses, nuts, whole grains, seafood
Copper	Cofactor for enzymes; necessary for iron metabolism; cross-linking of elastin	Liver, shellfish, whole grain cereals, legumes, nuts
Fluoride	Structural component in calcium hydroxyapatite of bones and teeth	Seafood, meat, fluoridated water
Iodide	A component of the thyroid hormone thyroxin, which helps regulate growth, development, metabolic rate	Iodized salt, seafood
Iron	Structural component of hemoglobin (carries oxygen in the blood) and myoglobin (makes oxygen available for muscle contraction) and other enzymes necessary for the utilization of energy	Red meats, fish, poultry, shellfish, legumes, dried fruits
Magnesium	One of the factors involved in bone mineralization, maintains electrical potential in nerves and muscle membranes, involved in building of proteins, enzyme action, normal muscular contraction, transmission of nerve impulses, maintenance of teeth	Widely distributed in most foods with nuts, fruits, vegetables, cereals as best sources
Manganese	Cofactor for enzymes	Whole grains, leafy green vegetables, wheat germ
Molybdenum	Xanthine oxidase, aldehyde oxidase	Legumes, whole grains, wheat
Phosphorus	Bone and teeth formation, regulation of acid-base balance, present in cell's genetic material as phospholipids, in energy transfer, and in buffering systems	Milk, poultry, fish, meat, carbonated beverages
Potassium	Regulation of osmotic pressure and acid-base balance, activation of a number of intracellular enzymes, nerve and muscle contraction	All whole foods; meats, milk, fruits, vegetables, grains, legumes

Continued.

B   FUNCTIONS AND FOOD SOURCES OF MINERALS AND TRACE ELEMENTS—cont'd

MINERAL NAME	CHIEF FUNCTIONS IN THE BODY	SIGNIFICANT SOURCES
Selenium	Part of glutathione peroxidase (an enzyme that breaks down reactive chemicals that harm cells), works with vitamin E	Seafood, organ meats, muscle meats, grains, vegetables (depending on soil conditions)
Sodium	Regulation of pH, osmotic pressure, and water balance; conductivity or excitability of nerves and muscles; active transport of glucose and amino acids	Salt, soy sauce, seafood, dairy products, processed foods
Zinc	Part of the hormone insulin and many enzymes; taste perception; wound healing, metabolism of nucleic acids	Red meat, seafood (especially oysters), beans

C   COMMERCIAL FOODS THAT FREQUENTLY CONTAIN UNEXPECTED ALLERGENS

FOODS CONTAINING MILK PROTEIN	FOODS CONTAINING EGG PROTEIN	FOODS CONTAINING WHEAT PROTEIN	FOODS CONTAINING SOY PROTEIN	FOODS CONTAINING PEANUT PROTEIN
Breads and bread crumbs	Egg beaters	Barbecue-flavored potato chips	Bagel, breads, and bread crumbs	Cakes, cookies, muffins, and chocolate bars
English muffin	Baby food spaghetti	Cereals	Bouillon cubes	Egg roll
Flavored crackers	Marshmallow cream	Gluten-free products (wheat starch)	Chicken hot dog	Frozen desserts
Nondairy creamer	Pasta	Low-fat beef franks	English muffin	Candies
Instant noodle cups	Waffles	Soy sauce	Reduced-fat peanut butter	Sauces and chili
Sorbets	Shiny baked goods (egg wash)	"Spelt"	Waffles	
Soy cheese	Wine (cleared with egg white)			
Waffles				
Canned fish				
Baby foods with mixed ingredients				
Most mammalian milks cross-react (e.g., sheep)				

D   LABEL INGREDIENTS/TERMS THAT INDICATE THE PRESENCE OF COMMON ALLERGENS

Milk

Artificial butter flavor, butter, buttermilk
Casein (rennet), caseinates (calcium, magnesium, potassium, and sodium)
Ghee
Hydrolysates (casein, milk, protein, and whey)
Lactalbumin, lactoglobulin, lactose (*may* contain), lactulose
Milk solids, milk powder, nonfat dry milk powder
Whey

Label ingredients that MAY indicate the presence of milk protein

Chocolate
Flavorings (artificial, caramel, and natural)
High-protein flour
Luncheon meats
Margarine

Egg

Albumin
Egg (white, yolk, dried, powdered, solids)
Mayonnaise

Label ingredients that MAY indicate the presence of egg protein

A shiny glaze or yellow baked goods
Flavorings (artificial and natural)
Lecithin

Wheat

Bran
Bread crumbs
Bulgur
Couscous
Cracker meal
Durum and durum flour
Farina
Flour (all-purpose, enriched, graham, high gluten, high protein, pastry, soft wheat)
Gluten
Kamut
Semolina
Spelt
Vital gluten
Whole-wheat berries
Whole-wheat flour

Label ingredients that MAY indicate the presence of wheat protein

Hydrolyzed protein
Flavorings (artificial and natural)
Modified food starch
Soy sauce
Starch (gelatinized, modified, vegetable)
Surimi

Soy

Hydrolyzed soy protein
Miso
Natto
Shoyu sauce
Soy (flour, grits, milk, nuts)
Soya
Soybean (granules, curd)
Soy protein isolate
Soy sauce
Tamari
Tempeh
Textured vegetable protein
Tofu

Label ingredients that MAY indicate the presence of soy protein

Flavorings (artificial and natural)
Vegetable broth, gum, starch

Peanut

Nuts (beer, ground, monkey, mixed)
Nu-Nuts flavored nuts
Peanut (butter, flour)
Peanut oil (cold pressed, expeller pressed, extruded)

Label ingredients that MAY indicate the presence of peanut protein

African, Chinese, Indonesian, Mexican, Thai, and Vietnamese dishes
Baked goods
Candy
Chili
Chocolate (candies, candy bars)
Egg rolls
Enchilada sauce
Flavorings (artificial and natural)
Marzipan
Nougat

Modified from The Food Allergy and Anaphylaxis Network: *How to read label cards,* Fairfax, Va, 2000, The Food Allergy and Anaphylaxis Network.

E   SUGGESTIONS ON FEEDING INFANTS WITH FOOD ALLERGY AND FOR DIETARY PREVENTION OF ATOPY: AMERICAN AND EUROPEAN PANEL REPORTS

SUMMARY RECOMMENDATIONS OF THE AMERICAN ACADEMY OF PEDIATRICS COMMITTEE ON NUTRITION, 2000[1]*

1. Breast milk is an optimal source of nutrition for infants through the first year of life or longer. Those breast-feeding infants who develop symptoms of food allergy may benefit from the following:
   a. maternal restriction of cow's milk, egg, fish, peanuts and tree nuts, and, if this is unsuccessful,
   b. use of a hypoallergenic (extensively hydrolyzed or, if allergic symptoms persist, a free amino acid–based formula) as an alternative to breast-feeding. Those infants with IgE-associated symptoms of allergy may benefit from a soy formula, either as the initial treatment or instituted after 6 months of age after the use of a hypoallergenic formula. The prevalence of concomitant allergy is not as great between soy and cow's milk in these infants as in those with non–IgE-associated syndromes such as enterocolitis, proctocolitis, malabsorption syndrome, or esophagitis. Benefits should be seen within 2 to 4 weeks and the formula continued until the infant is 1 year of age or older.
2. Formula-fed infants with confirmed cow's milk allergy may benefit from the use of a hypoallergenic or soy formula as described for the breast-fed infant.
3. Infants at high risk for developing allergy, identified by a strong (biparental; parent and sibling) family history of allergy, may benefit from exclusive breast-feeding or a hypoallergenic formula or possibly a partial hydrolysate formula. Conclusive studies are not yet available to permit definitive recommendations. However, the following recommendations seem reasonable at this time:
   a. Breast-feeding mothers should continue breast-feeding for the first year of life or longer. During this time, for infants at risk, hypoallergenic formulas can be used to supplement breast-feeding. Mothers should eliminate peanuts and tree nuts (e.g., almonds, walnuts) and consider eliminating eggs, cow's milk, fish, and perhaps other foods from their diets while nursing. Solid foods should not be introduced into the diet of high-risk infants until 6 months of age, with dairy products delayed until 1 year, eggs until 2 years, and peanuts, nuts, and fish until 3 years of age.
   b. No maternal dietary restrictions during pregnancy are necessary with the possible exception of peanuts.
4. Breast-feeding mothers on a restricted diet should consider the use of supplemental minerals (calcium) and vitamins.

*From The Commitee on Nutrition, American Academy of Pediatrics: *Pediatrics* 106:246-349, 2000.

SUMMARY RECOMMENDATIONS OF THE ESPACI COMMITTEE ON HYPOALLERGENIC FORMULAS AND ESPGHAN COMMITTEE ON NUTRITION, 1999[2]*

Treatment of Allergic Reactions to Food Proteins

- Infants with confirmed food protein allergy should be treated by complete exclusion of the causal protein.
- In exclusively breast-fed infants, a strict elimination of the causal protein from the diet of the lactating mother should be tried.
- Infants with cow's milk protein allergy who are not breast-fed should receive a dietary product with highly reduced allergenicity based on "extensively" hydrolyzed protein or, in selected cases, a product based on an amino acid mixture.
- In infants with adverse reactions to food proteins and malabsorptive enteropathy, the use of a formula with highly reduced allergenicity (extensively hydrolyzed formula or amino acid mixture) without lactose and with medium chain triglycerides might be useful until normal absorptive function of the mucosa is regained.
- For the treatment of most infants with food allergy whose digestive and absorptive functions show no major disturbances, products with highly reduced allergenicity based on extensively hydrolyzed protein or amino acid mixtures but whose other compositional characteristics meet the European Union criteria for infant formulas is recommended.
- Diets based on unmodified proteins of other species' milk (for example, goat's or sheep's milk) or so called partially hydrolyzed formulas should not be used for the treatment of cow's milk protein allergy.

Prevention of Adverse Reactions to Food Proteins

- Exclusive breast-feeding during the first 4 to 6 months of life might greatly reduce the incidence of allergic manifestations and is strongly recommended.
- Supplementary foods should not be introduced before the fifth month of life.
- In bottle-fed infants with a documented hereditary atopy risk (affected parent or sibling), the exclusive feeding of a formula with a confirmed reduced allergenicity is recommended because it can reduce the incidence of adverse reactions to food, especially to cow's milk protein.
- More studies comparing the preventive effects of formulas that have highly reduced allergenicity with formulas that have moderately reduced allergenicity are needed.
- Dietary products used for preventive purposes in infancy need to be evaluated carefully with respect to their preventive and nutritional effects in appropriate clinical studies.
- There is no conclusive evidence to support the use of formulas with reduced allergenicity for preventive purposes in healthy infants without a family history of allergic disease.

*From Host A, Koletzko B, Drebork S, et al: *Arch Dis Child* 81:80-84, 1999.

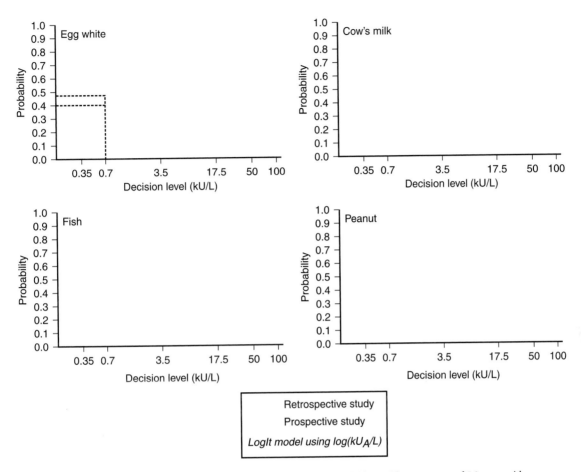

Summary of the results of a retrospective ($N = 196$ children with a mean age of 5.2 years with atopic dermatitis) and prospective ($N = 100$ children with a median age of 3.8 years, 61% with atopic dermatitis) study correlating the chance of an IgE-mediated clinical reaction (based upon blinded oral food challenges or convincing history) to the concentration of food-specific IgE antibody (measured in kU/L using the Pharmacia CAP System FEIA, Pharmacea & UpJohn Diagnostics, Uppsala, Sweden) for four foods. (From Sampson HA: *J Allergy Clin Immunol* 107:891-896, 2001.)

It is important to recognize that the clinical history is paramount, that allergen prick skin tests may add additional important predictive information, and that the curves may be shifted significantly to the left for patients younger than those studied (e.g., for infants, a concentration equal to and over 2 kU/L to egg and 5 kU/L to milk is 95% predictive of a reaction).[3,4] Based upon these studies, suggestions were made as summarized in Table F-1.

Food-Specific IgE Concentration Clinical Decision Points

	Egg	Milk	Peanut	Fish	Soy	Wheat
Reactive if ≥ (no challenge needed)	7	15	14	20	65	80
Possibly reactive (physician challenge*)	↓	↓	↓	↓	↓	↓
Unlikely reactive if less than (home challenged*)	0.35	0.35	0.35	0.35	0.35	0.35

*In patients with a strongly suggestive history of an IgE-mediated food allergic reaction, food challenges should be performed with physician supervision, regardless of food-specific IgE value. If the food-specific IgE level is less than 0.35 kU/L *and* the prick skin test is negative, the food challenge can be performed at home unless there is a compelling history of reactivity. ↓ = values between. (From Sampson HA: *J Allergy Clin Immunol* 107:891-896, 2001.)

G   FOOD ALLERGY ACTION PLAN FOR SCHOOLS/CAMPS

[PLACE CHILD'S PICTURE HERE]

Allergy To: _____

Student's Name: _____ DOB: _____ Teacher: _____

Asthmatic Yes*   No   * High risk for severe reaction

SIGNS OF AN ALLERGIC REACTION

SYSTEMS	SYMPTOMS
• MOUTH	Itching and swelling of the lips, tongue, or mouth
• THROAT*	Itching and/or a sense of tightness in the throat, hoarseness, and hacking cough
• SKIN	Hives, itchy rash, and/or swelling about the face or extremities
• GUT	Nausea, abdominal cramps, vomiting, and/or diarrhea
• LUNG*	Shortness of breath, repetitive coughing, and/or wheezing
• HEART*	"Thready" pulse, "passing out"

The severity of symptoms can quickly change.* All above symptoms can potentially progress to a life-threatening situation.

ACTION FOR MINOR REACTION

1. If only symptom(s) is(are): _____, give _____
                                                              (medication/dose/route)
Then call:

2. Mother _____, Father _____, or emergency contacts.

3. Dr. _____ at _____
If condition does not improve within 10 minutes, follow steps for Major Reaction below.

ACTION FOR MAJOR REACTION

1. If ingestion is suspected and/or symptom(s) is(are) _____, give

_____ IMMEDIATELY!
          (medication/dose/route)
Then call:

2. Rescue Squad (ask for advanced life support)

3. Mother _____, Father _____, or emergency contacts.

4. Dr. _____ at _____

DO NOT HESITATE TO CALL RESCUE SQUAD!

Patient's Signature _____ Date _____

Doctor's Signature _____ Date _____

EMERGENCY CONTACTS	**TRAINED STAFF MEMBERS**
1. _____ Relation: _____ Phone: _____	1. _____ Room: _____
2. _____ Relation: _____ Phone: _____	2. _____ Room: _____
3. _____ Relation: _____ Phone: _____	3. _____ Room: _____

EPI-PEN AND EPI-PEN JR DIRECTIONS

1. Pull off gray activation cap (Figure G-1).
2. Hold black tip near outer thigh (always apply to thigh) (Figure G-2).
3. Swing and jab firmly into outer thigh until Auto-Injector mechanism functions. Hold in place and count to 10. The Epi-Pen unit should then be removed and taken with you to the emergency room. Massage the injection area for 10 seconds.

For children with multiple food allergies, use one form for each food.

From Furlong AM, ed: *The School Food Allergy Program,* Fairfax, Va, 1995, The Food Allergy and Anaphylaxis Network.

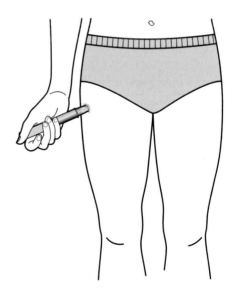

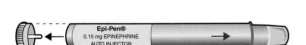

FIGURE G-1 Pulling off gray activation cap of Epi-Pen.

FIGURE G-2 Applying Epi-Pen to outer thigh.

H   EXAMPLE OF A "CHEF CARD" THAT CAN BE FASHIONED FOR USE IN RESTAURANTS

TO THE CHEF:

WARNING! I am allergic to PEANUTS. In order to avoid a life-threatening reaction, I must avoid eating all foods that might contain peanuts, including:

Peanut	Ground nuts
Peanut butter	Mandelonas
Peanut flour	Nu-Nuts
Peanut oil	Nut pieces
Artificial nuts	Monkey nuts
Beer nuts	Mixed nuts

Even a tiny amount of peanut can be dangerous to me. Please ensure any utensils and equipment used to prepare my meal, as well as prep surfaces, are thoroughly cleaned prior to use. Thanks for your cooperation.

From The Food Allergy and Anaphylaxis Network: *The food allergy training guide for restaurants and food services,* Fairfax, Va, 2001, The Food Allergy and Anaphylaxis Network.

REFERENCES

1. Committee on Nutrition, American Academy of Pediatrics: Hypoallergenic infant formulas, *Pediatrics* 106:346-349, 2000.
2. Host A, Koletzko B, Drebork S, et al: Dietary products used in infants for treatment and prevention of food allergy. Joint Statement of the European Society for Paediatric Allergology and Clinical Immunology (ESPACI) Committee on Hypoallergenic Formulas and the European Society for Paediatric Gastroenterology, Hepatology and Nutrition (ESPGHAN) Committee on Nutrition, *Arch Dis Child* 81:80-84, 1999.
3. Garcia-Ara C, Boyano-Martinez T, Diaz-Pena JM, et al: Specific IgE levels in the diagnosis of immediate hypersensitivity to cow's milk protein in the infant, *J Allergy Clin Immunol* 107:185-190, 2001.
4. Boyano MT, Garcia-Ara C, Diaz-Pena JM, et al: Prediction of tolerance on the basis of quantification of egg white—specific IgE antibodies in children with egg allergy, *J Allergy Clin Immunol* 110:304-309, 2002.

NOTE: Page numbers followed by *t* refer to tables, by *b* refer to boxes, and by *f* refer to figures.